9600553
WO200

£2-00

Clinical Anaesthesia

For Churchill Livingstone

Project Editor: Gavin Smith
Copy Editor: Liz Graham
Project Controller: Elspeth Masson, Nora Cameron
Design Direction: Sarah Cape
Marketing: Susan Jerdan-Taylor

Clinical Anaesthesia

Edited by

Alan R. Aitkenhead BSc MD FRCA
Professor of Anaesthesia,
University of Nottingham, UK

Ron M. Jones MD FRCA
Head, Department of Anaesthetics,
St. Mary's Hospital Medical School,
(Imperial College)
London, UK

CHURCHILL LIVINGSTONE

NEW YORK EDINBURGH LONDON MADRID SAN FRANCISCO TOKYO 1996

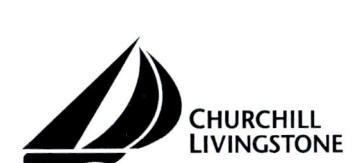

CHURCHILL LIVINGSTONE
Medical Division of Pearson Professional Limited

Distributed in the United States of America by Churchill Livingstone Inc., 650 Avenue of the Americas, New York, N.Y. 10011, and by associated companies, branches and representatives throughout the world.

© Pearson Professional Limited 1995

All rights reserved. No part of this publication may be reproduced, stored in a retrieval system, or transmitted in any form or by any means, electronic, mechanical, photocopying recording or otherwise, without either the prior permission of the publishers (Churchill Livingstone, Robert Stevenson House, 1-3 Baxter's Place, Leith Walk, Edinburgh, EH1 3AF), or a licence permitting restricted copying in the United Kingdom issued by the Copyright Licensing Agency Ltd, 90 Tottenham Court Road, London, W1P 9HE.

First published 1996

ISBN 0-443-04552-6

While great care has been taken to ensure the accuracy of the book's content when it went to press, neither the authors nor the publishers can be responsible for the accuracy and completeness of the information. If there is any doubt, the manufacturer's current literature or other suitable reference should be consulted

British Library Cataloguing in Publication Data
A catalogue record for this book is available from the British Library.

Library of Congress Cataloging in Publication Data
A catalog record for this book is available from the Library of Congress.

The publisher's policy is to use paper manufactured from sustainable forests

Printed in Singapore

Contents

1. Pre-operative assessment   1
   B. R. Baxendale, A. R. Aitkenhead
2. Influence of co-existing disease on anaesthetic management   31
   C. A. Marshall
3. Intercurrent medication   79
   S. Harding, R.M. Jones
4. Premedication   107
   R.S. Atkinson
5. Monitoring and monitoring equipment in clinical anaesthesia   115
   K. Merrett, R.M. Jones
6. Induction of anaesthesia   155
   J. Sear
7. The maintenance of anaesthesia   173
   D. C. White
8. Anaesthesia and abdominal surgery   189
   R. Ginsburg, L. Kaufman
9. Anaesthesia for vascular surgery   205
   S. Reiz, P. Coriat
10. Thoracic surgery   239
    J. W. W. Gothard
11. Anaesthesia for pelvic surgery   267
    B. J. Pollard
12. Anaesthesia for orthopaedic surgery   279
    L. H. D. J. Booij
13. Anaesthesia for dental, maxillofacial, thyroid and parathyroid surgery   287
    M. W. Platt
14. Anaesthesia for ENT and ophthalmological surgery   315
    A. W. A. Crossley
15. Obstetric analgesia and anaesthesia   329
    H. Breivik, D. Bogod
16. Anaesthesia for cardiac surgery   367
    M. Salmenperä, C. C. Hug Jr
17. Day-case surgery   413
    I. Smith, P. F. White
18. Anaesthesia for non-surgical interventions   439
    A. W. Harrop-Griffiths
19. Anaesthesia for plastic, microvascular and burns surgery   453
    D. W. Green
20. Anaesthesia for major organ transplantation   485
    R. A. Wilkund, J. A. Fabian, R. L. Keenan
21. Anaesthesia for the neurosurgical patient   513
    F. M. Borthwick, W. Fitch
22. Anaesthesia for paediatric surgery   533
    S. G. E. Lindahl
23. Local anaesthesia techniques   557
    T. M. Murphy, D. Fitzgibbon
24. Intra-operative complications   595
    A. J. Cunningham
25. Postanaesthesia care   619
    E. A. M. Frost
26. Postoperative pain relief   637
    R. Sharpe, A. Lawson, R. M. Jones
27. Cardiopulmonary resuscitation   667
    N. G. Bircher
28. Safety in clinical anaesthesia   685
    A. R. Aitkenhead
29. Audit and quality assurance   729
    W. B. Runciman
30. The quest for quality - how to keep up to date   749
    J. N. Lunn

Contributors

A.R. Aitkenhead BSc MD FRCA
Professor of Anaesthesia, University of Nottingham, Nottingham, UK

R. S. Atkinson OBE MA MB BChir FRCA
Honorary Consulting Anaesthetist, Hospital, Westcliff-on-Sea, Essex, UK

B. Baxendale FRCA
Research Fellow, University Department of Anaesthesia, University Hospital, Queen's Medical Centre, Nottingham, UK

N. Bircher
Safar Centre for Resuscitation, Pittsburgh, USA

D. Bogod FRCA
Consultant Anaesthetist, City Hospital, Nottingham, UK

L. H. D. J. Booij MD PhD FRCA
Professor and Chairman, Department of Anaesthesiology, University of Nijmegen, Nijmegen, The Netherlands

J. M. Borthwick BSc MB ChB FRCA
Consultant in Neuroanaesthesia and Intensive Care, Institute of Neurological Sciences, Southern General Hospital, Glasgow, UK

H. Breivik MD PhD FRCA
Professor and Chairman, Department of Anaesthesiology, University of Oslo, The National Hospital, Oslo, Norway

P. Coriat MD
Professor of Anesthesiology, Hôpital de la Pitie, Salpetrière, Université Paris VI, Paris, France

A. W. A. Crossley MB ChB FRCA
Senior Lecturer, University of Nottingham Hospital, Honorary Consultant Anaesthetist to Derby City General Hospital, Derbyshire Royal Infirmary, Derby, UK

A. J. Cunningham MD FFARCSI FACA FANZCA FRCPC
Professor of Anaesthesia, Beaumont Hospital, Royal College Of Surgeons in Ireland, Dublin, Ireland

J. A. Fabian MD
Associate Professor of Anesthesiology, University of New Mexico, Chief of Anesthesiology Service, Veterans Affairs Medical Center, Albuquerque, New Mexico, USA

W. Fitch BSc(Hons) MBChB PhD FRCA FRCP
Professor and Head of Department, University Department of Anaesthesia, University of Glasgow, Glasgow, UK

D. R. Fitzgibbon MB BcH BAO FFARCSI
Acting Assistant Professor, Multidisciplinary Pain Center, Department of Anesthesiology, University of Washington Medical Center, Seattle, Washington, USA

E. A. M. Frost MBChB
Professor and Chair, Department of Anesthesiology, New York Medical College, Valhalla, New York, USA

R. Ginsburg MB BS BSc FRCA
Consultant Anaesthetist, Department of Anaesthetics, King's College Hospital, London, UK

J. W. W. Gothard MB BS FRCA
Consultant Anaesthetist, Royal Brompton Hospital, London, UK

D. W. Green MB BS FRCA
King's College Hospital, London, UK

S. A. Harding MB BChir FRCA
Senior Registrar, Department of Anaesthetics, Royal Free Hospital, London, UK

W. Harrop-Griffiths MA FRCA
Consultant Anaesthetist, St Mary's Hospital, London, UK

C. C. Hug Jr MD PhD
Professor of Anesthesiology and Pharmacology, Emory University School of Medicine, Director Cardiothoracic Anesthesia, The Emory Clinic, Atlanta, Georgia, USA

R. M. Jones MD FRCA
Head, Department of Anaesthetics, St Mary's Hospital Medical School, (Imperial College), London, UK

L. Kaufman MD FRCA
Consulting Anaesthetist, University College Hospital and St Mark's Hospital, London, Honorary Senior Lecturer, Faculty of Clinical Sciences, University College London, UK

R. L. Keenan MD
Professor of Anesthesiology, Medical College of Virginia, Virginia Commonwealth University, Richmond, Virginia, USA

A. Lawson FFARCSI FANZCA
Consultant Anaesthetist, Chelsea & Westminster Hospital, Fulham Road, London, UK

S. G. E. Lindahl MD PhD
Professor and Chair, Department of Anesthesiology and Intensive Care, Karolinstea Hospital and Institute, Stockholm, Sweden

J. N. Lunn MD FRCA FANZCA
Senior Honorary Research Fellow, University of Wales College of Medicine, Honorary Consultant Anaesthetist, University Hospital of Wales, Cardiff, UK

C. A. Marshall MB BS MRCP FRCA
Consultant Anaesthetist and Honorary Senior Lecturer, Royal Free Hospital, London, UK

K. L. Merrett MB BS DA FFARACS FRCA
Lecturer in Anaesthetics, St Mary's Hospital Medical School, Imperial College of Science, Technology and Medicine, London, UK

T. M. Murphy MBChB FRCA
Professor of Anesthesiology and Clinical Pain Service, University of Washington, Seattle, Washington, USA

M. W. Platt MB BS FRCA
Senior Lecturer, Academic Department of Anaesthetics, St Mary's Hospital Medical School Imperial College, London, UK

B. J. Pollard B Pharm MD FRCA
Senior Lecturer in Anaesthesia, University of Manchester, Manchester Royal Infirmary, Manchester, UK

S. Reiz MD PhD
Professor of Anaesthesia and Intensive Care, University of Uveå, Uveå, Sweden

W. B. Runciman MB Bch FANCZA FFIANZA FHRCA FRCA PhD
Professor and Head, Department of Anaesthesia and Intensive Care, Royal Adelaide Hospital and University of Adelaide, Adelaide, South Australia

M. T. Salmenperä MD
Associate Professor of Anesthesiology, Department of Anaesthesia, Helsinki University Central Hospital, Helsinki, Finland

J. W. Sear MA MB BS PhD FFARCS
Reader in Anaesthetics, Nuffield Department of Anaesthetics, University of Oxford, Honorary Consultant Anaesthetist, Oxfordshire Health Authority, Oxford, UK

R. Sharpe BSc MB BS FRCA
Lecturer Academic Department of Anaesthetics, St Mary's Hospital Medical School, London, UK

I. Smith MB BS FFARCS
Department of Anesthesiology, Washington University School of Medicine, St Louis, Missouri, USA

D. White MB BS FRCA
Formerly Honorary Consultant Anaesthetist, Northwick Park Hospital, Harrow, Middlesex, UK

P. F. White PhD MD FFARCS
Professor and holder of the McDermott Chair, Department of Anesthesiology and Pain Management, University of Texas, Southern Medical Center, Dallas, Texas, USA

R. A. Wiklund MD
Assistant Professor of Anesthesiology, Yale University School of Medicine, New Haven, Connecticut, USA

Preface

Most anaesthetic textbooks either offer detailed discussion of an area of specialized practice, or attempt to provide a comprehensive overview of all aspects of anaesthesia, including physiology, pharmacology and other basic sciences. These comprehensive texts are intended for a variety of readers, and the level varies from the didactic, intended for new trainees, to the discursive, designed for the higher trainee or for established specialists. Inevitably, comprehensive textbooks, particularly those at the higher level, are large and very expensive.

We perceived a need for a more concise, yet detailed, text dealing primarily with the clinical practice of anaesthesia in the 1990s. We believe that most trainees in the later stages of their education will already have acquired and studied books which deal with the basic sciences. Established specialists may wish to update their knowledge of basic sciences, but will wish to do so usually, by acquiring a short book or monograph which discusses a specific area of interest in which knowledge has advanced since the subject was originally studied. Our book is intended to provide a detailed description of clinical aspects of anaesthesia, together with an insight into audit, safety and quality assurance, and we hope that it will be of value to experienced trainees, to specialists and to those involved in teaching clinical anaesthesia. A knowledge of the basic sciences is assumed, although specific topics are rehearsed, when necessary, to explain aspects of clinical management.

We have been fortunate in obtaining contributors from many countries, and are particularly indebted to those for whom English is not their native language, but who have produced chapters of outstanding quality not only in content but in style. The book is intended for an international readership, and we have attempted to provide alternative drug names where appropriate, although using the European generic name as the standard. Clearly, there are differences in clinical practice in various countries, but we have tried to ensure that the principles described in each chapter are of universal application.

Finally, we are grateful to the publishers, Churchill Livingstone, for their help and support in compiling the book, and to our wives for their patience and understanding.

Nottingham	A. R. Aitkenhead
London	R. M. Jones

1. Pre-operative assessment

B. R. Baxendale   A. R. Aitkenhead

The anaesthetic management of any patient due to undergo surgery begins with the pre-operative visit, which is arguably one of the most important aspects of the peri-operative process. In addition to being a courtesy which the patient has a right to expect, it may be used as one measure of the standard and quality of care offered by the anaesthetic department within an institution.

Usually, the decision to operate has already been taken, but the anaesthetist has a vital contributory role, particularly in respect of preparation of the patient and the timing of surgery. The perceived benefits of surgery must be balanced against any risks inherent to the peri-operative period. The anaesthetist's duty is to ensure that the patient is offered the best care, with anaesthesia and surgery taking place under conditions of maximum safety. The overall aims of assessment should be clear:

1. to anticipate difficulties;
2. to make advanced preparation regarding facilities, equipment and expertise;
3. to enhance patient safety and minimize the chance of errors;
4. to allay any relevant fears or anxieties perceived by the patient.

The process relies heavily on the anaesthetist possessing adequate knowledge and experience to predict the likely peri-operative progress of each patient. There is a need for education, so that factors of importance can be recognized in future by surgical and trainee anaesthetic staff.

WHO, WHEN AND WHERE?

There are numerous factors which influence the decision to operate on a patient (Table 1.1), some of which may place limitations on the process of pre-operative assessment. Just as there is pressure for the anaesthetic management to be optimized, there is also a demand to reduce inappropriate surgical intervention.[1,2] However, there appears to be little in the literature relating to critical evaluation of the appropriate indications for surgical intervention, and this remains a topic on which anaesthetists should keep themselves updated. The final emphasis must be on a team approach to patient care in order to provide the safest possible peri-operative management. As this may produce a conflict of opinions among the individuals concerned (i.e. anaesthetist, surgeon and patient), a thorough knowledge of factors affecting anaesthetic management and outcome is required.

The initial assessment of any patient is by surgical consultation, directed towards the presenting pathology and the need to operate. By implication, this should involve senior surgical staff. The first thorough assessment of general health occurs later when the patient is 'clerked', either on admission to hospital or shortly beforehand at a dedicated outpatient appointment; this is traditionally performed by one of the least

Table 1.1 Factors influencing the decision to operate

Institutional	Surgical	Patient
Adequate facilities appropriate to the procedure, including pre- and postoperative care	Nature of pathology	Intercurrent medical disease
Available support staff	Urgency of the procedure	Expectations
	Skill and experience of surgical and anaesthetic staff	Employment, social and family commitments
	Surgeon's usual practice	Likely benefit from intervention
	Availability of treatment	

experienced members of the surgical team. Recognition of problem cases has usually relied upon the general medical education and common sense of the medical staff concerned at this stage; access to a screening protocol for use by the surgical staff could easily improve this aspect of patient care, as well as providing a means of educating non-anaesthetic staff. The last point is essential, as clinical anaesthetic knowledge amongst junior surgical staff has been clearly demonstrated to be inadequate.[3]

Patients recognized as being at special risk should be 'flagged' for urgent anaesthetic assessment, particularly as this may result in some alteration to the proposed management of the patient. For this reason, the process must be designed to allow problem patients to be seen by an experienced anaesthetist well in advance of the proposed surgery. This is feasible for elective or scheduled operations, and it is not necessary at this stage for the anaesthetist ultimately responsible for the relevant operating list to be involved. However, this becomes more desirable after the patient has been admitted to hospital prior to operation, and should be obligatory if a patient requires urgent or emergency surgery to ensure continuity of management with enhanced safety for the patient. In addition, this procedure provides the opportunity to reassure the patient and explain the process of pre-operative and postoperative care.

Assessment in advance of hospital admission

The use of pre-admission clerking appointments has grown in popularity, driven by the need for more efficient hospital bed occupancy. These consultations can take place in the weeks preceding planned surgery, and allow the majority of the administrative details concerning hospital admission to be completed. It is an ideal time to include the anaesthetic assessment, as long as an experienced anaesthetist is available. When the patient is admitted, further assessment could be directed at excluding any acute changes in general condition. If an anaesthetic opinion is not available at the time of pre-clerking there must be guidelines for the surgical team to ensure that each patient is investigated adequately, and appropriate action taken if problems are discovered (see below).

Another change in practice involves the introduction of pre-operative questionnaires to be completed by patients in advance of their hospital admission (Fig. 1.1). Their use has gained popularity with the increasing demand for day-case surgery. They may predict the need for certain pre-operative laboratory tests or other investigations; an accompanying form sent to the patient may be used to provide basic information concerning details of hospital admission and routine. However, questionnaires cannot replace personal contact with hospital medical staff, and it is still essential for the surgical staff to have sufficient knowledge about pre-operative anaesthetic requirements to make appropriate responses when this information is presented to them.

OVERALL PROCEDURE OF PRE-OPERATIVE ASSESSMENT

Clinical skills are a vital attribute in medicine, and nowhere are they more important than in the anaesthetic assessment of a patient due to undergo surgery. These skills must be taught correctly in the first instance, and require a continuous process of practice and education regardless of individual experience. The usual procedure is for a detailed history to be taken and examination performed on all patients requiring hospital care in order to screen for the presence of disease, followed by investigations dictated by the findings. The anaesthetic assessment is then directed towards areas of particular relevance, searching out the important factors which will interact with anaesthesia. The fundamental aims remain to ensure that patients are in the best physical condition to undergo anaesthesia, and that the benefits of surgery will not be outweighed by perioperative risks.

History

The best source of information concerning the patient relevant to any subsequent anaesthesia is obtained by asking a series of questions which can be followed by more direct interrogation on receiving any positive responses. A questionnaire (Fig. 1.1) can still be given to the patient prior to clerking in order to provide a starting point.

Presenting condition and concurrent medical history

The indication for surgery can dictate the urgency for intervention and may influence anaesthetic management quite dramatically. The systemic effects of the presenting pathology must be quantified. For example, bowel cancer can be associated with anaemia, malnourishment or fluid and electrolyte imbalance. There are many diseases which can have a significant impact on anaesthetic management and outcome, particularly disease of the cardiovascular or respiratory systems. Their presence or absence is usually ascertained by

	Yes	No
1. Do you suffer or have you suffered from any of the following: Heart disease Palpitations High blood pressure Chest pains Swelling of ankles Shortness of breath on walking up a single flight of stairs Asthma Bronchitis Diabetes Epilepsy Ulcer trouble or hiatus hernia Jaundice or other liver disease Kidney disease Anaemia Arthritis Stroke		
2. Are you taking any tablets, pills, inhalers or medicines? If *yes*, please list:		
3. Have you any allergies? If *yes*, please list:		
4. Do you smoke? If *yes*, what or how many a day? ..../day		
5. Do you drink more than a moderate amount of alcohol? (more than 8 pints beer/week or 10 glasses wine/week)		
6. Do you bruise easily or bleed excessively?		
7. Have you had any operations or general anaesthetics before? If *yes*, please list, including approximate dates:		
8. Were there any complications? If *yes*, please give details:		
9. Have any members of your family had any problems with anaesthetics? If *yes*, please give details:		
10. Is there anything about yourself or your family's medical history you think we should know? If *yes*, please give details:		

Fig. 1.1 Pre-operative patient questionnaire. Spaces for the patient to give details of relevant points have been omitted in this example.

direct questioning, and the extent of any limitations imposed by them should be recorded carefully.

Anaesthetic history

Details of the administration and outcome of any previous anaesthetic exposure are important. This experience can form the basis for any pre-operative fears or preferences expressed by the patient, and often the patient uses minor sequelae (such as nausea, sore throat or headache) to judge quality of care. If previous problems were encountered, the anaesthetist must attempt to clarify their clinical significance in order to plan the next anaesthetic and avoid a repeat of the complication. Obtaining previous admission and anaesthetic records can prove invaluable in this respect. If general anaesthesia with halothane has been admistered during the previous 3 months, the Committee on Safety of Medicines recommends[4] that, in the absence of a clear, positive indication for its use, halothane should be avoided because of the increased risk of developing postoperative hepatotoxicity. There is not the same concern for repeat exposure to the other volatile anaesthetic agents, although the complication is not unknown with enflurane.[5]

Family history

There are a number of inherited conditions that have a significant influence on aspects of planned anaesthetic management, such as malignant hyperthermia, cholinesterase abnormalities, porphyria, certain haemoglobinopathies and dystrophia myotonica. Some of these disorders may have little impact on the patient's normal activities, but their peri-operative significance should be identified clearly for the patient. Details of these conditions are considered later. If such a condition is suspected, there has usually been a full investigation of relevant family members. Failing this, a careful history can usually help identify the likely problem if the diagnosis is unclear.

Drug history

Up to 42% of patients presenting for surgery are receiving regular drug therapy,[6,7] with potential either for interaction with anaesthetic agents and techniques, or for causing problems related to their sudden withdrawal during the peri-operative period[8] (Table 1.2). There are other substances taken habitually by some patients that can also have a significant influence on the process of anaesthesia. These include alcohol, tobacco and the use (or abuse) of non-prescription drugs.

Drug abuse.[9,10] Patients who have illicit drug habits can present to the anaesthetist in either an emergency or elective setting. A knowledge of national and local patterns of abuse is helpful, although these are liable to continual change. The most important drugs of abuse remain opioids and cocaine. The pre-operative features of significance concerning substance abuse are summarized in Table 1.3. In addition to these, there are increasing numbers of 'designer drugs' available, about which there is relatively little information regarding acute or chronic toxicity. One prominent example is the semisynthetic amphetamine Ecstasy (3,4-methylenedioxymethamphetamine or MDMA), the acute toxic effects of which are related to the parent compound, and which are becoming more widely known as cases of toxicity are reported.[11,12]

History of allergy

Patients may be aware of an allergy to specific sub-

Table 1.2 Drugs with potential anaesthetic interaction

Drug group	Comments
CARDIOVASCULAR *Angiotensin-converting enzyme inhibitors* Captopril Enalapril Lisinopril	Hypotensive effects may be potentiated by anaesthetic agents. Sudden withdrawal tends not to produce rebound haemodynamic effects, perhaps due to relatively long duration of action
Antihypertensives Clonidine Guanethidine Methyldopa Reserpine	Hypotension with all anaesthetic agents, requiring extreme care with dosage and administration. *Clonidine* (or *dexmedetomidine*) allows reduction in dosage of anaesthetic agents and opioids. Acute withdrawal of long-term treatment may result in a hypertensive crisis. *Guanethidine* potentiates effect of sympathomimetics. *Reserpine* depletes noradrenaline stores, so attenuating the action of any pressor agents acting via noradrenaline release
β-Blockers	Negative inotropic effects additive with anaesthetic agents to cause exaggerated hypotension. Mask compensatory tachycardia. Caution with concomitant use of any cardiovascular-depressant drugs. Acute withdrawal may result in angina, ventricular extrasystoles, or may even precipitate myocardial infarction
Ca^{2+} channel blockers Verapamil	Depresses atrioventricular conduction and excitability. Interacts with volatile anaesthetic agents leading to bradyarrhythmias and decreased cardiac output
Diltiazem Nifedipine	Negative inotropic effect and vasodilatation interact with volatile anaesthetic agents to cause hypotension. May augment action of competitive muscle relaxants. Acute withdrawal may exacerbate angina
Others Digoxin	Arrhythmias enhanced by calcium. Toxicity is enhanced by hypokalaemia, which must be corrected pre-operatively. Suxamethonium enhances toxicity, which should therefore be used with caution. Beware of bradyarrhythmias
Diuretics	Can cause hypokalaemia which may potentiate the effect of competitive muscle relaxants
Magnesium	Potentiates action of muscle relaxants, the dosage of which may need to be reduced

Table 1.2 (contd)

Drug group	Comments
Quinidine	Intravenous administration can produce neuromuscular blockade, particularly notable following suxamethonium
CENTRAL NERVOUS SYSTEM	
Anticonvulsants	Cause liver enzyme induction. May increase requirements for sedative or anaesthetic agents. Recommended to avoid enflurane. Sudden withdrawal may produce rebound convulsant activity
Benzodiazepines	Additive effect with many CNS-depressant drugs. Caution with dosage of intravenous anaesthetic agents and opioids. Additive effect with competitive muscle relaxants, causing potentiation of their action. Action of suxamethonium may be antagonized
Monoamine oxidase inhibitors	React with opioids causing coma or CNS excitement. Severe hypertensive response to pressor agents. Treatment of regional anaesthetic-induced hypotension can be difficult, especially as indirect sympathomimetics (e.g. ephedrine) are contra-indicated due to unpredictable and exaggerated release of noradrenaline. Adverse effects not guaranteed to occur, but recommended to withdraw drugs 2–3 weeks prior to surgery and use alternative medication
Tricyclic antidepressants	Inhibit the metabolism of catecholamines, increasing the likelihood of arrhythmias. *Imipramine* potentiates the cardiovascular effects of adrenaline
Phenothiazines *Butyrophenones*	Interact with other hypotensive agents, necessitating care with administration of all agents with potential cardiovascular effect
Others Lithium	Potentiates non-depolarizing muscle relaxants. Consider changing to alternative treatment 48–72 h prior to anaesthesia
L-Dopa	Risks of tachycardia and arrhythmias with halothane. Actions antagonized by droperidol. Augments hyperglycaemia in diabetes. Some suggest discontinuing on day of surgery, but this must be balanced against possible detrimental effects as a result
ANTIBIOTICS *Aminoglycosides*	Potentiation of neuromuscular block. Caution with the use of muscle relaxants. Effect may be partially antagonized with Ca^{2+}
Sulphonamides	Potentiation of thiopentone
NON-STEROIDAL ANTI-INFLAMMATORY DRUGS	Interfere with platelet function to varying degrees by inhibition of platelet cyclo-oxygenase. Possible effect on coagulation mechanism makes the use of regional anaesthesia controversial (see text)
STEROIDS	Potential adrenocortical suppression. Additional steroid cover may be required for the peri-operative period (see text)
ANTICOAGULANTS	Problems with minor trauma due to venous access, laryngoscopy and intubation (especially nasotracheal), intramuscular injections and the use of local anaesthetic blocks. Full anticoagulation is an absolute contra-indication to the use of regional anaesthetic techniques. Surgical haemorrhage more likely. Pre-operative management of anticoagulant therapy is discussed elsewhere
ANTICHOLINESTERASES *Ecothiopate eye drops* *Organophosphorus insecticides*	Rarely encountered nowadays. Inhibition of plasma cholinesterase. Caution should be exercised with the use of suxamethonium
ORAL CONTRACEPTIVE PILL	Increased risk of thrombo-embolic complications with oestrogen-containing formulations. Recommended that the pill is stopped 4 weeks prior to elective surgery or, if not possible, provide some form of prophylactic therapy, e.g. subcutaneous heparin
ANTIMITOTIC AGENTS	Inhibition of plasma cholinesterase. Caution should be exercised with the use of suxamethonium

CNS = Central Nervous System.

6 CLINICAL ANAESTHESIA

Table 1.3 Signs and symptoms of substance abuse

Substance	Comments
Opioids	Euphoria (most marked with heroin). Decreased conscious level or coma. Pinpoint pupils with overdose. Respiratory depression. Hypotension. Constipation. Chronic respiratory dysfunction (asthma, aspiration)
Cocaine and amphetamines	Sympathetic stimulation, excitement, delirium, hyperreflexia, tremors, convulsions, mydriasis, sweating, hyperpyrexia. Labile blood pressure; hypertension. Hallucinations (tactile = 'cocaine bugs'; visual = 'snow lights'), psychoses. Exhaustion and coma with overdose
Hypnotics: benzodiazepines and barbiturates	Central nervous system depression. Mood-calming. Overdose causes respiratory depression and coma. Hypothermia, cardiovascular depression
Hallucinogens; phencyclidine derivatives, LSD	Altered perception and judgement. High doses may progress to toxic psychosis. Sympathomimetic and weak analgesic effects. Phencyclidine produces dissociative anaesthesia with increasing doses
Volatile solvents	Altered perception. Euphoria. Overdose causes coma with progression similar to general anaesthesia. Respiratory and cardiovascular depression. Ventricular arrhythmias with halogenated hydrocarbons
Cannabis	Effects variable but dose-related. Euphoria. Occasional anxiety and panic reactions. Rarely psychosis. Tachycardia, labile blood pressure. Chronic use may produce poor memory and decreased motivation

From Wood & Soni,[9] with permission.
LSD = Lysergic acid diethylamide.

stances, or groups of substances, whether it be a drug, foods or adhesive tapes. The exact nature of the symptoms and signs must be sought, as the term allergy is not always understood accurately by patients. Most often, patients confuse predictable side-effects with true allergy. Drugs which are commonly quoted as having caused anaphylactoid reactions are antibiotics, especially co-trimoxazole and penicillin, and aspirin. Non-steroidal anti-inflammatory drugs (NSAIDs) are used commonly during the peri-operative period, and the risk of cross-sensitivity in patients allergic to aspirin must be considered. Patients who have a history of atopy do not necessarily have an increased risk of anaphylaxis, but may demonstrate greater sensitivity to released histamine or other vasoactive chemicals, with increased reactivity of the cardiovascular or respiratory systems on exposure to noxious stimuli.

A small proportion of patients describe an allergic reaction to a previous anaesthetic. The same principles as above apply when reviewing the precise history of the event, as an anaphylactoid reaction must be differentiated from malignant hyperthermia, plasma cholinesterase deficiency, incomplete reversal of neuromuscular blockade, or other predictable side-effects of various anaesthetic agents or other drugs administered in association with anaesthesia. The anaesthetic notes from the time of the incident must be obtained if possible, if only to exclude the occurrence of a serious adverse event; the postoperative history and investigations should also be reviewed. Although severe anaphylactoid reactions to anaesthetic drugs are rare, with an incidence of between 1 : 5000 and 1 : 25 000 anaesthetics,[13] they do represent an important cause of serious morbidity or mortality, and are usually investigated thoroughly in the postoperative period. Some drugs are associated with a relatively higher frequency of adverse reaction during general anaesthesia, although no drug is completely safe (Table 1.4).[14] Pre-operative screening of patients to predict likely anaphylactoid responses is not feasible at present due to difficulties with interpretation of results, risks and expense involved with the tests, the availability of certain forms of testing (e.g. radioallergosorbent tests) for only a limited

Table 1.4 Anaesthetic agents associated with serious anaphylactoid reactions. The agents are ranked within each group according to incidence of reported reactions, which therefore will be influenced by overall frequency of drug usage

Induction agents	Muscle relaxants	Local anaesthetic agents
Thiopentone Propofol Etomidate Methohexitone	Suxamethonium Alcuronium Atracurium Vecuronium Gallamine Tubocurarine Pancuronium	Bupivacaine Lignocaine Prilocaine

Adapted from Watkins,[14] with permission.

number of drugs,[15] and lack of any data validating any test as an accurate predictor of anaphylaxis in the absence of a previous reaction.

Smoking

Cigarette smoking has been identified as one independent factor for predicting adverse peri-operative outcome.[16] There are several potential mechanisms by which smoking may exert this effect. In the short term, both nicotine and carbon monoxide inhalation can be deleterious. The former contributes to an increase in myocardial oxygen demand by its effects on heart rate, blood pressure and peripheral vascular resistance. Carbon monoxide binds to haemoglobin to form carboxyhaemoglobin, resulting in a significant decrease in oxygen delivery to the tissues. The presence of carboxyhaemoglobin also produces an overestimation of oxygen saturation from pulse oximeter monitoring.[17] These effects are reversible if smoking is stopped for longer than 12 h, which is of particular relevance to patients at risk from decreased oxygen delivery, such as those with ischaemic heart disease. Longer-term problems from smoking, including depression of immune function, impaired clearance of secretions from the tracheobronchial tree and chronic airways disease, are less amenable to reversal.[18] Abstention for 6–8 weeks or longer is required before any beneficial effect is seen in these factors.[19] Ultimately, smoking is associated with a number of cardiovascular and respiratory diseases which are essentially irreversible and known to be associated with increased peri-operative risk. Although anaesthetists should give advice on the short-term benefits of not smoking, there is little evidence that it has any influence on patient's behaviour in the pre-operative period.[20]

Alcohol

Excessive alcohol intake (greater than 80g alcohol/day in men or 40 g/day in women) is a serious social issue, with considerable variation in incidence in different countries. Patients can present with acute intoxication or sequelae of chronic consumption, the majority of which are non-specific features of secondary organ damage (Table 1.5). Recognition of such a problem requires a high index of suspicion and is rarely straightforward. Once the diagnosis is established, it must be decided whether to allow continued alcohol consumption during admission to hospital or run the course of the withdrawal syndrome during the peri-operative period, which has its own risks of morbidity and mortality.

Physical examination

A full clinical examination should be performed on every patient by the admitting medical staff, and the findings must be documented in the hospital records. A suggested routine is detailed in Table 1.6. As with

Table 1.5 Alcohol-related illnesses

Organ	Syndromes caused by toxic effects	Syndromes caused by nutritional effects
Brain	Alcoholic dementia (cortical atrophy) Withdrawal seizures Delirium tremens	Wernicke–Korsakoff syndrome Cerebellar degeneration Central pontine myelinosis (secondary to electrolyte changes during therapy)
Nerves		Peripheral polyneuropathy (thiamine deficiency)
Heart	Alcoholic cardiomyopathy	Beriberi heart disease (thiamine deficiency)
Blood	Leucopenia, anaemia, thrombocytopenia, coagulopathies	Macrocytic hyperchromic anaemia (folic acid deficiency)
Gastro-intestinal tract	Acute and chronic gastritis Acute and chronic pancreatitis Oesophageal carcinoma	Poor oral hygiene Malabsorption syndrome (folic acid deficiency)
Liver	Fatty degeneration Acute hepatitis	Laennec's cirrhosis
Metabolic	Hyperlipidaemia Hyperuricaemia Hypoglycaemia	

Adapted from Kissen,[94] with permission.

Table 1.6 One routine for systematic clinical examination before anaesthesia

System	Points to examine
General	General well-being, nutritional state and build, fluid state. Colour of skin and mucous membranes for anaemia, perfusion and jaundice. Temperature
Cardiovascular	Pulse: rate, volume, rhythm. Jugular venous pressure and pulsations. Blood pressure. Cardiac impulses and auscultatory heart sounds. Carotid pulsations. Sacral or ankle oedema
Respiratory	Observation of dyspnoea. Auscultation of lung fields
Central nervous system	Confirm function of special senses, other cranial nerves, peripheral motor and sensory function
Airway	Mouth opening, neck movements, dental record

Adapted from Kissen B. Alcohol abuse and alcohol-related illness. In: Wyngaarden J B, Smith L H Jr (eds) Cecil Textbook of Medicine, 8th edn. Philadelphia, PA: W B Saunders, 1985: p 55.[94]

the history, there are areas of particular relevance to the anaesthetist, some of which may not be immediately apparent or easy to assess without experience. An important example of this is predicting difficulty with the airway during anaesthesia (see below).

It could be argued that there are certain situations in which a full physical examination is unnecessary, such as in young fit adults due to undergo short or minor procedures, because the likelihood of discovering an unsuspected and significant abnormality is small. However, clinical examination is a simple, safe and cheap method of confirming good health or otherwise, and provides important pre-operative information if unexpected morbidity or mortality occurs during or after anaesthesia. In addition, important abnormalities are found, from time to time even in young and apparently fit patients; appropriate treatment may reduce morbidity both in the peri-operative period and in the longer term. For these reasons we believe a truncated examination for specific situations is the first step along a potentially hazardous path.

Cardiovascular system

Previous myocardial infarction. Recent myocardial infarction increases the risk of re-infarction or other cardiac morbidity in the peri-operative period. This risk is related to how recently the infarct occurred, being greater during the first 3–6 months, and is also influenced by the degree of residual damage. The immediate post-infarct period carries the greatest risk, presumably because the majority of myocardial re-modelling and fibrosis occurs in the initial 6 weeks. Postinfarction subgroups have been identified based on electrocardiographic findings; for example, survivors of non-Q-wave infarcts are at greater risk of reinfarction than those who survive Q-wave infarction.[21] It is suggested that the former group have myocardial border zones related to the infarct which are at greater risk of subsequent damage. The introduction of thrombolytic therapy and angioplasty has significantly improved outcome following myocardial infarct,[22] presumably related to limitation of the acute injury. It may be necessary to re-examine much of the evidence concerning the risks of peri-operative cardiac morbidity following a recent myocardial infarct if such treatment has been provided. A more functional approach to the assessment of patients is suggested, looking carefully at the level of exercise capacity combined with ambulatory or exercise electrocardiography.[23] The risk of complication must be balanced against the benefit of surgery, and the traditional advice has been for surgery to be delayed by up to 6 months if feasible. If not, it has been suggested that invasive monitoring and aggressive control of haemodynamic parameters during the peri-operative period improve outcome;[24] these all need careful pre-operative planning. These data require careful prospective evaluation in the near future, if only because of the implications in terms of equipment and use of intensive care facilities.

Ischaemic heart disease. The cardinal symptom of ischaemic heart disease is angina, although its absence does not exclude disease. Consequently, known risk factors must be identified, such as smoking, hypertension, hyperlipidaemia and a positive family history. When angina is present, its relationship to exercise and position should be noted; the New York Heart Association classification is used widely for clinical grading (Table 1.7). Medication to prevent or treat symptoms gives another indication of severity, and any recent changes should be evaluated carefully. Up to 75% of all ischaemic episodes, defined by electrocardiography, echocardiography or nuclear imaging, occur without symptoms in patients with chronic stable angina,[25] which implies that patients presenting for surgery associated with a high degree of peri-operative stress (e.g. abdominal aneurysmectomy) should always undergo some form of objective pre-operative assessment of myocardial performance (see Chapter 16). Asymptomatic ischaemic heart disease

Table 1.7 New York Heart Association (NYHA) classification of angina

Grade	Symptoms
I	No limitation of ordinary physical activity, e.g. walking or climbing stairs does not cause angina. Angina is produced by strenuous or rapid prolonged exertion at work or recreation or with sexual relations
II	Slight limitation of normal activity, e.g. walking or climbing stairs rapidly, walking uphill, walking or stair-climbing after meals, or in cold, or in wind, or under emotional stress, or only during a few hours after awakening
III	Marked limitation of ordinary activity, e.g. after walking one or two blocks on the level or climbing one flight of stairs. 'Comfortable at rest'
IV	Inability to carry on any physical activity without discomfort, e.g. angina may be present at rest

This functional classification is adapted from the original,[95] and is useful for the purposes of pre-operative assessment. The NYHA have since updated their own classification to involve cardiac status and prognosis, which bears more relevance to the management of heart disease.

may be related to co-existing peripheral vascular disease or respiratory disease, which place their own limitations on exercise tolerance, reducing the opportunity for angina to present itself. Severity of stable pre-operative symptoms does not relate directly to likelihood of problems, although the number of peri-operative ischaemic episodes has been linked to the incidence of postoperative myocardial infarction.[26] However, patients with unstable angina have a higher long-term morbidity, and represent a prohibitive peri-operative risk; one study demonstrated a 28% incidence of peri-operative myocardial infarction or cardiac death.[27]

Hypertension. Newly diagnosed hypertension must be assessed for aetiological factors, which will be present in up to 10% of cases. These include renal disease, endocrine disease, pregnancy or the oral contraceptive pill, and aortic coarctation. These may easily be overlooked in otherwise asymptomatic patients, but they can have important implications for the patient's subsequent management. Long-standing hypertension is associated with an increased risk of cardiac disease, cerebrovascular events and renal impairment, all of which may interfere with the conduct and outcome of anaesthesia and surgery. The definition of hypertension has been a matter of some debate, particularly as treatment is long-term and requires good patient compliance. The presence of systolic hypertension may be as significant as diastolic hypertension in predicting long-term morbidity,[28] although less is known with regard to short-term peri-operative risk.

Poorly controlled or uncontrolled hypertension in the immediate pre-operative period is probably associated with increased cardiac peri-operative morbidity, and is certainly predictive of labile blood pressure intraoperatively.[29,30] Current opinion favours tolerating pre-operative diastolic blood pressures of up to 110 mmHg, provided that painstaking peri-operative monitoring is undertaken and pharmacological control of blood pressure is achieved, rather than instituting pre-operative therapy. Conversely, over-aggressive treatment of hypertension (diastolic pressure less than 85 mmHg) may itself increase morbidity or mortality in those with ischaemic heart disease, perhaps due to inadequate coronary artery perfusion pressures.[31] Evaluation of the hypertensive patient must include searching for evidence of left ventricular hypertrophy (clinical, radiographic or electrocardiographic), which is associated with an increased risk of peri-operative myocardial ischaemia due to imbalance of myocardial oxygen supply and demand, even in the absence of coronary artery disease.[32]

Valvular heart disease. The nature of any valvular heart disease must be evaluated carefully. Lesions may be congenital or acquired, and can be associated with other cardiac pathology. Some carry the risk of peri-operative arrhythmias, embolism or endocarditis (see below). Table 1.8 summarizes the significant points concerning assessment of patients with valvular lesions.

Arrhythmias and conduction defects. Any conduction pattern other than sinus rhythm, including the presence of premature supraventricular or ventricular beats, is associated with increased risk of cardiac morbidity.[33,34] This relates probably to the underlying pathology as much as the presence of the arrhythmia. Some conduction defects require insertion of a pacemaker pre-operatively, and this should be co-ordinated with the cardiologists (Table 1.9).[35] Patients who depend on a pacemaker are unable to increase heart rate intrinsically to alter cardiac output, highlighting the dangers of uncorrected pre-operative hypovolaemia or decreased systemic vascular resistance.

Table 1.8 Assessment of patients with valvular heart disease

Valvular pathology	Comments
Mitral stenosis	*Clinical:* Disease progression must be documented. Dyspnoea on exertion is a good guide, related to increased pulmonary venous pressure. Atrial fibrillation increases the risk of systemic embolization. An opening snap and diastolic murmur, the latter accentuated by exercise and lying on the left side. Drugs may include digoxin, diuretics and anticoagulants, and may need alteration to improve the patient's condition before surgery. Preoperative hypovolaemia must be carefully corrected *ECG:* 'p' mitrale, atrial fibrillation, right axis deviation or right bundle branch block *CXR:* Left atrial enlargement, upper venous congestion, and the valve if calcified *Echocardiography:* Investigation of choice, allowing quantification of the decreased valve closure rate *Cardiac catheterization:* Preoperative PAWP and LAP *Prothrombin time:* For patients on warfarin
Mitral regurgitation	*Clinical:* Often combined with rheumatic mitral stenosis. Disease progression is gauged by exertional dyspnoea. Left ventricular failure and subsequent right ventricular failure indicate more severe disease, especially if combined with atrial fibrillation. Drug treatment often includes diuretics and digoxin, and may need manipulation to improve symptoms preoperatively. Arterial hypertension increases the regurgitant flow, and can precipitate LVF *ECG:* 'p' mitrale, atrial fibrillation, or LVH *CXR:* Enlarged left atrium and ventricles *Echocardiography:* Demonstrates the increased diastolic closure rate *Cardiac catheterization:* Preoperative PAWP and LAP data, useful in those with most severe disease or if large fluid shifts are likely to occur peri-operatively
Mixed mitral valve disease	Assessment must be aimed at determining the dominant lesion, which then directs peri-operative management accordingly. If pulse volume is small and there is no LVH (in the absence of ventricular failure), mitral stenosis is more likely to be dominant. Cardiac catheterization may be necessary to clarify the situation
Aortic stenosis	*Clinical:* Disease of rheumatic origin is usually combined with mitral stenosis. Symptoms include angina, syncope on exertion, and dyspnoea (LVF), and usually indicate advanced disease. Onset of atrial fibrillation (usually in those with concomitant mitral stenosis) produces sudden deterioration *ECG:* LVH indicates marked stenosis *CXR:* Enlarged cardiac diameter only if ventricular dilatation has occurred *Echocardiography:* Shows restricted movement of the valve, and aids accurate diagnosis but not an assessment of severity *Cardiac catheterization:* Determines the true severity by quantifying the pressure gradient across the valve
Aortic regurgitation	*Clinical:* Usually rheumatic (chronic onset) or infective (acute onset); also occurs with chest trauma, Marfan's syndrome, ascending aortic aneurysms, and congenitally. Often asymptomatic until LVF or angina occurs, which indicates severe disease. Collapsing pulse. Atrial fibrillation: suspect co-existing mitral valve disease *ECG:* LVH and dilatation (chronic disease) *CXR:* Cardiomegaly ± aortic root dilatation *Echocardiography:* Indicates movement of valve leaflets, establishes presence of co-existing mitral valve disease, and the extent of regurgitation and ventricular dilatation. Regurgitant fraction > 0.6 is severe
Mixed aortic valve disease	Clinical evaluation of the pulse character may indicate the dominant feature, but cardiac catheterization is required to quantify the true contribution of each
Tricuspid stenosis	*Clinical:* Rare in isolation (e.g. carcinoid, SLE, congenital); usually rheumatic in origin with associated dominant mitral valve disease ± tricuspid regurgitation. Low cardiac output state with increased right atrial pressures resulting in peripheral oedema, jugular 'a' wave, and pulsating liver. Usually on diuretics *ECG:* Presence of 'p' pulmonale (lead II) *CXR:* Prominent right heart border because of enlarged right atrium
Tricuspid regurgitation	*Clinical:* Either rheumatic or following acute endocarditis (drug addicts). Can be secondary to valve ring dilatation with right ventricular failure. Jugular 'v' waves present, otherwise similar to tricuspid stenosis. Atrial fibrillation is common *ECG:* Right ventricular hypertrophy *CXR:* Cardiomegaly

Table 1.8 (contd)

Valvular pathology	Comments
Pulmonary stenosis	*Clinical*: Majority are congenital. 10% associated with ASD or VSD. Severe stenosis results in fatigue, angina (ischaemic right ventricle) and syncope due to low cardiac output. Further symptoms/signs related to right heart failure *ECG*: Right atrial and ventricular hypertrophy *CXR*: Prominent pulmonary artery because of poststenotic dilatation. Cardiomegaly *Cardiac catheterization*: Establishes pressure gradient
Pulmonary regurgitation	*Clinical*: Very uncommon, although can occur secondary to pulmonary hypertension. Usually asymptomatic and treatment is rarely necessary
Prosthetic valves	Valve replacement will help correct the direction and adequacy of blood flow, but ventricular hypertrophy or dilatation does not resolve as quickly. Residual ventricular performance becomes the main factor determining anaesthetic management. Other factors to be considered include concomitant anticoagulation and antibiotic prophylaxis against infective endocarditis

ECG = Electrocardiogram; CXR = chest X-rays; PAWP = pulmonary arterial wedge pressure; LAP = left atrial pressure; LVF = left ventricular failure; LVH = left ventricular hypertrophy; SLE = systemic lupus erythematosus; ASD = atrial septal defect; VSD = ventricular septal defect.

Respiratory system

Asthma. Increasing numbers of patients, and particularly children, are being diagnosed with asthma in the UK. The disease results in irritable airways with increased sensitivity to physical, chemical or endogenous vaso-active stimuli. Assessment should include enquiry regarding the severity and frequency of attacks, any hospital admissions, and the usual trigger stimuli. Records of previous anaesthetic history are useful if problems were encountered. The nature of relevant medication and any recent changes give further indications of the severity and stability of the disease process. Intermittent courses of steroids may be used for exacerbations, and some patients may be on longer-term therapy. Concurrent upper respiratory tract infections (URTIs) are likely to be associated with an increased risk of problems, and surgery should be postponed if possible until symptoms have cleared. On the day of surgery, patients should receive their usual medication. Anaesthetic drugs (including premedicants) associated with histamine release should be used with appropriate caution.

Table 1.9 Indications for placement of a cardiac pacemaker

Condition	Comments
Sick sinus syndrome	Commonest indication for a permanent pacemaker. Usually in the elderly, often *without* other evidence of heart disease
Second-degree atrioventricular block	
Type I (Wenckebach)	Progressive lengthening of the PR interval. Increased mortality now recognized if not paced
Type II	Consistently prolonged PR interval, often with broadened QRS. Frequently progresses to complete heart block
Complete heart block (CHB)	Unless *congenital* in origin
Bifascicular block	Right bundle branch block with left or right axis deviation. Pacemaker only indicated if symptomatic, as natural progression to transient or persistent CHB is rare
Postmyocardial infarction	Damaged myocardium usually recovers, but may require pacing whilst any of the above indications exist. Conduction defects secondary to an anterior myocardial infarction suggest extensive myocardial damage has occurred

Data from Bloomfield & Bowler.[34]

Chronic obstructive airways disease. Chronic bronchitis is defined clinically as the presence of a productive cough on most days for more than 3 months of at least 2 successive years. The peri-operative risks are related to atelectasis and the potential for infection. A number of patients have an element of reversible airways disease which can be improved pre-operatively with bronchodilators. It is useful to document this by formal lung function tests, for reference if post-operative problems arise or if there are future admissions. Some patients may rely on hypoxic ventilatory drive, whereby the respiratory stimulus of carbon dioxide has been diminished or lost due to the chronic disease process. It is essential to identify these patients, as delivery of oxygen-enriched gases can depress their ventilatory drive significantly. The diagnosis is aided pre-operatively by measuring arterial blood gases while breathing air and when breathing a higher concentration of oxygen. These patients will need careful postoperative management with respect to oxygen therapy. Other considerations are provision of physiotherapy and/or antibiotics if it is thought that an improvement in pre-operative condition can be achieved. For this reason, it is argued that elective surgery should be scheduled for those seasons of the year when the patient is least affected by the disease process.

Acute upper respiratory tract infection. The prevalance of URTIs, especially in children and during the winter months, means that many patients would have surgery postponed if this condition was taken routinely as an absolute contra-indication to anaesthesia. In children, there seems little doubt that providing general anaesthesia in the presence of a URTI increases the chance of peri-operative respiratory problems by up to seven times, particularly if the trachea has been intubated.[36] In minor procedures without tracheal intubation, the increased risk of complications is less clear.[37] The recommendations from these studies are that elective surgery should be postponed in children of less than 1 year old with mild URTI, and that older children should be considered individually, bearing in mind the benefit of the operation. If the surgery is major and tracheal intubation necessary, it is wise to postpone surgery for a few weeks until the infection has cleared. Similar recommendations seem reasonable for adults with any respiratory tract infection, especially as underlying chronic respiratory disease or other systemic illness increases the impact of peri-operative complications.

Gastro-intestinal and liver disease

Gastro-oesophageal reflux. There are a number of conditions which increase the risk of pulmonary aspiration of gastric fluid during anaesthesia. These include a history of hiatus hernia, any condition which decreases gastro-oesophageal sphincter tone such as pregnancy, or any condition which increases intra-gastric pressure, including obesity and pregnancy. Patients admitted with acute peritonitis, those who have recently eaten, are in pain, have suffered physical trauma, or have received opioid medication, are all at increased risk of regurgitation and aspiration because of delayed gastric emptying. The anaesthetist should never be complacent; many patients who present for elective surgery have significant volumes of gastric acid, although they rarely aspirate gastric fluid.[38]

Obesity. Morbid obesity is defined in a variety of ways such as comparison with population nomograms or a calculated body mass index greater than $30 kg.m^{-2}$. The condition is associated with many complications which increase the likelihood of peri-operative morbidity or mortality. These include cardiovascular and respiratory disease, gastro-oesophageal reflux, various liver diseases and alteration of normal drug phamacokinetics.[39] Obesity also presents numerous technical challenges including difficulty in managing the airway, obtaining venous access, monitoring blood pressure non-invasively, and performing many local anaesthetic techniques, in addition to the problems encountered by surgeons. All of these circumstances combine to produce a patient with considerable potential for peri-operative complications. Some patients will be receiving drugs aimed at appetite suppression, a number of which are amphetamine-related and have potential for interaction with anaesthetic drugs.

Liver disease. Significant liver disease implies that the majority of hepatic reserve has been exhausted by the pathological process. Manifestations of impairment reflect the multitude of functions performed by the liver, and include metabolic derangement, central nervous system toxicity, coagulation abnormalities, cardiac and respiratory dysfunction, nutritional disorders, and an increased risk of renal failure and sepsis. The cause of pre-operative jaundice should be pursued vigorously, and adequate fluid balance achieved to minimize the risk of consequent renal failure. The possibility of hepatitis B must always be considered, particularly in high-risk groups, and appropriate measures taken to minimize the risk of transmission to staff or other patients.

Renal disease

Chronic renal impairment is associated with a number of conditions affecting the kidney either directly or indirectly, including cardiac failure, hypertension, anaemia and diabetes. The end-result is disturbance of fluid and electrolyte balance, and impaired excretion of various drugs or their metabolites. This influences the choice of anaesthetic agents and the doses to be used. Severe uraemia can itself affect the cardiovascular, pulmonary, haematological, immunological and nervous systems. Development of acute renal failure in the peri-operative period is associated with increased mortality, and must be avoided wherever possible. Patients with established renal failure will be receiving dialysis via the peritoneal space or an extracorporeal system. Time of the most recent dialysis should be noted, and plasma electrolyte concentrations measured before commencing anaesthesia. Care must be taken when planning venous access for anaesthesia, in order to avoid potential arteriovenous fistula sites.

Metabolic and endocrine disease

Diabetes mellitus. Diabetes mellitus is the commonest endocrine disease encountered in anaesthesia. It is associated with several long-term complications which can influence the process of anaesthesia, including cardiac, renal and cerebral atherosclerotic disease, peripheral neuropathies and autonomic dysfunction. In the short term, patients are at risk of hypoglycaemia, especially whilst being kept 'nil by mouth', or may develop keto-acidosis or hyperosmolar states due to poor control of blood glucose concentration; this demands a logical, scientifically sound peri-operative management regimen to be instituted for each patient, aiming for stable, optimal control throughout. Several schemes have been described to achieve this, depending on the patient's usual pre-operative medication and its adequacy, the severity of surgery to be undertaken and the likely postoperative course.[40] The peri-operative management of the diabetic patient is described in detail on page 67. It is interesting to note that, although it seems wise to aim for close control of blood glucose concentration during the peri-operative period, there is no clear evidence that outcome is improved as a result.

Adrenocortical malfunction. The adrenal cortex is responsible for the secretion of glucocorticoids, mineralocorticoids and androgens. Excess secretion of androgens has no specific significance for anaesthesia, although the other hormones may cause problems. An excess production of glucocorticoids results in Cushing's syndrome, which can also arise from exogenous steroid therapy. The patient has thin, easily bruised skin resulting in difficulty in securing peripheral venous access, osteoporosis, hypertension, fluid retention, and occasionally peripheral neuropathies and diabetes mellitus. Pre-operative preparation must take these into account, with treatment aimed particularly at hypertension or fluid and electrolyte derangement.

Adrenocortical insufficiency may be primary to the adrenal gland (Addison's disease), or secondary to pituitary disease or reduced secretion of adrenocorticotrophic hormone. Patients can suffer an acute adrenal crisis if stressed sufficiently, leading to cardiovascular collapse. This can be minimized by providing adequate administration of steroids during the peri-operative period,[41] as well as correcting any pre-operative fluid and electrolyte problems, particularly hypovolaemia, hyponatraemia and hyperkalaemia. Patients on long-term steroid therapy for other conditions may display an iatrogenic adrenal suppression and should be managed in the same way.

Excess mineralocorticoid secretion (Conn's syndrome) is rare and produces a clinical picture which reflects the physiological effect of hyperaldosteronism. Hypertension is due to sodium and water retention, with expansion of blood volume. Hypokalaemia is associated with weakness, alkalosis and occasionally a nephropathy. The main pre-operative considerations are treatment of hypertension (usually with spironolactone) and correction of electrolyte imbalance.

Thyroid disease. Thyroid pathology can produce alteration in activity or enlargement of the gland, either of which may influence the conduct of anaesthesia. *Hyperthyroidism* produces weight loss despite a good appetite, increased bowel activity, intolerance to warm environments, tachyarrhythmias and, in severe cases, heart failure. Undiagnosed or undertreated patients are at risk of having a 'thyroid storm' — an overt life-threatening thyrotoxic crisis which may occur peri-operatively. *Hypothyroid* patients tend to show the converse symptoms and signs, although heart failure can also occur. It is a disease of rather insidious onset, and a high degree of suspicion is required to initiate the diagnosis, especially in the elderly. Pre-operative management relies on administering thyroid hormones until the patient is euthyroid. Without treatment, recovery from sedation or anaesthesia can be particularly prolonged. Patients with an *enlarged thyroid gland* can present problems with airway control peri-operatively, and the pre-operative assessment must seek symptoms or signs of tracheal compression. An X-ray of the thoracic inlet can be helpful in this respect.

Acromegaly. Excess secretion of growth hormone can produce impaired cardiac, respiratory and renal function, diabetes mellitus, and soft-tissue and bony deformities. Hypertension is common but, rarely, cardiomyopathy with heart failure can occur. Kyphoscoliotic changes tend to be responsible for respiratory impairment, but the main concern to anaesthetists relates to airway management, particularly tracheal intubation, in the presence of craniofacial bony deformity.

Neuromuscular disorders

Neuropathies and myopathies. Abnormalities of respiratory and cardiac function are associated with many of the inherited or acquired neuropathies and myopathies. Some drugs, particularly muscle relaxants, should be avoided or used with extreme caution because of unpredictable or prolonged effects. In Duchenne muscular dystrophy, the commonest of the familial dystrophies, administration of suxamethonium is contra-indicated because it results in marked release of potassium and myoglobin.

Nervous system

Patients with any neurological deficit secondary to a disease process should be assessed for current impairment, rate of progression of disease and relevant current medication. A full neurological examination is essential so that any subsequent deterioration in the post-operative period can be appraised, and the relationship to the anaesthetic technique ascertained. In epileptic patients, the manifestation of the convulsions, their frequency and the level of control on current medication should be documented accurately. Some anticonvulsants (e.g. phenytoin, phenobarbitone and carbamazepine) may interact with anaesthetic drugs, particularly the intravenous induction agents, causing profound alteration in the disposition of these agents. Methohexitone, propofol and enflurane are probably best avoided because of their potential for producing epileptogenic activity. Sudden withdrawal of anticonvulsant medication can result in rebound convulsions, and thought should be given to methods of maintenance of therapy, especially if delayed post-operative recovery of gastro-intestinal function is anticipated.

Psychiatric conditions. Patients may react to the prospect of anaesthesia and surgery quite unpredictably, with potential difficulties in communication and comprehension of the issues involved. The drug history must be evaluated carefully, as many antidepressants or antipsychotic drugs have great potential for interaction with anaesthetic agents (Table 1.2).

Inherited conditions

Malignant hyperthermia. This potentially fatal disorder of skeletal muscle can be triggered by a number of drugs used by the anaesthetist, particularly suxamethonium and the volatile agents. The long arm of chromosome 19 carries a defect which is transferred in autosomal dominant fashion, although its expression is not always complete. The reported incidence is 1:15 000 anaesthetics in children and 1:50 000 in adults; thus, it is rarely encountered by the majority of anaesthetists, and detection of new cases usually requires a high degree of suspicion. Its occurrence is more likely in the presence of muscular disorders such as strabismus, scoliosis, dystrophies, myotonia congenita and osteogenesis imperfecta. A family history of unexplained serious anaesthetic morbidity or mortality should be followed up with muscle biopsies to confirm the diagnosis. Affected members of the family should carry appropriate notification along with a Medic Alert type of bracelet.

Cholinesterase deficiencies. Abnormalities of plasma cholinesterase are not associated with any pre-operative symptoms or signs. Thus, only a family history or abnormal response to previous exposure to suxamethonium provides any pre-operative information to suggest the diagnosis. Pregnancy (third trimester) or impaired liver function is associated with an acquired deficiency (relative or absolute) of this enzyme. The only significance for anaesthesia is the prolonged effect of suxamethonium, although a similar effect may occur with the non-depolarizing relaxant mivacurium which is also broken down by plasma cholinesterase.

Haemoglobinopathies. Sickling disorders represent a significant proportion of known haemoglobinopathies which, as a whole, are the commonest inherited disorders throughout the world. Sickling of red blood cells in vivo is associated with several abnormal genotypes, including HbSS, HbAS and HbSC. The HbS gene is present in approximately 10% of the black population of the UK and USA, with HbC being found in about 2% of the same population. The sickle gene is also found in Indians, people of mixed race, Greeks and southern Italians. The homozygous state inevitably produces symptoms and signs secondary to a continuous process of sickling. These include bony deformities, chronic anaemia, jaundice, splenic infarcts, and possibly cardiac dysfunction secondary to myocardial fibrosis. Sickle-cell trait is frequently asymptomatic, but a sickling crisis can occur if provoked (e.g. by hypoxia or acidosis). Any family history of anaemia or blood disorder must be pursued, and haematological screening organized pre-operatively for all high-risk patients (see below). Deficiency of glucose-6-phosphate dehydrogenase is not uncommon in this population, and may be an alternative explanation for anaemia.

Porphyria. The porphyric patient has posed a

significant problem to anaesthetists in the past due to the potential for a number of anaesthetic drugs to provoke an acute episode.[43] Patients at risk can be clearly identified pre-operatively by a combination of family history, clinical examination and biochemical investigation. Subsequent anaesthesia must employ drugs which are considered safe; this list is updated as experience with new agents is gained.[43]

Muscular dystrophies. See the section on neuropathies and myopathies, above.

Haematological disorders

Anaemia can be acute or chronic, the latter being tolerated better due to physiological compensatory adjustment. The cause of chronic anaemia should be identified, as some causes may influence anaesthetic management in their own right. It has been common practice to transfuse patients pre-operatively if the haemoglobin concentration is less than 10 g.dl^{-1}. The choice of this threshold has been questioned, with a trend towards accepting a pre-operative haemoglobin concentration as low as 8 g.dl^{-1}, provided that significant peri-operative blood loss is unlikely.[44] However, patients with pre-existing cardiac or respiratory disease, or those who are subject to additional physiological stresses such as serious infection, are at increased risk of morbidity in the presence of anaemia, and the threshold for transfusion must take this into account. *Polycythaemia* (haemoglobin > 16 g.dl^{-1}) is associated with an increased risk of haemorrhage and thrombo-embolic phenomena, especially if major surgery is planned.

Table 1.10 Systemic complications of rheumatoid arthritis

System	Complication
Cardiovascular	Overall prevalence of cardiovascular involvement is up to 35% of patients[84]
Pericardium	Most common cardiac manifestation. Frequently asymptomatic, but can result in constrictive pericarditis or tamponade. Up to 50% of those with nodules have an effusion on echocardiography[85]
Myocardium	Diffuse interstitial myocarditis or granulomatous involvement occurs much less frequently (1–3%), although the latter may result in disruption of conduction pathways
Endocardium	Valvular endocardial disease is also less common, with the mitral valve being affected most frequently. Aortic incompetence is usually followed by rapid deterioration in the patient's condition
Respiratory	Pulmonary manifestations more common in men
Chest wall	Limitation of chest wall compliance can contribute to a reduction in lung volume and ventilatory efficiency[86]
Pleura	Pleural disease occurs in 3–12% of patients, usually producing small, asymptomatic effusions
Airways	Airflow obstruction has been estimated to occur in up to 38% of patients, associated especially with those who smoke. Rapidly worsening dyspnoea may be due to an obliterative bronchiolitis
Interstitium	Interstitial lung fibrosis can cause a restrictive lung disease, with a reduction in FVC and FEV$_1$
Haemopoietic	A mild normocytic normo- or hypochromic anaemia is common, with haemoglobin concentrations rarely below 10 g.dl^{-1}. Neutrophil and platelet counts can be raised, but concomitant drug therapy may produce the converse. *Felty's syndrome* describes the association of splenomegaly with anaemia, neutropenia and thrombocytopenia
Hepatic	Clinical hepatomegaly occurs in 11% of patients, often with normal biopsies. Altered serum protein concentrations are not uncommon, with reduced albumin and raised globulin levels
Renal	Subclinical renal dysfunction can be demonstrated commonly in patients with seropositive disease. This may be due to interstitial nephritis or amyloidosis, vasculitic lesions of renal vessels, or rarely an autoimmune nephropathy. Drug therapy aimed at disease modification or symptom relief also has a significant risk of nephrotoxicity
Special senses	*Sjögren's syndrome* can occur with rheumatoid arthritis, and will necessitate scrupulous care of the eyes intraoperatively

FEV$_1$ = forced expiratory volume in 1 s. FVC = forced vital capacity

16 CLINICAL ANAESTHESIA

Bone marrow failure. There are a number of conditions which can result in bone marrow failure, such as the leukaemias and aplastic anaemia. These vary in terms of aetiology, clinical presentation, prognosis and principles of treatment, the details of which can be sought elsewhere. The anaesthetic implications are similar and relate to the failure of function of the bone marrow. The most important features to assess are the degree of anaemia, the presence of any infection and the risk of bleeding due to thrombocytopenia. Some leukaemic patients may also present with symptoms secondary to mediastinal lymphadenopathy.

Rheumatoid arthritis

Rheumatoid arthritis (RA) is a disease which has serious articular and systemic manifestations, and patients are frequently receiving drug therapy which can affect the conduct of anaesthesia adversely.[45] Major problems secondary to musculoskeletal deformity include difficulty in securing venous access, positioning the patient during anaesthesia, and management of the airway. All of these may be minimized by appropriate pre-operative assessment and planning. Cervical spine involvement has been found at autopsy in up to 46% of patients with RA,[46] with radiological evidence of involvement in as many as 86%.[47] Atlanto-axial subluxation is the commonest deformity, usually resulting in the atlas moving forwards relative to the odontoid peg when the neck is flexed. More extensive rheumatoid damage results in subaxial subluxation and atlanto-axial impaction, when the odontoid peg can migrate into the foramen magnum. Neurological abnormalities from cervical spine involvement can be subtle and easily hidden by progressive arthritis, muscular atrophy and any associated neuropathy. Many patients remain asymptomatic, and a case can be made for mandatory cervical radiology in flexion and extension prior to general anaesthesia. The alternative is to manage patients with established RA cautiously, assuming all to have some degree of cervical spine instability. Further difficulty can arise with co-existing temporomandibular or crico-arytenoid joint involvement. *Systemic disease* is diffuse and quite common (Table 1.10), requiring clinical vigilance as well as appropriate investigation to detect and quantify significant problems. *Drug therapy* is either for symptomatic relief or aimed at modifying the course of the disease. Drugs intended to provide relief of symptoms are predominantly NSAIDs and steroids, the anaesthetic consequences of which are discussed elsewhere (see Table 1.2 and Chapter 3). Drugs used to treat RA are diverse and may have dramatic adverse effects which influence anaesthesia (Table 1.11).

Table 1.11 Adverse effects associated with drugs used to modify the course of rheumatoid arthritis

Drug	Adverse effects of possible relevance to the anaesthetist
Antimalarials	Chloroquine can rarely cause a neuromyopathy or cardiomyopathy. High plasma levels are associated with a late-stage irreversible retinopathy
Gold	Adverse effects are common (40%). Membranous glomerular nephropathy results in proteinuria and nephrotic syndrome. Other infrequent complications include pneumonitis, hepatitis, immune thrombocytopenia, agranulocytosis, marrow aplasia and gastro-intestinal side-effects. The presence of these adverse effects depends on the type of gold preparation being used
Sulphasalazine	Commonly results in gastro-intestinal intolerance. Haematological toxicity has been reported affecting all the cells lines. Eosinophilic pneumonitis and fibrosing alveolitis are also known to occur
Penicillamine	Nephrotoxicity occurs in 4% of patients. Haematological abnormalities (3%) include leukopénia, eosinophilia and thrombocytopenia. Rare autoimmune reactions include a myasthenia-like syndrome[87]
Azathioprine	Gastro-intestinal side-effects are frequent, and rarely may include pancreatitis. Cholestatic hepatitis can occur during institution of treatment. Leukopenia, thrombocytopenia and anaemia all occur
Methotrexate	Gastro-intestinal intolerance is most common. Bone marrow toxicity is usually associated with concomitant renal failure or folic acid depletion. Pulmonary toxicity occurs in up to 5% of patients, with progressive hypoxaemia due to interstitial and alveolar infiltrates and fibrosis. It has been postulated that nitrous oxide may compound the action of methotrexate at a cellular level.[88] Concomitant administration of salicylate or some other NSAIDs may increase the risk of methotrexate toxicity by causing displacement from plasma protein binding sites and decreasing renal excretion of the drug
Cyclosporin	Significant nephrotoxicity occurs with doses sufficient to cause any alteration in the disease process

NSAIDs = Non-steroidal anti-inflammatory drugs.

Investigations

Laboratory tests or imaging techniques are essential tools in forming a diagnosis and quantifying a disease process. The relevance of investigations to anaesthesia can be extended to provide pre-operative baseline data with which peri-operative changes can be compared. Where appropriate, screening tests can be offered to detect abnormalities which have a significant impact on the conduct of anaesthesia, but which may not be known or apparent to the patient during day-to-day activities.

In general, the results of many investigations may be predicted if a detailed history and examination are available. Therefore the aim should not be to offer a battery of tests as a matter of routine, but to pursue possible abnormalities which are of significance, and which may require changes to the patient's pre-operative management or the conduct of anaesthesia to facilitate a better outcome. It may be that the results of many tests are ignored without any adverse effect on outcome; this implies that the opportunity to provide more effective peri-operative treatment has been missed, or that the test was unnecessary. The likelihood of obtaining a clinically significant result must be balanced against other factors, including the risk attached to performing the investigation, the proportion of false-positive results and the cost involved (financial and time; Table 1.12).

Normal values and the recognition of abnormal results

Results of any investigation are reported with reference to a normal range which has been derived from performing that test on a large sample of 'normal' volunteers or patients. An abnormal value can be defined as lying outside the 2.5–97.5 percentile range, or being beyond a clinically significant physiological value. There are clear short-comings in this philosophy; for example, the sample group used to determine the normal range may not be representative of the population. There will always be a small proportion of normal subjects who lie outside the normal range, i.e. false positives (5% on the above description for a given test). The greater the number of tests performed on an individual, the higher the chance of producing an abnormal result. Within an institution, laboratory standards must be maintained, and variability of results acknowledged. The latter point is particularly pertinent with the increasing availability of ward-based, non-technician-operated laboratory investigations[48] where the risk of operator error will always be great and potentially undetectable, and individual sample quality control impractical.[49]

The use of guidelines

Rather than employing a battery of investigations for every surgical admission, it is becoming more common to request only those which will provide pertinent information. In the majority of situations this can be organized by following a set of guidelines, an example of which is shown in Table 1.13. It should be emphasized that this provides only a guide to the minimum level of investigation, not a set of firm rules. Each patient must be considered individually and more specialized tests organized if appropriate.

Specific investigations

There are several basic investigations which tend to be considered or even offered to the majority of patients attending hospital for surgery, such as urinalysis, blood chemistry and haematological profiles, electrocardiography and chest radiography. In addition, there are more specialized tests of respiratory function, blood coagulation, haemoglobinopathy and myocardial perfusion which are performed rather more selectively.

Urinalysis. This investigation is usually performed as a routine by nursing staff. It is cheap, easy and non-invasive, and is used to screen for conditions such as

Table 1.12 Factors influencing the decision to perform any investigation

Patient	Surgery	Investigation
Pre-existing medical disease	Confirmation or quantification of diagnosis	Clinical significance of result
Screening for specific conditions	Severity of proposed operation	Availability
		Reliability
		Inherent risk
		Cost

diabetes, renal disease or urinary tract infection. Its true value is debatable because of a high false-positive rate when used on its own,[50] which reduces its power to cause alteration in pre-operative management.

Full blood count. This provides information on the haemoglobin concentration, white blood cell count and platelet count, along with details of red-cell morphology. Deviations of haemoglobin concentration are of greatest practical interest to the anaesthetist (see above).

Blood chemistry. The range of measurements available includes urea, creatinine, electrolytes, glucose and liver function tests. There are specific conditions in which measurement of pre-operative values of some or all of these is regarded as mandatory, because the probability of an abnormal result of clinical significance is high (Table 1.13). Their value in pre-operative screening for all patients is much weaker, with the incidence of unexpected abnormality in apparently fit patients under 40 years of age being less than 1%,[51] but increasing with age[52] and American Society of Anesthesiologists (ASA) grade.[53] The age limit above which pre-operative biochemical screening becomes valid remains unclear. It has been argued that for healthy patients under 50 years, urinalysis is adequate.[51] Discovery of unexpected abnormalities

Table 1.13 Guidelines for pre-operative investigations

Investigations	Indication
Urinalysis	This should be performed on every patient. It will occasionally reveal an undiagnosed diabetic or urinary tract infection. Beware of false positives if not confirmed by other evidence of pathology
Urea, creatinine, and electrolytes	All patients over 65 years of age, or with a positive result from urinalysis All patients with cardiopulmonary disease, or taking cardiovascular active drugs, diuretics or steroids All patients with a history of renal or liver disease, diabetes or an abnormal nutritional state Any patient with a history of diarrhoea, vomiting or metabolic illness Patients who have been on intravenous fluid therapy for more than 24 h
Blood glucose	Unless a fasting sample is taken, this test is unlikely to be of benefit beyond confirming a one-off BM Stix reading
Liver function tests	Any history of liver disease, alcoholism, previous hepatitis or unexplained fever following a recent general anaesthetic Any patient with an abnormal nutritional state
Full blood count	All female adults, regardless of general health or reason for admission All male patients over 50 years of age, and all others with history suggestive of blood loss, previous anaemia or haematopoietic disease, cardiorespiratory disease or if surgery is likely to result in significant blood loss (i.e. any patient for whom blood is to be 'grouped and saved' or cross-matched)
Coagulation screen	Any patient with a history of coagulation disorder, significant chronic alcohol consumption, drug abuse or taking anticoagulant medication
Sickle screen	All patients belonging to an ethnic group at risk of carrying the sickle gene with previously unrecorded status (predominantly Afro-Carribbeans, but also includes Indians, those of mixed race and some southern Mediterranean countries)
Electrocardiogram	Male smokers > 45 years old; all others > 50 years old Any patient with a diastolic blood pressure greater than 95 mmHg during admission All patients with a history of heart disease (proven or suspected) or hypertension All patients on diuretics or cardiovascular active drugs Patients with symptomatic chronic or acute-on-chronic pulmonary disease
Chest X-ray	History suggestive of possible abnormality, e.g. trauma, cardiovascular disease, pulmonary disease with localizing chest signs, history suggestive of possible lung tumour (primary or secondary) A previously abnormal chest film Any patient with thyroid enlargement (*along with a thoracic inlet view*) This investigation will not be necessary if a chest X-ray from the previous 6 months is available, and the patient's medical condition is unaltered

may act as a spur for further enquiry and be a useful reference during the postoperative period, but abnormal findings often do not exert any direct influence on anaesthetic management, especially as the majority involve blood glucose or urea values. The final decision to perform the investigation must be based on clinical grounds, taking into account the likelihood of providing useful information for the peri-operative period. Our guidelines suggest a lower age limit of 65 years for screening (Table 1.13), but this figure is chosen arbitrarily based on the population data currently available.

Chest X-ray. The incidence of abnormalities detected by routine pre-operative chest radiographs has been estimated at 4%;[54] it is lower in patients under 40 years of age. The majority of these changes are predictable from a thorough history and examination, and few will impose any alteration to the plan for anaesthesia. Unlike many blood tests, a pre-operative X-ray is unlikely to be of use as a baseline as postoperative changes are treated mainly on the basis of their clinical significance. There is also a known false-positive rate, especially with conditions such as pneumonia, which may result in unnecessary postponement of surgery and needless further investigation.[55] It is clear that this investigation should be reserved for an older population (e.g. over 60 years), or those with a clear indication (Table 1.13).

Electrocardiography. The 12-lead electrocardiogram is capable of detecting many acute or longstanding pathological conditions affecting the heart, particularly changes in rhythm, myocardial perfusion or infarction, not all of which will be apparent from the history and examination. Such abnormalities are important, as many have been found to be associated with increased peri-operative morbidity, and alteration in the patient's pre-operative management can be beneficial. Of equal importance is the knowledge that the resting electrocardiogram is not a very sensitive test for coronary heart disease, being normal in up to 50% of patients with known disease. However, it does have value as a pre-operative baseline, and can be useful for subsequent hospital admissions.

In light of these considerations, it is valuable to perform stress or exercise electrocardiography in some patients; these tests have greater sensitivity for ischaemic changes and can be correlated directly with symptoms. Most cardiology departments are able to provide this form of assessment, usually following standard protocols.[56] The diagnostic sensitivity of exercise testing in coronary artery disease is related to the number of vessels involved, but a negative test does not exclude coronary disease, especially following a myocardial infarction. This places obvious limits on its use in screening asymptomatic patients for ischaemic heart disease. In addition, some surgical patients may be physically unable to perform an exercise test.

Screening for haemoglobinopathy. Screening for haemoglobin genotypes at risk of in vivo sickling should be performed on all individuals at risk of carrying such a gene. A positive Sickledex test, relying on the insolubility of HbS, should be followed by electrophoresis for accurate identification of the genotype. Thalassaemia is confirmed in susceptible patients by examination of a blood film and subsequent electrophoresis. Once these tests have been performed, the result must be documented correctly in the patient's medical records, and the patient made aware of the result. This will prevent needless repetition on subsequent hospital admissions.

Coagulation studies. These investigations should be reserved for specific situations indicated by the history and examination of the patient (Table 1.13).[57] Assessment of platelet function is becoming more important due to the more widespread use of NSAIDs, which can interfere with platelet function. Aspirin produces in vitro platelet function abnormalities lasting 7–10 days, as cyclo-oxygenase inhibition is irreversible. The majority of the other NSAIDs have a transient, reversible effect. Drug-related disturbance of platelet aggregation is another common cause of platelet dysfunction, along with immune disease and inherited defects. It has been suggested that measurement of bleeding time is the only practical in vivo test of platelet function, and that this test should be performed on all patients at risk of platelet dysfunction in whom a regional anaesthetic technique is proposed.[58] The reliability and reproducibility of this test have been questioned, and this has resulted in some confusion concerning its application in clinical practice. However, current opinion now accepts that low-dose aspirin therapy is not a contraindication to regional anaesthesia.

Respiratory function tests. For patients other than those scheduled to undergo lung resection, there is little evidence that pre-operative spirometry provides any significant information which is not already apparent from clinical assessment, nor does it help identify covert disease or influence outcome.[59] Nunn and colleagues[60] suggest that arterial blood gases are the most useful investigation to supplement clinical information (in particular the degree of dyspnoea at rest) with regard to the likelihood of requiring postoperative ventilation. This does not detract from the value of having a pre-operative baseline assessment of lung function which can be used for reference if postoperative problems arise. In patients with progressive disease, it also provides reference for future admissions.

Measurements of pulmonary vascular pressures and resistance, and estimation of shunt fractions, require invasive techniques with inherent risks as well as specialized equipment and facilities. For these reasons, they tend to be offered only to patients with specific indications.

Cardiac function tests. These include echocardiography, angiography and isotope tests which aim to provide specific information on myocardial perfusion and function. They are highly specialized and tend to be performed in relatively few centres. Echocardiography is more widely available, and is also non-invasive, which is encouraging its use. These tests are described in detail in Chapter 16.

PREDICTIVE SCORING OF PERI-OPERATIVE MORBIDITY OR MORTALITY

Scoring systems for determining the likelihood of adverse outcome can be divided into two groups:

1. those directed in general terms at predicting any undesirable events;
2. those which predict more specific morbidity, such as cardiac or respiratory events, or difficult intubation.

Prediction of non-specific adverse outcome

National Confidential Enquiry into Perioperative Death (NCEPOD) reports require assessors to judge whether any aspects of care in reported cases of postoperative death are substandard. From the information available in the medical notes it is often difficult to estimate how fit the patient was for the subsequent operation. True evaluation of characteristics of the patient and features of surgical and anaesthetic technique which have a significant bearing on final outcome are difficult to organize. This is because current standards of practice are high, and because there is a multiplicity of causes for adverse outcome, a relative paucity of untoward events, and great variability of patients' responses. Attempts have been made to classify or score patients pre-operatively in order to identify those at greater risk of suffering adverse outcome.

ASA physical status

Since the 1960s the ASA classification has used a clinical description of disability related to a patient's general health, along with an indication of whether surgery is elective or emergency (Table 1.14). This five-point scale correlates to some degree with the risks of peri-operative complication,[61,62] but unfortunately it is non-specific, poorly predictive of outcome when used alone,[63] and does not identify factors which can be altered pre-operatively to improve outcome. Neither does it necessarily take into account the severity of either the presenting disease or the proposed surgery.

APACHE scores

Acute Physiological and Chronic Health Evaluation (APACHE) scores have been studied rigorously as a means of predicting outcome in patients requiring critical care. The APACHE II system scores 12 physiological variables which have been found to be most discriminatory when rendered abnormal by acute illness, with additional scoring for serious chronic ill health and advancing age.[64] An APACHE III score has since been developed which aims to improve the prognostic estimate of outcome, primarily by re-evaluating the selection and weighting of physiological variables which are included.[65] Relatively few studies have evaluated APACHE scoring outside the intensive care setting. One study examined patients presenting with acute upper gastro-intestinal haemorrhage due to peptic ulceration. Use of APACHE II scores did suggest that

Table 1.14 American Society of Anesthesiologists (ASA) classification of physical status

ASA grade	Classification
I	A normal healthy patient
II	A patient with mild systemic disease
III	A patient with severe systemic disease that limits activity, but is not incapacitating
IV	A patient with incapacitating systemic disease that is a constant threat to life
V	A moribund patient not expected to survive 24 h with or without operation
E	Appended to any grade in the event of emergency surgery

From American Society of Anesthesiology,[96] with permission.

those at high risk of mortality related to surgery could be identified.[66] No comparison was made with a similar group of patients undergoing non-surgical management. Surgical staff were also found to prefer to rely on their expertise and experience than to use this prognostic score.

Pre-operative assessment of fitness score (PAFS)

This simple scoring method combines physiological information, demographic features and basic laboratory test results to obtain an objective assessment of the likelihood of peri-operative survival (Table 1.15).[67] The factors which contribute to the fitness score are similar to those used in APACHE II, but the information is more likely to be immediately available in the pre-operative setting. Prospective validation in patients undergoing emergency or major elective abdominal surgery demonstrated the score to be very sensitive at predicting mortality and major complications, but its specificity was only approximately 80%.

Any studies aiming to examine predictive factors of peri-operative risk must involve large numbers (almost inevitably being multicentre) and be designed scrupulously to allow meaningful conclusions to be drawn. Forrest and co-workers[16] have undertaken such a study, analysing independent predictors of severe peri-operative adverse outcome in over 17 000 patients. Table 1.16 summarizes the results. A history of some cardiovascular diseases, the need for abdominal and cardiothoracic surgery and specific demographic factors were found to be the most important predictors of severe cardiovascular or respiratory events.

Prediction of specific adverse events

The difficult airway

There are specific surgical or medical conditions which are known to be associated with potential airway

Table 1.15 Pre-operative assessment of fitness score (PAFS)

	Preoperative factor
Score 1 for each	Cardiac symptoms controlled by treatment Dyspnoea on climbing stairs Morning cough Stroke or myocardial infarction > 6 months ago Haemoglobin < 10 g.dl^{-1} Serum albumin 30–35 g.l^{-1} Plasma urea 10–19 mmol.l^{-1} Steroid treatment Controlled diabetes
Score 2 for each	Age 70–79 years Cardiac symptoms poorly controlled by treatment Dyspnoea on walking Persistent cough with sputum
Score 3 for each	Clinical jaundice Serum albumin < 30 g.l^{-1} Loss of 10% body weight in 1 month Plasma urea > 20 mmol.l^{-1} Dyspnoea at rest Myocardial infarction < 6 months ago Confusion Cytotoxic treatment
Score 4 for each	Age > 80 years Palliative operation for surgery Intestinal obstruction Perforation, pancreatitis and intraperitoneal abscess (excluding perforated appendix) Haemorrhage or anaemia requiring transfusion

From Playforth et al,[66] with permission.
A total score of less than 6 indicates low risk (10.0%) and a score of 6–10 high risk (84.4%) of postoperative death or major complication within 30 days of surgery. Major complication was defined as sepsis, pneumonia or non-infective organ failure. Validation was prospective on over 1500 consecutive patients undergoing major abdominal surgery.

Table 1.16 Prospective identification of independent predictors of severe peri-operative adverse outcomes

Predictor	Cardiovascular outcome ($n = 565$)	Respiratory outcome ($n = 120$)
Cardiac failure	ASCO	ASRO
Myocardial infarction < 1 year	ASCO	ASRO
Myocardial infarction > 1 year	Ventricular arrhythmia Tachycardia	
Myocardial ischaemia	Ventricular arrhythmia Bradycardia	Bronchospasm
Hypertension	Hypertension Tachycardia Bradycardia	
Ventricular arrhythmia	Ventricular arrhythmia	
COAD		ASRO
Obesity		ASRO (weak predictor)
Smoking	Hypertension Tachycardia	ASRO
ASA status	ASCO, particularly atrial arrhythmias hypertension hypotension	Respiratory failure (weak predictor)
Age > 50 years	ASCO (weak predictor)	
Male sex		ASRO (weak predictor)

Surgical category
  Abdominal
  Thoracic
  Cardiovascular
	ASCO	Abdominal surgery:
		ASRO

ASCO = Any severe cardiovascular outcome: hypotension, hypertension, tachycardia, bradycardia, ventricular arrhythmia, atrial arrhythmia, cardiac failure, myocardial ischaemia, myocardial infarction.
ASRO = Any severe respiratory outcome: bronchospasm, pulmonary secretions, respiratory failure. Number of severe respiratory events insufficient to draw strong conclusions about individual relationships with the predictive factors, although more information is given by Forrest et al.[15]
Pre-operative diseases found **not** to be significant predictors included diabetes, renal disease, asthma and cerebrovascular ischaemic episodes.
COAD = Chronic obstructive airways disease; ASA = American Society of Anesthesiologists.
The study sample was 17 201 and there were adverse outcomes in 847 patients (4.9%)
Adapted from Forrest et al.[15]

problems during general anaesthesia, including large neck or mediastinal tumours, obesity, the later stages of pregnancy or obvious faciomaxillary deformity. Beyond these, it would be inappropriate to expect non-anaesthetic staff to comment on the likelihood of airway difficulty. The trained anaesthetist's eye can identify a number of physical features which may herald difficulty with airway control or tracheal intubation. These include a short, thick neck, protruding premaxilla, a high arched palate, and any limitation of mouth opening or cervical spine movement. Unfortunately, difficult or impossible intubations still occur unexpectedly, and contribute to anaesthetic morbidity and mortality with regular frequency.[68-70]

Mallampati and colleagues devised a popular three-point classification of pharyngeal structures visible when the patient opens the mouth maximally and protrudes the tongue, which correlated with subsequent intubation difficulty;[71] a fourth class was subsequently added by Samsoon & Young (Table 1.17).[72] This

Table 1.17 Mallampati's modified classification

Grade	Description
I	Faucal pillars, soft palate and uvula visible
II	Faucal pillars and soft palate visible, but uvula masked by the base of the tongue
III	Only the soft palate visible
IV	Soft palate not visible

From Samsoon & Young[71] with permission.

grading is simple to perform at the bedside, but is not as reliable as had been hoped, with a high incidence of false positives.[73] To improve upon interobserver variability, other predictive scores have been described, such as that by Wilson and colleagues.[74] This identified five features which contributed towards a risk score: weight; movement of the head and neck; and jaw; mandibular recession; and the presence or absence of buck teeth. Unfortunately, this score still produces a significant number of false positives, especially if a high sensitivity is demanded.[73] It seems clear that various combinations of the features noted within these classifications need to be assessed rigorously and prospectively to identify which have the greatest predictive power. One simple attempt at such an assessment has suggested that any patient with a thyromental distance of less than 7 cm combined with a Mallampati grade III or IV is more likely to present intubation problems.[75]

The most sensitive predictor of difficult intubation is a past history of airway problems during anaesthesia. If the anaesthetic record can be traced, the episode should have been documented, allowing appropriate measures to be taken on the next occasion. One standard method of grading the view at laryngoscopy which should be familiar to all anaesthetists is that described by Cormack & Lehane (Table 1.18).[76]

Table 1.18 Cormack & Lehane's classification

Grade	Structures visible at laryngoscopy
I	Full glottic exposure
II	Only the posterior commisure of the glottis seen
III	No exposure of the glottis
IV	No exposure of the glottis, or of the corniculate cartilages

From Cormack & Lehane[76] with permission.

Adverse cardiac events

Goldman and colleagues[33] are renowned in the anaesthetic world for their retrospective identification of pre-operative risk factors which were associated with an adverse cardiac event in patients undergoing non-cardiac surgery (Table 1.19). Similar risk indices have been described more recently (Table 1.20),[34] although controversy persists about the most accurate predictors of serious peri-operative cardiac events.[77] One of the more contentious factors is the presence of pre-operative hypertension (treated or otherwise). Although studies have demonstrated a relationship with peri-operative lability of blood pressure and heart rate, there is little recent evidence supporting any relationship with adverse cardiac outcome.[16,77] The diversity of methods used to identify these factors, as well as the significant advances made in the understanding and management of cardiovascular pathology over the last 20 years, have certainly contributed to the conflicting opinions regarding identification of the most accurate predictors.

Respiratory complications

Despite the frequency of postoperative pulmonary complications, pre-operative respiratory function tests are not necessarily helpful in their prediction. Excluding patients undergoing pulmonary surgery, much of the existing literature on pre-operative testing does not include any reference to outcome, which makes interpretation of results from a predictive viewpoint impossible. One retrospective study by Nunn and colleagues[60] examined patients undergoing elective surgery who had a severely limited forced expiratory

Table 1.19 Goldman's multifactorial cardiac risk index

Risk factor	Points
Heart failure	11
Myocardial infarction < 6 months	10
Cardiac rhythm other than sinus	7
Ventricular ectopics > 5 min	7
Age > 70 years	5
Important aortic stenosis	3
Thoracic or abdominal surgery	3
Poor general medical condition	3
Emergency operation	4

From Goldman et al,[32] with permission.
The total point score relates to cardiac mortality or morbidity, with patients scoring > 25 found to be at significantly higher risk of life-threatening or fatal peri-operative cardiac event (myocardial infarction, cardiac failure or ventricular tachycardia).

Table 1.20 Detsky's multifactorial risk index

Variables	Points
Coronary artery disease	
MI < 6 months	10
MI > 6 months	5
Canadian Cardiovascular Society angina	
Class 3	10
Class 4	20
Unstable angina within previous 3 months	10
Alveolar pulmonary oedema	
Within 1 week	10
Ever	5
Valvular disease	
Suspected critical aortic stenosis	20
Arrhythmias	
Sinus plus atrial premature beats or rhythm other than sinus on last pre-operative electrocardiogram	5
More than 5 ventricular premature beats at any time prior to surgery	5
Poor general medical status *	5
Age > 70 years	5
Emergency operation	10

*Based on derangement of specific biochemical or arterial blood gas measurements, or if bed-ridden from non-cardiac causes.
MI = myocardial infarction
From Detsky et al,[33] with permission.
The calculated risk score for an individual patient is converted (using a nomogram) to obtain the probability of a significant peri-operative cardiac complication occurring (cardiac death, myocardial infarction or alveolar pulmonary oedema). This takes into account the type of surgical procedure being undertaken.

volume (FEV_1 < 1 l) on pre-operative assessment. They found the only useful predictors of the need for postoperative ventilation to be the combination of a pre-operative arterial oxygen tension of less than 9 kPa (or, more precisely, below the lower limit of the 95% reference range for the patient's age) and the presence of dyspnoea at rest.

PRE-OPERATIVE PREPARATION

After the presenting condition of the patient and any other relevant features have been assessed, a number of other factors require consideration in the final stage of preparation for theatre. These include pre-operative fasting, dental intervention and the oral contraceptive pill. In addition, any factors identified pre-operatively which are known to affect the risk of adverse outcome, and which could be improved to the patient's benefit before surgery, must be addressed. The time course of any improvement must then be balanced against the possible detriment of delaying surgery.

Pre-operative fasting

The time of last oral intake of solid and fluid must be established. One of the commonest causes of anaesthetic-related mortality and morbidity is aspiration of stomach contents. Placing restrictions on oral intake of solids or fluid aims to minimize this risk during anaesthesia, and reduce the incidence of postoperative vomiting. Numerous factors increase the likelihood of significant gastric content being present (see above). However, even starved patients do not necessarily have an empty stomach;[38] this is understandable, considering that the daily secretion of gastric fluid is approximately 2000 ml. Traditional practice has been to prohibit food and drink for at least 6 h pre-operatively. Normal physiology indicates that gastric emptying in normal adults has a half-life of 10–20 min;[78] subsequent clinical studies in adults and children have demonstrated that drinking clear fluids up to 2 h pre-operatively resulted in no significant difference in gastric volume or pH compared with patients starved for 6 h.[79] As a result, many departments are re-evaluating their pre-operative orders, reducing the period of clear fluid restriction accordingly. One word of caution is that gastric emptying may be delayed by premedication. Care should also be exercised before extrapolating these results beyond fit and healthy adults, on whom these studies were based.

Dental intervention

Dental trauma is often preventable, and is one of the commonest sources of litigation against the anaesthetist in the UK and USA.[80] Assessment of dental history and condition can be performed rapidly and must be documented accurately. The patient should be warned in advance that loose teeth may be removed during anaesthesia to prevent their accidental dislodgement, because of the potential for aspiration. If the dental condition is extremely poor, referral to an oral surgeon would be wise before undertaking anaesthesia.

Oral contraception

Thrombo-embolic phenomena are amongst the commonest causes of postoperative mortality.[68–70,81] Women taking an oral contraceptive pill which contains oestrogen appear to be at increased risk of developing postoperative venous thrombosis. The increased risk of venous thrombosis is small, and is related to the administration of ethinyloestradiol, the oestrogen component of combined oral contraceptives, which causes an increase in biological activity of several procoagulant factors such as II, VII, XII and fibrinogen. This has resulted in considerable debate over the best policy for women regarding discontinuation of this medication in the pre-operative period, although several points seem to have become clear.[82]

1. Medication should not be stopped, and heparin prophylaxis is not indicated, before minor surgical procedures, those in which early postoperative mobilization is possible, or in patients taking a progesterone-only pill.

2. For major elective surgery, surgery to the legs, or in patients with other risk factors for thrombo-embolic phenomena, any oestrogen-containing contraceptive pill should be stopped 4 weeks pre-operatively, and recommenced at the first menses postoperatively (provided that 2 weeks have elapsed since surgery).

3. In patients undergoing major surgery or who have additional risk factors, and in whom the oral contraceptive pill has not been stopped, prophylactic low-dose subcutaneous heparin or other measures must be employed.

Hormone replacement therapy (HRT) is becoming increasingly popular for women suffering menopausal symptoms, as well as to reduce the risk of osteoporosis in those with early natural or surgical menopause. Treatment involves replacement of natural oestrogen either orally or by depot release from patches or implants. The method of administration may be significant in terms of risk from thrombo-embolic complications, with oral oestrogens producing greater derangement of the coagulation/fibrinolytic system. Stopping non-oral HRT pre-operatively is probably illogical as it is designed to mimic the normal physiological state,[82] and the current recommendation in the UK is that no special precautions are required in patients who take HRT and who present for surgery.[83]

Providing information to the patient and obtaining consent

Patients are confronted with a barrage of information on arrival in hospital, as well as being introduced into an alien environment with its own routines and practices. It is very easy to overlook their lack of knowledge about theatre procedures, and there are many aspects of anaesthetic management which should not be left to non-anaesthetists to explain. Despite this, it is common for surgical consent forms to include consent to anaesthesia, which implies that the surgical team is capable of discussing this accurately with the patient. Therefore, during the pre-operative anaesthetic assessment, every effort should be made to provide sufficient information for the patient to feel comfortable about what is going to take place. Some will not wish to be told in great detail, but these patients usually make this clear during the consultation. If there are alternative techniques which are available (e.g. general versus regional anaesthesia, different local anaesthetic nerve blocks, methods of providing postoperative analgesia), then these should be explained fully, including the likely consequences, and the patient's view or preference should be obtained. A summary of the discussion should be documented in the anaesthetic record in case of future enquiry.

Rejection of advice

There are frequent occasions when ethical decisions are required regarding the delivery of health care to patients. The anaesthetist may become involved, for example:

- when surgery is considered for patients in whom there is a high risk of peri-operative mortality;
- in relation to provision of care to mentally handicapped patients or children without parental/custodial consent; and
- if adults reject one or other aspect of any proposed medical treatment (the commonest example of this is the use of blood transfusions in Jehovah's Witnesses[84]).

There are a number of principles which can be applied to help tackle most situations, but, if the anaesthetist is in doubt, higher authority should be obtained before administering treatment against the patient's consent. If a patient is suffering from a remediable state and is unable to make decisions regarding aspects of health care for himself/herself, then treatment should be administered if it will save life or prevent permanent harm. This is true for adults and minors; it is illegal for parents/custodians to expose those under their care to ill treatment or neglect, or to expose them to unnecessary suffering or ill health. If an adult of sound mind makes it clear that some or all aspects of proposed medical care are unacceptable, then this should be respected and documented accurately in the notes, with confirmation by an independent witness. A similar procedure should be followed if treatment is not offered for medical reasons.

Table 1.21 Prophylactic measures against specific complications

Complication	Methods of prophylaxis
Deep vein thrombosis[80,89,90]	Early postoperative mobilization Leg exercises (active/passive) Pneumatic compression of limbs Electrical stimulation of calf muscles Graduated stockings
	Low-dose subcutaneous heparin Warfarin anticoagulation Dextran-70 (Regional anaesthetic techniques, especially for orthopaedic lower-limb procedures)
Aspiration of gastric contents[91]	Nil by mouth Antacids: sodium citrate H_2-antagonists (Omeprazole) (Cisapride) Metoclopramide

Infection
  Surgical procedure
 	
  Infective endocarditis
	Directed by local or national practice with advice of microbiologists
	Follow guidelines of the Endocarditis Working Party[92]

Adrenocortical suppression Suggested for patients who have received exogenous systemic steroids during the 2 months preceding surgery[40]	Hydrocortisone 50 mg 4-hourly or 80 mg 4-hourly, or continue usual steroids if this is in excess of the current requirements (i.e. > 300 mg hydrocortisone equivalent, which is the maximum daily production in response to stress)

Premedication and consideration of prophylactic measures

The final part of pre-operative assessment is to consider premedication and the value of instituting or preparing prophylactic treatment for specific conditions. Premedication is discussed in detail in Chapter 4. A summary of some prophylactic considerations is shown in Table 1.21.

CONCLUSIONS

The standard of care in modern anaesthesia is high, but there are always areas in which improvement can be made. Pre-operative assessment is an essential element of peri-operative care, as many difficulties can be foreseen and addressed, with, benefit to the patient.

These include:

- ensuring that the proposed surgery is realistic in terms of benefit to the patient;
- ensuring that adequate facilities and staff with appropriate experience and expertise are available to perform the operation and to provide an appropriate level of postoperative care;
- ensuring that patients are prepared properly for the operation, and identifying and dealing with existing factors which place them at increased risk of adverse outcome; and
- providing prophylactic measures aimed at preventing the occurrence of some predictable serious complications, e.g. thrombo-embolic events, aspiration of gastric contents.

REFERENCES

1. Paterson-Brown S. Strategies for reducing inappropriate laparotomy rate in the acute abdomen. *Br Med J* 1991; 303: 1115–1118
2. Bates T. Avoiding inappropriate surgery: discussion paper. *J R Soc Med* 1990; 83: 176–178
3. Carnie J, Johnson RA. Clinical anaesthetic knowledge amongst surgical house staff. *Anaesthesia* 1985; 40: 1114–1117
4. British National Formulary, vol 26. London: British Medical Association and the Royal Pharmaceutical Society of Great Britain. 1993: p 457

5. Ray DC, Drummond GB. Halothane hepatitis. *Br J Anaesth* 1991; 67: 84–99
6. Duthie DJR, Montgomery JN, Spence AA, Nimmo WS. Concurrent drug therapy in patients undergoing surgery. *Anaesthesia* 1987, 42: 305–311
7. Corallo CE, Dooley M, Love JB. Failure to administer prescribed preoperative drugs. *Aust J Hosp Pharmacol* 1989; 19: 198–199
8. Wyld R, Nimmo WS. Do patients fasting before and after operation receive their prescribed drug treatment? *Br Med J* 1988; 296: 744
9. Wood PR, Soni N. Anaesthesia and substance abuse. *Anaesthesia* 1989; 44: 672–680
10. Frost EAM, Seidel MR. Preanesthetic assessment of the drug abuse patient. *Anesthesiol Clin North Am* 1990; 8: 829–842
11. Brown C, Osterloh J. Multiple severe complications from recreational ingestion of MDMA ('Ecstasy') *JAMA* 1987; 258: 780–781
12. Singarajah C, Lavies NG. An overdose of ecstasy. *Anaesthesia* 1992; 47: 686–687
13. Fisher MMcD, More DG. The epidemiology and clinical features of anaphylactic reactions in anaesthesia. *Anaesth Intens Care* 1981; 9: 226–234
14. Watkins J. Second report from anaesthetic reactions advisory service. *Anaesthesia* 1989, 44: 157–159
15. Noble DW, Yap PL. Screening for antibodies to anaesthetics; no case for doing it yet. *Br Med J* 1989; 2: 2–3
16. Forrest JB, Rehder K, Cahalan MK, Goldsmith CH. Multicenter study of severe perioperative outcomes. III: Predictors of severe perioperative adverse outcomes. *Anesthesiology* 1992; 76: 3–15
17. Ralston AC, Webb RK, Runciman WB. Potential errors in pulse oximetry. III: Effects of interference, dyes, dyshaemoglobin and other pigments. *Anaesthesia* 1991; 46: 291–295
18. Jones RM, Rosen M, Seymour L. Smoking and anaesthesia. *Anaesthesia* 1987; 42: 1–2
19. Warner MA, Divertie MB, Tinker JH. Preoperative cessation of smoking and pulmonary complications in coronary artery bypass patients. *Anesthesiology* 1984; 60: 380–383
20. Munday IT, Desai PM, Marshall CA, Jones RM, Phillips M-L, Rosen M. The effectiveness of pre-operative advice to stop smoking: a prospective controlled trial. *Anaesthesia* 1993; 48: 816–818
21. Benhorin J, Moss AJ, Oakes D et al. The prognostic significance of first myocardial infarction type (Q-wave versus non Q-wave) and Q-wave location. *J Am Coll Cardiol* 1990; 15: 1201–1207
22. ISIS-2 Collaborative Group. Randomised trial of intravenous streptokinase, oral aspirin, both or neither among 17 187 cases of suspected acute myocardial infarction. *Lancet* 1988; ii: 349–360
23. Fleischer LA, Barash PG. Preoperative cardiac evaluation for non-cardiac surgery: a functional approach. *Anesth Analg* 1992; 74: 586–598
24. Rao TLK, Jacobs KH, El-Etr AA. Reinfarction following anesthesia in patients with myocardial infarction. *Anesthesiology* 1983; 59: 499–505
25. Deanfield JE, Maseri A, Selwyn AP, Ribeiro P, Chierchia S, Krikler S. Myocardial ischaemia during daily life in patients with stable angina: its relation to symptoms and heart rate changes. *Lancet* 1983; ii: 753–758
26. Slogoff S, Keats AS. Does perioperative myocardial ischemia lead to postoperative myocardial infarction? *Anesthesiology* 1985; 62: 107–114
27. Shah KB, Kleinman BS, Rao TLK, Jacobs HK, Mestan K, Schaafsma M. Angina and other risk factors in patients with cardiac diseases undergoing non-cardiac operations. *Anesth Analg* 1990; 70: 240–247
28. Rosenman RH, Sholtz RI, Brand RJ. A study of comparative blood pressure measurements in predicting risk of coronary artery disease. *Circulation* 1976; 54: 51–58
29. Asiddao CB, Donegan JH, Whitesell RC, Kalbfleisch JH. Factors associated with perioperative complications during carotid endarterectomy. *Anesth Analg* 1982; 61: 631–37
30. Bedford RF, Feinstein B. Hospital admission blood pressure: a predictor for hypertension following endotracheal intubation. *Anesth Analg* 1980; 59: 367–370
31. Farnett L, Mulrow CD, Linn WB, Lucey CR, Tuley MR. The J-curve phenomenon and the treatment of hypertension: is there a point beyond which pressure reduction becomes dangerous? *JAMA* 1991; 265: 489–495
32. Yurenev AP, Dequattro V, Devereux RB. Hypertensive heart disease: relationship of silent ischemia to coronary artery disease and left ventricular hypertrophy. *Am Heart J* 1990; 120: 928–933
33. Goldman L, Caldera DL, Nussbaum SR et al. Multifactorial index of cardiac risk in noncardiac surgical procedures. *N Engl J Med* 1977; 297: 845–850
34. Detsky AS, Abrams HB, Forbath N, Scott JG, Hilliard JR. Cardiac assessment for patients undergoing non-cardiac surgery: a multi-factorial clinical risk index. *Arch Intern Med* 1986; 146: 2131–2134
35. Bloomfield P, Bowler GMR. Anaesthetic management of the patient with a permanent pacemaker. *Anaesthesia* 1989; 44: 42–46
36. Cohen MM, Cameron CB. Should you cancel the operation when a child has an upper respiratory tract infection? *Anesth Analg* 1991; 72: 282–288
37. Fennelly ME, Hall GM. Anaesthesia and upper respiratory tract infections. A non-existent hazard? *Br J Anaesth* 1990; 64: 535–536
38. Ong BY, Pahlniuk RJ, Cumming M. Gastric volume and pH in out-patients. *Can Anaesth Soc J* 1978; 25: 36–39
39. Shenkman Z, Shir Y, Brodsky JB. Perioperative management of the obese patient. *Br J Anaesth* 1993; 70: 349–359
40. Milaskiewicz RM, Hall GM. Diabetes and anaesthesia: the past decade. *Br J Anaesth* 1992; 68: 198–206
41. Napolitano LM, Chernow B. Guidelines for corticosteroid use in anesthetic and surgical stress. *Int Anesthesiol Clin* 1988; 26: 226–232
42. Savarese JJ, Ali HH, Basta SJ et al. The clinical neuromuscular pharmacology of mivacurium chloride. *Anesthesiology* 1988; 68: 723–732
43. Harrison GG, Meissner PN, Hift RJ. Anaesthesia for the porphyric patient. *Anaesthesia* 1993; 48: 417–421
44. Carson JL, Poses RM, Spence RK, Bonavita G. Severity of anaemia and operative mortality and morbidity. *Lancet* 1988; i: 727–729

45. Skeus MA, Welchew EA. Anaesthesia and rheumatoid arthritis. *Anaesthesia* 1993; 48: 989–997
46. Agarwal AK, Peppelman WC Jr, Kraus DR, Eisenbeis CH Jr. The cervical spine in rheumatoid arthritis. *Br Med J* 1993; 306: 79–80
47. Conlon PW, Isdale IC, Rose BS. Rheumatoid arthritis of the cervical spine. An analysis of 333 cases. *Ann Rheum Dis* 1971; 25: 120–126
48. Marks V. Clinical biochemistry nearer the patient. *Br Med J* 1983; 286: 1166–1167
49. Verma PK, Dhond G, Lawler PG. The interpretation of results by doctor technicians. *Anaesthesia* 1990; 45: 412
50. Lawrence VA, Kroenke K. The unproven utility of preoperative urinalysis. *Arch Intern Med* 1988; 148: 1370–1373
51. Campbell IT, Gosling P. Preoperative biochemical screening. *Br Med J* 1988; 297: 803–804
52. McKee RF, Scott EM. The value of routine preoperative investigations. *Ann R Coll Surg Engl* 1987; 69: 160-162
53. McCleane GJ. Urea and electrolyte measurement in preoperative surgical patients. *Anaesthesia* 1988; 43: 413–415
54. Royal College Working Party on the Effective Use of Diagnostic Radiology. Preoperative chest radiology. National study by the Royal College of Radiologists. *Lancet* 1979; ii: 83–86
55. Tape TG, Mushlin AI. The utility of routine chest radiographs. *Ann Intern Med* 1986; 104: 663–670
56. Bruce RA. Methods of exercise testing: step test, bicycle, treadmill, isometrics. *Am J Cardiol* 1974; 33: 715–720
57. Rohrer MJ, Michelotti MC, Nahrwold DL. A prospective evaluation of the efficacy of preoperative coagulation testing. *Ann Surg* 1988; 208: 554–557
58. Macdonald R. Aspirin and extradural blocks. *Br J Anaesth* 1991; 66: 1–3
59. Lawrence VA, Page CP, Harris GD. Preoperative spirometry before abdominal operations. A critical appraisal of its predictive value. *Arch Intern Med* 1989; 149: 280–283
60. Nunn JF, Milledge JS, Chen D, Dore C. Respiratory criteria of fitness for surgery and anaesthesia. *Anaesthesia* 1988; 43: 543–551
61. Hudson JC, Dawson KS, Kane FR, Tyler BL, Keenan RL. Are intraoperative complication rates influenced by ASA physical status, age, and emergency versus elective surgery? *Anesth Analg* 1990; 70: S166
62. Vacanti CJ, VanHouten RJ, Hill RC. A statistical analysis of the relationship of physical status to postoperative mortality in 68 388 cases. *Anesth Analg* 1969; 49: 564–566
63. Cohen MM, Duncan PG. Physical status score and trends in anesthetic complications. *J Clin Epidemiol* 1988; 41: 83–90
64. Knaus WA, Draper EA, Wagner D, Zimmerman JE. APACHE II: A severity of disease classification. *Crit Care Med* 1985; 13: 818–829
65. Knaus WA, Wagner DP, Draper EA et al. The APACHE III prognostic system: risk prediction of hospital mortality for critically ill hospitalized adults. *Chest* 1991; 100: 1619–1636
66. Schein M, Gecelter G. APACHE II score in massive upper gastro-intestinal haemorrhage from peptic ulcer: prognostic value and potential clinical applications. *Br J Surg* 1989; 76: 733–736
67. Playforth MJ, Smith GMR, Evans M, Pollock AV. Preoperative assessment of fitness score. *Br J Surg.* 1987; 74: 890–892
68. Buck N, Devlin HB, Lunn JN. *Report of the confidential enquiry into perioperative deaths.* London: Nuffield Provincial Hospitals Trust/King's Fund. 1987
69. Campling EA, Devlin HB, Hoile RW, Lunn JN. *Report of the national confidential enquiry into perioperative deaths.* London: NCEPOD. 1990
70. Campling EA, Devlin HB, Hoile RW, Lunn JN. *Report of the national confidential enquiry into perioperative deaths.* London: NCEPOD. 1991/2
71. Mallampati SR, Gatt SP, Gugino LD, Desai SK, Waraksa B, Freiberger D. A clinical sign to predict difficult tracheal intubation: a prospective study. *Can Anaesth Soc J* 1985; 32: 429–434
72. Samsoon GLT, Young JRB. Difficult tracheal intubation: a retrospective study. *Anaesthesia* 1987; 42: 487–490
73. Oates JDL, Oates PD, Pearsall RJ, Howie JC, Murray GD. Comparison of two methods for predicting difficult intubation. *Br J Anaesth* 1991; 66: 305–309
74. Wilson ME, Speighalter D, Robertson JA, Lesser P. Predicting difficult intubation. *Br J Anaesth* 1988; 61: 211–216
75. Frerk C. Predicting difficult intubation. *Anaesthesia* 1991; 46: 1005–1008
76. Cormack RS, Lehane J. Difficult tracheal intubation in obstetrics. *Anaesthesia* 1984; 39: 1105–1111
77. Mangano DT. Perioperative cardiac morbidity. *Anesthesiology* 1990; 72: 153–184
78. Hunt JN. Some properties of an alimentary osmoreceptor mechanism. *J Physiol (Lond)* 1956; 132: 267–288
79. Phillips S, Hutchinson S, Davidson T. Preoperative drinking does not affect gastric contents. *Br J Anaesth* 1993; 70: 6–9
80. Clokie C, Metcalf I, Holland A. Dental trauma in anaesthesia. *Can J Anaesth* 1989; 36: 675–680
81. Thromboembolic Risk Factors (THRIFT) consensus group. Risk of and prophylaxis for venous thromboembolism in hospital patients. *Br Med J* 1992; 305: 567–574
82. Whitehead EM, Whitehead MI. The pill, HRT, and postoperative thromboembolism: cause for concern? *Anaesthesia* 1991; 46: 521–522
83. British National Formulary, vol. 26, London: *British Medical Association and the Royal Pharmaceutical Society of Great Britain.* 1993: p 267
84. Benson KT. The Jehovah's Witness patient: considerations for the anesthesiologist. *Anesth Analg* 1989; 69: 647–656
85. Cathcart ES, Spodick DH. Rheumatoid heart disease: a study of the incidence and nature of cardiac lesions in rheumatoid arthritis. *N Engl J Med* 1962; 266: 959–964
86. Bacon PA, Gibson DG. Cardiac involvement in rheumatoid arthritis — an echocardiographic study. *Ann Rheum Dis* 1972; 31: 426
87. Begin R, Radoux V, Cantin A, Menard HA. Stiffness of the rib cage in a subset of rheumatoid patients. *Lung* 1988; 166: 141–148
88. Kay A. European league against Rheumatism: study of adverse reactions to D-penicillamine. *Br J Rheumatol* 1986; 25: 193–198

89 Nunn JF. Clinical aspects of the interaction between nitrous oxide and vitamin B_{12}. *Br J Anaesth* 1987; 59: 3–13
90 Goucke CR. Prophylaxis against venous thromboembolism. *Anaesth Intens Care* 1989; 4: 58–65
91 Dehring DJ, Arens JF. Pulmonary thromboembolism: disease recognition and patient management. *Anesthesiology* 1990; 73: 146–164
92 Joyce TH III. Prophylaxis for pulmonary acid aspiration. *Am J Med* 1987; 83 (suppl 6A): 46–52
93 Endocarditis Working Party of the British Society for Antimicrobial Chemotherapy. Antibiotic prophylaxis of infective endocarditis. *Lancet* 1990; 335: 88–89
94 Kissen B. Alcohol abuse and alcohol-related illness. In: Wyngaarden JB, smith LH Jr (eds) Cecil Textbook of Medicine, 8th edn. Philadelphia, PA: WB Saunders, 1992: p 45
95 New York Heart Association. *Diseases of the heart and blood vessels — nomenclature and criteria for diagnosis*, 6th edn. Boston, MA: Little, Brown. 1964
96 American Society of Anesthesiology classification of physical status. *Anesthesiology* 1963; 24: 111

2. Influence of co-existing disease on anaesthetic management

C. A. Marshall

HEART DISEASE

Pre-existing heart disease, whether diagnosed or not, remains the commonest cause of peri-operative morbidity and mortality. In developed countries, coronary artery disease accounts for the greatest proportion of conditions which damage the heart.

Coronary artery disease

Coronary artery disease is estimated to be present in 10 million adults in the UK, and is responsible for about one-third of all deaths in persons between 35 and 65 years of age.[1] It is likely that coronary artery disease is present in approximately 25% of patients who undergo anaesthesia and surgery and the presence of coronary artery disease is associated with increased postoperative morbidity and mortality.[2,3] Apart from rare congenital anomalies, most coronary artery disease is due to atheroma and its complications. There is increasing evidence that there may be different risk factors for angina as distinct from myocardial infarction. These factors are listed in Table 2.1.

Myocardial ischaemia may be asymptomatic or manifested by angina, arrhythmias and ventricular failure. A history of angina is the most important factor in making the diagnosis of coronary artery disease. This is usually described as a tightness around the middle of the chest and and may radiate down the arms and up to the throat. Situations precipitating angina include physical exertion, exposure to cold, heavy meals, intense emotion and even violent dreams. Physical examination is frequently negative, but evidence of contributing or concomitant diseases should be sought. These include hypertension, hyperlipidaemia, anaemia, obesity, diabetes mellitus, hypothyroidism and peripheral vascular disease. The presence of significant aortic valve disease, particularly aortic stenosis, should also be sought.

The electrocardiogram (ECG) may be normal in patients with coronary artery disease. The most convincing ECG evidence of ischaemia is the demonstration of reversible ST segment depression or elevation, with or without T-wave inversion, at the time the patient is experiencing symptoms. Some patients show ECG signs of established infarction. These include the presence of Q waves, and sometimes T-wave inversion. Formal exercise testing may be undertaken using a treadmill, and is a standard procedure which ensures a progressive and reproducible increase in workload. The amount of exercise which can be tolerated under these conditions is a useful guide to the extent of coronary disease.

Myocardial perfusion scanning using radioactive thallium may be helpful in evaluating the minority of patients with an atypical history, or the small group of patients with severe symptoms but no significant ECG abnormality on exercise testing. Echocardiography provides information about ventricular function and coronary arteriography provides detailed information about the coronary vessels and ejection fractions of the ventricles. The majority of patients are managed by drug treatment and the principal groups of drugs which are used in the control of angina are nitrates, β-adrenoceptor antagonists and calcium antagonists. Surgical treatment of ischaemic heart disease either

Table 2.1 Risk factors for angina and myocardial infarction

Risk factors for angina
Hypercholesterolaemia
Smoking
Hypertension
Diabetes mellitus
Sedentary lifestyle

Additional risk factors for myocardial infarction
Hypotriglyceridaemia
Hyperfibrinogenaemia
Polyunsaturated fatty acid deficiency
Increased plasma factor VII levels

involves coronary angioplasty or coronary artery bypass grafting.

Pathophysiology

The ischaemia is due to an imbalance between myocardial oxygen supply and demand, and the principal mechanism is an inadequate increase in myocardial oxygen delivery. Oxygen extraction from coronary blood is virtually maximal, leaving no room for increased delivery if flow rate remains steady. However, coronary blood flow can normally increase four- to fivefold to increase oxygen delivery. If the increase in flow is prevented by either static or dynamic occlusion of the coronary arteries, ischaemia may result.

Factors which influence oxygen delivery and demand are shown in Table 2.2. From this table, it can be surmised that tachycardia is a more important determinant of myocardial ischaemia than is systolic hypertension, and that an increased heart rate is more likely to produce ECG signs of ischaemia and angina.[4] This is logical because a tachycardia not only increases myocardial demand but, by shortening diastole, reduces coronary blood flow, whereas hypertension may actually increase coronary blood flow by increasing the perfusion pressure.

Factors influencing the incidence of peri-operative myocardial infarction

In conscious patients, angina occurs at a relatively constant rate-pressure product (RPP; the product of heart rate and systolic blood pressure.)[5] The amount of cardiac work which produces angina in the awake patient may differ from that which produces ischaemia in the anaesthetized patient. However, the RPP may still be of some value as it is the only simple clinical measure of cardiac work, although it must be appreciated that tachycardia is far more deleterious than systolic hypertension.

The most important predisposing factor for peri-operative myocardial infarction is history of a previous myocardial infarction. The incidence of myocardial re-infarction is related to the time elapsed since the previous infarction (Table 2.3);[2,3] 6 months after myocardial infarction, the incidence of peri-operative re-infarction was 5–6%, about 50 times greater than the incidence of approximately 0.1% in patients who underwent similar operations in the absence of a prior infarct. Mortality from myocardial re-infarction in both these studies was greater than 50%. The use of invasive monitoring, especially in centres with experience in dealing with high-risk patients, can reduce the incidence of re-infarction if therapeutic intervention is appropriate and aggressive. A single study has suggested that, if these conditions are met, the re-infarction rate may be no greater if surgery is performed within 6 months of a previous infarction than in patients undergoing surgery more than 6 months after infarction.[6] The incidence of re-infarction is greater in patients undergoing intra-thoracic or intra-abdominal operations lasting longer than 3 h.[3] Other adverse factors include intra-operative hypertension and tachycardia,[6] and patients with three vessel or left main stem coronary artery disease.[7] The risk of postoperative myocardial infarction following non-cardiac operations in patients with one- or two-vessel coronary artery disease appears to be relatively low, as it is in patients who have undergone prior coronary artery bypass operations.[7] Attempts to predict life-threatening postoperative complications by tabulating characteristics such as age, prior myocardial infarction,

Table 2.2 Factors affecting the balance between myocardial oxygen delivery and demand

Decreased oxygen delivery	Increased oxygen requirement
Decreased coronary blood flow	Increased sympathetic drive
Tachycardia	Tachycardia
Diastolic hypotension	Systolic hypertension
Coronary artery spasm	Increased myocardial contractility
	Increased afterload
Decreased coronary blood oxygen content	
Anaemia	
Arterial hypoxaemia	
Left shift of oxyhaemoglobin dissociation curve	
Increased preload	

Table 2.3 Incidence of peri-operative myocardial re-infarction

Time elapsed since prior myocardial infarction	Tarhan et al[2]	Steen et al[3]	Rao et al[6]
3 months	37%	27%	5.7%
3–6 months	16%	11%	2.3%
> 6 months	5%	6%	

aortic stenosis, evidence of congestive heart failure and cardiac arrhythmias has not proved to be superior to the American Society of Anesthesiologists (ASA) physical status classification.[8,9]

More recently, research has concentrated on the functional status of the autonomic nervous system. It has been demonstrated that the degree of impairment of autonomic reflexes can be correlated with the extent of haemodynamic instability after induction of anaesthesia.[10] Moreover, reduced autonomic function may be predictive of postoperative cardiac dysfunction,[11] and has been associated with an increased risk of adverse cardiac events after myocardial infarction.[12,13] It has also been implicated in prolonging episodes of myocardial ischaemia in patients with angina.[14] There are numerous diseases which are known to cause autonomic dysfunction, and these include diabetes, hypertension, congestive heart failure, myocardial infarction, chronic renal failure and the ageing process. It is noteworthy that this list has many diseases in common with the conditions which predispose to ischaemic heart disease. In addition, drugs, including anaesthetic drugs, have effects on the autonomic nervous system. The evaluation of the autonomic nervous system has been limited by the lack of an easily applied clinical measurement technique. One method which is at present purely a research tool, but has the potential to become a more routine clinical test, is power spectral analysis of heart rate variability. The beat-to-beat variation in heart rate consists of oscillations which are in phase with ventilation, and thought to result primarily from cardiac vagal mechanisms.[15] However, there are other periodic oscillations in heart rate, which are unrelated to ventilation, and which are usually slower than the respiratory frequency. By applying Fourier transformation to a time series of heart periods, the heart period oscillations can be described in a series of sine waves with different amplitudes and frequencies.[16] The analysis is complex, but some low-frequency oscillations (0.05–0.15 Hz) are thought to result primarily from changing levels of cardiac sympathetic activity.[17,18] A predominance of low-frequency power and a reduction in high-frequency power has been noted in patients shortly after myocardial infarction.[19,20] These data raise the possibility that power spectral analysis of heart period oscillations could serve as an early marker of myocardial ischaemia.

Anaesthetic management of patients with coronary artery disease for non-cardiac surgery centres on preventing peri-operative ischaemia. There is evidence that the presence of peri-operative myocardial ischaemia increases the risk of postoperative myocardial infarction.[21] More recently, research has concentrated also on the importance of the postoperative period in the generation of ischaemic events, and therefore of adverse outcome.

Large changes in heart rate and blood pressure must be avoided. A reasonable aim is to maintain heart rate and blood pressure within 20% of awake values. However, a significant proportion of new ischaemic episodes observed in patients before cardiopulmonary bypass are not preceded by significant changes in blood pressure or heart rate.[22] Forty-five per cent of patients also show evidence of myocardial ischaemia on thallium scan in the absence of haemodynamic changes, during intubation of the trachea.[22,23] These ischaemic changes are presumably due to coronary artery spasm.

It has been proposed that hypercoagulability after surgery might be an additional mechanism responsible for postoperative myocardial infarction. Epidural anaesthesia reduces the risk of deep venous thrombosis and pulmonary embolism in several patient populations subjected to major surgery.[24] This beneficial effect is explained in part by improved deep venous flow conditions, but in vitro studies have demonstrated that some local anaesthetics increase fibrinolytic activity and decrease platelet aggregation.[25] In 1991, Tuman and co-workers[26] published a study of 80 patients subjected to lower-limb revascularization, assigned randomly to receive general anaesthesia with or without associated epidural anaesthesia. In the epidural group, analgesia with bupivacaine and fentanyl was extended into the postoperative period, whereas the patients in the general anaesthesia group received parenteral opioid pain relief. Coagulation status was monitored by the thrombo-elastograph. An additional 40 patients without vascular disease, and undergoing non-cardiac surgery, served as controls for the coagulopathy studies. The authors found that hypercoagulability was significantly more common in patients with vascular disease than in control patients, and that epidural anesthesia reduced the incidence of thrombotic events. Stepwise logistic regression demonstrated that the only predictors of cardiac complications were previous congestive heart failure and general anaesthesia without epidural analgesia. These data on vascular surgery patients should not be extrapolated to other groups of patients. However, they provide an impetus for further studies on the influence of hypercoagulability during and after surgery upon thrombotic events and the modification of these effects by anaesthetic technique.

Management of anaesthesia

Adequate premedication is essential to avoid pre-induction ischaemia.[27] Most episodes of pre-induction ischaemia reported in the literature have been silent, i.e. detected by the ECG but not reported by the patients despite specific questioning.[27-29] A common regimen comprises administration of an oral dose of benzodiazepine on the night before surgery and again on the morning of surgery, followed by intramuscular administration of morphine and hyoscine 1 h before induction of anaesthesia. This regimen may produce considerable sedation, and supplementary oxygen should always be administered prior to and during transportation of the patient to the operating theatre. The patient's normal oral cardiac and antihypertensive medication should also be administered on the morning of surgery.

Induction of anaesthesia in patients with coronary artery disease can be accomplished using thiopentone, etomidate or intravenous alfentanil, fentanyl, or esmolol can be administered to minimize these haemodynamic changes. Continuous intravenous infusion of esmolol 100 $\mu g.kg^{-1}.min^{-1}$, before and during laryngoscopy, has been shown to be effective in reducing tachycardia.[30]

Patients with normal left ventricular function are likely to develop tachycardia and hypertension in response to surgical stimulation and are at risk of myocardial ischaemia. Consequently, a degree of myocardial depression from the use of a volatile anaesthetic agent may be beneficial. Both halothane and isoflurane produce similar changes in blood pressure and heart rate when administered to patients with coronary artery disease.[31] The mechanism for reduction in blood pressure is different, isoflurane producing predominantly peripheral vasodilatation, and halothane producing a reduction in cardiac output.[32] Isoflurane is a more potent coronary arterial vasodilator than halothane in patients with coronary artery disease.[33] This could theoretically lead to coronary artery steal, when drug-induced vasodilatation of normal coronary arterioles diverts blood flow from stenotic coronary arterioles which are unable to dilate. However, the administration of isoflurane to most patients with coronary artery disease is not associated with evidence of myocardial ischaemia, as long as any reduction in coronary perfusion pressure (mean arterial pressure) is minimized.[32,34,35] Patients with impaired left ventricular function may become hypotensive when anaesthesia is maintained with an inhalational agent due to depression of an already compromised ventricle. In these patients, large doses of short-acting opioids may be used as the predominant maintenance agent, with small doses of inhalational agents to guarantee unconsciousness. Nitrous oxide, particularly in the presence of opioids, may be associated with significant circulatory changes, including reductions in blood pressure and cardiac output.[36] However, nitrous oxide added to volatile anaesthetic drugs does not produce the same signs of myocardial depression.[37] Many centres now avoid the use of nitrous oxide in these patients.

Although regional anaesthesia can be used in conjunction with general anaesthesia in patients with coronary artery disease, any reduction in blood pressure due to reduced sympathetic tone, and the compensatory tachycardia, must not be allowed to persist, as these changes will reduce coronary perfusion pressure and increase myocardial oxygen demand. Prompt treatment with fluids and/or vasoconstrictors is imperative. A solution of dilute bupivacaine (0.25 or 0.125%) with an opioid provides effective blockade of sensory input, and therefore minimizes sympathetic stimulation, without excessive loss of systemic vascular resistance.

Muscle relaxants may affect the autonomic nervous system and have the ability to stimulate histamine release, and to produce significant changes in heart rate, cardiac output, blood pressure and myocardial oxygenation. These cardiovascular effects are influenced by choice of muscle relaxant, the haemodynamic status of the patient, pre-operative drug therapy, and by the sequence and speed of administration. The use of tubocurarine in clinical doses has a nicotine-like effect, and blocks both parasympathetic and sympathetic autonomic ganglia and pathways. It can also cause histamine release, which is mainly responsible for the peripheral vasodilatation and hypotension associated with the use of the drug.[38] Slow administration of tubocurarine and pretreatment with antihistamines attenuate its hypotensive effects.[39] Suxamethonium can precipitate cardiac arrhythmias because of autonomic stimulation, and muscle fasciculations have been reported to cause failure of cardiac pacemakers. Pancuronium has vagolytic effects and increases heart rate by 10–15%. Vecuronium has no effect on heart rate, blood pressure, α- or β-adrenoceptors, or baroreceptor reflex activity. It has a wide margin of safety between neuromuscular activity and autonomic ganglion blockade, and no haemodynamic effects in doses up to 20 times that required for neuromuscular blockade.[40] However, since vecuronium does not have the vagolytic effects of pancuronium, the vagotonic effect of opioids may become apparent, and severe bradycardia can occur. Atracurium also has a wide margin of safety between its neuromuscular blocking effects and its cardiovascular effects. Rapid administration of large doses of atracurium (four to eight times the ED_{95}) stimulate histamine release and cause tachycardia and hypotension. The use of relaxants free of cardiovascular side-effects has emphasized the side-effects of other drugs, such as the bradycardia caused by opioids. However, it is not appropriate to rely on a side-effect of a muscle relaxant to offset haemodynamic changes produced by other drugs. It is preferable to use muscle relaxants free of cardiovascular effects, such as vecuronium, and to use the appropriate therapy to treat haemodynamic changes as they occur. Reversal of neuromuscular blockade is best achieved using glycopyrronium as the anticholinergic drug administered with neostigmine, as it has less chronotropic effects than atropine.

Monitoring

In addition to the usual monitoring associated with the provision of safe anaesthesia, the aim of monitoring in patients with coronary artery disease is early detection of myocardial ischaemia and/or reduced myocardial contractility.

There is a predictable correlation between the ECG lead that best displays myocardial ischaemia, and the anatomical distribution of the diseased coronary artery in that patient. A V5 (precordial) lead will reflect myocardial ischaemia present in that portion of the left ventricle supplied by the left anterior descending coronary artery.[41] It is possible to obtain a V5 lead using a three-lead electrode system by placing the left arm lead in V5 position, and selecting aVL on the monitor. Lead II monitors the myocardium in the distribution of the right coronary artery. An oesophageal electrocardiogram is sometimes recommended, the advantage being that its position in the oesophagus just posterior to the atrium records augmented P waves, which may help in the diagnosis of arrhythmias, and has a secondary function in displaying early signs of posterior wall myocardial ischaemia. The ECG channel on continuous display during anaesthesia should be the lead covering the ischaemic area of the patient's myocardium, if that is known. Significant myocardial ischaemia is considered to be present when there is at least 1 mm depression of ST segments from the baseline on the ECG.

Use of a pulmonary artery catheter during anaesthesia may be helpful in a patient with left ventricular impairment, or when a large amount of blood loss is expected during the procedure. Acute increases in pulmonary artery occlusion (wedge) pressure, together with the appearance of abnormal wave forms, may reflect myocardial ischaemia.[42] In addition to providing a guide to intravascular fluid volumes and fluid replacement, and possibly providing early warning of ischaemia, the pulmonary artery catheter can be used to measure cardiac output and systemic and pulmonary vascular resistances. These measurements are useful in evaluating the response to inotropic or vasodilating drugs. With increasing emphasis on cost containment, and recognizing the morbidity attached to the insertion and use of pulmonary artery catheters, there has been much research into the indications for their placement. Central venous and pulmonary artery occlusion pressures have been shown to correlate closely in patients with coronary artery disease when ejection fraction is above 0.5 and there is no evidence of left ventricular dyskinesia.[43] However, when ejection fraction is below 0.5, the correlation is lost and a pulmonary artery catheter in this situation is therefore valuable.

In any patient with significant CAD in whom large volume blood losses are expected, direct arterial pressure monitoring is mandatory. At present, the goal of continuous non-invasive blood pressure measurement has not been achieved, although the Finapres monitor (Ohmeda, Denver, Colorado, USA), which uses finger photoplethysmography, has generated much interest. However, a recent study[44] comparing the Finapres device with intra-arterial blood pressure monitoring concluded that, although the device was accurate most of the time, there were discrepancies of significant magnitude and duration to limit the use of the device in clinical situations where this information is essential, e.g. significant arterial hypotension.

Intra-operative echocardiography is at present a research tool, but it offers the anaesthetist the ability to evaluate the function of the left and right ventricles continuously. It has been suggested that myocardial ischaemia may be detected as a reduction in ejection fraction before the ECG changes.[45] Continuous ejection fraction monitoring could also be used to assess the effect of volume loading and inotropic or vaso-active interventions. Valve competence under different fluid loads can be assessed with the use of Doppler colour flow imaging. In the future, the ability to perform continuous echocardiography may be an important tool in the anaesthetist's armamentarium.

Postoperative care

Postoperative management should be directed towards avoiding hypoxaemia during the time of excessive oxygen demand, avoiding sudden increases in peripheral vascular resistance and, above all, limiting postoperative tachycardia. If the patient is hypothermic on entering the recovery room, then anaesthesia and positive-pressure ventilation should ideally be continued until the patient achieves normal core and peripheral temperatures. The recovery period is characterized by elevated sympathetic tone with increased peripheral vascular resistance, tachycardia and hypertension. Calcium antagonists have been shown to be effective in controlling hypertensive episodes related to an increase in peripheral vascular resistance.[46] Anaesthetic care should be designed to produce a patient who is both warm and pain-free at the end of the operation, as this will minimize haemodynamic changes.

Tachycardia remains a common problem not just during recovery but in the extended postoperative period. Mangano and co-workers, who studied 474 abdominal or vascular surgical patients with evidence of coronary artery disease, recorded an intra-operative mean heart rate of 74 beats.min^{-1}, compared with a mean of 90 beats.min^{-1} postoperatively.[47] Tachycardia has been reported to persist for 7–10 days after surgery.[29] Although the causes of this tachycardia are undoubtedly multifactorial and also patient-dependent, it seems likely that effective pain relief is the single most important factor in providing haemodynamic stability. Postoperative thoracic epidural analgesia has been documented to limit postoperative haemodynamic alterations[48] and also to reduce cardiac complication rates in high-risk patients undergoing major non-cardiac surgery.[49]

Valvular heart disease

Anaesthesia for the patient with valvular heart disease requires an understanding of the pathophysiology of the valve lesion, and appraisal of its effects on the ventricular myocardium. The effect of the heart disease on pulmonary, hepatic and renal function must be assessed, and any underlying conditions such as connective tissue disease fully investigated.

Aortic stenosis

The likely aetiology of aortic stenosis varies with the age of the patient. The main causes are shown in Table 2.4. The clinical presentation may include exertional dyspnoea, angina, exertional syncope, pulmonary oedema and secondary right heart failure. In addition, the patient may be asymptomatic, even with tight aortic stenosis. Clinical features include an ejection systolic murmur, which radiates to the carotid arteries, and a slow rising carotid pulse. The ECG usually shows signs of left ventricular hypertrophy. The chest X-ray may be normal. As the disease progresses and the ventricle decompensates, an enlarged left ventricle may be seen, with a dilated ascending aorta on postero-anterior views. The calcified valve may be seen on the lateral view. Echocardiography shows an abnormal, usually heavily calcified valve and a hypertrophied left ventricle. The systolic gradient across the aortic valve should be assessed by Doppler cardiography, as crossing the aortic valve with a cardiac catheter may be dangerous. However, cardiac catheterization may be undertaken to assess the state of the coronary arteries.

Table 2.4 Causes of aortic stenosis (AS)

Children–adolescents
Congenital AS
Congenital subvalvular AS
Congenital supravalvular AS

Young adults–middle age
Calcification of bicuspid valve
Rheumatic

Middle age–elderly
Rheumatic
Calcification of bicuspid valve
Senile degeneration

Pathophysiology. Angina may be the presenting symptom in patients with aortic stenosis, even in the presence of normal coronary arteries. This is due to the increased myocardial oxygen requirements of the hypertrophied ventricular muscle. In addition, myocardial oxygen delivery, particularly to the sub-endocardium, is compromised by the increased left ventricular systolic pressure. Left ventricular filling in patients with aortic stenosis is dependent on atrial contraction, a normal heart rate and a normal intra-vascular fluid volume. Increases in heart rate reduce the time for left ventricular filling and ejection, and increase myocardial oxygen demand. Sudden reductions in heart rate can cause acute overdistension of the left ventricle.

Management of anaesthesia. The goal is to maintain a normal heart rate and rhythm, and avoid any excessive changes in circulating volume. A direct current defibrillator should be available to cardiovert a tachyarrhythmia, and to provide immediate defibrillation in the event of ventricular fibrillation. External cardiac massage is unlikely to be effective in these patients, as it is difficult to generate sufficient cardiac output across the stenosed valve, and the aortic root pressure is unlikely to be high enough to provide adequate flow to the myocardium. A study of the natural history of moderate aortic stenosis in 66 patients with early symptoms during a 4-year period revealed an overall mortality rate approaching that in patients with severe stenosis.[50] Therefore, all patients with moderate aortic stenosis are at significant risk of complications in the short term.

Pre-operative antibiotic prophylaxis should be given. A benzodiazepine premedication should not cause alteration in heart rate or peripheral vascular resistance. General anaesthesia is usually preferable to regional, as a reduction in peripheral vascular resistance and hence in aortic diastolic root pressure should be avoided. Anaesthesia should be induced in the presence of full monitoring. Although there are no specific recommendations for maintenance of anaesthesia, halothane is relatively contra-indicated because it depresses sino-atrial node automaticity and is associated with a high incidence of junctional rhythm. High doses of all the volatile anaesthetic agents produce myocardial depression, and a balanced technique with the addition of opioids is therefore preferable; a non-depolarizing muscle relaxant with minimal effects on blood pressure and heart rate, such as vecuronium, should be used. Intra-operative bradycardia must be treated promptly with an anticholinergic agent. Tachycardia should also be treated quickly, although it may be preferable to employ direct current cardioversion rather than pharmacological agents, which often have negative inotropic effects on the left ventricle. However, patients with aortic stenosis are prone to develop ventricular arrhythmias and a variety of anti-arrhythmic agents, including lignocaine, should be immediately to hand.

Aortic regurgitation

The valve may be congenitally abnormal or may have been damaged by rheumatic heart disease or infective endocarditis. Aortic regurgitation may also be due to dilatation of the first part of the aorta in cystic medial necrosis, Marfan's syndrome, ankylosing spondylitis, late syphilis or atheroma.

The patient usually presents with dyspnoea and sometimes an abnormal awareness of the heart beat, particularly when lying on the left side. The clinical diagnosis is made in the presence of a collapsing pulse with an early diastolic murmur of regurgitation, sometimes accompanied by an Austin Flint murmur in mid-diastole due to fluttering of the mitral leaflet in the regurgitant jet. A systolic flow murmur, due to the increased stroke volume, is common, and should not be regarded as signifying aortic stenosis without other evidence. The apex beat is displaced due to the enlarged left ventricle. The ECG is initially normal, but later shows signs of left ventricular hypertrophy and T-wave inversion. Chest X-ray shows cardiac dilatation and there may be associated aortic dilatation. Echocardiography shows a dilated left ventricle and associated fluttering of the anterior mitral leaflet.

Pathophysiology. The incompetent aortic valve produces a volume overload of the left ventricle. The ventricle initially compensates for the regurgitation by increasing stroke volume. This is associated with marked increases in ventricular muscle mass and, secondarily, myocardial oxygen requirements. The decreased aortic diastolic pressure has adverse effects on coronary artery blood flow, and subendocardial ischaemia may be present, even in the absence of coronary artery disease. The degree of regurgitation through the valve is reduced by tachycardia, and also by a lowered peripheral vascular resistance.

Management of anaesthesia. The aim of anaesthesia is to maintain forward left ventricular ejection by minimizing any increase in peripheral vascular resistance, or even decreasing it. This reduces impedance to ejection of the left ventricle. It must be remembered, however, that too low a diastolic pressure reduces coronary artery blood flow. Bradycardia must be avoided, and a mild tachycardia is preferable. Although regional anaesthesia may have desirable effects on peripheral vascular resistance, extensive blockade (for example, in Caesarean section) may produce catastrophic loss of peripheral vascular resistance combined with the need for fluid loading in a patient with an already distended left ventricle. These circumstances were implicated in a maternal death in a recent *Report on Confidential Enquiries into Maternal Deaths*.[51] There are no specific recommendations for induction and maintenance of anaesthesia, beyond avoiding bradycardia and left ventricular depression. An undesired increase in peripheral vascular resistance can be managed in these patients by an intravenous infusion of glyceryl trinitrate or sodium nitroprusside. However, a combination of pre-operative fluid loading and intravenous infusion of nitroprusside has been shown to produce more favourable changes to systemic vascular resistance and cardiac output than does vasodilator therapy alone.[52] Intra-operative monitoring should include use of an ECG lead which will reveal left ventricular ischaemia, and a pulmonary artery catheter may be helpful if large fluid shifts are expected.

Artificial aortic valves

The risk of cardiac death after aortic valve replacement has been studied prospectively in 100 patients, 58 of whom had aortic stenosis and 42 of whom had aortic regurgitation.[53] Mortality was higher in patients with pre-operative evidence of left ventricular dysfunction (irrespective of the underlying valve lesion), and also in those with ECG signs of left ventricular hypertrophy and repetitive premature ventricular beats after surgery. These findings have important implications for the peri-operative management and level of monitoring of these patients during subsequent operations.

Mitral stenosis

Mitral stenosis is almost always due to rheumatic fever, although there is a positive history of rheumatic fever or chorea in only 50% of patients. In severe mitral stenosis, the valve orifice is reduced from its normal 5 cm^2 to about 1 cm^2. Cardiac output is maintained by increases in left atrial, pulmonary venous and pulmonary capillary pressures, with a resulting loss of lung compliance. A sudden increase in pulmonary venous pressure, caused perhaps by the onset of atrial fibrillation, may precipitate pulmonary oedema. With a more gradual rise in pressure, there tends to be an increase in pulmonary vascular resistance, which protects against pulmonary oedema. The clinical features of mitral stenosis include a loud first heart sound (tapping apex beat), an opening snap and a mid-diastolic murmur. In addition, an abnormal pulsation is often felt to the left of the sternum; this may be due either to right ventricular hypertrophy or to forward displacement of the heart by a dilated left atrium. Pulmonary hypertension may cause a loud pulmonary component of the second heart sound, and right atrial hypertrophy may produce a prominent a wave of the jugular venous pulse. Tricuspid regurgitation, secondary to right ventricular dilatation, causes a systolic murmur and systolic waves in the venous pulse. The ECG may show left atrial hypertrophy or atrial fibrillation. There may also be evidence of right ventricular hypertrophy. Enlargement of the left atrium and its appendage, and of the main pulmonary artery, may be seen on the chest X-ray. There may be enlargement of the upper pulmonary veins and horizontal linear shadows in the costophrenic angles, indicating high left atrial and pulmonary venous pressures. Echocardiography is useful not only to confirm the diagnosis, but also to estimate its severity, as it provides information on the rigidity and state of calcification of the valve cusps, the size of the left atrium and the state of left ventricular function. The role of cardiac catheterization is principally to assess any associated mitral regurgitation and the condition of the coronary arteries.

Management of anaesthesia. Prophylactic antibiotics should always be given. Digitalis therapy for control of ventricular rate response during atrial fibrillation should be continued up until the time of surgery. Diuretic therapy should also be continued, although plasma potassium concentration should be measured pre-operatively. The need to continue anticoagulant therapy depends on the nature of the operation being contemplated; a cardiological opinion may be helpful in discussing this point. The aim of anaesthesia is to avoid excessive increases in heart rate, as this decreases diastolic filling of the left ventricle, whose filling is already impaired. A sudden decrease in peripheral vascular resistance in the face of a fixed cardiac output may produce severe hypotension. Furthermore, arterial hypoxaemia and acidosis, or administration of α-adrenergic agonists, can further increase an already elevated pulmonary vascular resistance. With these points in mind, a mild anxiolytic may be the best premedicant drug; anticholinergic drugs are contraindicated because of their chronotropic effect. Anaesthesia should be induced and maintained with minimal changes in heart rate and pulmonary and systemic vascular resistances. Full monitoring is therefore mandatory, and a combination of nitrous oxide, opioids and volatile agents is usually the most successful for minimizing haemodynamic changes. If reversal of muscle relaxation is required, glycopyrronium is a better choice than atropine to antagonize the muscarinic effects of neostigmine.

The need for invasive haemodynamic monitoring depends on the length and complexity of the surgery. However, patients who are symptomatic at rest, or who have persistent pulmonary hypertension with signs of right heart failure, are most at risk and warrant invasive haemodynamic monitoring. Intra-operative fluid replacement must be controlled carefully, as these patients are susceptible to excessive fluid replacement and pulmonary oedema. The head-down position is also not tolerated well, as the pulmonary vascular pressures are already raised. If light anaesthesia or pain leads to a further rise in pulmonary vascular resistance, intravenous infusions of glyceryl trinitrate or sodium nitroprusside may be required. Intra-operative hypotension can be counteracted with ephedrine or phenylephrine. The β-adrenergic activity of ephedrine or phenylephrine may be useful in increasing myocardial contractility, although its positive chronotropic effect may be a hindrance. Intra-operative tachyarrhythmias are probably best treated with direct current cardioversion, to avoid the negative inotropic effect of antiarrhythmic drugs. Due consideration must be given to keeping the patient warm during surgery, and providing adequate postoperative analgesia. These patients may benefit from continued cardiac monitoring, and monitoring of oxygen saturation during the postoperative period.

Postoperatively, pain and respiratory acidosis may cause further elevations in pulmonary vascular resistance, and precipitate right heart failure.

Mitral regurgitation

This condition can result from dilatation of the mitral

valve ring, in association with diseases such as rheumatic fever, myocarditis or cardiomyopathy. Muscle dysfunction or rupture may follow myocardial infarction. The valve cusps may be damaged by chronic rheumatic heart disease. A separate condition is that of mitral valve prolapse (floppy mitral valve). This is caused by a congenital abnormality or degenerative myxomatous change. It is sometimes a feature of connective tissue disorders such as Marfan's syndrome.

The patient usually presents with exertional dyspnoea; there may also be atypical chest pain. Clinical examination reveals an apical systolic murmur, which may radiate into the axilla. The apex beat is displaced to the left as a result of dilatation of the left ventricle. Increased forward flow through the mitral valve may give rise to a loud third heart sound, or a short mid-diastolic murmur. Mitral valve prolapse causes a mid-systolic click, due to the valve bulging back into the atrium during systole. The click may be followed by a late systolic murmur.

The chest X-ray and ECG show signs of left atrial or left ventricular hypertrophy. Atrial fibrillation is a common arrhythmia, as a consequence of atrial dilatation. Mitral valve prolapse is associated with an increased incidence of tachyarrhythmia.

Management of anaesthesia. Left atrial volume overload is the main change produced by mitral regurgitation. There is a decrease in the forward left ventricular stroke volume, because part of the stroke volume is regurgitated through the incompetent mitral valve into the left atrium. This regurgitant flow is responsible for v waves seen on recordings of the pulmonary artery occlusion pressures obtained from these patients. The amount of regurgitation is determined by the heart rate as well as the pressure gradient across the mitral valve. A bradycardia with a long duration of ventricular ejection can cause reduced forward flow, and a mild tachycardia is preferable. The pressure gradient across the mitral valve depends on the compliance of the left ventricle, and if this is reduced, then regurgitation increases. Conversely, a fall in systemic vascular resistance, mediated for example by vasodilator therapy, can improve cardiac output.

Anaesthesia is therefore directed towards producing a mild tachycardia and possibly a modest reduction in systemic vascular resistance. General anaesthesia is again thought to be more controllable than regional anaesthesia in these patients. Bearing these points in mind, the selection of agents for induction and maintenance of anaesthesia is not critical. Maintenance of intravascular fluid volume with prompt replacement of blood loss is important for maintaining cardiac filling. The intensity of invasive haemodynamic monitoring required depends on the severity of symptoms and the extent of the surgery contemplated. Minor surgery in patients with minimal symptoms does not require invasive monitoring. If manipulations of peripheral vascular resistance are contemplated, then a pulmonary artery occlusion catheter is indicated.

Tricuspid regurgitation

Tricuspid regurgitation is usually secondary to right ventricular dilatation, which may be caused by pulmonary hypertension or, rarely, right ventricular infarction. The tricuspid valve is occasionally involved in rheumatic heart disease, and is a common site of endocarditis in intravenous drug abusers. Isolated tricuspid regurgitation is well-tolerated and symptoms are non-specific. The most prominent clinical feature is a large systolic wave in the jugular venous pulse. Systolic hepatic pulsation may also be present. If right heart failure is severe, then liver function tests and clotting should be checked pre-operatively. Antibiotic prophylaxis must be given. During anaesthesia, intravascular volume must be well-maintained to create high-normal right heart pressures, and forward flow. Conditions which exacerbate pulmonary hypertension or increase pulmonary vascular resistance must be avoided. High airway pressures and positive end-expiratory pressure (PEEP) should also be avoided.

Disorders of cardiac conduction

First-degree heart block

The PR interval is prolonged beyond 0.2 s. In isolation, this condition is asymptomatic and can be diagnosed only by ECG. It requires no treatment prior to anaesthesia.

Second-degree heart block

In this condition, some impulses from the atria fail to reach the ventricles. In Mobitz type 1 second degree atrioventricular (AV) block, there is progressive lengthening of successive PR intervals, followed by a dropped beat (Wenckebach's phenomenon). This is due to progressive fatigue of the AV bundle, with recovery following the rest period when the dropped beat occurs. In Mobitz type II second-degree AV block, the PR interval of the conducted impulses remains constant, but some P waves are not conducted. This is usually caused by disease below the His bundle, and is more serious than Mobitz type I. When the atrial and ventricular contractions bear a simple ratio to one another, such as 2 : 1 or 3 : 1 block, the pulse is slow and regular. More complex ratios such as 3 : 2 or 4 : 3 block give rise to dropped beats on palpation of the pulse. As type II block frequently progresses to third-degree AV block, insertion of an artificial cardiac pacemaker is justified pre-operatively, even in the absence of symptoms such as syncope.

Unifascicular heart block (left anterior or left posterior hemiblock) and right bundle branch block, when occurring in isolation, do not have any particular significance for anaesthesia. The presence of left bundle branch block usually implies the presence of coronary artery disease, and may hide ECG evidence of myocardial infarction. The onset of left bundle branch block during surgery may signal an acute myocardial infarction.

Bifascicular heart block

Bifascicular heart block is present when right bundle branch block is associated with block of one of the fascicles of the left bundle branch. A theoretical concern in patients with bifascicular heart block is that peri-operative manipulation might compromise conduction of cardiac impulses in the one remaining fascicle, and third-degree heart block would ensue. However, several studies have found no evidence that either general or regional anaesthesia is likely to lead to the development of third-degree AV heart block.[54-56] These studies were based on asymptomatic patients with a normal PR interval, but even symptomatic patients have undergone uneventful surgery without the presence of a prophylactic artificial cardiac pacemaker.[57]

Trifascicular/atrioventricular heart block

This may be continuous or intermittent. The pulse is slow and, except in the case of congenital complete heart block, does not vary with exercise. Venous cannon waves may occur. Episodes of ventricular asystole (Adams–Stokes attacks) may occur, resulting in rapid loss of consciousness; the patient falls to the ground and may convulse. In contrast to epilepsy, recovery is rapid when the heart starts beating again. In patients with third-degree AV block, a cardiac pacemaker system should be inserted prior to induction of anaesthesia. In an emergency, an infusion of isoprenaline (1–4 µg.kg^{-1}.min^{-1}) may help to maintain an adequate ventricular rate until a pacemaker can be inserted.

Disorders of cardiac rhythm

Sick sinus syndrome

This is an inappropriate sinus bradycardia, caused by degenerative changes which result in a reduction in automaticity of the sino-atrial node. There may be episodes of sinus arrest, with either pauses or escape rhythms. Paroxysmal supraventricular tachycardia and paroxysmal atrial fibrillation are common features of sino-atrial disease. Insertion of an artificial cardiac pacemaker is justified only in patients with severe symptoms, or patients whose bradycardia has been exacerbated by the use of drugs required to prevent tachyarrhythmia.

Sinus bradycardia

This is defined arbitrarily as a sinus rate of less than 60 beats.min^{-1}. It may be a normal finding, and is common in athletes. It is also a feature associated with the use of β-adrenoceptor antagonists. However, it may occur in patients with myxoedema or raised intracranial pressure and, in some patients, after myocardial infarction; these conditions should be excluded prior to anaesthesia.

Sinus tachycardia

This is defined as a resting sinus rate of more than 100 beats.min^{-1}. It can be a feature of anxiety, hyperthyroidism and acute circulatory or cardiac failure.

Paroxysmal atrial tachycardia

This may occur with a rate of between 140 and 220 beats.min^{-1}, and is usually the result of a re-entry phenomenon, although it may occasionally be due to a rapidly firing ectopic focus in the atria or AV node. Coffee, alcohol, tobacco, anxiety or hyperthyroidism may be precipitating factors. It can often be terminated by application of carotid artery pressure; failing this, intravenous verapamil, a β-blocker or disopyramide may restore sinus rhythm, but should not be given together. Under anaesthesia, this tachycardia is usually easily terminated by direct current cardioversion.

Atrial flutter

This is a condition in which a rapid atrial rate of around 300 beats.min^{-1} is associated with varying degrees of AV block. The ECG shows characteristic saw-tooth flutter waves. Direct current cardioversion may be necessary if the arrhythmia is haemodynamically significant. Intravenous administration of digoxin, sometimes combined with propranolol, usually controls the heart rate.

Atrial fibrillation

This may be asymptomatic, particularly in the elderly.

Paroxysmal atrial fibrillation carries with it the risk of systemic embolization. Prior to surgery, the main consideration is to control the ventricular rate. Rates of 70–90 beats.min^{-1} probably reflect adequate therapeutic effects of digoxin. Direct current cardioversion may be required to treat atrial fibrillation that manifests for the for the first time during surgery.

Junctional rhythm

Junctional rhythm is often seen during anaesthesia, especially when halothane is being administered. Treatment with atropine or glycopyrronium is indicated if the rhythm becomes haemodynamically significant, or when bradycardia is undesirable for other reasons.

Premature ventricular contractions

These are associated with coronary artery disease, digitalis toxicity, arterial hypoxaemia, hypercapnia, hypertension or mechanical irritation of the ventricle. They are sometimes exacerbated by excessive tea, coffee or alcohol consumption. Hypokalaemia may cause ventricular ectopic beats, and potentiates other causes. Occasionally, they are a feature of mitral valve prolapse. Premature ventricular contractions in patients with an otherwise normal heart are often more prominent at rest, and tend to disappear with exercise. An attempt to treat them should be undertaken only when they are frequent (more than 6 per min), multifocal, occur in salvoes of three or more, or take place during the ascending part of the T wave (R-on-T phenomenon). These characteristics are all associated with an increased incidence of ventricular tachycardia or fibrillation. After eliminating any underlying causes, the drug of choice is lignocaine, administered as an initial intravenous dose of 1–2 mg.kg^{-1} and then continued as an infusion of 4 mg.kg^{-1}, reducing to 2 mg.kg^{-1} over a period of 2–4 h. The dose may need to be reduced in the elderly, the frail and those with liver disease.

Ventricular tachycardia

This is a grave arrhythmia because it is nearly always, associated with serious heart disease. The ventricular rate may be very rapid, and it may degenerate into ventricular fibrillation. The most common cause is acute myocardial infarction, but it may also be due to myocarditis, cardiomyopathy or chronic ischaemic heart disease, especially when the last is associated with a ventricular aneurysm. In a few individuals, a predisposition to ventricular tachycardia is associated with abnormal prolongation of the QT interval of the ECG, a trait which is sometimes hereditary. Prompt direct current cardioversion is the treatment of choice. Anti-arrhythmic agents which may be effective include lignocaine, mexilitine, flecainide, disopyramide and amiodarone. Hypokalaemia, hypomagnesaemia and acidosis must be corrected.

Pre-excitation syndromes

These are characterized by activation of a portion of the ventricles by cardiac impulses that travel from the atria via accessory AV conduction pathways. Three accessory pathways have been described in pre-excitation syndromes, and these are known as the Kent fibres, James fibres and Mahain fibres, of which the most common are the Kent fibres. These give rise to the Wolff–Parkinson–White syndrome (WPW). In normal sinus rhythm, conduction takes place partly through the AV node, and partly through the more rapidly conducting bypass tract. The ECG shows shortening of the PR interval and a slurring of the QRS complex, called a δ wave. Because the AV node and the bypass tract may have different conduction speeds and refractory periods, a re-entry circuit can develop, causing paroxysms of tachycardia. Because the bypass pathway lacks the rate-limiting properties of the normal AV node, patients are at risk from very rapid ventricular rates, and sometimes ventricular fibrillation and death. Treatment is aimed at reducing conduction rate, and increasing the refractory period of the bypass tract, using disopyramide, quinidine, sotalol or amiodarone. Atrial fibrillation may be terminated with direct current cardioversion, which is necessary if a rapid ventricular rate leads to severe hypotension. Digitalis and verapamil may decrease the refractory period of accessory pathways responsible for atrial fibrillation, and result in an increase in ventricular response. They should, therefore, be avoided.

The Lown–Ganong–Levine syndrome is due to accessory James fibres, and is characterized again by a short PR interval, but with a normal QRS complex duration and no δ wave. Mahain fibre pathways produce an ECG which resembles that in the WPW syndrome.

Prolonged QT syndrome

This is characterized by a QT interval longer than 0.44 s on the ECG, even when corrected for heart rate. It may be congenital (syncope may be manifest in early childhood and confused with seizures if an ECG is not obtained), or may be acquired due to anti-arrhythmic drugs, including quinidine and disopyramide. Phenothiazine, lithium, tricyclic antidepressants, hypokalaemia and hypocalcaemia may also prolong the QT interval of the ECG. Symptoms include syncope and, occasionally, sudden death, and are exacerbated or triggered by sympathetic nervous system stimulation. The mechanism of the congenital syndrome is thought to be an imbalance of the sympathetic innervation of the heart. Treatment consists of β-adrenoceptor blockade, which shortens the QT interval in affected patients, and reduces sympathetic nervous system activity. Phenytoin, verapamil and bretylium have also been used. Interestingly, a left stellate ganglion block successfully shortens the QT interval on ECG, although the effect is, of course, only transient. Anaesthesia must be undertaken only in the presence of an adequate degree of β-adrenoceptor blockade, or a prophylactic left stellate ganglion block. Factors known to increase sympathetic nervous system activity should be minimized. Thiopentone, volatile anaesthetic agents and opioids have all been used successfully in these patients. Pancuronium has been used successfully, despite its sympathomimetic activity, but vecuronium or atracurium are probably more acceptable alternatives. Pharmacological reversal of non-depolarizing neuromuscular blockade does not seem to affect the QT interval adversely in these patients. During anaesthesia, a defibrillator should be available. Propranolol is the drug of choice for treatment of acute ventricular arrhythmias developing intra-operatively; class 1 anti-arrhythmic drugs are not recommended, as they can prolong the QT interval.

Congenital heart disease

The incidence of haemodynamically significant congenital cardiac abnormalities is about 1% of live births. In most cases, the cause is unknown. Some defects are due to maternal infections during the early weeks of pregnancy, e.g. rubella. Increased rates of survival for children with congenital heart defects have resulted from earlier intervention and improved surgical techniques. However, in many cases there is still a significant level of cardiovascular morbidity after a palliative procedure. Anaesthetists are likely to be confronted with increasing numbers of children and adolescents with moderate to severe cardiovascular symptomatology, presenting for non-cardiac surgery. The haemodynamic problems may be exacerbated both by the drugs used and by positive-pressure ventilation, and a knowledge of the functional status of the patient's cardiovascular system is therefore very important.

Left-to-right intracardiac shunts

These may be due to atrial or ventricular defects, patent ductus arteriosus, or anomalous pulmonary venous return. They all result in increased pulmonary blood flow, with pulmonary hypertension, right ventricular hypertrophy and, eventually, congestive cardiac failure. With the rise in pulmonary vascular resistance, pulmonary artery pressure may increase until it equals or exceeds aortic pressure. The shunt through the defect may then reverse, causing central cyanosis.

Management of anaesthesia. Antibiotic prophylaxis is mandatory. A reduction in systemic vascular resistance, as produced by volatile anaesthetics, may improve systemic blood flow by decreasing the magnitude of the left-to-right shunt. Similarly, positive-pressure ventilation is well-tolerated, as increased airway pressure elevates pulmonary vascular resistance, reducing the left-to-right shunt. Persistent elevation of the systemic vascular resistance must be avoided.

Right-to-left intracardiac shunts

Defects producing right-to-left cardiac shunting include the tetralogy of Fallot, Eisenmenger's syndrome, Epstein malformation of the tricuspid valve, pulmonary atresia with a ventricular septal defect and tricuspid atresia. These patients are centrally cyanosed, and have varying degrees of polycythaemia.

Management of anaesthesia. Antibiotic prophylaxis is mandatory. The magnitude of the right-to-left shunt is increased by a reduction in systemic vascular resistance or an increase in pulmonary vascular resistance. Volatile anaesthetics and drugs which release histamine decrease systemic vascular resistance, and therefore increase the magnitude of the shunt. The shunt is increased further by the elevation of pulmonary vascular resistance produced by positive-pressure ventilation. It is important to maintain a good state of hydration pre-operatively, in view of the polycythaemia. Anaesthesia is often induced using intramuscular ketamine (3–4 mg/kg), despite the fact that ketamine has been alleged to increase pulmonary vascular resistance, which would be undesirable. Clinically, however, the use of ketamine is often associated with an improvement in arterial oxygenation. Inhalational induction of anaesthesia may be slow because of reduced pulmonary blood flow, and may precipitate hypercyanotic attacks in patients with Fallot's tetralogy. High inspired concentrations of oxygen are used and anaesthesia is usually maintained with a combination of opioids and a low concentration of an inhalational agent. Positive-pressure ventilation of the lungs is used, but it must be appreciated that excessive positive airway pressures reduce pulmonary blood flow, and PEEP should be avoided. Intravascular fluid volume must be strictly maintained, and it is crucial to avoid administration of any bubbles of air as these can lead to systemic, including cerebral, embolization.

Coarctation of the aorta

Although coarctation of the aorta should have been corrected in patients presenting for non-cardiac surgery, it is important to be aware that about 50% of patients who have had a postductal coarctation corrected also have a bicuspid aortic valve, which is vulnerable to the development of infective endocarditis. Therefore, these patients should be treated with antibiotics before undergoing surgical procedures. A recent review by Baum and Perloff[58] indicates that there is still significant morbidity in these patients even after correction with a 75% mortality by age 50. Causes include left ventricular failure, rupture of a cerebral aneurysm and dissection of the aorta. There is also an increased incidence of premature coronary artery disease which is the leading cause of death 11–25 years after the operation. As well as the known association with a bicuspid aortic valve, there are associated mitral valve abnormalities in up to 58% of patients with coarctation, and about 20% are functionally significant.

Corrected congenital defects

In any patient presenting for anaesthesia for non-cardiac surgery after total or partial correction of a congenital cardiac anomaly, it is essential to determine the functional anatomy of the correction. In some situations, there is an indication to increase rather than decrease pulmonary vascular resistance. Patients with truncus arteriosus, or any type of palliative shunt between the systemic and pulmonary arterial systems, are prone to develop myocardial ischaemia as these shunts may result in excessive aortic run-off, and therefore decreased systemic arterial diastolic pressure. Introduction of anaesthetic agents may further decrease diastolic pressure, compromising coronary perfusion. The pulmonary and systemic circulations of these patients are in parallel rather than in the form of a normal series circulation. Conventional treatments to increase systemic arterial diastolic pressure, such as administration of vasoconstrictors, may not have the desired effect. In this situation, it is occasionally necessary to institute temporary banding of the pulmonary artery.[59]

OTHER CARDIOVASCULAR DISEASES

Essential hypertension

It has been noted that there is a greater incidence of myocardial ischaemia on the ECG in patients whose hypertension is untreated prior to surgery.[60,61] It is therefore recommended that the diastolic blood pressure should not be above 110 mmHg prior to elective surgery. The patient's drug therapy should be reviewed, and the serum electrolytes measured (and corrected if necessary), if the patient is on diuretic therapy. There is some evidence of an interaction of angiotensin-converting enzyme inhibitors with volatile anaesthetic agents, producing profound hypotension, and a recommendation has been made to stop angiotensin-converting enzyme inhibitors prior to surgery.[62] The interaction of calcium antagonists with anaesthetic agents has been reviewed extensively.[63] Patients with hypertension may have evidence of other organ dysfunction, including cerebral vascular disease or peripheral vascular disease, renal dysfunction and coronary artery disease.

Induction and maintenance of anaesthesia

The patient's antihypertensive therapy should, in general, be maintained throughout the peri-operative period.[60,61] Anaesthesia can be induced with a barbiturate or etomidate, but it is probably wise to avoid a rapidly administered bolus of propofol in view of the greater haemodynamic changes sometimes experienced on induction with this drug.[64] The duration of time taken for laryngoscopy and intubation should be kept to a minimum, ideally less than 15 s.[65]

Intra-operative blood pressure may fluctuate more widely than normal due to the patient's drug therapy, especially if there were pre-operative symptoms of orthostatic hypotension. For this reason, close monitoring of blood pressure is important, and in all but the most minor surgery, intra-arterial monitoring of blood pressure is warranted. Intra-operative hypertension can often be managed by increasing the concentration of volatile anaesthetic agent, or by the addition of an opioid. An intravenous infusion of sodium nitroprusside is occasionally necessary. Hypotension during anaesthesia may respond to volume replacement, particularly if the ability to compensate for blood loss is compromised by the use of a β-blocker or calcium antagonist. Sympathomimetic agents, such as ephedrine, are sometimes necessary.

Regional anaesthesia may be hazardous, as hypertensive patients frequently have a reduced circulating volume; in the presence of coronary artery disease, a decrease in systemic vascular resistance may produce a significant reduction in coronary artery perfusion pressure.

Patients with transplanted heart and lungs

The success of the heart-lung transplant programme in

recent years has meant that there is an increasing likelihood of these patients presenting for elective or emergency surgery at a hospital distant from their transplantation centre. Initial assessment must include the reason for the organ transplantation, and identification of any residual disease process. For example, a patient with cystic fibrosis who has undergone a heart and lung transplant may still have abnormal liver function due to the ongoing cystic fibrosis. It has been noticed[66] that there is a higher incidence of general surgical complications in post-transplant patients, compared with other post-cardiopulmonary-bypass patients, and that these complications are associated with a greater than expected mortality rate. It is important during the pre-operative assessment to recognize a patient who is undergoing an episode of graft rejection. In this case, surgery should be postponed and the patient referred to the transplantation centre, as anaesthesia in the presence of ongoing rejection presents formidable management problems and may necessitate full inotropic and mechanical support. The patient with a denervated heart does not experience angina as a warning of myocardial ischaemia or rejection, but may complain of excessive tiredness and dyspnoea. Bradycardia and small ECG complexes, as well as an increased frequency of transient ischaemic attacks, should also alert the anaesthetist to the possibility of impending rejection.[67,68] In patients with heart and lung transplants, pulmonary rejection precedes cardiac rejection, and it is rare for cardiac rejection to occur in the absence of lung rejection. Symptoms may mimic those of a chest infection, with fatigue, dyspnoea, sudden arterial desaturation, pyrexia and leukocytosis. Perihilar infiltration or graft opacification on the chest X-ray may be preceded by a decrease in carbon monoxide transfer factor and forced expiratory volume in 1 s (FEV_1).[69,70] Obliterative bronchiolitis appears to be more common in lungs which have been rejected when the transplant was performed in conjunction with the heart.[71]

Transplanted organs are denervated, and therefore the normal sympathetic response to laryngoscopy and intubation is absent. Although the heart responds to circulating catecholamines, this response may take several minutes to manifest. Carotid sinus massage and Valsalva manoeuvres also have no effect on heart rate, and there is no tachycardia in response to light anaesthesia or hypovolaemia. An increase in cardiac output can be achieved only by increasing stroke volume. Care should therefore be taken to maintain normovolaemia and avoid significant peripheral vasodilatation. In patients with a single lung transplant, some of the airways distal to the carina are unable to initiate a cough reflex. Consequently, the trachea should not be extubated while the patient is deeply anaesthetized and, after surgery, it is necessary to encourage expectoration from the transplanted lung by postural drainage and physiotherapy.

Heart and lung transplant patients take a wide variety of drugs, which may include not only antirejection therapy but also diuretics, antihypertensive agents and antifungal and antiviral drugs. Although interactions and toxicity must be considered individually, common side-effects are nephrotoxicity and hepatotoxicity. All medication should be continued up to the day of operation. This is essential particularly for immunosuppressive therapy. An additional dose of steroid is usually given during anaesthesia. Medication must also be continued postoperatively, changing oral medication to intravenous where necessary.

Strict aseptic precautions must be observed while anaesthetizing these patients. Intravenous and intra-arterial lines must be inserted under sterile conditions. All intravenous infusions should be fitted with a bacterial filter, and injection points kept capped and sterile. During anaesthesia, it must be remembered that a peri-operative bradycardia will not respond to atropine, and so an infusion of isoprenaline should be available. Monitoring appropriate to the risk of the surgery and the fitness of the patient should be used. Invasive monitoring should not be used unnecessarily, to avoid the risk of infection. When central venous pressure monitoring is required, the catheter should be inserted through the left internal jugular vein, as the right internal jugular vein is used routinely for intracardiac biopsy.

During the postoperative period, care must be taken to maintain the patient's immunosuppressant regimen and to avoid infection. Urine, sputum and wound swabs should be sent daily and the help of microbiologists sought if there is any evidence of infection.

Disease of heart muscle

The myocardium may be involved in many systemic diseases. An international commission has recommended using specific terminology, e.g. sarcoid heart disease, when the cause of heart muscle disease is known, and using the term cardiomyopathy only if a cause cannot be identified. Some specific diseases of heart muscle are shown in Table 2.5. However, these specific heart muscle diseases are clinically indistinguishable from one of the three forms of cardiomyopathy. Connective tissue disorders, sarcoidosis, haemochromatosis and alcoholic muscle disease produce a clinical picture that is indistinguishable from dilated cardiomyopathy, and

Table 2.5 Specific diseases of heart muscle

Infections
Viral — coxsackie A and B, influenza
Bacterial — diphtheria, chickenpox
Protozoal — trypanosomiasis

Endocrine and metabolic disorders
Diabetes, thyroid disease, acromegaly, carcinoid syndrome, inherited storage disease

Connective tissue diseases
Scleroderma, SLE, polyarteritis nodosa

Infiltrative disorders
Haemochromatosis, haemosiderosis, sarcoidosis, amyloidosis

Endomyocardial fibrosis and eosinophilic heart disease

Toxins
Drugs, alcohol, irradiation

Neuromuscular disorders
Dystrophia myotonica, Friedreich's ataxia

SLE = Systemic lupus erythematosus.

anaesthesia can be approached in the same way. Amyloidosis and eosinophilic heart disease produce signs and symptoms similar to those found in restrictive cardiomyopathy, and Friedreich's ataxia produces a clinical picture resembling that of hypertrophic cardiomyopathy.

Dilated cardiomyopathy

In this condition, there is impaired ventricular contraction, often affecting both ventricles, and leading to progressive left-sided and later right-sided heart failure. Functional mitral and/or tricuspid regurgitation may occur, and arrhythmias are also common. Treatment is aimed at controlling heart failure, and managing arrhythmias that result in haemodynamic instability.

Management of anaesthesia. This is conducted in the same way as for any patient with congestive heart failure, the aims being to avoid drug-induced myocardial depression, maintain normovolaemia and prevent increases in ventricular afterload. Anticoagulation may be indicated because of the high incidence of systemic embolization, but benefits from this prophylactic policy have not been demonstrated[72] and the nature of the surgery may contra-indicate the use of anticoagulants.

Restrictive cardiomyopathy

In this condition, ventricular filling is impaired because the ventricles are 'stiff'. This leads to high atrial pressures with atrial hypertrophy and dilatation, and later atrial fibrillation. There may be pronounced signs of right heart failure, such as hepatosplenomegaly and ascites. There is no effective treatment. Management of anaesthesia in these patients may be very difficult.

Institution of general anaesthesia and positive-pressure ventilation of the lungs in the presence of a significant restrictive cardiomyopathy may lead to profound hypotension and even cardiac arrest. The reasons for this include drug-induced peripheral vasodilatation, direct myocardial depression and decreased venous return. Increased intrathoracic pressures due to straining or coughing during induction of anaesthesia, or to controlled ventilation of the lungs, may further reduce venous return. Consequently, spontaneous ventilation is to be preferred if possible. Ketamine is a useful drug for induction and maintenance of anaesthesia, as it increases myocardial contractility, systemic vascular resistance and heart rate; it may be supplemented with nitrous oxide and fentanyl. Pancuronium is a useful muscle relaxant if intermittent positive-pressure ventilation (IPPV) is used. Continuous monitoring of right-sided venous pressures indicated, preferably starting before induction of anaesthesia. The elevated right heart pressures should be maintained with appropriate intravenous fluids. An infusion of isoprenaline may be helpful to maintain myocardial contractility and heart rate.

Hypertrophic cardiomyopathy

Hypertrophic cardiomyopathy is characterized by obstruction to left ventricular outflow produced by asymmetrical hypertrophy of the interventricular septum. Additional obstruction is caused by anterior motion of the septal leaflet of the mitral valve during systole. The left ventricle hypertrophies to overcome the obstruction and muscle hypertrophy may be so massive that the volume of the left ventricular chamber is reduced. Diagnosis is usually made on echocardiography. Cardiac catheterization reveals the degree of obliteration of the ventricle, as well as the presence or absence of coronary artery disease. Symptoms include syncope, angina and congestive heart failure. However, a proportion of these patients are asymptomatic and present with sudden death; cardiac arrhythmias, especially ventricular tachycardia, are the most common cause. Although most patients show ECG changes consistent with left ventricular hypertrophy, as many as 15% of patients manifest no evidence of hypertrophy on the ECG, despite increased muscle mass. Q waves in patients with hypertrophic cardiomyopathy are most likely to be due to septal hypertrophy rather than evidence of a prior myocardial infarction. Ventricular premature beats and atrial fibrillation are common findings.

Management of anaesthesia. Management of anaesthesia in patients with hypertrophic cardiomyopathy is directed towards minimizing the pressure gradient across the left ventricular outflow. It must be realized that the obstruction is dynamic; obstruction is exaggerated by increased myocardial contractility, decreased preload and decreased afterload. However, obstruction is alleviated by decreased myocardial contractility, increased preload and increased afterload.

Pre-operative medication which results in a calm relaxed patients is ideal, but the use of anticholinergics is not advisable because of the accompanying tachycardia. Induction of anaesthesia should take place in the presence of full monitoring and adequate intravenous access, such that intravenous fluid can be given to minimize the effect of the fall in systemic vascular resistance during induction. Maintenance of anaesthesia should ideally produce mild depression of myocardial contractility, a normal or slow heart rate and a normal systemic vascular resistance. Halothane is a useful drug in these patients. Regional anaesthesia produces undesirable haemodynamic effects, and is not indicated. Non-depolarizing muscle relaxants such as vecuronium and atracurium, which have minimal haemodynamic effects, are preferable to pancuronium or curare. It is important that prompt replacement of blood loss occurs and that preload is well-maintained. If hypotension does occur due to a decrease in systemic vascular resistance, then a drug with predominant α-adrenergic agonist activity, such as phenylephrine, reliably increases blood pressure and decreases obstruction to left ventricular outflow. Drugs with β-adrenergic agonist activity (e.g. dopamine, dobutamine, ephedrine) are not recommended as increases in cardiac contractility and heart rate can increase obstruction to left ventricular outflow. Maintenance of sinus rhythm and avoidance of tachycardia are both vital. A short-acting intravenously administered β-blocker such as esmolol is useful for slowing persistent tachycardias.

RESPIRATORY DISEASE

Asthma

Bronchial asthma is characterized by paroxysms of breathlessness, chest tightness and wheezing, resulting from narrowing of the airways by a combination of muscle spasm, mucosal swelling and viscid bronchial secretions. The air flow obstruction, which characteristically fluctuates markedly, causes mismatch of alveolar ventilation and perfusion and increases the work of breathing. The obstruction is more marked during expiration and causes air to be trapped in the lungs. Mucus plugging of the smaller bronchi is a conspicuous finding at autopsy. Death may occur from alveolar hypoventilation and severe arterial hypoxaemia, culminating in cardiac arrest.

Asthma may have its onset in childhood in atopic individuals, who form immunoglobulin E antibodies to commonly encountered allergens. This is termed atopic asthma. It can also occur at any age in non-atopic individuals. The majority of these patients are adults and this form of the disease is often called late-onset asthma. It appears that external allergens play no part in the production of this form of the disease. Asthma attacks may therefore be triggered by exposure to allergens in atopic patients, but also by non-specific factors such as cold air, tobacco smoke, dust and fumes, respiratory viral infection and emotional stress. Physical signs of an asthma attack include tachypnoea and expiratory wheeze. There may be an unproductive cough and tachycardia, pulsus paradoxus and, in severe cases, central cyanosis. A chest X-ray during an acute attack may reveal only hyperinflation, but should be performed to exclude pneumothorax. Pulmonary function tests will reveal a reduced peak expiratory flow rate and spirometry will show an obstructive pattern with reduced FEV_1 and forced vital capacity (FVC), and a reduced FEV_1 : FVC ratio.

The mainstay of treatment is $β_2$-agonist drugs, which are usually inhaled. This treatment may be combined with an inhaled anticholinergic drug, oral aminophylline and/or corticosteroids. Sodium cromoglycate is used in atopic asthma for prophylaxis against acute attacks.

Management of anaesthesia

The patient's normal bronchodilator therapy should be continued up to the time of surgery. An anticholinergic premedication may dry secretions, increasing the likelihood of bronchial plugging, and benzodiazepine premedication is therefore recommended. If the patient has been on a significant dose of corticosteroids, including inhaled corticosteroids, then adrenal cortical suppression may be present and additional intravenous supplementation to cover the stress of surgery may be required. Regional anaesthesia may be an attractive choice when the site of operation is superficial or on the limbs. Barbiturates, etomidate or ketamine may be used for induction of anaesthesia. After loss of consciousness, the lungs are inflated with a gas mixture that includes a volatile anaesthetic, to ensure that an adequate depth of anaesthesia is present before laryngoscopy and tracheal intubation. It has been shown[73] that bronchoconstriction can be precipitated in patients with asthma by the introduction of a tube into the trachea without previously establishing sufficient depth of anaesthesia to suppress airway reflexes. Lignocaine 1–2 mg.kg^{-1} intravenously administered immediately before intubation of the trachea may also help prevent reflex bronchoconstriction.[74] Paralysis should be produced with a drug such as vecuronium which does not release significant quantities of histamine.

Mechanical ventilation of the lungs should be achieved using a slow respiratory rate with sufficient time for passive exhalation to occur, to prevent air trapping. Humidification should be included in the breathing system to reduce the risk of bronchoconstriction induced by cold air, and also to try to reduce the formation of thick secretions.

If there is an increase in airway pressure during the surgical procedure, it is important to exclude causes other than a worsening of the asthma. These include mechanical obstruction of the tracheal tube by secretions, kinking or overinflation of the tracheal tube cuff; inadequate anaesthesia or neuromuscular blockade resulting in active respiratory efforts; endobronchial intubation; and pneumothorax. If the rise in airway pressure is thought to be due to increased airway resistance, it may respond to deepening of anaesthesia with a volatile anaesthetic. Aminophylline administered intravenously at a rate of 0.5 mg.kg.h^{-1} may be administered after a loading dose of 5 mg.kg^{-1} if the patient has not previously been taking the drug. However, it is dangerous to administer aminophylline to a patient whose plasma concentration of the drug is already in the therapeutic range or if anaesthesia is being maintained with halothane. Intravenous salbutamol may also be given to treat bronchospasm, although its use may be limited by the resulting tachycardia. The use of mivacurium in doses less than $ED_{95} \times 3$ is not associated with histamine release, and with appropriate monitoring, allows for spontaneous recovery from paralysis; this obviates the need to administer an anticholinesterase, which may precipitate bronchospasm.

Chronic obstructive airways disease

Chronic bronchitis and emphysema are pathologically distinct, but they frequently co-exist and it may be difficult or impossible to determine the relative importance of each condition in an individual patient. Generalized air flow obstruction is the dominant feature of both diseases. They may be regarded as forming a spectrum with pure chronic bronchitis at one end and pure emphysema at the other. The same principles of management apply in both conditions.

Pre-operative evaluation

The most important aspects of the history are the patient's exercise tolerance and the smoking history. Cessation of smoking for 6 weeks pre-operatively produces considerable benefits; even stopping smoking for 24 h can reduce a patient's carboxyhaemoglobin levels, and improve oxygen delivery.[75]

Pre-operative pulmonary function tests are used to determine a baseline level (because virtually without exception, a patient's respiratory function will deteriorate immediately after operation), and to predict patients who may develop respiratory failure postoperatively.[76] One of the most helpful indices is the ratio of FEV_1 to vital capacity, and it has been shown that the risk of postoperative respiratory failure is increased if the measured ratio is less than 50%.[77] This ratio is also an excellent predictor of the ability to cough and clear secretions from the airways. However, clinical studies have shown widely different predictive values for the use of pulmonary function tests,[78,79] and with the possible exception of use before lung resection, no single value represents an absolute contraindication to general anaesthesia. Measurement of arterial blood gases and pH should be performed before major elective surgery in patients with severe dyspnoea and reduced exercise tolerance. It is unusual for carbon dioxide retention to occur until the ratio of FEV_1 to vital capacity is less than 0.35. Characteristically, patients with a predominantly emphysematous picture maintain normal arterial blood gases, with a high minute ventilation. Patients with a picture of predominantly chronic bronchitis are more likely to retain carbon dioxide. Evidence of carbon dioxide retention on pre-operative blood gases certainly increases the risk of postoperative respiratory failure.[80]

Management of anaesthesia

When any reversible components of the patient's condition, such as infection or bronchospasm, have been treated, management of anaesthesia is aimed predominantly at reducing postoperative complications. Regional anaesthesia is a suitable technique for operations that are on the body surface or lower extremities.[81,82] If general anaesthesia is indicated, there is no specific technique of choice. However, it should be remembered that nitrous oxide can cause expansion of bullae associated with pulmonary emphysema. This could conceivably lead to rupture of bullae and development of a tension pneumothorax.[83] Opioids should be given only in doses which are not likely to be associated with pronounced postoperative respiratory depression.

Humidification of inspired gases is important to prevent drying of secretions in the airways. In the patient who is retaining carbon dioxide, one option is to ventilate the lungs without reducing the carbon dioxide tension in an attempt to avoid postoperative loss of respiratory drive. Occasionally, ventilation may be dependent on hypoxic drive, but there is no reason to restrict the administration of oxygen intra-operatively if mechanical ventilation is employed.

Prevention of postoperative complications

The patient should be advised strongly to stop smoking, if possible when seen in the outpatient clinic. The most popular method to improve postoperative pulmonary function is incentive spirometry. This is taught by the chest physiotherapist pre-operatively. Conventional chest physiotherapy is obviously an important adjunct. Administration of continuous positive airways pressure (CPAP) can decrease the incidence of postoperative pulmonary complications.[84] However, some patients find the tight-fitting mask difficult to tolerate, and there is the potential for aspiration of gastric contents. Nasal CPAP is a useful alternative. Adequate pain relief is essential to allow not only deep breathing, but also early mobilization. Analgesia can be achieved either by a regional technique such as an epidural, or infiltration of the wound with local anaesthetic. The placement of an epidural catheter in the wound with continuous installation of a local anaesthetic may also be helpful. The patient should be encouraged when possible to remain in an upright position in bed, and to sit upright in a chair as soon as possible. Oxygen saturation should be monitored continuously in the postoperative period; however, carbon dioxide retention and respiratory failure may occur in the presence of a normal arterial oxygen saturation, if the patient is breathing added oxygen.

Bronchiectasis

This is characterized by permanent, abnormal dilatation of bronchi. This may be a congenital condition, associated with ciliary dysfunction syndromes or primary hypogammaglobulinaemia, or may be acquired, usually secondary to a pneumonia or an inhaled foreign body.

The treatment includes chest physiotherapy and postural drainage to facilitate elimination of secretions from the airways. Definitive treatment is by lung resection. Prophylactic antibiotic therapy should be started pre-operatively and anaesthetic management should include consideration of the use of a double-lumen tracheal tube to prevent spillage of purulent sputum into normal areas of the lung. Frequent bronchial suction should take place during anaesthesia, to maintain a patent airway. There is a high incidence of chronic sinusitis in patients with bronchiectasis; consequently, insertion of a nasotracheal tube should be undertaken only if absolutely necessary.

Cystic fibrosis

This is transmitted as an autosomal recessive disease with an incidence in Caucasian populations varying between 1 : 1500 and 1 : 15 000 live births. The basic abnormality in cystic fibrosis is a decreased chloride ion permeability in the cell membrane, but the precise mechanism of the increased bacterial affinity, which appears to be an important initial step in the pathogenesis of suppurative lung disease, is not understood. *Pseudomonas aeruginosa* is the predominant chronic pathogen, expressing altered phenotypes unique to cystic fibrosis. The host's response to bacterial antigens leads to tissue damage by lysosomal enzymes and oxygen radicals from stimulated neutrophils. Progressive airway obstruction occurs with airway collapse on exhalation. The major cause of death is respiratory failure, associated with pulmonary hypertension and cor pulmonale.[85,86]

The persistent bronchial infection is characterized by production of copious amounts of thick, greenish and purulent sputum. The development of bronchiectasis and diffuse parenchymal fibrosis causes reduced expiratory flow rates with increased airway resistance. Spontaneous pneumothorax is common in older children and adults. Blood gases show arterial hypoxaemia, hypercapnia and respiratory acidosis as the disease progresses.

Patients with cystic fibrosis generally have pancreatic insufficiency, and as well as progressive obstruction of bile ducts by mucus, they may develop hepatic cirrhosis and portal hypertension. Malabsorption of fat-soluble vitamins may cause vitamin K deficiency, with its related coagulation problems.

Elective surgery should be deferred if there is any evidence of acute infection. Vitamin K should be given if coagulation tests are abnormal. Humidification of inspired gases is important, as is very frequent suctioning of the trachea. Postoperatively, there must be early and very frequent chest physiotherapy, and the patient should be monitored with continuous pulse oximetry.

Kartagener's syndrome

This consists of dextrocardia, situs inversus of the abdominal organs, chronic sinusitis and bronchiectasis.

The principal defect is a generalized abnormality of ciliary function, and this extends to spermatozoa, rendering most males with the disease infertile. The incidence of congenital heart defects associated with dextrocardia is very low. Patients may present for surgery due to chronic otitis media or bronchiectasis, amongst other reasons. Management of anaesthesia is as described for bronchiectasis.

Interstitial lung disease

This may result from several different pathological processes, but all give rise to similar symptoms, physical signs, radiological changes and disturbances of pulmonary function. Thus, they may be considered collectively. Some causes of interstitial lung disease are shown in Table 2.6.

Progressive exertional dyspnoea is the presenting symptom in most patients, and may be accompanied by a persistent dry cough. There may be fine end-expiratory crackles audible over the lung bases. Pulmonary function tests show a restrictive ventilatory defect, with proportional reductions in FEV_1 and FVC. The carbon monoxide transfer factor is low, and there is an overall reduction in lung volume. Early in the disease there is arterial hypoxaemia on exercise, and this progresses to hypoxaemia and hypocapnia at rest.

Patients with interstitial lung disease should be assessed carefully prior to operation, concentrating not only on the severity of the pulmonary disease and the likelihood of postoperative complications, but also noting any extrapulmonary manifestations of the underlying disease process which may be influenced by anaesthesia, e.g. the presence of dry eyes in sarcoidosis. There are no specific drugs of choice in managing anaesthesia for patients with restrictive pulmonary disease; the technique must be directed towards a reduction of postoperative complications. Patients may need supplemental oxygen for a considerable time postoperatively, while the alterations in gas transfer that occur during anaesthesia revert back to the pre-operative state. The patient must also be able to maintain a normal hyperventilatory state and must not be limited by sedation or pain. The reduced lung volume makes it difficult to generate an effective cough for removal of secretions from the airway in the postoperative period.

Pulmonary arterial hypertension

The principal causes of pulmonary hypertension in adults are shown in Table 2.7. The clinical signs may include a left parasternal heave, either from right ventricular hypertrophy or from an enlarged pulmonary artery. There may be a loud second heart sound over the pulmonary valve, and pulmonary regurgitation may produce a soft early diastolic murmur. There may also be the signs of the associated condition. The ECG usually shows evidence of right atrial and right ventricular hypertrophy. The management is basically that of the underlying cause, if known. Domiciliary oxygen may be prescribed for these patients, and slows the progression of the disease. Vasodilator therapy, including calcium antagonists, has been tried, but the results are variable. Continuous infusion of prostacyclin has been successful in some patients.

Management of anaesthesia is directed towards optimizing the patient's condition prior to anaesthesia by correcting any reversible features such as an acute infection, or areas of pulmonary atelectasis. Pre-operative medication should avoid drugs likely to produce ventilatory depression, and it is also prudent to avoid anticholinergic drugs with their adverse effects on clearance of secretions. In a patient with severe pulmonary hypertension, induction of anaesthesia

Table 2.6 Causes of interstitial lung disease

Fibrosing alveolitis
Sarcoidosis
Extrinsic allergic alveolitis
Radiotherapy fibrosis
Drugs
  Bleomycin
  Busulphan
  Methotrexate
  Amiodarone
  Gold
Asbestosis
Idiopathic pulmonary haemosiderosis

Table 2.7 Causes of pulmonary hypertension in adults

Alveolar hypoxia
Destructive lung disease
  Emphysema
Thrombo-embolism
Disease affecting the pulmonary vessels
  Systemic sclerosis
  Schistosomiasis
Drugs
  Fenfluramine
Raised pulmonary capillary pressure
  Left heart failure
  Pulmonary veno-occlusive disease
Primary pulmonary hypertension

should take place in the presence of direct arterial pressure monitoring. Maintenance of anaesthesia is usually with a combination of nitrous oxide, a volatile anaesthetic agent and short-acting opioid. Reduction in systemic vascular resistance should be avoided, as this has adverse effects on venous return and right ventricular output. Fluid replacement should be prompt, and monitored by continuous right heart pressure monitoring. A pulmonary artery occlusion catheter may be helpful when left ventricular dysfunction accompanies pulmonary arterial hypertension. Positive-pressure ventilation is usually selected for these patients, because although positive pressure applied to the alveoli can increase pulmonary vascular resistance, this potentially adverse effect is more than offset by improved arterial oxygenation. This presumably reflects better distribution of ventilation/perfusion ratios within the lungs. A sudden rise in right ventricular pressures in the intra-operative period may indicate right ventricular dysfunction. Any treatable causes such as arterial hypoxaemia or hypoventilation should be sought. There is evidence from animal work that glyceryl trinitrate may provide some reduction in pulmonary vascular resistance in these circumstances.[87]

LIVER DISEASE

Some of the numerous causes of chronic liver disease are listed in Table 2.8. Chronic liver disease is a continuum of stages from an abnormality of liver function tests noted on routine biochemistry, with no adverse physiological consequences during anaesthesia, to severe end-stage liver disease, which results in an extreme anaesthetic risk. Risk assessment for patients with cirrhosis undergoing portocaval shunt was classified by Child & Turcotte[88] in 1964 (Table 2.9) and this risk assessment has been validated to include general surgical risk and also to score the level of liver dysfunction. The only important addition for the anaesthetist has been the observation that the prothrombin time is the most significant pre-operative predictor of mortality in patients undergoing surgery for variceal bleeding.[89]

Cardiovascular effects

A hyperdynamic circulatory state develops with progressive liver disease; this is characterized by increased cardiac output and oxygen consumption, increased blood volume and reduced systemic vascular resistance.[90] The blood volume increases due to sodium retention; the low systemic vascular resistance is due to vasodilatation and shunting. Although the mechanism of

Table 2.8 Causes of chronic liver disease

Infection
Hepatitis B or C virus

Toxins
Alcohol

Drugs

Biliary obstruction
Primary biliary cirrhosis
Secondary biliary cirrhosis
    Stricture
    Stone
    Neoplasm

Metabolism diseases
Haemochromatosis

Wilson's disease

α_1-*Antitrypsin deficiency*

Fibrocystic disease

Nutritional
Intestinal bypass surgery
Intravenous nutrition

Hepatic congestion
Budd–Chiari syndrome
Veno-occlusive disease
Cardiac failure

Unknown causes
Chronic active hepatitis
Cryptogenic cirrhosis

the vasodilatation is unknown, the systemic vasculature may be poorly responsive or unresponsive to vasoconstrictor agents, including noradrenaline.

Pulmonary shunting can (rarely) account for up to 70% of cardiac output, resulting in a high mixed venous oxygen content. An increase in pulmonary vascular resistance may be a feature of end-stage liver disease. If present, the degree of pulmonary hypertension and right ventricular function must be evaluated carefully. Moderate pulmonary hypertension with normal right ventricular function is an indication for combined lung and liver transplantation in end-stage liver disease; severe pulmonary hypertension is a contraindication to transplantation. Patients with alcohol cirrhosis, Wilson's disease or haemochromatosis may also have a cardiomyopathy.

Respiratory function

Hypoxaemia may occur in patients with liver disease due to intrapulmonary shunting, impaired hypoxic vasoconstriction and ventilation/perfusion mismatch.[91] Ventilation may also be impaired by poor nutrition,

Table 2.9 Child & Turcotte's risk grading for patients with hepatic cirrhosis

	Risk grade		
	A	B	C
Serum bilirubin (μmol.l^{-1})	< 40	40–50	> 50
Serum albumin (g l)	> 35	30–35	< 30
Ascites	Absent	Well controlled	Poorly controlled
Encephalopathy	Absent	Mild	Coma
Nutritional state	Excellent	Good	Poor
Mortality	5%	10%	> 50%

From Child & Turcotte,[88] with permission.

pleural effusions and basal atelectasis. Reversal of the pulmonary changes has been reported after liver transplantation.

Renal function

Although advanced liver disease is associated with an increased circulating blood volume, much of this is pooled in the systemic vasculature and the body behaves as if it were volume–depleted.[92] Glomerular filtration rate and cortical blood flow are decreased. There is increased renin-angiotensin activity, and antidiuretic hormone concentrations are decreased. Sodium and water are retained; the greater reduction is in free water clearance, resulting in dilutional hyponatraemia in some patients. Hypokalaemia is also common, with diuretic therapy and hyperaldosteronism enhancing potassium loss. It was observed in 1964[93] that hyperbilirubinaemia is associated with an increased risk of acute renal failure. Although the mechanism is not entirely clear, endotoxaemia probably plays an important role in the onset of acute renal failure in these patients. Adequate pre-operative rehydration, pre-operative antibiotics and maintenance of a peri-operative diuresis reduce its incidence significantly. The hepatorenal syndrome is a functional disorder of the kidneys which occurs late in the course of liver disease. It is characterized by low urine sodium concentration, uraemia and oliguria. Renal function can be restored to normal if liver disease resolves (for example, after liver transplantation). The prognosis of the hepatorenal syndrome is determined by the prognosis of the liver disease. Finally, some diseases which result in end-stage liver disease may also produce intrinsic renal disease, e.g. Wilson's disease or polycystic disease.

Coagulation abnormalities

Coagulation abnormalities may occur in patients with liver disease, due to a reduction in synthesis of clotting factors and the production of abnormal clotting factors. Furthermore, production of an abnormal fibrinogen (dysfibrinogenaemia) and a decrease in the clearance of activated clotting factors promote the development of disseminated intravascular coagulation. Production of the naturally occurring anticoagulants antithrombin III and proteins C and S may also be reduced. Platelet function is abnormal in patients with end-stage liver disease and platelet numbers may be reduced by sequestration. The involvement of the liver in both production and clearance of procoagulants, anticoagulants and fibrinolytic substances can result in a range of haemostatic abnormalities from hypercoagulation to hypocoagulation and hyperfibrinolysis.

Drug metabolism

The effects of drugs in patients with end-stage liver disease may be altered by both pharmacokinetic and pharmacodynamic factors. It has been recognized for many years that some patients with liver disease are particularly sensitive to the effects of some drugs, in particular sedatives such as benzodiazepines. This appears to result from altered pharmacological responsiveness, rather than derangement of pharmacokinetics.

Pharmacokinetic factors include a reduction in absorption of some drugs, abnormal volumes of distribution, altered drug binding due to the carriage of bilirubin and abnormal concentrations of plasma proteins.[94] Elimination of drugs is influenced by many factors, the most important of which are reduced liver blood flow, portasystemic shunting and impaired metabolic capacity. Drugs with a high first-pass metabolism are highly dependent on liver blood flow; in patients with liver disease, liver blood flow is generally reduced and portasystemic shunting allows blood draining from the splanchnic circulation to bypass the liver. These factors may lead to high peak drug concentrations with less effect on drug half-life. If such drugs are prescribed in patients with liver disease, the dose, rather than the frequency, should be reduced, otherwise high peak drug concentrations will result. Drugs with an extraction of less than 30% in a single pass through the liver depend more on the metabolic capacity of the liver. Even their elimination is not uniform; glucuronidation, which is carried out predominantly in the periportal area and is relatively well-preserved in most patients with end-stage liver disease, occurs relatively normally. Enzymes in the centrilobular area, which is more prone to hypoxia, are affected more severely. This area has the highest concentration of the cytochrome P-450 enzyme which is responsible for oxidation of drugs (a phase I reaction). Drugs with a low first-pass extraction do not show particularly high peak blood concentrations in liver disease, but have a prolonged half-life. The frequency of drug administration rather than the dose should be reduced. Not only is there a difference in the handling of various drugs depending on the metabolic pathways involved, but some drugs with relatively normal pharmacokinetics in patients with liver disease, for example lorazepam and morphine, should be prescribed with caution due to increased end-organ sensitivity.

Some drugs are handled relatively normally in liver disease; these include cimetidine, digoxin, spironolactone and frusemide.

Assessment of liver function

Although a battery of liver function tests is routinely available in most hospitals, chronic liver disease often produces little alteration in liver function, and may be clinically and biochemically undetectable. Only when some additional insult, for example surgery or infection, produces further deterioration in liver function does the underlying liver disease become clinically obvious as jaundice, ascites or encephalopathy.

Regardless of the cause of cirrhosis, the most useful information for the anaesthetist is an estimation of hepatic reserve, and thus by inference, the risk associated with operation. The schemes devised by Child & Turcotte (Table 2.9)[88] and Pugh (Table 2.10)[95] provide a guide to the risk of surgery. This may be useful in deciding whether to proceed with an elective procedure; for example, patients in Child & Turcotte group C should be considered only for emergency operation.

Management of anaesthesia

It is essential that very careful and thorough pre-operative investigation and preparation are carried out. Only then should the patient proceed to surgery. Regional anaesthesia can be used in patients with hepatic disease. However, there are severe restrictions placed upon this type of anaesthetic technique. Many surgical procedures in these patients are prolonged intra-abdominal operations, not amenable to regional anaesthesia, and inadequate correction of clotting abnormalities may preclude regional techniques. The mainstay of anaesthesia is the non-reactive halogenated inhalational drugs, such as isoflurane.[96] Both regional and general anaesthesia decrease total hepatic blood flow, usually in proportion to the reduction in cardiac output and systemic vascular resistance. The composition of hepatic artery and portal vein blood has profound effects on hepatic blood flow — a decrease in P_{CO_2} or alkalosis markedly decreases hepatic blood flow; it is essential that arterial P_{CO_2} is kept within normal limits to minimize effects on hepatic and mesenteric haemodynamics. Many studies have shown that the hepatic artery buffer response is less effective when assessed under anaesthesia than under more physiological conditions. Isoflurane is better than halothane at preserving flow through the hepatic artery; under

Table 2.10 Grading of severity of liver disease

Clinical and biochemical measurement	Points scored for increasing abnormalities		
	1	2	3
Encephalopathy (grade)	None	1 or 2	3 or 4
Bilirubin ($\mu mol.l^{-1}$)	< 25	25–40	> 40
Albumin ($g.l^{-1}$)	> 35	28–35	< 28
Prothrombin time (seconds prolonged)	1–4	4–6	> 6

4–6 points = Child and Turcotte group A;
7–9 points = Child and Turcotte group B;
10–12 points = Child and Turcotte group C.

From Pugh et al,[95] with permission.

anaesthesia, flow through the hepatic artery increases with isoflurane but decreases with halothane.[97] Recently it has been shown that isoflurane (but not halothane) also preferentially vasodilates human mesenteric vessels, compensating for the vasoconstriction caused by laparotomy. However, the changes induced by anaesthetic agents are relatively minor compared to those produced by surgery. Gelman's classic study in 1976[98] demonstrated a small decrease in total hepatic blood flow during anaesthesia, but a further fall with surgery; the extent of the decrease was related to the nature of the operation, its site and the degree of surgical trauma. Compared with baseline values (100%), blood flow decreased to 76% in patients undergoing hernia repair and to 42% in patients undergoing upper abdominal surgery.

Premedication comprises an oral benzodiazepine, together with ranitidine or omeprazole; cerebral depressant drugs should be omitted if encephalopathy is present. A rapid sequence induction is necessary if the patient has tense ascites or needs emergency surgery. Anaesthetic maintenance is with oxygen-enriched air, isoflurane, fentanyl and an atracurium infusion; nitrous oxide should be avoided because of the high risk of air embolism in these patients. Large tidal volumes and PEEP minimize basal atelectasis. Arterial $P\text{CO}_2$ should be kept within the normal range. Arterial blood gases, acid–base status, haematocrit, glucose and electrolytes should be measured at regular intervals. Active measures must be taken to prevent hypothermia, including heated cascade humidification and wrapping the peripheries, head and chest with thermally insulating drapes.

The degree of monitoring is determined by the extent of surgery and the risk category of the patient. In complex procedures, direct monitoring of arterial and central venous pressures is mandatory, as well as pulmonary artery catheterization to give information on left-sided filling pressures, cardiac output, systemic vascular resistance and oxygen supply. Third-space losses may be very large due to translocation of fluid, and re-accumulation of ascitic fluid which may be very rapid in cirrhotic patients. Renal doses of dopamine (e.g. 1–5 $\mu g.kg^{-1}.min^{-1}$) should be started to preserve renal function. Mannitol may also be used to preserve renal function in jaundiced patients.

Haemorrhage may be sudden and massive (a portal vein or inferior vena caval bleed can exceed 1000 ml.min^{-1}), and requires adequate venous access (8–10 French gauge cannulae), as well as the ability to deliver warmed, filtered, premixed transfusion fluids at rates of up to 1500 ml.min^{-1}. The Rapid Infusion System (Haemonetics) is ideal for this purpose.

Hypotension may occur due to surgical manipulation interfering with preload, ionized hypocalcaemia from citrate toxicity or venous air emboli.[99]

The coagulation status, which may already be abnormal, can deteriorate very rapidly due to dilutional coagulopathy and the onset of fibrinolysis. Serial monitoring of coagulation is essential to identify current problems and to ensure early and appropriate treatment, before irreversible coagulopathy and uncontrolled bleeding develop. Thromboelastography is ideally suited for this purpose, and gives information about clotting factor activity, platelet function and any clinically significant fibrinolytic process within 20–30 min.[100]

GASTRO-INTESTINAL DISEASE

Inflammatory bowel disease

The term inflammatory bowel disease comprises Crohn's disease and ulcerative colitis. Both are chronic disorders, characterized by unpredictable exacerbations and remissions. Crohn's disease may involve any part of the alimentary tract from the mouth to the anus, whereas ulcerative colitis is confined to the large bowel. There are a number of causes of malabsorption in Crohn's disease, shown in Table 2.11, and many patients suffer from malnutrition and weight loss. Malabsorption of iron, folic acid and vitamin B_{12} commonly leads to anaemia. In patients with chronic diarrhoea, sodium, potassium and water depletion are common and deficiency of magnesium and zinc may also occur. Urinary tract problems may be present if an inflammatory mass obstructs the ureter, leading to hydronephrosis; enterovesical fistulae may also develop. Intra-abdominal complications include abscess formation, which may discharge back into the

Table 2.11 Causes of malabsorption in Crohn's disease

Fat
Reduction in absorptive surface
Bacterial colonization of small intestine
Interruption of enterohepatic circulation of bile acids

Vitamin D
Interruption of enterohepatic circulation of bile acids

Protein
Protein loss through ulcerated mucosa

Carbohydrate
Lactose deficiency due to mucosal damage

Vitamin B_{12}
Diseased or resected terminal ileum

intestine, or through the bladder or vagina to create a fistula. Free perforation of the intestine may also occur. There is an increased incidence of carcinoma of the intestine in segments affected by Crohn's disease. There are a number of extra-intestinal complications of both Crohn's disease and ulcerative colitis, and these are listed in Table 2.12.

Ulcerative colitis always involves the rectum and may also involve various parts of the colon, or the entire colon. Strictures are uncommon, and fistula formation is absent. In severe ulcerative colitis, there is exhausting diarrhoea and dehydration. Toxic dilatation of the colon presents the most serious complication, with tachycardia, a high swinging temperature and abdominal distension and tenderness. The patient is at grave risk of dying from colonic perforation. Cancer of the colon in chronic colitis occurs with an increased frequency in patients with extensive or total colitis of more than 10 years' duration. The extrahepatic complications noted in Table 2.12 are common to both ulcerative colitis and Crohn's colitis, except that sclerosing cholangitis is much more common in ulcerative colitis.

Table 2.12 Extra-intestinal manifestations of inflammatory bowel disease

Hepatic
Cirrhosis
Abscess
Carcinoma of biliary tree
Sclerosing cholangitis

Skin
Erythema nodosum
Pyoderma gangrenosum

Aphthous stomatitis

Arthritis
Ankylosing spondylitis
Seronegative arthritis

Finger clubbing

Ocular lesions
Uveitis
Episcleritis
Conjunctivitis

Haematological disease
Auto-immune haemolytic anaemia
Thrombosis

Vasculitis

Cardiovascular disease

Renal disease
Pyelonephritis
Amyloidosis

Management of anaesthesia

Thorough pre-operative assessment is essential. The patients are frequently anaemic due either to malabsorption or blood loss. They are also frequently dehydrated and there may be severe deficiencies of sodium, potassium and magnesium. Hypo-albuminaemia may be present due to a combination of malnutrition and protein-losing enteropathy, and human albumin (administered with central venous pressure monitoring) may be the fluid of choice for resuscitation pre-operatively. Any manifestations of the disease outside the gastro-intestinal tract must also be assessed carefully; for example, arthritis may influence the management of the upper airway. Associated liver or renal disease must be sought, and great care should be taken with the patient's eyes if there is any ocular involvement. Patients with severe inflammatory bowel disease may be maintained on oral or intravenous corticosteroids, and the associated complications such as osteomalacia, susceptibility to infection, skin which is easily damaged and the need for steroid replacement therapy must all be borne in mind. Patients presenting as an acute emergency with toxic megacolon may be gravely ill. There must be adequate intravascular fluid replacement prior to anaesthesia, and direct monitoring of arterial and central venous pressures is helpful.

Reversal of non-depolarizing muscle relaxants with anticholinesterase drugs increases intraluminal pressures in the gastro-intestinal tract.[101] This has led to suggestions that they may pose an increased risk of dehiscence of a colonic anastomosis, but this effect has never been demonstrated convincingly. However, the use of mivacurium by infusion, with appropriate monitoring, makes reliance on spontaneous offset of paralysis a practical alternative to evoked offset.

Carcinoid syndrome

Carcinoid tumours arise from enterochromaffin tissues, and are most commonly found in the gastro-intestinal tract. They may sometimes arise in the bronchi, and occasionally in the ovaries. The syndrome is caused by the release of vaso-active substances, which include serotonin, prostaglandins, histamine and kallikreins. Kallikreins can activate a plasma factor (kininogen) which acts to produce a group of polypeptides (kinins), including bradykinin. These substances are normally inactivated in the liver, but symptoms occur either if the ability of the liver to metabolize these substances is overwhelmed, or when carcinoid tumours of the bronchus and ovary release the substances directly into the systemic rather than the portal circulation.

The symptoms of carcinoid syndrome include bronchoconstriction, episodic skin flushing, intermittent abdominal pain and diarrhoea, palpitations and supraventricular tachyarrhythmias. Other manifestations include tricuspid regurgitation, pulmonary stenosis, hepatomegaly and hyperglycaemia.

Management of anaesthesia

Patients with the carcinoid syndrome may present either for resection of the carcinoid tumour, or removal of hepatic metastases. Occasionally these patients may require replacement of a heart valve. It seems logical to treat the patient pre-operatively with drugs to counteract the effects of the vaso-active substances secreted by the tumour cells. Histamine H_1- and H_2-receptor blockers, for example diphenhydramine and cimetidine, are logical drugs to choose; there is a case report[102] of the use of ketanserin (a competitive serotonin-receptor antagonist) to attenuate the vasoconstrictor and bronchoconstrictor effects of serotonin. There is a further case report[103] of use of a somatostatin analogue during anaesthesia to reverse a carcinoid crisis. The patient may be intravascularly depleted pre-operatively, due to chronic secretion of vasoconstrictor substances and adequate pre- and intra-operative hydration is important. There are no specific drugs or techniques that have been proved to be especially beneficial in this situation, although morphine should be avoided as it may stimulate release of serotinin and histamine. Other drugs known to be associated with histamine release, for example tubocurarine and suxamethonium, should be avoided. Tachycardia and hypertension may occur intra-operatively, as may hypotension and bronchospasm. Bronchospasm may be very difficult to treat, as conventional therapy is not helpful. Corticosteroids are probably ineffective after the vaso-active substances have been liberated.[104]

Carcinoma of the oesophagus

Patients with this disease may present for resection of the oesophagus or for insertion of a feeding tube. They are often severely malnourished, not only due to the cachexia of the carcinoma, but also because of physical problems with swallowing. In addition, if there has been overflow of food substances above the oesophageal tumour, the patient may have recurrent chest infections from aspiration. The patient may be dehydrated prior to anaesthesia due to dysphagia, and careful correction of fluid balance should take place pre-operatively. Cricoid pressure may not stop spillage of contents on from the upper oesophagus into the larynx.

RENAL DISEASE

Chronic renal failure

Chronic renal failure is irreversible deterioration in renal function, and may be caused by any condition which destroys the normal structure and function of the kidney (Table 2.13). The condition may progress insidiously over a number of years, and frequently it is impossible to determine the underlying renal disease. In the UK, approximately 55 new patients per million of the adult population are accepted for long-term dialysis treatment each year. When renal function deteriorates slowly, it is not uncommon for patients to remain asymptomatic until the glomerular filtration rate is 15 ml.min^{-1} or less. However, because of the widespread effects of progressive renal failure, symptoms and signs are referable to almost every organ system (Table 2.14).

Pre-operative assessment

A normochromic, normocytic anaemia with a haemoglobin concentration in the range of 5–8 g.dl^{-1} is almost universal in patients with chronic renal failure. Several factors contribute:

1. reduced intake of iron and other haematinics due to anorexia and dietary restrictions
2. impaired intestinal absorption of iron
3. diminished erythropoiesis, due to toxic effects of uraemia on marrow precursor cells

Table 2.13 Causes of chronic renal failure

Congenital and inherited
Polycystic disease
Fabry's disease

Vascular disease
Arteriosclerosis
Vasculitis (PAN, SLE, scleroderma)

Glomerular disease
Glomerulonephritides

Interstitial disease
Chronic pyelonephritis
Vesico-ureteric reflux
Tuberculosis
Analgesic nephropathy
Nephrocalcinosis
Schistosomiasis

Obstructive uropathy
Calculus
Retroperitoneal fibrosis
Prostatic hypertrophy
Pelvic tumours

PAN = Polyarteritis nodosa;
SLE = systemic lupus erythematosus.

Table 2.14 Effects of renal failure

Anaemia
Metabolic bone disease
Neuropathy
Myopathy
Endocrine abnormalities
Hypertension and atherosclerosis
Acidosis
Susceptibility to infection

---

4. inappropriately low plasma erythropoietin concentration
5. reduced red-cell survival (erythrocyte half-life is 50% of normal), due to erythrocyte membrane fragility
6. increased blood loss due to capillary fragility and poor platelet function.

This chronic anaemia reduces oxygen-carrying capacity, which can result in tissue hypoxia. This is compensated for to an extent by a shift of the oxyhaemoglobin dissociation curve to the right and by increased tissue blood flow due to decreased blood viscosity. Recombinant human erythropoietin (rHuEpo) is now available for clinical use in anaemic patients with chronic renal failure.[105] Many thousands of anaemic haemodialysis patients have now been treated with erythropoietin, and in almost all patients the treatment has been effective in achieving target haematocrit or haemoglobin level, within 6–12 weeks after onset of therapy. There are a number of minor side-effects associated with therapy with rHuEpo; these include flu-like myalgias (5–7%), headaches (17–27%) and flank pain (14–30%).[106] However, there are two side-effects of more concern to the anaesthetist: increased blood pressure and grand mal seizures. An increase in blood pressure was observed in 35% of all patients during rHuEpo therapy, and in 25% of the patients, initiation of, or increase in, antihypertensive medication was necessary. A reversal of the peripheral vasodilatation occurring in anaemia, and a subsequent increase in peripheral resistance during rHuEpo treatment, are thought to cause the hypertension.[107] The incidence of seizure activity in rHuEpo-treated patients on haemodialysis was 8%, with approximately 50% of the seizures occurring within the first 12 weeks of treatment.

A coagulopathy is often present in patients with chronic renal failure. The most frequent coagulation defect is reduced platelet adhesiveness, and this may be detected by measuring the bleeding time. In addition to platelet abnormalities, patients requiring haemodialysis may also be given systemic or regional heparinization to maintain the patency of vascular shunts.

Renal osteodystrophy is a metabolic bone disease which accompanies chronic renal failure. It consists of a mixture of osteomalacia, hyperparathyroid bone disease, osteoporosis and osteosclerosis. Osteomalacia results from failure of the kidney to convert cholecalciferol to its active metabolite, 1,25-dihydroxycholecalciferol. A deficiency of the latter leads to diminished intestinal absorption of calcium, hypocalcaemia and a reduction in the calcification of osteoids. Hyperparathyroid bone disease results from secondary hyperparathyroidism, the parathyroid glands being stimulated by the low plasma calcium concentration and possibly also by hyperphosphataemia. These patients are vulnerable to pathological fractures, and great care must be taken when moving or positioning the unconscious patient during anaesthesia and surgery.

Patients with chronic renal failure may have a generalized myopathy, due to a combination of poor nutrition, hyperparathyroidism, vitamin D deficiency and disorders of electrolyte metabolism. Rarely, this is a cause of respiratory embarrassment postoperatively. A sensory and motor neuropathy may occur, causing paraesthesia and foot drop. An autonomic neuropathy may in part also explain development of disorders of gastro-intestinal motility and the onset of postural hypotension, in the absence of sodium and water depletion. These symptoms may improve or disappear when dialysis is started. Gastric fluid volume and acidity are likely to be increased in patients with chronic renal failure, and these changes, combined with delayed gastro-intestinal motility, may place these patients at increased risk of regurgitation and pulmonary aspiration.

Hypertension frequently co-exists with chronic renal failure either as a complication of the renal disease or as a cause of the renal failure. Sustained hypertension can lead to cardiomegaly and congestive cardiac failure, which may be aggravated by the AV fistula used for haemodialysis. The majority of patients with chronic renal failure require antihypertensive therapy.

Abnormalities in water and electrolyte balance frequently occur in chronic renal failure and the patient's volume status should be assessed prior to anaesthesia. Haemodialysis conducted in order to normalize serum electrolytes shortly before anaesthesia usually renders the patient hypovolaemic, and hypotension is likely to occur during induction of anaesthesia. Increased plasma magnesium concentrations may accompany chronic renal failure, and may potentiate the effects of depolarizing and non-depolarizing muscle relaxants.[108] A metabolic acidosis with a compensated respiratory alkalosis may occur, although haemodialysis is effective in restoring the arterial pH to near normal values.

Patients with chronic renal failure are extremely susceptible to infection, as both cellular and humoral immunity are impaired. In addition, the patient may be taking immunosuppressive drugs, including corticosteroids. Strict attention to asepsis is important when placing vascular cannulae and tracheal tubes. There is a high incidence of viral hepatitis, which reflects not only the frequent use of blood products, but also immunosuppression.

Management of anaesthesia

No induction agent is specifically indicated for patients with chronic renal failure, but there is increased vulnerability to hypotension and to gastric aspiration. Potassium release after administration of suxamethonium is not exaggerated in patients with chronic renal failure.[109] However, caution is necessary when the pre-operative plasma potassium concentration is already high. Atracurium is the non-depolarizing muscle relaxant of choice in patients with chronic renal failure. In one study, halothane, isoflurane and enflurane all caused a similar reduction in effective renal plasma flow in healthy patients, and this reduction was dose-dependent, being greater at 1.25 minimum alveolar concentration (MAC) than at 0.75 MAC.[110] There was no significant hypotension and no change in cardiac output, indicating that the reduction of effective renal plasma flow was caused by a direct effect on renal perfusion rather than by cardiovascular depression. Since renal blood flow may be affected independently or in concert by several extrinsic systems, including the sympathetic nervous system, antidiuretic hormone release, catecholamine release and the angiotensin system, further studies are needed to clarify whether anaesthetic agents themselves have significant effects on the regulation of renal blood flow. In view of its greater propensity for free fluoride ion release, enflurane should be avoided in patients with renal dysfunction. In a study of 15 patients in whom controlled hypotension was required (mean arterial pressure 60–70 mmHg) for dissection and clipping of a cerebral aneurysm, Zall et al[111] investigated renal function and renal haemodynamics when hypotension was induced either by adenosine or by an infusion of sodium nitroprusside. Adenosine induced marked decreases in glomerular filtration rate and renal plasma flow (90%), and a pronounced increase in renal vascular resistance. The decreases in glomerular filtration rate and renal plasma flow (24 and 36%) caused by sodium nitroprusside were significantly less. In view of these results, it is reasonable to suggest that controlled hypotension should not be induced by adenosine in patients with impaired renal function.

Regional anaesthesia may be used in patients with chronic renal failure and may prevent renovascular vasoconstriction by sympathetic efferent blockade. However, coagulopathy is a contra-indication to regional anaesthesia.

Impairment of renal function is increased by surgery more than by anaesthesia.[112] The extent of impairment depends on the nature of the surgery. For example, reduced cardiac output and utilization of extra-corporeal circulation are aggravating factors in cardiac surgery. Diminution in renal blood flow following clamping of the aorta results in cortical ischaemia which persists long after unclamping in aortic surgery.[113] Postoperative stress and pain stimulate secretion of catecholamines, antidiuretic hormone and renin, and blood loss may render the patient hypovolaemic.

Positive-pressure ventilation and PEEP have many effects on renal function, including reductions in renal blood flow, glomerular filtration rate, sodium excretion fraction and atrial natriuretic factor,[114] and stimulation of antidiuretic hormone, renin and noradrenaline secretion. Expansion of the plasma volume may reduce the severity of the renal effects.

Postoperative management

Postoperative analgesia with a regional technique may not be possible, due to the coagulopathy associated with chronic renal failure. Prolonged sedation and respiratory depression have been described in anephric patients after small doses of opioids,[115] and the intramuscular route of administration may be associated with haematoma formation. Recent attention has focused on non-steroidal anti-inflammatory drugs as a means of providing analgesia postoperatively. However, administration of these drugs to patients with renal dysfunction carries the risk of an acute ischaemic insult to the kidneys, because inhibition of synthesis of vasodilating prostaglandins allows uncontrolled renal vasoconstriction.[116] A recent prospective, randomized study using non-steroidal anti-inflammatory drugs demonstrated renal impairment in patients with mild but stable chronic renal failure,[117] and the study indicated that this might be dose-dependent. This class of drug should therefore be used with extreme caution, if at all, in the peri-operative period in patients with impaired renal function.

Polycystic kidney disease

This autosomal dominant congenital abnormality may present with chronic renal failure in middle age. The patients are frequently hypertensive. About one-third of patients have hepatic cysts, but disturbance of liver function is rare. Aneurysms of cerebral vessels occur and about 10% of patients have subarachnoid haemorrhage. Anaesthetic assessment and management are similar to those of any patient with chronic renal failure.

NEUROLOGICAL DISEASE

Cerebrovascular disease

Cerebrovascular accidents (CVAs) may be caused by cerebral thrombosis, cerebral embolism or intracranial haemorrhage. Nearly 50% of patients who experience cerebral thrombosis have had one or more previous transient ischaemic attacks. Symptoms of cerebral thrombosis depend on the cerebral vessel that becomes occluded; the middle cerebral artery, or one of its branches, is affected most frequently. When the main trunk is occluded, symptoms of hemiplegia, homonomous hemianopia and (if the dominant hemisphere is involved) an expressive and receptive dysphasia develop. Cerebral thrombosis is most likely to occur in patients who have atherosclerosis associated with essential hypertension or diabetes mellitus. The incidence of CVA has fallen with effective treatment of hypertension. Other causes of cerebral thrombosis include hypotension (e.g. following myocardial infarction or severe haemorrhage), inflammatory disease of the blood vessels (e.g. polyarteritis nodosa and systemic lupus erythematosus), and haematological disorders including polycythaemia, thrombotic thrombocytopenic purpura and sickle-cell anaemia. There is possibly an increased incidence with the use of oral contraceptive drugs.

Cerebral embolism is most commonly from the heart, in association with atrial fibrillation, prosthetic heart valves, infective endocarditis, intracardiac tumours and intracardiac thrombosis. Intracranial haemorrhage probably accounts for about 10% of all strokes; the most common cause is rupture of an intracranial aneurysm.

A recent study of 173 patients with a history of CVA, who underwent surgery and anaesthesia, found that the incidence of new CVAs was 2.9%.[118] The risk of a CVA did not correlate with age, sex, history of multiple CVAs, ASA physical status, use of aspirin, coronary artery disease, peripheral vascular disease, intra-operative blood pressure, time lapsed since the original stroke or cause of the original stroke. However, postoperative stroke was more common in patients given heparin pre-operatively. Thus the risk of postoperative recurrence of CVA is low, but not easily predictable. The risk continues beyond the first week of convalescence (average time of recurrence was 12.2 days after surgery). Finally, unlike myocardial infarction, it does not seem to depend on the length of time between the initial event and the subsequent anaesthesia and surgery.

Epilepsy

There are many different types of adult disorders, and the drugs used to treat these patients either singly or in combination depend on the type of seizure. It is important to consider not only the side-effects of these drugs, but also the effect that they may have on anaesthesia. Finally, it is important to consider how to maintain therapeutic drug levels during the peri-operative period in order to avoid uncontrolled postoperative seizures.

Phenytoin is the primary drug administered in treatment of all types of epilepsy with the exception of petit mal. Side-effects include gastro-intestinal irritation, megaloblastic anaemia and peripheral neuropathy. Phenytoin is metabolized in the liver and, rarely, is associated with hepatotoxicity. It may be administered either orally or intravenously.

The primary side-effect of phenobarbitone is sedation, but toxic plasma concentrations are associated with nystagmus and ataxia. Phenobarbitone is a potent hepatic microsomal enzyme inducer, resulting in enhanced metabolism of drugs. It is excreted mainly by the kidneys, and renal failure may result in unexpectedly high plasma concentrations of the drug.

Carbamazepine may cause bone marrow depression and hepatorenal dysfunction. Sodium valproate may also cause hepatotoxicity, but in addition may inhibit activity of hepatic microsomal enzymes.

When epileptic patients present for anaesthesia, it should be remembered that co-existing sedation produced by anticonvulsant drugs may have additive effects with anaesthetics, whereas drug-induced enzyme induction may alter responses to other drugs or even contribute to organ toxicity associated with administration of halothane or enflurane. Methohexitone, which may activate epileptic foci, is best avoided in these patients, as is propofol, which has also been associated with increased seizure activity. Although the central nervous system stimulating effects of laudanosine, a metabolite of atracurium, are probably only of theoretical importance in the majority of patients, it may be prudent to avoid this muscle relaxant. Enflurane predictably produces spike wave activity on the electroencephalogram, and this may be accompanied by visible skeletal muscle twitching. These changes occur in normal patients as well as those with known epileptic disorders. The likelihood of seizure activity is greatest when inspired concentrations of enflurane exceed 2.5%, and hypocapnia (less than 3.33 kPa; 25 mmHg) is present.[119] In addition, enzyme induction in these patients may increase free fluoride concentrations if enflurane is administered. There is no contra-indication to the use of opioids in epileptic patients.

Parkinson's disease

This is a degenerative disease of the central nervous system, characterized by loss of dopaminergic fibres in the basal ganglia of the brain. This results in diminished inhibition of the extrapyramidal motor system and an unopposed action of acetylcholine. Treatment of Parkinson's disease is designed to increase concentrations of dopamine in basal ganglia and/or to decrease neuronal effects of acetylcholine. The drugs most frequently used are levodopa, anticholinergics and antihistamines. Levodopa, the immediate precursor of dopamine, crosses the blood–brain barrier and is then converted to dopamine in the central nervous system. However, administration of levopoda results in total body increases in concentrations of dopamine as the decarboxylating enzyme responsible for the conversion of levopoda to dopamine is also present in the systemic circulation. For this reason, levodopa is administered with carbidopa, a drug that inhibits activity of decarboxylase enzyme in the systemic circulation and which reduces the dose-related adverse side-effects of this drug. These side-effects include increases in myocardial contractility and heart rate, and increased cardiac irritability. There is a chronic rise in peripheral vascular resistance, and it is likely that intravascular fluid volume is therefore decreased. Consequently, orthostatic hypotension is not uncommon in patients being treated with levodopa. In addition, there is decreased production of noradrenaline in the sympathetic nervous system nerve endings, due to the negative feedback inhibition of dopamine on the synthesis of catecholamines. This also contributes to orthostatic hypotension. These patients may be nauseated and vomit, due to stimulation of the chemoreceptor trigger zone by dopamine.

The patient's medication should be continued as usual on the day of surgery, and started as soon as possible after surgery; abrupt withdrawal may result in skeletal muscle rigidity, interfering with the maintenance of adequate ventilation. The possibility of orthostatic hypotension due to intravascular fluid depletion, and cardiac arrhythmias, should be borne in mind. Post-operatively, analgesia should be adequate to allow early mobilization and effective chest physiotherapy, as the immobility produced by Parkinson's disease contributes to postoperative atelectasis and pulmonary complications.

Multiple sclerosis

This is a disease of the central nervous system, characterized by random and multiple sites of demyelination of corticospinal tract neurones in the brain and spinal cord. The course of multiple sclerosis is characterized by unpredictable relapses and remissions over a period of years. The course is usually slowly progressive, with residual symptoms persisting during remission. There is no treatment that is curative, but administration of adrenocorticotrophic hormone or corticosteroids shortens the duration of an acute attack. Non-specific measures include avoidance of excessive fatigue, emotional stress and marked temperature changes. As the stress of surgery may produce a relapse, elective surgery should be undertaken only if absolutely necessary. The patient may also be receiving treatment for skeletal muscle spasticity in the form of diazepam, dantrolene or baclofen.

It is likely that multiple sclerosis will be exacerbated during the postoperative period, regardless of the anaesthetic technique and drugs selected for use. It is important that the patient is aware of this prior to anaesthesia and surgery. Subarachnoid anaesthesia has been implicated in exacerbations of multiple sclerosis, whereas epidural anaesthesia and peripheral nerve blocks have not.[120]

Resistance to the effects of non-depolarizing muscle relaxants has been observed in patients with multiple sclerosis, perhaps reflecting proliferation of extra-junctional cholinergic receptors characteristic of upper motor neurone lesions.[121] Great attention must be paid to avoid peri-operative increases in body temperature, as changes of even 1°C have been associated with deterioration of the disease. Infective foci must be identified and treated pre-operatively and appropriate measures taken to avoid postoperative infection (e.g. physiotherapy, prophylactic antibiotics if there is urinary stasis).

SKIN AND MUSCULOSKELETAL DISORDERS

Epidermolysis bullosa

Many skin disorders result in abnormal skin fragility, which can cause blister formation or bullae. Epidermolysis bullosa is a name given to a group of inherited disorders characterized by frictional separation of the epidermis, by a split at the lower epidermis or at the epidermal junction. It is transmitted as an autosomal recessive trait and has an incidence of approximately 1 in 3000 births. It is characterized by extensive bullous and dystrophic lesions which may develop spontaneously or at the sites of friction or trauma. Lateral friction to the skin is the most damaging, with pressure at right angles to the skin being less so. Abnormalities of the nails, conjunctiva, hair and teeth may occur. Lesions of the mucous membranes of the mouth, pharynx and oesophagus may lead to feeding difficulties, microstomia and the possibility of a difficult tracheal intubation.

There are numerous anaesthetic problems. Movement of the patient must be undertaken with extreme care. Simple monitoring may cause skin damage, and trauma to the skin from a face mask, or to the airway on intubation, may result in damage. This can lead to ulceration with increased risk of infection, fluid loss and scar formation in the long term. Adhesive strapping should be kept to a minimum and all pressure areas must be carefully padded. Sheets beneath the patient should be free from creases. Regional anaesthesia for patients with epidermolysis bullosa has been described,[122] as long as the skin on the back is free from lesions or infections. There is no contra-indication to the use of suxamethonium, unless there is extensive atrophy of the patient's muscles.[123] At laryngoscopy, great care should be taken to avoid damage to severely carious teeth and, obviously, to avoid damage to the delicate mucous membranes of the upper airway. It is wise to choose a tracheal tube smaller than usual to minimize contact with the laryngeal inlet.

Stevens–Johnson syndrome

This is a severe manifestation of erythema multiforme, associated with multisystem involvement. It may co-exist with fever, tachycardia and tachypnoea. Corticosteroids are used in its management. The problems of anaesthesia are similar to those encountered in patients with epidermolysis bullosa, but in addition, the patient may have pulmonary lesions which increase the risk of pneumothorax, especially in association with positive-pressure ventilation. Nitrous oxide is therefore best avoided.

Scleroderma

This is a multisystem disorder of unknown aetiology. It has characteristics of both a collagen disease and an auto-immune process. It is more common in women aged between 20 and 40 years at the time of onset. Significant manifestations may occur in the skin and musculoskeletal systems, peripheral nervous system, heart, lungs, kidneys and gastro-intestinal tract. Progression of the disease may be accelerated by pregnancy.

The skin exhibits a mild thickening and becomes taut as the disease progresses, leading to limited mobility and flexion contractures, especially of the fingers. Raynaud's phenomenon is common and the ability to sweat is reduced. Chest-wall involvement can cause respiratory failure.[124] A combination of calcinosis cutis, Raynaud's phenomenon, sclerodactyly and multiple telangectasia of the skin, lips, oral mucosa and gut is known as the CRST syndrome.

Cardiac involvement occurs in 80% of cases, and may result in cardiomegaly, pericarditis, pericardial effusions, conduction defects and arrhythmias. However, only 19% of patients have an abnormal rhythm if 24-h ECG monitoring is undertaken.[125] Intimal fibrosis of the pulmonary artery walls is associated with a high incidence of pulmonary hypertension, which may progress to cor pulmonale. Pulmonary hypertension is often present even in asymptomatic patients.[126] Pulmonary fibrosis causes decreased inspiratory capacity and vital capacity. Pulmonary compliance is diminished by fibrosis and arterial hypoxaemia is common even at rest.

Involvement of the gastro-intestinal tract may manifest as dryness of the mouth and microstomia. The patient may have noticed difficulty opening the mouth for dental treatment. Carious teeth are common as a consequence of the microstomia and the lack of saliva. Progressive fibrosis of the gastro-intestinal tract causes hypomotility of the lower oesophagus and small intestine. The patients often have dysphagia and gastric acid reflux, due to reduced lower oesophageal sphincter tone. Bacterial overgrowth occurs in the small intestine due to intestinal hypomotility, and produces a malabsorption syndrome. Malabsorption of the fat-soluble vitamins, including vitamin K, may result in a coagulation disorder. Broad spectrum antibiotics are effective in treating this.

Pre-operatively, mouth opening and the presence of carious teeth should be assessed. Assessment of all the organs affected by the disease should be carried out, and a chest X-ray, ECG, lung function tests and a clotting screen should be included amongst the pre-operative investigations. Steroid cover and pretreatment with vitamin K may be necessary. Venous access may be very difficult, rendering an inhalation induction necessary. A rapid-sequence induction technique is often not practical, because tracheal intubation may be difficult due to limited mouth opening and a fibrosed mandibular joint. Sellick's manoeuvre may also be effective if the oesophagus is fibrosed. Pre-operative prophylaxis with an H$_2$-receptor antagonist and antacid is indicated.

Intra-operatively, it may be necessary to ventilate the lungs with high inflation pressures due to decreased pulmonary compliance, and a high inspired oxygen content may be necessary to prevent arterial hypoxaemia. Respiratory acidosis and hypoxaemia should be avoided if possible, as they increase pulmonary vascular resistance and exacerbate any pre-existing pulmonary hypertension. Regional anaesthesia has been used, although it may be difficult because of skin and joint changes. However, regional techniques may be useful postoperatively in providing not only analgesia but peripheral vasodilatation to improve perfusion of the lower extremities. Measures should be taken intra-operatively to minimize peripheral vasoconstriction by maintaining the operating room temperature above 21°C, administering warm fluids, and placing the patient on a warming blanket.

Ehlers–Danlos syndrome

This inherited disorder of collagen synthesis is characterized by hypermobility of the joints and increased extensibility of the skin.[127] The skin is thin, fragile and easily torn. Joints are hyperextensible, and dislocations are common. Blood-vessel fragility leads to bruising, and at operation, bleeding may be profuse despite a normal clotting screen.[122] Aortic aneurysms, mitral regurgitation and cardiac conduction abnormalities are frequent. Pneumothorax and bowel perforation may occur. Premature labour and excessive bleeding with delivery are common obstetric problems.

Prophylactic antibiotics are indicated if mitral regurgitation is present. Intramuscular injections should be avoided, in view of the bleeding tendency. Likewise, nasotracheal intubation should not be undertaken unless absolutely necessary. Venous access may be difficult, but central venous cannulation is inadvisable because of the risk of bleeding.[122] Tracheal intubation should be gentle. Nitrous oxide should be avoided in view of the danger of pneumothorax formation. All skin surfaces should be padded and the same extreme care taken as with patients with epidermolysis bullosa. Because of the tendency of these patients to bleed and form haematomas, regional anaesthesia has traditionally not been recommended, but occasionally it may be the best compromise.[128]

Systemic lupus erythematosus

This is a multisystem disease of unknown aetiology and includes both arthritic manifestations involving the hands, wrists, elbows, knees and ankles, and systemic manifestations. The heart may be involved either by pericarditis, or myocarditis leading to conduction abnormalities and congestive heart failure. Pulmonary involvement may include diffuse fibrosis and arterial hypoxaemia. Renal abnormalities include a protein-losing nephropathy, resulting in hypoalbuminaemia and haematuria. The patient may have abnormal liver function tests with a lupoid hepatitis, which may occasionally be fatal. Treatment is usually with anti-inflammatory therapy, corticosteroids and sometimes immunosuppressive drugs. Management of anaesthesia must take into consideration the drugs used for the treatment of this condition, and an assessment of the organs affected by the disease.

Myotonic dystrophy

This is the most common form of adult muscular dystrophy. Onset is usually in the second to fourth decade, and the disease is slowly progressive; it is inherited as an autosomal dominant trait with variable penetrance. Death usually occurs from pneumonia or cardiac failure by the sixth decade. The disease is due to abnormal calcium metabolism in skeletal, smooth and cardiac muscle. There is failure of calcium adenosine triphosphatase to return calcium from the sarcoplasmic reticulum following depolarization of the muscle membrane. This allows continuing contraction following stimulation. Delayed relaxation after contraction is the hallmark of the condition. Classically, patients with the condition have facial weakness, ptosis, dysarthria, and an inability to relax the grip (myotonia). Other features are mental retardation, frontal baldness and cataract formation. There is an increased incidence of diabetes mellitus, hypothyroidism and adrenal insufficiency. Cardiac arrhythmias and conduction abnormalities are common, and reports of sudden death are probably due to arrhythmias. Weakness of the pharyngeal and thoracic muscles render these patients vulnerable to gastric acid aspiration. There are many reports of anaesthesia in patients with myotonic dystrophy.[129–132] They must be assumed to have a degree of cardiomyopathy, even if asymptomatic, and myocardial depression from volatile anaesthetic drugs may be exaggerated.[133] Cardiac conduction blockade may be exacerbated during anaesthesia, and require insertion of a temporary cardiac pacemaker. The use of suxamethonium is contra-indicated due to prolonged skeletal muscle contraction, which can be so severe as to make ventilation of the lungs difficult. The response to non-depolarizing muscle relaxants is normal. However, in patients with respiratory muscle weakness, a smaller dose than normal is required. The patients are very sensitive to the respiratory depressant effects of barbiturates, opioids and benzodiazepines, as there is an incidence of central sleep apnoea. Postoperative pain relief with regional anaesthesia is very useful and the patients should be kept in a highly staffed area for up to 24 h postoperatively.

Myasthenia gravis

This is a chronic auto-immune condition involving the neuromuscular junction. It is characterized by weakness and fatigue that is worsened by exercise. The condition most commonly affects the external ocular muscles, causing ptosis and diplopia. There is a decrease in the number of available receptors for acetylcholine at the postsynaptic neuromuscular junction.[134] Weakness of pharyngeal and laryngeal muscles results in dysphagia, dysarthria and difficulty in eliminating oral secretions. This renders patients at high risk of pulmonary aspiration of gastric contents. Skeletal muscle strength may be normal at rest, but weakens promptly with exercise. There is an association with other diseases of auto-immune origin, for example, decreased thyroid function is present in about 10% of patients with myasthenia gravis, and rheumatoid arthritis, systemic lupus erythematosus and pernicious anaemia also occur more commonly than in patients without myasthenia gravis. Aminoglycoside antibiotics can aggravate the skeletal muscle weakness. The mainstays of treatment include anticholinesterase drugs, corticosteroids, immunosuppressants, thymectomy and plasmapheresis.

Management of anaesthesia

At the pre-operative visit, respiratory function should be assessed carefully; blood gas analysis may be valuable. The presence and severity of any associated diseases should be evaluated. Respiratory infection should be treated prior to anaesthesia. Sedative or respiratory depressant premedication should be avoided. Suxamethonium may produce prolonged neuromuscular blockade, but patients with myasthenia are particularly sensitive to competitive neuromuscular blockade. Intubation of the trachea may be possible without resort to neuromuscular blockade, particularly if there has been omission of one of the prescribed anticholinesterases pre-operatively. Monitoring of neuromuscular blockade with a peripheral nerve stimulator is mandatory. Regional anaesthesia is not contra-indicated, but a high block above about T10 may precipitate respiratory failure. The facility to provide postoperative ventilation should be available, and should be employed after any major procedure.

Myasthenic syndrome (Eaton–Lambert)

This syndrome complicates approximately 1% of bronchogenic carcinomas and may predate the diagnosis of the primary malignancy by several years. The muscles most commonly affected are the proximal muscles of the limbs. Unlike myasthenia gravis, the disease is characterized by an increase in strength on activity. There is great sensitivity to suxamethonium and neuromuscular blocking drugs, causing prolonged weakness. If muscle paralysis is used during anaesthesia, monitoring with a peripheral nerve stimulator is essential. Occasionally, postoperative mechanical ventilation may be necessary.

Rheumatoid arthritis

This chronic inflammatory disease of unknown aetiology is characterized by symmetrical polyarthropathy, and also significant systemic involvement. There is a 3:1 female propensity and onset can be at any age, but occurs commonly in the 30s. The joint manifestations include the hands, wrists and knees, but of anaesthetic importance is disease of the cervical spine which may result in neurological complications and involvement of the atlanto-axial joint, with consequent subluxation. Involvement of the temporomandibular joint may lead to limitation of mouth opening. Crico-arytenoid arthritis may also occur, and is manifested by hoarseness, painful speech, dysphagia and stridor. The extra-articular manifestations of the disease are very common and include congestive heart failure, angina, diffuse pulmonary fibrosis, pleural effusion, pulmonary granulomata and fibrotic nodules in the lungs. A normochromic, normocytic anaemia is frequent. Twenty per cent of patients develop renal amyloidosis. Keratoconjunctivitis sicca occurs in about 10% of patients, and special care must be taken of the eyes. Drug treatment includes corticosteroids and immunosuppressants, as well as anti-inflammatory agents.

Thorough pre-operative assessment includes all the joints and all the organ systems which may be involved. Careful evaluation of the airway should take place, and the presence of atlanto-axial subluxation sought. Radiological demonstration that the distance from the anterior arch of the atlas to the odontoid process exceeds 3 mm confirms the presence of atlanto-axial subluxation. The importance of this lies in the fact that the displaced odontoid process can compress the cervical spinal cord or medulla, in addition to occluding the vertebral artery. Even minimal movement of the head during intubation of the trachea may cause further displacement of the odontoid process, and damage to the underlying spinal cord. Awake fibre-optic intubation is indicated in these patients.

Pre-operative pulmonary function tests and blood gas analysis should be performed, the severity of the anaemia assessed, and the need for corticosteroid supplementation considered. Some patients may be in need of postoperative ventilatory support if severe restrictive lung disease is present pre-operatively. Respiratory dysfunction may be exacerbated by the presence of costovertebral joint disease. If the patient is taking aspirin, then intramuscular premedication is best avoided as platelet dysfunction may lead to haematoma formation. The patient must be handled carefully during anaesthesia, particularly if prolonged corticosteroid therapy has been given, as this makes the patient vulnerable not only to skin tearing and bruising, but pathological fractures due to osteoporosis. The joints affected must be positioned carefully at an angle which produces the least strain. This is often best discussed with the patient prior to anaesthesia. Artificial tears should be used frequently in patients with dry eyes, or the eyes protected with ointment, and the lids taped closed. No specific anaesthetic drugs are contra-indicated.

ENDOCRINE DISEASE

Hyperthyroidism

This typically occurs between the ages of 20 and 40 years and is about four times more common in women than in men. The most common cause is diffuse toxic goitre (Graves disease). The signs and symptoms of hyperthyroidism include weight loss, diarrhoea, moist skin, heat intolerance, tachycardia, cardiac arrhythmias, high-output congestive heart failure and skeletal muscle weakness. Patients with a large obstructive goitre may be dyspnoeic or even stridulous. Exophthalmos may occur due to an infiltrative process involving the retrobulbar fat and eyelids. The retrobulbar oedema can be so severe that the optic nerve is compressed, with resultant blindness. Corneal damage can occur if the patient is unable completely to close the eyes. Thyroid 'storm' is a life-threatening illness brought on by stress such as surgery or infection. The patient becomes hyperpyrexic, tachycardic and cardiovascularly unstable.

The treatment of hyperthyroidism includes antithyroid drugs, β-adrenergic blockade, surgery and radio-active iodine. Whatever the method of treatment employed, elective surgery should never be considered until the patient has been rendered euthyroid. Anaesthesia in euthyroid patients does not pose an increased risk. For the euthyroid patient, concerns during anaesthesia centre on protection of the airway which may be compressed by haematoma formation during surgery on the neck; in addition injury to the laryngeal nerve during surgery may leave the patient with an adducted vocal cord after anaesthesia, and removal of a large goitre occasionally precipitates tracheal collapse.

If anaesthesia is essential while the patient is hyperthyroid, the aim must be to avoid administration of drugs that stimulate the already overactive sympathetic nervous system, and to provide sufficient anaesthetic depression to prevent exaggerated responses to surgical stimulation. Temperature should be monitored during anaesthesia as hyperthyroid patients may become hyperpyrexial. Invasive haemodynamic monitoring is necessary if there is any evidence of heart failure. β-Adrenergic blockade is effective in attenuating the end-organ effects of thyroid hormones but may precipitate heart failure with a sudden increase in pulmonary artery pressure in some patients. Glass[135] recommends the use of haemodynamic monitoring during the administration of β-blockers in thyrotoxic patients. The β-blocker is titrated according to heart rate, but administration should be avoided in patients with heart failure, bronchospasm or abnormalities of left ventricular function. Other drugs used perioperatively include reserpine and guanethidine. Both of these drugs decrease central nervous system stores of catecholamines. Dexamethasone may reduce thyroid hormone secretion in Graves' disease, and also reduces the peripheral conversion of thyroxine to tri-iodothyronine.

Amongst other peri-operative concerns is the proximal muscle weakness, although this does not usually involve respiratory muscles. However, the incidence of myasthenia gravis is increased in hyperthyroid patients, and it would therefore seem reasonable to reduce the initial dose of non-depolarizing muscle relaxant and to monitor its effects with a peripheral nerve stimulator. Pancuronium is best avoided because of its sympathomimetic effects. Anticholinergic drugs may interfere with the sweating mechanism and cause hyperpyrexia as well as tachycardia. Glycopyrronium should be used with neostigmine for reversal of muscle relaxation. There is some concern that the hyperthyroid state leads to an increase in anaesthetic requirement. Accelerated metabolism of drugs does not affect the partial pressure of inhaled agents in blood, but elevations in body temperature increase anaesthetic requirements, possibly by about 5% of MAC for each degree above 37°C. Before treatment of intra-operative hypotension, the possibility of an exaggerated response to catecholamines must be considered. A direct acting vasopressor such as phenylephrine (in a reduced dose) is a more logical choice than an indirect acting agent such as ephedrine.

Hypothyroidism

The patient with hypothyroidism may be hypothermic with slow mentation, slow movement, dry skin, depression of ventilatory responses to hypoxia and hypercapnia, impaired clearance of free water, slow gastric emptying, bradycardia and depressed myocardial contractility. Amyloidosis may occur, with the associated problems of cardiac conduction abnormalities, renal dysfunction and enlargement of the tongue, which may make intubation difficult. The patient may be rendered euthyroid by tri-iodothyronine or thyroxine supplementation, and a relatively euthyroid state as measured by heart rate, blood pressure, body temperature and resolution of hyponatraemia (caused by the decrease in free water clearance) can be established within 3–5 days. However, reduced left ventricular ejection fraction, which has been identified in patients with hypothyroidism, may not return to normal for at least 6 months.[136] This should be borne in mind when considering elective surgery. In severely hypothyroid patients, thyroid hormone replacement can precipitate angina, arrhythmias or even heart failure. As with the hyperthyroid patient, it is therefore inadvisable to proceed with elective surgery before the patient is biochemically and physiologically euthyroid, preferably for several months.

If surgery and anaesthesia must be undertaken in hypothyroid patients, the pre-anaesthetic assessment should take particular note of anaemia, hyponatraemia due to impaired free water clearance, hypoglycaemia and any evidence of primary adrenal insufficiency. Supplemental glucocorticoids and mineralocorticoids may be justified pre-operatively, as the stress of surgery may unmask the hypo-adrenalism that often accompanies hypothyroidism. During induction and maintenance of anaesthesia, it must be remembered that these patients will be extremely sensitive to cardiodepressant drugs. They have a hypodynamic cardiovascular system, with a reduced cardiac output due to reductions in both heart rate and stroke volume. Systemic vascular resistance is increased and blood volume decreased, with narrowing of the pulse pressure. Peripheral vasoconstriction is characteristic, leading to cold peripheries. The metabolism of many drugs, including opioids and benzodiazepines, may be slowed.[137] Hypothyroid patients may be extremely sensitive to the cardiodepressant effects of volatile anaesthetic agents, and in addition the vasodilatation produced may interact with the reduced circulating volume to produce hypotension. Hypothermia reduces anaesthetic requirements, and also impairs hepatic metabolism and renal excretion of drugs.

Monitoring must include invasive haemodynamic monitoring, both as a guide to central venous filling pressure and to give early warning of poor left ventricular function. Core temperature should be monitored and facilities must be available at least to maintain, if not raise, body temperature by warming intravenous fluids, humidifying and warming inhaled gases and wrapping the patient in thermal drapes. The patients may recover slowly from the sedative effects of anaesthesia, and may develop prolonged postoperative respiratory depression. It may be necessary to provide postoperative mechanical ventilation, and extubation should not occur until the body temperature is approaching 37°C.

Hyperparathyroidism

This is associated with hypercalcaemia due to increased bone resorption, increased calcium absorption from the gut, decreased renal calcium clearance and increased phosphate clearance in the proximal tubules. Hypercalcaemia may manifest itself in many organ systems. In the kidney, nephrolithiasis and renal calcification leading to renal failure may occur. There may also be renovascular hypertension. Neuromuscular dysfunction may occur, especially in proximal muscles. There may be skeletal demineralization with a history of frequent fractures and bone pain. The patient may develop memory impairment and depression. Peptic ulcer disease is common due to an increased production of gastrin and gastric acid; anorexia, vomiting and constipation may also be present. Other electrolyte abnormalities include hyperphosphataemia and hypomagnesaemia.

The treatment of hypercalcaemia includes plasma volume expansion, and the administration of loop diuretics to block calcium reabsorption in the thick ascending loop of Henle. Electrolyte abnormalities should be corrected. Mithramycin reduces the plasma calcium concentration by decreasing the responses of osteoclasts or parathyroid hormone. Side-effects include nausea, thrombocytopenia and hepatic and renal toxicity. Calcitonin or corticosteroids may also be used to reduce the calcium level. The pre-operative assessment of the patient should include examination of all the organ systems which could have been affected, and consideration of the drug therapy. An ECG may reveal shortening of the QT interval; however, changes in QT interval may not be a reliable index of changes in plasma calcium concentrations during anaesthesia.[138]

The patient should be handled and positioned carefully during anaesthesia, due to the generalized osteopenia. A high state of hydration and high urine output may help prevent further renal impairment. The response to non-depolarizing muscle relaxants is unpredictable, although there is a report of resistance to atracurium in a patient with hyperparathyroidism.[139]

Hyperadrenocorticism (Cushing's disease)

This may result from excess adrenocorticotrophic hormone production, excess production of cortisol or exogenous administration of corticosteroids. Patients may have hypertension, hypokalaemia, hypernatraemia, hyperglycaemia and skeletal muscle weakness. They are characteristically obese, with a centripetal fat distribution. They have osteoporosis and are prone to bacterial and fungal infections and thrombo-embolism. Their skin is fragile and prone to tearing by adhesive tapes or any shearing force. Anaesthesia must take into account all of these pathophysiological effects, and careful monitoring of electrolyte status and plasma glucose is indicated. They may have a proximal myopathy and if so, the dose of muscle relaxant used should be reduced. Hypokalaemia may also exaggerate the patient's response to muscle relaxants.

Phaeochromocytoma

Phaeochromocytoma is a catecholamine-secreting tumour, which originates in the adrenal medulla or in chromaffin tissue along the paravertebral sympathetic chain. Sympathetic ganglia in the wall of the bladder may be a site for phaeochromocytoma; however, over 95% are found in the abdominal cavity. It is usually an isolated finding, but can occur in conjunction with other endocrine tumours, including medullary thyroid carcinoma or parathyroid adenomas. Neurofibromatosis occurs in about 5% of patients with phaeochromocytoma.

Patients may present with headache and palpitations in association with hypertension. Orthostatic hypotension is a common finding and reflects decreases in intravascular fluid volume, associated with sustained hypertension. Hyperglycaemia may be present due to the excessive catecholamine production. A definitive diagnosis requires biochemical confirmation of excessive catecholamine production. The treatment is then surgical excision of the catecholamine-secreting tumour.

Management of anaesthesia

Pre-operative preparation includes not only full α- and β-blockade, but an attempt to return the intravascular fluid volume to as near normal as possible.[140]

Restoration of the circulating volume is associated with a much smoother intra-operative course and may be monitored by following the patient's haematocrit; however, it may require several weeks of normotension before the circulating volume increases. α-Receptor blockade is usually achieved using phenoxybenzamine, and only after this is established is β-blockade introduced with drugs such as atenolol, propranolol or even labetolol. α-and β-blockade is maintained up until the time of surgery. Adequate premedication, for example an oral benzodiazepine plus intramuscular morphine and hyoscine, is helpful to minimize anxiety-induced activation of the sympathetic nervous system. Intra-arterial monitoring should be instituted before induction of anaesthesia.

No specific anaesthetic drugs are indicated, but the anaesthetic must be geared towards reducing sympathetic nervous system activation. Halothane is not recommended because of the likelihood of cardiac arrhythmias in the presence of increased plasma concentrations of catecholamines. The vagolytic effect of pancuronium is generally unhelpful in this situation. Laryngoscopy should proceed only after establishment of an adequate depth of anaesthesia. An additional bolus of fentanyl or lignocaine immediately before laryngoscopy may help to attenuate blood pressure responses to intubation. An infusion of sodium nitroprusside should be immediately available if persistent hypertension accompanies intubation of the trachea. A regional technique in the form of a lumbar or thoracic epidural block in combination with general anaesthesia has been advocated.[140] This has the advantage of blocking the sympathetic nervous system during the dissection of the phaeochromocytoma. The disadvantage of this technique is that, following removal of the phaeochromocytoma, there is frequently a period of hypotension, and a reduction in systemic vascular resistance may be an added complication at this point. The reduction in blood pressure is treated by reducing the inhaled concentration of volatile anaesthetic and rapid infusion of crystalloid or colloid solution. Persistent hypotension may require intravenous infusion of noradrenaline, until the peripheral vasculature has adapted to the new level of α-adrenergic stimulation. Given the rapid haemodynamic changes anticipated in these patients and the fact that there may be a degree of left ventricular failure, even before the compromising effect of β-blocking drugs, a pulmonary artery catheter is essential for monitoring the status of intravascular fluid volume. The ability to measure cardiac output and ejection fraction is helpful in evaluating cardiac function and the need for intervention with inotropic or vasodilator drugs. The blood sugar level should be monitored closely in the peri-operative period, as hyperglycaemia is typical before excision of the tumour, and hypoglycaemia may occur after removal. The patient should be admitted to a high-dependence area or intensive care unit postoperatively to enable continuation of invasive haemodynamic monitoring until cardiovascular stability returns.

Acromegaly

This disease is due to excess secretion of growth hormone from an eosinophilic adenoma of the anterior pituitary gland. The manifestations include visual field defects, skeletal overgrowth, soft-tissue overgrowth (especially of the lips, tongue, epiglottis and vocal cords), peripheral neuropathy, glucose intolerance, osteoporosis and skeletal muscle weakness. A major problem during anaesthesia is the overgrowth of soft tissues in the upper airway, which may make maintenance of a patent airway difficult. In addition, involvement of the crico-arytenoid joints can result in alterations to the voice due to impaired movement of the vocal cords and the subglottic diameter of the trachea can be reduced.[141] Patients with acromegaly are also prone to hypertension and insulin-dependent diabetes mellitus. Pathological fractures may occur due to osteoporosis.

Obesity

Obesity is defined as a body weight 20% above ideal, and morbid obesity exists when body weight is twice the ideal weight. However, it has been proposed[142] that the definition of obesity should include the type of obesity which is more detrimental to the cardiovascular system, i.e. abdominal obesity. It has become evident that cardiovascular disease, cerebrovascular disease and non-insulin dependent diabetes mellitus (NIDDM) are closely associated with abdominal obesity and not with peripheral, gluteal–femoral obesity. This may reflect the fact that intra-abdominal adipose tissue has a very sensitive free fatty acid mobilizing system; the free fatty acids are extensively mobilized into the portal vein and liver, which then increases circulating concentrations of very low density lipoproteins, glucose and insulin.

A further study[143] has examined the relationship between obesity and hypertension, and suggested that it is related to activation of the sympathetic nervous system by hyperinsulinaemia. This in turn raises cardiac output and peripheral vascular resistance. Sympathetic stimulation also increases renal sodium reabsorption. This exacerbates hypertension by shifting the pressure–natriuresis relationship, such that higher renal perfusion pressures are required to maintain normal extracellular fluid volume.

The pulmonary effects of obesity have been well-described, and comprise predominantly decreased functional residual capacity and decreased expiratory reserve volume. These changes were thought to be entirely mechanical, caused by splinting of the diaphragm during normal tidal breathing. However, recent investigations[144] have suggested that the pulmonary function of obese people is abnormal. This study found that, in addition to the expected reductions in functional residual capacity, total lung capacity, expiratory reserve volume and forced exhaled volume, obese men also has a 20% reduction in expiratory flow rates at 50 and 75% of exhaled vital capacity. This indicated that non-smoking, morbidly obese men had peripheral airway obstruction.

Arterial oxygen saturation is reduced at rest in obese patients, presumably due to ventilation/perfusion mismatch related to the increased closing volume, which results in underventilation of dependent lung regions. These changes are reversible with weight loss.

One of the most obvious clinical effects of abnormal pulmonary function in the obese patient is the rapidity with which desaturation occurs in the presence of inadequate ventilation; this was confirmed by a recent study in which the time for a group of normal, obese and morbidly obese patients to desaturate from 100 to 90% was measured.[145]

The cardiac output and blood volume of obese patients are increased. It has been estimated that cardiac output increases by about $0.11.min^{-1}$ for every kg of weight gain related to adipose tissue. The risk of coronary artery disease is higher in obese patients. There is, as indicated above, a positive correlation between hypertension and obesity. This is not simply due to the use of inappropriately small cuffs for measuring blood pressure indirectly. Pulmonary artery pressure may also be high in obese patients, and may reflect the effect of chronic arterial hypoxaemia on the pulmonary vasculature.

There is some evidence that plasma fluoride concentrations increase more after enflurane administration to obese than to non-obese individuals.[146] There is no evidence of increased hepatocellular damage in obese patients receiving halothane, based on measurement of plasma concentrations of transaminase enzymes.[147] However, there is a high incidence of fatty infiltration of the liver in obese patients, and also an increased incidence of gall stones.

There are numerous practical difficulties associated with anaesthesia for the morbidly obese patient. Moving and lifting the patient are difficult; venous cannulation may be very challenging, as may be insertion of spinal or epidural needles. The patients are at increased risk of inhalation of gastric contents, as there are increased incidences of gastro-oesophageal reflux and hiatus hernia. An H_2-receptor antagonist and metoclopramide should be used pre-operatively, and rapid-sequence induction is favoured. Tracheal intubation may be difficult due to the large mass of soft tissue surrounding the jaw and neck. Arterial oxygenation decreases rapidly during apnoea, and the lungs of obese patients should always be pre-oxygenated prior to induction of anaesthesia. Isoflurane is a logical choice for maintenance of anaesthesia to avoid the high level of free fluoride ions associated with enflurane anaesthesia. Although it is theoretically possible that large quantities of lipid-soluble drugs may be stored in adipose tissue, resulting in delayed awakening, there is no evidence to corroborate that this presents a clinical problem.[148] The lungs should always be ventilated artificially, as induction of anaesthesia may further decrease the functional residual capacity and increase the perfusion of unventilated alveoli. The head-down position can further decrease chest-wall compliance, and increase the risk of passive regurgitation of gastric contents.

Obese patients are prone to develop hypoxaemia postoperatively; there is a higher incidence of deep venous thrombosis and pulmonary embolism, and wound infection and breakdown are also more common than in non-obese patients. The patient should be monitored for a prolonged period postoperatively, as the maximum reduction in arterial oxygenation typically occurs 2 or 3 days postoperatively.[149]

Anorexia nervosa

In addition to their very low body weight, patients who suffer from anorexia nervosa may have electrolyte disturbances, hypothermia, inability to concentrate urine and cardiac arrhythmias, including bradycardia. Spontaneous pneumomediastinum has been observed in patients with anorexia nervosa, possibly due to decreased lung elasticity.[150]

Diabetes mellitus

Primary diabetes mellitus may be type I (insulin-dependent mellitus: IDDM) or type II (NIDDM). Diabetes mellitus may also be secondary to other pathology, including pancreatic disease (cystic fibrosis, haemochromatosis); due to excess endogenous production of hormonal antagonist to insulin (phaeochromocytoma, Cushing's syndrome, pregnancy); secondary to medication (corticosteroids, thiazide diuretics); secondary to liver disease; or associated with genetic syndromes (muscular dystrophies, Friedreich's ataxia). There are several excellent reviews of management of surgical patients with diabetes mellitus in the literature.[151,152]

Insulin-dependent diabetes mellitus

It is believed that about 25% of the diabetic population in the UK have IDDM.[153] The IDDM patient is usually younger (less than 35 years) and is prone to develop keto-acidosis. The patient is unable to secrete insulin because of β-cell damage secondary to either an auto-immune defect, or viral injury altering human leukocyte antigen on chromosome 6. Given the large number of diabetic patients in the population (in the UK, the combined prevalence of diagnosed IDDM and NIDDM is just over 1% of the Caucasian population), the chances of encountering a diabetic patient on an operating list are quite high.[154] Studies from the Hammersmith Hospital[152] indicate that the mortality among diabetic patients undergoing cardiac surgery is 1.5 times that of the mortality for the general population.

Anaesthetic management for the diabetic patient concentrates on two areas: assessment of the organs involved in diabetic complications, and management of glycaemic control during the peri-operative period. There is a greatly increased risk of coronary artery disease in IDDM. While the incidence parallels that of the population in which diabetics occur, the presence of diabetes appears to amplify the risk.[155] At any given plasma lipid concentration, arterial pressure or level of cigarette consumption, the diabetic has twice the risk of the general population of developing coronary artery disease.[155] A useful screening test is the presence of micro-albuminuria, as it has been shown that the mortality from coronary artery disease increases in the presence of this abnormality.[156] This is not detected on routine tests, but the estimate should be made on a timed, overnight urine collection. A value exceeding 20 μg min in the absence of sepsis or congestive cardiac failure is significant. Apart from ischaemic heart disease, the cardiovascular system is also affected in diabetes by an increased incidence of hypertension, and atherosclerosis in both large and small vessels. There is some recent evidence that a diabetic cardiomyopathy may exist, and that this may relate to inadequate diastolic relaxation and therefore impaired ventricular filling.[157–159] There is some evidence in diabetic rats that prolongation of the action potential in ventricular muscle relates to impaired calcium channel function. This may contribute to altered diastolic function.[160]

The nervous system is involved in the disease; both peripheral and autonomic neuropathies may occur. An epidemiological study from Pittsburgh showed that hypertension is the strongest correlate of diabetic autonomic neuropathy, and was present in approximately 50% of patients with, but in fewer than 10% of patients without, neuropathy.[161] Peri-operative risk is 10 times higher in patients with both hypertension and diabetes than in those with diabetes without neuropathy and hypertension. Of interest to anaesthetists was a further large-scale epidemiological study in more than 11 000 subjects, which found that the onset of diabetes is preceded by a decline in FVC and FEV_1. It was approximately twice the decline in any normal patient, or in patients who have had diabetes for a period of years.[162] This was not thought to relate to a decrease in autonomic function, but possibly to an accumulation of abnormal connective tissue due to the non-enzymatic glycosolation of proteins.

The eyes are frequently involved in diabetes, causing retinopathy and blindness. The kidney is frequently involved in IDDM and end-stage renal disease develops in about 35% of patients.[163]

Given the high prevalence of cardiovascular disease in the diabetic population, it is not surprising that one series found the most common cause of peri-operative mortality to be coronary artery disease.[164] Pre-operative assessment should always include an ECG, but recent reports suggest that diabetic patients should also be screened for autonomic neuropathy prior to surgery, as this subpopulation is at a high risk for developing peri-operative hypotension,[165] and between 20 and 40% of insulin-dependent diabetics develop an autonomic neuropathy. Autonomic function may be tested by measuring the variation in the RR interval on an ECG during deep breathing and a Valsalva manoeuvre, and the blood pressure and heart rate response to standing.[166] Renal function should be assessed, including urinary dipstick determination for proteinuria. The existence of proteinuria even with a normal serum creatinine concentration should make the anaesthetist consider the use of drugs without a nephrotoxic potential, and avoid drugs such as aminoglycosides and possibly enflurane.

A final problem of interest to anaesthetists is stiff joint syndrome, which may cause difficulty with tracheal intubation.[167] This is seen in IDDM patients in association with rapidly progressive micro-angiopathy, a tight waxy skin and limited joint mobility. Cervical radiography demonstrates limited atlanto-axial extension.

Reasons to maintain tight control of plasma glucose concentration in the peri-operative period include the obvious dangers of ketosis and acidaemia, and the electrolyte abnormalities and volume depletion which result from osmotic diuresis; however, there is evidence[168] indicating impaired wound strength and wound healing when plasma glucose concentration exceeds 11.1 $mmol.l^{-1}$. In addition, hyperglycaemia interferes with leukocyte chemotaxis, opsonization and phagocytosis.[169]

There are many different approaches to the method of administration of insulin in the peri-operative period. The most frequently used methods involve giving intravenous insulin on the morning of surgery, either as a premixed bag with glucose or by infusion pump with a separate intravenous glucose infusion. The advantage of the second method is that the whole bag does not have to be discarded if the insulin requirements change. The patient's blood sugar should be checked hourly for the first 4 h after the insulin regimen is started, and thereafter, if stable, 4-hourly until the time of arrival in the operating theatre. The Alberti regimen, described in 1979, in which glucose, insulin and potassium are mixed in the same bag, is still in widespread use.[170] The extracellular potassium concentration may be changed both by changes in the serum insulin level, and by changes in acid–base balance. As only 2% of total body potassium is extracellular, a normal serum potassium concentration does not necessarily reflect a normal total body potassium content. In the normokalaemic diabetic patient with normal renal function, 20 mmol of potassium chloride should be added to each litre of glucose solution. Additional potassium may be required if the patient is insulin-resistant, and requires large doses of insulin. It is reasonable to check the potassium concentration 6–8 h after the infusion is started, and the glucose and electrolyte concentrations should always be measured when the patient is in the recovery room.

Non-insulin-dependent diabetes mellitus

Patients who maintain normoglycaemia by dietary control may require no additional measures during surgery. If surgery is minor and the patient will be eating again by the evening of operation, it may be adequate to omit the morning dose of oral hypoglycaemic agent and restart the medication when food is given. Patients who are undergoing major surgery will require conversion to an intravenous insulin infusion. These patients may be relatively insulin-resistant.

DISEASES OF THE BLOOD

Sickle-cell anaemia

Sickle-cell disease is an inherited disorder, which is

found predominantly, but not exclusively, in people of negroid origin. Sickle-cell disease (SS) patients are homozygotes, and have clinical symptoms; sickle-cell trait patients (AS) are heterozygotes and normally are asymptomatic. Erythrocytes of patients with the sickle-cell trait contain 20–40% haemoglobin S, with the remainder being haemoglobin A.

The molecular defect in haemoglobin S is a substitution of a single amino acid, valine, for glutamic acid at the sixth position on each of the β polypeptide chains of the globin molecule. This single change is responsible for the occurrence of polymerization of haemoglobin, with a resulting change in shape of the erythrocyte when it is desaturated. The shape change of the erythrocyte is a reversible process through which the cell may pass many times before it is irreversibly sickled. Factors which alter the sickling of cells are pH, temperature, 2,3-diphosphoglycerate concentration, percentage of haemoglobin S and presence of other haemoglobins.[171] In sickle-cell blood, the oxyhaemoglobin dissociation curve is shifted to the right, facilitating oxygen delivery and compensating for the anaemia. Intracellular polymerization starts when the oxygen saturation falls below 85%, and is complete at 38% saturation. However, the most dense cells, i.e. those with the highest mean corpuscular haemoglobin concentration, form significant polymers even at high oxygen saturations. Viscosity of sickle-cell blood is greater than that of normal blood and an increase in the viscosity can contribute to the pathogenesis of a sickle crisis.

Patients with sickle-cell trait usually have a normal life, and are generally not thought to be under increased risk during anaesthesia. However, there have been reports of occasional complications in this population, including complications following application of tourniquets, intravenous sickling after strenuous exertion and aortocaval compression during general anaesthesia for Caesarean section producing a sickling crisis and death.[172]

The manifestations of sickle-cell disease come under four main categories: chronic haemolytic anaemia, systemic manifestations, vaso-occlusive crises and organ damage as a result of multiple crises. The chronic anaemia is due to accelerated red-cell destruction; red-cell survival is 15% of normal. The bone marrow is unable to compensate, because the stimulus is blunted by the decreased affinity for oxygen, thus altering the erythropoietin-mediated control of red-cell production. This may be beneficial, because the decreased viscosity due to the anaemia reduces the occlusive manifestations. Bacterial infection is an important complication of sickle-cell disease, and may be life-threatening. The incidence of pneumococcal meningitis in children with sickle-cell disease is 300 times higher than normal.

An unpleasant feature of the disease is acute painful crises, which may be isolated to an individual organ or occur in several parts of the body. This specific end-organ damage begins to appear during childhood. Signs of heart failure, renal impairment and sometimes, if there have been sufficient pulmonary infarcts to increase pulmonary artery pressures, pulmonary hypertension and cor pulmonale, develop. Hepatic injury may occur from repeated infarcts and cholelithiasis is common due to the chronic haemolysis. A particularly serious complication of sickle-cell disease is cerebral infarction.

One of the mainstays of anaesthetic management is the use of exchange blood transfusion. The purpose of the transfusion is to remove irreversibly sickled cells and to provide normally deformable red blood cells, in order to decrease blood viscosity, to prevent vaso-occlusive stasis in the circulation, and expand to oxygen-carrying capacity.[173] Resistance to circulating blood flow is reduced in vitro when less than 40% of sickle cells are present in a well-oxygenated preparation. Most clinicians attempt to reduce the haemoglobin S concentration to less then 40%,[173] without increasing the haematocrit to more than 36%.[171] The benefits of transfusion are reduced if the post-transfusion haematocrit is greater than 36%.

Pre-operative preparation should also include correction of co-existing infection and of any pre-operative dehydration. During anaesthesia, great care must be taken to avoid acidosis, to maintain normal oxygenation, to prevent circulatory stasis due to awkward body positioning or use of tourniquets, and to maintain a normal body temperature. Close monitoring is helpful and should include measurement of arterial blood gases (to measure pH), oxygenation saturation, central venous pressure, preferably direct arterial pressure (to avoid frequent inflation of the blood pressure cuff), temperature, end-tidal carbon dioxide concentration and urine output.

Regional anaesthesia has been used successfully during surgery and to provide postoperative analgesia in patients with sickle-cell disease. However, it is important to provide adequate circulating volume.

Postoperatively, a high degree of analgesia should be provided, along with close monitoring. Supplemental oxygen, maintenance of intravascular fluid volume and maintenance of body temperature are all important goals. There is a high incidence of chest infections, which contributes to reduced arterial Po_2 postoperatively. Intensive physiotherapy is therefore also helpful.

ACQUIRED IMMUNODEFICIENCY SYNDROME (AIDS)

Between 1981 and 1990, 100 777 deaths from AIDS were reported to the Centers for Disease Control (CDC), in Atlanta, Georgia, USA. By the end of August 1992, there were 6431 known cases of AIDS in the UK, 6015 of which were men. 62% (3991) had died.[174] Human immunodeficiency virus (HIV) is an RNA retrovirus which causes depletion of the helper subset of T lymphocytes (T4 or CD4+ T cells) and profound immunosuppression. Since the T4 lymphocytes are critical effectors for a wide range of immunological responses, selective HIV-induced defects in function of this subset of cells result in a marked degree of overall immunosuppression. Patients presenting for surgery with HIV pose a twofold challenge to the anaesthetist: they not only constitute a source of infection, but they also have a compromised immune system which may be further altered by anaesthesia and which renders them vulnerable to opportunistic infections from the health care workers.

Figures released from the CDC suggest that 80% of all occupational exposures to HIV occur via a contaminated needlestick injury. The rate of HIV serum conversion after a needlestick exposure is approximately 0.5%, which is relatively low compared with hepatitis B virus, which has a needlestick transmission rate of 10–35%.[175] Although this figure appears relatively low, this conceals the fact that the magnitude of harm is enormous, since serum conversion is ultimately 100% fatal. The CDC therefore recommends that all patients be considered as potential hazards to health care workers, and that the following universal precautions be used with all patients. These are applicable not just to AIDS, but to other infectious diseases, especially hepatitis:

1. Precautions should be used when contact with blood or body fluid from any patient is anticipated.
2. Gloves should be worn when handling body fluids, mucous membranes or non-intact skin.
3. A mask and protective eye wear should be worn when droplets are formed.
4. Hand-washing is very important, and should be done frequently, and especially after patient contact.
5. Needles should be handled with great care and never recapped.
6. Mouth-to-mouth resuscitation should be minimized and adequate ventilatory equipment should always be available.
7. Health care workers with dermatitis, especially of the hands, should not be involved in direct patient care.
8. Pregnancy involves no special risk, but the pregnant health care worker should exercise all precautions.

The value of zidovudine for postexposure prophylaxis is still unclear. Zidovudine, a thymidine analogue, inhibits the replication of HIV by interfering with the RNA-dependent DNA polymerase (reverse transcriptase). A double-blind study by Burroughs Wellcome[176] investigated 84 health care workers who had undergone occupational exposure to HIV. Of the 84 exposed workers (of whom 49 received zidovudine), none had developed HIV infection after 6 months. However, this does not necessarily indicate the efficacy of the drug, since HIV transmission may not actually have occurred.

The patient with HIV infection may have a wide spectrum of clinical diseases or be completely asymptomatic. Infection may first demonstrate itself as the AIDS-related complex. This includes patients who have candidiasis, intermittent or continuous fevers for more than 1 month, repeated night sweats, debilitating fatigue, persistent diarrhoea and loss of body weight of 10% or more. However, these patients do not have a life-threatening opportunistic infection or a major tumour. The clinical manifestations of fully developed AIDS include opportunistic infection, Kaposi's sarcoma or other neoplasm, weight loss, diarrhoea, central and peripheral nervous system dysfunction, renal failure, cardiac arrhythmias or congestive cardiac failure, arthralgia, dementia and psychosis.

Involvement of the mouth and pharynx by candidiasis can cause such extensive erythema and oedema as to distort the anatomy of the upper airway, and make tracheal intubation very difficult. The larynx is involved in approximately 20% of patients with Kaposi's sarcoma and, although severe laryngeal obstruction is rare, the anaesthetist should be aware that these patients may present problems for tracheal intubation.[177] There has also been a case report in which an HIV-positive patient presented with laryngeal obstruction emanating from a non-Hodgkin's lymphoma, with additional evidence of laryngeal tuberculosis.[178]

Opportunistic infections within the lungs are important because of the respiratory inadequacy and failure associated with them. *Pneumocystis* pneumonia renders the lungs macroscopically grossly abnormal, and the alveoli are clogged with thick gummy exudate, limiting gas exchange. Tuberculosis is another common opportunistic infection in these patients. A non-specific interstitial pneumonitis, not related to an opportunistic infection, is also common and may be seen in as many as 32% of patients with AIDS.[179] Cytomegalovirus may be isolated from more than 90% of patients with AIDS, but does not usually cause a pneumonitis. However, when it does, it is almost universally fatal.

An autopsy study of 115 patients with AIDS or AIDS-related complex revealed a significant number of cardiac lesions, including pericardial effusion, fibrinous pericarditis, right ventricular hypertrophy, marantic endocarditis and dilated cardiomyopathy. In 7 cases, Kaposi's sarcoma was evident in the pericardium and myocardium.[180] On microscopic examination, the patients had interstitial oedema and evidence of perivascular and interstitial fibrosis. This emphasizes the need for thorough evaluation prior to surgery.

Electrolyte and fluid imbalance may occur following the extensive diarrhoea which often develops. Renal failure occurs in approximately 10% of patients hospitalized with AIDS and is progressive and generally unresponsive to therapy.[181] Involvement of both the central and peripheral nervous systems is common in AIDS. Peripheral neuropathies are frequently associated with ill-defined pain, and it may be difficult to achieve adequate pain relief. The question of the advisability of regional anaesthesia in a patient with an infected central or peripheral nervous system has been raised. There is so far no evidence of disease recrudescence or flare-up when regional anaesthesia is used, but it is difficult to evaluate this relationship as nervous system involvement is probably universally progressive anyway.

The final concern to the anaesthetist is that patients immunosuppressed by HIV may become further immunosuppressed by the administration of anaesthesia. A study in 1990 by Buehrer et al investigated the effect of invasive surgical procedures on wound infection rates in HIV serum-positive and HIV serum-negative haemophiliacs. The authors concluded that there was no increased risk of wound infections in the serum-positive patients.[182] However, the patients were in the early stages of the disease.

GERIATRIC PATIENTS

Age is not usually classed as a disease. However, organ function in the elderly patient is different to that in younger patients. In addition, the incidence of many diseases is highest among the elderly population, and these diseases may either precipitate the need for anaesthesia and surgery, or complicate anaesthesia required for other reasons. It is therefore appropriate to consider geriatric patients in this chapter.

Ageing is associated with decreased function in every organ, even if this is only manifest as a decreased margin of reserve. Of particular significance to anaesthetists are changes in general metabolism, cardiorespiratory physiology and liver and kidney function. Many important physiological functions decrease by about 1% per year after the age of 30 years. Thus, by age of 70 years, basal metabolic rate is about 40% of normal in young adults, and this in itself appreciably delays the excretion and metabolism of anaesthetic drugs. Cardiac output reduces by about 1% per year after the age of 30 years, and circulation time is prolonged. There is reduced autonomic and baroreceptor responsiveness and reduced arterial elasticity, leading to systolic hypertension. In the respiratory system, the vital capacity, maximum breathing capacity and total lung capacity are all decreased, whilst functional residual capacity is increased. Arterial Po_2 decreases with age, as do the ventilatory responses to hypercapnia and hypoxia. Renal blood flow and glomerular filtration rate also decrease by about 1% per year, as does liver blood flow. Therefore, drugs that undergo significant hepatic metabolism and/or renal excretion have a longer plasma half-life in the elderly. The decline in the plasma albumin concentration with age affects drugs that are significantly bound to albumin, such as fentanyl (80%). Barbiturates, opioids, local anaesthetics and muscle relaxants are all affected. For example, a 'sleep dose' of thiopentone is 1.8 mg.kg^{-1} in patients aged 65 years, but 2.8 mg.kg^{-1} in patients aged 20–40 years.[183] In the absence of any clinical evidence of hepatic or renal disease, the plasma concentration of propranolol after oral administration is five times higher in elderly than in younger patients.[184] The plasma half-life of diazepam increases with age, and its value in hours is approximately the same as the patient's age in years.[185]

With advancing age, multisystem disease and polypharmacy are the rule rather than the exception. The old have three times the incidence of unwanted drug side-effects,[186] are more prone to significant drug interactions and may be taking drugs which are no longer considered first-line therapy (e.g. reserpine for hypertension), with which the younger generation of anaesthetists may be unfamiliar.

In view if this, it is hardly surprising to find that approximately half of all intra-operative deaths occur in geriatric patients, in whom only about 5% of surgical procedures are performed.[187] With an increasingly elderly population, these statistics become even more relevant. At present, about 10% of the UK population is over 65 years of age, but by the year 2000, this figure will have risen to 12.5%. The anaesthetic management of this section of the population therefore deserves special attention.

Fractured neck of femur is a very common reason for elderly patients to require anaesthesia and surgery.

Although it has been said that early surgery leads to better bone union and a shorter hospital stay, a recent prospective study has shown that, if time is taken to treat concurrent medical conditions, there is no adverse effect on the short-term outcome of elderly patients with fracture of the proximal femur and associated medical problems, and that these patients do not create an extra workload for the orthopaedic or geriatric services.[188] Furthermore, an intervention programme with the collaboration of physicians and anaesthetists designed to reduce the incidence and severity of acute confusional states in elderly patients treated for femoral neck fractures has been assessed.[189] The programme consisted of pre- and postoperative geriatric assessments, oxygen therapy, early surgery, and prevention and treatment of decreases in perioperative blood pressure. There was a reduction in the incidence of acute confusional states from 61.3% in matched previously treated controls, at the same institution to 46.6% in the intervention study.

Another study demonstrated that there was no difference in terms of cognitive impairment between general and spinal anaesthesia in elderly patients undergoing transurethral resection of prostate, and whose mental state was evaluated 4 days and 3 months postoperatively.[190]

A study of the haemodynamic response to postural hypotension in 9 healthy elderly patients demonstrated stroke volume and cardiac index decreased because of an inability to reduce end-systolic volume.[191] mean arterial pressure was maintained through an increase in peripheral vascular resistance. In contrast, young people had reduced end-systolic volume and increased heart rate, while the peripheral vascular resistance remained unchanged.[191] In another study of left ventricular diastolic filling changes, there was a failure of relaxation in elderly patients, with a consequent impairment of early diastolic filling. These changes were reversed by the administration of diltiazam;[192] the use of calcium antagonists may be helpful in relieving myocardial dysfunction in the elderly.

Finally, thyroid dysfunction in elderly hospitalized patients is common. Simons et al[193] found a direct linear correlation between degree of illness as assessed by ASA physical status and degree of hypothyroidism. Assessment of thyroid function, and correction if necessary, should be essential in ASA grade III and IV elderly patients.

REFERENCES

1. Silverman KJ, Grossman W. Angina pectoris. N Engl J Med 1984; 310: 1712–1717
2. Tarhan S, Moffitt EA, Taylor WF, Guiliani ER. Myocardial infarction after general anesthesia. JAMA 1972; 220: 1451–1454
3. Steen PA, Tinker JH, Tarhan S. Myocardial reinfarction after anaesthesia and surgery. An update: incidence, mortality, and predisposing factors, JAMA 1978; 239: 2566–2570
4. Loeb HS, Saudye A, Croke RP et al. Effects of pharmacologically induced hypertension on myocardial ischemia and coronary hemodynamics in patients with fixed coronary obstruction. Circulation 1978; 57: 41–46
5. Cokkinos DV, Voridis EM. Constancy of pressure rate product in pacing-induced angina pectoris. Br Heart J 1976; 38: 39–42
6. Rao TLK, Jacobs KH, El-Etr AA. Reinfarction following anesthesia in patients with myocardial infarction. Anesthesiology 1983; 59: 499–505
7. Mahar IJ. Steen PA, Tinker JH et al. Perioperative myocardial infarction in patients with coronary artery disease with and without aorto-coronary artery bypass grafts. J Thorac Cardiovasc Surg 1978; 76: 533–537
8. Goldman I, Caldera DI, Nussbaum SR et al. Multifactorial index of cardiac risk in noncardiac surgical procedures. N Eng J Med 1977; 297: 845–850
9. Jeffrey C C, Kunsman J, Cullen D J, Brewster DC. A prospective evaluation of cardiac risk index. Anesthesiology 1983; 58: 462–464
10. Burgos LG, Ebert TJ, Asiddao CB et al. Increased intraoperative cardiovascular morbidity in diabetics with autonomic neuropathy. Anesthesiology 1980; 70: 591–597
11. Fleisher IA, Pincus SM, Rosenbaum SH. Approximate entropy (ApEn) as a correlate of postoperative cardiac dysfunction. In: Proceedings of the American Society of Critical Care Anesthesia. San Francisco, CA: 1991
12. Kleiger RE, Miller JP, Bigger JT Jr, Moss AJ. Decreased heart rate variability and its association with increased mortality after acute myocardial infarction. Am J Cardiol 1987; 59: 256–262
13. Rea RF, Martins JB, Mark AL. Baroreflex impairment and sudden death after myocardial infarction. Circulation 1988; 78: 1072–1074
14. Trimarco B, Chierchia S, Lembro G et al. Prolonged duration of myocardial ischemia in patients with coronary heart disease and impaired cardiopulmonary baroceptor sensitivity. Circulation 1990; 81: 1792–1802
15. Eckberg DI. Human sinus arrhythmia as an index of cardiac outflow. J Appl Physiol 1983; 54: 961–966
16. Malliani A, Pagani M, Lombardi F, Ceruti S. Cardiovascular neural regulation explored in the frequency domain. Circulation 1991; 84: 482–492
17. Inoue K, Miyake S, Kumashiro M et al. Power spectal analysis of blood pressure variability in traumatic quadriplegic humans. Am J Physiol 1991; 260: 842–847
18. Rinoldi O, Pierini S, Ferrari A et al. Analysis of short-term oscillations of R-R interval and arterial pressure in conscious dogs. Am J Physiol 1990; 258: 967–976
19. Bigger JT Jr, Kleiger RE, Fleiss JL et al. Components of

heart rate variability measured during healing of acute myocardial infarction. Am J cardiol 1988; 61: 208–215
20. Lombardi F, Sandrone G, Pernpruner S et al. Heart rate variability as an index of sympathovagal interaction after acute myocardial infarction. Am J Cardiol 1987; 60: 1239–1245
21. Slogoff K, Keats AS. Does perioperative ischemia lead to postoperative myocardial infarction? Anesthesiology 1985; 62: 107–22
22. Slogoff S, Keats AS. Further observations on perioperative myocardial ischemia. Anesthesiology 1986; 65: 539–542
23. Kleinman B, Henkin RE, Glisson SN et al. Qualitative evaluation of coronary flow during anesthetic induction using thallium-201 perfusion scans. Anesthesiology 1986; 64: 157–164
24. Modig J, Borg T, Karlstrom G et al. Thromboembolism after total hip hip replacement: role of epidural and general anesthesia. Anesth Analg 1983; 62: 174–180
25. Borg T, Modig J. Potential antithrombotic effects of local anaesthetics due to their inhibition of platelet aggregation. Acta Anaesthesiol Scand 1985; 29: 739–742
26. Tuman KJ, McCarthy RJ, March RJ et al. Effects of epidural anesthesia on coagulation and outcome after major vascular surgery. Anesth Analg 1991; 73: 696–704
27. Mangano DT. Perioperative cardiac morbidity. Anesthesiology 1990; 72: 153–184
28. Mangano DT, Hollenberg M, Fegert G et al. Perioperative myocardial ischemia in patients undergoing noncardiac surgery — 1: Incidence and severity during the 4 day perioperative period. J Am Coll Cardiol 1991; 17: 843–850
29. Mangano DT, Wong MG, London MJ et al. Perioperative ischemia in patients undergoing noncardiac surgery — II: Incidence and severity during the 1st week after surgery. J Am Coll Cardiol 1991; 17: 851–857
30. Menkhaus PG, Reves JG, Kisson I et al. Cardiovascular effects of esmolol in anesthetized humans. Anesth Analg 1985; 64: 327–334
31. Bastard OG, Carter JG, Moyers JR, Bross BA. Circulatory effects of isoflurane in patients with ischemic heart disease: a comparison with halothane. Anesth Analg 1984; 63: 635–639
32. Hess W, Arnold B, Schulte-Sasse U, Tarnow J. Comparison of isoflurane and halothane when used to control intraoperative hypertension in patients undergoing coronary artery bypass surgery. Anesth Analg 1983; 62: 15–20
33. Reiz S, Balfors E, Sorensenson MD et al. Isoflurane — a powerful vasodilator in patients with ischemic disease? Anesthesiology 1983; 59:91–97
34. O'Young J. Mastrocospoulos G, Hilgenberg A, Palacios I, Kyritsis A, Lappas DG. Myocardial circulatory metabolic effects of isoflurane and sufentanil during coronary artery surgery. Anesthesiology 1987; 66: 653–658
35. Smith JS, Cahalan MK, Benefiel DJ et al. Fentanyl versus fentanyl and isoflurane in patients with impaired left ventricular function. Anesthesiology 1985; 63: A18
36. Stoelting RK, Gibbs PS. Hemodynamic effects of morphine–nitrous oxide in valvular heart disease and coronary artery disease. Anesthesiology 1973; 38: 45–52
37. Smith NT, Calverley RK, Prys-Roberts C et al. Impact of nitrous oxide on the circulation during enflurane anesthesia in man. Anesthesiology 1978; 48: 345–394
38. Moss J, Rosow CE, Savarese JJ, Philbin DM, Kniffen KJ. Role of histamine in the hypotensive action of d-tubocurarine in humans. Anesthesiology 1981; 55: 19–25
39. Stoelting RK, McCammon RL, Hilgenberg JC. Changes in blood pressure with varying rates of administration of d-tubocurarine. Anesth Analg 1980; 59: 697–699
40. Marshall RJ, McGrath TC, Miller RD, Docherty JR, Lamar JC. Comparison of the cardiovascular actions of ORG NC45 with those produced by other non-depolarizing neuromuscular blocking agents in experimental animals. Br J Anaesth 1980; 52: 21–31
41. Kaplan JA, King SB. The precordial electrocardiographic lead (V_5) in patients who have coronary-artery disease. Anesthesiology 1976; 45: 570–574
42. Kaplan JA, Wells PH. Early diagnosis of myocardial ischemia using the pulmonary arterial catheter. Anesth Analg 1981; 60: 789–793
43. Mangano DT. Monitoring pulmonary artery pressure in coronary-artery disease. Anesthesiology 1980; 53: 364–370
44. Gibbs NM, Larach DR, Derr JA. The accuracy of noninvasive mean arterial pressure measurement in anesthetized patients. Anesthesiology 1991; 74: 647–652
45. Breisblatt WM, Weiland FL, McLain JR et al. Usefulness of ambulatory radionuclide monitoring of left ventricular function early after acute myocardial infarction for predicting residual myocardial ischemia. Am J Cardiol 1988; 62: 1005–1010
46. Turlapaty P, Vary R, Kaplan JA. Nicardipine, a new intravenous calcium antagonist: a review of its pharmacology, pharmacokinetics and perioperative applications. J Cardiothorac Anesth 1989; 3: 344–355
47. Mangano DT, Browner WS, Hollenberg M et al. SPI Research Group. Association of perioperative myocardial ischemia with cardiac morbidity and mortality in men undergoing noncardiac surgery. N Engl J Med 1990; 323: 1871–1788
48. Breslow MJ, Jordan DA, Christopherson R et al. Epidural morphine decreases post-operative hypertension by attenuating sympathetic nervous system hyperactivity. JAMA 1989; 261: 3577–3581
49. Yeager MP, Glass DD, Neff RK, Brinck-Johnsen T. Epidural anesthesia and analgesia in high-risk surgical patients. Anesthesiology 1987; 66: 729–736
50. Kennedy KD, Nishmura RA, Holmes DR, Bailey KR. Natural history of moderate aortic stenosis. J Am Coll Cardiol 1991; 17: 313–319
51. Report on confidential enquiries into maternal deaths in the United Kingdom 1985–1987. HMSO.London 1992
52. Stone JG, Hoar PF, Calabro JR, Khambatta HJ. Afterload reduction and preload augmentation improve the anesthetic management of patients with cardiac failure and valvular regurgitation. Anesth Analg 1980; 59: 737–742

53 Hoffman A, Burckhardt D. Patients at risk for cardiac death late after aortic valve replacement. Am Heart J 1990; 120: 1142–1146
54 Rooney SM, Goldiner PL, Muss E. Relationship of right bundle-branch block and marked left axis deviation to complete heart block during general anesthesia. Anesthesiology 1976; 44: 64–66
55 Venkataraman K, Madias JE, Hood WB. Indications for prophylactic preoperative insertion of pacemaker in patients with right bundle branch block and left anterior hemiblock. Br J Anaesth 1981; 53: 545–548
56 Coriat P, Harari A, Ducardonet A, Tarot J-P, Viars P. Risk of advanced block during extradural anaesthesia in patients with right bundle block and left anterior hemiblock. Br J Anaesth 1981; 53: 545–548
57 Belloci F, Santarelli P, Di-Gennaro M et al. The risk of cardiac complications in surgical patients with bifascicular block: a clinical and electrophysiologic study in 98 patients. Chest 1980; 77: 343–348
58 Baum VC, Perloff JR. Anesthetic implications of adults with congenital heart disease. Anesth and Analg: 76; 1342–1358
59 Wong RS, Baum VC, Sangwan S. Truncus arteriosus: recognition and therapy of intraoperative cardiac ischemia. Anesthesiology 1991; 74: 38–380
60 Prys-Roberts C. Anaesthesia and hypertension. Br J Anaesth 1984; 56: 711–724
61 Prys-Roberts C, Meloche R, Foex P. Studies of anaesthesia in relation to hypertension. I Cardiovascular responses to treated and untreated patients. Br J Anaesth 1971; 43: 122–137
62 Coriat P, Reiz S. Cardiac outcome after non-cardiac surgery in patients with coronary artery disease. Baillière's Clin Anaesthesiol 1992; 6: 491–513
63 Jones RM. Calcium antagonists. In Atkinson RS, Adams AP, eds. Recent advances in anaesthesia and analgesia, vol 15. Churchill Livingstone, 1985: pp 89–106
64 McCollum JSC, Dundee JW. Comparison of induction characteristics of four anaesthetic agents. Anaesthesia 1986; 41: 995–100
65 Stoelting RK. Blood pressure and heart rate changes during short duration laryngoscopy for tracheal intubation: influence of viscous or intravenous lidocaine. Anesth Analg 1978; 57: 197–199
66 Steed DL, Brown B, Reilly JJ et al. General surgical complications in heart and heart–lung transplantation. Surgery 1985; 98: 739–744
67 Chomette G, Auriol M, Cabrol C. Chronic rejection in human transplantation. J Heart Transplant 1988; 7: 292–297
68 Hotson JR, Pedley TA. Neurological complications of cardiac transplantation. Brain 1976; 99: 673–694
69 Conacher ID. Isolated lung transplantation: a review of problems and guide to anaesthesia. Br J Anaesth 1988; 61: 468–474
70 Higginbottom T. Physiology of the transplanted lung and results. In: Wallwork J, ed. Heart and lung transplantation. Philadelphia, PA: W.B. Saunders, 1989: pp 533–544
71 Dark J, Cooper JD. Transplantation of the lungs. Br J Hosp Med 1987; 35: 443–445
72 Johnson RA, Palacios I. Dilated cardiomyopathies of the adult. N Engl J Med 1982; 307: 1051–1058
73 Shnider SM, Papper EM. Anesthesia for the asthmatic patient. Anesthesiology 1961; 22: 886–892
74 Downes H, Gerber N, Hirshman CA. IV lignocaine in reflex and allergic bronchoconstriction. Br J Anaesth 1980; 52: 873–878
75 Pearce AC, Jones RM. Smoking and anesthesia: preoperative and perioperative morbidity. Anesthesiology 1984; 61: 576–584
76 Stein M, Koota GM, Simon M et al. Pulmonary evaluation of surgical patients. JAMA 1982; 181: 765–770
77 Stein M, Cassara EL. Preoperative pulmonary evaluation and therapy for surgery patients. JAMA 1970; 211: 878–890
78 Milledge IS, Nunn JF. Criteria of fitness for anaesthesia in patients with chronic obstructive lung disease. Br Med J 1975; 3: 670–673
79 Nunn JF, Milledge IS, Chen D, Dore C. Respiratory criteria of fitness for surgery and anaesthesia. Anaesthesia 1988; 43: 543–551
80 Pietak S, Weenig CS, Hickey RF, Fairley HB. Anesthetic effects on ventilation in patients with chronic obstructive pulmonary disease. Anesthesiology 1975; 42: 160–166
81 Tarhan S, Moffitt EA, Sessler AD et al. Risk of anesthesia and surgery in patients with chronic bronchitis and chronic obstructive pulmonary disease. Surgery 1973; 74: 720–726
82 Ravin MB. Comparison of spinal and general anesthesia for lower abdominal surgery in patients with chronic obstructive airway disease. Anesthesiology 1971; 35: 319–322
83 Gold MI, Joseph SI. Bilateral tension pneumothorax following induction of anesthesia in two patients with chronic obstructive airway disease. Anesthesiology 1973; 38: 93–96
84 Ricksten SE, Bengtsson A, Soderberg C et al. Effects of periodic positive airway pressure by mask on post-operative pulmonary function. Chest 1986; 89: 774–781
85 Neijens HJ, Sinaasappel M, De Groot R, De Jonste JC, Overteek SE. Cystic fibrosis, pathophysiological and clinical aspects. Eur J Pediatr 1990; 149: 742–751
86 Elborn IS, Shale DJ. Lung injury in cystic fibrosis. Thorax 1990; 45: 970–973
87 Pearl RG, Rosenthal MH, Ashton JPA. Pulmonary vasodilator effects of nitroglycerin and sodium nitroprusside in canine oleic acid-induced pulmonary hypertension. Anesthesiology 1983; 58: 514–518
88 Child CG, Turcotte JG. The liver and portal hypertension. In: Child CG, ed. Major Problems in Clinical Surgery, vol 1. Philadelphia, PA: W.B. Saunders, 1964: pp 50–59
89 Jacobs S, Chang RWS, Lef B, Al Rawaf A, Pace NC, Salan I. Prediction of outcome in patients with acute variceal haemorrhage. Br J Surg 1989; 76: 123–126
90 DiCarlo V, Staudacher C, Chiesa R et al. The role of cardiovascular hemodynamics and liver histology in evaluating bleeding cirrhotic patients. Ann Surg 1979; 190: 218–226
91 Agasti AGN, Roca J, Bosch J, Rodriguez-Roism R. The lung in patients with cirrhosis. J Hepatol 1990; 10: 251–257
92 Schrier RW. Pathogenesis of sodium and water retention in high output and low output cardiac failure,

93. Dawson JL. Jaundice and anoxic renal damage: protective effect of mannitol. Br Med J 1964; 1: 810–811
94. Hayes PC. Liver disease and drug disposition. Br J Anaesth 1992; 68: 459–461
95. Pugh RNH, Murray-Lyon IM, Dawson JL. Transection of the oesophagus for bleeding oesophageal varices. Br J Surg 1973; 60: 646–649
96. Bader JM. Hepatoxicity and metabolism of isoflurane in rats with cirrhosis. Anesth Analg 1989; 68: 214–218
97. Gelman S, Fowler KC, Smith LR. Liver circulation and function during isoflurane and halothane anesthesia. Anesthesiology 1984; 61: 726–730
98. Gelman S. Disturbances in hepatic blood flow during anesthesia and surgery. Arch Surg 1976; 111: 881–883
99. Hatano Y, Murakawa M, Segawa H et al. Venous air embolism during hepatic resection. Anesthesiology 1990; 73: 1281–1285
100. Mallet SV, Cox DJA. Thrombelastography. Br J Anaesth 1992; 69: 307–313
101. Aitkenhead AR. Anaesthesia and bowel surgery. Br J Anaesth 1984; 56: 95–101
102. Casthely PA, Tablons M, Griepp RB, Arisanergin M, Goodman R. Ketanserin in the preoperative and intraoperative management of a patient with carcinoid tumor undergoing tricuspid valve replacement. Anesth Analg 1986; 65: 809–811
103. Marsh HM, Martin JK, Kvols LK et al. Carcinoid crisis during anaesthesia. Successful treatment with a somatostatin analogue. Anesthesiology 1987; 66: 89–91
104. Miller R, Boulukos PA, Warner RRP. Failure of halothane and ketamine to alleviate carcinoid syndrome-induced bronchospasm during anesthesia. Anesth Analg 1980; 59: 621–623
105. Nissenson AR, Nimer SD, Wolcott DL. Recombinant human erythropoietin and renal anemia: molecular biology, clinical efficacy, and nervous system effects. Ann Intern Med 1991; 114: 402–416
106. Eschbach, JW, Abdulhadi MH, Browne JK et al. Recombinant human erythropoietin (rHuEpo) in anemic patients with end-stage renal disease: results of a phase III multicenter trial. Ann Intern Med 1989; 111: 992–1000
107. Satoh K, Masuda, T, Ikeda Y et al. Hemodynamic changes by recombinant erythropoietin therapy in hemodialyzed patients. Hypertension 1990; 15: 262–266
108. Ghoneim MM, Long JP. The interaction between magnesium and other neuromuscular blocking agents. Anesthesiology 1970; 1970; 32: 23–27
109. Powell DR, Miller RD. The effect of repeated doses of succinylcholine on serum potassium in patients with renal failure. Anesth Analg 1975; 54: 746–748
110. Groves ND, Leach KG, Rosen M. Effects of halothane, enflurane and isoflurane anaesthesia on renal plasma flow. Br J Anaesth 1990; 65: 796–800
111. Zall S, Eden E, Winso I et al. Controlled hypotension with adenosine and sodium nitroprusside during cerebral aneurysm surgery: effects on renal hemodynamics, excretory function and renin release. Anesth Analg 1990; 71: 631–636
112. Thomsen K, Zanoni MK, Christensen S. Effects of recovery from anesthesia and surgery on renal sodium handling in conscious rats. Renal Physiol Biochem 1988; 11: 316–324
113. Myers BD. Nature of postischaemic renal injury following aortic or cardiac surgery. In: Bihari D, Neild G, eds. Acute renal failure in the intensive therapy unit. Berlin: Springer-Verlag, 1990: pp 167–180
114. Kharasch ED, Kiang Teck Yeo, Kenny MA, Buffington CW. Atrial natriuretic factor may mediate the renal effects of PEEP ventilation. Anesthesiology 1988; 69: 862–869
115. Don HF, Dieppa RA, Taylor P. Narcotic analgesics in anuric patients. Anesthesiology 1975; 42: 745–747
116. Murray MD, Brater DC. Adverse effects of nonsteroidal anti-inflammatory drugs on renal function. Ann Intern Med 1990; 112: 559–560
117. Whelton, A, Stout RL, Spilman PS, Klassen DK. Renal effects of ibuprofen, piroxicam, and sulindac in patients with asymptomatic renal failure. Ann Intern Med 1990; 112: 568–576
118. Landercaspar J, Merz BJ, Cogbill TH et al. Peri-operative stroke risk in 173 consecutive patients with a past history of stroke. Arch Surg 1990; 125: 86–989
119. Lebowitz MH, Blitt CB, Dillon JB. Enflurane induced nervous system excitation and its relation to carbon dioxide tension. Anesth Analg 1972; 51: 355–363
120. Crawford JS, James FM, Nolte H et al. Regional anesthesia for patients with chronic neurological disease and similar conditions. Anaesthesia 1981; 36: 821–828
121. Brett RS, Schmidt JH, Gage IS, Schartel SA, Poppers PJ. Measurement of acetylcholine receptor concentration in skeletal muscle from a patient with multiple sclerosis and resistance to atracurium. Anesthesiology 1987; 66: 837–839
122. Smith GB, Shribman AJ. Anaesthesia and severe skin disease. Anaesthesia 1984; 39: 443–455
123. Smith RB. Hyperkalaemia following succinylcholine administration in neurological disorders: a review. Can Anaesth Soc J 1971; 18: 199–201
124. Russell DC, Maloney A, Muir AL. Progressive generalised scleroderma: respiratory failure from primary chest wall involvement. Thorax 1981; 36: 219–220
125. Clements PJ, Furst DE, Cabeen W et al. The relationship of arrhythmias and conduction disturbances to other manifestations of cardiopulmonary disease in progressive systemic sclerosis (PSS). Am J Med 1981; 71: 38–46
126. Young RH, Mark GJ. Pulmonary vascular changes in scleroderma. Am J Med 1978; 64: 998–1000
127. Dolan P, Sisko F, Riley E. Anesthetic considerations for Ehlers–Danlos syndrome. Anesthesiology 1980; 52: 266–269
128. Abouleish E. Obstetric anaesthesia and Ehlers–Danlos syndrome. Br J Anaesth 1980; 52: 1283–1286
129. Mitchell MM, Ali HH, Savaresse JJ. Myotonia and neuromuscular blocking agents. Anesthesiology 1978; 49: 44–48
130. Mudge BJ, Taylor PB, Vanderspek AFL. Perioperative hazards in myotonic dystrophy. Anaesthesia 1980; 35: 492–495
131. Aldridge ML. Anaesthetic problems in myotonic dystrophy. A case report and review of the Aberdeen

experience comprising 48 general anaesthetics in a further 16 patients. Br J Anaesth 1985; 57: 1119–1130

132 Cope DK, Miller JN. Local and spinal anesthesia for cesarean section in a patient with myotonic dystrophy. Anesth Analg 1986; 65: 687–690

133 Meyers MB, Barash PG. Cardiac decompensation during enflurane anesthesia in a patient with myotonia atrophica. Anesth Analg 1976; 55: 433–436

134 Drachman DB. Myasthenia gravis. N Engl J Med 1978; 298: 136–142

135 Glass AR. Use of betablockers in thyrotoxic patients with heart failure (letter). Am J Med 1991; 90: 136–137

136 Lee RT, Plappert M, Sutton MGS. Depressed left ventricular systolic ejection force in hypothyroidism. Am J Cardiol 1990; 65: 526–527

137 Sonne J, Boesgaards S, Poulsen HE et al. Pharmacokinetics and pharmacodynamics of oxazepam and metabolism of paracetamol in severe hypothyroidism. Br J Clin Pharmacol 1990; 30: 737–742

138 Drop LJ, Cullen DJ. Comparative effects of calcium chloride and calcium gluconate. Br J Anaesth 1980; 52: 502–505

139 Al-Mohayas, Naguib M, Abdelatif M, Farag H. Abnormal responses to muscle relaxants in a patient with primary hyperparathyroidism. Anesthesiology 1986; 65: 554–556

140 Hull CJ. Phaeochromocytoma. Diagnosis, preoperative preparation and anaesthetic management. Br J Anaesth 1986; 58: 1453–1468

141 Hassan SZ, Matz G, Lawrence AM, Collins PA. Laryngeal stenosis in acromegaly. Anesth Analg 1976; 55: 57–60

142 Bjorndorp P. How should obesity be defined? J Intern Med 1990; 227: 147–149

143 Landsberg L. Obesity, metabolism and hypertension. Yale J Biol Med 1989; 62: 511–519

144 Rubenstein I, Zamel N, DuBarry L, Hoffstein V. Airflow limitation in morbidly obese, nonsmoking men. Ann Intern Med 1990; 112: 828–832

145 Jense HG, Dublin SA, Silverstein PI, O'Leary-Escolas U. Effect of obesity on safe duration of apnea in anesthetized humans. Anesth Analg 1991; 72: 89–93

146 Bentley JB, Vaughan RW, Miller MS, Calkins JM, Gandolfi AJ. Serum inorganic fluoride levels in obese patients during and after enflurane anesthesia. Anesth Analg 1979; 58: 409–412

147 Nawaf K, Stoelting RK. SGOT values following evidence of reductive biotransformation of halothane in man. Anesthesiology 1979; 185–186

148 Cork RC, Vaughan RW, Bentley JB. General anesthesia for morbidly obese patients — an examination of postoperative outcomes. Anesthesiology 1981; 54: 310–313

149 Vaughan RW, Wise L. Postoperative arterial blood gas measurements in obese patients: effect of position on gas exchange. Ann Surg 1975; 705–709

150 Donley AJ, Kemple TJ. Spontaneous pneumomediastinum complicating anorexia nervosa. Br Med J 1978; 2: 1604–1605

151 Hirsch IB, McGill JB, Cryer PED, White PF. Perioperative management of surgical patients with diabetes mellitus. Anesthesiology 1991; 74: 346–359

152 Milaskiewicz RM, Hall GM. Diabetes and anaesthesia: the past decade. Br J Anaesth 1992; 68: 198–206

153 Laing W, Williams R. Diabetes — a model for health care management. London: Office of Health Care Economics. 1989

154 Byyny RL. Management of diabetes during surgery. Postgrad Med 1980; 68: 191–201

155 Keen H, Ashton CE. Mechanisms of excess cardiovascular mortality in diabetes. Postgrad Med J 1989; 65 (suppl 1): S26–S29

156 Borch-Johnsen K, Kreiner S. Proteinuria: value as a predictor of cardiovascular mortality in insulin-dependent diabetes mellitus. Br Med J 1987; 1651–1654

157 Weise F, Heydenreich F, Gehrig W, Runge U. Heart rate variability in diabetic patients during orthostatic load — a spectral analytic approach. Klin Wochenschr 1990; 68: 26–32

158 Jermendy G, Khoor S, Koltai MZ, Pogatsa G. Left ventricular diastolic dysfunction in type 1 (insulin-dependent) diabetic patients during dynamic exercies. Cardiology 1990; 77: 9–16

159 Starling MR. Does a clinically definable diabetic cardiomyopathy exist? J Am Coll Cardiol 1990; 15: 1518–1520

160 Nobe S, Aomine M, Arita M, Ito S, Tataki R. Chronic diabetes mellitus prolongs action potential duration of rat ventricular muscles. Circumstantial evidence for impaired Ca^{2+} channel. Cardiovasc Res 1990; 24: 381–389

161 Maser RE, Pfeifer MA, Dorman JS et al. Diabetic autonomic neuropathy and cardiovascular risk. Pittsburgh epidemiology of diabetes complications study III. Arch Intern Med 1990; 150: 1218–1222

162 Lange P, Groth S, Mortensen J et al. Diabetes mellitus and ventilatory capacity: a five year follow-up study. Eur Respir J 1990; 3: 288–292

163 Reddi AS, Camerini-Davalos RA. Diabetic nephropathy: An update. Arch Intern Med 1990; 150: 31–43

164 Galloway JA, Shuman CR. Diabetes and surgery. Am J Med 1963; 34: 177–191

165 Burgos LG, Ebert TJ, Asiddao C et al. Increased intraoperative cardiovascular morbidity in diabetics with autonomic neuropathy. Anesthesiology 1989; 70: 591–597

166 Ewing DJ, Clarke BF. Diagnosis and management of diabetic autonomic neuropathy. Br Med J 1982; 285: 916–918

167 Salzarulo HH, Taylor LA. Diabetic 'stiff joint syndrome' as a cause of difficult endotracheal intubation. Anesthesiology 1986; 64: 366–368

168 Rosen RB, Enquist IF. The healing wound in experimental diabetes. Surgery 1961; 50: 525–528

169 Rayfield EJ, Ault MJ, Keusch GT et al. Infection and diabetes: the case for glucose control. Am J Med 1982; 72: 439–450

170 Alberti KGMM, Thomas DJB. The management of diabetes during surgery. Br J Anaesth 1979; 51: 693–710

171 Esseltine DW et al. Sickle cell status and the anaesthetist. Can J Anaesth 1988; 35: 385–403

172 Dunn A et al. Intraoperative death during Caesarian section in a patient with sickle-cell trait. Can J Anaesth 1987; 34: 67–70

173. Luban NLC, et al. Sickle cell disease and anesthesia. In: Eckenhoff JE, ed. Year book of anaesthesia. Chicago, IL: Year Book 1984: pp 289–336
174. Communicable Disease Report. AIDS and HIV-1 infection in the United Kingdom: monthly report. 1993; 38: 175
175. Gerberding JL. Transmission of HIV to health care worker: risk and risk reduction. Bull NY Acad Med 1988; 64: 491–497
176. CDC: Public Health Service statement of management of occupational exposure to human immunodeficiency virus, including considerations regarding zidovudine post-exposure use. MMWR 1990; 39: 1–4
177. Greenberg JE, Fishe MA, Berger JR. Upper airway obstruction to acquired immunodeficiency syndrome related Kaposi's sarcoma. Chest 1985; 88: 638–640
178. Bullingham A, Mackenzie S. Laryngeal obstruction in HIV infection. Anaesthesia 1989; 44: 1003–1004
179. Suffredini A F, Ognibene F P, Lack EE et al. Nonspecific interstitial pneumonitis: a common cause of pulmonary disease in the acquired immunodeficiency syndrome. Ann Intern Med 1987; 107: 7–13
180. Lewis W. AIDS: cardiac findings from 115 autopsies. Prog Cardiovasc Dis 1989; 32: 207–215
181. Rao TKS, Friedman EA, Nicastri AD. The types of renal disease in the acquired immunodeficiency syndrom. N Engl J Med 1987; 316: 1062–1068
182. Buehrer JL, Weber DJ, Meyer AA et al. Wound infection rates after invasive procedures in HIV-1 seropositive versus HIV-1 seronegative hemophiliacs. Ann Surg 1990; 211: 492–498
183. Muravchick S, Mandel J. Thiopental sleep dosages in geriatric patients. Anesthesiology 1982; 57: A327
184. Castelden CM, Kaye CM, Parsons RL. The effect of age on plasma levels of propranolol and practolol in man. Br J Clin Pharmacol 1975; 2: 303–306
185. Mclesky CH. Anesthesia for the geriatric patient. In: Stoelting RK, Barash PG, Gallagher TJ, eds. Advances in anesthesia, vol 2. Chicago, IL: Year Book, 1985: pp 31–68
186. Hurwitz N. Predisposing factors in adverse reactions to drugs. Br Med J 1969; 1: 536–539
187. Davenport HT. Anaesthesia for the geriatric patient. Can Anaesth Soc J 1983; 30: s51–s55
188. Harries DJ, Eastwood H. Proximal femoral fractures in the elderly: does operative delay for medical reasons affect short term outcome? Age Ageing 1991; 20: 41–44
189. Gustafson Y, Brannstorm B, Berggren D et al. A geriatric anesthesiologic program to reduce acute confusional states in elderly patients treated for femoral neck fractures. J Am Geriatr Soc 1991; 39: 655–662
190. Haan J, Van Kleef JW, Bloem BR et al. Cognitive function after spinal or general anaesthesia for transurethral prostatectomy in elderly men. J Am Geriatr Soc 1991; 39: 596–600
191. Shannon RP, Maher KA, Santiga JT, Royal HD, Wei JY. Comparison of differences in the hemodynamic response to passive postural stress in healthy subjects > 70 years and < 30 years of age. Am J Cardiol 1991; 67: 1110–1116
192. Manning WJ, Shannon RP, Santiga JA et al. Reversal of changes in left ventricular diastolic filling associated with normal aging using diltiazem. Am J Cardiol 1991; 67: 894–896
193. Simons RJ, Simon JM, Demers LM, Santen RJ. Thyroid dysfunction in elderly hospitalized patients. Effects of age and severity of illness. Arch Intern Med 1990; 1249–1253

3. Intercurrent medication

S.A. Harding   R.M. Jones

Concurrent drug therapy, acutely or chronically administered, may profoundly alter the patient's response to anaesthesia and surgery. This may have implications for the type of anaesthetic, and on occasion the type of surgery planned. During the pre-operative visit it is essential that the anaesthetist obtains a complete drug history from the patient, including both prescribed and over-the-counter medicines. This may alert the anaesthetist to the nature and severity of medical disorders previously undisclosed. The anaesthetist requires a thorough understanding of the pharmacology of the many agents which may be taken pre-operatively in order to predict and modify potentially significant interactions with agents used during anaesthesia. Indeed, the anaesthetist may deliberately employ combinations of drugs which have complementary effects. The likelihood of a significant drug interaction increases with the number of medications taken. Drug interactions may be considered to fall into two main groups: *pharmacokinetic*, where one drug affects the absorption, distribution, metabolism or excretion of another agent; and *pharmacodynamic*, when the effects caused by the drugs are similar and complementary or antagonistic when one drug inhibits the effect of the other.

Pharmacokinetic interactions

Examples of pharmacokinetic interactions include the displacement of a highly protein-bound drug such as a sulphonylurea by another highly protein-bound agent such as aspirin; the risk with this combination is of hypoglycaemia. Hepatic metabolism may be increased by enzyme-inducing drugs which include barbiturates, phenytoin and other factors such as cigarette smoking and high alcohol intake. The clearance of drugs which are metabolized in the liver is increased and when a drug has a toxic metabolite, toxicity may be enhanced. For example, liver damage may be more likely following large doses of paracetamol. Hepatic enzyme induction with barbiturates increases the development of halothane-associated hepatotoxicity in animal experiments[1] and increased metabolism of fluorinated volatile anaesthetic agents may increase the risk of renal damage from the effects of inorganic fluoride on the renal tubule. Cimetidine inhibits hepatic cytochrome P-450 iso-enzymes. It also decreases liver blood flow and may precipitate toxicity of other drugs, including theophylline, warfarin and lignocaine. The monoamine oxidase inhibitors are non-specific enzyme inhibitors and they also inhibit hepatic enzymes which metabolize many other drugs. The effects of opioids and other sedative agents may be dangerously potentiated. Several agents are known to inhibit the enzyme plasma cholinesterase and cause a prolongation of the effects of suxamethonium or mivacurium, which are broken down by this enzyme. Ecothiopate iodide is a long-acting cholinesterase inhibitor used as eye drops in the treatment of glaucoma. Systemic absorption may be associated with a decrease in cholinesterase activity. Organophosphorus pesticides and some cytotoxic alkylating agents, including cyclophosphamide, mustine, tretamine and thiotepa, have caused a similar effect. The oral contraceptive pill may reduce hepatic production of plasma cholinesterase but there is unlikely to be prolonged apnoea following suxamethonium or mivacurium unless an abnormal cholinesterase variant is present.

Pharmacodynamic interactions

These are seen frequently in anaesthetic practice. For example, the sedative effects of hypnotic agents, opioids and phenothiazines may potentiate anaesthetic agents and decrease requirements. Drugs used in the treatment of hypertension and ischaemic heart disease may be potentiated by the cardiovascular effects of inhaled anaesthetic agents. Several groups of drugs have been found to possess some neuromuscular blocking activity. These include some antibiotics, calcium antagonists, lithium, quinidine, procainamide and magnesium.

Muscle power is not reduced in normal individuals but there may be weakness if neuromuscular transmission is already compromised. Thus, the requirement for muscle relaxants may be reduced as their action is potentiated.

It has been reported that 44% of a surgical population were receiving regular medication before admission and in those aged over 70 years the proportion increased to 70%.[2] Cardio-active medication accounted for the greatest proportion of drugs administered. Results from the 1993 *Report of a Confidential Enquiry into Perioperative Deaths*[3] show that in 89% of the deaths evaluated, the patient was receiving some form of medication before operation, compared with 37% of index cases. Although some drugs may be discontinued peri-operatively with little adverse effect, others should be continued throughout the peri-operative period because sudden discontinuation may be harmful. Notably, it has been demonstrated that patients receiving medication for hypertension and ischaemic heart disease may suffer rebound hypertension and myocardial ischaemia if treatment is suddenly withdrawn. Clear guidelines should be given to nursing staff regarding which medications must be continued when a patient is unable to take oral preparations pre- and post-operatively. An alternative route of administration may be required or an alternative agent substituted if the return of gastro-intestinal function is delayed.

CARDIOVASCULAR DRUGS

Pre-existing cardiovascular disease is probably the major medical cause of peri-operative morbidity and mortality and thus the drugs used in the treatment of cardiovascular disease are of major significance to the anaesthetist. Ischaemic heart disease and systemic arterial hypertension are the most common indications for treatment and the agents used have profound effects on cardiovascular physiology including vasodilatation, negative inotropy and altered impulse initiation and conduction, which may compromise the patient's ability to respond to peri-operative stresses. Anaesthetic agents have additional cardiovascular effects and awareness of potential drug interactions during anaesthesia is essential if the risk of adverse effects due to drug interactions is to be minimized. The sudden withdrawal of cardiovascular medication may precipitate hypertension or myocardial ischaemia which could result in peri-operative myocardial infarction. Such medication should be continued up to the morning of surgery and re-introduced at the earliest opportunity after surgery. If the return of gastro-intestinal function is delayed, alternative routes of administration should be considered.

β-Adrenoceptor antagonists

These agents are used for the treatment of hypertension, angina and certain arrhythmias. They may also be used in the treatment of anxiety and migraine and to reduce the systemic effects of thyrotoxicosis. β-Adrenoceptor antagonists are competitive antagonists of the naturally occurring β-agonists adrenaline and noradrenaline and inhibit the effects of sympathetic stimulation on β-receptors in many tissues of the body. Beneficial effects are obtained in ischaemic heart disease by decreasing heart rate and contractility and thus myocardial oxygen demand. The precise mechanism of the antihypertensive action of β-blockers is unclear but is likely to involve the inhibition of renin release from the kidney and presynaptic inhibition of noradrenaline release, in addition to the effects on the heart.

Cardioselective agents have greater potency for blocking β_1-receptors and cause less undesirable effects, such as bronchoconstriction and worsening of peripheral vascular disease. However, with increasing drug concentration, the β_2-receptors also become blocked. Some β-adrenoceptor antagonists have a local anaesthetic or quinidine-like membrane-stabilizing activity. The membrane-stabilizing potency of propranolol is equal to that of lignocaine, although the concentration range at which this occurs is much higher than that required for β-blockade. It is likely that the predominant anti-arrhythmic activity is due to removal of sympathetic stimulation. Others have partial agonist activity in addition to their β-adrenoceptor antagonist properties. Thus, a decrease in cardiac output may be avoided at rest, whereas the sympathetic response to exercise or stress will still be inhibited. This property is known as intrinsic sympathomimetic activity and may be beneficial for patients in whom β-blockers may precipitate cardiac failure or bronchoconstriction. Some of the commonly used β-adrenoceptor antagonists are shown in Table 3.1.

Side-effects

The side-effects of β-blockers may be predicted with a knowledge of the effects of β-adrenergic stimulation. Cardiac failure may be precipitated in patients with impaired cardiac reserve who rely on increased sympathetic drive to the heart to maintain adequate cardiac output. Peripheral vascular disease and Raynaud's phenomenon can be exacerbated by the inhibition of β_2-mediated vasodilatation. The blockade of β_2-receptors in the bronchi can precipitate bronchospasm in patients with asthma or chronic obstructive pulmonary disease. Although β_1-selective agents are less likely to

Table 3.1 Properties of commonly used β-adrenoceptor antagonists

Drug	β₁-Selectivity	MSA	ISA
Acebutolol	+	+	+
Atenolol	+	0	0
Esmolol	+	0	0
Labetalol	0	+	0
Metoprolol	+	+/−	0
Nadolol	0	0	0
Oxprenolol	0	+	+
Penbutolol	0	+	+
Pindolol	0	+/−	+
Propranolol	0	+	0
Sotalol	0	0	0
Timolol	0	0	0

MSA = Membrane-stabilizing activity; ISA = intrinsic sympathomimetic activity.

have this effect, all β-adrenoreceptor antagonists must be avoided or used with care in this group of patients. In diabetics, β-blockers may mask the symptoms and signs of hypoglycaemia and, by inhibiting the hyperglycaemic actions of catecholamines, may prolong the period of hypoglycaemia. The β₁-selective compounds are less likely to delay recovery from hypoglycaemia and are preferred in the treatment of unstable diabetics. β-Adrenoceptor antagonists cause elevation of plasma triglycerides and lower the concentrations of high-density lipoproteins — an effect which may be undesirable in patients with arterial disease.

Implications for anaesthesia

Sudden withdrawal of β-blockers can precipitate angina, ventricular arrhythmias and myocardial infarction.[4] Following withdrawal, there is hypersensitivity to circulating catecholamines, possibly due to an increase in the receptor population. Administration of a β-adrenoceptor antagonist to hypertensive patients under anaesthesia has been shown to attenuate the hypertensive response to laryngoscopy and intubation and reduce the incidence of peri-operative arrhythmias without causing a reduction in cardiac output.[5] It is therefore recommended that β-blockade is continued throughout the peri-operative period. During anaesthesia, the myocardial-depressant effects of inhaled anaesthetic agents may be increased by the presence of a β-adrenoceptor antagonist. In addition, halothane has a marked influence on impulse initiation and conduction and, if used in higher concentrations for anaesthesia, may precipitate complete heart block. (Halothane also significantly decreases liver blood flow and this influences the kinetics of acutely administered intra-operative β-blockers, which should be used with great caution during halothane anaesthesia.) When a patient has been treated with a β-blocker, the pulse rate is unreliable as a monitor of hypovolaemia or light anaesthesia. Vascular volume should be monitored carefully and hypovolaemia corrected. The continuation of β-blockade throughout the peri-operative period is desirable for the reasons outlined above. Many agents are available as intravenous preparations but the dose may be considerably lower than the oral dose because of the low bio-availability of many of these agents when given orally (propranolol, for example, undergoes extensive first-pass metabolism in the liver and the oral dose required for a given response is much greater than the intravenous dose). The intravenous dose is titrated to obtain the desired effect. Thus, if a β-blocker is to be administered before surgery to inhibit the pressor response to laryngoscopy and tracheal intubation, small aliquots of the drug are given at intervals in order to decrease the resting pulse rate by a predetermined amount, such as 10 beats.min^{-1}.

Calcium antagonists

The calcium antagonists comprise a structurally dissimilar group of agents which are used for the treatment of hypertension, angina pectoris and the control of supraventricular arrhythmias. They have a similar spectrum of application to the β-adrenoceptor antagonists but have a different mechanism of action and may be used safely in patients with obstructive airways disease and peripheral vascular disease. The main action of the calcium antagonists is to inhibit the slow inward calcium current of voltage-operated calcium channels in cardiac and smooth-muscle cells. The intracellular calcium ion concentration is reduced and excitation–contraction coupling of cardiac and smooth muscle is inhibited. The cardiac action potential — which is slow channel-dependent — is also affected, causing an increase in the effective refractory period of conducting tissue; there is slowing of the sinus rate and of atrio-ventricular nodal conduction. Calcium antagonists do not block calcium channels directly but interact with receptors functionally linked with the calcium channels (dihydropyridine receptors) to reduce calcium flux. The structurally dissimilar calcium antagonists act at different receptor sites and exhibit selectivity between cardiac and smooth-muscle calcium channels; thus, they exhibit different profiles of action. The action of calcium antagonists is not confined to inhibiting the slow calcium current; they also affect other ion currents, and may inhibit the binding of calcium with binding proteins such as calmodulin.

Nifedipine and the other dihydropyridines, nicardipine and nimodipine, are potent vasodilators. This effect occurs at significantly lower concentrations than those required for direct effects on the heart. The reduction in systemic vascular resistance is due to relaxation of the smooth muscle of the arteriolar resistance vessels and may induce sympathetic reflexes such that cardiac output and heart rate are modestly increased. Verapamil is a synthetic papaverine derivative which has less effect on the peripheral vasculature and more direct myocardial action; this results in depression of contractility, reduced rate of sinus discharge and slowing of atrioventricular conduction. Diltiazem has rather fewer effects on cardiac rate and conduction and causes less depression of contractility and vasodilatation than does verapamil. The different spectra of activity explain the different clinical applications for the use of these agents. The dihydropyridines are used in the treatment of hypertension, whereas verapamil and diltiazem are effective in the treatment of supraventricular tachycardias. All the agents are beneficial in the treatment of myocardial ischaemia, particularly when coronary artery spasm may play a role. Side-effects of nifedipine and other agents with similar actions are due to vasodilatation and include dizziness, hypotension, headache, flushing and nausea. Peripheral oedema may occur. Verapamil and diltiazem may cause bradycardia and transient asystole, particularly in patients with preexisting conduction disturbances. Verapamil may cause exacerbation of heart failure and the combination of verapamil and β-blockers should be avoided because of the possibility of severe depression of ventricular function and risk of atrioventricular block.

Implications for anaesthesia

As with other long-term cardiac therapy, the calcium antagonists should be continued up until the time of surgery. The volatile anaesthetics may be considered to be non-specific calcium antagonists and may have additive effects on the cardiovascular system when used in patients who are treated with these agents.[6] The cardiovascular effects of isoflurane are similar to those of nifedipine with markedly reduced systemic vascular resistance but little effect on contractility and conduction; a combination of these agents may cause profound systemic hypotension. Similarly, verapamil and halothane both have greater effects on myocardial contractility and conduction and the combination of these agents might be expected to lead to significant myocardial depression and severe conduction disorders. If a clinically significant effect occurs, the administration of calcium may reverse, to some extent, additive negative inotropic effects but has little influence on decreased vascular resistance. This probably reflects the greater reliance of the heart on extracellular calcium for excitation–contraction coupling, compared with vascular muscle. Careful observation of blood pressure and the electrocardiogram (ECG) is essential during anaesthesia, and agents for resuscitation must be readily available.

Calcium antagonists have an effect on the neuromuscular junction because presynaptic mobilization and release of acetylcholine are triggered by calcium ions. When calcium flux is decreased, less acetylcholine is released and the margin of safety for neuromuscular transmission is reduced. Verapamil and nifedipine have been shown to increase the potency of neuromuscular blocking agents.[7,8] The requirement for muscle relaxants may be reduced and neuromuscular function should be monitored. There is some evidence that, if a prolonged block occurs, edrophonium may antagonize the residual paralysis more effectively than neostigmine;[8] this presumably reflects the greater presynaptic effect of edrophonium.

Diuretics

Thiazide diuretics

These agents increase urine formation and create a negative fluid balance resulting in a reduction in extracellular volume and mobilization of oedema fluid. The thiazides are moderately potent diuretics which also have an antihypertensive action and they are commonly used as first-line treatment for hypertension and in the treatment of oedema due to mild heart failure. The diuretic action is due to inhibition of sodium transport in the early distal convoluted tubule. The precise mechanism for the blood pressure-lowering effect is not known but long-term therapy results in reduced vascular resistance. It is postulated that a small reduction in total body sodium gives rise to a decrease in intracellular vascular smooth-muscle Na^+ concentration that in turn reduces intracellular Ca^{2+} concentration. This would reduce the response to contractile stimuli, including vasoconstrictor hormones.[9] The antihypertensive effect is seen at low doses. Higher doses cause more metabolic disturbance with no advantage in blood pressure control. The thiazides enhance the antihypertensive action of most other antihypertensive drugs and are thus frequently part of a combination antihypertensive regimen (the traditional 'step' approach to antihypertensive therapy). An apparently paradoxical use of thiazides is in the treatment of nephrogenic diabetes insipidus, where they cause a reduction in the urine volume.

Adverse effects are dose-related and include reduced plasma concentrations of potassium and magnesium, hypochloraemic metabolic alkalosis, raised plasma uric acid concentrations, impaired glucose tolerance and raised plasma lipid concentrations. Rarely, hypercalcaemia and hypophosphataemia occur, simulating hyperparathyroidism. Rashes, photosensitivity, neutropenia and thrombocytopenia are also rare.

Loop diuretics

This group includes frusemide, bumetanide and ethacrynic acid. These are less effective antihypertensive agents than the thiazides but very potent diuretics. The main site of action of the loop diuretics is the thick ascending limb of the loop of Henle where they inhibit the sodium–potassium–chloride co-transport mechanism. Up to 30% of filtered sodium may be excreted, causing a rapid and profound diuresis. These agents are effective in the treatment of oedema due to cardiac failure or of hepatic and renal origins. In chronic renal failure, much higher doses may be required to produce an equivalent effect. Because of the rapid and profound action, this group of drugs is used in the treatment of pulmonary oedema. When given intravenously, there is an increase in the systemic venous capacitance, causing a reduction in left ventricular filling pressure which is beneficial before the onset of diuresis. The majority of adverse effects caused by this group of drugs are due to fluid and electrolyte imbalance. The profound diuresis can cause hypovolaemia with postural hypotension. The increase in potassium excretion is greater than that seen with the thiazides, and hypokalaemia often occurs. Other metabolic changes in common with the thiazides are hypomagnesaemia, hypochloraemic metabolic alkalosis and increased concentrations of uric acid. Impaired glucose tolerance is less severe. Unlike the thiazides, loop diuretics increase calcium excretion and they may be used in the treatment of hypercalcaemia. Other adverse effects include gastro-intestinal disturbance (more common with ethacrynic acid), skin rashes, neutropenia and thrombocytopenia. Frusemide and bumetanide are structurally related to the sulphonamides and cross-sensitivity may occur. Allergic interstitial nephritis has been reported as a cause of reversible renal failure. Deafness and tinnitus are rare complications of treatment with loop diuretics in high doses. They are most common with ethacrynic acid and are due to a disturbance of the electrolyte composition of the endolymph of the middle ear. To reduce the incidence of this serious complication, large intravenous doses of frusemide should be infused at a maximum rate of 4 mg.min^{-1} and the concurrent use of other ototoxic drugs such as the aminoglycoside antibiotics should be avoided.

Potassium-sparing diuretics

Spironolactone, an aldosterone antagonist, triamterine and amiloride are potassium-sparing diuretics. Weak diuretics when used alone, they are most commonly prescribed in combination with a thiazide or loop diuretic to prevent excessive losses of potassium. Spironolactone is a competitive antagonist of aldosterone and thus inhibits the mineralocorticoid effect of sodium retention and potassium secretion in the late distal tubule and collecting duct. It is particularly effective in clinical situations such as congestive heart failure, nephrotic syndrome and hepatic cirrhosis where there is secondary hyperaldosteronism. Amiloride and triamterine directly inhibit sodium reabsorption by the late distal tubule and collecting duct and have a similar effect to spironolactone. The most important toxic effect of these drugs is hyperkalaemia, which is most likely to occur if patients have chronic renal insufficiency, are taking potassium supplements or are receiving angiotensin-converting enzyme (ACE) inhibitors, which also have a potassium-sparing effect. Spironolactone can cause gynaecomastia and minor gastro-intestinal symptoms.

Implications for anaesthesia

Before surgery, serum urea and electrolyte concentrations should be measured in any patient who is receiving diuretics. Chronic hypokalaemia is common in those taking thiazides or loop diuretics. There is a risk of increased peri-operative arrhythmias, and this is exacerbated by a reduction in serum magnesium concentrations. Hypokalaemia also enhances the toxicity of digoxin and causes increased sensitivity to non-depolarizing muscle relaxants. Hyperkalaemia may occur in patients taking a potassium-sparing diuretic; there is a risk of cardiac arrhythmias and a further increase in serum potassium concentration associated with the use of suxamethonium may be particularly dangerous. The contraction of the circulating blood volume caused by diuretic therapy can enhance the hypotensive effects of anaesthetic agents and vasodilators. The impaired glucose tolerance associated with the use of thiazides may result in the precipitation of frank diabetes mellitus with the additional stress of surgery and the blood glucose concentrations should be monitored peri-operatively. Some patients, particularly those who are taking moderately large doses of loop diuretics, are dependent on continued diuretic therapy to maintain adequate fluid balance. It is important that the usual maintenance dose is recommenced as soon as possible following surgery or an equivalent intravenous dose administered. Drug interactions occur between diuretics and lithium. The renal clearance of lithium is reduced when chronic sodium and water depletion are induced by diuretic therapy and lithium toxicity may be precipitated. Indomethacin and other non-steroidal anti-inflammatory drugs (NSAID) inhibit the natriuretic and antihypertensive effects of loop diuretics and concurrent administration increases the nephrotoxicity associated with NSAIDs.

Angiotensin-converting enzyme inhibitors

Captopril, the first available ACE inhibitor, was introduced in 1976. This group of agents acts by inhibiting the conversion in the lung of angiotensin I to the potent vasoconstrictor angiotensin II and consequently the formation of aldosterone is reduced. The drugs also inhibit the degradation of the vasodilator bradykinin, which is broken down by the same enzyme, and thus increase the formation of vasodilatory prostaglandins. ACE inhibitors are effective in the treatment of hypertension and congestive cardiac failure. They may cause a profound decrease in blood pressure when used in volume-depleted patients in whom plasma renin activity is high. The antihypertensive action of ACE inhibitors is enhanced by the addition of a thiazide diuretic, whereas the combination with a β-blocker is not as effective because part of the action of β-blockers depends on the inhibition of renin release. As a class, they are increasingly used for the treatment of hypertension, as their administration appears not only to arrest the deleterious effects of sustained high arterial pressure but also to reverse some of the changes (unlike thiazides and β-blockers, which have a deleterious influence on plasma lipid profile). With calcium antagonists, and more recently some of the newer α-adrenoceptor antagonists, they are part of the modern tailored approach to antihypertensive therapy.

In congestive cardiac failure, ACE inhibitors reduce both afterload and preload by causing arteriolar and venodilation. Natriuresis occurs as a result of reduced secretion of aldosterone. There is an improvement in cardiac output and an increased exercise tolerance. Captopril is eliminated by the kidneys and has a half-life in the plasma of about 2 h, although the duration of clinical effect is longer and captopril is usually prescribed two or three times a day. Enalapril is a *prodrug* which is metabolized by a serum esterase to the active compound, enalaprilat. The onset is more gradual than that of captopril, and the duration of action is more prolonged, allowing single daily dosage. Other agents of this group include lisinopril, cilazapril, fosinapril and quinapril. Unlike β-blockers and thiazide diuretics, ACE inhibitors do not cause adverse effects on plasma lipid concentrations, or impaired glucose tolerance. The inhibition of aldosterone produces a mild potassium-sparing effect and they should not be used with other potassium-sparing diuretics. Adverse effects include a dry cough, skin rash and loss of the sense of taste. These effects disappear on discontinuation of the drug. Renal failure may be induced in patients with renal artery stenosis who rely on a high perfusion pressure and the presence of angiotensin II to constrict the efferent arterioles in order to maintain adequate glomerular filtration. Proteinuria may also occur, particularly in patients with pre-existing renal parenchymal disease. Concomitant treatment with NSAIDs increases the risk of renal damage. Neutropenia and thrombocytopenia occur rarely.

Implications for anaesthesia

Pre-operatively, renal function should be checked and the plasma concentration of potassium should be measured. There is the possibility of profound hypotension peri-operatively[10,11] and comprehensive cardiovascular monitoring should continue in the postoperative period. During therapy with ACE inhibitors, the renin response to haemorrhage or hypotension is greatly attenuated and therefore normal homeostatic reflexes are impaired. Hypotension is more likely if the patient is salt- and volume-depleted and may be anticipated where there has been prolonged pre-operative fasting. The use of ACE inhibitors contributes to the hypotensive effects, and reduces the requirement for agents such as sodium nitroprusside when controlled hypotension is desirable.

Nitrates

Glyceryl trinitrate is an effective agent for the relief of acute myocardial ischaemia. Isosorbide dinitrate and isosorbide mononitrate are longer-acting preparations which may be used for prophylaxis of angina or in the treatment of congestive cardiac failure. Nitrates are potent vasodilators which act through the production of nitric oxide. Smooth muscle is relaxed in both veins and arteries, but the effects are predominantly on the venous side of the circulation, producing an increase in venous capacitance and a reduction in ventricular filling pressures. This results in decreased myocardial wall tension and a reduction in myocardial oxygen requirements. Although nitrates have been shown to cause coronary vasodilatation, this is not thought to be the principal mechanism for their beneficial effect in myocardial ischaemia. Glyceryl trinitrate is also available as a sustained-release buccal preparation and as a topical patch for prophylaxis of angina. However, as with the longer-acting oral nitrate preparations, tolerance to the haemodynamic effects can occur and it is advisable to have a drug-free period, usually overnight, to retain the beneficial effect. Side-effects of nitrates include headache and dizziness due to postural hypotension. Peri-operatively, there may be decreased vascular responsiveness due to vasodilatation and it should be remembered that antimuscarinic drying agents used for premedication reduce the absorption of sublingual nitrates. A defibrillator paddle should not be placed over a glyceryl trinitrate patch as there is the risk of explosion.

α-Adrenoceptor antagonists

Prazosin and the newer agents doxazosin and terazosin are selective α_1-blocking agents which are effective in the treatment of hypertension. Unlike the non-selective agents phentolamine and phenoxybenzamine, there is little reflex tachycardia which is the result of antagonism at the presynaptic α_2-receptors. These receptors are normally stimulated by noradrenaline to produce negative feedback of its own release; consequently, blockade produces a reflex increase in sympathetic stimulation. The α_1-blockers may cause symptomatic postural hypotension with the first dose. They have beneficial effects on plasma lipids, causing a reduction in triglycerides and LDL-cholesterol and an increase in HDL-cholesterol (LDL and HDL are low- and high-density lipoproteins). During anaesthesia, decreased vascular responsiveness is likely.

α-Adrenoceptor agonists

Clonidine

Clonidine is a centrally acting α_2-agonist which is an effective antihypertensive agent. The *stimulation* of central α_2-receptors causes a *decrease* in sympathetic outflow. This apparent paradox — stimulation causing a decrease in activity — is explained by the fact that α_2-receptors are linked to an *inhibitory* G-protein. G-proteins act as signal transduction molecules and serve to link receptors on the cell surface with intracellular second messengers. It is these second messengers, for example cyclic adenosine monophosphate (cAMP) and Ca^{2+}, that bring about the alteration in cellular function consequent upon the interaction of receptor with ligand. (It should be noted here that α_1, β_1 and β_2-adrenoceptors are linked to *stimulatory* G-proteins and generally bring about an increase in cellular activity by increasing the activity of cell second messengers.)

The decrease in central sympathetic outflow consequent upon agonist activity at α_2-receptors causes a reduction in plasma renin activity and a fall in blood pressure. Sudden discontinuation of clonidine can result in rebound hypertension and tachycardia; thus, care must be taken in the peri-operative period to continue therapy. A side-effect of clonidine is sedation and the drug has been used as a premedicant before general anaesthesia, when it also reduces the requirement for anaesthetic agents and opioids, and obtunds the cardiovascular response to intubation and surgery.[12] Applied spinally, it potentiates the analgesic effects of local anaesthetic agents and opioids (α_2-receptors modulate the onward transmission of nociceptive impulses at the spinal cord level). Use during anaesthesia may be associated with an increased incidence of systemic arterial hypotension. Clonidine has some α_1-activity and recently a more α_2-specific agonist, dexmedetomidine, has undergone trials specifically for use as an anaesthetic- and analgesic-sparing agent.[12] Its potential role in anaesthetic practice remains to be defined.

Methyldopa

Methyldopa is metabolized in the brain to methylnoradrenaline which produces its antihypertensive effect by stimulating α_2-receptors in the brainstem. As with clonidine, sedation is a frequent side-effect; depression and decreased mental acuity may also occur. Methyldopa may also cause haemolytic anaemia, neutropenia, thrombocytopenia, drug-induced lupus syndrome and acute hepatitis; any evidence of these complications necessitates immediate discontinuation of the drug. Because of the frequent side-effects, methyldopa is now rarely used, but occasionally patients, usually elderly, who have been taking it for many years, present for surgery. Methyldopa is also used in the treatment of pregnancy-induced hypertension, a condition in which it has a long history of safe use.

Anti-arrhythmic drugs

A large number of anti-arrhythmic drugs are available but many have significant side-effects. In addition, all may have a pro-arrhythmic effect in specific circumstances, and all exhibit some degree of negative inotropism. Before treatment of an arrhythmia, it is necessary to consider carefully the relative danger of the arrhythmia and the toxicity of the agents used for its treatment. The Vaughan-Williams classification of anti-arrhythmic drugs is based on the cellular electrophysiological effects of the agents and they are divided into four main classes, I–IV (Table 3.2).

Other classes have been added to the original classification. Digitalis alkaloids are sometimes referred to as class V; anticholinesterases, such as edrophonium, which slow the heart rate, have occasionally been included as a separate class.

A more clinically relevant classification is the division of these agents into groups according to their clinical use[13] (Table 3.3).

β-Blockers

This group exhibits anti-arrhythmic effects as a result of sympathetic blockade. Excitability and conduction are depressed, especially at the sinus and atrioventricular nodes, and the drugs are effective in the treatment of supraventricular arrhythmias and other catecholamine-mediated arrhythmias. A more detailed description of these drugs is given above. β-Blockers should be avoided in patients with congestive cardiac failure and significant cardiac depression can occur if other cardiodepressant agents are used concurrently. Sotalol is frequently used as an anti-arrhythmic. In addition to its antisympathetic activity, it has a class III effect, with prolongation of the QT interval.

Table 3.2 The Vaughan-Williams classification of anti-arrhythmic drugs

Class	Effects	Examples
Ia	Membrane stabilization Prolonged action potential duration	Quinidine Procainamide Disopyramide
Ib	Membrane stabilization Shortened action potential duration	Lignocaine Mexiletine Tocainide
Ic	Membrane stabilization Variable action potential duration	Flecainide Propafenone
II	β-Blockade	Propranolol Metoprolol
III	Action potential prolongation	Amiodarone Bretylium Sotalol
IV	Calcium antagonism	Verapamil Diltiazem

Table 3.3 Anti-arrhythmic drugs classified according to clinical use

Main site of action	Uses	Examples
Atrioventricular node	Supraventricular arrhythmias	Digoxin β-Blockers
Ventricle	Ventricular arrhythmias	Lignocaine Mexiletine Tocainide Phenytoin
Atria and ventricles	Supraventricular or ventricular arrhythmias	Quinidine Disopyramide Flecainide Amiodarone Procainamide

From Mason,[13] with permission.

Calcium antagonists

Verapamil and diltiazem are calcium antagonists with anti-arrhythmic action. The main effect is to prolong atrioventricular nodal refractoriness and this is beneficial in the treatment of supraventricular tachycardias. Where the atrioventricular node merely transmits an atrial tachycardia to the ventricles, the ventricular response rate is slowed (for example, atrial tachycardia, atrial flutter and fibrillation). Where the atrioventricular node is important in maintaining the tachycardia, as in junctional re-entry tachycardia, the arrhythmia is usually terminated. Verapamil should not be used in the treatment of re-entry tachycardias in association with the Wolff–Parkinson–White syndrome because it may shorten the refractoriness of the accessory pathway and increase the ventricular response rate. As is the case with propranolol, verapamil undergoes extensive first-pass metabolism and thus the intravenous dose of 5–10 mg is considerably smaller than the oral dose. Following intravenous administration, the onset of effect is seen at 2 min, peaking at 10 min. After oral administration, onset is at 2 h with a peak effect at 5 h. The half-life is 3–7 h and verapamil is usually prescribed three times a day. Intravenous verapamil should not be used in patients concurrently taking β-blockers, because the myocardial-depressant effects of the drugs are additive and inhibition of conduction can lead to asystole.[14] Other contraindications include sick sinus syndrome and atrioventricular block. Diltiazem produces less arterial vasodilatation and depresses the myocardium less than verapamil. It is only available as an oral preparation. Side-effects are less troublesome but the same contraindications apply.

Lignocaine

Lignocaine is used as the first-choice drug in the short-term treatment of ventricular arrhythmias. It is only active when given parenterally because of extensive first-pass metabolism. The half-life is approximately 1.5 h and a continuous infusion is required after the initial bolus to maintain the clinical effect. Toxic side-effects are dose-related and are predominantly central nervous effects: drowsiness, anxiety and convulsions. Lignocaine possesses a negative inotropic effect and must be used cautiously in patients with impaired left ventricular function. In addition, lignocaine clearance is reduced in congestive cardiac failure, during treatment with propranolol and during halothane anaesthesia as a result of a reduction in liver blood flow. Therapeutic lignocaine concentrations reduce the minimum alveolar concentration (MAC) value of anaesthetic agents.

Mexiletine and tocainide

These agents have similar actions to lignocaine but have longer half-lives and are active after oral administration. They are indicated for the chronic treatment of ventricular arrhythmias, including torsade de pointes. Side-effects, including nausea and vomiting, tremor and ataxia, are dose-related; haematological abnormalities, including agranulocytosis, occur rarely. The use of local anaesthetics in a patient receiving chronic mexiletine or tocainide therapy may result in additive local anaesthetic toxicity.

Phenytoin

Phenytoin is more commonly used as an anti-convulsant but it is also effective in the treatment of ventricular arrhythmias. It is of particular value in the treatment of arrhythmias caused by digoxin toxicity because it can enhance atrioventricular nodal conduction. Its use should be considered also in the treatment of lignocaine-resistant ventricular arrhythmias. When required parenterally, phenytoin should be administered as a loading dose of 10–15 mg.kg^{-1} undiluted as a slow intravenous bolus at a maximum rate of 50 mg/min. Rapid intravenous administration can result in hypotension and cardiac conduction abnormalities, including heart block or asystole. Intramuscular administration is not recommended because the drug may crystallize in tissue and absorption is unreliable.

Quinidine

Quinidine is the dextro-isomer of the antimalarial agent quinine and has been used as an anti-arrhythmic agent for many years. It is effective in the treatment of both atrial and ventricular arrhythmias but has a low toxic to therapeutic ratio and this has led to decreased use as safer drugs have been developed. Unwanted side-effects are common and include gastro-intestinal disturbances such as nausea and vomiting, thrombocytopenia, haemolytic anaemia and pro-arrhythmic activity. Conduction disturbances may develop with prolongation of the QRS and QT durations; ventricular arrhythmias, including torsade de pointes and ventricular fibrillation, may occur at high plasma concentrations. Quinidine is metabolized in the liver and has some active metabolites. Its clearance is increased by drugs which induce hepatic mixed-function oxidase, such as phenytoin, rifampicin and phenobarbitone. Quinidine itself inhibits one of the hepatic cytochrome iso-enzymes. In particular, it decreases digoxin clearance significantly, necessitating a reduction in dosage of digoxin by half when quinidine is administered to a digitalized patient. Quinidine can potentiate the neuro-muscular-blocking effects of suxamethonium and non-depolarizing muscle relaxants.[15] It may provoke weakness in patients with myasthenia gravis.

Procainamide

Procainamide is structurally related to the local anaesthetic drug procaine. It is available as both oral and parenteral preparations. Its spectrum of anti-arrhythmic activity is identical to that of quinidine and it causes similar pro-arrhythmic side-effects. It may also potentiate neuromuscular block and should be avoided in myasthenia gravis.

Disopyramide

Disopyramide has similar anti-arrhythmic effects to quinidine and procainamide. It may be given orally or intravenously and has a plasma half-life of about 7 h. This is prolonged in renal impairment and following myocardial infarction. There are cardiodepressant effects and disopyramide should be avoided in the presence of heart failure. The commonest side-effects are anticholinergic actions (dry mouth, constipation, urinary retention and blurred vision) which frequently limit tolerance of the agent. Disopyramide should be avoided in patients with narrow-angle glaucoma and symptoms of prostatism. Ventricular arrhythmias may also occur, including ventricular fibrillation and sudden death.

Flecainide and encainide

Flecainide is a newer anti-arryhthmic agent with a wide spectrum of activity. It is a membrane-stabilizing agent which dissociates slowly from cardiac sodium channels and has little effect on action potential duration. Electrocardiographic effects are prolongation of PR and QRS durations. Flecainide is effective in the suppression of both atrial and ventricular arrhythmias. It may be given either orally or intravenously, and has a half-life of about 13 h. Oral administration is usually twice a day. It has a potent negative inotropic effect which necessitates care in patients with impaired left ventricular function. Patients with impaired ventricular function and coronary artery disease are more prone to develop conduction abnormalities and serious ventricular arrhythmias. Flecainide should be used with caution in patients with known conduction system disturbances because profound bradycardia may develop.[16] Pacing thresholds are significantly elevated by flecainide, and to a greater extent than occurs with other anti-arrhythmics. Encainide has similar effects to flecainide but is less likely to exacerbate cardiac failure.

Since the report of the Cardiac Arrhythmia Suppression Trial in 1989,[17] the use of this group of drugs has altered. In this study, patients with ventricular arrhythmias following myocardial infarction were randomized to receive flecainide, encainide or placebo. Mortality was increased in the treatment groups, possibly as a result of the pro-arrhythmic effects of these agents. As a result, flecainide and encainide are less widely used and there is greater reluctance to use anti-arrhythmic agents in general in the treatment of non-sinister ventricular arrhythmias.

Amiodarone

Amiodarone is structurally similar to tri-iodothyronine and is an effective anti-arrhythmic agent against a wide range of supraventricular, junctional and ventricular arrhythmias. It blocks cardiac sodium and calcium currents and produces a moderate non-competitive block of both α- and β-adrenergic receptors. The major electrophysiological effect is prolongation of the action potential duration and refractory period in atrial and ventricular tissue. It has been postulated that the mechanism of the anti-arrhythmic effect may be due to a direct inhibition of the action of thyroid hormone on the heart.[18] A major advantage of amiodarone compared with other anti-arrhythmic agents is that it is not usually associated with a negative inotropic effect and can therefore be used in patients with impaired ventricular function. However, there are other important side-effects which limit its use. Between 5 and 10% of patients develop pulmonary fibrosis during the first year of treatment. This can be reversed if recognized early, the amiodarone withdrawn and steroid treatment given, but the condition may be rapidly progressive and fatal. Corneal microdeposits are detectable in all patients, but rarely interfere with vision. Hyper- and hypothyroidism may occur, as can a peripheral neuropathy which may be irreversible unless the drug is stopped promptly. Insomnia and nightmares occur commonly, as do photosensitivity and bluish discoloration of exposed areas of skin.

Amiodarone is extremely lipid-soluble; it has a volume of distribution estimated at about 5000 l and a half-life of 7–40 days.[19] The extremely long half-life allows daily dosage but a disadvantage is that the effects are prolonged if discontinuation is required due to the development of an adverse effect. Because of the large volume of distribution, a loading regimen is required when treatment is started. When a rapid onset of effect is required, a high-dose intravenous loading regimen has been used — 5 mg.kg^{-1} over 60 min followed by 15 mg.kg^{-1} over 24 h. The maintenance dose is usually 200 mg daily.

Implications for anaesthesia. When used intravenously, amiodarone may cause hypotension due to ventricular depression[20] and there is the potential for additive effects with β-blockers and calcium antagonists on the depression of sinus node function and myocardial contractility and conduction. During anaesthesia there is the possibility of development of an atropine-resistant bradycardia, myocardial depression and hypotension due to peripheral vasodilatation in patients on chronic amiodarone treatment. The presence of pulmonary fibrosis should be sought pre-operatively. Drug interactions frequently occur due to inhibition of hepatic enzymes; notably, the clearance of warfarin is reduced, with a risk of bleeding. The clearances of digoxin, quinidine, procainamide and flecainide are also reduced.

Bretylium

Bretylium is an adrenergic-neurone blocker with a class III anti-arrhythmic effect. It is used in the treatment of ventricular arrhythmias which are refractory to lignocaine, and is given intravenously. The anti-arrhythmic effects are independent of the adrenergic neurone-blocking effects which cause vasodilatation that may be beneficial in impaired left ventricular function. Bretylium displaces noradrenaline from adrenergic neurones and inhibits its re-uptake. An initial increase in blood pressure is followed by orthostatic hypotension. The effect of exogenous catecholamines is magnified because of the re-uptake inhibition, whereas the effects of indirectly acting sympathomimetic agents, such as ephedrine, are inhibited.

Cardiac glycosides

The extracts of the foxglove have been recognized for many centuries as having beneficial effects in medicine. Digoxin and digitoxin are the only agents in common use; they are used to slow the ventricular rate in atrial fibrillation and flutter, and for their positive inotropic effects in the treatment of congestive cardiac failure. Digoxin exerts its effects both directly on the heart and indirectly via the autonomic nervous system. The mechanism for the positive inotropic effect is inhibition of the myocardial membrane-bound enzyme, Na^+-K^+-ATPase. This leads to an increase in intracellular sodium concentration, which in turn influences transmembrane Na^+–Ca^{2+} exchange, resulting in a rise in intracellular calcium. There is an increased store of calcium in the sarcoplasmic reticulum, and with each depolarization, a greater release of calcium to activate the contractile apparatus. The direct effects of digitalis on the electrophysiological activity of the heart cause an increase in excitability. The resting potential is decreased, which brings the resting potential closer to the threshold and also causes voltage-dependent inactivation of fast Na^+ channels with a decrease in the rate of phase 0 depolarization and a reduction in conduction velocity. The action potential duration is reduced, resulting in a shortening of the effective refractory period. Automaticity is enhanced due to an increase in the rate of phase 4 depolarization and the appearance of calcium-dependent after-depolarizations. Whilst these direct effects are pro-arrhythmic, the beneficial anti-arrhythmic effects of digitalis result from increased vagal tone, which slows conduction through the atrioventricular node, prolonging the effective refractory period of nodal tissue and slowing the ventricular response rate in atrial fibrillation and flutter. As a result of improved cardiac performance, there is also a reflex reduction in sympathetic tone, which may further reduce heart rate.

The toxic effects of digoxin occur when plasma concentrations are high ($>3\,\mu g.l^{-1}$) and include nausea, anorexia, visual disturbances and arrhythmias. Any arrhythmia can be provoked by digoxin toxicity, although heart block and ventricular arrhythmias are particularly common. Hypokalaemia potentiates the effects of digoxin and may cause toxic effects to be seen at therapeutic levels (0.8–$2.2\,\mu g.l^{-1}$). Elimination is mainly by the kidney, with a half-life of about 36 h; dosage should be reduced in the elderly and in the presence of renal impairment. The treatment of digoxin toxicity comprises withdrawal of the drug and correction of hypokalaemia and other electrolyte disturbances. In severe cases, the widespread inhibition of Na^+-K^+-ATPase can cause a dangerous increase in the plasma potassium concentration. Thus, potassium should not be administered until the plasma concentration is known to be low. Lignocaine or phenytoin can be used to treat ventricular arrhythmias, and temporary pacing may be required for severe bradycardia. In life-threatening cases, digoxin-specific antibodies can be administered; these bind both digoxin and digitoxin and decrease the concentration of the free drug in the plasma. The antibody–digoxin complex is eliminated in the urine.

Implications for anaesthesia

In the peri-operative period, the long half-life of digoxin allows omission of a single dose with little adverse consequence. If the return of gastro-intestinal function is delayed, digoxin may be given intravenously, allowing for the fact that oral bio-availability is around 60%. In some patients, digoxin is metabolized by gut bacteria. Treatment with broad-spectrum antibiotics may result in increased plasma concentrations and precipitate toxicity. It is often claimed that cardioversion is contra-indicated in a digitalized patient because of the risk of producing ventricular fibrillation. This is unlikely unless the digoxin concentration is in the toxic range.[21] During anaesthesia, the risk of arrhythmias may be increased, and the patient should be monitored carefully. Calcium must be given with great caution, as it potentiates the arrhythmogenic effects of digoxin.

RESPIRATORY DRUGS

The agents used to treat respiratory disease are of less significance to the anaesthetist than is the underlying disorder. Asthma and chronic obstructive airways disease commonly present as incidental findings in the pre-operative interview. Together with the clinical history, pulmonary function tests and other investigations, the extent of drug treatment often provides a clue to the severity of the disease.

β_2-Adrenoceptor agonists

Bronchodilators may be used in the treatment of acute attacks of bronchospasm. The selective β_2-agonists such as salbutamol, terbutaline, pirbuterol and rimiterol act on bronchial smooth-muscle receptors causing relaxation and bronchodilation. These agents may be given by aerosol inhalation, allowing maximal bronchodilation at lower systemic concentrations with fewer adverse effects. At high systemic concentrations, these agents have β_1 effects and may cause tachycardia, arrhythmias and tremor. Prolonged use can result in tolerance due to receptor down-regulation and patients with more severe disease are usually receiving additional therapy.

Anticholinergics

Ipratropium is an anticholinergic agent which causes bronchodilation. The drug is particularly useful in chronic obstructive airways disease, when it is given by metered dose inhaler or nebulizer. It is a quaternary anticholinergic agent which causes minimal systemic side-effects and, unlike atropine, does not cause thickening of bronchial secretions and inhibition of mucociliary clearance.

Theophylline

Theophylline is a methylxanthine which is closely related to caffeine and is a bronchodilator. Theophylline itself has low solubility in water and it is administered as the ethylenediamine salt, aminophylline, which is water-soluble. The mechanism of theophylline-induced bronchodilation is not clear. At higher concentrations than occur in vivo, theophylline inhibits the enzyme phosphodiesterase. This increases the intracellular concentration of the second messengers AMP and cyclic guanosine monophosphate (GMP), which give rise to smooth-muscle relaxation. Other possible mechanisms of action are the potentiation of catecholamine release and competitive antagonism at adenosine receptors. The latter effect occurs at concentrations within the therapeutic range.

The methylxanthines have significant effects on many other systems. Theophylline and caffeine are potent central nervous system stimulants. As the plasma concentration increases, anxiety, restlessness, insomnia, tremor and convulsions occur. The sensitivity of the respiratory centre to carbon dioxide is increased and theophyllines have been used in the treatment of neonatal apnoea. There is an increase in myocardial contractility, and at higher concentrations, tachycardia and other arrhythmias can occur. The effect on peripheral vascular resistance is variable and may be modified by autonomic reflexes, but cerebrovascular resistance is increased, with a decrease in cerebral blood flow. Theophylline has a diuretic effect.

The therapeutic index of theophylline is low. The effective plasma concentration range is 10–20 mg.l^{-1} and serious central nervous system and cardiac toxicity can occur at levels above 20 mg.l^{-1}. Clearance is reduced in cirrhosis, cardiac failure, cor pulmonale and following treatment with drugs which inhibit hepatic enzymes including cimetidine, erythromycin and the oral contraceptive pill. Infusion rates and dosage may need to be reduced in these situations. Nausea and vomiting, anorexia, anxiety and tremor are signs of mild toxicity; arrhythmias and convulsions occur at higher plasma concentrations. The measurement of plasma concentration is a useful guide to determining optimal dosage.

Corticosteroids

Asthma is an inflammatory disease and corticosteroids are useful in the treatment of acute attacks and for long-term control of the disease. For long-term use, administration by inhalation is effective and avoids the side-effects of long-term systemic steroids. Oral *Candida* infection and hoarseness are side-effects of inhaled steroid therapy. This route of administration is unlikely to cause adrenal suppression but consideration should be given to providing peri-operative steroid cover for patients who are receiving high-dose inhaled steroid (greater than 1.5 mg beclomethasone per day).

Implications for anaesthesia

Patients should take their normal medication up to the time of surgery and should be asked to bring their normal inhaler to theatre with them on the day of surgery. All the volatile anaesthetics are bronchodilators to a similar degree but instrumentation of the upper airway and some adjuvant drugs given during anaesthesia, for example tubocurarine, may result in an increase in airway resistance. If a β_2-agonist or theophylline is administered acutely during anaesthesia, it is safer to avoid halothane, which potentiates the arrhythmic effects of these agents. Ketamine is also a bronchodilator, but its sympathomimetic effects may give rise to arrhythmias in the presence of β_2-agonists or theophylline. Chronic oral steroid ingestion requires steroid cover for the operative period.

CENTRAL NERVOUS SYSTEM

It is not surprising that drugs prescribed for their effect on the central nervous system often have significant interactions with anaesthetic agents. Hypnotics and other sedative agents may potentiate the anaesthetic effect, although long-term use of these agents may produce some degree of tolerance to anaesthetic agents. Many of the drugs used in psychiatric practice affect neuronal transmission involving catecholamines, and have significant cardiovascular side-effects.

Antidepressants

Tricyclic antidepressants

Imipramine was the first drug with a three-ring (*tricyclic*) molecular structure found to be effective in depression. Other structurally related compounds with similar action include amitriptyline, dothiepin, doxepin, desipramine, clomipramine, trimipramine and lofepramine. Some antidepressants which do not have a tricyclic structure have similar effects; these include mianserin, maprotiline and trazodone. These agents are thought to exert their clinical effect by blocking the re-uptake of noradrenaline and/or serotonin (5-hydroxytryptamine; 5-HT) into nerve terminals in the central nervous system. There is immediate blockade of amine uptake but the antidepressant effect is not apparent for several weeks and appears to correlate with changes in adrenergic receptor population and sensitivity. Tricyclic antidepressants also have antimuscarinic effects, weak α_1-antagonist activity and some antihistamine effects. The side-effect profile of the individual agents is determined by the potency of these other effects.

Common side-effects resulting from the antimuscarinic action of the tricyclics are dry mouth, blurred vision, constipation and urinary retention. Rarely, glaucoma can be precipitated. Sedation is a feature of several of these agents, notably amitriptyline. Confusion or delirium can occur and is more common in the elderly. A fine tremor is common, and the seizure threshold is reduced. Postural hypotension occurs and a sinus tachycardia results from the antimuscarinic action and inhibition of noradrenaline re-uptake. There is a quinidine-like prolongation of intracardiac conduction, and direct myocardial depression. The ECG may show flattening or inversion of the T waves and prolongation of the PR interval, QRS and QT times. This may be particularly dangerous in the presence of pre-existing conduction defects, when ventricular arrhythmias may be precipitated.

Overdose of tricyclic antidepressants is common and life-threatening. Symptoms include agitation, delirium, seizures, coma, respiratory depression, hypotension and cardiac arrhythmias. Ventilation may be required. Digoxin and drugs which prolong cardiac conduction, such as quinidine and procainamide, are contraindicated. Phenytoin, propranolol and lignocaine have been used safely for the treatment of tricyclic-induced arrhythmias. Temporary pacing may be required for bradyarrhythmias.

Implications for anaesthesia. During anaesthesia, there may be increased potential for the development of ventricular arrhythmias, particularly if halothane is used. The ECG should be monitored and hypercapnia avoided. Inhibition of neuronal uptake may cause the effects of exogenous adrenaline and noradrenaline to be dangerously potentiated, resulting in severe hypertension and arrhythmias. It is possible that tricyclics will block the entry of indirectly acting sympathomimetics such as ephedrine into the nerve terminal, with inhibition of the vasopressor effects. If a vasopressor is required, methoxamine is the drug of choice. Felypressin can be used for topical vasoconstriction with local anaesthesia. The antihypertensive effect of guanethidine is blocked, as is the centrally mediated antihypertensive effect of clonidine.

Selective serotonin re-uptake inhibitors

Fluoxetine, fluvoxamine and paroxetine belong to a newer class of antidepressant with similar efficacy to the tricyclic antidepressants.[22] They are often better tolerated because they cause fewer anticholinergic side-effects and less sedation than the tricyclics. The commonest side-effect is nausea, which is usually self-limiting. They have fewer cardiovascular effects, and are less toxic in overdose. Serious drug interactions have been reported between selective serotonin uptake inhibitors and monoamine oxidase inhibitors (MAOIs — see below), tryptophan and lithium.[23]

Monoamine oxidase inhibitors

MAOIs have been used for the treatment of depression since 1957 after it was noticed that the antituberculous agent iproniazid had mood-elevating effects. Iproniazid was withdrawn because of hepatotoxicity, but the related agents phenelzine, isocarboxazid and tranylcypromine are in current use. These drugs have dangerous and unpredictable interactions with other drugs and food-derived amines and became used less frequently when other effective, less dangerous antidepressants were developed. MAOIs are used when tricyclics have not been effective or cannot be tolerated. They are also useful in anxiety states, phobias and neurotic conditions. The enzyme monoamine oxidase (MAO) is located in mitochondrial membranes of neuronal and most other tissues, where it acts to regulate the monoamine levels. Lung, liver and kidney have high MAO content so the intestine and liver play an important role in inactivating food-derived monoamines such as tyramine and phenylethanolamine, which have an indirect sympathomimetic action. Inhibition of MAO can result in dangerous hypertension if foods containing these substances are ingested. Patients who are taking MAOIs are issued with a treatment card and advised to avoid cheese, pickled herring, broad beans, yeast extracts, game and alcoholic drinks. Cough mixtures and cold remedies often contain sympathomimetics and must also be avoided.

There are two types of monoamine oxidase (A and B) based on their relative affinity for different substrates. The MAOIs in current use are non-selective, irreversible inhibitors which form a stable covalent complex with the enzyme. It is the inhibition of MAO-A which appears to be necessary for the antidepressant action; selegiline, a selective MAO-B inhibitor used in the treatment of Parkinson's disease, has no antidepressant activity. Within a few hours of administration of an MAOI, the brain content of noradrenaline and dopamine approximately doubles and the synthesis of byproducts, such as octopamine, increases by up to 30 times. However, the therapeutic effect is delayed by 2 or more weeks, probably as a result of adaptation to the raised monoamine levels by changes in the receptor numbers and sensitivity. There is down-regulation of β-receptors, both in number and functional activity, and also α_1 and α_2-adrenoceptors and 5-HT receptors. The overall effect is a reduction in sympathetic outflow, with lower blood pressure and postural hypotension. However, the increased cytoplasmic concentrations of amines may give rise to dangerous hypertensive crises if they are displaced from neurones by an indirectly acting sympathomimetic. Toxicity due to overdosage of an MAOI can cause agitation, hallucinations, hyperpyrexia, hyperreflexia, convulsions and hypo- or hypertension. Hepatic parenchymal damage can occur at normal dosage but is rare with currently used agents. Postural hypotension, dizziness, headache, fatigue, dry mouth and constipation are common side-effects. The MAOIs also inhibit hepatic microsomal enzymes which are involved in the metabolism of many other drugs and this can cause significant potentiation of the effects of central nervous system-depressant agents including anaesthetic agents, opioids and anticholinergic drugs.

Implications for anaesthesia

There have been many reports of serious and sometimes fatal drug interactions with MAOIs, including some with drugs commonly used during anaesthesia. The tricyclic antidepressants, selective serotonin re-uptake inhibitors and pethidine have been reported to interact with the MAOIs to produce a life-threatening excitatory response characterized by hyperpyrexia, agitation, convulsions and coma. Either hyper- or hypotension may occur. The likely mechanism for this reaction is an increase in cerebral 5-HT content which is potentiated by the antidepressants and pethidine which have a 5-HT re-uptake blocking action. Because of the irreversible nature of enzyme inhibition by MAOIs, the danger of interaction persists for 2 weeks after treatment has been discontinued. It is recommended that other antidepressants are not given during this period. A fatal hyperpyrexic reaction has been reported with dextromethorphan, an opioid which also blocks neuronal 5-HT uptake, and which is found in some cough mixtures.[24] As well as the excitatory MAOI–opioid interaction, a reaction may occur, consisting of respiratory depression, hypotension and coma which is due to the inhibition of the hepatic enzymes responsible for degradation of the opioid, causing an exaggeration of the opioid effect. This is less dangerous, and can be treated with naloxone and supportive measures. It should be avoided by using small incremental doses of opioid. Morphine has not been reported to cause an excitatory response but has been associated with prolonged action in patients receiving MAOIs. Fentanyl has been used during anaesthesia, and postoperatively, with no problems. Methadone has been given safely with tranylcypromine for a period of 3 months. Papaveretum has caused a depressive response when given as premedication and is probably best avoided as it contains a mixture of narcotic alkaloids and offers little advantage over morphine. Centrally acting anticholinergic agents are potentiated by MAOIs and hyperpyrexia has been reported in animals. These agents are best avoided as premedicants.

Induction of anaesthesia with thiopentone has been used safely, although animal studies have demonstrated potentiation of the effects of barbiturates as a result of hepatic enzyme inhibition. Phenelzine, but not other MAOIs, may reduce serum cholinesterase concentrations, causing prolongation of the effect of suxamethonium. No interactions have been reported with non-depolarizing relaxants. Indirectly acting sympathomimetic agents used during anaesthesia may cause serious hypertension. Hypertensive reactions have been reported with ephedrine, metaraminol, methylamphetamine, phenylephrine, levodopa, dopamine and phenylpropranolamine. Directly acting sympathomimetic amines do not provoke such a severe hypertensive response but their effects may be enhanced by receptor hypersensitivity and reduced breakdown. If treatment is required for anaesthetic-induced hypotension which does not respond to intravenous fluids, a directly acting agent such as methoxamine should be used in reduced dosage of about one-third of normal, with careful titration to effect. Hypertensive crises should be treated with intravenous phentolamine, an α-adrenoceptor antagonist.

Hydralazine or sodium nitroprusside may also be used. Chlorpromazine, an α-blocker, has antihypertensive, antipyretic and cerebral depressant actions, and has been used in the treatment of excitatory reactions. The serious and unpredictable nature of interactions between MAOIs and other drugs, notably opioid analgesics and sympathomimetics, has led to the recommendation that MAOIs should be discontinued at least 2 weeks before surgery. However, this practice also carries risks; the severely depressed patient may not tolerate withdrawal of medication and the effects of MAOIs may take longer than 2 weeks to resolve.

Given a full understanding of the actions of MAOIs and possible drug interactions which may occur, the peri-operative period can be managed safely.[25,26] General guidelines include the absolute avoidance of pethidine. Fentanyl and morphine can be used with an awareness that their effects may be potentiated. Frequent monitoring of blood pressure should be employed. Regional techniques are alternative methods of providing analgesia but hypotension caused by spinal or epidural anaesthesia may be a problem; this should be treated with intravenous fluids initially, and if necessary with small doses of a directly acting drug such as methoxamine.

Antipsychotic drugs

Agents used in the treatment of schizophrenia and other psychiatric disorders include the phenothiazines, thioxanthines and butyrophenones. They relieve psychotic symptoms such as hallucinations, delusions and agitation and cause emotional flattening, indifference and psychomotor slowing by blockade of central dopaminergic receptors. Action at the chemoreceptor trigger zone produces an anti-emetic effect. The butyrophenones, haloperidol and droperidol, are also used in combination with a potent opioid to produce neuroleptanalgesia and neuroleptanaesthesia. These agents also have variable degrees of antihistamine activity, anticholinergic actions and α_1-antagonist properties which may be used if desirable, but which may cause troublesome side-effects. The dopamine antagonism often gives rise to extrapyramidal side-effects which consist of drug-induced parkinsonism, acute dystonia, akathisia (motor restlessness) and tardive dyskinesia. The seizure threshold is lowered and fits may be precipitated in poorly controlled epileptics. α-blockade can result in orthostatic hypotension and increased susceptibility to hypothermia. There is a quinidine-like action on the heart which may produce ECG changes and exacerbate pre-existing conduction disturbances. Hyperprolactinaemia can cause galactorrhoea, gynaecomastia and amenorrhoea. Chlorpromazine has caused cholestatic jaundice and there is a risk of blood dyscrasias, including agranulocytosis. Skin reactions can occur and there is often photosensitivity.

The neuroleptic malignant syndrome (NMS) is a rare but potentially fatal side-effect of these agents.[27] It has been reported in association with a large number of neuroleptics, including haloperidol, chlorpromazine and flupenthixol. NMS consists of a state of hyperthermia, fluctuating consciousness, muscular rigidity and autonomic instability which develops over 24–72 h. It differs from malignant hyperpyrexia in that the syndrome is centrally mediated and not due to a defect in skeletal muscle calcium ion control. NMS has been reported in an intensive care patient who was receiving chlorpromazine.[28] It should be considered in the differential diagnosis of severe pyrexia when the patient is receiving neuroleptics or anti-emetic therapy. The characteristic rigidity is masked if the muscles are paralysed to facilitate ventilation. Dantrolene has been used in the treatment of NMS to reduce muscle tone, together with the centrally acting dopamine agonist bromocriptine and discontinuation of the antipsychotic agent.

Despite the large number of side-effects, antipsychotic agents generally cause few problems during anaesthesia. There may be potentiation of the sedative and hypotensive effects of anaesthetics. The α-blockade may produce increased liability to hypothermia and reduced ability to compensate for hypovolaemia. When taken as an overdose, the drugs are rarely lethal because the therapeutic index, or ratio of toxic dose to therapeutic dose, is very high.

Lithium

Lithium is used for the treatment of acute mania, and the prevention of recurrent manic-depressive illness, although the mechanism of action is unknown. Lithium has a very low therapeutic index and plasma concentrations must be monitored carefully during initiation of treatment, and regularly during maintenance. Plasma concentration should be 0.8–1.2 mmol.l^{-1} for the treatment of mania, although 0–4–0.8 mmol.l^{-1} is effective for prophylaxis. Toxicity occurs at concentrations above 1.5 mmol.l^{-1}. The drug is given in the form of lithium carbonate or lithium citrate tablets or syrup, which are well-absorbed orally; usual doses range from 900 mg to 2 g per day. Slow-release preparations are given to avoid high peak plasma concentrations.

Symptoms of mild toxicity include nausea and vomiting, abdominal pain, diarrhoea, sedation and fine tremor; at high plasma concentrations confusion occurs, progressing to hyperreflexia, seizures, focal neurological signs, coma and cardiac arrhythmias, which can be fatal. A diffuse goitre may develop due to inhibition of the synthesis of thyroxine. Rarely, hypothyroidism occurs. The goitre regresses after discontinuation of lithium or with the administration of thyroxine. Polyuria and polydipsia may occur and are caused by inhibition of the effect of antidiuretic hormone on the kidneys, inducing a nephrogenic diabetes insipidus. The ECG may show T-wave depression and widening of the QRS complex. There may be an increase in the number of circulating neutrophils.

Implications for anaesthesia

Lithium prolongs the action of suxamethonium and some non-depolarizing neuromuscular blockers, possibly by inhibiting presynaptic acetylcholine synthesis or release.[29] Neuromuscular function must be monitored closely with a nerve stimulator when these drugs are used in a patient who is taking lithium. The fluid restriction and hormonal changes associated with anaesthesia and surgery may precipitate lithium toxicity. Lithium is conserved with sodium during dehydration and if lithium-induced polyuria is present, dehydration may occur in the peri-operative period. Intravenous fluids should be given while oral intake is restricted. It is recommended that lithium is stopped 48–72 h before elective surgery to reduce the risk of toxicity and avoid interaction with muscle relaxants. If lithium therapy is stopped for a long period following surgery acute mania may occur; consequently, it should be restarted as soon as possible provided that fluid and electrolyte balance are stable. Acute toxicity is treated with intravenous saline to encourage diuresis. An osmotic diuretic such as mannitol increases excretion, and in severe cases haemodialysis may be required.

Benzodiazepines

The benzodiazepines have sedative, anxiolytic, anticonvulsant and muscle-relaxant effects. They are widely used as hypnotics, as premedicants, in the treatment of acute anxiety and for muscle spasm associated with musculoskeletal injury. Intravenous preparations are used to induce anaesthesia or to provide sedation during regional anaesthesia or endoscopic procedures, when their amnesic effect is valuable. Benzodiazepines act at a specific receptor in the central nervous system and potentiate the effect of the inhibitory neurotransmitter γ-hydroxybutyric acid (GABA). The nature and function of the natural ligand for the benzodiazepine receptor are not known.

The benzodiazepines have been classified into three groups according to their duration of action:

1. long-acting, including diazepam, flunitrazepam, nitrazepam and chlordiazepoxide;
2. medium-acting, including lorazepam, temazepam and oxazepam;
3. short-acting, including midazolam, triazolam and lormetazepam.

Diazepam and several other agents have a common active metabolite, desmethyldiazepam (nordiazepam), which has a prolonged half-life of up to 200 h; this may be responsible for the hangover effect often seen with these agents and for accumulation after repeated doses.

The longer-acting drugs are used in the treatment of anxiety and dependence can occur after several weeks. Withdrawal symptoms include anxiety, agitation, irritability, confusion, sweating, tremors and convulsions if large doses have been taken over prolonged periods. Because of the problems of dependence, it is recommended that anxiolytic treatment is limited to the lowest possible dose for the shortest possible time.[30] Chronic benzodiazepine therapy should be weaned gradually.

When taken in overdose, the benzodiazepines do not cause severe respiratory or cardiovascular depression and are rarely fatal unless other agents are taken at the same time. They are relatively safe drugs and have virtually replaced the barbiturates for use as sedative–hypnotics. Zopiclone is structurally distinct from benzodiazepines but has a similar spectrum of therapeutic applications. It also acts at the GABA receptor, but apparently at a site distinct from that of benzodiazepines; it is this mechanistic distinction that has led to the suggestion that zopiclone is less likely to cause dependence.

Anticonvulsants

Phenytoin, carbamazepine and sodium valproate are the first-line drugs for the treatment of generalized or partial seizures. Phenobarbitone, primidone, clonazepam and vigabatrin are also effective but tend to cause more sedative side-effects. Absence seizures or petit mal respond best to ethosuximide or sodium valproate. The mechanism of action of anticonvulsants is not fully understood. Some, like the benzodiazepines, potentiate the action of GABA, the main inhibitory neurotransmitter in the central nervous system. Others, including phenytoin, phenobarbitone and sodium valproate, cause membrane hyperpolarization by altering ion gradients. Most anticonvulsants have a narrow therapeutic range and care must be taken to achieve control of the epilepsy without producing toxicity.

Phenytoin, sodium valproate and carbamazepine are highly protein-bound. Thus, reduction in plasma protein concentrations or competition for binding sites with other agents such as aspirin, sulphonamides, warfarin and sulphonylureas can precipitate toxicity. Metabolism of the anticonvulsant agents occurs in the liver. Several of these agents are potent enzyme inducers which can reduce their own plasma half-life and those of other agents, causing a reduction in clinical effect. The addition of agents such as cimetidine, chloramphenicol, erythromycin and allopurinol, which inhibit hepatic enzymes, may give rise to higher, potentially toxic levels of anticonvulsant agent. Several haematological abnormalities may be associated with anticonvulsant therapy. Phenytoin and phenobarbitone can cause depletion of folate and lead to megaloblastic anaemia or peripheral neuropathy. During pregnancy, vitamin K deficiency may develop and cause bleeding at delivery or in the neonate. Leukopenia and, rarely, agranulocytosis can occur with phenytoin, carbamazepine, ethosuximide and sodium valproate. Sodium valproate can cause thrombocytopenia and inhibition of platelet aggregation, giving rise to prolongation of the bleeding time.

Implications for anaesthesia

Abrupt withdrawal of anticonvulsant therapy has a high risk of precipitating convulsions and it is important to continue treatment throughout the peri-operative period. If it is not possible to restart oral therapy, phenytoin, phenobarbitone and sodium valproate may be given intravenously. Conversely, the disruption during the operative period may precipitate anticonvulsant toxicity. Drug interactions or temporary hepatic dysfunction may cause an increase in plasma concentration, leading to delayed recovery from anaesthesia and other signs of toxicity. Phenytoin and carbamazepine cause resistance to the action of non-depolarizing muscle relaxants;[31] the mechanism for this is unclear.

Antiparkinsonian drugs

Parkinson's disease is caused by a deficiency of dopaminergic transmission in the basal ganglia. There is a resulting excess of cholinergic activity. The two main strategies for therapy aim to increase dopaminergic transmission or to reduce muscarinic cholinergic activity with cholinergic antagonists.

Levodopa is the most effective treatment for Parkinson's disease. Dopamine does not cross the blood–brain barrier, but levodopa, which is its immediate precursor, does, and is converted to dopamine by L-amino acid decarboxylase. A peripherally acting decarboxylase inhibitor is usually given in conjunction with levodopa, allowing a reduction in dose and significantly reducing peripheral side-effects. Decarboxylase inhibitors include carbidopa and benserazide and are combined with levodopa as Sinemet and Madopar. Levodopa is started gradually to allow the development of tolerance to unwanted side-effects. It produces significant reductions in bradykinesia, tremor and rigidity and improves overall functional ability. Abnormal involuntary movements and psychiatric disturbance may limit dosage or necessitate discontinuation of treatment. Nausea and vomiting commonly occur. Postural hypotension is due to a central effect of dopamine, but if levodopa is given without a decarboxylase inhibitor, the peripheral action of dopamine can cause hypertension, cardiac arrhythmias and increased cardiac contractility. These cardiac effects can be inhibited with a β-blocker, although tolerance does occur with chronic levodopa therapy.

Dopamine agonists, such as bromocriptine and lisuride, are centrally acting dopamine agonists which exert their effect at surviving dopamine receptors. They are used when levodopa alone is not effective or cannot be tolerated. Side-effects of nausea and vomiting, postural hypotension and involuntary movements may be troublesome. Amantadine has modest antiparkinsonian effects and, although only a minority of patients derive significant benefit from it, the drug is relatively free from side-effects.

Selegiline is an MAO-B inhibitor. It increases central nervous system levels of dopamine and is used in conjunction with levodopa. It does not exhibit the dangerous interactions with certain drugs and foodstuffs that occur with the non-specific MAOIs.

Anticholinergic agents used in the treatment of Parkinson's disease include benzhexol, orphenidrine, benztropine and procyclidine. They are less effective than levodopa when used alone, but may be used in patients with mild symptoms or in conjunction with levodopa, when they produce further improvement. These drugs are also used in the treatment of the parkinsonian syndrome caused by antipsychotic drugs, and in acute dystonic reactions. Mental confusion may occur, and peripheral side-effects include dry mouth, cycloplegia, constipation and urinary retention.

Implications for anaesthesia

Peripheral side-effects of dopamine are minimized by the co-administration of a decarboxylase inhibitor with levodopa but cardiac arrhythmias and hypertension may occur. Phenothiazines, butyrophenones and other agents such as metoclopramide, which have an anti-dopaminergic effect, can exacerbate Parkinson's disease and should be avoided.[32] Medication should be re-started as soon as possible after surgery to avoid deterioration in mobility. L-Dopa is available as an intravenous preparation if the return of gastro-intestinal function is delayed but there is no intravenous formulation of a peripheral decarboxylase inhibitor.

ENDOCRINE

Corticosteroids

Patients may be taking replacement doses of corticosteroids if they have adrenal or pituitary failure but more commonly take a glucocorticoid for its anti-inflammatory or immunosuppressive effect. These agents are used in a wide range of clinical conditions. Equivalent doses of the commonly used corticosteroids are shown in Table 3.4.

Physiological levels of adrenal corticosteroids are essential for normal homeostasis and are met by the secretion of 20–30 mg of cortisol (hydrocortisone) per 24 h. At times of stress, secretion is increased up to 150 mg per day. The administration of exogenous corticosteroids in a dose exceeding 7.5 mg prednisolone for longer than a week can cause suppression of the hypothalamo–pituitary–adrenal axis which may persist for several months after cessation of treatment. Sudden withdrawal of steroid treatment may precipitate acute adrenal insufficiency and there is an inability to mount increased levels of secretion at times of stress, such as surgery or infection. Deaths attributed to adrenal insufficiency have been reported in the peri-operative period.[33] Consequently, it is important to provide peri-operative corticosteroid cover.

Patients who are on long-term corticosteroid therapy usually have a medical disorder of significance to the anaesthetist. In addition, side-effects of treatment should be considered. Most corticosteroids have a mild mineralocorticoid effect, causing sodium and water retention, potassium loss and metabolic alkalosis. There is impaired glucose tolerance, and diabetes mellitus may be precipitated. With long-term use, osteoporosis and muscle wasting may develop and the skin and veins become extremely fragile. Peptic ulceration is associated with corticosteroid therapy, and clinical signs of peritonism and sepsis are often masked. The immunosuppression leads to increased susceptibility to infection. A suitable regimen for peri-operative steroid cover should mimic the cortisol response to surgery in normal subjects. Following major surgery, cortisol secretion increases to 75–150 mg per day and returns to normal levels after 72 h unless there are post-operative complications. Minor surgery produces a minimal increase in cortisol levels on the day of surgery. A regimen utilizing hydrocortisone 100 mg intramuscularly pre-operatively and 100 mg intramuscularly every 6 or 8 h for 3 days following major surgery has been widely used.[34] Such a regimen is effective in avoiding adrenal insufficiency, but these large doses may have undesirable effects, including increased susceptibility to infection, impaired wound healing, hyperglycaemia and electrolyte disturbances. A low-dose regimen of hydrocortisone 25 mg intravenously on induction followed by 100 mg infused over 24 h produces cortisol levels similar to those which occur in normal subjects undergoing major surgery.[35] Napolitano & Chernow recommend a protocol using smaller doses of intravenous hydrocortisone — 25 mg pre-operatively, 100 mg intra-operatively, 50 mg every 8 h for the first 24 h postoperatively and 25 mg every 8 h subsequently, tapering down to the usual dose of oral corticosteroid when gastro-intestinal function returns.[36] For minor surgery, a single dose of hydrocortisone is sufficient. Signs of adrenocortical insufficiency include vomiting and cardiovascular collapse. Larger doses of hydrocortisone should be given if this is suspected. Full anti-inflammatory doses may be required for treatment of the primary condition if it deteriorates during the peri-operative period.

Oral hypoglycaemic agents

The oral hypoglycaemic agents are used in conjunction with diet to control hyperglycaemia in non-insulin-dependent diabetes mellitus. The most commonly used agents are the sulphonylureas, whose half-lives and dosage ranges are shown in Table 3.5. Metformin is a biguanide which is available in the UK and Europe.

Table 3.4 Equivalent doses of corticosteroids

Drug	Equivalent anti-inflammatory dose (mg)	Mineralocorticoid effect
Hydrocortisone	100	Weak
Cortisone acetate	125	Weak
Prednisolone	25	Very weak
Methylprednisolone	20	Very weak
Betamethasone	4	Negligible
Dexamethasone	4	Negligible
Fludrocortisone	8	Very strong

Table 3.5 Half-lives and daily doses of the sulphonylureas

Drug	Half-life (h)	Daily dose
Chlorpropamide	33	100–500 mg o.d.
Glibenclamide	5–8	5–15 mg o.d.
Glicazide	12	40–160 mg o.d.
Glipizide	2–4	2.5–40 mg divided doses
Gliquidone	1.5	15–18 mg divided doses
Tolazamide	7	100 mg–1 g divided doses
Tolbutamide	5	500 mg–2 g divided doses
Metformin	1.5–3	500 mg–1 g 8-hourly

o.d. = once daily

The sulphonylureas act mainly by increasing insulin secretion from the pancreas. During long-term administration, they also increase the sensitivity of peripheral tissues to insulin. They have no hypoglycaemic action if there is no pancreatic β-cell function. These agents are metabolized by the liver and the metabolites are excreted by the kidney. Care must be taken to avoid precipitating hypoglycaemia in hepatic or renal impairment. A significant fraction of chlorpropamide is excreted unchanged by the kidney and this drug is therefore contra-indicated in renal failure.

Common side-effects include nausea and vomiting, headaches and a transient rash which may rarely progress to erythema multiforme or exfoliative dermatitis. Very rarely, blood dyscrasias such as thrombocytopenia, agranulocytosis and aplastic anaemia may occur. Chlorpropamide causes unpleasant facial flushing with alcohol and can enhance the effect of antidiuretic hormone on the renal collecting duct, causing hyponatraemia. Hypoglycaemia may be precipitated by an overdose of the sulphonylureas, by drug interactions with agents which inhibit hepatic enzymes or interactions with other highly protein-bound drugs such as aspirin, sulphonamides and warfarin which transiently increase the free concentration of hypoglycaemic agent.

Metformin is the only available biguanide. Phenformin was withdrawn because it was associated with an increased incidence of lactic acidosis. Metformin inhibits hepatic gluconeogenesis, increases peripheral utilization of glucose and inhibits the absorption of glucose by the gut. It does not cause hypoglycaemia in normal subjects. Metformin is completely excreted by the kidney and is contra-indicated in renal failure, when lactic acidosis may occur.

Implications for anaesthesia

Patients who are taking oral hypoglycaemic agents are at risk of developing hypoglycaemia during a period of peri-operative starvation. This risk is especially great with long-acting drugs such as chlorpropamide. For minor surgery, the oral hypoglycaemic agent should be omitted on the morning of surgery and in the case of chlorpropamide, also on the day before surgery. The blood sugar concentration must be monitored regularly to detect hypoglycaemia, and solutions containing glucose should not be infused because they cause hyperglycaemia. The oral hypoglycaemic agent can be restarted when the patient starts to eat. For major surgery when a more prolonged period of fasting is anticipated, the oral hypoglycaemic is omitted as above and the diabetes is managed peri-operatively with short-acting insulin and an infusion of glucose.

Insulin

Insulin is essential for the treatment of type 1 diabetics (insulin-dependent diabetes mellitus) and is also used in non-insulin-dependent diabetes mellitus when oral hypoglycaemic agents are unable to produce good control, or to cope with the disturbances which accompany acute illnesses or the peri-operative period.

In the past, insulin was only available from animal pancreatic extract. Bovine insulin has three amino acid differences and porcine insulin has one amino acid difference from human insulin. Human insulin can be produced by enzymatic modification of porcine insulin or by recombinant DNA techniques. Preparations of insulin may be classified as short-, intermediate- or long-acting. Short-acting insulins are soluble, regular or neutral insulin. When injected subcutaneously, onset of action occurs in about 30 min, with the peak effect at 2–4 h. It may also be given intravenously, when the onset is immediate, the half-life is 5 min and its effect disappears after 30 min. Longer-acting insulin preparations are designed to dissolve more gradually when injected subcutaneously. Intermediate-acting preparations include isophane insulin, a suspension of insulin with protamine, and lente insulin or insulin zinc suspension. After subcutaneous administration onset of action occurs in 1–2 h with a peak effect at 6–12 h. Long-acting insulins are insulin zinc suspension (crystalline) or ultralente, and protamine zinc insulin. The long duration of action makes them suitable for daily administration and they are particularly suitable for elderly patients. These longer-acting insulin preparations are cloudy and cannot be given intravenously. Most patients receive a combination of a longer-acting insulin with soluble insulin to cover meals. In the UK, all insulin preparations are presented in a strength of 100 units.ml^{-1} to avoid confusion over dosage. Human insulin is less immunogenic than other insulins but allergic reactions may occur to minor contaminants or to protamine or zinc used in the formulation. Antibody formation may result in insulin resistance, requiring extremely large doses for treatment.

During the peri-operative period, it is necessary to maintain insulin treatment to allow peripheral glucose metabolism to continue. Without insulin, fat is employed as an alternative energy source and the production of ketones causes acidosis. Hyperglycaemia produces an osmotic diuresis, with dehydration and electrolyte depletion. A regimen for peri-operative management should provide insulin, with an infusion of glucose to prevent hypoglycaemia; the blood sugar concentration must be monitored closely. The insulin and glucose may be given separately or combined in the same bag as in the Alberti regimen.[37]

Thyroxine and antithyroid drugs

Patients with hypothyroidism receive replacement therapy with thyroxine. The usual maintenance dose is 100–200 µg daily. Thyroxine is highly bound to plasma proteins and has a half-life of 6–7 days, so that a brief interruption of therapy during the peri-operative period is insignificant. Before elective surgery, plasma thyroxine and thyroid-stimulating hormone concentrations should be measured to ensure that there is adequate replacement. L-tri-iodothyronine is more potent than thyroxine, has a quicker onset of action and a shorter half-life. A dose of 20 µg is equivalent to 100 µg of thyroxine. It is indicated for the treatment of severe hypothyroid states when a rapid response is required. It can be given orally or by intravenous injection in the treatment of hypothyroid coma.

Patients with hyperthyroidism should be rendered clinically euthyroid with antithyroid drugs or radioactive iodine before they undergo surgery — otherwise there is the danger of precipitating a thyrotoxic crisis. The antithyroid drugs in use are the thioureas, propylthiouracil and carbimazole. They inhibit the synthesis of thyroid hormones by interfering with the iodination of the tyrosyl residues of thyroglobulin and the coupling of the iodotyrosyl residues. There is a delay in onset of clinical effect until stores of thyroid hormone are depleted. When a euthyroid state has been achieved, the dose is reduced to approximately one-third and maintained for 12–18 months unless surgery is planned. Hypothyroidism may be induced, and thyroxine replacement is then required. These sulphur-containing drugs commonly cause an urticarial rash, which often disappears spontaneously but may necessitate a change to another drug. A more serious side-effect, occurring in 0.1–0.5% of patients, is the development of agranulocytosis. Patients should be warned to report any sore throat or fever immediately. The drug should be discontinued immediately if there is clinical or laboratory evidence of neutropenia.

Iodide has a temporary effect on the thyroid gland, inhibiting synthesis and release of thyroxine. It can be used in hyperthyroidism when its effect is seen within 24 h and is maximal in 10–15 days, after which the symptoms gradually return. Lugol's solution is iodine 5% and potassium iodide 10% in water. It is given most often for 10 days before surgery after a euthyroid state has been attained using antithyroid drugs; it reduces the vascularity of the gland and makes surgery technically easier. Iodide is also given in conjunction with propranolol and antithyroid drugs in the treatment of thyrotoxic crisis. Propranolol should be used to control the symptoms of hyperthyroidism if urgent surgery is required.

Oral contraceptive and hormone replacement therapy

There is laboratory and clinical evidence which suggests that women taking the combined oestrogen–progestogen oral contraceptive pill (OCP) are at increased risk of developing postoperative venous thrombo-embolism.[38] The synthetic oestrogen, ethinyloestradiol, causes an increased activity of coagulation factors II, VII, X, XII and fibrinogen and a reduction in the activity of the naturally occurring anticoagulant antithrombin III. For this reason, it is recommended that the OCP be discontinued 4 weeks before major elective surgery or any surgery to the legs, and alternative contraceptive arrangements be made.[39] This is not necessary for minor surgery where early ambulation is anticipated or for women taking the progestogen-only pill, which does not affect coagulation. In the event of a patient requiring emergency surgery whilst taking the OCP, prophylaxis against venous thrombo-embolism should be employed using subcutaneous heparin and elastic stockings.

The position regarding postmenopausal women taking hormone replacement therapy (HRT) is less clear.[40] HRT may be taken orally as the synthetic ethinyloestradiol in smaller doses than that contained in the contraceptive pill, or as a preparation based on a natural oestrogen. There are also non-oral delivery systems, patches and implants which produce similar plasma concentrations of oestradiol to those seen in premenopausal women. The changes in activity of the coagulation factors with oral HRT are similar but to a smaller degree than those seen with the OCP. Non-oral administration has been shown to have no effect on coagulation. It appears that continuation of HRT carries little risk but a clinical trial would be required to confirm this. At present, there is no evidence to suggest that women receiving HRT are at increased risk of thrombo-embolic complications related to surgery, and no special precautions are recommended.

MUSCULOSKELETAL

Non-steroidal anti-inflammatory drugs

Aspirin and the other NSAIDs are the most commonly prescribed group of drugs, and are used for their analgesic and anti-inflammatory properties in inflammatory joint disease and other musculoskeletal disorders. The NSAIDs act peripherally by inhibiting the enzyme cyclo-oxygenase which converts arachidonic acid to the prostaglandin endoperoxides. The prostaglandins act locally at the site of tissue damage to potentiate the inflammatory process, and promote the pain and hyperalgesia associated with inflammation. NSAIDs also have an antipyretic action by inhibiting the formation of prostaglandin E_2 in the hypothalamus. Side-effects occur as a result of the inhibition of prostaglandin synthesis. In the gastric mucosa, prostaglandins inhibit acid secretion and promote the secretion of protective mucus. Aspirin-like drugs can precipitate gastric or intestinal ulceration which may frequently be silent and present with chronic blood loss, acute gastro-intestinal haemorrhage or perforation. NSAIDs may have adverse effects on renal function. In normal kidneys, administration of an NSAID has no significant effect on renal function, but in conditions of decreased renal perfusion, prostaglandins play an important role in modulating renal haemodynamics. The production of vasodilator prostaglandins by the kidney overcomes renal vasoconstriction, stimulates renin release and maintains the glomerular filtration rate. In conditions of reduced circulatory volume, congestive cardiac failure, hepatic cirrhosis with ascites, pre-eclampsia, chronic renal failure, renal artery stenosis and toxic renal damage, the administration of an NSAID may precipitate a severe decline in renal function.[41] Inhibition of cyclo-oxygenase also causes salt and water retention. This effect is rarely significant, but may cause oedema in some patients, and aspirin-like drugs may inhibit the effectiveness of thiazide diuretics and other antihypertensive therapy.

Normal haemostasis is dependent on the formation of thromboxanes and prostaglandins. Platelet aggregation is induced by the formation of thromboxane A_2, which is inhibited by the cyclo-oxygenase inhibitors. Aspirin causes irreversible acetylation of the cyclo-oxygenase enzyme, and because platelets cannot synthesize new enzyme, there is a prolongation of the bleeding time for 12–15 days until new platelets are produced. Other NSAIDs are reversible inhibitors and inhibit platelet aggregation only for as long as they remain in the circulation. This property of aspirin is used in the treatment of coronary and cerebrovascular disease but may cause problems with increased bleeding during surgery and increase the risk of haemorrhagic complications during the performance of spinal and epidural blockade. Aspirin intolerance occurs in some individuals and is more common in those who suffer from asthma, nasal polyps or chronic urticaria. Symptoms range from rhinitis, urticaria and angioneurotic oedema, to bronchospasm and shock. The response may occur with any NSAID and a history of hypersensitivity to aspirin is a contra-indication to treatment with any agent of this group.

Implications for anaesthesia

Treatment with aspirin should be stopped approximately 2 weeks before surgery associated with a significant risk of bleeding. Other NSAIDs may be continued until 1–2 days pre-operatively. The haemoglobin concentration should be estimated to screen for silent gastro-intestinal blood loss, and renal function should be assessed. There is a potential risk of the development of a significant extradural haematoma when epidural anaesthesia is performed in a patient who has ingested drugs which inhibit platelet function and cause a prolongation of the bleeding time. Ideally, aspirin should be stopped 10–14 days before such a procedure. It has been recommended that estimation of the bleeding time should be performed, and the use of extradural anaesthesia avoided if it is longer than 10 min, the upper limit of normal.[42] Low–dose aspirin (50–150 mg daily) is used in obstetric practice as prophylaxis against pre-eclampsia; in this dose range, aspirin is probably not a contra-indication to the use of extradural anaesthesia.

ANTICOAGULANTS

Anticoagulants are drugs which inhibit the clotting of blood and are used in the treatment and prophylaxis of thrombo-embolic disease (including deep vein thrombosis and pulmonary embolism) and cardiac thrombus associated with atrial fibrillation, myocardial infarction and artificial and rheumatic heart valves. Oral anticoagulants include the coumarin derivatives (warfarin and nicoumalone) and phenindione, which has a faster onset of action and shorter half-life but which is less commonly used because it has a greater incidence of serious side-effects, particularly sensitivity reactions and agranulocytosis. All the oral anticoagulants are structurally similar to vitamin K and act by inhibiting the hepatic synthesis of the vitamin K-dependent clotting factors, II, VII, IX and X. Thus, they have no effect on coagulation in vitro and the onset of their anticoagulant effect is delayed for 12–24 h until the existing clotting factors are depleted.

Warfarin

Warfarin is the most commonly used oral anticoagulant. It is completely absorbed after oral administration and is 97% bound to plasma albumin. The half-life is approximately 48 h and the drug is metabolized in the liver. The dose of warfarin is determined by monitoring the prothrombin time and the results are expressed as the international normalized ratio (INR). An INR of 2.0–3.0 is therapeutic for the prophylaxis and treatment of deep vein thrombosis and pulmonary embolism, and from 3.0 to 4.0 for recurrent deep vein thrombosis and pulmonary embolism, for cardiac prostheses and for thrombosis prophylaxis following myocardial infarction. The most common adverse effects are due to bleeding. Drug interactions are frequent; other highly protein-bound drugs including salicylates and sulphonamides may displace warfarin, resulting in an increase in the free concentration of drug and a temporary enhancement of effect. Agents which inhibit hepatic metabolism, including chloramphenicol, cimetidine and the MAOIs, can also enhance the anticoagulant effect. Warfarin inhibits hepatic enzymes and may increase the effect of oral hypoglycaemic agents and anticonvulsants. It crosses the placenta freely and is teratogenic when taken in the first trimester of pregnancy. In late pregnancy it may cause fetal or neonatal haemorrhage and should therefore be avoided throughout pregnancy.

Implications for anaesthesia

Due to the prolonged action of warfarin, it is preferable to convert an anticoagulated patient to heparin in the pre-operative period so that anticoagulation may be rapidly reversed if necessary. For minor operations with negligible risk of bleeding, warfarin may be continued. In an emergency, deficient clotting factors may be replaced with administration of fresh frozen plasma. Vitamin K stimulates the synthesis of new clotting factors within 24–36 h but may render the patient refractory to warfarin for several weeks and this should be considered when oral anticoagulation is to be resumed following surgery.

Heparin

Heparin was discovered in 1916 by a medical student at Johns Hopkins University. It is a naturally occurring complex mucopolysaccharide which occurs in the body in the granules of mast cells. Commercial preparations are obtained from animal tissues and contain a wide range of molecular weights from 3 to 30 kDa. Anticoagulant activity is measured in units, a unit being that amount which prevents 1 ml of citrated sheep plasma from clotting for 1h after the addition of 0.2 ml of a 1 : 100 $CaCl_2$ solution. The standard preparations contain 100–120 units.mg^{-1}. Heparin is a co-factor for the plasma molecule antithrombin III and enhances its ability to inactivate thrombin and the activated factors X, XII, XI, and IX. In addition to its effects on coagulation factors, heparin inhibits platelet function and increases the permeability of blood vessel walls — effects which may contribute to heparin-induced bleeding.[43] Heparin is poorly absorbed from the gastro-intestinal tract and is therefore given by intravenous or subcutaneous injection. Following intravenous injection the plasma half-life is 1–2 h and a continuous infusion of 24 000–40 000 units per 24 h, after a bolus dose of 5000 units, is usually required to maintain the activated partial thromboplastin time (APTT) in the therapeutic range. The effect of heparin is monitored by the measurement of the APTT, which should be prolonged to 60–100 s or 1.5–2.5 times the control by therapeutic doses of heparin. Smaller doses of heparin, 5000 units every 12 h subcutaneously, are effective for the prophylaxis of thrombo-embolic disease but may not cause a prolongation of the APTT and laboratory control is not required. Low-molecular-weight heparin contains only the fraction of heparin with a molecular weight below 7 kDa. At doses producing an equivalent antithrombotic effect, these heparins cause fewer haemorrhagic complications and are effective in the prevention of venous thrombo-embolism in medical and surgical patients who are at high risk. The mechanism of action is predominantly to catalyse the inhibition of factor Xa by antithrombin III, with little activity against thrombin. The APTT is not prolonged and, although laboratory control is rarely required, anticoagulant activity may be monitored by the measurement of factor Xa activity. Low-molecular-weight heparins have a relatively long plasma half-life and may be administered once daily by subcutaneous injection.

The most common side-effect of heparin is haemorrhage, the incidence of which increases with the dose of heparin. Thrombocytopenia may occur and is more common with bovine heparin than with that of porcine origin. It has an immunological aetiology and may be associated with arterial thrombotic complications. Osteoporosis occurs rarely, but is a particular problem during long-term treatment with heparin, such as may be required during pregnancy.

Implications for anaesthesia

The short half-life of heparin allows discontinuation with reversal of anticoagulation within hours if bleeding occurs. Protamine sulphate 1 mg per 100 units heparin may be given if rapid reversal is required. The risk of neurological damage by an extradural haematoma is increased in a patient who is receiving systemic anticoagulation and who undergoes spinal or extradural anaesthesia. It is not yet apparent whether low-dose heparin prophylaxis confers such a risk. An extradural catheter should not be inserted or removed if the coagulation times are prolonged.

ANTIBIOTICS

Antibiotics are frequently given to the surgical patient either in the treatment of a known or suspected infection, or for prophylaxis. Most antibiotics are relatively non-toxic drugs, although indiscriminate use of powerful broad-spectrum agents can lead to the development of resistant strains of organisms and pseudomembranous colitis.

Penicillins

The most serious side-effects of the penicillins are hypersensitivity reactions, which may be delayed in the form of a rash, or immediate life-threatening angioneurotic oedema and anaphylaxis. The hypersensitivity is to the basic penicillin structure. Thus, all members of the group must be avoided if a history of penicillin allergy is given. Very high doses or impaired excretion in the presence of renal failure can give rise to cerebral irritation and encephalitis. Penicillin must never be given by intrathecal injection.

Cephalosporins

These are structurally related to the penicillins and 10% of penicillin-sensitive patients exhibit hypersensitivity to these agents. They are potentially nephrotoxic at high doses or in the presence of pre-existing renal disease, especially when given in combination with aminoglycosides or other nephrotoxic agents.

Aminoglycosides

This group includes gentamicin, amikacin, netilmicin, streptomycin and tobramycin. They are active against Gram-negative and some Gram-positive organisms but relatively toxic and not absorbed after oral administration; consequently, they are only given by injection for serious systemic infections. Ototoxicity is manifest as hearing loss or tinnitus and the incidence is increased if there is prolonged treatment, high plasma concentrations or concurrent administration of frusemide or ethacrynic acid. Nephrotoxicity causes a reduction in glomerular filtration and is likely if there is pre-existing renal impairment and concurrent administration of other nephrotoxic agents such as amphotericin, cyclosporin and cisplatin. If there is impairment of renal function, the interval between doses must be increased. Plasma concentrations should be monitored during therapy.

The aminoglycosides potentiate the effects of neuromuscular-blocking agents. They act predominantly presynaptically, reducing the amount of acetylcholine released by a nerve impulse. At higher concentrations, they also act at the postsynaptic membrane. Other groups of antibiotics which exhibit a neuromuscular blocking effect are the polymyxins, the tetracyclines and the lincosamines, although the main site of action of these agents is postjunctional.[44] Due to the high margin of safety of neuromuscular transmission, the neuromuscular-blocking action of these antibiotics is rarely significant unless transmission is already compromised (as in myasthenia gravis, muscular dystrophies or in the presence of muscle relaxants). There can be potentiation of both depolarizing and non-depolarizing relaxants. Although the block is often resistant to reversal with neostigmine, calcium may be effective; however, it is probably safer to continue ventilation until normal muscle function returns.

Chloramphenicol

This is a potent broad-spectrum antibiotic used for life-threatening infections caused by *Haemophilus influenzae* and for typhoid fever. It can cause irreversible bone marrow depression and its use has diminished as resistant organisms have evolved and other less toxic drugs have been developed.

Antituberculous therapy

The treatment of tuberculosis requires a combination of drugs for at least 6 months. First-line agents are isoniazid, rifampicin and pyrazinamide. Ethambutol or streptomycin may be added if resistance to any of these agents is suspected or if side-effects necessitate discontinuation.

Isoniazid is highly effective. It may cause a peripheral neuropathy, especially in the presence of diabetes mellitus, alcoholism, chronic renal failure or malnutrition. Pyridoxine 10 mg daily should be given prophylactically. Hepatitis, psychosis and drug-induced systemic lupus erythematosus syndrome occur rarely. Rifampicin should also be given unless there is a specific contra-indication. It may cause a transient disturbance of liver function but rarely needs to be discontinued. It induces liver enzymes, and an increase in the metabolism of drugs such as warfarin, oral hypoglycaemics, steroids, phenytoin and the oral contraceptive pill may reduce their clinical effect. Rifampicin can also cause thrombocytopenia, gastro-intestinal disturbance, an influenza-like syndrome and respiratory symptoms, including breathlessness. It colours urine, saliva and other body secretions orange-red. Pyrazinamide is given for the first 2 months of treatment. It is particularly useful in tuberculous meningitis because it has good meningeal penetration. It can cause hepatotoxicity, nausea and vomiting, and sideroblastic anaemia. Streptomycin is used if the organism is known to be resistant. It is given by intramuscular injection and has the same potential ototoxicity and nephrotoxicity as the aminoglycosides. Plasma concentrations should be monitored. Ethambutol can cause optic neuritis. The visual changes are reversible on discontinuation of the drug. It should be avoided in young children and others unable to report visual disturbances.

DRUG TREATMENT IN AIDS

The acquired immunodeficiency syndrome (AIDS) is a relatively recent disease. The first cases were reported in the USA in 1981 and the causative agent, the human immunodeficiency virus (HIV), was discovered in 1983. Much energy is going into research in an attempt to find a cure for this fatal disease. Current treatment involves agents directed at the virus itself and against the infections and tumours which result from the profound immunodeficiency that it causes. Because of the nature of the condition, many of the drugs used are required for prolonged periods and their potential side-effects and toxicity become prominent.[45]

Antiretroviral therapy

As yet, there is no cure for AIDS. The agents currently under investigation are designed to interfere with the life cycle of HIV. Since the brain is a site of replication, therapeutic agents must be capable of crossing the blood–brain barrier. Strategies against HIV include blocking antibodies to prevent the virus entering target cells, viral enzyme inhibitors and agents which prevent viral budding.[46] *Zidovudine* (AZT) was the first antiviral agent licensed for use in AIDS. It is a nucleoside analogue which acts as a reverse transcriptase inhibitor and DNA chain terminator. A multicentre clinical trial in 1986 in patients with AIDS or AIDS-related complex demonstrated significantly reduced mortality and reduced incidence of opportunistic infection in the treated group.[47] It is now widely used in patients with symptomatic disease and trials are being conducted in seropositive asymptomatic patients in the hope that it will delay the progression to AIDS and AIDS-related complex. It is not known whether the benefits will outweigh the drug's significant toxicity. The dose of zidovudine is 3.5 mg.kg^{-1} orally every 4 h.

Adverse reactions include nausea, vomiting, severe headaches and myalgia. It also causes bone marrow depression, with macrocytic anaemia, neutropenia and thrombocytopenia occurring in approximately 50% of patients. Toxicity is worse in patients with more severe disease. The use of any other therapy toxic to the bone marrow, such as co-trimoxazole for treatment or prophylaxis against *Pneumocystis* pneumonia, exacerbates bone marrow depression. Some patients develop a transfusion-dependent anaemia.

Dideoxycytidine (DDC) is another nucleoside analogue that is undergoing clinical trials. In vitro it is more potent than AZT and it exhibits less bone marrow toxicity. Unfortunately, its use has been limited by a painful peripheral neuropathy. *Anti-CD4* antibodies and *AL721* are agents designed to inhibit HIV attachment and entry into target cells. They remain at the experimental stage. *Ampligen* is a mismatched double-stranded RNA molecule which blocks viral RNA cleavage and inhibits HIV replication in vitro. *Foscarnet* is a reverse transcriptase enzyme inhibitor which also has activity against herpes viruses and cytomegalovirus. It reduces virus activity in HIV and may have a role during acute opportunistic viral infection. *Ribavirin* interferes with viral messenger RNA production and is currently used in the treatment of respiratory syncytial virus infections. As yet, there are no conclusive data regarding its effect in HIV infection.

Another approach is to stimulate residual immune

function. α-*Interferon* has antiviral and immunostimulatory actions. It is thought to inhibit budding of new virus particles from the cell surface. When used in the treatment of Kaposi's sarcoma, it can cause significant regression of the tumour but with a high incidence of side-effects, including severe influenza-like symptoms, hepatic dysfunction, neurological symptoms and bone marrow suppression.

Treatment of opportunistic infections

Most of the infections seen in AIDS are due to reactivation of latent organisms in the host or common, normally non-pathogenic, organisms. Treatment can control these infections but they often relapse when treatment is stopped. The side-effects of many of the agents make long-term treatment difficult. Agents used in the common infections associated with AIDS are shown in Table 3.6.

Antitumour therapy

Kaposi's sarcoma is a common presentation of AIDS, when it may run an aggressive course. Treatment depends on the staging and clinical appearance of the lesions. In widespread disease, systemic chemotherapy may be successful in shrinking tumour mass but must be weighed against worsening of the immunosuppression. Surgical excision may be used for small lesions and radiotherapy can be used for isolated lesions. More widespread disease can be treated with single-agent chemotherapy using vinblastine, vincristine, bleomycin or etopiside, with close monitoring of the neutrophil count. Highly toxic combination chemotherapy may be considered for severe Kaposi's sarcoma when the patient is otherwise well, but carries considerable morbidity and mortality. α-Interferon has been used in the treatment of disseminated disease. It is a very expensive drug and produces a high incidence of side-effects. Treatment is by daily intramuscular injection. Side-effects include severe influenza-like symptoms with high fever and bone marrow suppression.

Patients with AIDS may also develop a high-grade B-cell lymphoma. Treatment with multiple agent regimens of chemotherapy can induce remission but there is a high relapse rate and survival is usually less than 1 year. If the lymphoma presents early in the course of HIV disease, full remission may be obtained.

CYTOTOXICS

Immunosuppressive agents

Modification of the immune response has greatly enhanced the success of organ transplantation and is also used in the treatment of auto-immune and inflammatory conditions. The cytotoxic agents given continuously and in lower doses than those used for cancer chemotherapy cause suppression of the lymphoid cells in the bone marrow, resulting in immune suppression. Corticosteroids and cyclosporin are the other main agents used. A combination of prednisolone and cyclosporin or azathioprine is usually started immediately before organ transplantation and must be continued indefinitely in order to prevent rejection. Patients receiving immunosuppressive agents are at increased risk of infection with viral, bacterial and fungal organisms. Particular care should be taken to reduce the risk of infection; invasive monitoring should be avoided where possible and postoperative ventilation minimized to avoid nosocomial pneumonia.

Cyclosporin selectively inhibits the activation of T lymphocytes. It does not cause significant bone marrow suppression but has a high incidence of nephrotoxicity. Following renal transplantation, cyclosporin nephrotoxicity may be confused with acute rejection. Hypertension is a common side-effect; hepatic failure and neurological toxicity in the form of tremor or convulsions can also occur. Toxicity may be precipitated by concurrent administration of agents which inhibit hepatic enzymes, including erythromycin, ketoconazole and amphotericin B. Conversely, acute rejection has occurred due to increased metabolism induced by anticonvulsant agents, rifampicin or co-trimoxazole. *Azathioprine* is a cytotoxic agent which has been used for many years to suppress rejection of transplanted organs. It is also used in the treatment of severe refractory rheumatoid arthritis. Bone marrow suppression is the major side-effect and hepatic fibrosis can also occur. *Prednisolone* in a dose of 5–10 mg daily is used as prophylaxis against rejection and carries the problems of long-term steroid administration. During acute graft rejection high doses of intravenous methylprednisolone are given. A full blood count must be performed to exclude leukopenia and thrombocytopenia if surgery is planned in a patient who is taking immunosuppressive agents. Renal and hepatic function should also be assessed. Patients on corticosteroids may require peri-operative supplementation (see p. 96).

Table 3.6 Drugs used in the treatment of infections associated with acquired immunodeficiency syndrome (AIDS)

Infection	Drug	Comments/toxicity
Pneumocystis carinii pneumonia		
Treatment	Co-trimoxazole	Nausea, fever, rash, Stevenson-Johnson syndrome Bone-marrow suppression Given orally for prophylaxis
	Pentamidine isethionate	Hypotension, hypoglycaemia, renal failure, hepatitis Bone marrow suppression Or by nebulizer in less severe pneumonia and fortnightly for prophylaxis Can cause bronchospasm but fewer other side-effects
Investigational	Dapsone and trimethoprim	Rash, nausea, methaemoglobinaemia, bone-marrow suppression
	Clindamycin and primaquine	Rash, nausea, bone-marrow suppression
	High-dose steroids	Additional immune suppression
Salvage therapy	Trimetrexate and folinic acid	Raised transaminases, bone-marrow suppression
	Eflornithine	Bone-marrow suppression
Toxoplasmosis	Pyrimethamine plus sulphadiazine or clindamycin	Rash, nausea, bone-marrow suppression Dose reduced for maintenance therapy
Cryptosporidiosis	Spiramycin Erythromycin	Poor response to treatment
Herpes simplex	Acyclovir	Give in reduced dose for prophylaxis
Cytomegalovirus	Gancyclovir	Anaemia, neutropenia, intravenous preparation only, high toxicity
	Foscarnet	Nausea, renal failure
Candidiasis	Nystatin oral suspension Miconazole oral gel Amphoteracin lozenges	
Systemic treatment	Ketoconazole Fluconazole	Nausea, hepatitis, thrombocytopenia Nausea
Cryptococcus	Amphotericin B and flucytosine Fluconazole	Nausea, rash, bone-marrow suppression, renal impairment, hypocalcaemia
Mycobacterium tuberculosis	Conventional antituberculosis therapy	
Atypical *Mycobacterium* (*Mycobacterium avium-intracellulare*)	Amikacin Clofazimine Rifampicin Cycloserine Isoniazid — ethambutol, streptomycin	Ototoxicity, nephrotoxicity Often resistant to treatment
Bacterial pneumonias Skin infections Salmonella	Conventional antibiotics	
Gum and periodontal disease	Metronidazole	

REFERENCES

1. Eger EI II, Johnson BH, Strum DP, Ferrel LD. Studies of the toxicity of I653, halothane, and isoflurane in the enzyme-induced, hypoxic rats. Anesth Analg 1987; 66: 1227–1229
2. Duthie DJR, Montgomery JM, Spence AA, Nimmo WS. Concurrent drug therapy in patients undergoing surgery. Anaesthesia 1987; 42: 305–306
3. Buck N, Devlin HB, Lunn JN. The report of a confidential enquiry into perioperative deaths. London: Nuffield Provincial Hospitals Trust and King's Fund Publishing Office. 1993
4. Miller RP, Olsen HG, Amsterdam EA, Mason DT. Propranolol withdrawal rebound phenomenon. N Engl J Med 1975; 293: 416–418
5. Prys-Roberts C, Foex P, Biro GP, Roberts JG. Studies of anaesthesia in relation to hypertension. V. Adrenergic beta-receptor blockade. Br J Anaesth 1973; 45: 671–681
6. Jones RM. Calcium antagonists. Anaesthesia 1984; 39: 747–749
7. Bikhazi GB, LeungI, Fouldes FF. Ca-channel blockers increase potency of NMBs in vivo. Anesthesiology 1983; 59: A269
8. Jones RM, Cashman JN, Casson WR, Broadbent MP. Verapamil potentiation of neuromuscular blockade: failure of reversal with neostigmine but prompt reversal with edrophonium. Anesth Analg 1985; 64: 1021–1025
9. Insel PA, Motulsky HJ. A hypothesis linking intracellular sodium, membrane receptors and hypertension. Life Sci 1984; 34: 1009–1023
10. Russel RM, Jones RM. Postoperative hypotension associated with enalapril. Anaesthesia 1989; 44: 837–838
11. McConachie I, Healy TEJ. ACE inhibitors and anaesthesia. Postgrad Med J 1989; 65: 273–274
12. Maze M, Tranquilli W. Alpha-2 adrenoceptor agonists: defining the role in clinical practice. Anesthesiology 1991; 74: 581–605
13. Mason RA. Antiarrhythmic drugs. In: Anaesthesia databook. London: Churchill Livingstone, 1990: pp 356–362
14. Krikler D, Spurrell R. Asystole after verapamil. Br Med J 1972; 2: 405
15. Miller RD, Way WL, Katzung BG. The potentiation of neuromuscular blocking agents by quinidine. Anesthesiology 1967; 28: 1036–1041
16. Roden DM, Woolsey RL. Flecainide. N Engl J Med 1986; 315: 36–41
17. The CAST investigators (cardiac arrhythmia suppression trial). Preliminary report; effect of encainide and flecainide on mortality in a randomised trial of arrhythmia suppression after myocardial infarction. N Engl J Med 1989; 321: 406–412
18. Teasdale S, Downar E. Amiodarone and anaesthesia. Can J Anaesth 1990; 37: 151–155
19. Holt DW, Tucker GT, Jackson PR, Storey GCA. Amiodarone pharmacokinetics. Am Heart J 1983; 106: 840–847
20. Kosinski EJ, Albin JB, Young E, Lewis SM, Leland OS. Hemodynamic effect of intravenous amiodarone. J Am Coll Cardiol 1983; 146: 848–856
21. Lown B. Cardioversion and the digitalised patient. J Am Coll Cardiol 1985; 5: 889–890
22. Edwards JG. Selective serotonin reuptake inhibitors. Br Med J 1992; 304: 1644–1646
23. Committee on Safety of Medicines. Fluvoxamine and fluoxetine — interaction with monoamine oxidase inhibitors, lithium and tryptophan. Curr Prob 1989; 26: 61
24. Rivers N, Horner B. Possible lethal reaction between nardil and dextromorphan. Can Med Assoc J 1970; 103: 408
25. Wells DG, Bjorksten AR. Monoamine oxidase inhibitors revisited. Can J Anaesth 1989; 36: 64–74
26. Stack CG, Rogers P, Linter SPK. Monoamine oxidase inhibitors and anaesthesia. Br J Anaesth 1988; 60: 222–227
27. Abbott RJ, Loizou LA. Neuroleptic malignant syndrome. Br J Psychiatry 1986; 148: 47–51
28. Montgomery JN, Ironside JW. Neuroleptic malignant syndrome in the intensive therapy unit. Anaesthesia 1990; 45: 311–313
29. Hill GE, Wong KC, Hodges MR. Lithium carbonate and neuromuscular blocking agents. Anesthesiology 1977; 46: 122–126
30. British national formulary. London: British Medical Association and British Pharmaceutical Society, 1992: p 136
31. Desai P, Hewitt PB, Jones RM. Influence of anticonvulsant therapy on doxacurium and pancuronium-induced paralysis. Anesthesiology 1989; 71: A784
32. Severn AM. Parkinsonism and the anaesthetist. Br J Anaesth 1988; 61: 761–770
33. Lewis L, Roblasol RF, Yee J, Hacker LA, Eisen G. Fatal adrenal cortical insufficiency precipitated by surgery during prolonged continuous cortisone treatment. Ann Intern Med 1953; 39: 116–126
34. Plumpton FS, Besser GN, Cole PV. Corticosteroid treatment and surgery 2. The management of steroid cover. Anaesthesia 1969; 24: 12–18
35. Symreng T, Karlberg BE, Kagedal B, Schildt B. Physiological cortisol substitution of long term steroid treated patients undergoing major surgery. Br J Anaesth 1981; 53: 949–954
36. Napolitano LM, Chernow B. Guidelines for corticosteroid use in anesthetic and surgical stress. Int Anesthesiol Clin 1988; 26: 226–232
37. Alberti KG. Diabetes and surgery. Anesthesiology 1991; 74: 209–211
38. Stadel BV. Oral contraceptives and cardiovascular disease. N Engl J Med 1981; 305: 612–618
39. Guillebaud J. Surgery and the pill. Br Med J 1985; 291: 498–499
40. Whitehead EM, Whitehead MI. The pill, HRT and postoperative thromboembolism: cause for concern? Anaesthesia 1991; 46: 521–522
41. Harris K. The role of prostaglandins in the control of renal function. Br J Anaesth 1992: 69: 233–235
42. Macdonald R. Aspirin and extradural blocks. Br J Anaesth 1991; 66: 1–3
43. Hirsh J. Heparin. N Engl J Med 1991; 324: 1565–1574
44. Singh YN, Marshall IG, Harvey AL. Pre- and postjunctional blocking effects of aminoglycoside, polymyxin, tetracycline and lincosamine antibiotics. Br J Anaesth 1982; 54: 1295–1306
45. Adler MW. ABC of AIDS, 2nd edn. London: British Medical Journal. 1991
46. Youle M, Clarbour J, Wade P, Farthing C. AIDS therapeutics in HIV disease. Edinburgh: Churchill Livingstone. 1988
47. Richman DD, Fischl MA, Grieco MH et al. The toxicity of azidothymidine (AZT) in the treatment of patients with AIDS and AIDS-related complex. N Engl J Med 1987; 317: 192–197

4. Premedication

R.S. Atkinson

The development of premedication in the UK has been described by Shearer.[1,2] For the first 50 years medication prior to anaesthesia was employed infrequently. The Section of Anaesthetics of the Royal Society of Medicine was the forum in which from 1911 to 1915 the value of the administration of drugs such as morphine, hyoscine and atropine before anaesthesia was discussed by the leading anaesthetists of the day. Foremost among these were Dudley Buxton[3] and Blomfield.[4] By 1920 the word 'premedication' was not yet in general use, although the subject was being aired in the current textbooks.[5,6] It was 1928 before the *Lancet* published an annotation entitled 'Premedication with anaesthesia'.[7] Similar changes were taking place in the USA where McMechan used the word as a paragraph-heading in 1920 in the *American Year Book of Anesthesia and Analgesia*[8] and also described the results of a questionnaire on the use of premedication.[9]

In due couse, and for many years, pre-operative medication came to be regarded as mandatory. Morphine became the most commonly prescribed drug, in combination with atropine or hyoscine, although there was some interest in the use of barbiturates,[10] often administered to children per rectum.[11] Then, more recently, with the declining use of ether, which promoted salivation, the routine use of pre-operative medication came to be questioned.[12,13] A recent questionnaire[14] showed that 93% of anaesthetists used sedative-hypnotic drugs in adults and 83% in children. Benzodiazepines were used in adults by 74% of anaesthetists, the remainder preferring opioids. In children, 6% used trimeprazine, 12% diazepam and 6% temazepam. Combinations of drugs were also used. Anticholinergic drugs have also declined in use; they were employed routinely in this survey by only 36% of anaesthetists in adults and 56% in children.

ADVANTAGES OF PRE-OPERATIVE MEDICATION

Drugs have been given before induction of anaesthesia for a number of reasons. Sedative drugs are often prescribed in order to allay anxiety, to promote a smooth induction of anaesthesia, and as an integral part of the anaesthetic itself by reducing the doses of anaesthetic agents required. Specifically, pre-operative medication can be used to provide analgesia, to diminish the chances of awareness, and to provide amnesia and anti-emesis. All these are valid reasons, but the anaesthetist of today assesses the need for all these effects at the pre-operative visit and may prefer to administer drugs him- or herself either in the anaesthetic room or during surgery. In this way he or she can be sure that they are given and can observe their effects with the benefit of direct observation and monitoring.

Similar observations can be applied to the use of anticholinergic drugs administered intramuscularly or orally. Routine use is uncomfortable for the patient who suffers a dry mouth, but has the advantage over intravenous administration that a significant tachycardia is seldom encountered. Routine use for the drying of secretions is often not justifiable with modern anaesthetic drugs and techniques, although it can still be advantageous before procedures such as surgical dental extractions or diagnostic endoscopy of the upper airway. If difficult tracheal intubation is envisaged, salivation can create an additional hazard, whether in passage of the laryngoscope or tracheal tube, or when suxamethonium, especially in repeated doses, may be required.

Another reason for the administration of an anticholinergic drug is to prevent vagally induced bradycardia. Complete abolition of vagal action requires large doses of atropine, perhaps as much as 3 mg, but it should be remembered that partial vagal block is all that is required in clinical practice. For example, when the heart rate is considered to be unacceptably low during surgery, a dose of atropine as low as 0.1 mg may increase the heart rate significantly. It is not just the reflex vagal responses which should be considered. Drugs such as suxamethonium can cause vagal slowing of the heart, especially when given in repeated doses. Anticholinergic drugs can be given in a number of other specific circumstances to anticipate unopposed vagal action. These include traction on the extra-ocular muscles during squint surgery, in patients on medication with β-adrenergic receptor blocking drugs and in patients with partial heart block.

CONTRA-INDICATIONS TO SEDATIVE PREMEDICATION

It is unwise to administer sedative premedication if the patient is in a critical condition. Not only is the usual dose a possible overdose for that patient, but its absorption to the general circulation may be delayed unless the drug is given intravenously. Sedative premedication is particularly unwise when the respiratory function of the patient is critical. This may be the case in advanced emphysema or whenever the patient depends on the accessory muscles of respiration to maintain gas exchange. Particular care is necessary in the presence of respiratory obstruction, which may be latent or manifest in the presence of laryngeal tumours, and which is usually life-threatening in infective conditions such as epiglottitis.

CONTRA-INDICATIONS TO ANTICHOLINERGIC DRUGS

These are not nearly so clear-cut. They may be withheld when the heart rate is already high, but it is not always clear what effect they will have if vagal tone is already ineffectual. Intravenous atropine has a much greater effect on heart rate than atropine administered intramuscularly or orally and it can be argued that atropine given by these latter routes might obviate the need for intravenous use. Hyoscine and glycopyrronium are much less likely to give rise to tachycardia, but this cannot be guaranteed. Other unwanted side-effects of atropine include abolition of sweating, which may be deleterious in hot climates or in pyrexial patients, and the possible activation of the central anticholinergic syndrome. The latter is more likely to occur in elderly patients receiving hyoscine and does not occur with glycopyrronium.

DRUGS USED FOR PREMEDICATION

Opioid analgesics

Traditionally, opioid drugs led the field for many years; they still have advantages. In many patients, they provide a pleasant euphoria with analgesia. The potent analgesic properties may help in the minimization of stress responses and form an integral part of the anaesthetic technique. Potent analgesics may be particularly valuable in patients in pain before surgery. As recently as the 1950s, morphine tablets had to be dissolved in sterile water over a spirit flame and then drawn up into a sterile syringe for injection. The introduction of a convenient ampoule containing papaveretum 20 mg and hyoscine 0.4 mg in 1ml did much to popularize this combination because the premedication injection could be given in a small volume. Papaveretum contains a mixture of alkaloids, 20 mg being clinically equivalent to 13.3 mg morphine. Other popular opioid alternatives to morphine (10 mg) include pethidine (100 mg) and diamorphine (5 mg). Pethidine (meperidine) was preferred by some anaesthetists because of its atropine-like effect and its bronchodilator action. However, others found that the side-effects, which include sweating, hypotension and vertigo, made it unreliable, especially in elderly patients.

Benzodiazepines

Benzodiazepines can be given by mouth[15] and have been recommended for night sedation.[16] Diazepam was the first drug of this group to be used commonly, and the first to be associated with anterograde amnesia[17] but temazepam (10–30 mg) is now often preferred[18] because of its shorter duration of action, and has some popularity before day surgery. Lorazepam (1–5 mg) has a longer duration of action and provides appreciable anterograde amnesia;[19] it has an attraction before inpatient surgery because all patients on the operating list can be given their tablets at the same time. It has advantages over diazepam in inpatients.[20] The benzodiazepines can be given by injection but there is evidence that oral administration gives better results.[21] The use of these compounds avoids some of the undesirable side-effects of opioids, notably respiratory depression and the increased incidence of nausea and vomiting. They are useful when these side-effects must be avoided and potent analgesia is not required. One disadvantage of oral premedication is that patients may not realize they have been given a potent sedative/amnesic agent and may be reluctant to stay quietly in bed. The choice of benzodiazepine is often a personal preference and other drugs used include nitrazepam (5–10 mg), flurazepam (15–30 mg) and flunitrazepam (1 mg).

Benzodiazepines act by enhancing the action of γ-aminobutyric acid (GABA), a major inhibitory neurotransmitter in the central nervous system. Two receptors for this neurotransmitter have been characterized: $GABA_A$ and $GABA_B$. Benzodiazepines act at specific binding sites on the $GABA_A$ receptor. Barbiturates (see below) are thought to act at a separate binding site, possibly the chloride channel itself.

Barbiturates

Barbiturates were once popular, given by mouth, per rectum or sometimes intramuscularly. They have fallen out of favour because of a general desire to avoid drugs which can cause death if taken in deliberate overdose and because of fears that they may have an anti-analgesic action.[22]

Phenothiazines

Phenothiazine derivatives are also less popular than formerly, except for the use of oral trimeprazine in children. Their attraction lies in their anti-emetic and antihistamine effects combined with sedation. Different phenothiazine drugs exhibit these properties in varying degrees. Chlorpromazine and promethazine used to be popular in combination with pethidine as part of the lytic cocktail which has lost favour, partly because of the prolonged periods of sleep which sometimes accompanied its use and partly because hypotension could occur. The sedative response to a single premedication dose was also variable and difficult to predict.

Phenothiazines mediate their sedative and anti-emetic effects by acting at dopamine (D_2), cholinergic (muscarinic) and histamine (H_1) receptors.

Neuroleptanalgesia

The neurolept drugs were popular in some centres. Butyrophenones, such as droperidol, provided good anti-emetic effects while combination with the short-acting synthetic analgesics provided a quiet and co-operative patient. It has since been realized that, although patients appeared calm and tranquil, they often felt deeply disturbed. The analgesic action might be short but the butyrophenones were long-acting.

Butyrophenones predominantly act at D_2 receptors but have some action at H_1 and serotonin (5-HT) receptors.

Clonidine

There has been recent interest in clonidine which decreases the anaesthetic requirements for inhaled agents[23,24] and for propofol,[25] although recovery times may be somewhat prolonged.

Clonidine is an α_2-agonist and it appears to potentiate anaesthetics by decreasing central noradrenergic activity. Dexmedetomidine has a more specific action at α_2-receptors and may have a place as a premedicant.

Non-steroidal anti-inflammatory drugs

These drugs may reduce opioid requirements following surgery[26] and may therefore have a use in pre-operative medication.

Anticholinergic agents

Hyoscine and atropine have been in common use for many years. They inhibit salivary secretions and block vagal nerve endings in the heart. The drugs can be given intramuscularly or subcutaneously in doses of about 0.5 mg in the adult, in similar dosage intravenously and in doses of 1–2 mg by mouth. The disadvantages of this medication are the pain occasioned by intramuscular injection, the dry mouth which results from their use and the tendency to produce tachycardia. The last is much more common when atropine is given intravenously, but does not always occur in the elderly.

Inhibition of sweating is also a consequence of the administration of anticholinergic drugs, and may be significant in pyrexial patients. Hyoscine produces some sedation and has amnesic and anti-emetic effects. It principally acts at muscarinic reptors but has some D_2 and H_1-antagonist actions. It is often feared that anticholinergic drugs may precipitate acute glaucoma in susceptible individuals, but there is no real evidence that these drugs are dangerous unless they are applied directly into the conjunctival sac. The central anticholinergic syndrome can result on rare occasions (see below).

Glycopyrronium (0.4 mg) has advantages over atropine in that tachycardia is less common and its effect on inhibition of salivary secretions is more potent and longer-lasting. It does not cross the placental or blood–brain barriers.

The central anticholinergic syndrome

This is seen particularly in elderly patients following administration of anticholinergic drugs which cross the blood–brain barrier. Clinical manifestations include restlessness, drowsiness and, occasionally, coma. Treatment comprises administration of intravenous physostigmine 2 mg cautiously, repeated if necessary. This drug is effective but neostigmine is not, because the latter does not cross the blood–brain barrier. The syndrome does not occur when glycopyrronium is used because it does not cross the blood–brain barrier.

Other drugs

It is usually wise to continue chronic medication, although drugs such as insulin, lithium, the contraceptive pill, anticoagulants and monoamine oxidase inhibitors require special consideration, beyond the scope of this chapter. In particular, the β-blockers should not be discontinued; indeed they have been advocated as part of a premedication routine to protect the heart from adrenergic stimulation.[27]

H_2-receptor blockers may be administered pre-operatively to patients with hiatus hernia, who may regurgitate acid stomach contents during anaesthesia. Cimetidine may be used as a single oral dose of 400 mg,[28] although ranitidine is favoured because of its greater potency, longer duration of action and absence of effects on hepatic drug metabolism.[29] It has been given in a dosage of 150–300 mg orally the night before surgery. These drugs reduce secretion of gastric acid but do not affect acid already present in the stomach; thus, in emergency surgery (e.g. obstetrics), antacids are administered immediately before anaesthesia to increase the pH of gastric fluid.

ROUTE OF ADMINISTRATION

By the alimentary tract

Drugs given orally are easy to administer and the patient is spared the discomfort of a hypodermic needle. However, they are absorbed more slowly than when given by injection and the rate of absorption may be variable. Unco-operative patients may reject some or all of the dose. Oral medication is usually inappropriate in the presence of pathology of the gastro-intestinal tract and is contra-indicated in the presence of vomiting or gastric stasis. Rectal administration is an alternative portal of entry but some patients are unaccustomed to this route and may find it unacceptable. It is not commonly used in UK practice, but is more common in other European countries.

Subcutaneous and intramuscular

Hypodermic injection has the advantage that the dose is seen to have been given. Traditionally, many premedicant drugs were given by the subcutaneous route, but the better blood supply of muscles means that absorption is likely to be more uniform when intramuscular injection is used.

Intravenous

Many anaesthetists now prescribe only oral premedication or no pre-operative drugs to be given on the ward, and prefer to give more potent agents intravenously when the patient arrives in the anaesthetic room. Monitoring equipment can be attached, the drugs can be titrated against clinical observations, and changes in heart rate and oxygen saturation can be assessed. This applies particularly in the emergency situation, when absorption from intramuscular injection may be erratic and unreliable.

SPECIAL SITUATIONS

Emergencies

There is sometimes little time for the administration of drugs on the ward. Some patients are aware of their acute condition and are anxious to have corrective surgery as soon as possible. Others require a period of pre-operative preparation and it is the responsibility of the anaesthetist to assess the premedication requirement as a part of overall management. The anesthetist must bear in mind the need for analgesia pre-operatively and the anaesthetic sequence he or she intends to employ.

Obstetrics

Whether the procedure is elective or emergency, the anaesthetist must avoid depression of the fetus and it is therefore usual to avoid opioid analgesics in premedication. The problem is then one of avoiding maternal awareness by giving the correct dose of induction and maintenance agents in patients who are young and able to clear anaesthetic drugs rapidly from the cerebral circulation.

Children

The pre-operative visit is more important than the type of pharmacological medication in relieving anxiety. Most anaesthetists would agree that the presence of a parent at the time of induction is usually, though not always, helpful. In any event, most children dislike injections and oral premedication is often preferred, though in an unco-operative patient this can be difficult.

Examples of popular oral regimens include trimeprazine (Vallergan syrup) 2–3 mg.kg^{-1} up to a maximum of 100 mg 2 h pre-operatively, sometimes combined with droperidol 0.2 mg.kg^{-1} to a maximum of 5 mg. The child who is not disturbed often falls asleep. Restlessness sometimes occurs postoperatively, paticularly in the presence of pain. Temazepam (0.3 mg.kg^{-1}) is also available as a syrup and has a shorter duration of action than diazepam (0.2 mg.kg^{-1}).

Anticholinergic drugs can also be given by mouth. Hyoscine has not been as popular as atropine, possibly because it is less well absorbed by the oral route.[30]

The intramuscular route is preferred when it is important to obtain a reliable pharmacological effect. This may be the case in certain sick children when reduced doses of other agents are advantageous (e.g. cardiac surgery) and in mentally handicapped patients or those unable to co-operate. Examples of suitable doses are morphine 0.2 mg.kg^{-1}, pethidine 1.5 mg.kg^{-1}, atropine, 0.015 mg.kg^{-1}, hyoscine, 0.015 mg.kg^{-1}, and glycopyrronium 5 µg.kg^{-1}.

Rectal administration is not popular in the UK, but is used in other countries. Thiopentone 40 mg.kg^{-1} or methohexitone 20 mg.kg^{-1} ensure a sleeping child, but nursing observation must be close as respiratory obstruction can result in the presence of large tonsils. Atropine is also satisfactorily absorbed from the rectum.[31]

The elderly

The pensionable age population in the UK has grown considerably during the 20th century, but by the first decade of the 21st century, the post-1945 rise in birth rate will be reflected in a substantial increase in the number of elderly patients.[32] Anaesthetists are cautious about prescribing sedative drugs and opioid analgesics in the elderly, while anticholinergic agents are often thought to be unnecessary and the central anticholinergic syndrome more likely to occur. The pre-operative visit can help allay anxiety in elderly patients who are outside their normal environment.

There is a need to assess physical status in a group of patients likely to suffer intercurrent disease, to be on chronic medication and also to have irregular compliance with therapy. For example, reduced ventilatory capacity, an increase in closing capacity to encroach on tidal volume especially in the supine position, a degree of upper and lower airway obstruction and impaired control of ventilation are likely to result in a low 'normal' arterial oxygen saturation. For premedication, benzodiazepines such as temazepam are popular, although traditionally, small doses of morphine have been used with success. Studies of ventilatory responses to intravenous morphine before surgery in elderly subjects suggest that care is needed,[33] and this may be more significant in the presence of renal insufficiency.[34]

Ophthalmic surgery

Many patients are in the older age groups and many are suitable for management under local analgesia. It is desirable to avoid increases in intra-ocular pressure when intra-ocular surgery is undertaken, and opioid analgesics, which may cause postoperative nausea and vomiting, are best avoided. The benzodiazepines are often used; for example, lorazepam 1–2.5 mg orally provides sedation and amnesia. Traction on the extra-ocular muscles often causes vagal slowing of the heart during squint operations in children and this can be counteracted by use of atropine; however, intravenous atropine administered at induction is much more effective. Atropine is not contra-indicated before operations for the relief of glaucoma, because it has a minimal effect on pupil size unless given directly into the eye and a surgical drainage system is being created at operation.

Mental handicap

Mentally handicapped patients are managed relatively easily when they are small, but can become increasingly difficult as they grow. Patients must be approached with understanding, and frightening or unfamiliar situations avoided as far as possible. Premedication is often helpful, but the difficulty lies in its administration. Oral drugs are often not potent enough and may be rejected. Careful intramuscular injection ensures that the drug has entered the body. The need for premedication in this difficult field requires individual assessment and sympathetic handling. Some handicapped patients also have physical problems and it may be unwise to prescribe potent drugs with potential side-effects.

Drug addiction

Drug addicts form a difficult group and the history may be unreliable. Withdrawal symptoms may occur if their drug has been discontinued for any reason. Sedative drugs may be needed in large doses if tolerance has developed. Requirements for premedication need individual assessment.

Day patients

In many centres, medication is withheld in the interests of speedy recovery and early discharge from the unit. Children are an exception because parents maintain supervision. Young adult patients are often anxious.[35] Temazepam has enjoyed some popularity,[36] and is preferable to other benzodiazepines.[37] Its use has been recommended in doses of up to 40 mg.[38] Older patients are less likely to require pre-operative sedation, which should only be prescribed in small doses. The volumes and acidity of gastric contents are higher in day-care patients than in inpatients,[39] and it has been suggested that oral antacids may have a place in premedication.

Local or regional techniques

Patients who are to have a local, regional or central neurological block may have some anxiety about the procedure itself, which is not always without discomfort. When multiple injections are required, an analgesic component in premedication is a kindness which should not be withheld in the absence of a contra-indication. However, heavy premedication which prevents co-operation is not helpful. Sometimes a patient may be asked to sit, for example to facilitate spinal analgesia, and it must be possible for him or her to do this without support or hypotension. Intravenous titration of a sedative or analgesic drugs is often helpful before an extensive or difficult block.

In summary, it must be emphasized that each patient is an individual. Premedication is no longer a routine procedure, delegated to the house surgeon or to another anaesthetist colleague. It is something to be prescribed after a pre-operative visit at which all relevant factors have been taken into account. It may begin with night sedation given the evening before surgery, continue in association with the appropriate psychological environment and be part of the pharmacology of the anaesthetic procedure itself, even extending into the postoperative period. Good premedication practice is helpful to the patient and satisfying to the anaesthetist who obtains a good result.

REFERENCES

1. Shearer WM. The evolution of premedication. Br J Anaesth 1960; 32: 554–562
2. Shearer WM. The evolution of premedication (II). Br J Anaesth 1961; 33: 219–225
3. Buxton D. The use of morphine and scopolamine, atropine and similar drugs before inhalation anaesthesia. Proc R Soc Med 1911; 4: 53
4. Blomfield J. The influence of preliminary narcotics on the induction, maintenance and after effects of anaesthesia. Proc R Soc Med 1915; 8: 15
5. Buxton D. Anaesthetics, 6th edn. London: Lewis, 1920
6. Robinson H. Revision of Hewitt's anaesthetics and their administration, 5th edn. London: Frowde. 1922
7. Lancet. Annotation. Lancet 1928; 2: 1252
8. McMechan FH. (ed) The American year book of anesthesia and analgesia, vol 2. New York: Surgery Publishing, 1920: p 245
9. McMechan FH. Results of a survey by the National Anesthesia Research Society of a selected group of hospitals to determine the status of anesthetic service. Am J Surg, Q Suppl 1920; 34: 123
10. Boyd AM. The use of nembutal as a basal hypnotic before general anaesthesia based upon over 1000 cases. St Bart's Hosp Rep 1932; 65: 283
11. Burnap RW, Gain EA, Watts EH. Basal anaesthesia in children using sodium pentothal by rectum. Anesthesiology 1948; 9: 524
12. Holt AT. Premedication with atropine should not be routine. Lancet 1962; ii: 984–985
13. Inglis JM, Barrow MEH. Premedication: a reassessment. Proc R Soc Med 1965; 58: 29–32
14. Mirakhur RK. Preanaesthetic medication: a survey of current usage. J R Soc Med 1991; 84: 481–483
15. Kanto J. Benzodiazepines as oral premedicants. Br J Anaesth 1981; 53: 1179–1188
16. Sjövall S, Kanto J, Kangas L, Pakkanen A. Comparison of midazolam and flunitrazepam for night sedation. A randomised double-blind study. Anaesthesia 1982; 37: 924–928
17. Clarke PRF, Eccersley PS, Frisby JP, Thornton JA. The amnesic effect of diazepam (Valium). Br J Anaesth 1970; 42: 690–697
18. Ratcliff A, Indalo AA, Bradshaw EG, Rye RM. Premedication with temazepam in minor surgery. The relationship between plasma concentration and clinical effect after a dose of 40 mg. Anaesthesia 1989; 44: 812–815
19. Gale G, Galloon S. Lorazepam as a premedication. Can Anaesth Soc J 1976; 23: 22–29
20. Galloon S, Gale GD, Lancee WJ. Comparison of lorazepam and diazepam as premedicants. Br J Anaesth 1977; 49: 1265–1269
21. Gale GD, Galloon S, Porter WR. Sublingual lorazepam: a better premedication? Br J Anaesth 1983; 55: 761–765
22. Dundee JW. Alterations in response to somatic pain associated with anaesthesia II: The effect of thiopentone and pentobarbitone. Br J Anaesth 1960; 32: 407–414
23. Bloor BC, Flacke WE. Reduction in halothane anesthetic requirement by clonidine, an alpha-adrenergic agonist. Anesth Anal 1982; 61: 741–745
24. Woodcock TE, Millard RK, Dixon J, Prys-Roberts C. Clonidine premedication for isoflurane-induced hypotension. Sympathoadrenal responses and a computer-controlled assessment of vapour requirement. Br J Anaesth 1988; 60: 388–394
25. Richards MJ, Skeus MA, Jarvis AP, Prys-Roberts C. Total i.v. anaesthesia with propofol and alfentanil: dose

requirements for propofol and the effect of premedication with clonidine. Br J Anaesth 1990; 65: 157–163
26 Hodsman NBA, Burns J, Blyth A, Kenny GNC, McArdle CS, Rotman H. The morphine sparing effects of diclofenac sodium following abdominal surgery. Anaesthesia 1987; 42: 1005–1008
27 Prys-Roberts C, Meloche R. Management of anaesthesia in patients with hypertension or ischaemic heart disease. Int Anesthesiol Clin 1980; 18: 181–217
28 Husemeyer RP, Davenport HT, Rajasekaran T. Cimetidine as a single oral dose for prophylaxis against Mendelson's syndrome. Anaesthesia 1978; 33: 775–778
29 Gallagher EG, White M, Ward S, Cottrell J, Mann SG. Prophylaxis against acid aspiration syndrome. Single oral dose of H_2-antagonist on the evening before elective surgery. Anaesthesia 1988; 43: 1011–1014
30 Gupta RK, Blades HR, Hatch DJ. Oral premedication in children. Atropine or hyoscine with triclofos. Anaesthesia 1972; 27: 32–36
31 Olsson GL, Bejersten A. Feychting H, Palmer L, Pettersson B-M. Plasma concentrations of atropine after rectal administration. Anaesthesia 1983; 38: 1179–1182
32 Warnes AM. The demography of ageing. In: Davenport HT, ed. Anaesthesia and the aged patient. Oxford: Blackwell, 1988: p 9
33 Arunasalam K, Davenport HT, Painter S, Jones JG. Ventilatory response to morphine in young and old subjects. Anaesthesia 1983; 38: 529–533
34 McQuay H, Moore H. Beware of renal function when prescribing morphine. Lancet 1984; 2: 284–285
35 Norris W, Baird WLM. Pre-operative anxiety: a study of the incidence and aetiology. Br J Anaesth 1967; 39: 503–509
36 Beechey APG, Eltringham RJ, Studd C. Temazepam as premedication in day surgery. Anaesthesia 1976; 31: 10–15
37 Greenwood BK, Bradshaw EG. A comparison between oxazepam and temazepam. Br J Anaesth 1983; 55: 933–937
38 O'Boyle CA, Harris D, Barry H. Sedation in outpatient oral surgery. Br J Anaesth 1986; 58: 378–384
39 Millar M, Wishart HY, Nimmo WA. Gastric contents at induction of anaesthesia. Br J Anaesth 1983; 55: 1185–1188

5. Monitoring and monitoring equipment in clinical anaesthesia

K. Merrett   R.M. Jones

Over recent years, a number of groups have introduced guidelines for minimal standards of monitoring during surgery and anaesthesia. In 1986, the Harvard Medical School's Anesthetic Department drew up guidelines[1] based on information from their own anaesthesia-related claims and incidents in an attempt to reduce morbidity and mortality by more attention to peri-operative monitoring. The American Society of Anesthesiologists followed with the publication of their 'Standards for basic intra-operative monitoring'[2] (amended subsequently in 1990 to mandate the use of pulse oximetry). In July 1988, the Association of Anaesthetists of Great Britain and Ireland published their *Recommendations for Standards of Monitoring during Anaesthesia and Recovery*,[3] and in the same year in Australia, the document 'Minimal monitoring standards'[4] was produced. The World Federation of Societies of Anaesthesiologists (WFSA) in June 1992 adopted the 'International standards for a safe practice of anaesthesia'[5] developed over 2 years by an International Task Force on Anaesthesia Safety comprising representatives from 10 countries.

The scientific basis underlying the evolution, acceptance and implementation of these standards remains the subject of much interest and debate. Their adoption has certainly resulted in a significant alteration to anaesthetic practice and they have without doubt led to an increased awareness by anaesthetists and others of the importance of monitoring. There is a subjective impression that with an increased level of monitoring and earlier detection of subtle degrees of change in physiological parameters, the incidence of minor anaesthetic-related incidents resulting in serious morbidity and mortality has decreased. However, there are few well-controlled studies or objective data confirming this. The use of pulse oximetry has been shown in a recent, relatively large (20 802 patients), prospective multicentre trial predictably to increase the detection of critical incidents such as hypoxaemia, but had no statistically significant effect on outcome.[6,7] Demonstrable improvement in outcome as a result of the adoption of minimal monitoring standards remains to be clearly shown and it is unlikely that such studies, providing objective statistical proof will be performed in the near future.

Despite the widespread propagation of standards of monitoring, many instances still arise where the standards are not implemented or the monitoring equipment is not available. The application to anaesthesia of quality management and continuous quality improvement strategies may improve this situation. A further problem remains, however, because there is clear evidence that human error[8,9] (e.g. wrong drug, dosage error, alarms immobilized, monitor not used, etc.) plays a major part in adverse outcomes after critical anaesthetic incidents. Monitoring is useful only if it is used correctly and the response by the anaesthetist to the information is appropriate. Comprehensive training and appropriate supervision remain vital.

With the widespread adoption of increased levels of monitoring, new problems have arisen. There is less direct contact with the patient, and perhaps a false sense of security and complacency is encouraged if the monitors are not sounding an alarm. Many anaesthetists resent the imposition of dogmatic guidelines and the subsequent loss of professional autonomy. The standards have medicolegal implications, and malpractice liability may be enhanced. A lack of knowledge of the benefit/risk profile, limitations, accuracy and correct use of monitoring devices may result in major errors of measurement and a risk of patient safety. It remains wise to have a healthy suspicion of the accuracy of the recorded data, and to seek clinical signs to corroborate the values displayed. Technology is no substitute for the continuous presence of a vigilant, well-trained anaesthetist displaying good clinical judgement. The simple act of applying monitors will not improve patient safety.

Alarm systems are also important. Frequently, the anaesthetist is faced with a selection of diverse devices that are fitted with non-descriptive alarm sounds without a visual display to indicate the source. There is a clear need for integration and more meaningful alarms.[10] Alarms should perhaps provide early warning of trends rather than of single values in isolation. Degrees of warning should exist, with the level of the alarm dependent on the severity of the problem and the degree of deviation from the baseline values. Trend analysis and display should exist, separate from the real-time display. A high incidence of false alarms often leads to the hazardous practice of inactivating the alarm systems.

Comprehensive monitoring is an accepted part of contemporary anaesthetic practice. In this chapter, monitoring will be discussed with reference to individual physiological systems but it should be borne in mind that each system is inseparably related to the others. At any specific time in the anaesthetic and peri-operative periods, a judgement concerning the welfare of the patient must be made by reviewing all the system monitors in use, and integrating this information with the clinical status of the patient. It is especially important that major clinical decisions and interventions are not made on the basis of data from a single monitor viewed in isolation.

In many respects, the welfare of the patient depends on optimum tissue oxygenation. The state of the cardiovascular and respiratory systems is therefore of prime importance in the evaluation of welfare and safety in the operative and peri-operative periods. It is important to emphasize that monitoring is often — indeed usually — continued into the postoperative period. It should be discontinued only when the patient has regained all homeostatic reflexes. It is increasingly appreciated that certain types of monitoring, such as pulse oximetry, should be continued for much longer after surgery than has hitherto been usual practice. Indeed, pulse oximetry may be advisable for a number of days postoperatively, especially at night and in vulnerable groups such as the elderly or the obese. Specific at-risk groups may also benefit from continuous pre-operative monitoring (e.g. continuous Holter monitoring of the electrocardiogram (ECG) in patients with a history of ischaemic heart disease for a number of days prior to surgery). However, the value of extensive pre- and postoperative monitoring remains to be clearly defined in well-designed, sufficiently powerful studies using appropriate (not intermediate) outcome measures such as functional status, quality of life, length of stay, cost-effectiveness and patient satisfaction, as well as death.

Although this chapter will review cardiovascular monitoring first, the respiratory and cardiovascular systems are so intimately interrelated that some monitors, for example the pulse oximeter, could reasonably be reviewed under either heading. For convenience, pulse oximetry is reviewed with respiratory monitors.

MONITORING OF THE CARDIOVASCULAR SYSTEM

CLINICAL EVALUATION

Palpation of the pulse, capillary refill, the presence or absence of cyanosis and the colour of the blood in the surgical field are simple measures which require no special equipment. They are subjective and hard to quantify but are useful, in conjunction with monitoring equipment, to provide an overall picture of the cardiovascular status of the patient and to corroborate the values displayed on the monitors. Clinical information does not suffer from artefacts such as electrical interference from diathermy.

ELECTROCARDIOGRAPHY

ECG monitoring is universally accepted as a routine, minimum standard of intra-operative monitoring.[1–5] Modern machines provide a continuous display of the ECG, a numerical indication of heart rate and identification and elimination of artefact. Sophisticated instruments are available which will also provide ST segment and arrhythmia analysis.

Basic requirements for ECG monitoring

1. *Display*. Although a screen display is invariably present, it is useful to have some form of hard-copy recorder. This may help in establishing a diagnosis and, of increasing importance, provides a permanent record. A display also enables the identification of artefact to be made more clearly.

2. *Diagnostic or monitoring mode*. Monitoring mode has a narrower frequency response (0.5–40 Hz), which helps to eliminate baseline drift and motion artefacts. Diagnostic mode has a wider frequency range (0.05–100 Hz), and gives a more accurate representation of the original signal. Diagnostic mode is used for ST segment analysis as monitoring mode provides greater filtering of the ECG signal at the lower end of the frequency range, and this distorts the ST segment changes associated with ischaemia. The filtering may cause a spurious shift of the ST segment, i.e. the iso-electric baseline may be increased or decreased; similarly, an elevated or depressed ST segment may appear to be iso-electric. Not all operating room

machines are equipped with both modes; basic machines offer only the monitoring mode. A monitor equipped with diagnostic mode should be used in all at-risk cases.

3. The machine should be calibrated correctly such that 1 mV = 10 mm. Paper speed should be 25 mm/s so that 1 mm corresponds to 0.04 s.

4. The leads should be placed correctly, with good electrode contact.

Lead systems

Unipolar leads measure the voltage at the electrode relative to a zero point, whereas bipolar leads measure the voltage difference between two electrodes. Leads I, II and III are bipolar. They represent permutations of two leads from electrodes on the right arm, left leg and left arm, and from Einthoven's triangle. If these bipolar leads are connected to a 5000 Ω resistance, a common central point is formed with a zero potential. If this zero point is then used with an active or exploring electrode, the potential at the exploring electrode is recorded, forming a unipolar lead system. Precordial leads V1–6 are unipolar. Leads V1 and V2 'look' at the right ventricle, V3 and V4 at the anteroseptal region of the left ventricle, and V5 and V6 the lateral aspect of the left ventricle. They are useful indicators of ischaemia and of left ventricular hypertrophy.

The augmented limb leads aVR, aVL and aVF are so called because they are augmented in height by disconnecting the right arm, left arm and left leg electrodes respectively from the common terminal; they are thus unipolar. They increase the available range of views of the heart in the frontal plane. Leads II, III and aVF give information regarding the inferior region of the myocardium.

Ideally, a full 12-lead system (leads I, II, III, V1–6, aVR, aVL, aVF) should be monitored. However, this is not usually practical in the theatre environment. A five-lead system, comprising leads I, II, III, aVR, aVL, aVF and V5, has been recommended,[11] allowing comprehensive monitoring of both rhythm and anterior and inferior wall ischaemia. Most ECG monitors used intra-operatively have a three-lead system. Therefore, various lead systems have been devised to form *modified bipolar limb leads* in an attempt to gain more information and alternative views of the heart from the basic three-lead system geometry. An example, the CM5 configuration, involves setting the monitor to the lead I position and then placing the right arm electrode on the manubrium, the left arm electrode in the V5 position, and using the left leg as a ground or indifferent lead. It is useful as a monitor of anterior ischaemia. The modified central lead (MCL1), in which the left leg lead is moved to the V1 position and lead III is recorded, provides good P-wave deflection as well as good views of the QRS complex. The CB5 lead system has the right arm lead centred on the right scapula, the left arm in the V5 position and lead I is recorded. It provides good definition of the P wave, and detects anterior ischaemia. Many other combinations are available, e.g. CS5, CC5, CL3, etc. All modified limb leads represent some form of compromise of the various specific leads of the 12-lead ECG used to monitor changes in rhythm or the presence of ischaemia.

Additional lead positions, and therefore different views of the heart, are available by placing electrodes in the oesophagus, the trachea, or within the myocardium itself (with an appropriately isolated monitor). The oesophageal electrode records a prominent P wave and may be particularly useful in defining atrial contraction and its relationship to ventricular activity and the QRS complex. It may also be of value in the measurement of ischaemia in the posterior region of the myocardium, which is poorly defined with conventional leads.[12] Intramyocardial electrodes (e.g. via a pulmonary artery flotation catheter with three atrial and two ventricular electrodes) produce the atrial and ventricular electrogram (AEG and VEG), and can be useful in helping to characterize complex atrial arrhythmias.

Arrhythmia monitoring

The detection and diagnosis of arrhythmias has become the most important use of the ECG since its introduction to anaesthesia in the early 1960s. The incidence of arrhythmias reported in anaesthetized patients ranges from 15 to 84%.[13–17] Clearly, the incidence varies according to the population studied, the type of surgery being undertaken and the criteria used to define a change of rhytm as an arrhythmia.

An increased incidence of peri-operative arrhythmias is associated with:

- patients with pre-existing cardiovascular disease, including coronary artery disease
- the elderly
- abnormal arterial blood gases and electrolytes, e.g. hypoxaemia, hypercapnia, hypokalaemia and hyperkalaemia
- specific types of concurrent medication, e.g. cardiac glycosides, tricyclic antidepressants
- the use of various vaso-active drugs, e.g. cocaine, adrenaline, aminophylline
- light levels of anaesthesia

- the use of some anaesthetic drugs, e.g. halothane, ketamine
- laryngoscopy and intubation, especially if prolonged or performed during light levels of anaesthesia
- more invasive surgery, especially cardiothoracic, major vascular and intracranial
- various peri-operative reflexes, e.g. vagal and ocular–cardiac
- during the passage of wires and catheters through the heart, e.g. pulmonary artery flotation catheter.

If a disturbance of cardiac rhythm occurs, it is important to determine its nature and possible cause or causes. Factors involved in diagnosing a specific rhythm disturbance include establishing whether the rhythm is regular or irregular, and defining the nature of the QRS complex and its relationship to the P wave. It is then usually possible to determine if it is a potentially dangerous disturbance that requires treatment (these would include those resulting in circulatory compromise, a sustained tachycardia, or those with the potential to lead to ventricular fibrillation (VF) and/or ventricular tachycardia (VT)). Treatment should include the correction of any physiological or pharmacological imbalance that may be contributing to the arrhythmia.

Lead selection for arrhythmia detection

A lead which provides the maximum definition of the P wave and its relationship to the QRS complex is the most appropriate. Lead V1 gives good P-wave definition and is also useful in diagnosing the origin of any ventricular premature complexes but cannot usually be monitored with most equipment available during surgery. Leads II or MCL1 are the most appropriate for a three-lead system.

Automated analysis of arrhythmias is available; however, due to technical constraints, it is more accurate for ventricular than for atrial arrhythmias, and accuracy is enhanced if more than one lead is analysed.[18] Movement and diathermy can also cause interference. Automated analysis does not obviate the need for vigilance and corroboration by the anaesthetist.

Monitoring of ischaemia

All patients have a potential risk of peri-operative myocardial ischaemia. This risk has been demonstrated to be greater if:

- there is pre-existing coronary artery disease,[19,20] especially if the patient has had a myocardial infarction within 6 months;[21]
- adverse peri-operative haemodynamic events occur, such as tachycardia, hypotension and hypertension;[21,22]
- thoracic and intra-abdominal surgery,[23] and perhaps other prolonged procedures, are undertaken.

In the absence of pro-arrhythmic drugs, such as halothane, anaesthetic technique per se appears to have little effect on the incidence of ischaemia, provided that normal haemodynamic parameters are maintained.[23]

Peri-operative ischaemia has been clearly shown to increase morbidity and mortality[19,24] It is important to note that ECG detection of ischaemia is not as sensitive as other measures available. The most sensitive are probably measures of ventricular compliance such as an increase in left ventricular end-diastolic pressure (ischaemic endocardium is less compliant).[25] These precede the development of regional wall motion abnormalities (RWMAs) as seen on transoesophageal echocardiography, and changes in contractility. Only with continuing ischaemia do ECG changes become apparent.

Increasing the number of leads monitored increases the sensitivity of ischaemia detection.[26] In general, monitoring of the precordial leads provides most information concerning myocardial ischaemia. Of the various lead systems available, V5 is probably the most sensitive single lead for detecting ischaemia.[26] The modified bipolar lead CM5 (or CC5) is the next most sensitive for the detection of anterior ischaemia (it also benefits from being less sensitive than V5 to electrical interference).[27] Leads II, III, and aVF are the best for inferior ischaemia. Ideally, the choice of leads monitored should be guided by the results of pre-operative coronary angiography or exercise stress testing, if these are available.

ST segment analysis

The majority of the information concerning ST segment changes and their relationship to myocardial ischaemia comes from exercise ECG stress testing. Myocardial ischaemia is first evidenced by depression of the J-point (the J-point identifies the junction of the S wave and the ST segment) and an up-sloping ST segment. If ischaemia continues, progressive depression of the ST segment develops (this is deemed to be significant if there is >1 mm depression 0.06 s from the J-point)[28] which may be convex, horizontal or down-sloping. The more severe the depression, the more severe the ischaemia. ST segment elevation of >1 mm indicates severe transmural myocardial ischaemia.

Computerized ST segment analysis has been developed in an attempt to improve the detection of ischaemia. It has proven useful in exercise ECG testing.[29] The accuracy is improved if more than one lead is monitored. However, errors can occur with ectopic beats, conduction defects and with electrical interference.

The risk of ECG monitoring is slight, but burns from faulty or poorly insulated machines and from small electrodes have been reported.[30] Protection is afforded with modern machines by electrical isolation from the patient and the presence of a line isolation monitor in the circuitry of the theatre power supply.

BLOOD PRESSURE MONITORING

Arterial blood pressure is a fundamental cardiovascular parameter representing the driving force available for organ and tissue perfusion, and gives some indication of the workload imposed on the heart (i.e. afterload). Its measurement, along with other physiological variables such as heart rate, is used as a guide in adjusting the depth of anaesthesia. It is an essential component of minimal standards of monitoring during anaesthesia.[1-5] Blood pressure may be measured non-invasively or invasively.

Non-invasive blood pressure measurement

The underlying principle of all systems of non-invasive blood pressure measurement involves the inflation of a pneumatic cuff enclosing a peripheral artery to the point at which blood flow is occluded, and then measuring the sequence of physiological changes that occur as the cuff is deflated. The measurement may be achieved by palpation, pulse oximetry[31] (recording systolic blood pressure only), by auscultation (listening for Korotkoff sounds I–V), ultrasound, Doppler, measurement of arterial wall motion or by the oscillometric method. The latter is the method used in most current automatic blood pressure devices, e.g. the Dinamap (Device for Indirect Non-invasive Automated Mean Arterial Pressure) and the Accutor.

The modern automatic devices allow consistent, reasonably reliable, 'hands-free' measurement of blood pressure. Many are equipped with alarms for high and low pressure as well as a recorder, printer and facility for trend analysis. They display a numerical value for the systolic, diastolic and mean blood pressure along with a value for heart rate. The majority use the oscillometric method, which relies on the variation in cuff pressure resulting from the arterial pulsation during deflation to determine the blood pressure. The peak deflection is equivalent to the mean blood pressure, and the systolic and diastolic pressures are calculated from the rate of change of the pressure pulsation. The systolic is taken to be somewhere between 25 and 50% of the increasing pulsation, and the diastolic is taken at 80% of decline from the maximum.[32] There is a good correlation with invasive techniques at normal ranges of blood pressure. However, at lower levels (<80 mmHg), an overestimation of blood pressure occurs.[33]

A number of factors can affect the measured value. It is important to match the cuff size to the size of the patient's arm, for if the cuff is too small it will cause an over-reading, and if it is too big it may underestimate the blood pressure. It is recommended that the cuff width should be 30–40% of the arm circumference.[34] The pneumatic balloon should be centred over the artery. An adequately slow deflation rate is required and a rate of 3 mmHg/s or 2 mmHg per heart beat has been suggested.[35] The actual location on the body for measurement is probably unimportant. Complications are infrequent, but nerve damage, petechiae, superficial thrombophlebitis, skin necrosis and compartment syndrome have been reported when the measurements were repeated with excessive frequency.[36-38]

An alternative method of non-invasive blood pressure measurement comprises the use of a finger-cuff system. The device is known as the Finapres, and it uses the method described by Penaz in 1973;[39] a pressurized cuff is applied to a finger and a constant digital arterial size is maintained during each pulse cycle by varying the pressure within the cuff. The digital artery size is determined by photoplethysmography. The rapidly varying cuff pressure tracks the arterial pressure throughout the pulse cycle and provides a continuous readout of the arterial pressure wave form. However, it is affected by a number of factors; these include cuff size, movement, haemodynamic disturbances, vasoactive drugs, sympathetic stimulation, hypovolaemia, arterial spasm and the presence of an intra-arterial catheter in the same hand.[40] There is a tendency for a downward drift of readings with time, although this may be corrected by repeated calibration. Studies comparing it with direct and oscillometric methods suggest that it has reasonable correlation with values obtained with the oscillometric method,[41,42] but that the technique requires further refinement before it can be relied upon as a measure comparable with invasive methods.

Two newer technologies are being developed for continuous, non-invasive blood pressure measurement. Both are calibrated with standard oscillometric techniques. The first, arterial tonometry, involves the use of arterial microtransducers to produce partial compression of a superficial artery against bone and thereby record the intra-arterial force and hence the arterial pressure.[43] It has shown good correlation with invasive measures in both normotensive and hypotensive patients.[44] It is subject to inteference from movement, and transducer compression. The second method measures the delay in the propagation of the arterial pulse wave by comparing the pulse detected with photodiode sensors at two different sites (e.g. finger and forehead). The measured delay is related to the blood velocity, which in turn is related to the arterial blood pressure.

Invasive blood pressure measurement

Direct intravascular monitoring is accepted to be the 'gold standard' for blood pressure measurement. It provides beat-to-beat blood pressure monitoring and inspection of the displayed waveform can provide some information on myocardial contractility, afterload (the impedance to left ventricular ejection) and the significance of any disturbances of cardiac rhythm. For example, changes in the waveform with intermittent positive-pressure ventilation (IPPV) may suggest a decrease in preload (left ventricular end-diastolic pressure). It requires arterial cannulation, a pressure transducer and flush system as well as a signal-processing and display unit. A suggested list of indications for invasive blood pressure monitoring is given in Table 5.1.

The radial artery is used most commonly for direct blood pressure monitoring because it is usually superficial and readily palpable, and has a good collateral circulation via the ulnar artery. A test of this collateral circulation is Allen's test. Allen's test was described in 1929 for assessing collateral flow in patients with thrombo-angitis obliterans.[45] It has been modified somewhat for testing the integrity of the palmar arch before radial artery cannulation. After clenching the fist, both the radial and ulnar arteries are occluded by firm digital pressure. Then, with the hand open, the ulnar artery pressure is released and the time for return of normal colour to the palm is noted. If the recorded time is >15 s, ulnar collateral flow is said to be impaired and it is suggested that cannulation of the radial artery

Table 5.1 Indications for invasive blood pressure monitoring

Continuous blood pressure measurement
Cardiovascular instability, deliberate hypotension or hypothermia

Severe cardiovascular or pulmonary disease

Major fluid shifts, blood loss, multiple trauma

Inability to record blood pressure non-invasively (e.g. the very obese, or patients with extensive burns)

Direct manipulation of the cardiovascular sytem, e.g. cardiac surgery, inotropic therapy, aortic surgery

Intracranial procedures

Thoracic surgery

Liver transplantation

Frequent arterial blood sampling
Blood gas measurement

Acid–base disturbances

Electrolyte or metabolic derangements

Coagulopathies

in that hand should be avoided. Its predictive role has been challenged, with complications occurring in the presence of a normal Allen's test,[46,47] and none being reported in patients with an abnormal test.[48,49] Hand dominance may be of some relevance in the decision on which side to cannulate. Alternative cannulation sites include the ulnar, brachial, axillary, femoral, dorsalis pedis and the posterior tibial arteries.

Complications of arterial cannulation include haemorrhage, haematoma formation, vascular insufficiency and embolic phenomena, skin necrosis, catheter site infection and possible source for systemic sepsis, and inaccurate pressure measurement resulting in errors of treatment. Important features in reducing thrombosis and other complications include aseptic technique and a narrow (20-gauge) parallel-sided cannula made of a non-thrombogenic material such as Teflon with a continuous flush system of heparinized saline at 4 ml/h. The incidence of complications increases with time, and the duration of cannulation should be as short as possible.

CARDIAC FILLING PRESSURES

The filling pressure of the heart is one of a number of factors involved in determining cardiac performance and output because of its relationship to left ventricular end-diastolic volume and contractility. The pressures that can be measured clinically include central venous pressure (CVP), pulmonary artery pressure (PAP) and the pulmonary artery occlusion pressure (PAOP) or pulmonary capillary wedge pressure. Central venous cannulation is a prerequisite for monitoring these pressures, although left atrial pressure is occasionally monitored after cardiac surgery through a catheter introduced directly into the atrium during surgery. The indications for central venous cannulation are listed in Table 5.2.

Various sites of cannulation are available, including the internal jugular, subclavian, external jugular, cephalic, basilic and femoral veins. The right internal jugular vein is selected most often because it has a well-defined anatomical location associated with clear landmarks (the carotid artery and the sternomastoid muscle). In addition, it is often ballottable or visible when the patient is placed in the head-down position, it is straight and valveless, and it offers direct access to the superior vena cava with a high success rate of cannulation and low incidence of complications. The right side is technically easier for the majority of operators (who are right-handed), and the absence of a thoracic duct on that side eliminates another potential complication.

The incidence and type of complications of central venous cannulation (Table 5.3) vary with the experience of the operator and the site of cannulation.

Central venous pressure measurement

CVP measurement gives some indication of the intravascular blood volume, venous return and right ventricular function. CVP measurement is of value only if it is used in combination with other measures and clinical observations (e.g. blood pressure, heart rate,

Table 5.2 Indications for central venous cannulation

Measurement of central venous pressure

Insertion of a pulmonary artery flotation catheter (measurement of pulmonary artery pressure, pulmonary artery occlusion pressure, cardiac output)

Insertion of a pacing wire

Administration of fluids, blood, chemotherapy, vaso-active drugs or sclerosant drugs

Total parenteral nutrition

Inability to obtain peripheral venous access

Treatment of air embolism

Plasmapheresis

Haemofiltration and haemodialysis

Table 5.3 Complications of central venous cannulation

Trauma to artery, e.g. carotid, subclavian
Trauma to nerves, e.g. brachial plexus, stellate ganglion
Trauma to lung and pleura, e.g. pneumothorax, haemothorax, pleural effusion
Haematoma
Chylothorax (on the left)
Mediastinal effusion
Emboli: air, catheter, wire
Cardiac perforation and tamponade
Arrhythmias and heart block
Thrombosis and thrombo-embolism
Infection, endocarditis
Extravasation and extravascular migration
Catheter knotting and fracture
Microshock

urine output, skin temperature). The trend of values and the response to intervention are of much more relevance than the absolute value itself. The importance of the precise location of the cannula tip depends on the reason for the insertion of the cannula. If the indication is rapid transfusion, the precise location of the tip is of limited importance. However, if inserted for the measurement of right atrial pressure or for aspiration of air emboli, then its location should be at the junction of the superior vena cava and the right atrium.

The most simple method of measurement is with a water manometer. However, a major disadvantage of this technique is that the information that can be gained from inspection of the waveform is lost. The use of a pressure transducer system provides this information. The normal wave form consists of three waves, the *a*, *c* and *v* waves. The *a* wave represents atrial contraction, the *c* wave the bulging of the tricuspid valve during systole, and the *v* wave right atrial filling against a closed tricuspid valve. Observation of the waveform may be useful in the diagnosis of specific cardiac conditions (e.g. absence of *a* waves may represent atrial fibrillation or flutter, cannon *a* waves appear with complete heart block and large *v* waves are seen in association with tricuspid incompetence). Regardless of the method of measurement, CVP should be measured at the end of expiration with the reference point at the junction of the superior vena cava and the right atrium.

Pulmonary artery pressure measurement

In 1970, Swan, Ganz and their colleagues described a catheter that could be floated into the pulmonary artery without the use of radiography or fluoroscopy.[50] Subsequent results from many studies have shown that there is poor bedside assessment by clinicians of the haemodynamic status of critically ill patients,[51] and this has, amongst other factors, contributed to the widespread use of the pulmonary artery flotation catheter (PAFC) in operating theatres and the intensive care unit (ICU). A number of studies have suggested that invasive monitoring with cardiac output measurement reduces the incidence of peri-operative ischaemia and improves outcome,[21,52] and that optimization of cardiac output and oxygen delivery reduces mortality in ICU patients.[53,54] However, there is also a body of opinion that suggests that PAFCs are overused, and result in unnecessary complications with no demonstrated improvement in morbidity and mortality; large prospective studies in patients undergoing elective coronary artery bypass grafts[55] or abdominal aortic reconstructive surgery[56] have shown no difference in outcome with PAFC monitoring. Similarly, no improvement in mortality was found in a large group of patients with acute myocardial infarction.[57]

The PAFC does allow:

- measurement of right- and left-sided cardiac filling pressures (CVP, PAP and PAOP)
- measurement of cardiac output and the calculation of other haemodynamic variables
- sampling of mixed venous blood
- measurement of partial pressures of oxygen and carbon dioxide in samples of mixed venous blood
- differential arrhythmia diagnosis
- cardiac pacing
- continuous mixed venous pulse oximetry
- instantaneous and continuous pulmonary blood flow measurements
- blood temperature measurement.

The measurement of PAOP gives an estimation of the LVEDP and, indirectly, of left ventricular end-diastolic volume (LVEDV), or preload, which is a determinant of left ventricular contractility. A number of assumptions are made in relating the PAOP to the LVEDV, and factors such as left ventricular compliance, mitral valve function, airway pressure and location of the tip in different West lung zones (the tip should be ideally in West zone III where venous pressure > arterial pressure > alveolar pressure) can affect the validity of such assumptions.

However, with the exception of direct measurement of left atrial pressure (LAP), measurement of the PAOP remains the best estimate of the filling pressure of the left ventricle. CVP measurement has been shown to be a poor indicator of left ventricular filling in many circumstances[58-60] and pulmonary artery diastolic pressure is also a poor correlate in situations of raised pulmonary vascular resistance[61] (e.g. hypoxaemia, hypercapnia, hypothermia, chronic lung disease and tachycardia >120 beats/min).

Measurement of PAOP has also been suggested as a monitor of myocardial ischaemia.[62] Ischaemia results in a decrease in ventricular compliance because ischaemic myocardium is stiffer,[25] and subsequently there is an increase in LVEDP. This rise in the LVEDP has been shown to be a sensitive and early indicator of ischaemia. However, the estimates of LVEDP obtained from measuring PAOP and pulmonary artery diastolic pressure are too insensitive to be of value in the detection of ischaemia.[63]

Indications for pulmonary artery flotation catheter

In the absence of large, well-controlled and appropriate outcome studies, it is difficult to give precise indications for the insertion of a PAFC. In general, PAFC monitoring is used to assess volume status, to measure cardiac output and give some indication of myocardial function, to measure mixed venous oxygen saturation and to derive haemodynamic parameters. A suggested list of clinical indications is shown in Table 5.4.

The PAFC is passed through a sheath (typically 8–8.5 French gauge) placed into a large, usually central vein. The distal end of the catheter is connected to a pressure transducer system, thereby continuously identifying the location of the tip in its passage through the superior (or inferior) vena cava, right atrium, right ventricle, pulmonary artery, and finally to its 'wedged' position when the PAOP is recorded. A detailed description of the technique of insertion has been reviewed elsewhere.[64] Measured values obtained include the CVP, PAP, PAOP and mixed venous oxygen saturation with a fibre-optic PAFC. Calculated values include cardiac output and cardiac index, stroke volume and index, systemic vascular resistance (SVR) and pulmonary vascular resistance (PVR), left ventricular stroke work (LVSW) and index (Table 5.5), and oxygen delivery and oxygen consumption. The index equivalent is obtained by dividing the value by the body surface area (m^2).

Measurement and calculation may allow tailoring of treatment to the various forms of circulatory failure. It may also improve the accuracy of diagnosis and allow the construction of left ventricular function curves.

Complications of pulmonary artery catheters

Complications include all those listed previously for central venous cannulation and catheterization. In

Table 5.4 Clinical indications for pulmonary artery flotation catheter monitoring

Non-cardiac surgery

Cardiac disease: severe coronary artery disease, recent acute myocardial infarction, right and left ventricular failure, aortic and mitral valvular disease, cardiomyopathies, uncontrolled arterial hypertension

Pulmonary disease: severe chronic obstructive pulmonary disease, adult respiratory distress syndrome, pulmonary emboli, pulmonary hypertension

Shock: septic, hypovolaemic, cardiogenic

Major fluid shifts and/or losses, e.g. multiple trauma, major burns

Aortic surgery involving cross-clamping

Intravascular volume assessment

Inotropic therapy and intra-aortic balloon counterpulsation

High-risk patients, e.g. ASA 4 and 5, especially those undergoing complicated surgery

Liver transplantation, porto-systemic shunt surgery

Patients receiving assisted ventilation with high levels of positive end-expiratory pressure

Cardiac surgery

Poor left ventricular function (ejection fraction < 0.5, left ventricular end-diastolic pressure > 15 mmHg, cardiac index < 21/min)

Significant aortic or mitral valve disease

Severe ischaemic heart disease

Recent (< 6 months) acute myocardial infarction

ASA = American Society of Anesthesiologists.

addition, there are some complications which are specific to PAFCs:

- pulmonary haemorrhage
- pulmonary infarction
- pulmonary artery rupture
- pulmonary and tricuspid valve trauma
- tricuspid incompetence
- balloon rupture
- transient hypotension and hypoxaemia with balloon inflation.

Relative contraindications to the insertion of a PAFC include:

- tricuspid or pulmonary valve disease/replacement
- recent pacemaker insertion
- ventricular arrhythmias/complete heart block
- coagulopathy.

Table 5.5 Derived haemodynamic variables

CO = HR × SV (1/min)
SVR = (MAP − RAP) × 80 / CO (dyne.s per cm^5)
LVSW = (MAP − MPAOP) × SV × 0.0136 (g/m)
PVR = (MPAP − MPAOP) × 80 / CO (dyne.s per cm^5)

CO = cardiac output; HR = heart rate; SV = stroke volume; SVR = systemic vascular resistance; MAP = mean arterial pressure; RAP = right atrial pressure; LVSW = left ventricular stroke work; MPAOP = mean pulmonary artery occlusion pressure; PVR = pulmonary vascular resistance; MPAP = mean pulmonary artery pressure.

Left atrial pressure measurement

Direct monitoring of LAP is usually restricted to patients undergoing cardiac surgery. It is a definitive measurement of the LAP, unlike the estimation made from the PAFC, and therefore a much more accurate index of LVEDV. The cannula is inserted directly by the surgeon either through the right atrium or through the right pulmonary vein. There is the potential risk of air embolism (in this situation, directly to the systemic circulation), catheter shearing and bleeding.

CARDIAC OUTPUT MONITORING

Adequate cardiac output is fundamental to tissue perfusion as it provides the driving force for delivery of oxygen and substrate, and the removal of carbon dioxide and waste. CO is normally 5–6/1 min in an adult and is adjusted and regulated to meet global requirements and local tissue needs. Normally, it can be increased by up to five times if required. It is used with other measurements in the calculation of SVR and other derived haemodynamic variables. It can be measured either invasively (Fick principle, indicator dilution method, thermodilution method), or non-invasively (Doppler and transthoracic impedance plethysmography).

Invasive cardiac output measurement

These methods are generally more expensive, require access to the central circulation and often repeated blood sampling.

Fick cardiac output measurement

In 1870, Fick described a method in which blood flow was calculated from the oxygen consumption and the difference between arterial and mixed venous oxygen contents:[65]

$$Q = \frac{Vo_2}{(Cao_2 - Cvo_2) \times 10} \quad \text{(equation 1)}$$

where Q = cardiac output (l/min); Vo_2 = oxygen consumption (ml/min); Cao_2 = oxygen content of arterial blood (ml/dl); Cvo_2 = oxygen content of mixed venous blood (ml/dl).

Interest in this method has been rekindled by recent developments in continuous measurement of mixed venous oxygen saturation by PAFC oximetry and continuous respiratory gas analysis with infrared and mass spectrometry.[66] If steady-state haemodynamics exist and there are no errors in sampling and analysis, the Fick method gives highly reproducible results.[67]

Indicator dilution cardiac output measurement

This is a variant of the Fick principle in which a known quantity of indicator (e.g. the dye indocyanine green) is injected and the changes in concentration are measured. It allows for fairly rapid cardiac output measurement, but requires repeated continuous blood sampling, and problems exist with accumulation of dye and recirculation effects. A more recent method involves the detection of the dye by a fibre-optic densitometer placed on the ear, negating the need for repeated blood sampling.[68] Its role remains to be clarified.

Thermodilution cardiac output measurement

Thermal indicators were first used in dogs in 1954 and introduced into cardiac output measurement in humans in 1968.[69] A thermistor is located in the tip of the PAFC, allowing repeated measurements of cardiac output with a non-toxic, non-cumulative and non-recirculating dye, i.e. cold liquid. It requires a computation constant to be entered manually into the computer (this constant is affected by the catheter size, the injected volume, the thermal properties of the injectate and temperature). Accuracy and reproducibility are improved by taking the average of three measurements, thereby approximately doubling the confidence limits. Usually an injectate volume of 10 ml is used; ice-cold injectate has not been shown to confer a major advantage over fluid at room temperature, and carries with it the risk of bradycardia and other arrhythmias.

Non-invasive cardiac output measurement

Doppler techniques

In 1843, Doppler described a change or shift in the frequency of a transmitted wave when it is reflected from a moving object. Ultrasound waves of frequencies ranging from 1 to 10 MHz are produced from piezoelectric crystals. The Doppler shift of the reflected waves is processed to produce a measure of blood velocity.

Cardiac output may be measured using the Doppler principle with a probe positioned in the suprasternal notch, the oesophagus or in the trachea. It can also be applied to the measurement of regional organ perfusion. An implantable Doppler microprobe technique has been developed, and has been used to measure portal vein and hepatic artery blood flow in volunteers[70] and in patients following liver transplantation,[71] and to measure saphenous vein graft flow after coronary artery bypass graft surgery.[72]

Cardiac output equals the average blood velocity multiplied by the cross-sectional area of the vessel multiplied by the time period of ejection multiplied by the heart rate. Thus, regardless of the location of the Doppler probe, the measurement of cardiac output requires a value for the cross-sectional area of the blood vessel that does not change throughout the cardiac cycle, an ultrasonic beam closely parallel to the direction of the blood flow and the ability to integrate the blood flow velocity over the period of ejection to provide an average velocity. Potential sources of error include the miscalculation of the average velocity from the measured values and inaccuracy in obtaining a value for the cross-sectional area of the vessel.

The suprasternal location gives a measure of the blood flow velocity in the ascending aorta at the aortic valve level. It allows positioning of the beam parallel to the blood flow and measures total cardiac output minus the coronary artery blood flow. The aortic root diameter is measured by precordial echographic imaging or via a monogram using the patient's height and weight. The probe positioning is critically important and is a source of error with intermittent measurements. There is reasonably good correlation with thermodilution measurement.[73]

Transoesophageal positioning allows continuous unattended measurement. An ultrasound transducer is placed on the tip of a standard oesophageal stethoscope. It measures the blood flow velocity in the descending thoracic aorta and therefore requires some correction or calibration factor to give a value of the total cardiac output. This calibration involves using a suprasternal probe to give an initial value for the total cardiac output and comparing that with the value obtained from the oesophageal probe. One source of error is that the relationship between the two measured cardiac outputs can change; further error is introduced because the beam is directed at 45° to the direction of blood flow. The cross-sectional area of the aorta is determined by ultrasonic imaging or from a nomogram. Consequently, the absolute values of cardiac output measured by transoesophageal echocardiography are less reliable than those obtained by other methods, but the technique provides information concerning trends in cardiac output.[74] It can reasonably detect an increase in cardiac output of more than 15%, but is not as accurate in the detection of a decrease in cardiac output.[75] With further development, analysis of the Doppler waveform itself may give information on hypovolaemia, myocardial contractility and other disease states.

Transtracheal measurement involves the use of a special tracheal tube with an ultrasound transducer located at its tip and a specially shaped cuff to hold the probe against the anterior wall of the trachea. It measures the aortic diameter and the ascending aortic blood flow continuously, with no requirement for calibration. However, the beam is not parallel to the direction of blood flow, being at an angle of approximately 52°. There is a poor agreement with thermodilution measurements and with other techniques.[76] Optimal placement of the tracheal tube can be difficult.

A PAFC has been equipped with multiple transducers and has been used to determine instantaneous and continuous pulmonary blood flow.[77] This should allow assessment of right ventricular function and right ventricular–pulmonary vascular coupling, and give some indication of the output from the left ventricle. Early studies are encouraging, showing good correlation with thermodilution measurements, although the exact role of the technique is still not clear.

Impedance plethysmography

The technique was described in 1966, originally to measure cardiac performance in astronauts.[78] It relates changes in electrical impedance to the flow of current through the thoracic cavity to the ejection of blood during the cardiac cycle. Four pairs of skin electrodes are placed on the neck and lower thorax. A small current is passed across the chest and the impedance measured. The height, weight and sex of the patient are entered into the computer, allowing an estimate of the volume of the thoracic cavity. There is a reasonably good correlation with other measures,[79] but it is not as accurate at higher heart rates or in situations of sepsis and haemodilution when blood flow is less pulsatile.[80] Impedance plethysomography is presently neither sufficiently accurate nor reliable enough to replace invasive techniques. Further development with improved thoracic cavity estimates and mathematical algorithms may lead to an improvement in performance.

ECHOCARDIOGRAPHY

Echocardiography uses reflected ultrasound waves from various tissue interfaces to construct a spatial image of the reflecting surface. By incorporating a facility to measure the Doppler shift of the reflected waves, flow velocities can be recorded.

Transoesophageal echocardiography provides a continuous, stable view of the heart during anaesthesia and surgery and can therefore be used as a perioperative monitor of myocardial function. The oesophageal approach offers the benefit of close proximity of the probe to the heart, with fewer problems of image degradation. It also results in less interference from bone and lung and gives a clearer image in the obese or emphysematous patient.

Initial devices were equipped with M-mode imaging, in which a narrow, single beam is used to display the structure and movement of the tissues in the line of the beam.[81] This is displayed against time to give a continuously changing unidimensional image of the tissue section. It provides good temporal resolution and accurate information on rapidly moving objects.

Two-dimensional echocardiography was subsequently developed. It uses multiple, repetitive scans in a fan-shaped pattern to give an image that resembles more closely an anatomical section of the tissues being scanned. It gives improved axial and lateral image resolution as well as real-time imaging, further increasing the amount of information obtained. Most devices incorporate a Doppler blood flow velocity measurement capability. Colour flow Doppler[82] uses a real-time image of the heart with colour coding, which demonstrates the direction and the velocity of blood flow. The three primary colours are used. Red indicates that the flow is directed towards the transducer, blue that it is directed away from the transducer, and green indicates that there is rapidly accelerating or turbulent flow, regardless of direction. Various combinations of the three colours are possible, representing the range of flow patterns seen.

The transoesophageal echocardiograph consists of a transducer attached to the tip of a standard 110 cm flexible gastroscope. The distal 10 cm can be deflected around 180° in two planes. The newer instruments contain a thermistor for temperature measurement, which guards against overheating and therefore prevents any risk of thermal injury. The instrument is guided to the correct position by use of the ultrasound image.

Two views are described, the long-axis and the short- or minor-axis view. The long axis visualizes all four chambers of the heart and the atrioventricular valves. The short axis shows a cross-section of the ventricle and is usually positioned at midpapillary muscle level. From both views, a qualitative estimate of the end-diastolic volume and the end-systolic volume can be made and therefore ejection fraction can be estimated. The use of transoesophageal echocardiography requires a well-trained operator with expertise in interpretation of the various views and measures. Reported risks include aspiration, arrhythmias, bleeding and oesophageal damage.[83]

Clinical uses

Assessment of global cardiac function

Preload. Measures of volume and area of the left ventricle can be made at the end of diastole. The short axis measure of LVEDV may be a better indicator of preload and predictor of cardiac output than is PAOP.[84] There is less correlation between the midpapillary short-axis measurement of left ventricular end-diastolic area and radionuclide studies.[85]

Afterload. Calculations of end-systolic ventricular wall stress can be made by measurement of ventricular size, wall thickness and arterial blood pressure. The place of wall stress measurement is not yet clear, but it may provide a better measure of afterload than does SVR. There is a strong association between ventricular wall stress and myocardial oxygen consumption.

Contractility. A number of measures are available, all requiring a comparison of an end-diastolic and end-systolic measurement. These include fractional shortening, ejection fraction, ejection fraction area and computer-assisted estimates of cardiac output.

Regional cardiac function/myocardial ischaemia detection

It has been demonstrated that myocardial contractile function is very sensitive to ischaemia. Inadequate myocardial perfusion is reflected in regional disturbances of activity, e.g. wall thickening and RWMAs, as evidenced by transoesophageal echocardiography. These RWMAs have been shown to precede ECG changes during the development of myocardial ischaemia, and can be used as a sensitive measure of ischaemia.[86,87] However, ischaemia is not the only cause of RWMAs; other factors, such as changes in afterload, heart rate and anaesthetic drugs, can alter wall motion.

Assessment of cardiac anatomy

The long-axis view demonstrates the mitral and aortic valves and may reveal evidence of calcification or vegetations. Its intra-operative use in adult and paediatric cardiac surgery can give valuable information concerning, for example, the function of repaired and prosthetic valves, and the presence of intracardiac shunts and the efficacy of their repair.[88–90] The left atria can be visualized and a myxoma or intramural thrombus can be diagnosed.

Intracardiac air

This application may be particularly relevant during neurosurgery[91] or open-chamber cardiac surgery.[92] Bubbles between 2 and 100 μm can be detected. It has been shown to be more sensitive than precordial Doppler monitoring in the detection of air bubbles and clearly gives more information regarding the possibility of paradoxical air embolism in patients with a patent foramen ovale.

Echocardiography has also been used in the diagnosis of thoracic aortic pathology,[93] e.g. acute dissection.

MONITORING OF THE RESPIRATORY SYSTEM

MEASURES OF OXYGENATION

One of the fundamental responsibilities of the anaesthetist is to ensure that the patient's tissues are adequately oxygenated. The consequences of even a temporary interruption to oxygen supply can result in major morbidity and mortality. Most commonly, oxygenation of blood is measured, either indirectly by measurement of the degree of saturation of haemoglobin or directly as oxygen tension; however, methods are also available to measure oxygenation of specific tissues. The varying techniques provide information regarding oxygenation at different points on the oxygen cascade. Each method has its advantages and limitations, and data from one source usually complement the information gained from another.

Measures of oxygen saturation

Pulse oximetry

Pulse oximetry is a non-invasive technique used to estimate the percentage saturation of haemoglobin with oxygen in arterial blood. An estimation of the partial pressure of oxygen can be made with knowledge of the oxygen dissociation curve. The oxygen content can be derived. The technique was developed initially in the 1940s[94] but early devices were impractical, and pulse oximeters were not introduced into clinical practice until 1983. Since then, the technique has gained widespread use and acceptance, and it is now regarded as a basic minimum standard of monitoring.[3-5] Introduction of pulse oximetry has been a major advance in monitoring, not only in the operating theatre but also in the post-anaesthetic care unit (PACU), ICU, accident and emergency department and, in some circumstances, the general ward environment.

Pulse oximeters have the disadvantage of being rather insensitive to large changes in arterial Po_2 at the upper end of the oxygen dissociation curve where a small change in oxygen saturation may signify a large change in partial pressure. No information concerning trends in the Pao_2 is given until it falls below about 11 kPa (83 mmHg). In addition, as the pulse oximeter monitors only arterial oxygen saturation, it provides no direct information regarding oxygen delivery to the tissues. However, its clear advantages are that it provides continuous information, that the measurements are reasonably reliable (particularly in the range 80–100%), that it is non-invasive and that it is easy to use. It enables detection of incipient and unsuspected arterial hypoxaemia, so that early treatment and intervention may be instituted and disastrous consequences avoided. It requires no special training and carries minimal risk.

A large number of studies have demonstrated clearly that the clinical detection of cyanosis is poor and unreliable, and that transient episodes of desaturation, and more severe hypoxic episodes, are much more frequent in the peri-operative period than was appreciated previously.[95,96] The use of pulse oximetry has been shown to reduce the frequency of peri-operative hypoxic episodes[95] and in a retrospective study has resulted in a significant decrease in the number of unexpected admissions to the ICU.[97]

Principles of pulse oximetry. The basic physical principles are based on the laws of Beer and Lambert. Beer's law relates the amount of light absorbed to the concentration of solute in the solution. Lambert's law relates absorbance of light to the thickness of the absorbing layer.

One wavelength is required for each substance measured and therefore, to measure oxyhaemoglobin and deoxyhaemoglobin, two different wavelengths are used. Clinically, the choice of wavelengths is restricted to between approximately 550 and 1300 nm, because wavelengths less than 550 nm are absorbed by the skin and those greater than 1500 nm are absorbed by body water. The pulse oximeter uses monochromatic light-emitting diodes, one with a wavelength in the red range (660 nm; the same as that used in the display of an electronic calculator), and the other in the infrared band (940 nm; the wavelength used routinely in remote-control handsets). These two wavelengths provide good sensitivity as there is a marked difference in the absorption of oxyhaemoglobin and deoxyhaemoglobin at these two values; 805 nm is one of the isobestic points of oxyhaemoglobin and deoxyhaemoglobin.

Absorption is measured by a silicone photodiode which changes the incident light into an electrical signal. Light is emitted in a rapidly repeating triplet sequence of red, infrared, and then off (400 Hz in the UK, 480 Hz in the USA — these represent multiples of mains frequency and are selected so as to minimize interference from background illumination). The off sequence allows a baseline measurement for any changes in ambient lighting. The voltage output from the silicone diode represents the optical changes in the tissue between the light source and the transducer, and it is presumed that these changes are due to the pulsatile arterial flow. It is this detection of a pulsatile absorbance signal that generates the name 'pulse' oximeter.

The signal from the detection of both the red and the infrared spectra can be divided into two parts, a stable component (DC) and a rapidly changing (AC) component. Absorbance in the DC component is from tissue, venous and capillary blood, and non-pulsatile arterial blood, whilst that of the AC component is from the pulsatile arterial blood flow. One of the main determinants of the accuracy of the device is the proportion of total signal coming from the AC component in comparison with that coming from the DC component. Usually, the AC component comprises approximately 0.5% of the total signal. Newer devices have lower limits for signal strength, and if the AC component falls below this level, an error message is displayed. The red and infrared values are then equalized by dividing the DC signal by the AC signal. The resulting values are then converted into numerical values and the ratios of these are used to calculate saturation of oxygen by an algorithm within the device. The mathematical calculation is represented in equation 2, where S = oxygen saturation, and AC_n and DC_n represent the AC and DC components at the two frequencies.

$$S = (AC_{660}/DC_{660})/(AC_{940}/DC_{940}) \quad \text{(equation 2)}$$

Simple machines use the difference between the peak and the trough of the signal, or a proportion of it, to calculate the saturation; this difference is presumed to be due to the arterial blood. However, problems arise with unstable data, and more sophisticated machines calculate instantaneous values which are then averaged over a few seconds and displayed. This allows rejection of poor-quality signals, and a more rapid and accurate response. However, they remain vulnerable to the effects of perfusion and motion.

Two methods of refinement have been developed. The first involves averaging 10 or more values to calculate a single value for display, and attaching a weight to each value; a poor-quality signal has a low weighted value and a good-quality signal has a higher one. The resultant figures are then averaged to reduce the sensitivity to motion and low perfusion. The second method involves using the ECG signal to time the oximetric signal, thereby reducing interference and improving performance in conditions of low perfusion or interference.

For the Beer–Lambert law to be applicable, there is a requirement for monochromatic light to pass in a parallel and perpendicular path of known length through a non-interfering solution, with only one unknown compound in solution. The light path should be short, and the solution non-turbid. Clearly, these conditions are not easily applicable to clinical in vivo measurements. The major problem encountered is the scattering of light in its passage through blood and other tissues. While all devices are theoretically based on the Beer–Lambert law, different manufacturers used different algorithms for the calculation of saturation. These are determined by comparing the predicted values obtained from the pulse oximeter with simultaneous in vitro measurements of saturation, either by manometric or by spectrophotometric methods. The accuracy of each device depends on the range of saturations compared and the number of values compared at each saturation. All machines are more accurate in the 80–100% range than when saturation is <70%. In addition, algorithms are based on measurements made under stable conditions, and the dynamic responses of different devices vary. Quoted accuracies are of the order of ±2% oxygen saturation from in the range 100–70%, ±3% in the range 70–50%, and unspecified below 50%.[98]

Interference can come from optical shunting, a phenomenon which occurs if the probe slowly comes off the finger; there is then an artefactual decrease in the saturation as the light starts to bypass the finger and be shunted to the photodiode. Other causes of interference include movement, hypothermia, vasoconstriction, diathermy, optical cross-talk, low perfusion, pulsatile flow not due to arterial inflow and variation in wavelength output from the light-emitting diodes.

Differing species of haemoglobin can also affect the accuracy of the reading. In most current devices, only two wavelengths are used and absorption is related only to two species of haemoglobin — adult deoxyhaemoglobin and adult oxyhaemoglobin. The wavelengths required to differentiate accurately between HbA and other haemoglobins (e.g. HbF, COHb, metHb and sulphHb) are in the range of less than 550 nm and are therefore limited to in vitro oximeters. Different haemoglobins affect the values obtained differently. HbF has an absorption spectrum similar to adult haemoglobin over the range of wavelengths used and it therefore causes no significant clinical error.[99] MetHb is normally present in concentrations less than 1%, but may rise to levels of greater than 8% after intravenous regional anaesthesia with prilocaine. MetHb simulates deoxyhaemoglobin at 660 nm, and the presence of high concentrations of MetHb drives the measured value of oxygen saturation towards 85% irrespective of the true proportion of oxyhaemoglobin in blood.[100] COHb is present in levels of approximately 3% in urban dwellers but may increase up to as much as 15% in heavy smokers; in carbon monoxide poisoning (e.g. smoke inhalation from conflagrations), COHb concentrations may approach 50%. COHb absorbs minimally at 940 nm, but at 660 nm absorbance is similar to that of oxyhaemoglobin. Its presence results in an overestimation of the saturation[101] so that a hypoxic patient may appear to have a normal oxygen saturation. Bench oximetry (where five wavelengths are available) is required to measure the carboxyhaemoglobin concentration in at-risk patients. SulphHb rarely presents a problem clinically.

A number of other factors may influence measured saturation. The presence of a raised level of bilirubin results in no clinically significant error. However, various dyes can affect the reading.[102] Methylene blue has its peak absorbance around 660 nm and its presence results in a decrease in the recorded saturation. Indocyanine green has a similar but smaller effect. Fluorescein has no clinical effect. Atrial fibrillation may cause errors, with unstable beat-to-beat measurements of oxygen saturation. Venous pulsation, such as that which occurs in severe right heart failure or tricuspid incompetence, may cause a spuriously low value since the pulsatile component is not solely due to arterial inflow. Blue nailpolish has a minimal effect. Pigmented skin gives minimal, if any, error. The potential problems and errors in pulse oximetry have been reviewed recently.[103–105]

Pulse oximetry is a remarkably safe procedure. However, there have been a number of reports of tissue damage from the probe.[106,107] Theoretically, the elderly and neonates are at greatest risk due to delicate or poorly perfused skin. There have also been instances of awareness during anaesthesia when spurious low oxygen saturation values have prompted the anaesthetist to increase the inspired oxygen concentration, delivering inadequate concentrations of anaesthetic agents.

Mixed venous haemoglobin saturation measurement

Pulmonary artery oximetry allows continuous monitoring of the mixed venous oxygen saturation (SvO_2). This measurement was first used in humans in 1973 with a dual-wavelength system.[108] In the late 1970s, a three wavelength (670, 700 and 800 nm) system was introduced, providing greater accuracy. The catheter contains fibre-optic bundles which transmit the incident and reflected light, and a value of SvO_2 is calculated. SvO_2 is related to SaO_2, oxygen consumption, cardiac output and haemoglobin concentration (equation 3).

$$SvO_2 = SaO_2 - \frac{VO_2}{1.38 \times Q \times [Hb] \times 10} \quad \text{(equation 3)}$$

where VO_2 = oxygen consumption, 1.38 = value for the combining power of oxygen with Hb (ml per g of Hb), Q = cardiac output and [Hb] = Hb concentration in g dl.

Thus a decrease in SvO_2 may result from decreases in arterial oxygen saturation, cardiac output or haemoglobin concentration, or from an increase in oxygen consumption. Alternatively, if oxygen consumption and content remain the same, then changes in SvO_2 are proportional to changes in cardiac output. Thus, continuous monitoring of SvO_2 can detect changes in the relationship between oxygen delivery and oxygen consumption. However, the technique cannot identify the cause of the imbalance or detect regional ischaemia.

Despite the theoretical link between cardiac output and SvO_2, a number of studies have failed to demonstrate any direct relationship between the two, probably because other variables in the equation do not remain constant.[109,110] It appears that the value of SvO_2 may be difficult to interpret and does not always represent global oxygenation. Moreover, little or no effect on outcome has yet been demonstrated by monitoring SvO_2 and it is probably not justified for routine use on cost/benefit grounds.[111,112]

Measures of oxygen tension

Continuous arterial blood gas monitoring

As noted above, pulse oximetry gives little information regarding trends in PaO_2 when the value is greater than 11 kPa (83 mmHg), as this represents the flat section of the oxygen dissociation curve. However, intermittent arterial blood gas sampling may miss significant and dramatic changes in PaO_2. Technology is now available to monitor continuously PaO_2, $PaCO_2$ and pH via an indwelling intra-arterial catheter.

The first continuous intra-arterial measurement of PO_2 was performed with a miniaturized Clark electrode (an electrical cell with a platinum cathode and a silver anode), but problems of interference with blood pressure monitoring and blood sampling, and poor accuracy, were reported. This system was improved upon, when the photoluminescence PO_2 sensor or optode was described.[113] The sensor is based on the principle that oxygen can reduce (or quench) the fluorescence intensity of various dyes adsorbed by certain inorganic chemicals. It is much simpler and smaller than the Clark electrode sensor.

With the use of a triple fluorescence catheter it is now possible to make in vivo measurements of PO_2, PCO_2 and pH (carbon dioxide and H^+ increase the fluorescence of the dyes) with approximately the same accuracy as laboratory blood gas analysis.[114] There have been problems with in vivo biocompatibility (sensors are now heparin-coated) and artefactual reductions in the recorded values. The system has been used in the ICU and operating theatre[115] and involves the insertion of an 18- or 20-gauge radial artery cannula. Results to date have been encouraging; catheters have been reported to be of value in the detection of air embolism, in detecting hypoxaemia during one-lung ventilation, and in monitoring of the extracorporeal circuit during cardipulmonary bypass.

Miniature oximetry catheters (which measure oxygen saturation rather than partial pressure) have also been developed for intravenous and intra-arterial use;[116] these are expected to have a significant impact.

Transcutaneous oxygen and carbon dioxide tensions

Transcutaneous measurement of oxygen and carbon dioxide was developed in the 1970s to provide a continuous, relatively non-invasive measure of tissue oxygenation. The basic principle is that in an area of skin where local blood flow is greater than the amount required for local oxygen consumption, the capillary partial pressure of oxygen approximates to the arterial oxygen tension. If the skin is heated, thereby increasing blood flow, the correlation is enhanced. Oxygen and carbon dioxide diffuse through the hyperaemic skin and the partial pressure is measured by surface electrodes. The electrodes are similar to those used for standard blood gas analysis, i.e. a Clark oxygen electrode (an electrical cell composed of a platinum cathode and a silver anode), and a Severinghaus carbon dioxide electrode (a pH-sensitive glass electrode in an electrolyte cell enclosed in a membrane permeable to carbon dioxide). They are placed on the skin surface, which is heated to 41–45°C (ideally ≥ 43°C). The values obtained are termed $PtcO_2$ and the $P_{tc}CO_2$. They reflect changes in local gas tension and/or changes in local blood flow.

It was shown in 1972 that a good correlation (within 10%) existed between PtcO$_2$ and PaO$_2$ in haemodynamically stable infants.[117] PtcO$_2$ measures peripheral tissue oxygenation over a wide range of PaO$_2$ values, and may detect deficits in perfusion when compared with the measurement of PaO$_2$ itself.

Problems with transcutaneous measurements include:

- inter-individual variability of up to 10%
- site-to-site variability (i.e. peripheral versus central location of the sensor)
- impaired reliability under conditions of haemodynamic instability, low cardiac output, skin hypoperfusion and peripheral vasoconstriction
- variation with increasing age; in newborn infants, PtcO$_2$ is almost identical to PaO$_2$, in young adults PtcO$_2$ is approximately 80% of the PaO$_2$, while in the elderly, this proportion decreases to approximately 70%
- a reduction in the recorded values in the presence of hypocapnia
- an upward drift of values caused by halothane; halothane can be electrochemically reduced and the resulting electrical current can cause interference with the oxygen electrode.

The instruments currently available have a warm-up time of 10–15 min and need regular calibration. Maintenance of electrodes is expensive, requiring regular replacement, and they have a slow response time. There is the potential for skin burns and these have been reported, particularly at temperatures of 45°C for longer than 4 h. Burns have not been reported when the temperature is less than or equal to 43°C and the site is changed every 4–8 h (more frequently in the newborn).

Transcutaneous devices may be superior to pulse oximetry in patients with carbon monoxide poisoning, because they continue to measure oxygen tension accurately. The ratio of distal limb to central PtcO$_2$ correlates with peripheral vascular disease[118] and has been used to determine limb viability. PtcO$_2$ measurement is also useful in the detection of venous air embolism in neurosurgery.

PtcCO$_2$ electrodes measure carbon dioxide tension in the tissues; thus, normal values of PtcCO$_2$ are greater than simultaneous measurements of PaCO$_2$ (e.g. 8 compared with 5.3 kPa, or 60 compared with 40 mmHg), and due to local heating, values are even greater than the venous carbon dioxide tension. Despite these discrepancies, there is a constant relationship between PtcCO$_2$ and PaCO$_2$[119] and various correction factors have been incorporated into the devices (most commonly either multiplying the measured value by 0.66, or using the formula PtcCO$_2$ × 0.75 − 3 mmHg). The relationship between PtcCO$_2$ and PaCO$_2$ is more consistent than that between PaCO$_2$ and end-tital carbon dioxide.

Limitations are the same as those of PtcO$_2$ measurement, but PtcCO$_2$ measurement also requires a more complex two-point calibration every 4–6 h. However, the technique is less sensitive than P_{tc}O$_2$ to the effects of age and perfusion. There tends to be some drift of values, which appears to be due to movement of water in and out of the electrode layers.

Conjunctival oxygen tension

In an attempt to improve the response time, a conjunctival PO$_2$ (PcjO$_2$) electrode has been developed. It consists of Clark electrode in a polymethylmethacrylate ring which rests against the conjunctiva. It does not require heating, equilibrates in 60 s, and has a more rapid response time. However, readings are still consistently lower (50–80%) than PaO$_2$.[120] As with PtcO$_2$ measurement, measured values are affected by cardiac output, age, halothane and hypovolaemia. There have been no reports to date of eye damage.

Measures of regional oxygenation

The presence of an adequate arterial oxygen tension does not, of itself, guarantee an adequate oxygen tension in the tissues (e.g. in situations of altered blood flow through the microcirculation in sepsis). More information concerning oxygen delivery and oxygen consumption can be gained if the oxygen tension is measured at tissue level. Four methods are currently available for the measurements of regional tissue oxygenation.

Intravascular and subcutaneous oximetry

Minature oximetry catheters are available for intra-arterial, intravenous and subcutaneous use. The use of subcutaneous oximetry in patients undergoing colorectal surgery has suggested a relationship between clinical outcome and oximetric signs of tissue hypoperfusion.[121] Catheters have also been placed in the suprahepatic vein and used to detect and measure liver ischaemia during hepatic surgery.[122]

Tissue Po$_2$ electrode

This technique involves the direct measurement of

oxygen tension by the insertion of microneedle sensors through the skin into the tissues. There is some suggestion in specific circumstances that their use may provide an earlier indication of an adverse event or trend regarding oxygenation than does the measurement of the arterial or venous Po_2.[123] However, a number of problems exist, including sterilization, biocompatibility, the requirement for regular calibration both immediately before and during use, the possibility of tissue damage, a large distribution of 'normal' values, and cost. Further development is required before they are introduced into regular clinical practice.

Cerebral oximetry

Cerebral oximetry is based on the principle of near infrared spectroscopy, which is similar to the principle of pulse oximetry, except that all wavelengths are in the infrared spectrum (typically wavelengths of 775, 805, 845 and 905 nm are used), as wavelengths in the visible spectrum will not penetrate the cranium. The maximum interoptode distance is 8 cm, allowing transmission spectroscopy in neonates and reflectance spectroscopy in adults.

There is absorption of the infrared light by the specific chromophores Hb and cytochrome Aa3, and this absorption changes with the redox state of the individual chromophores.[124] Reduction of oxygen to water occurs at the end of the cytochrome chain and therefore Aa3 absorption measurement theoretically gives some indication of oxygen availability at the cellular level. Unfortunately, the signal received from cytochrome Aa3 is overshadowed by that from Hb and there is some doubt regarding the accuracy of the values of cerebral oxygenation which are obtained. By assuming that the patient's haematocrit remains constant, values for cerebral blood volume can also be derived.

Cerebral oximetry has found experimental applications in a number of areas including fetal monitoring in labour, measurement of cerebral blood flow and oxygenation in paediatric patients,[125] myocardial oxygenation and blood flow in healing fractures. There is at least one commercial monitor currently available for clinical use, although its role is yet to be clearly defined.

Gastric intraluminal tonometry and pH measurement

Splanchnic tissue acidosis may be an early sign of decreased perfusion. The technique of intraluminal pH measurement presumes that intraluminal Pco_2 is equivalent to the Pco_2 in the wall of the stomach, and that the concentration of bicarbonate ions in the tissues is equivalent to the concentration in the arterial blood. As perfusion decreases, tissue Pco_2 increases. Carbon dioxide diffuses into the gut lumen and then equilibrates with a saline-filled Silastic tonometry balloon, permeable to carbon dioxide, which is placed in the stomach. By measuring separately the arterial bicarbonate concentration and using the Henderson–Hasselbalch equation (equation 4), a value for the mucosal pH can be calculated.

$$pH = 6.1 + \log \frac{[HCO_3^-]}{0.03\, Pco_2} \qquad \text{(equation 4)}$$

where 6.1 = pKa of the H_2CO_3 system, 0.03 = solubility coefficient of carbon dioxide in blood, Pco_2 = partial pressure of carbon dioxide and $[HCO_3^-]$ = plasma bicarbonate ion concentration.

This measurement has been shown to be a useful early predictor of mortality in critically ill adult patients,[126] but is less reliable under conditions of low perfusion pressure (e.g. cardiogenic shock) and in sepsis. In some centres, the measurement is used to guide resuscitation, and specific measures (e.g. dopexamine infusion) are taken if more general measures fail to improve mucosal pH.

In animals intramucosal pH correlates well with intestinal oxygen consumption, falling linearly with Vo_2 after oxygen delivery has been reduced to a critical level.

Measures of expired gas concentrations

In 1961, it was demonstrated that the continuous measurement of expired carbon dioxide could provide early detection of many adverse events.[127] Since then, there has been increasing awareness that preventable respiratory anaesthetic mishaps are a major contributor to peri-operative morbidity and mortality.[128,129] Capnography is now accepted in many countries as an essential monitor.

Capnometry and capnography

The capnometer measures non-invasively the concentration of carbon dioxide in the inspiratory and expiratory gases, giving a breath-by-breath analysis, and representing this diagrammatically in the form of the capnograph. Inspection of the waveform in terms of the height, frequency, rhythm, baseline and shape gives more information than simple inspection of the numerical values alone, and permits validation of the recorded value. Capnography does not provide only respiratory monitoring; information is gained also on aspects of the function of the cardiovascular system as well as some indication of metabolism and of the functioning of the anaesthetic and breathing system.

A number of methods are available for measurement of carbon dioxide, including mass spectrometry and Raman analysis. However, the majority of devices rely on the use of infrared light absorption. This involves the passage of monochromatic infrared light through a gas sample and also through a reference cell containing a known concentration of carbon dioxide. The amount of light absorbed is proportional to the concentration of carbon dioxide according to the laws of Beer and Lambert. A correction must be made if nitrous oxide is present as it has a similar absorption pattern to that of carbon dioxide. Measurement with this technique is also affected by the presence of water vapour, and water traps and filters are required.

The gas exhaled initially originates in the anatomical dead space, which is not involved in gas exchange and therefore contains no carbon dioxide. There is then a sudden increase in carbon dioxide concentration as alveolar gas enters the capnograph. The slope of this rapid rise gives some indication of the uniformity of alveolar emptying. The plateau phase is then reached; the plateau has a small upward slope, and ends at a peak value known as the end-tidal carbon dioxide tension (normally 4.5–6.0 kPa or 35–45 mmHg). This end-tidal carbon dioxide value is used as an estimate of the alveolar, and thus arterial, P_{CO_2}. There is then a sudden decrease in the carbon dioxide concentration as fresh gas replaces the alveolar gas during inspiration. During anaesthesia, the partial pressure of inspired carbon dioxide depends on the breathing system employed and the fresh gas flow rate. The normal capnograph therefore has a baseline at zero, a sharp upstroke, an almost horizontal alveolar plateau, and a sharp downstroke returning to the baseline.

There are two methods of sampling respiratory gases for capnography:

1. *Side-stream analyser.* A sampling tube continuously aspirates gas from the breathing system and conducts it to a distant measuring cell. The optimal sampling rate in adults is approximately 200 ml/min (with a range of 50–500 ml/min). Difficulties exist with low expired gas flows (where there is a tendency to under-read if fresh gas dilutes the carbon dioxide from the expired gas) and also with the potential for multiple leakage sites. There is a transport time delay which may amount to several seconds, depending on the volume of tubing and the sampling flow rate.

2. *Main stream.* The measuring cell is positioned between the cathether mount and the end of the tracheal tube in the breathing system. There is no aspiration of gas from the circuit, no transport delay and the signal changes almost immediately, with a typical response time of 50–150 ms. The measuring head is relatively heavy and is often heated to prevent water condensation; consequently, it must be supported, and it must not be placed in direct contact with the patient's skin.

The relationship between end-tidal and arterial P_{CO_2}

A correlation exists between end-tidal and arterial carbon dioxide tensions.[130] In a healthy adult with a normal lung, the end-tidal partial pressure of carbon dioxide is approximately 0.3–0.6 kPa (2.5–5 mmHg) less than that of arterial blood (the difference is decreased if the lungs are ventilated with a large tidal volume, and also in pregnancy[131]). However, there are many situations in which the relationship between end-tidal and arterial carbon dioxide tension is less clear. These include the following.

1. Failure to obtain an alveolar sample. This may occur when tidal volume is very low, if there is obstruction of the sampling catheter, or if the sample is obtained from an inappropriate position within the breathing system. These problems exist particularly in paediatric anaesthetic practice.[132]

2. Ventilation/perfusion (*V/Q*) mismatch. *Ventilation with no perfusion* (e.g. severe respiratory failure, pulmonary embolus, lateral decubitus position, systemic hypoperfusion, air embolism, cardiac arrest) results in increased alveolar deadspace. The excretion of carbon dioxide is from perfused alveoli only and the alveolar plateau recorded by the capnograph gives a value significantly below the actual partial pressure of arterial carbon dioxide. The magnitude of the difference between the end-tidal and the arterial carbon dioxide partial pressures provides some quantitative information on the size of the alveolar dead space.[133] *Perfusion with no ventilation* (e.g. endobronchial intubation, mucus plug, foreign body) causes a smaller increase in the difference between the arterial and the end-tidal carbon dioxide partial pressures.

3. Uneven emptying of alveoli (e.g. chronic obstructive airways disease) results in a sloping trace with no plateau. The lung units which empty last are those with poorest ventilation, the lowest *V/Q* ratio and therefore the highest partial pressure of carbon dioxide. During IPPV, expiration may not be complete when the next breath is delivered. Consequently, the end-tidal P_{CO_2} is significantly less than the arterial value; the difference may be exceed 2 kPa (15 mmHg).

4. An increase in apparatus dead space may allow

rebreathing, which results in an increase in end-tidal $P\text{CO}_2$ along with a rise in the inspired carbon dioxide concentration. However, in this instance, the relationship between arterial and end-tidal carbon dioxide tensions is not affected.

The clinical uses of capnography are shown in Table 5.6.

Anaesthetic agent monitoring

Ideally, all constituents of the breathing system should be measured, including the concentrations of oxygen, nitrous oxide, nitrogen and the volatile anaesthetic agent. Volatile agent monitoring is of particular importance, as excessive concentrations of volatile anaesthetic agents may result in hypotension, cardiac depression and cardiac arrest. Inadequate concentrations may result in awareness, pain and recall of intra-operative events. Vaporizer output may not equal the dial setting and clinically significant errors in dosage are possible, even with modern vaporizers. In addition, vaporizer output may vary with changing concentrations of nitrous oxide in the carrier gas. Agent monitoring also serves to detect leaks, air entrainment, contamination and errors of cross-filling.

There are two main methods available for monitoring the concentration of anaesthetic agent:

1. *Mass spectrometry* measures gas concentrations using a technique which depends largely on their molecular weight. Gas samples from the breathing system, obtained from a source as close as possible to the patient, are passed through an ionizer and then accelerated through magnetic fields; they are then separated according to the charge/mass ratio, allowing the concentrations of the different gases in the sample to be measured simultaneously. Problems arise if two molecules have the same molecular weight (e.g. carbon dioxide and nitrous oxide). In this instance, the products of ionization, and not the primary molecules, are measured. Corrections are also required for the measurement of

Table 5.6 Clinical uses of expired carbon dioxide measurement

Respiratory system
Non-invasive breath-by-breath *estimation* of $P\text{aCO}_2$
Provides some information on V/Q ratio and dead space
Measures respiratory rate
Aids detection of:
  Apnoea/ventilator failure
  Breathing system disconnection
  Oesophageal intubation
  Endobronchial intubation
  Airway obstruction
  Hyper-/hypoventilation (and allows ventilation to be adjusted to maintain normocapnia)
  Rebreathing
  Decline of neuromuscular blockade
  Spontaneous respiratory efforts

Cardiovascular system
Provides indication of:
  Changes in blood flow to the lungs (and thus indirect estimates of cardiac output, venous return, hypovolaemia, myocardial depression, cardiac arrest and adequacy of cardiac massage and resuscitation)
  Changes in blood flow through the lungs (altered by embolic phenomena, e.g. air, thrombus, fat, methylmethacrylate)
  Right-to-left shunts

Anaesthetic machine and equipment
May be used to detect:
  Inadequate fresh gas flow
  Faulty unidirectional or non-rebreathing valves
  Exhausted or bypassed carbon dioxide absorber
  Increased dead space

Metabolism
May be used to detect:
  Increased carbon dioxide production (e.g. malignant hyperthermia, seizures, fever)
  Decreased carbon dioxide production (e.g. hypothermia, muscle paralysis)
  Carbon dioxide absorption from peritoneum during carbon dioxide insufflation (e.g. laparoscopy)
  Bicarbonate administration
  Release of tourniquets and reperfusion

halogenated anaesthetic agents. Early mass spectrometers were big, bulky and expensive, with distal analysis and intermittent sampling and display. Modern monitors are available for individual operating room use which allow the simultaneous measurement of concentrations of oxygen, carbon dioxide, nitrogen, air, nitrous oxide and volatile anaesthetic agents, with a response time in the order of 100–200 ms.

2. *Mono- and polychromatic non-dispersive infrared spectrometry* measures the transmission and absorption of infrared light through a gas sample cell and a reference cell. The use of multiple wavelengths in the polychromatic analyser allows the measurement of a number of agents simultaneously, with no requirement for agent pre-selection (cf. monochromatic analyser). These devices are able to measure the concentrations of carbon dioxide, nitrous oxide, oxygen and the volatile anaesthetic agents.

Monitoring the anaesthetic machine and breathing system

Monitoring of the anaesthetic machine and breathing system complements many of the other patient monitors in helping to ensure the adequacy of ventilation, oxygenation and anaesthetic agent delivery. It serves to give early detection and warning of a fault in the machine and/or the breathing system before the patient is at risk, and also supplies valuable information concerning the possible aetiology of the problem.

Measurement of inspired oxygen concentration

Oxygen monitoring in the breathing system allows rapid detection of a hypoxic mixture at source, thus preventing its delivery to the patient and thereby preventing the potentially catastrophic sequelae of damage to the brain and other organs. The central nervous system is damaged irreversibly after only 3–5 min of severe hypoxia, making rapid detection of a hypoxic mixture essential. It is an accepted minimum standard of monitoring.[1-5]

Irrespective of the type of device used, calibration should be performed daily against known concentrations of oxygen (usually 21% (room air) and 100%). Accuracy in the lower range is particularly important, as oxygen values in the range 30–50% are used commonly in clinical practice. The ideal location of the oxygen sensor is dependent on its response time. If there is a slow response time, it should be sited on the inspiratory limb of the breathing system. A monitor with a fast response time is best located on the patient connection limb, where it allows monitoring of the inspiratory and expiratory oxygen concentration and the inspiratory : expiratory gradient.

Two types of analyser are used commonly:

1. *Paramagnetic oxygen analyser.* Oxygen measurement is based on the principle that, if oxygen molecules are introduced into a non-uniform magnetic field, they experience a force which is proportional to the partial pressure of oxygen, provided that the temperature is constant.

2. *Fuel cell (polarographic and galvanic cells) analyser.* A polarographic fuel cell consists of an electrochemical cell formed by an anode (e.g. silver) and a cathode (e.g. gold) immersed in an electrolyte solution and covered by a permeable membrane. A voltage of 0.7–0.75 V is applied between the two electrodes and the current flow is proportional to the partial pressure of oxygen surrounding the membrane. The device requires an external power source and regular replacement of the sensor cell. The 95% response time is of the order of 15 s. A galvanic fuel cell is similar, except that, by changing the material forming the anode (lead), no voltage is required for oxygen reduction. However, a battery is still required to power the alarms and displays. These devices have a slower response time (of the order of 2–3 min) and are disposable.

Other measures available to prevent delivery of a hypoxic mixture to the patient include oxygen supply alarms, a reserve supply of oxygen, a device to shut off the supply of nitrous oxide in the event of failure of the oxygen supply, and an oxygen : nitrous oxide ratio controller.

Airway pressure

A pressure gauge incorporated within the anaesthetic machine or breathing system monitors instantaneous pressure changes during spontaneous ventilation and IPPV. This provides information concerning changes in lung and chest wall compliances, as well as problems with the breathing system and the ventilator. It should possess audible and visible high and low alarms. High-pressure monitoring of peak airway pressure serves to detect obstruction in the airway, tracheal tube or breathing system, and may help to prevent barotrauma. Low-pressure monitoring may detect a disconnection, leak or inadequacy of the fresh gas flow. A resting positive pressure in the circuit (e.g. due to increased resistance in the expiratory limb) can also be detected.

Spirometry

Spirometry measures expired tidal volume and detects a disconnection or an abnormal change in ventilation.

Tidal volume should not be measured on the inspiratory limb, as a disconnection or obstruction between the device and the patient makes the recorded value meaningless in terms of the ventilation received by the patient. Gas flow and volume can be measured directly (e.g. Wright's respirometer) or indirectly by integration of a flow signal (e.g. hot wire flowmeter, electronic respirometer or pneumotachograph).

The Wright's respirometer measures expired volume and is a modified vane anemometer. The gas flow turns a vane connected by a system of gears to a calibrated dial, enabling measurement of tidal volume and minute volume. Problems exist with accumulation of moisture and foreign materials, inertia and momentum causing over-reading at high flows and under-reading at low flows and small tidal volumes. It is also affected by changes in the composition of the gas mixture and instantaneous rates of gas flow. The instruments are prone to damage by rough handling.

The pneumotachograph is a form of constant orifice flowmeter. Gas passes through an area of linear resistance, resulting in a small pressure drop which is proportional to flow rate. This decrease in pressure is measured and used to calculate the gas flow. There is a rapid response time.

Ventilator alarm

When a mechanical ventilator is employed, the valuable information gained from the 'feel of the bag' is lost. A ventilator should never be used without a monitor of airway pressure; this is accepted as a minimum standard of monitoring.[1-5] The ventilator alarm should, ideally, be switched on automatically and have both audible and visible alarms. The low-pressure or disconnection alarm detects a failure to achieve a predetermined pressure within a predetermined time interval. The level should be set just below the peak inspiratory pressure. The device should be located as close as possible to the patient connection. The expiratory limb is preferred to the inspiratory. The ventilator alarm detects major leaks, disconnections and ventilator failure. High-pressure monitoring detects airway obstruction, a kinked or blocked tracheal tube, occlusion of the breathing system and the patient coughing or straining against the tracheal tube. It may serve to prevent pulmonary and cardiovascular barotrauma.

Monitoring of the central nervous system

Monitoring of the central nervous system is performed routinely in virtually every anaesthetic by assessing the response of the autonomic and motor systems to the surgical stimulus. In addition to giving information concerning depth of anaesthesia, central nervous system monitoring aims to improve outcome by identifying the state of neurological structures which are at potential risk, and thereby allowing therapeutic intervention to prevent irreversible brain damage. In the general surgical population, the incidence of serious neurological sequelae after anaesthesia and surgery is small, with a quoted rate of 0.44–0.7 per 1000 anaesthetics,[134,135] the clear majority of which occur in the postoperative period. The risk of neurological damage is higher in some procedures (e.g. carotid endarterectomy,[136] open ventricle cardiac surgery and scoliosis surgery[137]), and central nervous system monitoring may be considered a minimal standard of care only during specific high-risk procedures (e.g. seventh nerve surgery and during cerebropontine angle tumour resection).

New developments and research are aimed at improving the ability to monitor the functional status and the physiological environment of the central nervous system. Adequate studies of outcome are not available but central nervous system monitoring does provide information that may facilitate the potential for improved neurological outcome in high-risk procedures.

Methods available for central nervous system monitoring during anaesthesia and in the ICU can be subdivided into six broad categories:

1. clinical assessment
2. electroencephalogram
3. evoked potentials
4. cerebral blood flow
5. cerebral metabolism
6. monitoring depth of anaesthesia.

Clinical assessment

Monitoring of pupillary signs and the loss of various reflexes is employed in virtually every anaesthetic procedure. This is supplemented by monitoring movement and changes in respiratory rate if muscle relaxants are not employed. More refined tests include intra-operative functional testing. For example, in carotid artery surgery performed under regional anaesthesia, the patient may be asked to respond to a verbal command after clamping of the carotid artery, and contralateral motor function is assessed (this is performed typically before, and then 1 and 2 min after, occlusion). If a deficit is noted, the vessel is unclamped and a temporary shunt is inserted before proceeding with the operation. The incidence of reversible deficits is of the order of 10%.[138,139] It has been perceived as a sensitive and reliable measure, with the added advantages of being inexpensive and simple.

Another example is the 'wake-up' test during anaesthesia for the surgical correction of scoliosis, in which the spinal artery and spinal cord are at risk from manipulation. This test allows direct, intra-operative assessment of the anterior spinal cord motor pathways.

Electroencephalogram

An electrical field results from the background and intrinsic electrical activity of the central nervous system. This electrical activity can be recorded by measuring either electrical or the magnetic fields. The first measurement of the electrical activity of the central nervous system in humans was made in 1929. The activity comes from the pyramidal neurons in laminae I, II and V within the cerebral cortex. The summation of the excitatory and inhibitory postsynaptic potentials in the neuronal pathways results in the recorded waveforms. These waveforms, beta, alpha, theta and delta, are classified according to their amplitude and frequency (Table 5.7). Also of relevance is their degree of organization, and information regarding their symmetry, rhythm and reactivity. The waveforms are all of low voltage, and there is the potential for interference from leakage currents, muscle activity, diathermy or induced currents.

The recording electrodes are either silver chloride surface electrodes or platinum needles, and they are arranged in what is termed a montage. In the neurophysiological department, this is classically a 10–20 lead system involving 21 electrodes and providing a 16-channel record of voltage (y axis) against time (x axis). This montage is too cumbersome for use in the operating room or the ICU. It produces large quantities of paper, it is bulky and it requires specialist training for its interpretation. Normally, only electrodes P3 and P4 (even numbers overlie the right hemisphere, odd numbers the left) are used for intraoperative monitoring as these monitor the electrical activity of an area of the brain supplied by the anterior, middle and posterior cerebral arteries. By using four electrodes (C3, P3, C4 and P4), the right and left hemispheres can be monitored and compared.

A number of methods of signal-processing and computer-assisted data analysis have been developed which compress the data and make interpretation easier and more acceptable. These include the following.

Cerebral function monitor (CFM)

The CFM was introduced in 1969.[140] It records only frequencies between 2 and 25 Hz; those between 4 and 10 Hz are amplified selectively and all other frequencies are filtered. It prints the product of the mean frequency and the log of the amplitude. The CFM requires only one pair of recording electrodes and gives a basic indication of the total electric activity from that part of the brain from which the recordings are taken.

Cerebral function analysing monitor (CFAM)

Developed in 1984[141] as a refinement of the CFM, this instrument provides analysis of both the amplitude and frequency in 2-s periods. The minimum, 10th percentile, mean, 90th percentile, and maximum amplitude are displayed on a logarithmic scale. The frequency display gives some indication of interference.

Compressed spectral array (CSA)[142]

The CSA uses a Fourier transformation and shows the processed electroencephalogram (EEG) as a series of peaks and troughs, with time displayed along the vertical axis and frequency along the horizontal axis. The relative power at any given frequency is shown by the height of the peak and the range of low to high frequencies is displayed from left to right in periods of 2-s analyses or epochs. As time passes, further epochs are progressively displayed. The display of the high peaks may hide subsequent decreases in activity at that frequency.

Density spectral array (DSA)[143]

The DSA represents the amount of activity in 2-s epochs at each frequency by a line running across the paper from low to high frequencies. The greater the activity at any frequency, the thicker the line.

Spectral edge frequency (SEF)

The SEF is the EEG frequency below which 95% of activity is present.

Table 5.7 Classification of electroencephalographic waveforms

	Frequency (Hz)	Amplitude (μV)
beta	14–30	<20
alpha	8–13	20–50
theta	4–7	20–50
delta	1–4	>50

General anaesthetic agents have effects on central nervous system activity and therefore the EEG. Not all agents produce identical EEG changes. For example, isoflurane causes a progressive reduction in voltage and frequency of the EEG, with burst suppression at 2 minimum alveolar concentration (MAC) and an isoelectric EEG at higher concentrations.[144] Desflurane has similar effects.[145] In contrast, administration of enflurane may result in epileptiform activity and grand mal seizure patterns[146] which are exacerbated by hypocapnia. Barbiturates, opioids and benzodiazepines all have different effects on the EEG. Thiopentone in low doses causes initial activation of the EEG. With increasing doses, there is a progression from slower waves of higher amplitude to burst suppression.[147]

Many physiological variables (e.g. hypoxia, hypercapnia, hypocapnia, temperature, hypotension), can also affect the EEG. In addition, the EEG is significantly influenced by varying levels of stimulation (e.g. surgical incision, physiotherapy).

The uses of EEG monitoring during anaesthesia include the following:

1. *Detection of cerebral ischaemia and adequacy of cerebral blood flow* (e.g. during carotid endarterectomy, cardiopulmonary bypass and deliberate hypotension). As cerebral blood flow decreases to less than 18–20 ml/min per 100 g of brain tissue, there is progressive loss of activity, initially affecting the faster frequencies. There is a decrease in the EEG voltage and the SEF. The role of EEG monitoring during carotid endarterectomy has not been clearly defined. DSA monitoring has been shown to be effective in identifying patients who do not require insertion of a shunt;[148] however, postoperative ischaemic lesions have occurred when there has been no change in the SEF.[149,150] The incidence of EEG changes at the time of cross-clamping is greater than changes seen clinically in awake patients in whom a regional anaesthetic technique is employed.[138] The EEG appears to be excessively sensitive, and its use could result in unnecessary insertion of a shunt with the accompanying risk of cerebral ischaemia secondary to embolic phenomena.

2. *As a monitor of depth of anaesthesia*. None of the commonly derived parameters from the EEG has been shown to predict imminent arousal.[151] However, the processed EEG (SEF) has been used with moderate accuracy to predict haemodynamic responses of anaesthetized patients to surgical stimuli and to the stimuli of laryngoscopy and tracheal intubation; when SEF was <14 Hz, blood pressure increased by an average of 12%, but if SEF was >14 Hz, blood pressure increased by 40%.[152] In one study, 1.3 MAC isoflurane was associated with an EEG median frequency of less than 5 Hz and adequate intra-operative anaesthesia.[153] A complex mathematical approach with bispectral analysis has been developed recently in an attempt to predict responsiveness. It may be more accurate than routine spectral analysis and it appears to be less sensitive to the anaesthetic technique.[154] There is currently considerable interest in the role of mid-latency auditory evoked potentials (see below).

3. *Titration of 'cerebral protective' agents* to achieve burst suppression or electrical silence.

4. *Management of patients with status epilepticus* and presurgical evaluation of epileptic patients prior to resection.

5. *Indication of severity and prediction of outcome after head injury*.

An alternative method of recording the EEG is to measure the magnetic field generated by electrical activity in the brain (magnetoencephalography).[155] This measurement has relied on the development of super conducting quantum interference devices (SQUIDs). These sensitive devices can detect the very small magnetic fields associated with brain activity. However, they are very expensive and more studies on large numbers of patients are required to evaluate their clinical applications and usefulness.

Evoked potentials

Evoked potential monitoring records the electrical signal generated in the central nervous system by a series of specific, repetitive stimuli, and indicates the functional integrity of the neural pathways stimulated. The repeated stimulation enables the background EEG activity to be subtracted, allowing the display of only the evoked potential. The response is recorded by monitoring the electrical activity in the central nervous system at the level of the spinal cord, the brainstem or the cerebral cortex. The stimuli may be flashes of light or changing high contrast patterns, e.g. checker-board (visual evoked potential; VEP), repeated clicking noises (auditory evoked potential; AEP), electric shocks over a peripheral nerve (somatosensory evoked potential; SSEP), or cortical stimulation and distal recording (motor evoked potential; MEP).

The evoked potential from any stimulus can be subdivided on the basis of the different latencies of the response. Long-latency (recorded >100 ms after the stimulus) potentials are suppressed by anaesthesia and therefore have limited value in intra-operative monitoring. Middle-latency (10–100 ms) potentials are affected less, but still remain sensitive to the effects of anaesthetic drugs. The short-latency (<10 ms) responses are the most robust and least affected by anaesthetic drugs.

Anaesthetic agents (especially >0.25 MAC) cause a dose-related decrease in amplitude and increase in the latency (conduction time) of evoked responses; enflurane and isoflurane have fewer effects on SSEPs than halothane.[156] A decrease in amplitude, an increase in latency or a complete loss of waveform is seen with ischaemia or surgical trespass. Ideally, the end-tidal concentration of the volatile anaesthetic agent should be kept at a constant level during critical periods of monitoring. The responses are also affected by changes in blood pressure, cerebral blood flow, temperature, haematocrit, carbon dioxide and oxygen tensions, blood glucose and diathermy.

Visual evoked potentials

VEPs, especially those of middle latency, are the most sensitive of all to the effects of anaesthetic agents.[157] They are also affected by the changes in pupillary size and eye position which accompany anaesthesia, despite the use of mydriatic eye drops. They are the least useful for intra-operative monitoring but have been used during anaesthesia for surgery involving the optic nerve and chiasma, pituitary and thalamic tract.

Auditory evoked potentials

These may be divided into brainstem auditory evoked potentials (BAEPs) and cortical AEPs, the latter recording the later responses to auditory stimulation occurring outside the brainstem (i.e. a latency of 50–400 ms compared with 0–10 ms for the BAEP).

BAEPs are the simplest to produce and interpret. They are recorded by electrodes placed over the vertex and the mastoid process, and monitor activity in the pons and mesencephalon. The brainstem responses are less sensitive to the effects of anaesthetic drugs and benefit from a stable and reproducible waveform. They have proved to be useful in posterior fossa and brainstem surgery[158] (e.g. cerebropontine angle, cerebellar tumour resection, acoustic neuroma,[159] eighth nerve surgery). BAEPs have also been used in comatose patients for monitoring brain stem function, and in conjunction with SSEP monitoring have some predictive value in patients with severe head injury.[160] Cortical AEPs have also been used in predicting outcome after head injury, and show promise as a measure of depth of anaesthesia.[161,162]

Somatosensory evoked potentials

SSEPs record the response to repeated electrical stimulation (square waveform, 100–200 ms duration at 1–2 Hz) of a peripheral nerve with surface electrodes or fine-needle electrodes. The nerve selected is usually the posterior tibial in the lower limb, or the median nerve in the upper limb, although others such as the common peroneal, trigeminal and pudendal nerves have also been used. The responses are recorded by surface electrodes and reveal components from the peripheral nerve and plexus, the spinal nerve roots, spinal cord, thalamus and the frontoparietal sensory cortex. Recordings can be made at various levels, from the level of the cortex, the epidural space, or over the peripheral nerves themselves. SSEPs monitor the neural pathways in the dorsal column and give little if any information on the function and integrity of the anterior column of the spinal cord. The shorter-latency SSEPs are most commonly used intra-operatively as they are less influenced by anaesthetic agents.

Despite their use in the operating room for many years, the exact role and usefulness of SSEP monitoring remain somewhat controversial. There is no clear consensus concerning their exact role. They have been used in the following circumstances.

1. *Scoliosis and corrective spinal surgery*. Scoliosis surgery carries with it a relatively high incidence (364 in 60 000 patients) of neurological injury.[137] Lower-limb SSEP monitoring, using the posterior tibial nerve, has been used to detect cord ischaemia and in one study predicted true positives in 72% of cases.[137] However, there were relatively high incidences of false-positive and false-negative results, which may be due in part to the inability of SSEPs to monitor the anterior spinal cord. Another study, in which epidural recording electrodes were used during spinal corrective surgery, found SSEP monitoring to be an accurate predictor of postoperative motor function.[163] SSEP monitoring has been recommended for all cases of spinal cord corrective surgery where the cord is at risk of damage.[137,164] SSEP monitoring can be combined with MEP monitoring.

2. *Abdominal and thoraco-abdominal aortic surgery*. As in scoliosis surgery, SSEP monitoring has some predictive value,[165] but may fail to detect anterior cord ischaemia, which is at more risk from compromise of its blood supply via the anterior spinal artery in the operative period.

3. *Resection of spinal cord tumours or atrioventricular malformations*.

4. *Brachial plexus exploration after injury*.

5. *Carotid endarterectomy.* SSEP monitoring using the median nerve has been shown to be a useful monitor of cerebral ischaemia during anaesthesia for carotid endarterectomy, but does not predict all adverse neurological outcomes.[166]

6. *Middle cerebral artery aneurysm surgery.*[167]

7. *Predictor of outcome after head injury.*[168]

Technical problems with SSEP monitoring have been reported; these include artefact, abnormal pre-operative SSEPs, inaccessible electrodes during the operative period, electrical interference in the hostile environment of the theatre and effects of other variables (e.g. anaesthetic agents, temperature, blood pressure and oxygen and carbon dioxide tensions).

Motor evoked potentials

Measurement of MEPs involves stimulation of the motor nervous system and recording of the distal responses. The motor pathway may be stimulated at various locations from the motor cortex itself down to peripheral nerve level. Transcutaneous stimulation of the motor cortex may be achieved either by direct application of an electrical current, or by induction of electrical currents by the a magnetic field (transcranial magnetic MEP; tcMMEP).[169] This indirect cortical stimulation is more sensitive to the effects of anaesthetic agents than direct stimulation, with different agents causing different effects.[170] In addition, there is considerable inter- and intrapatient variability, making its use as in the intra-operative period more difficult.[170] There are also problems with the attraction of nearby metallic objects. No induction of seizures was seen in 58 epileptic patients.[171]

The distal responses can be recorded from surface electrodes overlying the spinal cord, the peripheral motor nerve or the muscle. As with SSEP monitoring, ischaemia decreases the amplitude and increases the latency of the recorded potential. This may be preceded by an initial transient increase in amplitude and decrease in latency. Some animal studies have shown MEPs to be more sensitive than SSEPs to a reduction in spinal cord blood flow and to correlate better with postoperative motor function.[172,173] This is not surprising, as MEPs monitor the motor pathway in the anterior column of the spinal cord; these pathways may be more vulnerable to the effects of ischaemia and are generally more important functionally to the patient.

MEPs are more sensitive than SSEPs to the effects of anaesthetic agents and are affected by the concurrent use of muscle relaxants. They need more refinement and assessment before they are introduced into routine clinical practice.

Cerebral blood flow

A number of direct and indirect measures of cerebral blood flow are available. These all measure flow in the larger vessels and do not necessarily reflect regional or local blood flow. Theoretically, measurement of changes in cerebral blood flow might identify patients at risk of ischaemia, allowing intervention prior to irreversible neurological damage. A number of methods are available:

1. *Indicator methods.* Xenon washout is generally accepted as the 'gold standard' of cerebral blood flow measurement. However, it is too cumbersome for intra-operative use and requires repeated blood sampling for 10–15 min under relatively stable conditions. Xenon itself has anaesthetic properties, with a MAC value of 75 kPa. During carotid endarterectomy, a radio-active tracer can be injected into the carotid artery both before and after clamping, and after unclamping, of the artery; cerebral blood flow is measured with a radio-activity counter.[174] A new indicator dilution method for measuring regional tissue perfusion with an ultrasound contrast agent has been described.[175] It provides better spatial and temporal resolution than xenon, but is not yet available for routine use. A number of problems need to be overcome before it replaces xenon measurements.

2. *Transcranial Doppler (TCD).* TCD records the blood flow velocity in the major vessels at the base of the brain. It is being used increasingly in the operating theatre and intensive care environments. The measurements correlate well with distal stump pressure in carotid arterectomy, and can detect embolic phenomena (air or particulate) which frequently accompany the procedure.[176] It can also be used to detect post-endarterectomy hyperaemia.[177] TCD is also a sensitive indicator of carotid emboli during cardiopulmonary bypass.[178] However, the measurements correlate poorly with xenon flow studies, especially in the presence of hypocapnia.[179] TCD has been studied to define patterns consistent with brain death.[180]

3. *Stump pressure.* The measurement of distal stump pressure after clamping of the carotid artery during carotid endarterectomy provides some indication of collateral flow and perfusion pressure in the circle of Willis, and is often a major determinant of the need for inserting a temporary shunt. It is measured with a pressure transducer connected to a needle which is inserted into the distal common carotid artery. A high

incidence of false positives (low stump pressure, adequate cerebral blood flow and normal EEG) and false negatives (adequate stump pressure, ischaemic EEG) occur.[181] The role and significance of routine stump pressure monitoring are unclear. A method of manual palpation has been described; palpation of an appreciable distal pulse correlated with a measured stump pressure of at least 42 mmHg.[182]

Cerebral metabolism

Near infrared spectroscopy provides a non-invasive, non-quantitative assessment of the oxygen saturation of haemoglobin in a volume of brain tissue, and may also provide an indication of the redox state of mitochondrial cytochrome Aa3, thereby revealing more direct information on oxygen supply and demand.[124]

Cerebral magnetic resonance imaging spectroscopy

Magnetic resonance imaging spectroscopy provides global cerebral metabolic monitoring with detection of functional activation[183] and of cerebral blood flow.[183] There are many practical difficulties. The technique currently has diagnostic value, but no role as a routine peri-operative monitor.

Monitoring depth of anaesthesia

Currently there is no uniformly applicable or consistently reliable measure of anaesthetic depth. Part of the problem stems from the difficulty in clearly defining what is meant by 'depth of anaesthesia'. Clinically, anaesthetists rely on observing autonomic responses (blood pressure, heart rate, heart rate variability, sweating and lacrimation), movement if muscle relaxants have not been given (or by using the isolated forearm technique), and changes in the respiratory rate in the spontaneously breathing patient. However, these signs are not always reliable in detecting an inadequate level of anaesthesia in the unstimulated patient, which may be associated with awareness if a strong surgical stimulus is applied. When inhaled anaesthetic agents are employed, the end-tidal concentrations can be measured; end-expiratory values equivalent to a total of 0.8 MAC are usually sufficient to ensure lack of awareness.

A number of electrophysiological methods have been investigated as possible adjuncts to clinical monitoring of depth of anaesthesia:

1. *EEG*. With increasing doses of anaesthetic agents, there is a decrease in the frequency of the recordings, progressing with some, but not all anaesthetic agents, to an iso-electric EEG. Many derived measures of the EEG have been investigated. These include the median frequency, the 95% spectral edge, the total power or voltage, the frequency band power ratio, the ratio of frontal to occipital power and bispectral analysis. None has been shown to predict depth of anaesthesia accurately.[151]

2. *Middle-latency AEPs*. These are the 10–100 ms latency responses to repetitive auditory stimulation, and arise from the hippocampus and auditory cortex. They are affected by anaesthetic agents (more so than shorter-latency potentials which are too robust to be used as a monitor of anaesthetic depth, and less so than the late cortical responses which are too sensitive to the effects of anaesthetic agents). The amplitude of the signal decreases, and the latency increases, as the cerebral concentration of anaesthetic agent increases. There is a consistent response to different anaesthetic drugs. The changes induced by anaesthetic drugs are partly reversed by surgical stimulation, indicating that the technique should be sensitive to the factors which determine depth of anaesthesia during surgery. At present, measurement of mid-latency auditory evoked responses is probably the most promising technique for determining depth of anaesthesia. However, further evaluation is required.

3. *Frontalis muscle electromyogram*. Anaesthesia reduces power in the electromyogram recording from the frontalis muscle but in a non-linear fashion. The technique can predict imminent arousal and return of consciousness with reasonable accuracy. However, it is affected by neuromuscular blocking drugs, which limits the use of the technique during anaesthesia.

4. *Lower oesophageal contractility*. The oesophagus is composed of non-striated smooth muscle and therefore not affected by neuromuscular blocking agents. Spontaneous and provoked oesophageal contractions can be measured with an oesophageal balloon. With a total intravenous anaesthesia technique of propofol and alfentanil, the absence of spontaneous lower oesophageal contractions equates with the absence of muscle movement.[185] The relationship of this to awareness is less well-defined.[186] It has proved to be of little value in predicting depth of anaesthesia.

5. *Respiratory sinus arrhythmia*. The degree of respiratory sinus arrhythmia reflects the parasympathetic tone inhibiting the heart via the vagus nerve, and is mediated by activity in the brainstem. Using spectral analysis of heart rate variability, a technique has been developed which analyses respiratory sinus arrhythmia continuously.[187] Preliminary data suggest that increasing depth of anaesthesia reduces respiratory sinus arrhythmia.

Neuromuscular function monitoring

Monitoring of neuromuscular transmission provides:

- an objective assessment of the attainment of sufficient muscle paralysis to allow atraumatic tracheal intubation
- information which assists in determining the optimal time to administer an incremental bolus or to alter the rate of infusion of muscle relaxants in order to provide appropriate surgical relaxation
- the ability to determine when residual paralysis is amenable to reversal with an anticholinesterase, and whether the block is sufficiently reversed either by spontaneous effect or after administration of an anticholinesterase
- the ability to differentiate between depolarizing and non-depolarizing block.

There is a degree of interpatient variability in response to relaxants and an individual's response can be unpredictable due to many factors (e.g. concurrent medications, temperature, acid–base balance and co-existing neuromuscular disease).

Many clinical measures are available to test the strength of voluntary muscle in the conscious patient. These include the ability to protrude the tongue, lift the head for 5 s, grip strength and measures of respiratory function such as vital capacity, tidal volume and inspiratory force. They require a patient who is both conscious and co-operative, and are therefore neither appropriate nor possible during anaesthesia. Neuromuscular block should be monitored whenever non-depolarizing agents are administered or depolarizing relaxants are given by infusion or repeated incremental injection.

The principle of neuromuscular monitoring is that a peripheral nerve is stimulated electrically, via surface electrodes or subcutaneous needles, and the evoked muscular response recorded in order to test transmission of impulses across the neuromuscular junction. The muscular response can be assessed electrically, mechanically, by measures of acceleration or with the visual or tactile senses. Commonly, the ulnar nerve at the wrist is used and the response of adductor pollicis is measured. There are alternative sites of stimulation and measurement of response, such as the facial nerve to stimulate the orbicularis oculi muscle, or the lateral popliteal nerve to stimulate the evertors of the foot.

A supramaximal stimulus is required to ensure that all muscle fibres supplied by the stimulated nerve will react to provide a maximal response. Any decrease in response to nerve stimulation will then parallel the degree of block at the neuromuscular junction. A supramaximal stimulus is ensured by stimulating at a current at least 25% greater than that needed for a maximal response. The nerve impulse should be a square wave with a duration of 0.2–0.3 ms; if the stimulus lasts for longer than 0.5 ms, there may be direct muscle stimulation.

There are five commonly used patterns of stimulation:

1. single twitch
2. train-of-four stimulation
3. tetanic stimulation
4. post-tetanic count
5. double-burst stimulation.

Single twitch

Single twitch (ST) stimulation consists of a supramaximal stimulus with a frequency of between 1 and 0.1 Hz. It provides a measure of the onset of neuromuscular block (time to abolition of response) and depth of blockade (percentage inhibition of twitch response); it can also be used to indicate the relative potencies of neuromuscular blocking drug by assessment of the dose required to produce 95% twitch depression. The duration of neuromuscular block is assessed from the time for twitch response to return to a percentage of its initial height (e.g. 10, 25 and 75%). It requires a pre-relaxant baseline or control value. Because of its simplicity and reliability, it is often used in clinical studies of muscle relaxants.

Train-of-four stimulation

Train-of-four stimulation consists of four supramaximal twitches at a frequency of 2 Hz, repeated no more often than every 12 s, and was first described in 1970.[188] The neurotransmitter acetylcholine is depleted by successive stimulation. In the presence of a non-depolarizing neuromuscular block, there is a decrease in the height of the successive twitches. Train-of-four stimulation allows the calculation of the *train-of-four ratio*, which is the height or amplitude of the fourth twitch divided by the height or amplitude of the first twitch. It is more sensitive than ST stimulation in detecting residual block as there may be some degree of fade present when the ST height has recovered to 100%. The train-of-four response also allows the extent of non-depolarizing block to be determined directly, with no requirement for a baseline pre-relaxant value.

In the presence of a depolarizing block, the height of all twitches is reduced equally and the train-of-four ratio is 1. It is a less painful stimulus than tetanic stimulation and does not influence the degree of neuromuscular block in the stimulated muscle (post-tetanic facilitation; see below).

Tetanic stimulation

Tetanic stimulation can be applied for varying periods and at varying frequencies, although commonly it comprises a 5-s stimulation at 50 Hz. The intense stimulation gives continued release of acetylcholine at the neuromuscular junction. In the presence of a non-depolarizing block, the phenomenon of fade appears, whilst with a depolarizing block or with normal neuromuscular transmission there is no fade and the response is sustained. The fade seen with a non-depolarizing neuromuscular block is explained by a reduction in the release of acetylcholine, and perhaps a presynaptic impairment of mobilization of acetylcholine within the nerve terminals. The appearance of fade also depends on the length and frequency of the applied stimulus, and how often the stimulation is repeated.

Immediately after tetanic stimulation, there is an increase in the stores of acetylcholine immediately available at the nerve terminal, due to increased mobilization and increased synthesis of the transmitter, and any subsequent twitch responses are therefore enhanced. This gives rise to the phenomenon of post-tetanic facilitation. The degree and duration of post-tetanic facilitation depend on the degree of neuromuscular blockade and on the frequency of application of the tetanic stimulus. Frequently repeated stimulation affects the response of the stimulated muscle and may lead to an underestimation of the general degree of block. Stimulation frequencies in excess of 100 Hz may give fade in the absence of any neuromuscular block.[189]

The phenomenon of post-tetanic facilitation is used in performing a post-tetanic count when there is profound degree of neuromuscular block with no detectable response to train-of-four stimulation (see below). Tetanic stimulation is painful and not tolerated by the conscious patient.

Post-tetanic count

This technique quantifies intense neuromuscular blockade. A tetanic stimulus is applied at 50 Hz for 5 s, and the response to repetitive single twitch stimulation at 1 Hz, starting 3 s after the end of tetanic stimulation, is observed. With very intense non-depolarizing neuromuscular block, there is no post-tetanic count, no single twitch response and no response to train-of-four stimulation. As the intensity of the block decreases, but before the return of a response to tetanic stimulation, the post-tetanic twitches occur. The post-tetanic count is related inversely to the time needed for the return of a response to train-of-four or single twitch stimulation. The actual count and time of appearance vary with different agents and with the degree of neuromuscular blockade; for example, post-tetanic twitches appear approximately 37 min before train-of-four elicits movement when pancuronium 0.1 mg/kg has been administered,[190] whereas the time difference is 4–14 min with atracurium 0.5 mg kg or vecuronium 0.1 mg/kg.[191,192] Post-tetanic count also varies with the frequency and duration of tetanic stimulation, the time from the end of tetanic stimulation to the start of the single twitches, and the frequency of the single twitches. If atracurium or vecuronium is used, then in general, a post-tetanic count of 8–10 usually correlates with the return of the first response to train-of-four stimulation.[191,192] The interval is increased with longer-acting drugs.

Double-burst stimulation

Compared with train-of-four stimulation, double-burst stimulation allows a more accurate manual detection of residual neuromuscular block (fade). It comprises two short bursts (0.2 ms) of 50 Hz tetanic stimulation separated by 750 ms (750 ms allows complete relaxation of the muscle between bursts).[193] In a partly paralysed muscle, the second response is weaker than the first. If measured by a quantitative method, the double-burst stimulation ratio can be calculated; this is the height or amplitude of the second burst divided by the height or amplitude of the first. Double-burst stimulation fade is easier to detect manually than fade with train-of-four stimulation; however, it may not be detected manually with a train-of-four ratio of 0.5–0.6[194] and its presence may not be detected visually when the double-burst stimulation ratio is as low as 0.41.[195]

The nerve stimulator

There are various requirements for the performance and output of a nerve stimulator. It must be able to deliver a monophasic stimulus with a rectangular waveform with a duration of 0.2–0.3 ms. At a given setting, the stimulation should be at a constant current, not at a constant voltage, and there should ideally be a current output display. It should have the ability to generate 60–80 mA if required and for this current output to remain constant over a range of impedances up to 5 kΩ. It should be battery-operated, with provision for a battery check. The polarity should be indicated (generally less current is required to depolarize the nerve if the negative electrode is placed nearer the nerve). It should possess the ability to deliver single twitch stimulation at frequencies between 0.1 and 1 Hz, a train-of-four stimulus either singly or repeatedly at intervals of 10–12 s or more, tetanic stimulation at 50 Hz, and an ability to perform a post-tetanic count and double-burst stimulation.

Stimulating electrodes

A small conducting area is required, of the order of 7–8 mm in diameter. The skin should be clean, dry and ideally gently roughened to reduce the impedance. Subcutaneous needle electrodes may be used; these should be placed near the nerve to be stimulated, never within the nerve itself.

Site of nerve stimulation

Accessibility and convenience are important determinants in the choice of a nerve. The ulnar nerve on the volar aspect of the wrist, on the medial site of the tendon of flexor carpi ulnaris, is used most commonly, and the response of the adductor pollicis muscle recorded. The electrodes are placed approximately 1 and 4 cm proximal to the flexion crease. The polarity is not important if electrodes are placed close together. Alternative sites include the median nerve, the posterior tibial nerve, the common peroneal nerve and the facial nerve. Different muscle groups have different sensitivities to neuromuscular blockers. The diaphragm is most resistant (1.4–2 times less susceptible than adductor pollicis to the effects of neuromuscular blockers[196,197] consequently, it has a slower onset time and more rapid recovery from neuromuscular blockers.[198] The laryngeal muscles are comparable with the diaphragm in their response.[199,200] It is therefore apparent that, even if there is no response in the adductor pollicis muscle, this does not exclude the possibility of diaphragmatic movement. Conversely, if the train-of-four ratio measured in the adductor pollicis is greater than 0.7, one can safely assume that diaphragmatic and laryngeal adductor muscle function have recovered.

Recording of evoked responses

As indicated above, the muscle response to nerve stimulation may be assessed either qualitatively (by the visual or tactile senses, the latter being more sensitive) or by quantitative measures.

Visual and tactile

This is the easiest and least expensive method for monitoring the response. However, it is of limited accuracy, with failure to detect fade when the train-of-four ratio is as low as 0.3.[194,201] Fade with double-burst stimulation can be detected more easily. A sustained response to a tetanic stimulation of 50 Hz for 5 s correlates clinically with a 5-s head lift.

Mechanical (mechanomyography)

Mechanomyography records the changes associated with excitation–contraction coupling and muscle contraction. For accurate measurement, the muscle contraction must be isometric, which requires the application of a preload of 200–300 g. The measurement is made with a force-displacement transducer (possessing a linear response to loads up to 10 kg), where the force of contraction is converted into an electrical signal which is processed, displayed and recorded. The arm and hand must be immobilized and the transducer is required to be in the line of contraction. It is generally accurate and reliable. However, there are problems with changes in the contractile response of the muscle and drift from baseline values. It is applicable to only one muscle and requires some skill in setting up. It is regarded as the 'gold standard', and is the method most often used in clinical research.

Electrical (electromyography)

Electromyography records the changes in electrical activity in the muscle subsequent to nerve stimulation. Technological advances now make it possible for rapid analysis (rectification and integration) and graphic representation or numerical display of the electromyographic response. It is becoming increasingly popular. The median or ulnar nerves are commonly used, with measurement of the evoked response from the thenar or hypothenar eminence or from the first dorsal interosseous muscle using surface or needle electrodes. Electrical activity in the thenar eminence muscle correlates well with mechanical measures of the adductor pollicis muscle.[202] This does not necessarily hold true for other muscle groups, in which there is a tendency for the electromyogram to underestimate the degree of neuromuscular block.[203] The electromyogram can be applied to a larger range of muscles than a force transducer, is easier to set up, less bulky and is usually accurate and reliable. However, it is expensive and subject to electrical interference, e.g. from diathermy. The electromyogram is not intended for tetanus, double-burst stimulation or post-tetanic count stimulation.

Measures of acceleration

The acceleration of the thumb after peripheral motor nerve stimulation may be measured. Newton's law states that force is equal to mass multiplied by acceleration and therefore if the mass is held constant, then force is proportional to acceleration. A piezo-electric wafer is used to generate an electrical voltage proportional to acceleration. The signal is then analysed and recorded. It is a simple method, less bulky and expensive than mechanomyography, with reasonably good correlation with the train-of-four ratio and with mechanical measurements.[204,205] However, the correlation is less satisfactory in the presence of small degrees of neuromuscular blockade as the response exceeds (up to 120%) that obtained with a force transducer.[205] It is suitable for single twitch and train-of-four stimulation only.

Clinical correlates and non-depolarizing block

With an intense block, there is no measured response to a single twitch or train-of-four stimulation. There is a correlation between the post-tetanic count and the time of re-appearance of the first response to train-of-four stimulation.[190–192] With a moderate degree of block or 'surgical block', the first response to train-of-four stimulation is seen; this progresses to the appearance of all four twitches as the block declines. The appearance of the first response correlates with approximately 90–95% receptor block. By the appearance of the fourth response, the percentage of neuromuscular block has decreased to between 60 and 85%.[206] The presence of one or two responses to train-of-four stimulation is usually deemed adequate for most surgical procedures. Reversal of the block is possible if two (atracurium and vecuronium), or three (pancuronium) responses are present. In the recovery phase, the return of the fourth twitch occurs and the train-of-four ratio can be calculated. This correlates well with clinical observations of neuromuscular function. If the train-of-four ratio is 0.4 or less, the patient is unable to lift the head; the tidal volume may be adequate, but vital capacity and inspiratory force are reduced. With a train-of-four ratio of 0.6, the patient is able to sustain a head lift for 3 s, but vital capacity and inspiratory force remain reduced. By the time that the ratio has risen to 0.7–0.75, the patient can maintain a head lift for 5 s, and is able to cough, open the eyes and stick out the tongue.[207] This has been generally accepted as an adequate level of recovery of neuromuscular function; however, at this train-of-four ratio, the ventilatory response to hypoxaemia is still impaired, and it is not until the train-of-four ratio has returned to 0.8 or more that vital capacity and inspiratory force return to normal. Full neuromuscular function does not return in all patients until a ratio of 0.85–0.9 has been reached.[208]

Phase I and phase II block

If a patient with normal levels of the enzyme pseudocholinesterase is given suxamethonium in a dose of between 0.5 and 1.0 mg/kg, a *phase I block* occurs, in which there is no evidence of fade and no post-tetanic facilitation. However, if the patient has abnormal enzyme activity, if the dose is increased, or if a prolonged infusion is administered, then *phase II block* develops, which has the characteristics of block with a non-depolarizing agent. Neostigmine reverses a phase II block if pseudocholinesterase is present in normal amounts and with normal activity, but if pseudocholinesterase is abnormal, then neostigmine has unpredictable effects. The precise cause of phase II block is uncertain. One theory is that it is related to hyperactivity of the membrane sodium pump. Suxamethonium has a dynamic relationship with the nicotinic receptor and this results in a block with the characteristics of a non-depolarizing block; the effect is blocked by digoxin, which supports the theory. Suxamethonium may also have a presynaptic effect resulting in a decrease in transmitter mobilization and release. Both factors may be involved.

Monitoring of temperature

Abnormal temperature can cause numerous adverse effects on many organ systems and it is therefore important in at-risk patients to monitor the patient's temperature and to aim to maintain normothermia in the peri-operative period. Detection of surface skin temperature changes may also be of interest when determining the integrity of vascular repairs, vasodilatation in response to a local anaesthetic block, or the state of the circulation after cardiopulmonary bypass. Guidelines from the Harvard Medical School[1] include temperature as a minimum standard of monitoring. The Association of Anaesthetists of Great Britain and Ireland recommend that it should be used when indicated.[3]

Heat production comes from cellular metabolism (which is related to the basal metabolic rate, muscular activity, sympathetic nervous system and hormonal activity) and endogenous sources. Heat loss occurs by four mechanisms: radiation (this is the major source clinically, accounting for over 60% of total heat loss), conduction, convection and evaporation (which comprises 10–25% of heat loss, including insensible losses from lung). Infants are at increased risk of hypothermia because they have a large surface area to volume ratio, with less body fat (and hence insulation), and reliance on non-shivering thermogenesis. The elderly are also at increased risk, with a tendency towards greater intra-operative decreases in temperature and a longer time to rewarm postoperatively.[209].

Hypothermia is an extremely common accompaniment to anaesthesia — 75% of patients undergoing surgery involving body cavities have a core temperature of less than 36°C on arrival in the recovery area.[210] A number of anaesthetic and surgical factors contribute to this decrease in body temperature. These include low ambient temperature (especially if the theatre temperature is <21°C), cold, dry inhaled gases, cold intravenous and irrigation fluids, and prolonged exposure of body cavities. Anaesthetic agents cause vasodilatation, a slowing of the basal metabolic rate with a reduction in metabolic heat production and direct interference with the hypothalamus and central thermoregulation. They also inhibit the behavioural responses to a fall in temperature and cause alterations in heat redistribution within the body.

Hypothermia causes a decrease in the basal metabolic rate and oxygen consumption (6–9% for each degree Celsius) and may therefore provide some protection against tissue ischaemia and hypoxia. The anaesthetic requirement is reduced (decreased MAC values), and there is decreased metabolism in the liver and the kidneys, resulting in decreased metabolism and excretion of drugs. There is impairment of immune function and platelet function,[211] and plasma potassium concentration may decrease. Pulse oximeters may malfunction, and the solubility of gases in blood is increased, influencing the measurement of arterial blood gases. Twitch tension in the adductor pollicis muscle decreases.[212] There is vasoconstriction and increased peripheral vascular resistance. Blood viscosity increases, as does the blood glucose concentration.

On rewarming, the patient mounts a thermoregulatory response as the effects of the anaesthetic agents and neuromuscular block wear off. Shivering and tremor can double the metabolic rate[213] and increase oxygen consumption by up to 4–5 times,[214] necessitating increased oxygen delivery and cardiac output. This imposed stress may result in hypoxaemia, an increase in lactic acid production and myocardial ischaemia in at-risk patients. Shivering is maximal when the temperature is in the range of 34–35°C. There may be hypertension and arrhythmias due to the increased SVR and PVR and the increase in circulating levels of adrenaline and noradrenaline. There may be increases in intracranial pressure and intra-ocular pressures with shivering. Pain may be aggravated and the integrity of the wound may be threatened. As the patient continues to rewarm, there is vasodilatation with a subsequent reduction in preload and possibly blood pressure.

Prevention includes the use of radiant heat lamps, warming mattress, blankets, covering of exposed skin surfaces, heated humidification of inspired gases (or, less effectively, a heat and moisture exchanger), increasing the ambient temperature (ideally the ambient temperature should be >21°C for adults, higher for neonates), warming irrigation and intravenous fluids, and the use of a circle breathing system.

Although it is less common, hyperthermia may be recorded, warning of infection, thyroid overactivity or crisis, or malignant hyperthermia, a life-threatening condition requiring early diagnosis and prompt treatment.

Methods of temperature monitoring

Methods of temperature monitoring include the use of a thermistor, thermocouple, mercury-in-glass thermometer, infrared or liquid crystals.[215] A thermistor measures temperature by change in electrical resistance. A thermocouple measures temperature change using two dissimilar metals and recording the potential developed between them. Liquid crystals change their molecular structure with temperature changes.

Temperature may be monitored centrally or peripherally.

Central

Tympanic membrane. This is performed easily and is thought to reflect hypothalamic temperature. It can be used if the patient is awake, and is perhaps the best index of core temperature. Problems include the potential for bleeding and perforation, although this is reduced by the use of modern, soft, flexible thermometers. Any wax in the external auditory meatus or canal interferes with the measurement.

Nasopharyngeal temperature. This approximates to brain temperature. However, the thermometer is easily displaced and may be affected by inspiratory gases. There is potential for nasal bleeding and trauma.

Oesophageal temperature. This reflects approximately the temperature of the heart and great vessels. However, it may be difficult to position the probe accurately in the distal one-third of the oesophagus.

Rectal temperature. This route tends not to be tolerated well in the awake patient and is affected by the presence of faeces. It has a slow response time.

Bladder temperature. This is affected by urinary flow and is obviously not possible in genito-urinary procedures. It is expensive and carries with it a risk of introducing infection.

Pulmonary artery temperature. Pulmonary artery catheters used for measurement of cardiac output by thermodilution can be used to measure blood temperature in the pulmonary artery.

Peripheral

Measurement of skin temperature can be used as an indicator of tissue perfusion. It is not a measure of core temperature and the value is affected by many factors, particularly vasoconstriction and environmental temperature.

In the conscious subject, tympanic membrane, pulmonary artery, rectal, nasopharyngeal and oesophageal temperatures are all approximately equal.[216] Oral temperature is less reliable. During cardiopulmonary bypass or deliberate cooling, tympanic membrane, pulmonary artery and oesophageal temperatures change more rapidly than rectal temperature.

It might be supposed that hypothermia would result in an increased risk of morbidity during the postoperative period, especially in neonates, the elderly and patients with cardiorespiratory or cerebrovascular disease. However, there is very limited evidence to support this assertion. Nevertheless, it would seem logical to monitor temperature in patients who are at risk of temperature change in the peri-operative period. These would include patients at the extremes of age, those undergoing long surgical procedures (especially if body cavities are exposed or if large fluid volume shifts are anticipated), those with cardiorespiratory or cerebrovascular disease, those suspected of susceptibility to malignant hyperthermia, and perhaps when combining regional and general anaesthetic techniques.

Coagulation monitoring

Anticoagulants are used increasingly in clinical practice, both intra-operatively (e.g. during cardiopulmonary bypass, vascular procedures) and also in the ICU (e.g. neonatal extracorporeal membrane oxygenation, haemofiltration). There is also a growing awareness of the risks of administration of blood and blood products, as well as the problems of availability and cost of these products, making monitoring of coagulation in at-risk patients essential. A suspected disorder of coagulation can no longer be treated empirically.

A number of tests are available which reflect different aspects of the complex process of coagulation. The majority of these are static tests concerned with specific aspects of the coagulation system. There is a small number of dynamic tests (e.g. thromboelastography), which determine the functioning of the coagulation system in a more global manner. The tests continue to become more refined. They are summarized in Table 5.8.

Heparin

Clinical trials with heparin commenced in 1938.[219] It comprises a group of negatively charged mucopolysaccharides (6–30 kDa) and acts by binding and activating antithrombin III, affecting thrombin, factors Xa, XIa, IXa, XIIa and plasmin, and thus the intrinsic pathway. It is derived from bovine and porcine sources and shows marked variation in its activity, along with enormous variability in the responsiveness of individual patients to a given dose. Peri-operative measures of its activity are perhaps the most important for anaesthetists.

Table 5.8 Tests of coagulation

Platelets
Count and morphology
Bleeding time: first described in 1910 by Duke[217] and modified by Ivy et al in 1941,[218] it determines the haemostatic effectiveness of platelets. There are at least three commercially available devices. The normal range is 3.5–8.5 min
Petechiometer test: the appearance of more than 10 petechiae cm^2 after suction at a pressure of 50 cmH$_2$O for 1 min suggests a platelet or vascular abnormality.

Common pathway
Thrombin time
Fibrinogen concentration
Reptilase time

Intrinsic pathway
Partial thromboplastin time
Activated partial thromboplastin time
Activated clotting time

Extrinsic pathway
Prothrombin time
International normalized ratio

Tests of fibrinolysis
Fibrinogen degradation products and D-dimers
Euglobulin lysis time

Visco-elastic clot strength
Thromboelastography
Sonovet coagulation analyser

Three intra-operative tests of coagulation are used commonly.

Activated clotting time (ACT)

The ACT is simple, reliable, effective and inexpensive. It was described first by Hattersly[220] in 1966. The test involves placing 2 ml of blood into a tube with an activator (12 mg of diatomaceous earth, kaolin or glass particles) which provides a large surface area to accelerate the conversion of factor XII to factor XIIa, and then seeking evidence of clot formation. Diatomaceous earth is the standard activator because of its excellent activating properties; however, it may be affected by aprotinin, whereas kaolin is not.[221] In its automated form, ACT is measured by the Haemochron. The sample is heated to 37°C, and as the clot forms, a small magnet is pulled from the base of the machine, halting a timer and activating an audible alarm. The elapsed time is displayed (normal range 105–167 s).

The ACT is prolonged by hypothermia, haemodilution, cardioplegic solutions, platelet dysfunction, hypofibrinogenaemia and other coagulopathies. It is related linearly to heparin dose up to an ACT value of 500–600 s. A value of more than 400 s is generally accepted to be safe for cardiopulmonary bypass and this usually requires the administration of 300 units (3 mg) of heparin per kilogram body weight. There is up to a fourfold variation in both patient sensitivity and the rate at which heparin disappears from the blood. Underdosage may lead to thrombosis in the extracorporeal circuit and overdosage may lead to dangerous bleeding. Heparin resistance may be seen in the presence of antithrombin III deficiency, previous heparin therapy, concurrent administration of the oral contraceptive pill, old age and errors of dosage.

Activated partial thromboplastin time (APTT)

Unlike ACT, APTT is not related linearly to heparin doses of more than 200 units/kg. Multiple reagents and instrumentation are required, and it is not therefore a bedside test. The APTT is almost invariably more than 600 s during cardiopulmonary bypass and the test is therefore a poor guide to the effect of heparin in this setting.

Thromboelastography

Thromboelastography was developed in 1948.[222] It enables a global assessment of haemostatic function, and indicates the dynamic process of coagulation rather than isolated static functions. It measures clot formation from the initial reaction of platelets with the coagulation cascade, through to platelet aggregation and fibrin strengthening of clot, and finally clot lysis. Information is gained on in vivo platelet activity, clotting factor function and the interrelationship between the two, as well as data relating to fibrinolysis. The test takes 20–30 min and is available for use in the operating room and the ICU. The blood sample (0.35 ml) is placed in a heated cup and clot formation is sensed by a pin suspended from a torsion wire attached to an amplifying and recording system detailing the thromboelastography trace on moving paper. Various measurements can then be made from the tracing, with each representing a different component of the coagulation system. Thromboelastography has been shown to be particularly useful in liver transplantation[223,224] (coagulopathies and fibrinolysis) and *cardiopulmonary bypass*[225,226] (defects in platelet function and coagulopathies). It has been shown to reduce blood product utilization in paediatric cardiac patients[227] and during orthotopic liver transplantation.[223]

REFERENCES

1. Eichorn JH, Cooper JB, Cullen DJ, Maier WR, Philip JH, Seeman RG. Standards for patient monitoring during anesthesia at Harvard Medical School. JAMA 1986; 256: 1017–1020
2. Standards for basic intra-operative monitoring. Am Soc Anesthesiol Newslett 1986; 50: 12–13
3. Recommendations for standards of monitoring during anaesthesia and recovery. London: Association of Anaesthetists of Great Britain and Ireland. 1988
4. Cass NM, Crosby WM, Holland RB. Minimal monitoring standards. Anaesth Intensive Care 1988; 16: 110–113
5. The International Task Force on Anaesthesia Safety. Eur J Anaesth 1993; 10 (suppl 7): 1–44
6. Moller JT, Pedersen T, Rasmussen LS et al. Randomized evaluation of pulse oximetry in 20 802 patients: I. Design, demography, pulse oximetry failure rate and overall complication rate. Anesthesiology 1993; 78: 436–444
7. Moller JT, Johannessen NW, Espersen K et al. Randomized evaluation of pulse oximetry in 20 802 patients: II Perioperative events and postoperative complications. Anesthesiology 1993; 78: 445–453
8. Wang LP, Hagerdal M. Reported anaesthetic complications during an 11-year period. A retrospective study. Acta Anaesthesiol Scand 1992; 36: 234–240
9. Cheney FW. ASA closed claims project progress report: the effect of pulse oximetry and end-tidal CO_2 monitoring on adverse respiratory events. ASA Newslett 1992; 56: 6–10

10 Weinger MB, Englund CE. Ergonomic and human factors affecting anesthetic vigilance and monitoring performance in the operating room environment. Anesthesiology 1990; 73: 995–1021
11 Kaplan JA, King SB. The precordial electrocardiographic lead (V_5) in patients who have coronary artery disease. Anesthesiology 1976; 45: 570
12 Trager M, Feinberg BI, Kaplan JA. Right ventricular ischemia diagnosed by an esophageal ECG and right atrial tracing. J Cardiothorac Anesth 1987; 1: 123
13 Dodd RB, Sims WA, Bone DJ. Cardiac arrhythmias observed during anesthesia. Surgery 1962; 51: 440
14 Kuner J, Enescu V, Utsu F et al. Cardiac arrhythmias during anesthesia. Dis Chest 1967; 52: 580
15 Vanik PE, Davis HS. Cardiac arrhythmias during halothane anesthesia. Anesth Analg 1968; 47: 299
16 Russel PH, Coakley CS. Electrocardiographic observation in the operating room. Anesth Analg 1969; 48: 784
17 Bertrand CA, Steiner NV, Jameson AG, Lopez M. Disturbances of cardiac rhythm during anesthesia and surgery. JAMA 1971; 216: 1615
18 Weinfurt PT. Electrocardiographic monitoring: an overview. J Clin Monit 1990; 6: 132–138
19 Slogoff S, Keats AS. Does perioperative myocardial ischemia lead to postoperative myocardial infarction? Anethesiology 1985; 62: 107
20 Coriat P, Harari A, Daloz M, Viars P. Clinical predictors of intraoperative myocardial ischemia in patients with coronary artery disease undergoing non-cardiac surgery. Acta Anaesthesiol Scand 1982; 26: 287
21 Rao TLK, Jacobs KH, El-Etr AA. Reinfarction following anesthesia in patients with myocardial infarction. Anesthesiology 1983; 59: 499
22 Kaplan JA. Cardiac anesthesia, 2nd edn. Orlando, FL: Grune & Stratton. 1987
23 Steen PA, Tinker JH, Tarhan S. Myocardial reinfarction after anesthesia and surgery. JAMA 1978; 239: 2566
24 Mangano DT, Browner W, Hollenberg M et al. Prediction of cardiac morbidity and mortality in patients undergoing noncardiac surgery. N Engl J Med 1990; 323: 1787–1788
25 Bourdillon PD, Lorell BH, Mirsky I et al. Increased regional myocardial stiffness of the left ventricle during pacing-induced angina in man. Circulation 1983; 67: 316–323
26 London MJ, Hollenberg M, Wong MG et al. Intra-operative myocardial ischemia: localization by continuous 12-lead electrocardiography. Anesthesiology 1988; 69: 232–241
27 Fortuin NJ, Weiss JL. Exercise stress testing. Circulation 1976; 56: 699
28 Ellestad MH, Cooke BM, Greenberg PS. Stress testing: clinical application and predictive capacity. Prog Cardiovas. Dis 1979; 21: 431
29 Davies CT, Kitchin AH, Knibbs AV. Computer quantitation of ST segment response to graded exercise in untrained and trained normal subjects. Cardiovasc Res 1971; 5: 201
30 Finlay B, Couchie D, Boyce L, Spencer E. Electrosurgery burns resulting from use of miniature ECG electrodes. Anesthesiology 1974; 41: 263–269
31 Talke P, Nichols RJ, Traber DL. Does measurement of systolic blood pressure with a pulse oximeter correlate with conventional methods? J Clin Monit 1990; 6: 5–9
32 Gorback MS. Consideration in the interpretation of systemic pressure monitoring. In: Lumb PD, Bryan-Brown CW, eds. Complications in critical care medicine. Chicago, IL: Yearbook Medical Publishers. 1988
33 Gourdeau M, Martin R, Lamarche Y et al. Oscillometry and direct blood pressure: a comparative clinical study during deliberate hypotension. Can Anaesth Soc J 1986; 33: 300
34 American Heart Association. Recommendations for human blood pressure determination by sphygmomanometers. Circulation 1980; 62: 1146A
35 Yong PG, Geddes LA. The effect of cuff pressure deflation rate on accuracy in indirect measurement of blood pressure with the auscultatory method. J Clin Monit 1987; 3: 155
36 Celoria G, Dawson JA, Teres D. Compartment syndrome in a patient monitored with an automated blood pressure cuff. J Clin Monit 1987; 3: 139
37 Showman A, Belts EK. Hazards of automatic noninvasive blood pressure monitoring. Anesthesiology 1981; 55: 1981
38 Bickley PE, Schapera A, Bainton CR. Acute radial nerve injury from use of an automatic blood pressure monitor. Anesthesiology 1990; 73: 186–188
39 Penaz J. Photoelectric measurement of blood pressure, volume, and flow in the finger. In: Digest of the 10th International Conference on Medical and Biological Engineering. Dresden, 1973: p 104
40 Kurki TS, Smith NT, Head N et al. Noninvasive continuous blood pressure measurement from the finger. Optimal measurement conditions and factors affecting reliability. J Clin Monit 1987; 3: 6–13
41 Gibbs NM, Larach DR, Deer JA. The accuracy of Finapres noninvasive mean arterial pressure measurements in anesthetized patients. Anesthesiology 1991; 74: 647–652
42 Epstein RH, Huffnagel S, Barkowski RR. Comparative accuracies of a finger blood pressure monitor and an oscillometric blood pressure monitor. J Clin Monit 1991; 7: 161–167
43 Kemmotsu O, Ueda M, Otsuka H et al. Arterial tonometry for noninvasive, continuous blood pressure monitoring during anesthesia. Anesthesiology 1991; 75: 333–340
44 Kemmotsu O, Ueda M, Otsuka H et al. Blood pressure measurement by arterial tonometry in controlled hypotension. Anesth Analg 1991: 73: 54–58
45 Allen EV. Thromboangitis obliterans. Methods of diagnosis of chronic obstructive lesions distal to the wrist with illustrative cases. Am J Med Sci 1929; 178: 237
46 Mangano DT, Hickey RF. Ischemic injury following uncomplicated radial artery catheterization. Anesth Analg 1979; 58: 55
47 Thompson SR, Hirshberg A. Allen's test re-examined (letter). Crit Care Med 1988; 16: 915
48 Slogoff S, Keats AS, Arlund C. On the safety of radial artery cannulation. Anesthesiology 1983; 59: 42–47
49 Davis FM, Stewart JM. Radial artery cannulation: a prospective study in patients undergoing cardiothoracic surgery. Br J Anesth 1980; 52: 42

50. Swan HJC, Ganz W, Forrester J, Marcus H, Diamond G, Chonette D. Catheterization of the heart in man with the use of a flow-directed balloon-tipped catheter. N Engl J Med 1970; 283: 447–451
51. Connors AF Jr, Dawson NV, Shaw PK, Montenegro HD, Nara AR, Martin L. Hemodynamic status in critically ill patients with and without acute heart disease. Chest 1990; 98: 1200–1206
52. Moore CH, Lombardo TR, Allums JA, Gordon FT. Left main coronary artery stenosis: hemodynamic monitoring to reduce mortality. Ann Thorac Surg 1978; 26: 445–451
53. Bland RD, Shoemaker WC, Abraham E et al. Hemodynamic and oxygen transport patterns in surviving and nonsurviving postoperative patients. Crit Care Med 1985; 13: 85
54. Shoemaker WC, Kram HB, Appel PL, Fleming AW. The efficacy of central venous and pulmonary artery catheters and therapy based upon them in reducing mortality and morbidity. Arch Surg 1990; 125: 1332–1337
55. Tuman KJ, McCarthy RJ, Speiss BD et al. Effect of pulmonary artery catheterization on outcome in patients undergoing coronary artery surgery, Anesthesiology 1989; 70: 199–206
56. Isaacson IJ, Lowdon JD, Berry AJ et al. The value of pulmonary artery and central venous monitoring in patients undergoing abdominal aortic reconstructive surgery: a comparative study of two selected, randomized groups. J Vasc Surg 1990; 12: 754–760
57. Zion MM, Balkin J, Rosenmann D et al. Use of pulmonary artery catheters in patients with acute myocardial infarction. Analysis of experience in 5841 patients in the SPRINT registry. Chest 1990; 98: 1331–1335
58. Swan HJC. Central venous pressure monitoring is an outmoded procedure of limited practical value. In: Ingelfinger FJ, Ebert RV, Finland M et al eds. Controversies in internal medicine. Philadelphia, PA: WB Saunders, 1974: p 185
59. Bell H, Stubbs D, Pugh D. Reliability of central venous pressure as an indicator of left atrial pressure. Chest 1971; 59: 169
60. Toussaint GPM, Burges JS, Hampson LG. Central venous pressure and pulmonary capillary wedge pressure in critical surgical illness. Arch Surg 1974; 109: 265
61. Vender JS. Pulmonary artery catheter monitoring. In Barash PG, ed. Cardiac monitoring. Philadelphia, PA: WB Saunders, 1988: p 743
62. Kaplan JA, Wells PH. Early diagnosis of myocardial ischemia using the pulmonary arterial catheter. Anesth Analg 1981; 60: 789–793
63. van Deale MERM, Sutherland GR, Mitchell MM et al. Do changes in pulmonary capillary wedge pressure adequately reflect myocardial ischaemia during anesthesia? A correlative preoperative hemodynamic electrocardiographic, and transesophageal echocardiographic study. Circulation 1990; 81: 865–871
64. Wheatley S, Pollard B. Inserting a pulmonary artery flotation catheter. In: Pollard BJ (ed) Current anaesthesia and critical care, vol. 3. Edinburgh: Longman, 1992: 108–116
65. Fick A. Uber die messung des blutquantums in den herzventrikeln. Verh Dtsch Phys-med Ges Wurzburg 1870; 2: 16
66. Rieke H, Weyland A, Hoeft A et al. Continuous measurement of cardiac output based on the Fick principle in cardiac anesthesia. Anaesthetist 1990; 39: 13–21
67. Selzer A, Sudrann RB. Reliability of the determination of cardiac output in man by means of the Fick principle. Circ Res 1958; 6: 485
68. Robinson PS, Crowther A, Jenkins BS et al. A computerized dichromatic earpiece densitometer for the measurement of cardiac output. Cardiovasc Res 1979; 13: 420
69. Branthwaite MA, Bradley RD. Measurement of cardiac output by thermal dilution in man. J Appl Physiol 1968; 24: 434
70. Horn JR, Zierler B, Bauer LA, Reiss W, Strandness DE. Estimation of hepatic blood flow in branches of hepatic vessels utilizing a non invasive, duplex Doppler method. J Clin Pharmacol 1990; 30: 922–929
71. Payen DM, Fratacci MD, Dupuy P et al. Portal and hepatic arterial blood flow after human liver transplantation using implantable doppler flow probe: pathophysiological data of early complications and nutrition. Surgery 1990; 107: 417–427
72. Beloucif S, Laborde F, Beloucif I, Piwnica A, Payen D. Determinants of systolic and diastolic flow in coronary bypass graft under inotropic stimulation. Anesthesiology 1990; 73: 1127–1135
73. Nishimura RA, Callahan MJ, Schaff HA et al. Noninvasive measurement of cardiac output by continuous-wave Doppler echocardiography: initial experience and review of the literature. Mayo Clin Proc 1984; 59: 484
74. Perrino AC, Fleming J, LaMantia KR. Transesophageal Doppler ultrasonography for improved cardiac output monitoring. Anesth Analg 1990; 71: 651–665
75. Muhludeen IA, Kuecherer HF, Lee E, Cahalan MK, Schiller NB. Intraoperative estimation of cardiac output by transesophageal pulsed Doppler echocardiography. Anesthesiology 1991; 74: 9–14
76. Siegel C, Fitzegerald DC, Engstrom RH. Simultaneous intraoperative measurement of cardiac output by thermodilution and transtracheal Doppler. Anesthesiology 1991: 74: 664–669
77. Segal J, Nassi M, Ford AJ, Schuenemeyer TD. Instantaneous and continuous cardiac output in humans obtained with a Doppler pulmonary catheter. J Am Coll Cardiol 1990; 16: 1398–1407
78. Kubicek WG, Karnegis JN, Patterson RP et al. Development and evaluation of a impedance cardiac output system. Aerospace Med 1966; 37: 1208
79. Wong DH, Tremper KK, Stemmer EA et al. Noninvasive cardiac output: simultaneous comparison of two different methods with thermodilution. Anesthesiology 1990; 72: 784–792
80. Appel PL, Kram HB, MacKabee J. Comparison of measurements of cardiac output by bioimpedance and thermodilution in severely ill surgical patients. Crit Care Med 1986; 14: 933
81. Thys DM, Hillel Z. How it works: basic concepts in echocardiography. In: de Bruijn NP, Clements F, eds. Intraoperative use of echocardiography. Philadelphia, PA: JB Lippincott. 1991

82. Kisslo J, Adams DB, Belkin RN. Doppler color flow imaging. New York: Churchill Livingstone. 1988
83. Daniel WG, Erbel R, Kaspar W et al. Safety of transesophageal echocardiography, a multicenter survey of 10 419 examinations. Circulation 1991; 83: 817–821
84. Thys DM, Hillel Z, Goldman ME et al. A comparison of hemodynamic indices by invasive monitoring and two-dimensional echocardiography. Anesthesiology 1987; 67: 630–634
85. Urbanowicz JH, Shaaban MJ, Cohen NH et al. Comparison of transesophageal echocardiographic and scintigraphic estimates of left ventricular end-diastolic volume index and ejection fraction in patients following coronary artery bypass grafting. Anesthesiology 1990; 72: 607–612
86. Hauser AM, Gangadharan V, Ramos RG et al. Sequence of mechanical, electrocardiographic and clinical effects of repeated coronary artery occlusion in human beings: echocardiographic observations during coronary angioplasty. J Am Coll Cardiol 1985; 5: 193–197
87. Wohlgelernter D, Cleman M, Highman HA et al. Regional myocardial dysfunction during coronary angioplasty: evaluation by two-dimensional echocardiography and 12 lead electrocardiography. J Am Coll Cardiol 1986; 7: 1245–1254
88. Sheikh KH, de Bruijn NP, Rankin JS et al. The utility of transosephageal echocardiography and Doppler color flow imaging in patients undergoing cardiac valve surgery. J Am Coll Cardiol 1990; 15: 363–372
89. Hagler DJ, Seward JB, Tajik J et al. Intraoperative two-dimensional color flow imaging. Circulation 1986; 74: II-36
90. Maurer G, Czer L, Bolger A et al. Intraoperative color Doppler flow mapping for repair of congenital heart disease. Circulation 1986; 74: II-37
91. Cucchiara RF, Nugent M, Seward JB et al. Air embolism in upright neurosurgical patients; detection and localization by two-dimensional transesophageal echocardiography. Anesthesiology 1984; 60: 353
92. Oka Y, Boriwaka K, Hong Y et al. Detection of air emboli in the left heart by M-mode transesophageal echocardiography following cardiopulmonary bypass. Anesthesiology 1985; 63: 109
93. Freeman WK, Khanderia BK, Oh JK et al. Thoracic aortic pathology by transesophageal echocardiography. Circulation 1988; 78: II-298
94. Severinghaus JW, Astrup PB. History of blood gas analysis. Int Anesth Clin 1987; 25: 167–199
95. Cote CJ, Goldstein EA, Cote MA et al. A single blind study of pulse oximetry in children. Anesthesiology 1988; 68: 184–188
96. Morris RW, Buxchman, A, Warren DI et al. The prevalance of hypoxaemia detected by pulse oximetry during recovery from anesthesia. J Clin Monit 1988; 4: 16–20
97. Cullen DJ, Nemeskal AR, Cooper JB, Zaslavsky A, Dwyer MJ. Effect of oximetry, age and ASA physical status on frequency of patients admitted unexpectedly to a postoperative intensive care unit and the severity of their anesthesia-related complications. Anesth Analg 1992; 74: 181–188
98. Nellcor N100 Technical manual. Hayward, CA: Nellcor. 1985
99. Harris AP, Sendak MJ, Donham PT et al. Absorption characteristics of human fetal hemaglobin at wavelengths used in pulse oximetry. J Clin Monit 1988: 4: 175–177
100. Barker SJ, Tremper KK, Hyatt J, Zaccari J. Effects of methemoglobin on pulse oximetry and mixed venous oximetry. Anesthesiology 1983; 50: 349–352
101. Barker SJ, Tremper KK. The effect of carbon monoxide inhalation on pulse oximetry and transcutaneous Po_2. Anesthesiology 1987; 66: 677–679
102. Scheller MS, Unger RJ, Kelner MJ. Effects of intravenously administered dyes on pulse oximetry readings. Anesthesiology 1986; 65: 550–552
103. Ralston AC, Webb RK, Runciman WB. Potential errors in pulse oximetry I: pulse oximeter evaluation. Anaesthesia 1991; 46: 202–206
104. Webb RK, Ralston AC, Runciman WB. Potential errors in pulse oximetry II: effects of changes in saturation and signal quality. Anaesthesia 1991; 46: 207–212
105. Ralston AC, Webb RK, Runciman WB. Potential errors in pulse oximetry III: effects on interference, dyes, dyshaemoglobins and other pigments. Anaesthesia 1991; 46: 291–295
106. Murphy KG, Secunda JA, Rockoff MA. Severe burns from a pulse oximeter. Anesthesiology 1990; 73: 350–352
107. Sobel DB. Burning of a neonate due to a pulse oximeter — arterial saturation monitoring. Pediatrics 1992; 89: 154–155
108. Martin WE, Cheung PW, Johnson CC, Wong KC. Continuous monitoring of mixed venous oxygen saturation in man. Anesth Analg 1973; 52: 784–793
109. Richard C, Thuillez C, Pezzano M, Bottineau G, Giudicelli JF, Auzepy P. Relationship between mixed venous oxygen saturation and cardiac index in patients with chronic congestive heart failure. Chest 1989; 95: 1289–1294
110. Vaughan S, Puri VK. Cardiac output changes in continous mixed venous oxygen saturation measurement in the critically ill. Crit Care Med 1988; 16: 495–498
111. Larson LO, Kyff JV. The cost-effectiveness of oximetrix pulmonary artery catheters in the post-operative care of coronary artery bypass graft patients. J Cardiothorac Anesth 1989; 3: 276–279
112. Jastremski MS, Chelluri M, Beney KM, Bailly RT. Analysis of the effects of continuous on-line monitoring of mixed venous oxygen saturation on patient outcome and cost effectiveness. Crit Care Med 1989; 17: 148–153
113. Lubbers DW, Opitz N. Die Pco_2/Po_2 Optode. Eine Neue Pco_2 bzw. Po_2-Messonde zur Messung des Pco_2 oder Po2 von Gasen und Flussigkeiten. Z Naturforsch (C) 1975; 30: 532–533
114. Mahutte CK, Sassoon CSH, Muro JR et al. Progress in the development of a fluorescent intravascular blood gas system in man. J Clin Monit 1990; 6: 147–157
115. Barker SJ, Hyatt J. Continous measurement of intra-arterial pH, $Paco_2$ and Pao_2 in the operating room. Anesth Analg 1991; 73: 43–48
116. Haessler R, Brandl F, Zeller M, Briegel J, Finsterer U. Intra-arterial catheter oximetry and pulse oximetry

compared to co-oximetry in cardiac anesthesia. Anaesthetist 1991; 40: 602–607
117 Huch A, Huch R, Meinzer K et al. Eine scheulle, behitze Ptoberflachenelektrode zur kontinuierlichen Uberwachung des Po_2 beim Menschem: Elecktrodenaufbau und Eigenschaftern (Abstr.) Medizin technik (Stuttgart) 1972; 26
118 Cheatle TR, Stibe ECL, Shami SK, Scurr JH, Coleridge Smith PD. Vasodilatory capacity of the skin in venous disease and its relationship to transcutaneous oxygen tension. Br J Surg 1991; 78: 607–610
119 Reid CW, Martineau RJ, Miller DR, Hull KA, Baines J, Sullivan PJ. A comparison of transcutaneous end-tidal and arterial measurements of carbon dioxide during general anesthesia. Can J Anaesth 1992; 39: 31–36
120 Chapman KR, Liu FLW, Watson RM, Rebuck AS. Conjunctival oxygen tension and its relationship to arterial oxygen tension. J Clin Monit 1986; 2: 100–104
121 Gys T, Van Esbroeck G, Hubens A. Assessment of perfusion in peripheral tissue beds by subcutaneous oximetry and gastric intramucosal pH-metry in elective colorectal surgery. Intensive Care Med 1991; 17: 78–82
122 Kainuma M, Fujiwara Y, Kimura N, Shitaokoshi A, Nakashima K, Shimada Y. Monitoring hepatic venous hemoglobin oxygen saturation in patients undergoing liver surgery. Anesthesiology 1991; 74: 49–52
123 Kessler M, Hoper J, Krumme BA. Monitoring of tissue perfusion and cellular function. Anaesthesia 1976; 45: 184–196
124 Jobsis-VanderVliet FF, Fox E, Sugioka K. Monitoring of cerebral oxygenation and cytochrome aa$_3$, redox state. Int Anesthesiol Clin 1987; 25: 209–230
125 Brazy JE. Cerebral oxygen monitoring with near infrared spectroscopy: clinical application to neonates. J Clin Monit 1991; 7: 325–334
126 Doglio GR, Pusajo JF, Egurrola MA et al. Gastric mucosal pH as a prognostic index of mortality in critically ill patients. Crit Care Med 1991; 19: 1037–1040
127 Leigh M, Jones J, Motley H. The expired carbon dioxide as a continuous guide of the pulmonary and circulatory systems during anaesthesia and surgery. J Thorac Cardiovasc Surg 1961; 41: 597–610
128 Cooper J, Newbower R, Kitz R. An analysis of major errors and equipment failures in anesthesia management: consideration for prevention and detection. Anesthesiology 1984; 60: 34–42
129 Caplan RA, Posner KL, Ward RJ, Cheney FW. Adverse respiratory events in anesthesia. A closed claim analysis. Anesthesiology 1990; 72: 826–833
130 Fisher D, Swedlow D. Estimating $PaCO_2$ by end-tidal gas sampling in children. Crit Care Med 1981; 9: 287
131 Shankar KB, Moseley H, Kumar Y, Vemula V. Arterial to end-tidal carbon dioxide tension difference during Caesarean section anaesthesia. Anaesthesia 1986; 41: 698–702
132 Sasse FJ. Can we trust end-tidal carbon dioxide measurements in infants? J Clin Monit 1985; 1: 147–148
133 Yamanaka M, Sue D. Comparison of arterial end-tidal PCO_2 difference and dead space/tidal volume ratio in respiratory failure. Chest 1987; 92: 832–835
134 Forrest JB, Cahalan MK, Rehder K, Goldsmith CH et al. Multicenter study of general anaesthesia. II. Results. Anesthesiology 1990; 72: 262–268
135 Hart R, Hindman B. Mechanisms of perioperative cerebral infarction. Stroke 1982; 13: 766–773
136 Wong DH. Perioperative stroke. Part I: general surgery. Carotid artery disease and carotid endarterectomy. Can J Anaesth 1991; 38: 347–373
137 Dawson EG, Sherman JE, Kanim LE, Nuwer MR. Spinal cord monitoring results of the scoliosis research society and the European Spinal Deformity Society survey. Spine 1991; 16: 361–364
138 Silbert BS, Koumoundouros E, Davies MJ, Cronin KD. Comparison of the processed electroencephalogram and awake neurological assessment during carotid endarterectomy. Anaesth Intensive Care 1989; 17: 298–304
139 Davies MJ, Murrell GC, Cronin KD et al. Carotid endarterectomy under cervical plexus block — a prospective clinical audit. Anaesth Intensive Care 1990; 18: 219–223
140 Maynard D, Prior PF, Scott DF. Device for continuous monitoring of cerebral activity in resuscitated patients. B Med J 1969; 4: 545–546
141 Maynard DE, Jenkinson JL. The cerebral function analysing monitor. Initial clinical experience, application and further development. Anaesthesia 1984; 39: 678–690
142 Bickford RG, Fleming NI, Billinger TW. Compression of EEG data by isometric power spectral plots. Electroencephal Clin Neurophysiol 1971; 31: 631P
143 Fleming RA, Smith NT. An inexpensive device for analysing and monitoring the electroencephalogram. Anesthesiology 1979; 50: 456–461
144 Eger EI II, Stevens WC, Cromwell TH. The electroencephalogram in man anesthetized with Forane. Anesthesiology 1971; 35: 504
145 Rampil IJ, Lockhart SH, Eger EI II et al. Human EEG dose response to desflurane. J Neurosurg Anesth 1990; 2: S14
146 Wollman H, Smith AL, Hoffman JC. Cerebral blood flow and oxygen consumption in man during electroencephalographic seizure patterns induced by anesthesia with Ethrane. Fed Proc 1969; 28: 356
147 Hudson RJ, Stanski DR, Saidman LJ. A model for studying depth of anesthesia and acute tolerance to thiopental. Anesthesiology 1983; 59: 301–308
148 Bloom MJ, Schwartz DM, Berkowitz HD et al. DSA processing of EEG is an effective monitor in carotid endarterectomy. J Neurosurg Anesth 1990; 2: s 13
149 Bowdle TA, Rooke A, Kaziners A. Intraoperative stroke during carotid endarterectomy without a change in the spectral edge frequency of the compressed spectral array. J Cardiothorac Anaesth 1988; 2: 204–206
150 Kresowik TF, Worsey MJ, Khoury MD et al. Limitations of electroencephalographic monitoring in the detection of cerebral ichemia accompanying carotid endarterectomy. J Vasc Surg 1991; 13: 439–443
151 Drummond JC, Brann CA, Perkins DE, Wolfe DE. A comparison of median frequency, spectral edge frequency, a frequency band power ratio, total power, and dominance shift in the determination of depth of anesthesia. Acta Anaesthesiol Scand 1991: 35: 693–699
152 Rampil IJ, Matteo RS. Change in EEG spectral edge frequency correlate with the hemodynamic response to

laryngoscopy and intubation. Anesthesiology 1987; 67: 139–142
153. Schwö dem H, Stoeckel H. Quantitative EEG analysis during anaesthesia with isoflurane in nitrous oxide at 1.3 and 1.5 MAC. Br J Anaesth 1987; 59: 738–745
154. Kearse L, Saini V, DeBros F, Chamoun N. Bispectral analysis of EEG may predict anesthetic depth during narcotic induction. Anesthesiology 1991; 75: 175
155. Sato A, Balish M, Muratore R. Principles of magnetoencephalography. J Clin Neurophysiol 1991; 8: 144–156
156. Pathak KS, Ammadio M, Kalamchi A et al. Effects of halothane, enflurane and isoflurane on somatosensory evoked potentials during nitrous oxide anesthesia. Anesthesiology 1987; 66: 753
157. Cedzich C, Schramm J, Fahlbusch R. Are flash-evoked visual potentials useful for intraoperative monitoring of visual pathway function? Neurosurgery 1987; 21: 709–715
158. Grundy BL, Jannetta PJ, Procopia PT, Lina A, Boston JR, Doyle E. Intraoperative monitoring of brain-stem auditory evoked potentials. J Neurosurg 1982; 57: 674–681
159. Yingling CD, Gardi JN. Intraoperative monitoring of facial and cochlear nerves during acoustic neuroma surgery. Otolarying Clin North Am 1992; 25: 413–448
160. Barelli A, Valente MR, Clemente A, Bozza P, Proietti R, Della CF. Serial multimodality-evoked potentials in severely head-injured patients: diagnostic and prognostic implications. Crit Care Med 1991; 19: 1374–1381
161. Thornton C, Konieczko K, Jones JG, Jordon C, Dore CJ, Henegan CP. Effect of surgical stimulation on the auditory evoked response. B J Anaesth 1988; 60: 372–378
162. Schwender D, Keller I, Schlund M, Klasing S, Madler C. Acoustic evoked potentials of medium latency and intraoperative wakefulness during anesthesia maintenance using propofol, isoflurane and flunitrazepam/fentanyl. Anaesthetist 1991; 40: 214–221
163. Forbes HJ, Allen PW, Waller CS et al. Spinal cord monitoring in scoliosis surgery: experience with 1168 cases. J Bone Joint Surg 1991; 73: 487–491
164. Apel DM, Marrero G, King J, Tolo VT, Bassett GS. Avoiding paraplegia during anterior spinal surgery. The role of somatosensory evoked potential monitoring with temporary occlusion of segmental spinal arteries. Spine 1991; 16 (suppl): 365–370
165. Drenger B, Parker SD, McPherson RW et al. Spinal cord stimulation evoked potentials during thoracoabdominal aortic aneurysm surgery. Anesthesiology 1992; 76: 689–695
166. Lam AM, Manninen PH, Ferguson GG, Natau W. Monitoring electrophysiological function during carotid endarterectomy: a comparison of somatosensory evoked potentials and conventional electroencephalogram. Anesthesiology 1991; 75: 15–21
167. Friedman WA, Chadwick GM, Verhoeven FJS, Mahla M, Day AL. Monitoring of somatosensory evoked potentials for middle cerebral artery aneurysms. Neurosurgery 1991; 29: 83–88
168. Hutchison DO, Frith RW, Shaw NA, Judson JA, Cant BR. A comparison between electroencephalography and somatosensory evoked potentials for outcome prediction following severe head injury. Electroencephalogr Clin Neurophysiol 1991; 58: 228–233
169. Barker AT, Freeston IL, Jalinous R et al. Magnetic stimulation of the human brain and peripheral nervous system: an introduction and results of an initial clinical evaluation. Neurosurgery 1987; 20: 100–109
170. Schmid UD, Boll J, Liechti S, Schmid J, Hess CW. Influence of some anaesthetic agents on muscle responses to transcranial magnetic cortex stimulation: a pilot study in humans. Neurosurgery 1992; 30: 85–92
171. Tassinari GA, Michelucci R, Forti A et al. Transcranial magnetic stimulation in epileptic patients: usefulness and safety. Neurology 1990; 40: 1132–1133
172. Owen JH, Naito M, Bridwell KH, Oakley DM. Relationship between duration of spinal cord ischaemia and postoperative neurologic deficits in animals. Spine 1990; 15: 846–851
173. Owen JH, Masatoshi N, Bridwell KH. Relationship among level of distraction, evoked potentials spinal cord ischaemia and integrity, and clinical status in animals. Spine 1990; 15: 852–857
174. Waltz AG, Sundt TM Jr, Michenfelder JD. Cerebral blood flow during carotid endarterectomy. Circulation 1972; 45: 1091–1096
175. Rampil IJ. Cerebral perfusion mapping with ultrasound contrast. Anesthesiology 1991; 75: A1006
176. Naylor AR, Wildsmith JA, McClure J, Jenkins AM, Ruckley CV. Transcranial Doppler monitoring during carotid endarterectomy. Br J Surg 1991; 78: 1264–1268
177. Powers AD, Smith RR. Hyperperfusion syndrome after carotid endarterectomy: a transcranial Doppler evaluation. Neurosurgery 1990; 26: 56–60
178. Van Der Linden J, Casmir-Ahn H. When do cerebral emboli appear during open heart operation? A transcranial study. Ann Thorac Surg 1991; 51: 237–241
179. Hartmann A, Ries F, Tsuda Y, Lagreze H, Seiler R, Grolimund P. Correlation of regional cerebral blood flow and blood velocity in normal volunteers and patients with cerebro-vascular disease. Neurochirurgia (Stuttg) 1991; 34: 6–13
180. Werner C, Kochs E, Rau M, Schulte AM, Esch J. Transcranial Doppler sonography as a supplement in the detection of cerebral circulatory arrest. J Neurosurg Anesthesiol 1990; 2: 159–165
181. McKay RD, Sundt TM, Michenfelder JD et al. Internal carotid artery stump pressure and cerebral blood flow during carotid endarterectomy. Anesthesiology 1976; 45: 390–399
182. Ammar A D, Pauls DG. Correlation of carotid argery stump pressure with a palpable carotid artery pulse. J Cardiovasc Surg (Torino) 1992; 33: 59–61
183. Belliveau JW, Kennedy DJ, McKinstry RC et al. Functional mapping of the human visual cortex by magnetic resonance imaging. Science 1991; 254: 716–719
184. Detre JA, Leigh JS, Williams DS, Koretsky AP. Perfusion imaging. Magn Reson Med 1992; 23: 37–45
185. Richards MJ, Skeus MA, Jarvis AP, Prys-Roberts C. Total IV anaesthesia with propofol and alfentanil: dose requirements for propofol and the effect of premedication with clonidine. Br J Anaesth 1990; 65: 157–163

186 Isaac PA, Rosen M. Lower eosophageal contractility and detection of awareness during anaesthesia. Br J Anaesth 1990; 65: 319–324

187 Pomfrett CJD, Barrie JR, Healy TEJ. Respiratory sinus arrhythmia: an index of light anaesthesia. Br J Anaesth 1993; 71: 212–217

188 Ali HH, Utting JE, Gray TC. Stimulus frequency in the detection of neuromuscular block in humans. Br J Anaesth 1970; 42: 967

189 Stanec A, Heyduh J, Stanec G et al. Tetanic fade and post-tetanic tension in the absence of neuromuscular blocking agents in anesthetized man. Anesth Analg 1978; 57: 102–110

190 Viby-Mogensen J, Howardy-Hansen P, Chraemmer-Jorgensen B et al. Posttetanic count (PTC): a new method of evaluating an intense nondepolarizing neuromuscular blockade. Anesthesiology 1981; 55: 458

191 Sonsu AK, Viby-Morgensen J, Fernando PUE et al. Relationship of post-tetanic count and train-of-four response during intense neuromuscular blockade caused by atracurium. Br J Anaesth 1987; 59: 1089

192 Mucchal KK, Viby-Morgensen J, Frenando PUE et al. Evaluation of intense neuromuscular blockade caused by vecuronium using a posttetanic count (PTC). Anesthesiology 1987; 66: 846

193 Engbaek J, Ostergaard D, Viby-Morgensen J. Double burst stimulation (DBS): a new pattern of nerve stimulation to identify residual neuromuscular block. Br J Anaesth 1989; 62: 274–278

194 Gill SS, Donati F, Bevan DR. Clinical evaluation of double burst stimulation: its relationship to train-of-four stimulation. Anaesthesia 1990; 45: 543–548

195 Brull SJ, Silverman DG. Visual assessment of train-of-four and double burst-induced fade at submaximal stimulating currents. Anesth Analg 1991; 73: 627–632

196 Laycock JRD, Donati F, Smith CE, Bevan DR. Potency of atracurium and vecuronium at the diaphragm and the adductor pollicis muscle. Br J Anaesth 1988; 61: 286–291

197 Smith CE, Donati F, Bevan DR. Potency of succinylcholine at the diaphragm and at the adductor pollicis muscle. Anesth Analg 1988; 67: 625–630

198 Pansard JL, Chauvin M, Lebreault C et al. Effect of an intubating dose of succinylcholine and atracurium on the diaphragm and adductor pollicis in humans. Anesthesiology 1987; 66: 117–122

199 Meistelman C, Plaud B, Donati F. Neuromuscular effects of succinylcholine on the vocal cords and adductor pollicis muscles. Anesth Analg 1991; 73: 278–282

200 Donati F, Meistelman C, Plaud B. Vecuronium neuromuscular blockade at the adductor muscles of the larynx and adductor pollicis. Anesthesiology 1991; 74: 833–837

201 Viby-Morgensen J, Jensen NH, Engbaek J et al. Tactile and visual evaluation of the response to train-of-four nerve stimulation. Anesthesiology 1985; 63: 440–443

202 Katz RL. Electromyographic and mechanical effects of suxamethonium and tubocurarine on twitch, tetanic and posttetanic responses. Br J Anaesth 1973; 45: 849–859

203 Kopman AF. The relationship of evoked electromyographic and mechanical responses following atracurium in humans. Anesthesiology 1985; 63: 208

204 Viby-Morgensen J, Jensen E, Werner M, Kirkegaard-Nielsen H. Measurement of acceleration: a new method of monitoring neuromuscular function. Acta Anaesthesiol Scand 1988; 32: 45

205 Werner MU, Kirkegaard-Nielsen H, May O, Djernes M. Assessment of neuromuscular transmission by the evoked acceleration response: an evaluation of the accuracy of the acceleration transducer in comparison with a force displacement transducer. Acta Anaesthesiol Scand 1988; 32: 395

206 Gibson FM, Mirakhur RK, Clarke RSJ, Brady MM. Quantification of train-of-four responses during recovery of block from nondepolarizing muscle relaxants. Acta Anaesthesiol Scand 1987; 31: 655

207 Brand JB, Cullen DJ, Wilson NE, Ali HH. Spontaneous recovery from nondepolarizing neuromuscular blockade: correlation between clinical and evoked responses. Anesth Analg 1977; 56: 55

208 Engbaek J, Ostergaard D, Viby-Morgensen J, Skovgaard LT. Clinical recovery and train-of-four ratio measured mechanically and electromyographically following atracurium. Anesthesiology 1989; 71: 391–393

209 Carli F, Gabrielczyk M, Clark MM, Aber VR. An investigation of factors affecting postoperative rewarming of adult patients. Anaesthesia 1986; 41: 363–369

210 Vaughan MS, Vaughan RW, Randall CC. Postoperative hypothermia in adults; relationship of age, anesthesia and shivering to rewarming. Anesth Analg 1981; 60: 746–751

211 Valeri RC, Cassidy G, Khuri S et al. Hypothermia induced reversible platelet dysfunction. Ann Surg 1987; 205: 175–181

212 Heier T, Caldwel JE, Sessler DI, Miller RD. The effect of local surface and central cooling on adductor pollicis twitch tension during nitrous oxide/isoflurane and nitrous oxide/fentanyl anesthesia. Anesthesiology 1990; 72: 807–811

213 Hovarth SM, Spurr GB, Hutt BK, Hamilton LH. Metabolic cost of shivering. J Appl Physiol 1956; 8: 595–602

214 Bay J, Nunn JF, Prys-Roberts C. Factors influencing arterial Po_2 during recovery from anaesthesia. Br J Anaesth 1968; 40: 398–407

215 Vale RJ. Monitoring of temperature during anaesthesia. Int Anesthesiol Clin 1979: 61–83

216 Cork RC, Vaughan RW, Humphrey LS. Precision and accuracy of intraoperative temperature monitoring. Anesth Analg 1983; 62: 211–214

217 Duke WW. The relation of blood platelets to hemorrhagic disease: description of a method for determining the bleeding time and coagulation time and report of three cases of hemorrhagic disease relieved by transfusion. JAMA 1910; 55: 1185–1192

218 Ivy AC, Nelson D, Bucher G. The standardization of certain factors in the cutaneous "venostasis" bleeding time technique. J Lab Clin Med 1941; 26: 1812–1822

219 Chargoff F, Olson KB. Studies on the chemistry of blood coagulation. VI: Studies on the action of heparin and other anticoagulants: The influence of protamine on the anticoagulant effect in vivo. J Biol Chem 1938; 122: 153

220 Hattersley PG. Activated coagulation time of whole blood. JAMA 1966; 196: 440
221 Wang JS, Lin CY, Hung WT, Thisted RA, Karp RB. In vitro effects of aprotinin on activated clotting time measured with different activators. J Thorac Cardiovasc Surg 1992; 104: 1135–1140
222 Hartert H. Blutgerninnungstudien mit der Thrombelastrographic, Einen neuen Untersuchingsver Fahren. Kln Wochenschr 1948; 16: 257
223 Kang YG, Martin DJ, Marquez JM et al. Intra-operative changes in blood coagulation and thromboelastographic monitoring in liver transplantation. Anesth Analg 1985; 64: 888–896
224 Kang Y, Lewis JH, Navalgund A et al. Epsilon-amino caproic acid for treatment of fibrinolysis during liver transplantation. Anesthesiology 1987; 66: 766–773
225 Kang Y, Martin LK, Marquez J, Lewis JH, de Wolf A. Thromboelastographic monitoring of coagulation during cardiac surgery. Anesthesiology 1989; 71: A8
226 Speiss BD, Tuman KJ, McCarthy RJ, DeLaria GA, Schillo R, Ivankovitch AD. Thromboelastography as an indicator of post-cardiopulmonary bypass coagulopathies. J Clin Monit 1987; 3: 25-30
227 Greeley WJ, Quill TJ, Greenberg CS. Blood coagulation and thromboelastogram changes during and after pediatric cardiovascular surgery. In: Annual Meeting-Society of Cardiovascular Anesthesiologists, 1987: A146

6. Induction of anaesthesia

J. W. Sear

Induction of anaesthesia is usually accomplished by either the intravenous (i.v.) or the gaseous route; however, in specific circumstances (see below), drug administration may be by the intramuscular, oral or rectal route.

The aim of the induction phase is to produce unconsciousness, and then to increase the depth of central nervous suppression to a plane such that the normal autonomic, somatic and sensory responses to noxious stimulation are obtunded. In an editorial in 1987, Prys-Roberts[1] defined anaesthesia as 'drug-induced unconsciousness when the patient neither perceives nor recalls noxious stimuli'. Thus, he considered anaesthesia as an all-or-none phenomenon, and his view differed from the concept of a continuum, as proposed by Jones & Konieczko.[2] Secondary aims to the successful induction of anaesthesia are the provision of an unobstructed airway; prevention of laryngospasm; avoidance of the accumulation of excessive secretions; prevention of vomiting or regurgitation of gastric contents; and the avoidance of iatrogenic problems such as gastric distension following manual inflation of the stomach, myalgia, sore throat and facial or dental trauma.

Although the clinical anaesthetist requires knowledge of the pharmacokinetics and pharmacodynamics of the frequently used intravenous and inhaled agents, induction of anaesthesia is achieved normally by titration of these drugs to specific pharmacological end-points. For many of the i.v. drugs, there are narrow therapeutic margins. Thus the barbiturates (thiopentone and methohexitone), midazolam and propofol have therapeutic indices of 4–6 (therapeutic index = lethal dose in 50% of animals/anaesthetic dose in 50% of animals). Greater therapeutic indices are associated with the steroidal anaesthetic drugs (e.g. Althesin, 5β-pregnanolone).[3]

The aims of the successful induction of anaesthesia have been summarized by Willenkin.[4] He defined anaesthesia as the onset of a clinically appropriate level of central nervous system depression to allow surgical intervention. He then defined five levels of anaesthesia-induced depression from loss of consciousness to deep anaesthesia. Thus, light anaesthesia was defined as:

- respiratory depression, but response to maximal stimulation
- hypotension in the absence of surgical stimulation
- minimal haemodynamic response to surgical stimulation
- an absence of significant somatic response to surgical stimulation.

Although Guedel[5] described the classical signs of alterations in the depth of anaesthesia, modern anaesthesia (involving an i.v. induction technique) often masks the early stages (I and II) which he defined. Many anaesthetists utilize the loss of eyelash reflex as an indicator of successful i.v. induction of anaesthesia; this may have been appropriate for the barbiturates, but using this end-point with the newer agents (propofol and 5β-pregnanolone) may result in overdosing.[6,7] Similarly, pupillary size and movement, and the rate and depth of ventilation, are poor indices of induction of anaesthesia, especially if a combination of i.v. and inhaled agents is used.

However, some signs are useful. The pattern of spontaneous breathing does provide one monitor. With loss of consciousness, the duration of each breath varies, as does the inspiratory-to-expiratory ratio. Inspiratory and expiratory flow rates change, as do the pauses at the ends of inspiration and expiration. As the depth of anaesthesia increases, expiration becomes active and involves the use of the accessory respiratory muscles. With the attainment of the plane of surgical anaesthesia, ventilation becomes regular again both in pattern and rate, with expiration being a passive process, coupled with loss of the end-inspiratory pause.

Changes in heart rate and arterial blood pressure are much more agent-specific. Thus, *most* agents cause a decrease in heart rate with increasing depth of anaesthesia, *but* with isoflurane and ketamine, the heart rate may increase. Blood pressure similarly decreases with induction of anaesthesia; the decrease in arterial pressure is of the order of 15–20% compared with the value in the resting individual. With the three commonly used inhaled agents, arterial pressure decreases with increasing depth of anaesthesia.

When i.v. agents are employed, increasing depth of anaesthesia and the associated decrease in arterial pressure are less clearly dose-dependent. The minimum infusion rate (MIR) for i.v. agents has been compared with the minimum alveolar concentration (MAC) value for inhaled agents.[8] However, there are few data available for multiples of the MIR for individual intravenous anaesthetic agents. The same general premise probably applies, although the cardiovascular safety of the steroid hypnotic agents (coupled with their high therapeutic indices) suggests that they may differ from some of the volatile agents, and also from propofol.[8-12]

KINETICS AND DYNAMICS OF I.V. DRUGS FOR INDUCTION OF ANAESTHESIA

The efficacy and duration of action of an i.v. induction agent depend largely on its physicochemical and pharmacological properties. To achieve unconsciousness in one arm–brain circulation time, agents should be lipophilic (or solubilized in emulsions to act as if lipid-soluble) and hence able to cross the blood–brain barrier to interact with one or more receptor subtypes in the central nervous system. The exact site of action is still unknown, but there is growing evidence that many i.v. induction agents interact with the benzodiazepine receptor–γ-aminobutyric acid (GABA) receptor–chloride channel complex, as well as with acetylcholine receptors and voltage-dependent sodium channels.[13,14]

The duration of effect of an induction agent is not limited by its rate of metabolism in the liver (or other possible drug-metabolizing organs), but by its redistribution within the body. Thus, in the case of thiopentone, recovery to awakening occurs within 15–20 min following a single bolus dose of 3–5 mg.kg^{-1}. At the time of awakening, only about 18% of the injected dose has undergone metabolism, compared with about 38% of a dose of methohexitone and nearly 70% of propofol.

The differences in the rates of initial recovery (to opening eyes or ability to give a verbal response to a simple command) are small; the choice of one drug or another in ambulatory surgery relates more to the speed at which patients achieve intermediate recovery indices as assessed by psychometric testing (e.g. critical flicker fusion, choice reaction time, pegboard test, p-deletion test, post-box test, Trieger dot test). These tests probably provide a guide to the suitability (or not) for discharge of the patient from an area of high nursing dependence, to a lower one. Such end-points are influenced more by rates of clearance and/or metabolism of i.v. induction agents than by redistribution alone.

The pharmacokinetics of the different i.v. induction agents show some similarities and some differences. They all have similar distribution half-lives, but vary greatly in their clearance rates and in the fraction of drug eliminated during the distribution phases (Table 6.1). Present clinical data indicate that induction of anaesthesia with propofol is associated with a more rapid recovery profile than for the other i.v. agents, and this is clearly in agreement with the known kinetics of the i.v. hypnotic agents.

Because the duration of action of induction agents is perfusion-dependent, any decrease in blood flow (e.g. hypovolaemia, circulatory shock) affects drug redistribution, and thus increases the time to recovery.

KINETICS OF GASEOUS INDUCTION OF ANAESTHESIA

With inhaled agents, as with i.v. agents, induction of anaesthesia can be achieved only if the brain tension of the anaesthetic agent exceeds the tension associated with hypnosis. For inhaled induction of anaesthesia, there are three main factors which influence the rate at which the alveolar concentration, and thus brain tension, approaches the inspired value: the inspired concentration itself, alveolar ventilation and cardiac output.[15]

Inspired concentration

This determines the ultimate alveolar concentration and thus *tension* of the anaesthetic agent, and hence the arterial blood tension and, in turn, the brain tension. The state of anaesthesia is related to the *tension* of an inhaled anaesthetic at the active site(s) in the brain. The time to induction depends on the time taken for the brain tension to reach the effect threshold. Increasing the inspired concentration (and thus tension) therefore quickens the induction period as long as breath-holding, laryngospasm and coughing are avoided. In current clinical practice, halothane and enflurane are the most appropriate drugs for inhaled induction; high concentrations of isoflurane and desflurane are pungent and irritant to the laryngeal mucosa and nitrous oxide alone cannot always induce hypnosis in

Table 6.1 Disposition parameters for intravenous hypnotic agents used for induction of anaesthesia

Agent	$T_{1/2}\alpha$ (min)	$T_{1/2}\beta$ (min)	$T_{1/2}\gamma$ (h)	Systemic clearance (ml.min^{-1}.kg^{-1})	%AUCγ
Thiopentone	2–7	42–59	5.1–11.5	2.2–3.5	0.72
Methohexitone	6	2–58	1.62–3.9	8.2–12.0	0.66
Etomidate	1–3	12–29	2.9–5.5	11.6–25	0.64
Propofol	1–4	5–69	1.62–63.0	23.2–32.9	0.29
Ketamine	1–3	8–18	2.2–3.0	14.0–19.1	0.68
Midazolam	5–15	25–30	1.5–3.0	5.0–7.0	
5β-Pregnanolone	?	9–17	0.78–6.3	20.8–39.0	0.42

$T_{1/2}$ α, β, and γ = three half-lives for data described by a three-compartment model; %AUC γ = area under the curve during the terminal elimination phase as a percentage of the total area under the concentration–time curve (zero to infinity).

the absence of hypoxaemia. Inspired concentrations of between 1 and 3% halothane or between 2 and 4% enflurane in oxygen are needed to induce anaesthesia.

Alveolar ventilation

The anaesthetic agent in the inspired gas mixture is diluted by functional residual air. When using a non-rebreathing system, circuit equilibration (i.e. inspired to alveolar equilibration) takes about 3 min for a gas which is completely insoluble in blood. The time can be decreased by increasing alveolar ventilation, and decreased by rebreathing, by respiratory depression and respiratory obstruction.

Cardiac output

An alteration of cardiac output has an apparently paradoxical influence on the rate of uptake of inhaled anaesthetics and thus the rate of induction of anaesthesia. An increase in cardiac output does not increase the speed of induction (as an increase in alveolar ventilation does), but decreases it. This is because, at any moment, the tension in the alveolus is the balance between the amount of anaesthetic delivered to the alveolus and the amount taken away in the alveolar capillary blood. An increase in cardiac output, and thus in alveolar capillary blood flow, has the effect of decreasing alveolar tension. It is common clinical observation that inhaled induction of anaesthesia in shocked patients is rapid.

Note that the rate of increase of alveolar tension to meet that of inspired gas is most rapid for agents of low solubility. Thus, the speed of induction with agents which possess a relatively low solubility in blood, such as the newer agents desflurane and sevoflurane, is more rapid than with agents which are more soluble, such as halothane.

The factors which increase the speed of induction are listed in Table 6.2.

An alternative technique for rapid inhaled induction (RII) of anaesthesia was described by Ruffle et al[16] in

Table 6.2 Factors which increase the speed of induction of anaesthesia with inhaled agents

Factor	Notes
Concentration and solubility of the inhaled anaesthetic	Either by addition of carbon dioxide or by assisting ventilation
Hyperventilation	Reduces flow to the non-vital organs in conditions such as hypovolaemic shock, dehydration, in the elderly and in malnutrition
Decreased circulating blood volume	High flow aids the speed of equilibration; thus non-rebreathing systems offer a faster induction than do closed or rebreathing systems
High gas flow systems	Enhanced uptake of poorly soluble gases increases the alveolar concentration of the second gas in the mixture.
Second gas effect	This is only of significance when nitrous oxide is administered, and the clinical importance of this phenomenon is not great
Uptake and elimination of anaesthetic agents	More rapid in infants because of their relatively greater alveolar ventilation and smaller functional residual capacity per unit body weight

volunteers and by Wilton & Thomas[17] in patients. A 4 L reservoir bag is filled with 67% nitrous oxide and 4% halothane in oxygen and the mix delivered using a Mapleson A breathing system at a flow rate of 6 l.min^{-1}. The patient exhales to residual volume, and then takes a breath to maximal inspiration and holds his/her breath. The technique differs from the older method of inhaled induction in requiring the patient's co-operation. Loper et al[18] used the technique to compare RII with halothane and isoflurane, suggesting that the latter may be faster.

The efficacy and general utility of the method need to be evaluated further; the technique might be particularly appropriate for use with the new inhalational agents (desflurane and sevoflurane) because of their low blood/gas solubilities.

Although studies comparing the cardiorespiratory effects of different anaesthetic drugs at induction have been conducted for the i.v. agents, similar data for the inhaled agents are largely missing.

INTRAMUSCULAR AND RECTAL DRUG ADMINISTRATION

Although the intramuscular route has been described for induction of anaesthesia with ketamine, peak levels are not achieved for 22 min.[19] The size of the necessary injected dose precludes this route for most other i.v. hypnotic agents.

The administration by the rectal route of lipid-soluble i.v. anaesthetic agents for premedication, sedation or induction of anaesthesia in children has been described for thiopentone, methohexitone, etomidate, benzodiazepines and ketamine.

Rectal methohexitone (in doses of 20–25 mg.kg^{-1}) has been used for induction of anaesthesia in healthy children.[20-22] However, kinetic studies show a sixfold variation in bio-availability, making the effective induction dose unpredictable. Induction doses of ketamine[23,24] vary between 6.7 and 10.6 mg.kg^{-1}. Linton & Thornington[25] have described the use of rectal etomidate. The use of midazolam by the rectal route for induction of anaesthesia (in doses up to 5 mg.kg^{-1}) is unreliable, and cannot be recommended.[26]

AGENTS USED FOR INDUCTION OF ANAESTHESIA

The main factors which influence the usefulness of an intravenous or inhaled induction drug are the effects on the cardiovascular and respiratory systems. Other adverse or side-effects include their influence on the liver and other organs with respect to toxicity, their venous tolerance and their liability to allergic reactions.

Unconsciousness may be induced by the use of a variety of i.v. hypnotics alone or in combination with other agents (e.g. opioids or benzodiazepines). In general, hypnotics do not possess analgesic properties, nor do they relax skeletal muscle. The most widely used agents are listed in Table 6.3.

Thiopentone

This thiobarbiturate continues to be a popular choice for i.v. induction of anaesthesia. When given intravenously, the barbiturates all achieve onset of hypnosis within one arm–brain circulation time; this relates to their high lipid-solubility and rapid uptake into the brain. The maximum effect of thiopentone depends on circulation time but in healthy adults usually occurs within about 1 min of a single induction dose of 3–6 mg.kg^{-1}.

There is then a rapid decline in the brain concentration of the barbiturates due to their redistribution into the lean body tissue, so that the duration of effect of an induction dose is about 5–10 min. Lower induction doses of thiopentone are required in the pre-medicated patient; in patients with severe anaemia or burns; in malnourished patients; in patients with uraemia or liver failure; and in the hypovolaemic individual, irrespective of the cause. Circulatory failure and hypothermia slow the circulation time and prolong the induction period. Moreover, the total dose needed in such patients is also reduced.

Absolute contra-indications to the use of thiopentone are airway obstruction, shock with cardiovascular collapse, status asthmaticus and porphyria (see below).

Thiamylal has a similar pharmacological profile to thiopentone with regard to potency, incidence of laryngospasm and respiratory depression, cardiac toxicity and recovery time.[27]

Methohexitone

This oxybarbiturate is accompanied by a faster recovery

Table 6.3 Intravenous drugs used commonly for induction of anaesthesia (see text for details)

Thiopentone and thiamylal
Methohexitone
Etomidate
Propofol
Midazolam
Ketamine
Newer agents

profile than thiopentone due to its greater clearance (700–800 ml.min⁻¹) and shorter elimination half-life (420–460 min). Its main metabolite has no pharmacological activity; consequently, in contrast to thiopentone, it may be given by continuous infusion to maintain anaesthesia or for sedation. Methohexitone has two asymmetrical carbon atoms, and can therefore exist as four optimal isomers. The α-dl pair produce hypnosis, while the β-pair appear to be responsible for the excessive motor activity.

Induction of anaesthesia requires a dose of 1–2 mg.kg⁻¹ (the potency of methohexitone is 2.7 times that of thiopentone). Side-effects after methohexitone administration are more frequent than after thiopentone, and include pain on injection, a tendency to venous thrombophlebitis and exaggerated involuntary movements (especially in unpremedicated patients). Inadequate induction doses can also cause excitatory phenomena because the inhibitory areas of the brain are thought to be depressed at lower drug concentrations.

Etomidate

This carboxylated imidazole compound has a number of important advantages over the barbiturates. These include haemodynamic stability, minimal respiratory depression and a virtual absence of any propensity to release histamine from mast cells and basophils. The drug has a wider margin of safety in animals, with a therapeutic index of 26.4 (compared with thiopentone — 4.6).

Induction doses of 0.2–0.4 mg kg provide hypnosis for between 5 and 15 min, with only minor alterations in cardiovascular parameters in both healthy patients and in those with valvular or ischaemic heart disease (see below). However, etomidate alone does not obtund the sympathetic responses to laryngoscopy and tracheal intubation.[28] For a smooth haemodynamic profile, the drug should be combined with an opioid or an inhaled anaesthetic agent.

However, its use is associated with a number of minor disadvantages: pain on injection, thrombophlebitis, myoclonia and a high incidence of postoperative nausea and vomiting. There is also the well-documented effect of etomidate (when given either as a single induction dose or by infusion) in suppressing adrenal steroidogenesis.[29–31] Although the low plasma cortisol concentrations in patients receiving etomidate by infusion for sedation in the intensive care unit were associated with increased mortality,[32] there are no data to support this association when the drug is used as a single bolus to induce anaesthesia.

Etomidate has been given by the rectal route for induction of anaesthesia in children in doses of 6–7 mg.kg⁻¹; the onset of hypnosis occurs in about 4 min. There are no significant haemodynamic effects, and recovery is still rapid.

Propofol

This is a water-soluble hindered phenol which is presently formulated in soya oil (Intralipid) as an emulsion.[33] It has a neutral pH, and a pK$_a$ in water of 10.96. At physiological pH, there is extensive protein binding (>97–98%). Propofol is a highly lipophilic compound, which is broken down rapidly to inactive metabolites (the glucuronide, and corresponding quinol glucuronide and sulphate) in the liver and possibly other organs. The parent compound[34–37] has a long elimination half-life (up to 45 h), an apparent volume of distribution of 1000–3940 l, and a systemic clearance of 1.0–1.8 l.min⁻¹. Thus, propofol shows flow-dependent clearance characteristics.

Doses of 1–2.5 mg.kg⁻¹ (depending on patient age, physical status and premedication) induce anaesthesia in about 30 s.[6,38] Lower induction doses should be used in elderly patients or those with cardiovascular disease (see below). Loss of the eyelash reflex is not a reliable end-point for propofol anaesthesia, and may not be seen until overdosing has occurred. The potency of propofol has been compared with that of thiopentone in a number of studies;[38,39] the dose ratio of propofol : thiopentone is 1 : 1.6–1.9. After a dose of 2.5 mg.kg⁻¹, recovery to eye opening occurs in approximately 5 min, and is faster[40] than after methohexitone 1.5 mg.kg⁻¹ or thiopentone 5.0 mg.kg⁻¹.

Pain on injection is a feature of induction of anaesthesia with propofol, with incidences of up to 50% when administered into the small veins on the dorsum of the hand. The incidence may be reduced by use of large veins, by mixing with lignocaine (10–20 mg) and by pretreatment with fentanyl or alfentanil.[41,42] Other side-effects of induction include excitatory myoclonic phenomena and respiratory upsets; these tend to be short-lived.

The incidence and duration of apnoea can be reduced by slow administration of the drug, and the careful titration of dose to clinical effect.[43–45] One apparent advantage of propofol is that of more effective depression of pharyngeal and laryngeal reactivity than that associated with thiopentone;[46] this may be of benefit during upper-airway instrumentation or insertion of the laryngeal mask airway.

More recently, there have been reports of convulsions and opisthotonus following propofol anaesthesia (although in experimental animals, propofol has been shown to have anticonvulsant activity).[47,48] Another important central nervous system effect of propofol is its reduction of the duration of the seizure, compared with methohexitone, during electroconvulsive therapy.[49]

Propofol appears to have in vitro potential for inhibition of adrenal steroidogenesis,[50,51] but this appears not to be relevant in clinical anaesthetic practice.[30]

Maintenance of anaesthesia with propofol requires blood propofol concentrations of between 2 and 8 µg.ml^{-1} (infusion rates 2–10 mg.kg^{-1}.h^{-1}) when administered with either 70% nitrous oxide or an opioid infusion. Higher blood concentration (>10 mg.ml^{-1}) are necessary when propofol is used as the sole anaesthetic agent. Recovery occurs rapidly after cessation of an infusion, at blood concentrations[35,52,53] of about 1.0 µg.ml^{-1}.

Benzodiazepines

Midazolam is the only benzodiazepine suitable for induction of anaesthesia. It has a faster onset, and lower incidence of venous complications, than either diazepam or lorazepam. Induction of anaesthesia (as is the case with the barbiturates) co-incides with loss of the eyelash reflex.

Induction doses of 0.1–0.2 mg.kg^{-1} midazolam are given over 20–30 s; smaller doses are sufficient in premedicated patients, in the elderly and in patients of American Society of Anesthesiologists (ASA) groups III–V. Emergence from midazolam-induced anaesthesia is often prolonged.[54] However, induction with midazolam has some advantages compared with thiopentone, including improved peri-operative amnesia and haemodynamic stability, as well as decreased intra-operative requirements for inhaled anaesthetic agents. In contrast to some other i.v. hypnotic agents, the benzodiazepines are comparatively free from allergic reactions, and in single doses do not suppress the adrenal gland.[55] However, high doses of midazolam prevent the increase in plasma cortisol concentrations in response to surgical stress.[56,57]

A specific antagonist to the benzodiazepines (flumazenil) is also available. This antagonist is devoid of any intrinsic effects on the respiratory or cardiovascular systems, but reverses the respiratory-depressant effects of an agonist.[58] However, its effect is of short duration, with the peak occurring within 1–3 min of i.v. injection. Because it has a shorter elimination half-life (40–70 min) and faster clearance rate (5–20 ml.kg^{-1}.min^{-1}) than midazolam, flumazenil may produce an initial arousal from sedation, followed by re-sedation.[59] When larger doses of midazolam have been used for induction and maintenance of anaesthesia, the antagonist should be given as a loading dose followed by a continuous infusion in order to maintain a plasma drug concentration in excess of 20–40 ng.ml^{-1}.

Ketamine

This phencyclidine derivative is a racemic mixture, and is unique among the induction agents in that it produces both dose-related unconsciousness and analgesia. In addition, patients have no recall of surgery or anaesthesia, although the amnesia is not as pronounced as with the benzodiazepines.[60]

Ketamine has a pK$_a$ close to physiological pH, is lipid-soluble, and hence crosses the blood–brain barrier to produce rapid induction of anaesthesia when given by the i.v. route. Its effects on the cardiovascular system differ from the other hypnotic agents, as its use is accompanied by increases in heart rate, blood pressure and cardiac output, leading to increased cardiac work and myocardial oxygen consumption. These effects occur both in healthy patients and in those with heart disease. As it increases pulmonary vascular resistance (as well as systemic vascular resistance), ketamine is best avoided in patients with pre-existing elevated pulmonary arterial pressures (e.g. some congenital heart lesions, and patients with mitral valve disease). The hyperdynamic effects on the circulation are mediated via central mechanisms, as ketamine blocks the re-uptake of noradrenaline by both the uptake$_1$ (extra-neuronal) and uptake$_2$ (intraneuronal) mechanisms. It also causes the release of noradrenaline from the sympathetic ganglia. In vitro studies have shown it to have mild intrinsic myocardial depressant effects on the isolated heart.

The in vivo effects can be obtunded by use of adrenergic antagonists (both α- and β-), vasodilators, and also by pretreatment with benzodiazepines.

The main uses of ketamine for induction are in poor-risk patients (ASA classes IV and V), in patients with chronic obstructive respiratory disease, and patients with hypovolaemia or myocardial disease. It is also useful for field anaesthesia in disasters and in trauma medicine. It is not widely used for induction or maintenance of anaesthesia in industrial nations as administration is usually accompanied by unpleasant psychological side-effects, including nightmares and hallucinations.

Current interest extends to investigation of the relevant potency of the two stereo-isomers [R (−) and S (+)].[61,62] The potency ratio for anaesthesia and analgesia is approximately 4:2:1 for S ketamine: ketamine racemate: R ketamine. There are also some data to show that administration of S ketamine (compared with the racemate) is accompanied by a lower median electroencephalogram (EEG) power spectrum, a greater increase in blood pressure and heart rate, decreased locomotor activity, shortened recovery times, fewer psychological side-effects and equipotent analgesia.[62-65]

New i.v. hypnotic agents

A number of new formulations of some i.v. hypnotic agents are currently undergoing laboratory and/or clinical investigation. These include emulsion formulations of propanidid, methohexitone and etomidate, as well as etomidate solubilized in 2-hydroxypropyl, β-cyclodextrin and a liposomal preparation of propanidid. Whether these offer advantages over current formulations remains to be determined.

One new hypnotic agent, the steroid 5β-pregnanolone (eltanolone), has been investigated in humans. It has a high therapeutic index (>40) and, when given to rats, caused minimal cardiovascular depression. Recovery is intermediate between propofol and thiopentone.[66] Initial clinical studies with this water-insoluble agent (which is therefore formulated in Intralipid) indicate a median anaesthetic dose (AD_{50}) induction of 0.44 mg.kg^{-1} in subjects premedicated with an opioid.[7] Cardiovascular effects are similar to those seen previously with Althesin. Side-effects include short periods of apnoea following induction, and some involuntary muscular movements, but no pain on injection. Recovery after 5β-pregnanolone appears to be less rapid than after propofol.[67] Kinetic studies indicate an elimination half-life of between 47 and 376 min, and a clearance of 1.25–2.34 l.kg^{-1}.h^{-1}.

Effects of i.v. induction agents on central haemodynamics in healthy patients

Barbiturates, etomidate and propofol

Induction of anaesthesia with a sleep dose of a hypnotic drug decreases arterial blood pressure due to both myocardial depression and peripheral vasodilatation. The decreases in systolic and diastolic pressures are maximal within 1 min of injection, and are sustained for at least 5 min. The magnitude of response varies among patients and with the different i.v. agents. With either of the barbiturates, the decrease in systolic pressure is accompanied by a compensatory tachycardia, resulting in maintenance of cardiac output.[68-70]

Compared with the barbiturates, etomidate causes less haemodynamic perturbation when used for induction of anaesthesia. In a dose of 0.3 mg.kg^{-1}, there are no significant changes in systemic or coronary haemodynamics either in healthy patients or in those with ischaemic heart disease.[71-73] Maximum decreases in systolic and diastolic pressures are between 12 and 20%, with a smaller reduction in cardiac output. In the hypertensive patient, the responses to induction of anaesthesia are similarly obtunded, but there may be significant increases in heart rate and blood pressure following laryngoscopy and intubation.[28,74]

Most studies to investigate induction of anaesthesia with propofol in unpremedicated patients have shown only minimal increases in heart rate. As a result of this and the decrease in stroke volume (10–15%), blood pressure and cardiac output fall in both normotensive and hypertensive patients.[9,75,76] These decreases are more pronounced in patients concurrently receiving opioids, and in hypertensive patients receiving β-adrenoceptor-blocking drugs.[75,77] These haemodynamic responses may be attenuated[78] by induction of anaesthesia with the combination of a subhypnotic bolus dose (1 mg.kg^{-1}) and a low-dose infusion (1 mg.kg^{-1} per min) instead of the usual induction dose of 2 mg.kg^{-1}.

Laryngoscopy and intubation evoke potent sympathomimetic responses which are suppressed to a variable extent by different anaesthetics; the extent relates to the blood concentration achieved at the time of laryngoscopy. Propofol appears to be effective in suppressing the haemodynamic consequences of laryngoscopy and intubation, in contrast to anaesthetic doses of induction agents such as thiopentone, methohexitone and etomidate.[28,69,70,79] The addition of fentanyl 2 μg.kg^{-1} prior to induction of anaesthesia results in arterial pressures lower than those observed with the induction agent alone, and attenuation — although not abolition — of the response to laryngoscopy and intubation. These changes in blood pressure are accompanied by comparable increases in intra-ocular pressure which, on occasions, can have disastrous consequences.[80,81] Compared with thiopentone and etomidate, propofol causes a greater decrease in intra-ocular pressure and, following a second smaller dose, propofol is more effective in preventing the increases in intra-ocular pressure secondary to administration of suxamethonium and tracheal intubation.

Benzodiazepines

In healthy patients, there are no significant differences between the cardiovascular effects of midazolam and thiopentone for induction of anaesthesia.[54,82] The decrease in blood pressure following induction is principally due to a decrease in systemic vascular resistance.

Although the intravenous benzodiazepines are considered by many anaesthetists as the ideal drugs for induction of anaesthesia in the sick patient, significant reductions in both cardiac output and systemic vascular resistance occur after administration of either diazepam or midazolam (just as with thiopentone), the effects of the latter being more marked.[83] The cardiovascular effects of midazolam are not influenced by addition of 50% nitrous oxide in oxygen,[84] but addition of nitrous oxide to diazepam may cause significant increases in right atrial pressure, indicating some degree of myocardial depression.[85]

Ketamine

Induction of anaesthesia with ketamine (2–10 mg.kg^{-1} i.v.) is almost always associated with hypertension, tachycardia, an increase in cardiac output and an increased left ventricular force of contraction.[86] In the absence of premedicant drugs, the systolic pressure increases by 20–40 mmHg, with a smaller diastolic increase. These effects are probably mediated through sympathomimetic stimulation and may be obtunded by a number of other i.v. drugs, including thiopentone, diazepam, flunitrazepam and midazolam. The effects of ketamine during induction of anaesthesia are similar in patients with healthy and impaired myocardium.[87]

Effects of i.v. induction agents on ventilation

Induction of anaesthesia by i.v. drugs is frequently followed by a period of apnoea (the incidence of 4–30% varying with drug and the rate of administration). The rate is increased in patients premedicated with a benzodiazepine or an opioid.[83,88] In addition, bronchospasm and laryngospasm have both been reported after administration of the barbiturates, probably due to the attempted early instrumentation of a lightly anaesthetized patient.

With propofol, the incidence and duration of apnoea are dose-related and may be exacerbated by ventilation with 100% oxygen prior to induction. Most comparative studies of ventilatory effects of thiopentone and propofol show similar depression of tidal volume and ventilation rate. Apnoea and respiratory upsets occur also in patients induced with midazolam, and are more pronounced and of longer duration in the patient with chronic obstructive airways disease.

In contrast, ketamine has a minimal effect on central respiratory drive, with an unaltered ventilatory response to carbon dioxide. It also acts as a smooth-muscle relaxant, resulting in bronchodilation and improved pulmonary compliance. These effects are mediated by both a sympathomimetic action and a direct antagonism of carbachol and histamine-induced bronchoconstriction. One adverse effect on the airway, especially in the unpremedicated patient and in children, is increased salivation. This may result in upper-airway obstruction or laryngospasm. Although the majority of upper-airway reflexes are maintained, silent aspiration has been reported during ketamine anaesthesia.

Effects of i.v. induction agents on cerebral haemodynamics and cerebral pressures

The barbiturates (either by bolus dosing or continuous infusion) have been shown to reduce intracranial pressure effectively.[12,89] and have other potential advantages in terms of improving outcome after cardiopulmonary bypass, and in affording protection after regional ischaemia (e.g. during aneurysm clipping, and in the control of post-hypoxic convulsive activity). However, their use is associated with prolonged recovery (especially after thiopentone) and liability to seizures (after large doses of methohexitone).

Induction agents all affect cerebrospinal fluid pressure, which depends normally on the balance between its rate of formation and its rate of re-absorption. Thiopentone, midazolam and etomidate all reduce cerebrospinal fluid formation when used in high doses,[90] but have little effect on re-absorption.

In patients who present with severe head injuries, these three agents increase cerebrovascular resistance and therefore reduce intracranial pressure, presumably due to a decrease in cerebral blood flow, and a consequent decrease in cerebral blood volume. They also decrease cerebral oxygen consumption.

There are few data on the efficacy of i.v. induction agents in patients with raised intracranial pressure. Thiopentone and etomidate reduce intracranial pressure. Some studies of propofol suggest that it acts to reduce intracranial pressure through a simple reduction in arterial pressure[91,92] while others show maintenance of autoregulatory responsiveness to changes in arterial pressure.[93] Propofol has been reported to have no effect on cerebral vascular reactivity in response to changes in carbon dioxide tension.[94]

Thiopentone is a satisfactory agent for use during somatosensory evoked potential monitoring; the evoked responses persist even after administration of large doses of thiopentone, which result in a silent EEG. However, thiopentone does cause a dose-dependent change in the brainstem and cortical auditory evoked responses.

Propofol also affects brainstem auditory evoked potentials. In one study, the latency was increased but there was no change in amplitude.[95] However, this observation has not been confirmed by studies from workers at Northwick Park Hospital[96] who found both increased latency and decreased amplitude. Etomidate bolus doses increase the latency and amplitude of early somatosensory evoked potentials in patients anaesthetized with isoflurane in oxygen.[97]

There are few outcome studies of the protective properties of hypnotic agents against cerebral ischaemia. Nussmeier et al[98] investigated postoperative neurological sequelae in 182 patients undergoing cardiopulmonary bypass. Eighty-nine of the patients received thiopentone (39.5 mg.kg^{-1}) during bypass to maintain EEG silence; the other 93 patients received fentanyl alone. Enflurane was used in both groups to control intra-operative hypertension. Neurological sequelae occurred in both groups when assessments were made on the first postoperative day; however, by the 10th postoperative day, there was evidence of persistent dysfunction in 7 out of 93 patients in the control group, but none in the thiopentone-treated group. The use of thiopentone resulted in longer sleeping times, delayed tracheal extubation and increased postoperative sedation.

In a follow-up study, Metz et al[99] compared thiopentone by infusion during cardiopulmonary bypass with a smaller bolus (16 mg.kg^{-1}) of the barbiturate given just prior to aortic declamping. The latter regimen afforded the same protection, and reduced the awakening time. However, it did not alter the need for inotropic support during weaning from bypass.

It is still uncertain whether other presently available intravenous agents (such as propofol and midazolam) afford any cerebral protection in humans.

INFLUENCE OF I.V. INDUCTION AGENT ON RECOVERY

Comparisons of thiopentone, methohexitone, etomidate and propofol as induction agents, followed by maintenance with enflurane or isoflurane in nitrous oxide, indicate improved immediate recovery in the etomidate and propofol groups.[4,100-103] In premedicated patients undergoing urological surgery with enflurane–nitrous oxide anaesthesia, Mackenzie & Grant[40] showed propofol to be associated with the most rapid recovery to eye opening on command and to giving the correct date of birth. Psychomotor testing using critical flicker fusion showed no decrement in performance at 30, 60, 90 or 120 min after surgery in the propofol groups, while patients who had received methohexitone showed impaired ability at 30 min and thiopentone was accompanied by an effect persisting to 90 min. Other data comparing propofol and etomidate show little difference between the drugs when followed by maintenance with a volatile agent.

COMPLICATIONS OF INDUCTION OF ANAESTHESIA WITH I.V. DRUGS

Minor sequelae associated with i.v. agents

These occur to differing extents with all hypnotic agents.

Induction complications

Excitatory phenomena (involuntary movements, hypertonus) are associated with all drugs when given to the unpremedicated patient. However, the incidence varies greatly among agents; the incidence associated with the use of thiopentone is about 8%, while muscle movements with etomidate and methohexitone are considerably more common (up to 90%, and 30–35% respectively). For all drugs, the incidence appears to be related principally to the dose administered, and not to the rate of administration.

Tissue irritation

All i.v. induction agents are liable to cause pain on injection, and postoperative venous sequelae. The incidence of pain on injection varies with the individual drugs, as well as the site and speed of injection.

Major complications of i.v. hypnotic agents

Allergic reactions

Between 1964 and 1984, about 1000 reports of hypersensitivity reactions to i.v. anaesthetic agents were cited in the French and English-language literature; about 50% were due to neuromuscular relaxant drugs, 40% to the hypnotic agents, and the remainder to opioids (3%), benzodiazepines (2%) and neuroleptic agents (<1%).

Thiopentone and other barbiturates. There are over 300 cases reported in the literature of allergic reactions to the barbiturates. Most relate to thiopentone, although the quoted incidences of adverse reactions to thiopentone and methohexitone are 1 : 14 000 and 1 : 7000 respectively.

The classical features of the allergic response to thiopentone were first described in 1943 by Hunter.[104] Cutaneous and cardiovascular manifestations predominate (65 and 56% respectively) with respiratory side-effects in about 35% (laryngospasm or difficulty in ventilating the lungs). At least 10 patients have died following allergic reactions to thiopentone. Postoperatively, many affected patients give a history of atopy, allergy or a previous general anaesthetic (presumably including one of the barbiturates). The rate of reactions to thiopentone appears fairly constant.

Laboratory testing after a suspected reaction usually shows a significant immediate decrease in the plasma concentration of immunoglobulin E (IgE) with no significant change in the concentrations of complement proteins C_3 and C_4. The incidence of IgE-mediated reactions to the thiobarbiturate has been estimated[105] to be about 1 in 23 000. In those rare cases in which both IgE and complement are involved, secondary complement activation occurs, probably as a result of hypotension leading to metabolic derangement. Cutaneous manifestations of induction with thiopentone (histaminoid wheal and flaring) are seen in many patients. Whether these represent true reactions is uncertain; they may represent a local response to the extreme alkalinity of thiopentone in patients who are often nervous and peripherally vasoconstricted.

Other cases of anaphylaxis to thiopentone (with positive detection of specific IgE antibodies supported by a positive intradermal test in 2 out of 3) have been described by Fisher et al[106] One interesting feature of this article was that all three patients had postoperative gastro-intestinal symptoms. These are generally observed in only about 10% of patients who experience anaphylaxis during anaesthesia. However, all three had received anaesthesia of short duration (<10 min) and it is possible that involvement of the gastro-intestinal system occurs more frequently than was realized previously, but that symptoms are usually masked by the continuation of anaesthesia during the resuscitative phase of the adverse reaction.

Moneret-Vautrin et al[107] reported two cases of simultaneous immune reactions to thiopentone and a neuromuscular-blocking drug. The presence of specific IgE antibodies to thiopentone has been demonstrated on the basis of positive passive cutaneous anaphylaxis, basophil degranulation, leukocyte histamine release and radio-immunoassay.[108]

Clarke[88] summarized data from 15 cases of suspected hypersensitivity to methohexitone, and two cases following thiamylal. Other cases may also have occurred but the incidence is undoubtedly low and no deaths have been reported. Most patients show peri-orbital and facial oedema, with no history of allergy. The possibility that the response to methohexitone is a passive sensitization to a thiobarbiturate should be considered, as cross-sensitivity may exist between the two barbiturates.

Etomidate. There are few reports of allergic reactions to etomidate. Five cases were studied beween 1978 and 1982;[109] all involved widespread cutaneous flushing or urticaria, and the occurrence of postoperative vomiting. None of the patients showed complement activation. Another two patients exhibited anaphylactoid responses, with signs of cyanosis, marked hypotension and, in one case, oedema. Whether these are due to etomidate is difficult to decide, as the drug was administered concurrently with suxamethonium or alcuronium. Nevertheless, complement C_3 activation was shown in one of the cases.

Another case report[110] described a reaction to etomidate, with generalized erythema, urticaria, tachycardia and hypotension. A similar picture has been described in a patient scheduled for coronary artery surgery;[111] positive skin tests supported etomidate as the causative agent of this anaphylactoid reaction. Fazackerley et al[112] described a patient with urticaria and severe bronchospasm leading to hypoxic cardiac arrest following induction of anaesthesia with etomidate; there was no complement activation, but the patient had a raised plasma IgE level, consistent with atopy. This is the first report of severe bronchospasm in response to etomidate but, unlike many of the other reports, direct release of histamine or other immune mediators by the i.v. hypnotic agent seems the most likely explanation. In two other cases, etomidate was given at induction of anaesthesia with other i.v. drugs (lignocaine and vecuronium respectively).[113,114] Studies suggest that these other drugs were the probable causative agents.

These 12 cases represent the only documented adverse reactions to a drug which has been used over 4 000 000 times for induction of anaesthesia. This is a very low incidence compared with those reported for the other i.v. hypnotic agents (Table 6.4).

Ketamine. This phencyclidine derivative has been associated with only two reports of allergic reactions;[115,116] one probably had a non-immune basis, and the other involved IgE.

Propofol. This hypnotic agent was solubilized originally in Cremophor EL, and, as a result, at least 5 cases of hypersensitivity were reported among the 1131 patients who received the drug. One of these patients[117] showed classical complement pathway activation (with C_3 conversion and C_4 consumption). As the patient had not received propofol previously, this probably resulted from re-exposure to the Cremophor solvent.

Propofol is now formulated in soya oil–egg phosphatide emulsion (Intralipid). Data from the Committee for Safety of Medicines (to August 1991) indicate 22 reports categorized as 'allergic, anaphylactoid or anaphylactic', with one associated death.

Table 6.4 Incidence of adverse hypersensitivity reactions to intravenous hypnotic agents

Drug	Incidence
Thiopentone	1 : 14 000–1 : 20 000
Methohexitone	1 : 1600–1 : 7000
Propofol (as Cremophor formulation)	5 in 1131
Etomidate	10+ cases (estimate 1 : 50 000–1 : 450 000)
Propofol as emulsion	40+ cases (estimate 1 : 80 000–1 : 100 000)
For comparison:	
Althesin (in Cremophor)	1 : 400–1 : 11 000
Propanidid (in Micellophor)	1 : 500–1 : 17 000
Neuromuscular-blocking drugs	(overall) 1 : 5000
Penicillin	1 : 2500–1 : 10 000
Dextrans	1 : 3000
Gelatins	1 : 900
Hydroxyethyl starch	1 : 1200

Several of these have appeared in the literature as case reports.[118-121] More recently, another 16 cases of anaphylactoid/anaphylactic reactions to the drug have been reported.[122-124]

Other side-effects which occur with a high incidence (possibly related to histamine or other mediator release) include erythematous rashes, bronchospasm, flushing and hypotension. Although the frequency of reports of allergic-type responses to propofol seems to be increasing, the concurrent administration of neuromuscular-blocking drugs may be a significant causative factor. When all of these hypersensitivity reactions are taken together, the manufacturers believe that the overall incidence for propofol is probably between 1 in 80 000 and 1 in 100 000 administrations.

Benzodiazepines. There have been few reports of clinically overt adverse reactions to diazepam when formulated in propylene glycol (Valium).[125] However, five reactions (pronounced cardiovascular collapse in three patients, and minor cutaneous sequelae in the other 2) to a Cremophor formulation of the drug (Stesolid) were reported in a total of 5200 administrations.[126] A further case report of two more reactions to Stesolid describes rash, bronchospasm and hypotension in one patient, and erythema, facial oedema and cardiovascular collapse in the other. These reactions involved probable alternative pathway activation in one of the patients, with C_3 consumption and conversion and a normal C_4 concentration.[127]

More recently, Brogger-Nielsen[128] reported the case of a 20-year-old female patient who received Diazemuls (an emulsion formulation) as sedation for gastroscopy, and developed flushing, urticaria and upper-body oedema. This histaminoid picture was not associated with activation of either complement pathway. Thus, all three present formulations of this commonly prescribed benzodiazepine have been implicated in adverse reactions.

There are no reports of allergic reactions to any other of the benzodiazepines commonly used in anaesthetic practice (midazolam, lorazepam, temazepam).

Other adverse effects of i.v. induction agents

Porphyrias. Drugs are among the commonest of the exogenous factors that precipitate acute attacks of porphyria. It is thought that the basic problem in porphyria is one or more enzyme defect in the biosynthetic pathway of haem from succinyl co-enzyme A and glycine, which condense to form 5-aminolaevulinic acid (ALA) in the mitochondria in the presence of the enzyme ALA-synthetase. This enzyme is readily inducible by a number of substances (especially barbiturates, but also other i.v. induction agents; Table 6.5). The overall pathways of haem synthesis (with the individual enzymes identified) are shown in Figure 6.1. The rate-limiting step is the first enzyme reaction (ALA synthetase) which is regulated by the end-product, haem, so that only trace amounts of the intermediate metabolites are normally present.

In healthy subjects, the levels of plasma protoporphyrins are $<3 \mu g.ml^{-1}$, with undetectable amounts of other precursors. Urinary excretion of ALA is $<2.5 mg.day^{-1}$, porphobilinogen (PBG) $<1.0 mg.day^{-1}$, uropophyrins $5–30 \mu g.day^{-1}$ and coproporphyrins $1–160 \mu g.day^{-1}$. In the faeces, there are variable amounts of coproporphyrins ($0–250 \mu g.day^{-1}$) and protoporphyrins ($0–1 mg.day^{-1}$). Larger amounts of the type I byproducts are excreted compared with the type III isomers which are incorporated into haem.

Two types of porphyria exist — hepatic and erythropoietic. A number of inherited hepatic enzyme defects are of importance to the anaesthetist:

- porphobilinogen deaminase (acute intermittent porphyria)
- coproporphyrinogen oxidase (hereditary coproporphyria)
- protoporphyrin oxidase (variegate porphyria).

There are other porphyrias which result from red-cell enzyme defects, but these are rare autosomal recessive diseases.[129]

Table 6.5 Presently available drugs known to induce porphyric crises acute: (a); cutaneous: (c), drugs demonstrated experimentally to have porphyrinogenic potential (e) and anaesthetic drugs safe to use in susceptible patients (s)

Analeptics
Nikethamide (e)

Anticonvulsants
Barbiturates (a)
Hydantoins (a)
Succinimides (a)
Sodium valproate (s)

Analgesics
Amidopyrine (a)
Aspirin (s)
Fentanyl (s)
Morphine (s)
Paracetamol (s)
Pentazocine (a)
Pethidine (s)

Anti-infective drugs
Cephalosporin (s)
Chloramphenicol (e)
Chloroquine (c)
Griseofulvin (a)
Sulphonamides (a, e)
Tetracyclines (s)

Endocrine drugs
Androgens (a, c, e)
Dexamethasone (s)
Metyrapone (e)
Oestrogens (a, c, e)
Oral contraceptive pill (a)
Progestogens (a, c, e)
C19 or C21 steroids with A/B *cis* configuration (a, e)

Sulphonylureas
Chlorpropamide (c)
Tolbutamide (a, c)

Hypnotics and anaesthetics
Barbiturates (a, c, e)
Chloral hydrate (s)
Chloridiazepoxide (a)
Diazepam (e)
Droperidol (s)
Ethanol (a, c)
Etomidate (e)
Flunitrazepam (a, c)
Glutethimide (e)
Ketamine (? s in humans; e)
Propofol (probably s)

Other drugs and chemicals
Allylisopropylacetamide (e)
Atropine (s)
Ergot alkaloids and derivatives (a)
Gallamine (s)
Hexachlorobenzene and other chlorobenzenes (c)
Inorganic mercurials (c)
α-Methyldopa (a)
Nitrous oxide (s)
Organochlorine insecticides (e)
Pancuronium (s)
Procaine (s)
Prochlorperazine (a)
Promethazine (s)
Propranolol (s)
Suxamethonium (s)
d-Tubocurarine (s)

In each condition, there are increased plasma and urinary concentrations of the precursors (or their metabolites) to the individual enzymes blocked.

Acute intermittent porphyria. This is due to enzyme defects in both the hepatocyte and red blood cell. The reduction in haem synthesis stimulates increased activity of ALA synthetase, with resulting increased plasma and urinary levels of ALA and PBG. The disease is inherited as an autosomal dominant condition, and has an incidence of about 1/100 000 live births. It is common in Northern Europe, especially Sweden. The main clinical features are vague gastro-intestinal symptoms (nausea and vomiting, colicky abdominal pains) and central and peripheral demyelination. Acute exacerbations may be precipitated by a low carbohydrate intake, infection, pregnancy, menstruation or lead exposure. Some drugs (including alcohol) can also precipitate acute episodes (see Table 6.5). Many of the drugs are inducers of hepatic cytochrome P-450, which is the main consumer of haem produced by the liver. Induction of cytochrome P-450 therefore depletes the haem pool, with the loss of a negative feedback on ALA synthetase. Evaluation of anaesthetic drugs for porphyrinogenic potential may be made using either an in vitro rat liver model[130] or the 3,5-diethoxycarbonyl-1,4-dihydrocollodine (DDC)-primed rat.[131] Of all episodes induced by i.v. anaesthetic drugs, over 30% are initiated by thiopentone.

Variegate porphyria. This arises because of a separate enzyme defect to acute intermittent porphyria (protoporphyrin oxidase, which is responsible for conversion of protoporphyrin IX to haem). It is found most commonly among the white population of South Africa. There is increased excretion of coproporphyrin and protoporphyrin in the faeces, and increased urinary excretion of ALA and PBG during acute attacks. The disease is less severe than acute intermittent porphyria

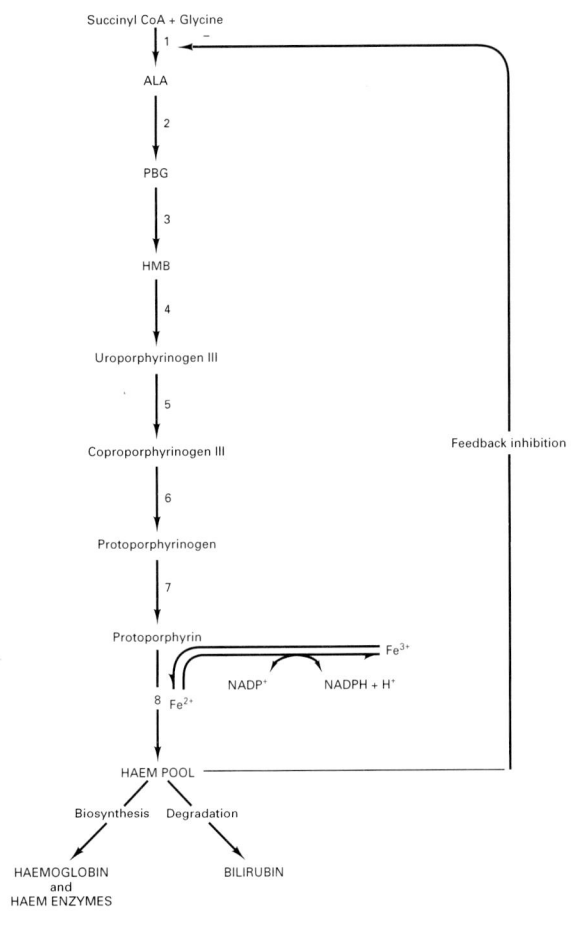

Fig. 6.1 Pathways of haem synthesis. COA = co-enzyme A; ALA = δ-aminolaevulinate; PBG = porphobilinogen; HMB = hydroxymethylbilan. *Enzymes:* 1 = aminolaevulinate synthetase; 2 = aminolaevulinate dehydratase; 3 = porphobilinogen deaminase; 4 = uroporphyrinogen III cosynthetase; 5 = uroporphyrinogen decarboxylase; 6 = coproporphyrinogen oxidase; 7 = protoporphyrinogen oxidase; 8 = ferrochelatase.

whilst the liver remains capable of the biliary excretion of porphyrins. However, if excretion becomes impaired, the patient develops increased plasma bilirubin concentrations and porphyrinaemia. Eighty per cent of patients have cutaneous lesions (sensitivity, skin fragility and blistering), as well as the gastro-intestinal and central nervous system symptoms. The same drugs which precipitate acute intermittent porphyria may cause an acute episode of variegate porphyria.

Hereditary coproporphyria. This is a very rare autosomal dominant condition (fewer than 50 documented cases) leading to excretion of increased amounts of ALA and PBG in the urine together with increased faecal (and urinary) concentrations of coproporphyrins.

Most of the patients are asymptomatic, but acute episodes are precipitated by the same factors as for acute intermittent porphyria.

Porphyria cutanea tarda. Unlike the other porphyrias, this is due to a partial enzyme deficiency of uroporphyrinogen decarboxylase (resulting in excessive hepatic synthesis and urinary excretion of uroporphyrin I). Urinary concentrations of ALA and PBG are not increased. Acute attacks are not precipitated by drugs.

Safe induction of anaesthesia in porphyria-susceptible patients may be achieved with etomidate, ketamine, midazolam or propofol, although the first two have been reported to be porphyrinogenic in the DDC-primed rat. An increase in excreted porphyrins has been reported 24 h after induction with propofol in a patient with known variegate porphyria.[132] However, this may have been triggered not by the induction agent but by the concomitant use of lignocaine.

Malignant hyperpyrexia. There are no data to suggest that any of the i.v. induction agents can trigger an episode of malignant hyperpyrexia in susceptible patients. Barbiturates, opioids and ketamine are safe to use as induction agents. In vitro muscle contracture tests and in vivo studies in the malignant hyperpyrexia-susceptible pig model[133] suggest the safety of etomidate and propofol, although there are few reports of their use in susceptible patients.

Induction of anaesthesia by the inhalational route is contra-indicated in all susceptible patients, although there are no data at present (1994) on the safety or otherwise of desflurane or seroflurane in humans.

Effects of i.v. induction agents on liver function tests. As a generality, single induction doses of i.v. hypnotic agents (thiopentone, etomidate, midazolam and propofol) have no significant effect on hepatic integrity as assessed by routine liver function tests. However, single infusions of ketamine given to healthy patients undergoing minor gynaecological surgery have caused increases in alanine aminotransferase and γ-glutamyl transpeptidase.[134]

Measurement of the plasma activities of liver isoenzyme lactate dehydrogenase$_V$ (LDH$_V$) have shown increases above 16% total activity in some postoperative samples for 4 of 6 patients who received methohexitone by infusion, but this was not accompanied by increases in the plasma activity of the liver-specific enzyme ornithine carbamoyl transpeptidase.[79] It must be concluded therefore that methohexitone (in total doses between 767 and 1531 mg) was not associated with hepatocellular dysfunction. This is in contrast to the earlier observations of Bittrich et al[135] and Dundee[136] for methohexitone and thiopentone respectively.

REFERENCES

1. Prys-Roberts C. Editorial. Anaesthesia: a practical or impractical construct? Br J Anaesth 1987; 59: 1341–1345
2. Jones JG, Konieczko K. Hearing and memory in anaesthetised patients. Br Med J 1986; 292: 1291–1293
3. Hogskilde S, Wagner J, Carl P, Bredgaard-Sorensen M. Anaesthetic properties of pregnanolone emulsion. A comparison with alphaxalone/alphadolone, propofol, thiopentone and midazolam in a rat model. Anaesthesia 1987; 42: 1045–1050
4. Willenkin RL. Management of general anesthesia. In: Miller RD, ed. Anesthesia, vol 2, 3rd ed New York: Churchill Livingstone, 1990: pp 1335–1346
5. Guedel AE. Inhalational anesthesia, a fundamental guide. New York: Macmillan. 1937
6. Cummins CG, Dixon J, Kay NH et al. Dose requirements of ICI 35868 (propofol; Diprivan) in a new formulation for induction of anaesthesia. Anaesthesia 1984; 39: 1168–1171
7. Powell H, Morgan M, Sear JW. Pregnanolone: a new steroid intravenous anaesthetic. Dose-finding study. Anaesthesia 1982; 47: 287–290
8. Sear JW, Prys-Roberts C. Dose-related haemodynamic effects of continuous infusions of althesin in man. Br J Anaesth 1979; 51: 867–873
9. Coates DP, Monk CR, Prys-Roberts C, Turtle M. Hemodynamic effects of infusions of the emulsion formulation of propofol during nitrous oxide anesthesia in humans. Anesth Analg 1987; 66: 64–70
10. Becker KE, Tonneson AS. Cardiovascular effects of plasma levels of thiopental necessary for anesthesia. Anesthesiology 1978; 48: 197–200
11. Christensen JH, Andreasen F, Kristoffersen MD. Comparison of the anaesthetic and haemodynamic effects of chlormethiazole and thiopentone. Br J Anaesth 1983; 55: 391–397
12. Todd MM, Drummond JC, U HS. The hemodynamic consequences of high-dose thiopental anesthesia. Anesth Analg 1985; 64: 681–687
13. Pocock G, Richards CD. Cellular mechanisms in general anaesthesia. Br J Anaesth 1991; 66: 116–128
14. Halsey MJ. How do intravenous anaesthetics work. In: Dundee JW, Sear JW, eds. Intravenous Anaesthesia — what is new? Baillière's Clinical Anaesthesiology: International Practice and Research, vol 5, no. 2. London: Baillière Tindall, 1991: pp 303–325
15. Eger EI II. Uptake and distribution. In: Miller RD, ed. anesthesia, vol 1, 3rd edn. New York: Churchill Livingstone, 1990: pp 85–104
16. Ruffle JM, Latta W, Snider MT. Single breath halothane oxygen induction in man. Anesthesiology 1982; 57: A461
17. Wilton NCT, Thomas VL. Single breath induction of anaesthesia using a vital capacity breath of halothane, nitrous oxide and oxygen. Anaesthesia 1986; 41: 472–476
18. Loper K, Reitan J, Bennett H, Benthuysen J, Snook L. Comparison of halothane and isoflurane for rapid anesthetic induction. Anesth Analg 1987; 66: 766–768
19. Grant IS, Nimmo WS, Clements JA. Pharmacokinetics and analgesic effect of i.m. and oral ketamine. Br J Anaesth 1981; 53: 805–810
20. Quaynor H, Corbey M, Bjorkman S. Rectal induction of anaesthesia in children with methohexitone. Br J Anaesth 1985; 57: 573–577
21. Bjorkman S, Gabrielsson J, Quaynor H, Corbey M. Pharmacokinetics of i.v. and rectal methohexitone in children. Br J Anaesth 59: 1987; 59: 1541–1547
22. Kestin IG, McIlvaine WB, Lockhart CH, Kestin KJ, Jones M. Paediatric rectal methohexitone induction with and without rectal suctioning after sleep — a pharmacokinetic and pharmacodynamic study. Anesthesiology 1987; 67: A493
23. Idvall J, Holasek J, Stenberg P. Rectal ketamine for induction of anaesthesia in children. Anaesthesia 1983; 38: 60–64
24. Pedraz JL, Calvo MB, Lanao JM, Muriel C, Santos Lamas J, Dominguez-Gil A. Pharmacokinetics of rectal ketamine in children. Br J Anaesth 1989; 63: 671–674
25. Linton DM, Thornington RE. Etomidate as a rectal induction agent. Part II: a clinical study in children. S Afr Med J 1983; 64: 309–310
26. Spear RM, Yaster M, Deshpande JK, Wetzel RC, Nichols DG. Rectally administered midazolam for preinduction sedation and induction of general anesthesia in small children. Anesthesiology 1989; 69: A742
27. Tovall RM. A comparative clinical and statistical study of thiopental and thiamylal in human anesthesia. Anesthesiology 1965; 16: 910–913
28. Harris CE, Murray AM, Anderson JM, Grounds RM, Morgan M. Effects of thiopentone, etomidate and propofol on the haemodynamic response to tracheal intubation. Anaesthesia 1988; 43: (suppl): 32–36
29. Fragen RJ, Shanks CA, Molteni A, Avram MJ. Effects of etomidate on hormonal responses to surgical stress. Anesthesiology 1984; 60: 652–656
30. Fragen RJ, Weiss HW, Molteni A. The effect of propofol on adrenocortical steroidogenesis: a comparative study with etomidate and thiopental. Anesthesiology 1987; 66: 839–842
31. Moore RA, Allen MC, Wood PJ, Rees LH, Sear JW. Perioperative endocrine effects of etomidate. Anaesthesia 1985; 40: 124–130
32. Watt I, Ledingham IMcA. Mortality amongst multiple trauma patients admitted to an intensive therapy unit. Anaesthesia 1984; 39: 973–981
33. Glen JB, Hunter SC. Pharmacology of an emulsion formulation of ICI 35868. Br J Anaesth 1984; 56: 617–626
34. Kay NH, Sear JW, Uppington J, Cockshott ID, Douglas EJ. Disposition of propofol in patients undergoing surgery. A comparison in men and women. Br J Anaesth 1986; 58: 1075–1079
35. Shafer A, Doze VA, Shafer SL, White PF. Pharmacokinetics and pharmacodynamics of propofol infusion during general anesthesia. Anesthesiology 1988; 69: 348–356
36. Cockshott ID, Douglas EJ, Prys-Roberts C, Turtle M, Coates DP. The pharmacokinetics of propofol during and after intravenous infusion in man. Eur J Anaesthesiol 1990; 7: 265–275
37. Morgan DJ, Campbell GA, Crankshaw SP. Pharmacokinetics of propofol when given by intravenous infusion. Br J Clin Pharmacol 1990; 30: 144–148

38 Grounds RM, Moore M, Morgan M. The relative potencies of thiopentone and propofol. Eur J Anaesthesiol 1986; 3: 11–17
39 Leslie K, Crankshaw DP. Potency of propofol for loss of consciousness after a single dose. Br J Anaesth 1990; 64: 734–736
40 Mackenzie N, Grant IS. Comparison of the new emulsion formulation of propofol with methohexitone and thiopentone for induction of anaesthesia in day cases. Br J Anaesth 1985; 57: 725–731
41 Stark RD, Binks SM, Dutka VN, O'Connor KM, Arnstein MJA, Glen JB. A review of the safety and tolerance of propofol (Diprivan). Postgrad Med J 1985; 61 (suppl 3): 152–156
42 Helmers JHJH, Kraaijenhagen RJ, Van Leeuven L, Zuurmond WWA. Reduction of pain on injection caused by propofol. Can J Anaesth 1990; 37: 267–270
43 Rolly G, Versichelen L, Huyghe L, Mungroop H. Effect of speed of injection on induction of anaesthesia using propofol. Br J Anaesth 1985; 57: 743–746
44 Peacock JE, Lewis RP, Reilly CS, Nimmo WS. Effect of different rates of infusion of propofol for induction of anaesthesia in elderly patients. Br J Anaesth 1990; 65: 346–352
45 Venn PJH, Loach AB, Collins PD. Effect of speed of injection on the dose required to induce anaesthesia with propofol. Br J Anaesth 1990; 65: 199–200
46 McKeating K, Bali IM, Dundee JW. The effects of thiopentone and propofol on upper airway integrity. Anaesthesia 1988; 43: 638–640
47 Lowson S, Gent JP, Goodchild CS. Anticonvulsant properties of propofol and thiopentone: comparison using two tests in laboratory mice. Br J Anaesth 1990; 64: 59–63
48 Lowson S, Gent JP, Goodchild CS. Convulsive thresholds in mice during the recovery phase from anaesthesia by propofol, thiopentone, methohexitone and etomidate. Br J Pharmacol 1991; 102: 879–882
49 Rampton AJ, Griffin RM, Stuart CS, Durcan JJ, Huddy NC, Abbott MA. Comparison of methohexital and propofol for electroconvulsive therapy: effects of hemodynamic responses and seizure duration. Anesthesiology 1989; 70: 412–417
50 Kenyon CJ, McNeil LM, Fraser R. Comparison of the effects of etomidate, thiopentone and propofol on cortisol synthesis. Br J Anaesth 1985; 57: 509–511
51 Lambert A, Mitchell R, Robertson WR. Effect of propofol, thiopentone and etomidate on adrenal steroidogenesis in vitro. Br J Anaesth 1985; 57: 505–508
52 Sear JW, Shaw I, Wolf A, Kay NH. Infusions of propofol to supplement nitrous oxide–oxygen for the maintenance of anaesthesia. A comparison with halothane. Anaesthesia 1988; 43 (suppl.) 18–22
53 Sear JW. Should propofol infusion rate be related to body weight? In: Prys-Roberts C, ed. Focus on infusion: intravenous anaesthesia. London: Current Medical Literature, 1991: pp 100–101
54 Nilsson A, Lee PFS, Revenas B. Midazolam as induction agent prior to inhalational anaesthesia: a comparison with thiopentone. Acta Anaesthesiol Scand 1984; 28: 249–251
55 Dawson D, Sear JW. Influence of induction of anaesthesia with midazolam on the neuroendocrine response to surgery. Anaesthesia 1986; 41: 268–271
56 Crozier TA, Beck D, Wuttke W, Kettler D. Endocrinological changes following etomidate, midazolam or methohexital for minor surgery. Anesthesiology 1987; 66: 628–635
57 Desborough JP, Hall GM, Hart GR, Burrin JM. Midazolam modifies pancreatic and anterior pituitary hormone secretion during upper abdominal surgery. Br J Anaesth 1991; 67: 390–396
58 Brogden RL, Goa KL. Flumazenil: a preliminary review of its benzodiazepine antagonist properties, intrinsic activity and therapeutic use. Drugs 1988; 35: 448–467
59 Nilsson A, Persson P, Hartvig P. Effects of the benzodiazepine antagonist flumazenil on postoperative performance following total intravenous anaesthesia with midazolam and alfentanil. Acta Anaesthesiol Scand 1988; 32: 379–382
60 White PF, Way WL, Trevor AJ. Ketamine — its pharmacology and therapeutic uses. Anesthesiology 1982; 56: 119–136
61 White PF, Ham J, Way WL, Trevor AJ. Pharmacology of ketamine isomers in surgical patients. Anesthesiology 1980; 52: 231–239
62 White PF, Schuttler J, Shafer A, Stanski DR, Horai Y, Trevor AJ. Comparative pharmacology of the ketamine isomers. Br J Anaesth 1985; 57: 197–203
63 Schuttler J, Stanski DR, White PF et al. Pharmacodynamic modelling of the EEG effects of ketamine and its enantiomers in man. J Pharmacokin Biopharm 1987; 15: 241–253
64 Schuttler J, Kloos S, Ihmsen H, Pelzer E. Pharmacokinetic-dynamic properties of S (+) ketamine v. racemic ketamine: a randomised double-blind study in volunteers. Anesthesiology 1992; 77: A330
65 Pfenninger E, Baier Ch, Claus S. Analgesia and psychic side effects under ketamine racemate vs. S (+) ketamine in analgesic doses. Anesthesiology 1992; 77: A412
66 Carl P, Hogskilde S, Nielsen JW et al. Pregnanolone emulsion. A preliminary pharmacokinetic and pharmacodynamic study of a new intravenous anaesthetic agent. Anaesthesia 1990; 45: 189–197
67 Kallela H, Haasio J, Korttila K. Comparison of eltanolone and propofol in anesthesia for termination of pregnancy. Anesthesiology 1992; 77: A15
68 Etsten B, Li TH. Hemodynamic changes during thiopental anesthesia in humans. J Clin Invest 1955; 34: 500–510
69 Forbes AM, Dally FG. Acute hypertension during induction of anaesthesia and endotracheal intubation in normotensive man. Br J Anaesth 1970; 42: 618–624
70 Sanders DJ, Jewkes CF, Sear JW, Verhoeff F, Foex P. Thoracic electrical bioimpedance measurement of cardiac output and cardiovascular responses to the induction of anaesthesia and to laryngoscopy and intubation. Anaesthesia 1992; 47: 736–740
71 Kettler D, Sonntag H, Donath U, Regensburger D, Schenk HD. Hemodynamics, myocardial mechanics, oxygen requirement, and oxygenation of the human heart during induction of anesthesia with etomidate. Anaesthesist 1974; 23: 116–121
72 Colvin MP, Savege TM, Newland PE et al. Cardiorespiratory changes following induction of

anaesthesia with etomidate in patients with cardiac disease. Br J Anaesth 1979; 51; 551–556
73. Criado A, Maseda J, Navarro E, Escarpa A, Avello F. Induction of anaesthesia with etomidate: haemodynamic study of 36 patients. Br J Anaesth 1980; 52: 803–806
74. Gooding KM, Dimick AR, Tavakoli M, Corrsen G. A physiologic analysis of cardiopulmonary response to etomidate anesthesia in noncardiac patients. Anesth Analg 1977; 56: 813–816
75. Coates DP, Monk CR, Prys-Roberts C, Turtle M. Haemodynamic responses of hypertensive patients to an infusion of propofol to supplement nitrous oxide anaesthesia. In: Bergman H, Kramer H, Steinbereithner K, eds. Abstracts of VII European Congress of Anaesthesiology, vol. 16. Vienna: Verlag Wuhelm Maudrich, 1986: p 136
76. Noble DW, Maclean D, Power I, Spence AA, Weatherill D. Haemodynamic responses of hypertensive patients to induction of anaesthesia with propofol. A preliminary report. In: proceedings of scientific session: the haemodynamic effects of propofol, mechanisms and implications. 9th World Congress of Anesthesiologists, Washington. ICI, 1988
77. Van Aken H, Meinshausen E, Prien T, Brussel T, Heinecke A, Lawin P. The influence of fentanyl and tracheal intubation on the hemodynamic effects of anesthesia induction with propofol/N_2O in humans. Anesthesiology 1988; 68: 157–163
78. Roberts FL, Dixon J, Lewis GTR, Tackley RM, Prys-Roberts C. Induction and maintenance of propofol anaesthesia. A manual infusion scheme. Anaesthesia 1988; 43 (suppl): 14–17
79. Prys-Roberts C, Sear JW, Low JM, Phillips KC, Dagnino J. Hemodynamic and hepatic effects of methohexital infusion during nitrous oxide anaesthesia in humans. Anesth Analg 1983; 62: 317–323
80. Mirakhur RK, Shepherd WFI, Darrah WC. Propofol or thiopentone: effects on intraocular pressure associated with induction of anaesthesia and tracheal intubation (facilitated with suxamethonium). Br J Anaesth 1987; 59: 431–436
81. Mirakhur RK, Shepherd WFI, Elliott P. Intraocular pressure changes during rapid sequence induction of anaesthesia: comparison of propofol and thiopentone in combination with vecuronium. Br J Anaesth 1988; 60: 109–111
82. Lebowitz PW, Cote ME, Daniels AL et al. Comparative cardiovascular effects of midazolam and thiopental in healthy patients. Anesth Analg 1982; 61: 771–775
83. Reves JG, Fragen RJ, Vinik HR, Greenblatt DJ. Midazolam pharmacology and uses. Anesthesiology 1985; 62: 310–324
84. Samuelson PN, Reves JG, Kouchoukos NT, Smith LR, Dole KM. Hemodynamic responses to anesthetic induction with midazolam or diazepam in patients with ischemic heart disease. Anesth Analg 1981; 60: 802–809
85. McCammon RL, Hilgenberg JC, Stoelting RK. Hemodynamic effects of diazepam and diazepam–nitrous oxide in patients with coronary artery disease. Anesth Analg 1980; 59: 438–441
86. Virtue RW, Alanis JM, Mori M, Lafargue RT, Vogel JHK, Metcalf DR. An anesthetic agent: 2-orthochlorophenyl 2-methylamine cyclohexanone HC1 (CI-581). Anesthesiology 1967; 28: 823–833
87. Tweed WA, Minuck M, Mymin D. Circulatory responses to ketamine anesthesia. Anesthesiology 1972; 37: 613–619
88. Clarke RSJ. Adverse effects of intravenously administered drugs used in anaesthetic practice. Drugs 1981; 22: 26–41
89. Todd MM, Drummond JC, U HS. The hemodynamic consequences of high-dose methohexital anesthesia in humans. Anesthesiology 1984; 61: 495–501
90. Artru AA. Dose-related changes in the rate of cerebrospinal fluid formation and resistance to reabsorption of cerebrospinal fluid following administration of thiopental, midazolam, and etomidate in dogs. Anesthesiology 1988; 69: 541–546
91. Ravussin P, Guinard JP, Ralley F, Thorin D. Effect of propofol on cerebrospinal fluid pressure and cerebral perfusion pressure in patients undergoing craniotomy. Anaesthesia 1988; 43 (suppl): 37–41
92. Van Hemelrijck J, Van Aken H, Plets C, Goffin J, Vermaut G. The effects of propofol on intracranial pressure and cerebral perfusion pressure in patients with brain tumours. Acta Anaesthesiol Belg 1989; 40: 95–100
93. Fitch W, Van Hemelrijck J, Mattheussen M, Van Aken H. Responsiveness of the cerebral circulation to acute alterations in mean arterial pressure during administration of propofol. J Neurosurg Anesthesiol 1989; 1: 375–376
94. Stephan H, Sonntag H, Schenk HD, Kohlhausen S. Einfluss von Disoprivan (Propofol) auf die durchblutung und den sauerstoffverbrauch des gehirns und die CO_2-reaktivitat der hirngefabe beim menschen. Anaesthesist 1987; 36: 60–65
95. Chaussard D, Joubard A, Colson A, Guiraud M, Dubreuil C, Banssillon V. Auditory evoked potentials during propofol anaesthesia in man. Br J Anaesth 1989; 62: 522–526
96. Thornton C, Konieczko KM, Knight AB et al. Effect of propofol on the auditory evoked response and oesophageal contractility. Br J Anaesth 1989; 63: 411–417
97. McPherson RW, Levitt R. Effect of time and dose on scalp-recorded somatosensory evoked potential wave augmentation by etomidate. J Neurosurg Anesthesiol 1989; 1: 16–21
98. Nussmeier NA, Arlund C, Slogoff S. Neuropsychiatric complications after cardiopulmonary bypass: cerebral protection by a barbiturate. Anesthesiology 1986; 64: 164–170
99. Metz S, Slogoff S, Keats AS. Single dose thiopental compared to infusion for central nervous system protection during cardiopulmonary bypass. Anesth Analg 1990; 70: s266
100. Gold MI, Sacks DJ, Grosnoff DB, Herrington CA. Comparison of propofol with thiopental and isoflurane for induction and maintenance of general anesthesia. J Clin Anesth 1989; 1: 272–276
101. Heath PJ, Kennedy DJ, Ogg TW, Gilks WR. Which intravenous agent for day surgery? A comparison of propofol, thiopentone, methohexitone and etomidate. Anaesthesia 1988; 43: 365–368

102 Heath PJ, Ogg TW, Gilks WR. Recovery after day-case anaesthesia. A 24-hour comparison of recovery after thiopentone or propofol anaesthesia. Anaesthesia 1990; 45: 911–915

103 Sanders LD, Isaac PA, Yeomans WA, Clyburn PA, Rosen M, Robinson JO. Propofol induced anaesthesia. Double-blind comparison of recovery after anaesthesia induced by propofol or thiopentone. Anaesthesia 1989; 44: 200–204

104 Hunter AR. Dangers of pentothal sodium anaesthesia. Lancet 1943; i: 46–48

105 Beamish D, Brown DT. Adverse responses to i.v. anaesthetics. Br J Anaesth 1981; 53: 55–58

106 Fisher MM, Ross JD, Harle DA, Baldo B. Anaphylaxis to thiopentone: an unusual outbreak in a single hospital. Anaesth Intensive Care 1989; 17: 361–365

107 Moneret-Vautrin DA, Widmer S, Gueant J-L et al. Simultaneous anaphylaxis to thiopentone and a neuromuscular blocker: a study of two cases. Br J Anaesth 1990; 64: 743–745

108 Harle DG, Baldo BA, Smal MA, Wajon P, Fisher MM. Detection of thiopentone reactive IgE antibodies following anaphylactoid reactions during anaesthesia. Clin Allergy 1986; 16: 493–498

109 Watkins JA. Etomidate: an 'immunologically safe' anaesthetic agent. Anaesthesia 1983; 38 (suppl): 34-38

110 Krumholz W, Muller H, Gerlach H, Russ W, Hempelmann G. Ein fall von anaphylaktoider reaktion nach gabe von etomidat. Anaesthesist 1984; 33: 161–162

111 Sold M, Rothhammer A. Lebensbedrohliche anaphylaktoide reaktion nach etomidat. Anaesthesist 1985; 34: 208–210

112 Fazackerley EJ, Martin AJ, Tolhurst-Cleaver CL, Watkins J. Anaphylactoid reaction following the use of etomidate. Anaesthesia 1988; 43: 953–954

113 Bricker SRW, Raitt DG. Angioneurotic oedema following etomidate/lignocaine. Anaesthesia 1987; 42: 323–324

114 Farrell AM, Gowland G, McDowell JM, Simpson KH, Watkins J. Anaphylactoid reaction to vecuronium followed by systemic reaction to skin testing. Anaesthesia 1988; 43: 207–209

115 Mathieu A, Goudsouzian N, Snider MT. Reaction to ketamine: anaphylactoid or anaphylactic. Br J Anaesth 1975; 47: 624

116 Laxenaire M-C, Moneret-Vautrin D, Vervloet D. The French experience of anaphylactoid reactions. Int Anesthesiol Clin 1985; 23: 145–160

117 Briggs LP, Clarke RSJ, Watkins J. An adverse reaction to the administration of disoprofol (Diprivan). Anaesthesia 1982; 37: 1099–1101

118 Laxenaire M-C, Gueant JL, Bermejo E, Mouton C, Navez MT. Anaphylactic shock due to propofol. Lancet 1988; ii: 739–740

119 Jamieson V, Mackenzie J. Allergy to propofol? Anaesthesia 1988; 43: 80

120 Dold M, Konarzewski WH. Delayed allergic response to propofol. Anaesthesia 1989; 44: 533

121 Kumar CM, McNeela BJ. Ocular manifestation of propofol allergy. Anaesthesia 1989; 44: 266

122 Laxenaire M-C, Mata-Bermejo E, Moneret-Vautrin DA, Gueant J-L. Life-threatening anaphylactoid reactions to propofol ('Diprivan'). Anesthesiology 1992; 77: 275–280

123 McHale SP, Konieczko K. Anaphylactoid reaction to propofol. Anaesthesia 1992; 47: 864–865

124 de Leon-Casasola OA, Weiss A, Lema MJ. Anaphylaxis due to propofol. Anesthesiology 1992; 77: 384–386

125 Falk RH. Allergy to diazepam. Br Med J 1977; i: 287

126 Schou Olesen A, Huttel MS. Circulatory collapse following intravenous administration of Stesolid MR. Ugeskr Laeger 1980; 140: 2644

127 Huttel MS, Schou Olesen A, Stofferson E. Complement mediated reactions to diazepam with Cremophor as solvent (Stesolid MR). Br J Anaesth 1980; 52: 77–79

128 Brogger-Nielsen F. Anaphylactoid reaction to diazemuls. Br J Anaesth 1984; 56: 1179

129 Moore M, McColl K, Rimmington C, Goldberg A. Disorders of porphyrin metabolism. New York: Plenum. 1987

130 Parikh RK, Moore MR. Effect of certain anaesthetic agents on the activity of rat hepatic-5-aminolaevulinate synthetase. Br J Anaesth 1978; 50: 1099–1103

131 Blekkenhorst GH, Harrison GG, Cooke ES, Eales L. Screening of certain anaesthetic agents for their ability to elicit acute porphyric phases in susceptible patients. Br J Anaesth 1980; 52: 759–762

132 Weir PM, Hodkinson BP. Is propofol a safe agent in porphyria? Anaesthesia 1988; 43: 1022–1023

133 Raff M, Harrison GG. The screening of propofol in MHS swine. Anesth Analg 1989; 68: 750–751

134 Dundee JW, Fee JP, Moore J, McIlroy PD, Wilson DB. Changes in serum enzyme levels following ketamine infusions. Anaesthesia 1980; 35: 12–16

135 Bittrich NM, Kane AV, Mosher RE. Methohexital and its effects on liver function tests. Anesthesiology 1963; 24: 81–90

136 Dundee JW. Thiopentone as a factor in the production of liver dysfunction. Br J Anaesth 1955; 27: 14–20

7. The maintenance of anaesthesia

D. C. White

The maintenance of general anaesthesia, although a subject of clinical importance, is not usually awarded a whole chapter in textbooks of anaesthesia. It is understandable that the rapid and critical events occurring during induction of anaesthesia should be closely studied. The slower and less controllable reverse changes during eduction of anaesthesia are now receiving more attention, largely as a result of the greater interest in day-case surgery. It is now desirable to complete the picture by detailed consideration of the maintenance of anaesthesia.

The state of anaesthesia is brought about when the partial pressure of an inhalation agent reaches the necessary level at the site of action, which is within the central nervous system. In the case of intravenous agents, it is the concentration of agent at the site of action which is significant and this at once indicates a potentially adverse feature of intravenous anaesthesia which will be considered in detail later. Briefly, the concentration of intravenous agent at the site of action during maintenance of anaesthesia cannot be known with the degree of precision with which the partial pressure of an inhalation agent can be known. The site of action of anaesthetic agents is no more accurately known than is the locus of consciousness, but most would agree that it lies within the central nervous system.

INHALATION ANAESTHESIA

The brain is part of the vessel-rich group (VRG) of tissues which receive 75% of the cardiac output.[1] It can be calculated that one time constant for nitrous oxide uptake by the VRG is 1.3 min [compared with, perhaps, 100 min for the fat group (FG) of tissues]. Thus, maintenance of anaesthesia relies upon keeping the partial pressure of agent constant in the brain, where uptake will have ceased after 5–15 min. However, anaesthetic must still be delivered; although the brain and other VRG organs are in equilibrium with the blood, the remaining tissues continue to take up anaesthetic at varying rates which depend on their perfusion and solubility characteristics (tissue/blood partition coefficient).

This state of affairs is shown graphically in Figure 7.1. This figure uses the computer program NARKUP[2] to plot the uptake into brain (which is part of the VRG of tissues), muscle and skin (muscle group: MG), the vessel-poor group (VPG) of tissues which comprises bone, cartilage and ligaments, and finally the FG of tissues. The first three tissue groups have similar solubility characteristics, but widely different perfusions. The VRG (brain, heart, kidney, liver, gut and endocrine glands) comprise 9% of body weight but receive 75% of cardiac output. Muscle and skin constitute half the body weight but are perfused (at rest) by rather less than 29% of the cardiac output. The fatty tissue differs from the other tissue groups in having a much greater capacity for anaesthetic agents. Although its rate of perfusion is about 75% of that of resting muscle, the solubility of agent in the fat is so great that, in the case

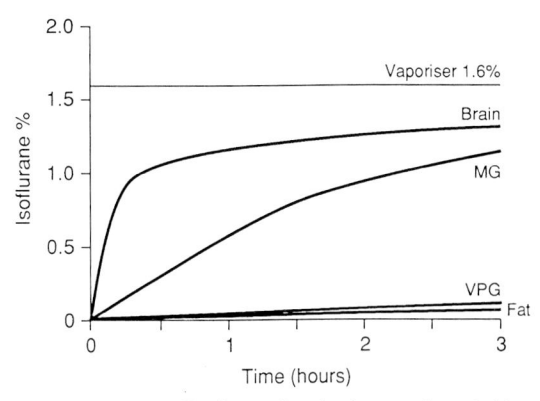

Fig. 7.1 Uptake of isoflurane into brain, muscle and skin (muscle group: MG), bone, cartilage and ligaments (vessel-poor group: VPG) and fatty tissues (fat group: FG). Inspired concentration 1.6%. Computer simulation in a 70-kg subject.

Table 7.1 Characteristics of four body compartments (see text) and their rate of equilibration with five anaesthetic agents

	Compartment			
	VRG	MG	VPG	FG
Body mass (%)	9	50	19	20
Volume (l), 70-kg person	6	33	14.5	12.5
Perfusion (% of cardiac output)	75	18	5.4	1.5
Perfusion (l.min^{-1} with cardiac output = 6 l.min^{-1})	4.5	1.1	0.3	0.1
τ (min) nitrous oxide	1.3	30	160	100
τ (min) desflurane	5.8	49	300	1350
τ (min) sevoflurane	9.2	82	437	2230
τ (min) isoflurane	8.7	80	480	2110
τ (min) halothane	9.3	85	550	2550

VRG = Vessel-rich group; MG = muscle group; VPG = vessel-poor group; FG = fat group.
τ = elimination time constant.
Modified from Eger[1] and Yasuda et al.[4,5]

of halothane, it would take 45 h to reach 63% of full saturation.[3] Table 7.1 shows data on this subject for a number of anaesthetic agents.

The administration of an anaesthetic can be divided into three periods: induction, maintenance and education (or recovery). The period of maintenance begins when the required partial pressure of agent is reached at the site of action in the brain and ends when this partial pressure is allowed to fall to permit the patient to wake up. The rate at which induction takes place (i.e. the speed with which the partial pressure or concentration of agent in the brain can be made to rise) is dependent on the solubility of the agent but it is also under the control of the anaesthetist since he or she can (within limits) adjust the concentration gradient down which the anaesthetic moves to reach the brain. This gradient for isoflurane is shown in Figure 7.2.[6]

Maintenance of anaesthetic concentration is also under the control of the anaesthetist. Having a knowledge of the gradients shown in Figure 7.2, he or she has to deliver sufficient anaesthetic to the patient to maintain the brain partial pressure at the necessary level. It could be argued that such detailed knowledge is not necessary if the patient is not paralysed; all that is needed under these circumstances is to give enough anaesthetic to stop the patient moving in response to the surgeon's activities.

When the desired partial pressure is achieved in the brain, no further uptake is needed in that organ, but uptake continues into other compartments, as shown in Figure 7.1. The anaesthetist does not need to consider this if an open circuit is used because the supply of anaesthetic is, for practical purposes, unlimited. The patient can be said to 'sample' from a stream of anaesthetic gas whose composition is regulated by the anaesthetist. The patient takes from the gas the amount of agent required to maintain the arterial concentration (and thus brain concentration) at the required level and the rest is wasted by passing out of the overflow valve.

During the induction phase, a large quantity of anaesthetic is taken up but this becomes less as the compartments become progressively saturated. The time taken to reach the anaesthetizing partial pressure in the brain can be reduced by increasing the

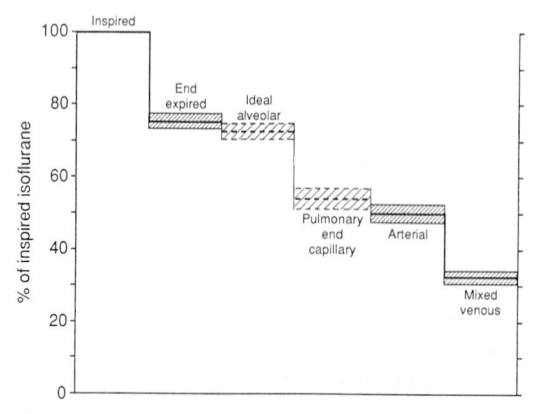

Fig. 7.2 Cascade of isoflurane partial pressures from inspired gas to mixed venous blood expressed as a percentage of inspired partial pressure. Experimental data from 6 patients (Landon et al, unpublished observations).

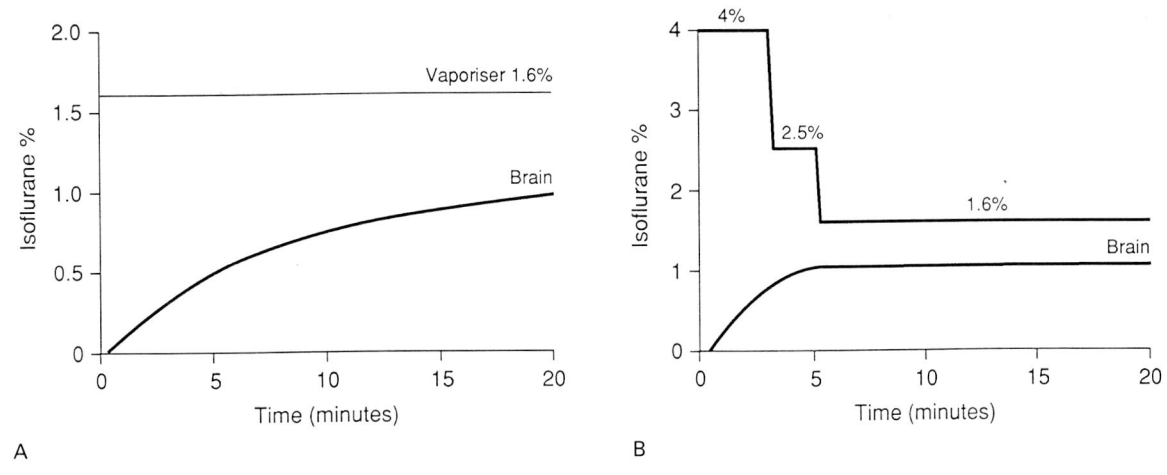

Fig. 7.3 (a) Change of brain concentration of isoflurane with time at constant inspired concentration. (b) Change of brain concentration of isoflurane with use of over-pressure.

concentration gradient which drives anaesthetic into the tissues. This is achieved by over-pressure — increasing the inspired concentration of agent considerably above that required for maintenance. Over-pressure is an almost essential procedure in routine inhalation anaesthesia and, without it, soluble agents such as trichloroethylene could not be used. Figure 7.3(a) shows how the brain isoflurane concentration rises if the inspired concentration is constantly at 1.6% and contrasts with Figure 7.3(b), which shows the more rapid rise in brain concentration when over-pressure is employed. A servo-controlled system into which anaesthetic is injected to produce a preset end-expiratory anaesthetic concentration automatically produces over-pressure in a most efficient manner.[7] Over-pressure is still required with the newer agents sevoflurane and desflurane, although because of their very low blood : gas partition coefficients, less over-pressure is required, and for a shorter period, than with the conventional volatile anaesthetics.

To ensure anaesthesia, the partial pressure of an inhalational agent in the brain must be known or predictable with confidence. Table 7.2 shows that this can be achieved with inhalational agents. The end-expired partial pressure of agent can be measured continuously and Table 7.2 shows that this provides a measure of the arterial partial pressure once a near-equilibrium state has been reached, which is the case

Table 7.2 Partial pressures and concentrations of three volatile anaesthetic agents equilibrated with minimum alveolar concentration (MAC) atmosphere absolute (ATA).

	Gas	Blood	Brain (grey matter)
Halothane (MAC = 0.75%)			
Partial pressure (kPa)	0.75	0.75	0.75
Concentration (vol %; 1 ATA)	0.75	1.80	3.80
Concentration (mmol.l^{-1})	0.29	0.71	1.50
Enflurane (MAC = 1.68%)			
Partial pressure (kPa)	1.68	1.68	1.68
Concentration (vol %; 1 ATA)	1.68	3.20	4.78
Concentration (mmol.l^{-1})	0.66	1.26	1.91
Isoflurane (MAC = 1.16%)			
Partial pressure (kPa)	1.16	1.16	1.16
Concentration (vol %; 1 ATA)	1.16	1.61	2.99
Concentration (mmol.l^{-1})	0.45	0.63	0.74

Note that partial pressures remain constant in all phases, while the concentration within each phase is determined by solubility. Anaesthetic activity is related to partial pressure. Solubilities taken from Fiserova-Bergerova.[8]

during maintenance. However, with intravenous agents, the blood concentration cannot be predicted with accuracy and the relationship between arterial and brain concentration is complex, depending on relative solubilities (see below).

During closed-circuit anaesthesia, the anaesthetic in the expired gas is rebreathed and therefore affects the inspired concentration. The factors regulating uptake depend therefore on the mode in which the anaesthetic system is operated (open or closed), or states between those two extremes. Also affecting the behaviour of the system is the way in which anaesthetic vapour is introduced into the system, e.g. vaporizer in the circle (VIC) or in the fresh gas flow (vaporizer outside the circle: VOC). This subject is considered in detail by Lockwood & White.[2]

If uptake of anaesthetic is measured continuously during induction and maintenance of anaesthesia, a curve such as that shown in Figure 7.4 is obtained. Total body uptake of anaesthetic can be measured by using a servo-controlled closed circuit;[9] after a short period of high uptake, the rate of uptake settles to an almost steady rate for a long period. The biggest single component of the rapidly changing uptake in the first few minutes of anaesthesia is the wash-in of anaesthetic to the functional residual capacity (FRC) of the lungs and then the uptake by the VRG. Because of its high blood flow, the VRG equilibrates quickly with the arterial blood and, after this has taken place, maintenance of anaesthesia continues with a constant brain partial pressure and a rising level in tissues of other groups.

The gradients of tissue partial pressures of isoflurane shown in Figure 7.2 were obtained after about 50 min of anaesthesia. It can be seen from Figure 7.4 that these relationships will be maintained for a long period, i.e. uptake will continue at an almost constant rate. However, if anaesthesia is continued for a long enough period, then equilibrium should be achieved and uptake will cease. It is unlikely that this is of clinical importance with the conventionally used anaesthetics; it can be calculated that at a constant inspired concentration of halothane, more than 5 days of anaesthesia would be required to produce 95% saturation of the FG of tissues. There are other reasons for believing that equilibrium (i.e. whole-body saturation) would not actually occur. Measurable losses of agents occur by diffusion through skin, although these are very small. It has been established that percutaneous loss of nitrous oxide through the intact skin is less than 10% of the amount delivered to the skin, and of ether and halothane less than 1% of the amount delivered. In the case of nitrous oxide, it has been estimated that losses through the skin may amount to 5–10 ml.min^{-1} when the alveolar concentration is 70%.[10] Losses of desflurane, isoflurane and halothane through the skin are 0.16, 0.20 and 0.23% respectively.[11] However, it is likely that losses by diffusion through mucous membranes are greater than this. Significant concentrations of anaesthetic agents can be measured in the pharynx of intubated anaesthetized patients[12] and losses from the open abdominal or thoracic cavities may be considerable, although not easy to quantify.[13] The rate of loss through skin or mucous membrane correlates with blood or tissue solubility of the agent. The effect is too small to be of importance under normal circumstances.

The other major factor which could affect the rate of equilibration of anaesthetic agents is metabolism. Significant metabolism of some agents occurs during anaesthesia, and has the effect of slowing equilibration. Once equilibrium has been attained, the only effect of metabolism is to increase the uptake required to maintain equilibrium.

In the case of halothane, anaesthetic metabolism becomes independent of concentration when the concentration exceeds 2–10% of minimum alveolar concentration (MAC).[14] It is not clear whether halothane inhibits its own metabolism at higher concentrations or whether the enzyme systems involved become saturated. Halothane is metabolized more than any of the other agents in current use and even at subanaesthetic concentrations it has not been possible to demonstrate any effect of metabolism on the maintenance of alveolar concentrations.[15] Thus it seems that metabolism of agents can be ignored in considering maintenance of anaesthesia. This may not be the case for recovery. Elimination of agents from the body is regulated by solubility in the same way as

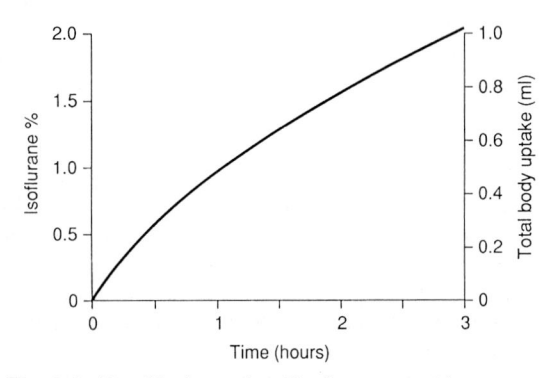

Fig. 7.4 Total body uptake of isoflurane over 3 h at constant inspired concentration (1.5%). Computer simulation: 70-kg subject.

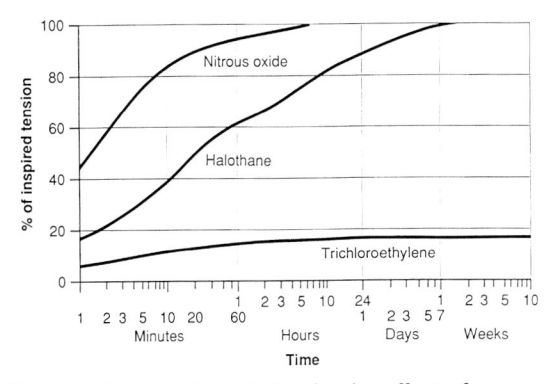

Fig. 7.5 Computed simulation showing effects of metabolism of trichloroethylene on the inspired/expired partial pressure ratio. A 25% clearance of trichloroethylene was assumed.[16]

uptake, but metabolism significantly accelerates the elimination of halothane from the body.

Although metabolism does not appear to have any influence on maintenance with agents in current use, this is not true for some older drugs. This is shown to an extreme degree in Figure 7.5, in which arterial partial pressure of agent as a percentage of inspired partial pressure is plotted against time.[16] It can be seen that the arterial concentration of trichloroethylene never reaches even 20% of the inspired concentration. The plot is a computed simulation based on measurements made during trichloroethylene anaesthesia in human subjects. To account for the measured values, it was necessary to assume that 25% of the cardiac output was cleared of trichloroethylene, presumably by metabolism in the liver.

The trend in the development of modern inhalation drugs has been towards agents with greater chemical stability. While this trend continues, it seems that metabolism can be ignored when considering maintenance. There is no evidence that drugs administered during the course of anaesthesia affect metabolism of anaesthetic agents. However, chronic administration of enzyme-inducing drugs such as phenytoin may affect metabolism. Once again, an example may be given involving trichloroethylene, an agent which is now of greater interest than use. Trichloroethylene is unusual in that one of its metabolites, trichloroethanol, is pharmacologically active. Cases have been reported in which patients in whom enzyme induction had taken place relapsed into unconsciousness after awakening from trichloroethylene anaesthesia.[17] High blood levels of trichloroethanol were found. In these cases, there was recovery from anaesthesia before the pharmacological action of the metabolite was seen; this supports the view that most of the metabolism of inhalational agents takes place after recovery and that the agent being metabolized is that portion of the total uptake which went into fatty tissues and which is being released slowly in low concentrations into the circulation.

Duration of anaesthesia

A feature of the action of many, but not all, drugs is that, at a constant dose level, their action declines with time. This is called tachyphylaxis or acute tolerance and it is clearly important to know if this occurs with anaesthetic agents. The subject was investigated in the course of the first experimental work on MAC,[18] with the results shown in Figure 7.6. No change in MAC is seen in up to 10 h of anaesthesia. This finding supports the general impression gained in clinical practice and has been confirmed with the newer agent desflurane.[19] However, recent work has shown a 19% decrease in isoflurane MAC after 3–4 hours of anaesthesia and surgery.[29]

There may also be an exception in the case of nitrous oxide. This agent was used at subanaesthetic concentrations postoperatively in many hospitals to produce analgesia for periods of 24 h or more, particularly in patients needing mechanical ventilation. Under these circumstances, the development of tolerance to nitrous oxide was sometimes noted and the effect has been described[20] and demonstrated experimentally in human subjects.[21]

Experimentally, both acute and chronic tolerance to nitrous oxide can be demonstrated in mice.[22,23] Exposure to subanaesthetic concentrations of nitrous oxide for 14 days increases the righting reflex ED_{50} for nitrous oxide by about 16%, together with cross-tolerance to other inhalational agents.[24] Comparable exposure in the human subject cannot be investigated easily. Perhaps the nearest circumstance is that of the chronic alcoholic in whom it is well known that there is an increased anaesthetic requirement. In mice, the chronic administration of ethanol increases MAC by 30–45%.

Nitrous oxide has a substantial analgesic action, which is separable from its anaesthetic action by naloxone in experimental animals.[24] In the human subject, it is acute tolerance to the analgesic effect of nitrous oxide that has been demonstrated rather than its anaesthetic action. This point may be of more than theoretical interest, as in the fully paralysed patient whose lungs are ventilated with oxygen, nitrous oxide 67% and an inhalational agent, nitrous oxide may represent a substantial proportion of the anaesthetizing

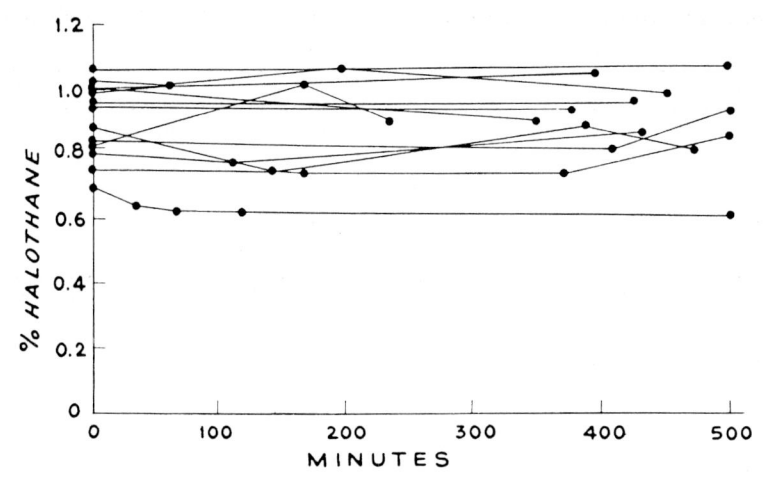

Fig. 7.6 Repeated halothane minimum alveolar concentration (MAC) determinations in 7 dogs. Time 0 was between 1 and 2 h after induction of anaesthesia. No change in MAC is seen in up to 10 h of anaesthesia. From Eger et al,[18] with permission.

gas mixture. If the development of acute tolerance caused a significant fall in the contribution of the nitrous oxide to anaesthesia then awareness could result. There is as yet no evidence of this occurring during anaesthesia in humans.

Experimental evidence for the development of tolerance after intermittent exposure to anaesthetics is inconclusive and in clinical practice patients receiving repeated anaesthetics do not appear to become tolerant to inhalational agents. Acute tolerance to opioids in humans is of considerable interest to anaesthetists. It has been little studied.[25]

INTRAVENOUS ANAESTHESIA

The calibrated vaporizer allows the anaesthetist to establish stable conditions with, usually, relatively few changes in delivered concentration of volatile anaesthetic agent during an operation. This is largely because the patient tends to come into equilibrium with the delivered concentration, irrespective of body size or physiological variations; the total dose of drug taken up by the body is variable, but is, to a large extent, unimportant, and it is determined by the characteristics of the patient and the drug rather than by the anaesthetist. The task of achieving equilibrium with intravenous anaesthetic agents is more complex, as delivery must be matched to the size of the patient as well as to the expected rates of distribution and metabolism of the drug. Unlike the situation pertaining during inhalation anaesthesia, conventional methods of delivering intravenous agents result in the total dose of drug being determined by the anaesthetist, and the concentration achieved in tissues depends on the volume and rate of distribution, the solubility of the drug in each tissue and the rate of elimination of the drug in the individual patient.

Minimum infusion rate (MIR)

Because of the difficulties in inferring brain concentration of intravenous agents, the concept of MIR was introduced to determine the relative potencies of the different drugs.[26] The MIR is the minimum infusion rate of an intravenous anaesthetic which prevents movement in response to an initial skin incision in 50% of patients. Although in theory this should be equivalent to the use of MAC to compare potencies of inhaled agents, the two are not strictly comparable because of the difficulty in securing steady-state conditions during intravenous infusion. Nevertheless, the data available indicate that the variability of MIR is very much greater than that of MAC (Table 7.3),[18,26-28] reflecting the greater variation in brain concentration of intravenous agents resulting from wide variability in distribution and elimination of a fixed dose of the drug. There is also a relatively imprecise relationship between infusion rate of an intravenous agent and the resultant plasma concentration because the concentration is related to the balance between infusion rate and clearance of the drug and, at least with some agents, clearance varies with infusion rate. In contrast, there is a linear relationship between alveolar concentration and brain concentration for the inhaled anaesthetics. Further, the relationship between blood concentration and brain concentration (and thus anaesthetic effect) depends on the relative solubility of the drug in the brain.

Not only does MIR vary more than MAC, but some

Table 7.3 Mean and standard deviation of ED_{50} values, ED_{95} values, and ratio of $ED_{95} : ED_{50}$ for intravenous and inhalational anaesthetics

Agent	ED_{50}*	95% CI*	ED_{95}*	$ED_{95} : ED_{50}$
Halothane	0.74	0.45–1.03	0.90	1.21
Enflurane	1.69	1.36–2.02	1.88	1.11
Isoflurane	1.16	0.59–1.73	1.63	1.41
Propofol	130	106–167	348	2.68
Althesin (as alphaxolone)	18.4	1.1–38.6	24.2	1.31
Methohexitone	66.0	24.4–108.9	80.7	1.22

*Data in end-tidal concentration (vol %) for volatile anaesthetic agents and as the infusion rate ($\mu g.kg^{-1}.min^{-1}$) for intravenous agents.
CI = Confidence interval
Modified from Sear et al,[26] Turtle et al[27] and de Jong & Eger.[28]

of the intravenous agents also have a flatter dose–response curve than the inhaled agents. For example, the ratio of $ED_{95} : ED_{50}$ for propofol is more than 2,[27] compared with a ratio of 1.21 for halothane (Table 7.3).[28]

Calculation of dose

Adult patients can have a body fat content ranging from 15 to 80% of total body weight (TBW). One of the reasons for the wide variability in effect of

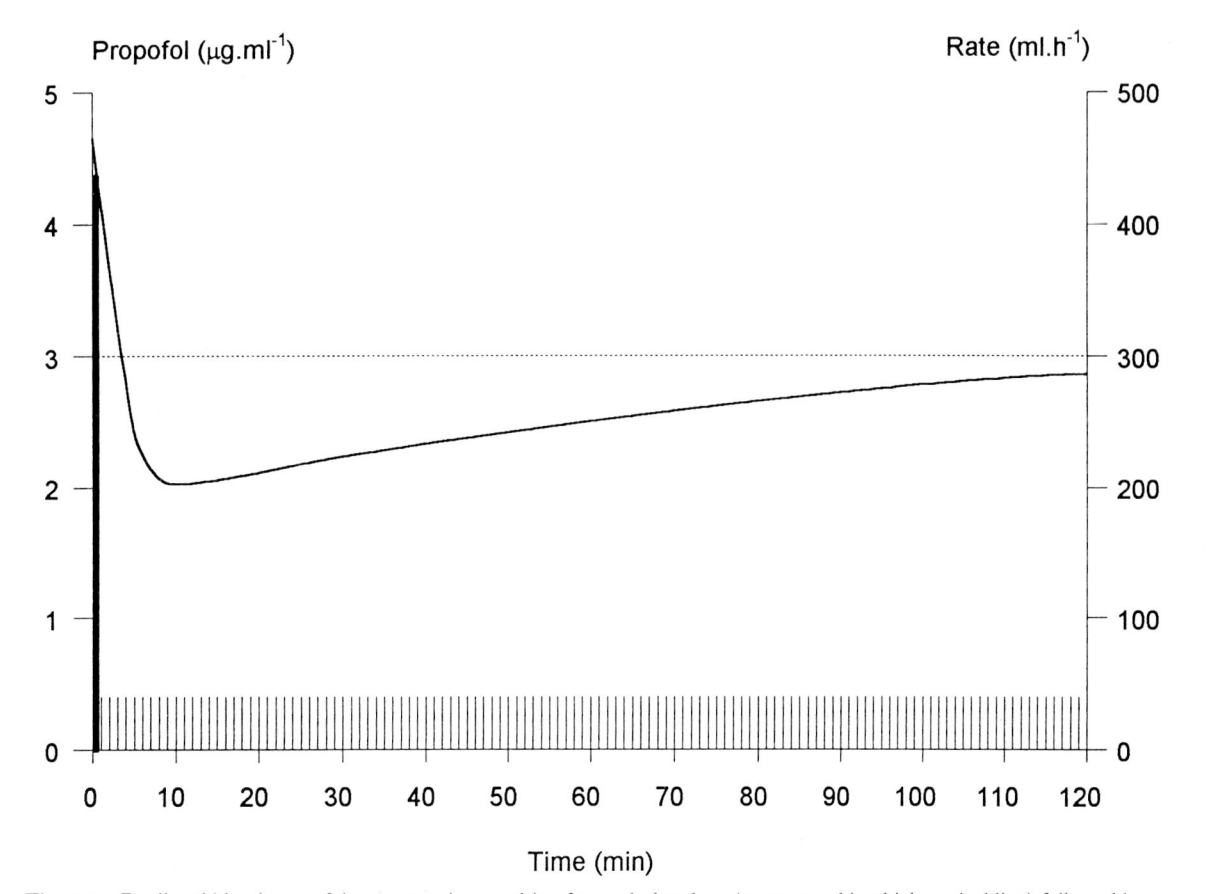

Fig. 7.7 Predicted blood propofol concentration resulting from a bolus dose (represented by thick vertical line) followed by a continuous infusion (infusion rate shown by narrow vertical lines). Redrawn from White & Kenny.[29]

intravenous agents is that they are usually administered in a dose or infusion rate based on TBW, whereas the 'pharmacologically active' mass of the patient may be reflected more accurately by lean body mass (LBM). There is evidence that variability in response is reduced if the infusion rate is calculated on the basis of LBM,[30] but most infusion schemes continue to be based on TBW.

Techniques of administration

Intermittent injection

Although some anaesthetists are skilled in the delivery of intravenous anaesthetic agents by intermittent bolus injection, the plasma concentrations of drug, and the anaesthetic effect, vary widely, and the technique is acceptable only for procedures of short duration in unparalysed patients.

Manual infusion techniques

The infusion rate required to achieve a predetermined plasma concentration of an intravenous drug can be calculated if the clearance of the drug from plasma is known [infusion rate (μg.min^{-1}) = steady-state plasma concentration (μg.ml^{-1}) × clearance (ml.min^{-1})]. One of the difficulties is that clearance is variable, and it is possible only to estimate the value by using population kinetics; depending on the patient's clearance in relation to the average, the actual plasma concentration achieved may be higher or lower than the intended concentration.

A fixed-rate infusion is inappropriate because the serum concentration of the drug increases only slowly, taking 4–5 times the elimination half-life of the drug to reach steady state. A bolus injection followed by a continuous infusion results in achievement of an excessive concentration (with an increased incidence of side-effects) initially, and this is followed by a prolonged dip below the intended plasma concentration (Fig. 7.7). In order to achieve a reasonably constant plasma concentration (other than in very long procedures), it is necessary to use a multistep infusion regimen, a concept similar to that of over-pressure for inhaled agents, as described above. Roberts et al[31] devised a three-stage infusion scheme for propofol which proved effective in unparalysed patients who also received nitrous oxide and fentanyl. The intended (target) plasma concentration of propofol was 3 μg.ml^{-1}, and this was achieved using a bolus dose of 1 mg.kg^{-1} followed by infusion at a rate of 10 mg.kg^{-1}.h^{-1} for 10 min, 8 mg.kg^{-1}.h^{-1} for the next 10 min, and a maintenance infusion rate of 6 mg.kg^{-1}.l^{-1} thereafter. The predicted blood concentrations in an average patient receiving such a regimen are shown in Figure 7.8. However, a wide range of infusion rates is required to produce satisfactory anaesthesia in clinical practice. Spelina et al[32] reported that the infusion rate of propofol required to abolish movement on incision in 95% of patients premedicated with morphine and given 67% nitrous oxide ranged from 5.1 to 18.4 mg.kg^{-1}.l^{-1}, and Turtle et al[27] found that, in patients premedicated with lorazepam, the ED$_{95}$ of propofol was 20.3 mg.kg^{-1}.l^{-1} with 95% confidence intervals of 13.9–77.9 mg.kg^{-1}.l^{-1}. Other disadvantages of manual infusion schemes are that there is obvious scope for error in calculating the infusion rate if a fixed multistep infusion scheme is employed, and that a modest change in the infusion rate achieves only a very slow change in plasma concentration.

Computer-driver infusion techniques

By programming a computer with appropriate pharmacokinetic data and equations, it is possible at frequent intervals (several times a minute) to calculate the appropriate infusion rate required to produce a preset target plasma concentration of drug. The drug is infused by a syringe driver. To produce a step increase in plasma concentration, the syringe driver infuses drug very rapidly (a slow bolus), and then delivers drug at a progressively decreasing infusion rate (Fig. 7.9). To decrease the plasma concentration, the syringe driver stops infusing until the computer calculates that the target concentration has been achieved, and then infuses drug at an appropriate rate to maintain a constant level.[33,34] The anaesthetist is required only to enter the desired target concentration, and to change it if clinically indicated, in the same way as a vaporizer might be manipulated according to clinical signs of anaesthesia.

The potential advantages of such a system are its simplicity, the rapidity with which plasma concentration can be changed (particularly upwards) and avoidance of the need for the anaesthetist to undertake any calculations (resulting in less potential for error). However, the actual concentration achieved may be >50% greater than or less than the predicted concentration,[33] because the computer is programmed with population kinetics which may be very different from the kinetics of the drug in an individual patient. This may not be a major practical disadvantage provided that the anaesthetist adjusts the target concentration according to clinical signs relating to adequacy of anaesthesia rather than assuming that a

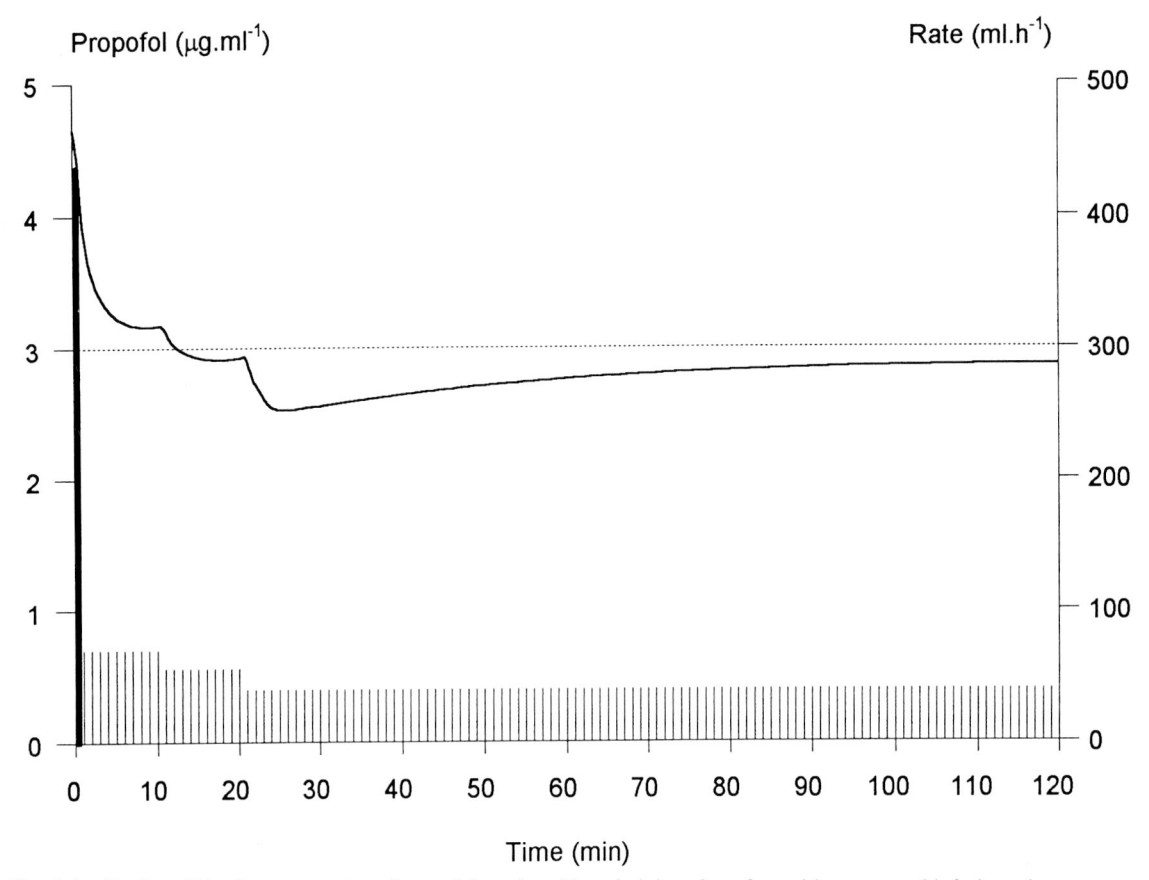

Fig. 7.8 Predicted blood concentration of propofol produced by administration of a multistep manual infusion scheme as described by Roberts et al.[31] Redrawn from White & Kenny.[29]

specific target concentration will always result in the desired effect.

Although these devices have been used widely, published evaluation of the technique is sparse. There is evidence that the use of infusion techniques rather than rapid bolus doses improves haemodynamic stability with propofol,[35] fentanyl[36] or alfentanil.[37] A target-controlled system for infusing propofol has been used by a number of anaesthetists.[38] No data were presented regarding outcome, but 27 of 30 participants increased their use of propofol for maintenance, the main reasons being ease of use and more confidence in predicting anaesthetic effects of the drug in comparison with a manual infusion system. The median target concentration selected by these anaesthetists was 6.6 µg.ml^{-1}.

Target-controlled infusion systems can also be employed to identify the potency of intravenous agents, and to assess the effect of administration with other anaesthetic agents. Using a target-controlled infusion system in female patients, the EC_{50} (to prevent movement in response to surgical incision) of propofol was estimated to be 6 µg.ml^{-1} when patients breathed oxygen, compared with 4.5 µg.ml^{-1} when 67% nitrous oxide was administered;[39] mean measured blood concentrations were 8.1 and 5.4 µg.ml^{-1} respectively. The relatively small reduction in EC_{50} for propofol resulting from administration of 0.65 MAC of nitrous oxide is both interesting and potentially important. A much greater reduction occurs when volatile anaesthetic agents are administered with nitrous oxide; for example, simultaneous administration of 70% nitrous oxide reduces the MAC of halothane from 0.75 to 0.29%.[40]

Effect site concentration

One of the disadvantages of target-controlled infusion systems based purely on pharmacokinetic modelling is that they do not take account of delays in transfer of drug from the blood to the effect site in the central

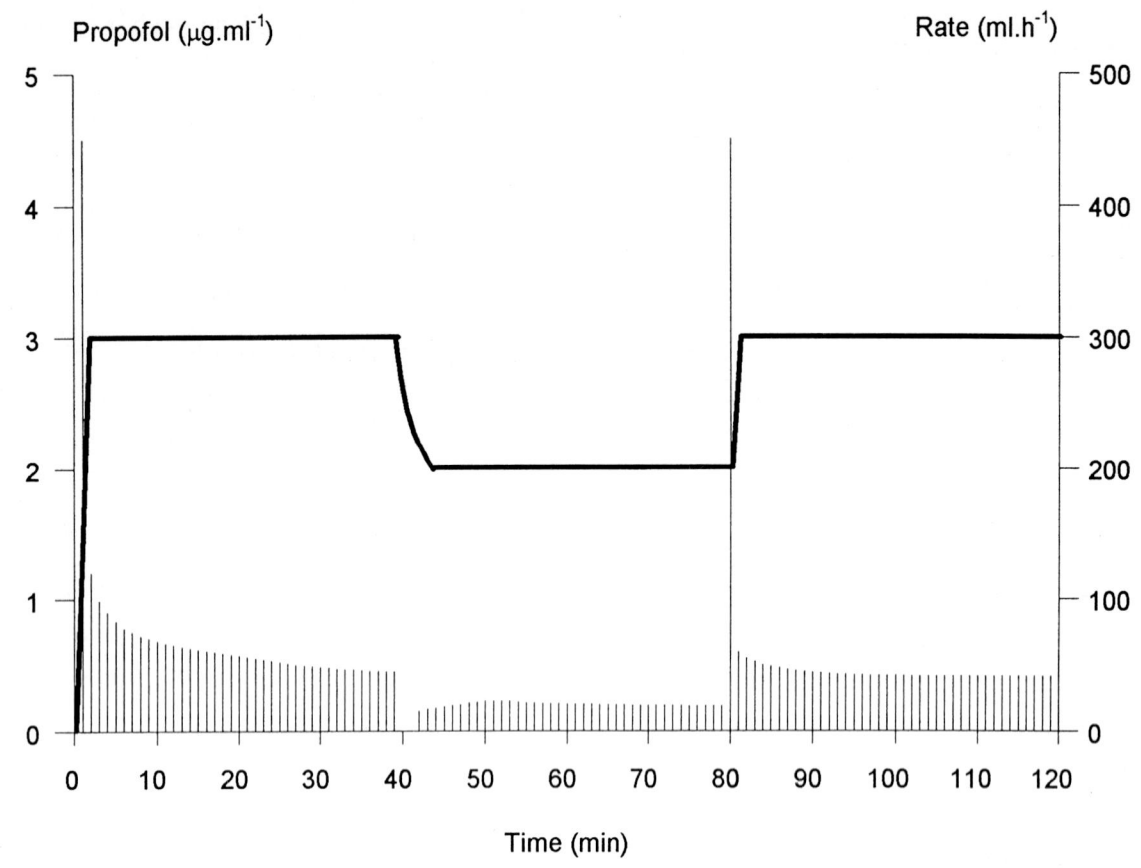

Fig. 7.9 Blood concentrations of propofol and infusion profiles produced by a computer-controlled system to achieve and maintain different target concentrations. Redrawn from White & Kenny.[29]

nervous system. With some intravenous drugs, equilibration is slow, and although a target-controlled infusion system may achieve a rapid increase in blood concentration, there is a delay in achieving a satisfactory depth of anaesthesia. Pharmacodynamic aspects of drug behaviour can be programmed into computer-controlled infusion systems to take account of this delay, which is related to the concentration gradient between blood and brain. Thus, sophisticated programs can infuse the drug in such a way that a rapid step change in predicted effect site concentration is produced (by 'over-pressure'), with a reduction in blood concentration to the required steady-state level when it is predicted that equilibrium has been achieved.

Closed-loop systems

Target-controlled infusion systems may be used as part of a closed-loop system to control depth of anaesthesia. Because there is no method of measuring blood concentrations of intravenous anaesthetics on-line, it is necessary to use some form of monitor of depth of anaesthesia on the input side of the system. A control system (using enflurane and morphine) based on arterial pressure measurement was described by Robb et al,[41] and although the system was used successfully in a small number of fit patients undergoing elective gynaecological surgery, problems were foreseen in attempting to use arterial pressure as the only input to a control system in less fit patients, or during surgery in which major cardiovascular disturbances might be superimposed by the nature of the procedure.

Median frequency of the electroencephalogram (EEG) has been used in a closed-loop control system for infusion of propofol,[42] but the resulting depth of anaesthesia in volunteers would have been insufficient to permit surgery to take place. The auditory evoked response (AER) appears to be a more robust index of depth of anaesthesia, and a system using a 'level of arousal' score, based on continuous AER recordings, has been used together with a target-controlled infusion system with propofol to maintain anaesthesia.[43] This index is passed automatically every few seconds to a controller device which compares the index with that requested by the anaesthetist, and which then adjusts the target concentration of propofol delivered by the infusion pump to minimize the discrepancy between the desired and measured effects. The infusion rate automatically decreases slowly over time to prevent accumulation of drug, but this decrease is overridden by the system if the index shows that the level of arousal is becoming higher.

Indications for intravenous maintenance of anaesthesia

There are a number of situations in which intravenous anaesthesia (IVA; the use of an intravenous anaesthetic to supplement nitrous oxide) or total intravenous anaesthesia (TIVA) may offer advantages over the traditional inhalational techniques. In the doses required to maintain clinical anaesthesia, intravenous agents cause minimal cardiovascular depression. In comparison with the most commonly used volatile anaesthetic agents, IVA with propofol (the only currently available IVA with an appropriate pharmacokinetic profile; offers rapid recovery of consciousness and good recovery of psychomotor function, although the newer volatile anaesthetics desflurane and sevoflurane are also associated with rapid recovery and minimal hangover effects. The use of TIVA allows the use of a high inspired oxygen concentration in situations where hypoxaemia may otherwise occur, such as one-lung anaesthesia or in the severely ill or traumatized patient, and has obvious advantages in procedures such as laryngoscopy or bronchoscopy, when delivery of inhaled anaesthetic agents to the lungs may be difficult. TIVA can also be used to provide anaesthesia in circumstances where there are clinical reasons to avoid nitrous oxide, such as middle-ear surgery, prolonged bowel surgery and in patients with raised intracranial pressure. There are few contraindications to the use of IVA, provided that the anaesthetist is aware of the wide variability in response. For surgical anaesthesia, it is desirable either to use nitrous oxide supplemented by IVA, or to infuse an opioid as well as an intravenous anaesthetic drug; target-controlled systems for opioid infusion have also been described.[44] However, at a time when there is increasing concern about the risk of awareness during anaesthesia, the wide variability in plasma concentration with intravenous techniques, combined with the increased availability of monitors of end-tidal inhalation anaesthetic concentrations, is likely to result in intravenous maintenance techniques remaining less popular than maintenance by inhaled anaesthetic drugs.

OPIOIDS

The use of opioids as supplements to general anaesthetic agents, particularly nitrous oxide, entered routine practice following the paper by Neff et al.[45] Nitrous oxide (MAC 105%) is not a sufficiently potent agent to guarantee anaesthesia routinely and opioid supplements clearly met a need. Techniques which employed incremental doses of, for example, pethidine (meperidine) 25 mg every 25–30 min during anaesthesia with 66% nitrous oxide and relaxant achieved widespread use. Pethidine may be particularly useful for this purpose since its use reduces postoperative shivering.[46] Whether or not opioids are themselves able to produce a state of general anaesthesia remains a matter of controversy. However, in an exhaustive review of the subject,[47] with over 900 references, it is stated that to date there is no study demonstrating that an opioid alone can reliably produce anaesthesia in the absence of any supplements. Techniques involving nitrous oxide and modest doses of opioid are associated with an incidence of awareness of 1–2%.

The reasons for using opioids in current practice include the obtunding of the sympathetic response to laryngoscopy and tracheal intubation, and of the metabolic response to surgery; both, to be effective, require very large doses of opioids. In this connection, the classical works of George Crile[48] on anoci-association and Lundy[49] on balanced anaesthesia are often cited. However, both authors advocated local anaesthetics to produce the analgesic component in their balanced anaesthetic techniques. Local anaesthetics do block the metabolic response to surgery more effectively than opioids, but only while their local anaesthetic action persists.

Of greater importance in the maintenance of routine anaesthesia is the general anaesthetic agent-sparing effect of opioids. It was noticed by Claude Bernard in 1869 that the administration of morphine to dogs reduced by half the amount of chloroform required to produce surgical anaesthesia; similar observations during cyclopropane anaesthesia were reviewed by Robbins in his monograph on cyclopropane.[50] Morphine 10 mg given to patients 10 min before ether anaesthesia was found to reduce by 15% the blood ether concentration required for a given clinical depth of anaesthesia or to produce a similar change in electroencephalography.[51]

More recent work on this subject has concentrated on the reduction of MAC which can be produced by opioids in experimental animals. There are difficulties in applying much of this work to the human subject, partly because of the considerable difference in response to opioids found in different species (e.g. dogs, cats, rats and mice). This is in contrast to the small differences in MAC for inhalational agents among not only different species of mammal but also in fish amphibia[1] and even luminous bacteria.[52]

In dogs, MAC for enflurane or isoflurane cannot be reduced by more than 60–70% irrespective of the dose of opioid employed. In rats, a greater reduction in MAC is found (up to 90%) but a ceiling effect still appears to be present, although this is disputed by some workers. The maximum reduction of MAC which can be obtained from mixed agonist–antagonist drugs such as nalbuphine and butorphanol is only about 10%. For further details of this subject the reader is referred to the review by Bailey & Stanley.[47] The doses of opioid required to produce substantial reductions in MAC are sufficiently high to require artificial ventilation.

There is a further difficulty in considering this subject which illustrates the limitations of animal models. The MAC for inhalational agents is determined by observing the presence or absence of a motor response to a painful stimulus such as a tail clamp. It is not surprising that powerful analgesics reduce the effect of this painful stimulus. However, while measuring the reduction of MAC by sufentanil during enflurane anaesthesia in dogs, Hall et al[53] observed that there was little difference in the haemodynamic response to the stimulus whether or not movement resulted. This indicates that the apparent potency of agents depends on the end-point used to measure that potency. MAC remains the standard in this field. In its favour it can be argued that if an anaesthetized, unparalysed patient does not move on skin incision, then awareness of pain is not occurring.

It should be remembered that inhalational agents also block the haemodynamic response to painful stimuli. Roizen et al,[54] using a group of unpremedicated patients, found that the alveolar concentration of halothane required to block the cardiovascular response to skin incision in 50% of the group (MAC-BAR) was 1.1% (147% of MAC). The dose of morphine needed to achieve the same result was 1.13 mg.kg^{-1} (79 mg in a 70-kg man). It can be concluded that opioids are not very effective in blocking haemodynamic responses to painful stimuli.

Another objection to relying too heavily on opioids for maintenance of anaesthesia is that accurate prediction of plasma concentration after a dose of opioid is not possible; a variation by a factor of 5 may be found in pharmacokinetics between patients, and pharmacodynamics may be equally or even more variable.[47] This contrasts with the small variation (s.d. ≈ 10%) found with MAC determinations.

Thus, for routine maintenance of anaesthesia, greater reliance can be placed on inhalational agents than opioids and the introduction of newer inhalational agents with more rapid actions (both onset and offset) further increases this advantage.

Intra-operative opioids do have the advantage, if their analgesic action is sufficiently long, of providing analgesia in the postoperative period. There may be advantages in 'pre-emptive analgesia'.[55] Clearly, opioids such as fentanyl and alfentanil are unsuitable for this purpose unless they are given by continuous infusion.

BODY TEMPERATURE DURING MAINTENANCE OF ANAESTHESIA

The thermoregulatory centre in the hypothalamus is controlled by signals indicating the temperature of a variety of tissues in the body, including the skin, the brain and other deeply seated tissues. These signals taken together, in a weighted manner (15% from skin and 85% from the central nervous system and deep tissues), constitute the mean body temperature and when a threshold temperature (hot or cold) is passed, thermoregulatory mechanisms are activated.

The extent to which general anaesthesia depresses the thermoregulatory threshold depends on the depth of anaesthesia, i.e. the concentration of inhalation agent.[56] During normal surgical anaesthesia, a depression of the threshold from 37°C to about 34.5°C occurs;[57] consequently, a decrease in core temperature of between 0.7 and 1.5°C usually occurs in the first hour of surgery, with a slower fall to not lower than 33°C after this. This decrease in temperature can be reduced by various measures such as a warming mattress, humidification of inspired gases, heating infused fluids, etc.

MAC declines with body temperature and the extent of the fall of MAC is related to the change of lipid solubility of the agent with temperature.[1] This change differs among agents; for example, MAC decreases by 5% per degree Celsius for halothane and 2% per degree Celsius for cyclopropane. The fall in MAC with temperature appears to be linear and the extent to which it is taken into account in determining the anaesthetic concentration for maintenance depends on the degree of hypothermia (core temperature). The chief factors determining the degree of hypothermia are the duration of the operation, the size of the incision, the volume of cold fluids transfused and the operating theatre temperature. Clearly, it is desirable to monitor core temperature during prolonged and major surgery, and in patients at the extremes of age.

FLUID REQUIREMENTS DURING MAINTENANCE OF ANAESTHESIA

Intra-operative fluid requirements are determined by consideration of a number of factors. First, there is the need to make good any pre-operative fluid deprivation and provide basal metabolic requirements during the operative period. Second, there is the need to replace intra-operative fluid loss, particularly of blood, but also evaporative loss from exposed tissues. Third, there is the more difficult question of compensating for fluid shifts which occur intra-operatively.

The normal (basal) intake of water by a 70-kg subject at rest in a temperature climate averages 100 ml.h^{-1}. A 6-h period of pre-operative fluid deprivation, 1 h of anaesthesia and a 3-h postoperative period without imbibing represents a water deficit of about 1 l. The total extracellular fluid (ECF) volume is about 15 l and in a normal healthy patient it is not necessary to administer fluid to make good this deficit, provided that the patient is able to do so by normal drinking and eating after the immediate peri-operative period.

When anaesthesia last for many hours, the situation is rather different for a number of reasons. More careful assessment of fluid requirements for metabolism may be necessary. The basal metabolic rate of a 70-kg man in about 2000 kcal.day^{-1} (there are a number of pathological conditions commonly found in surgical practice in which this may be considerably increased). Anaesthesia reduces metabolism by an amount related to the depth of anaesthesia: 30% at 1 MAC, 40% at 2 MAC.[58,59] In addition, oxygen uptake is reduced by about 6% by artificial ventilation.[60] The fall in oxygen uptake with core temperature is non-linear but figures of between 6 and 8% per degree Celsius are quoted commonly and are in agreement with experimental observations in the range 37–30°C. A fall of 2°C in core temperature therefore reduces oxygen uptake by a further 14%. Consequently, during prolonged anaesthesia, the basal metabolic rate may be reduced by as much as 50% and the metabolic requirement for water by a similar factor. Clearly, metabolic water is a very minor component of fluid requirements during most surgical operations.

The next component of the intra-operative fluid requirement to consider is the replacement of fluid loss, particularly blood. There is now considerable evidence that oxygen delivery to the tissues is facilitated by haemodilution, which reduces the viscosity of the blood, so that, for a given amount of cardiac work, more blood is pumped through the tissues. There is therefore an optimal haematocrit value, in the region of 25–30% (i.e. 60–75% of normal) at which oxygen delivery, or more accurately oxygen transport capacity, is greater that at 'normal' haematocrit values. It is, of course, necessary that normovolaemia and blood oxygenation are maintained.

It is fortunate that this work has become known at the same time as a decrease in the availability of whole blood, so that, at the present time, large intra-operative losses of blood may be treated by a combination of plasma substitutes or 'expanders' and packed red cells to maintain an optimal haematocrit. The subject is reviewed by Laubenthal et al.[61]

Finally, there is the question of intra-operative fluid shifts. The body fluids (40 l) are normally partitioned into 25 l of intracellular fluid and 15 l of ECF, of which 3 l are plasma. The intra- and extracellular volumes can be measured only by tracer techniques; these techniques are slow because of the time taken to equilibrate the tracer, and thus cannot be repeated quickly to measure trends. Information on fluid shifts between compartments during anaesthesia and surgery is therefore limited. The well-known work on this subject is that of Shires and colleagues.[62] His group, using radioactive sodium sulphate, found deficits of up to 28% in ECF volume when measured 2 h after major surgical operations and considered that the fluid had entered a 'third space' where it was unavailable to maintain the intravascular volume and should therefore be replaced by a crystalloid solution of composition similar to ECF, such as compound sodium lactate.

The view that quite large amounts of crystalloid solution should be given to all major surgical patients was contrary to previous orthodoxy[63] that fluid should be restricted intra- and postoperatively because water and sodium retention were unavoidable responses to surgery. More recently, the argument has centred on whether colloids or crystalloids should be used to maintain plasma volume.[64] A balanced view seems more likely to be correct and a ratio of crystalloids to colloids of 2–3 : 1 has been suggested as optimal.[65] Rather than follow pre-ordained routines, fluid therapy in major surgery should be regulated by observation of central venous pressure, urine output, haematocrit, etc.

The fluid imbalances referred to above have all been ascribed mostly to surgery; there is almost no information relating to prolonged anaesthesia (for obvious reasons) except in the case of the kidney, where direct depressant effects on function are produced by all the standard anaesthetic agents.

The increase in the number of lengthy operations such as vascular and neurosurgical procedures using microscopes may provide the opportunity to gain new knowledge on the maintenance of anaesthesia. The surgical stimulus during many such procedures is minimal, giving opportunities to study the effects of anaesthesia unconfused by surgery.

REFERENCES

1. Eger E I. Anesthetic uptake and action. Baltimore: Williams & Wilkins, 1974
2. Lockwood G G, White D C. Effect of ventilation and cardiac output on the uptake of anaesthetic agents from different breathing systems: a theoretical study. Br J Anaesth 1991; 66: 519–526
3. Webster N R, White DC. Study of the uptake of inhalational agents by modelling. In: Kaufman L (ed) Anaesthesia review 6. Edinburgh: Churchill Livingstone, 1989
4. Yasuda N, Lockhart S H, Eger E I, Weiskopf R B, Liu J, Laster M, Taheri S, Peterson N A. Comparison of kinetics of sevoflurane and isoflurane in humans. Anesth Analg 1991; 72: 316–324
5. Yasuda N, Lockhart S H, Eger E I, Weiskopf R B, Johnson B H, Freiere B A, Fassoulaki A. Kinetics of desflurane, isoflurane and halothane in humans. Anesthesiology 1991; 74: 489–498
6. Landon M J, Matson A M, Royston B D, Hewlett A M, White D C, Nunn J F. Components of the inspiratory–arterial isoflurane partial pressure difference. Br J Anaesth 1993; 70: 605–611
7. Ross J A S, Wloch R T, White D C, Hawes D W. Servo controlled closed circuit anaesthesia. Br J Anaesth 1983; 55: 1053–1059
8. Fiserova-Bergerova V. Modelling of inhalational exposure to vapors: uptake, distribution and elimination. CRC Press Florida, 1983.
9. O'Callaghan A C, Hawes D W, Ross J A S, White D C. Uptake of isoflurane during clinical anaesthesia. Br J Anaesth 1983; 55: 1061–1064
10. Stoelting R K, Eger E I II. Percutaneous loss of nitrous oxide, cyclopropane, ether and halothane in man. Anesthesiology 1969; 55: 278–283
11. Fassoulaki A, Lockhart S, Freire B A et al. Percutaneous loss of desflurane, isoflurane and halothane in humans. Anesthesiology 1991; 74: 479–483
12. Mostert J W. Cuffs do not seal the trachea airtight. Anesthesiology 1977; 46–309
13. Laster M J, Taheri S, Eger IS II, Lin J, Rampil I J, Dwyer R. Visceral losses of desflurane, isoflurane and halothane in swine. Anesth Analg 1991; 73: 209–212
14. Sawyer D C, Eger E I, Bahlam S H et al. Concentration dependence of hepatic halothane metabolism. Anesthesiology 1971; 34: 230–245
15. Cahalan M K, Johnson B H, Eger E I II. Relationship of concentrations of halothane and enflurane to their metabolism and elimination in man. Anesthesiology 1981; 54: 3–8
16. Mapleson W W. Quantitative prediction of anesthetic concentrations. In: Papper E M, Kitz R J (eds) Uptake and distribution of anesthetic agents. New York: McGraw-Hill, 1963
17. Hewlett A M. Personal communication 1992
18. Eger E I II, Saidman L J, Brandstater B. Minimum alveolar anesthetic concentration: a standard of anesthetic potency. Anesthesiology 1965; 26: 756–763
19. Eger E I II, Johnson B H. MAC of I.653 in rats including a test of the effect of body temperature and anesthetic duration. Anesth Analg 1987; 66: 974–976
20. Whitwam J G, Morgan M, Hall G M, Petrie H. Pain during continuous nitrous oxide administration. Br J Anaesth 1976; 48: 425–429
21. Rupreht J, Dworacek J, Bonke B, Dzologic M R, van Eindhoven J H, de Vrieger M. Tolerance to nitrous oxide in volunteers. Acta Anesthesiol Scand 1985; 29: 635
22. Smith R A, Winter P M, Smith M, Eger E I II. Rapidly developing tolerance to acute exposures to anesthetic agents. Anesthesiology 1979; 59: 496–500
23. Koblin D D, Doug D E, Eger E I II. Tolerance of mice to nitrous oxide . J Pharmacol Exp Ther 1979; 211: 317
24. Smith R A, Winter P M, Smith M, Eger E I II. Tolerance to and dependence on inhalational anesthetics. Anesthesiology 1979; 50: 505–509
25. McQuay H J, Bullingham R E, Moore R A. Acute opiate tolerance in man. Life Sci 1981; 28: 2513–2517
26. Sear J W, Phillips K C, Andrews C J H, Prys-Roberts C. Dose–response relationships for infusions of Althesin or methohexitone. Anaesthesia 1983; 38: 931–936
27. Turtle M J, Cullen P, Prys-Roberts C, Coates D, Monk C R, Faroqui M H. Dose requirements of propofol by infusion during nitrous oxide anaesthesia in man. II: Patients premedicated with lorazepam. Br J Anaesth 1987; 59: 283–287
28. de Jong R H, Eger E I. MAC expanded: ED_{50} and ED_{95} values of common inhalational anesthetics in man. Anesthesiology 1975; 42: 384–389
29. White M, Kenny G N C. Intravenous anaesthetic agents: delivery systems. In: Nimmo WAS, Rowbotham D J, Smith G (eds) Anaesthesia, 2nd edn. Oxford: Blackwell Scientific Publications, 1994; pp 106–118
30. Crankshaw D P, Beemer G H. How should we administer intravenous anaesthetic drugs? Baillière's Clin Anaesthesiol 1991; 5: 327–351
31. Roberts F L, Dixon J,. Lewis G T R, Tackley R M, Prys Roberts C. Induction and maintenance of propofol anaesthesia: a manual infusion scheme. Anaesthesia 1988; 43: S14–S17
32. Spelina K R, Coates D P, Monk C R, Prys-Roberts C, Norley I, Turtle M J. Dose requirements of propofol by infusion during nitrous oxide in anaesthetic man. I: Patients premedicated with morphine sulphate. Br J Anaesth 1986; 58: 1080–1084
33. White M, Kenny G M C. Intravenous propofol infusion using a computerised infusion pump. Anaesthesia 1990; 45: 204–209
34. Glass P S A, Jacobs J R, Reves J G. Intravenous anaesthetic delivery. In: Miller R D (ed) Anesthesia, 4th edn. New York: Churchill Livingstone, 1994
35. Peacock J E, Lewis R P, Reilly C S, Nimmo W S. Effect of different rates of infusion of propofol for induction of anaesthesia in elderly patients. Br J Anaesth 1990; 65: 346–352
36. Alvis J M, Reves J G, Govier A V, Menkhaus P G, Hanling C E, Spain J A, Bradley E. Computer-assisted continuous infusions of fentanyl during cardiac anesthesia: comparison with a manual method. Anesthesiology 1985; 65: 41–49
37. Ausems M E, Vuyk J, Hug C C, Stanski D R. Comparison of a computer-assisted infusion versus intermittent bolus administration of alfentanil as a supplement to nitrous oxide for lower abdominal surgery. Anesthesiology 1988; 68: 851–861
38. Taylor I, White M, Kenny G N C. Assessment of the

value and pattern of use of a target-controlled propofol infusion system. Int J Clin Monit Comput 1993; 10: 175–180
39 Davidson J A H, McLeod A D, Howie J C, White M, Kenny G N C. The effective concentration$_{50}$ for propofol with and without 67% nitrous oxide. Acta Anaesthesiol Scand 1993; 36: 458–464
40 Eger E I. Nitrous oxide. New York: Elsevier, 1985
41 Robb H M, Asbury A J, Gray W M, Linkens D A. Towards a standardised anaesthetic state using enflurane and morphine. Br J Anaesth 1991; 66: 358–364
42 Schwilden H, Stoeckel H, Schüttler J. Closed-loop feedback control of propofol anaesthesia by quantitative EEG analysis in humans. Br J Anaesth 1989; 62: 290–296
43 Kenny G N C, MacFadzean W, Mantzaridis H, Fisher A C. Closed-loop control of anesthesia. Anesthesiology 1992; 77: 328A
44 Schüttler J, Kloos S, Schwilden H, Stoeckel H. Total intravenous anaesthesia with propofol and alfentanil by computer-assisted infusion. Anaesthesia 1988; 43 (suppl): 2–7
45 Neff W, Mayer E C, De La Luz A, Perales M. Nitrous oxide and oxygen anesthesia with curare relaxation. Californian Med 1947; 66: 67–69
46 Panca A L, Savage R T, Simpson S, Roy R C. Effect of pethidine, fentanyl and morphine on postoperative shivering in man. Acta Anaesthesiol Scand 1984; 28: 138–143
47 Bailey P L, Stanley T H. Narcotic intravenous anesthetics in anesthesia, 3rd edn. Miller R D (ed) New York: Churchill Livingstone, 1990: pp 281–366
48 Crile G W. Phylogenetic association in relation to certain medical problems. Boston Med Surg 1910; 163: 893–894
49 Lundy J S. Balanced anaesthesia. Minnesota Med 1926; 9: 399–404
50 Robbins B H. Cyclopropane anesthesia, 2nd edn. Baltimore: Williams & Wilkins, 1958
51 Taylor H E, Doerr J C, Gharib A. Effect of pre-anesthetic medication on ether content of arterial blood required for surgical anesthesia. Anesthesiology 1957; 18: 849–856
52 White D C, Dundas C R. Effect of anaesthetics on emission of light by luminous bacteria. Nature 1970; 266 : 456
53 Hall R I, Murphy M R, Hug C C Jr. The enflurane sparing effects of sufentanil in dogs. Anesthesiology 1987; 67: 518–525
54 Roizen M F, Horrigan R W, Fraser B M. Anesthetic doses blocking adrenergic (stress) and cardiovascular responses to incision MAC-BAR. Anesthesiology 1981; 54: 390–398
55 McQuay H J. Pre-emptive analgesia. Br J Anaesth 1991; 69: 1–3
56 Støen R, Sessler D I. The thermoregulatory threshold is inversely proportional to isoflurane concentration. Anesthesiology 1990; 72: 822–827
57 Sessler D I, Olofsson C I, Rubinstein E H et al. The thermoregulatory threshold in humans during anesthesia. Anesthesiology 1988; 68: 836–842
58 Eger E I II, Smith N T, Stoelting R K, Cullen D J, Kadis L B, Whitcher C E. Cardiovascular effects of halothane in man. Anesthesiology 1970; 32: 396–409
59 Stevens W C, Cromwell T H, Halsey M J, Eger E I II, Shakespeare T F, Bahlman S H. The cardiovascular effects of a new inhalation anesthetic, Forane, in human volunteers at constant arterial carbon dioxide tension. Anesthesiology 1971; 35: 8–16
60 Nunn J F. Applied respiratory physiology. London: Butterworths, 1977: p 181
61 Laubenthal H, Peter K, Haessler R. Fluid therapy. In: Nunn J F, Utting J K, Brown B R (eds) General anaesthesia, 5th edn. London: Butterworths, 1989; pp 549–650
62 Shires T, Williams J, Brown F. Acute changes in extracellular fluids associated with major surgical procedures. Ann Surg 1961; 154: 803–810
63 Moore F D, Ball M R. The metabolic response to surgery. Philadelphia: W B Saunders, 1952
64 Tingley A J, Hillman K M. The end of the crystalloid era? Anaesthesia 1985; 40: 860–871
65 Modig J. Effectiveness of Dextran 70 versus Ringer's acetate in traumatic shock and adult respiratory distress syndrome. Crit Care Med 1985; 14: 454–457

8. Anaesthesia and abdominal surgery

R. Ginsburg   L. Kaufman

LOWER ABDOMINAL SURGERY

Colonic surgery

Elective operations on the bowel are performed for malignancy, inflammatory bowel disease, diverticulitis, polyposis, Hirschsprung's disease, megacolon, volvulus and intestinal obstruction from malignancy or from previous surgery. Anaesthesia for large-bowel surgery has been reviewed on many occasions[1-3] and the most important aspects of the subject will be reviewed here.

Pre-operative preparation

In addition to routine investigations, attention should be paid to the fact that the bowel is prepared 1 or 2 days before surgery by purgation and this may result in loss of fluids and electrolytes, and occasionally renal failure. The presence of an ileostomy from previous surgery may lead to chronic water and salt depletion. Pre-existing electrolyte imbalance and low plasma protein concentrations, especially albumin, are not infrequent in Crohn's disease and there is often a large total body potassium deficit which is not reflected in the serum concentration.

Lung function in patients with inflammatory bowel disease may be compromised; Heatley et al[4] have demonstrated that 50% of patients have abnormal pulmonary function tests, 25% have a reduction in lung transfer factor and 6% have fibrosing alveolitis. It has also been found that many patients treated with broncho-alveolar lavage have a high lymphocyte count and an increase in dead space in the upper part of the lung.[5] Oedema of the nasopharynx and epiglottis, arytenoids and vocal cords has been reported as well as granulations on the trachea and bronchi, which appear to respond to steroid therapy.[6] Respiratory function may also be compromised by the presence of distended bowel from intestinal obstruction, megacolon or Hirschsprung's disease, resulting in elevation of the diaphragm with pulmonary collapse.

Chronic inflammatory bowel disease results in fibrosis of the intestines which may hinder absorption, including that of orally administered drugs. Disturbances of glucose metabolism, including insulin resistance, may occur in patients with colorectal carcinoma.[7] Villous adenomas of the rectum are reputed to cause a loss of potassium but it is estimated that this is only significant in 4% of patients. An additional hazard may be the prior administration of β-adrenergic blocking agents for the management of hypertension, which may cause constriction of the large bowel and mask the cardiovascular response to haemorrhage.

Premedication

Some authorities prefer the use of oral benzodiazepines, although others prefer to administer drugs by intramuscular injection, usually an opioid and an anticholinergic agent; the latter not only has antisialogogue properties but also inhibits gastro-intestinal activity during operation. For patients with diverticular disease, it has been suggested that morphine is contra-indicated because of the increase in intraluminal pressure;[8] indeed following resection of bowel the remaining colon can still exhibit an abnormal response to morphine.[9] A study of 80 patients failed to reveal an increased incidence of disruption of the intestinal anastomosis,[10] while other studies have demonstrated that increased intraluminal activity had little effect on the outcome of the anastomosis.[11] High-fibre diet has reduced the need for surgical treatment for diverticular disease.

Posture

Most operations on the right colon are performed with the patient in a supine position but those on the left colon, rectum and anal canal are performed with the patient in the Lloyd-Davies position which allows ready access to the abdomen and perineum, especially for low anterior resection and synchronous combined excision of the rectum. Steep Trendelenburg posture is no longer necessary and has in the past caused complications such as cerebral oedema and retinal haemorrhage. It may also make adequate ventilation more difficult, necessitating increased inspiratory pressure. The patient's arms are positioned by the sides, thus avoiding possible neuropathy associated with excessive arm abduction. Special attention should be paid to ensure that peripheral infusions are well-sited.

Some operations are performed using a transanal approach with the patient in the prone jack-knife position. This position may lead to serious respiratory embarrassment and depression of cardiac function unless the pelvis and chest are supported to allow free movement of the abdomen. Although the initial positioning of the patient may result in a significant decrease in cardiac index, this tends to return to previous levels following some degree of Trendelenburg tilt.[12]

Techniques

In the UK, most centres prefer general anaesthesia for colonic surgery and this involves the use of an intravenous induction agent, muscle relaxant and mechanical ventilation with nitrous oxide, oxygen and either inhaled or intravenous agents plus supplemental analgesic. The technique which has evolved over a period of 25 years in the management of over 5000 patients in our institutions includes etomidate and suxamethonium for anaesthetic induction, spraying the larynx and vocal cords with lignocaine, intubating the trachea with a sterile disposable tube and ventilating the lungs with nitrous oxide, oxygen and enflurane to near normocapnia. Muscle relaxation is obtained by the use of an initial bolus of atracurium 0.5 mg.kg^{-1} followed by increments or an infusion of atracurium according to the response to nerve stimulation. Analgesia is supplemented with intermittent doses of alfentanil, the initial dose being administered prior to the incision.

Alternatively, analgesia may be obtained by the use of extradural or intraspinal opioids which not only provide adequate analgesia but also attenuate the endocrine response to surgery as assessed by blood glucose, plasma cortisol, adrenocorticotrophic hormone and antidiuretic hormone.[13]

It is planned to administer the last dose of atracurium not less than 30 min before skin closure in an attempt to obviate the need for reversal of the muscle relaxant. Atropine is more effective than glycopyrrolate in inhibiting the gastro-intestinal effects of neostigmine.[14] However, there is little evidence that neostigmine influences the incidence of anastomotic breakdown in the colon. The endotracheal tube is left in situ until the patient's airway reflexes are completely restored and then oxygen is administered by a face-mask. While the patient is being transferred to the recovery area, Smith & Crul[15] have demonstrated that oxygen saturation can readily fall below 90% unless supplemental oxygen is administered at this time. There may be a place for administering oxygen for a few days postoperatively, as Rosenberg et al[16] have shown that there are many episodes of sudden desaturation and cardiac arrhythmias, even in the third postoperative day and this may be related to the loss of rapid eye movement sleep.[17]

Monitoring

Essential monitoring at operation includes electrocardiogram with rate meter, intermittent non-invasive blood pressure measurement, oxygen saturation, end-tidal carbon dioxide, oesophageal temperature and urinary output.

Two intravenous lines are set up — a peripheral line and a central line, usually inserted in the internal jugular vein to measure central venous pressure, which is kept between 5 and 7 cm H_2O. Intravenous fluids (initially compound sodium lactate) are administered through a heat-exchanger at the rate of 5–7 ml.kg^{-1}.h^{-1}. Losses of blood and plasma are replaced initially by colloids and, when necessary, by blood. Antibiotics are administered before surgery commences; these may include metronidazole and gentamicin, the latter being an aminoglycoside which can potentiate the action of competitive neuromuscular-blocking agents. Essential monitoring is continued in the postoperative period, care being taken to maintain body temperature with the possible use of a space blanket.

Postoperative care

Oral fluids are prohibited initially, and intravenous therapy is continued in the postoperative period. A stomach tube is not usually required, and fluid balance is maintained by intravenous infusion until bowel sounds are present. It is important to provide adequate pain relief. A number of regimens are suitable, but the authors favour the use of intrathecal diamorphine[13] or an intravenous infusion of morphine at the rate of 1–5 mg.h^{-1}, although an initial bolus dose may be required. There is some evidence that morphine increases the risk of anastomotic breakdown, and the use of pethidine may be preferable.[18]

Nausea and vomiting

The management of nausea and vomiting is not entirely satisfactory in that many of the traditionally used anti-emetics display side-effects involving the extrapyramidal system and also hypotension. This is because many of the traditionally used agents are dopamine antagonists and dopamine is a transmitter at many sites in the central nervous system (e.g. the basal ganglia). The serotonin antagonists appear to have a promising role in the control of postoperative nausea and vomiting.

Temperature

The physiology and pharmacology of sweating and thermoregulation during anaesthesia has been reviewed recently.[19] Hypothermia can occur readily during prolonged surgery and this may affect the elimination of muscle relaxants. However, another important consideration is postoperative shivering, which results in a marked increase in oxygen demand.[20] Normothermia decreases, but does not eliminate, protein breakdown and nitrogen loss following surgery.[21]

Cardiovascular complications

Untoward cardiovascular complications during operation may include hypotension and tachycardia due to blood loss tachycardia, sweating and hypertension due to inadequate analgesia and bradycardia, often associated with hypotension, due to traction on viscera resulting in stimulation of parasympathetic nerves; the bradycardia responds readily to intravenous atropine.

Comments on drugs and techniques

There are many techniques of anaesthesia for abdominal surgery and the reasons for those adopted by the authors are briefly summarized below. Etomidate is short-acting, maintains cardiovascular stability and suppresses the endocrine response to surgery reflected in cortisol concentrations. Suxamethonium allows easy intubation while enflurane and isoflurane preserve splanchnic blood flow better than halothane.[22] Atracurium is intermediate-acting and with careful timing does not require reversal with anticholinesterases. Mivacurium is shorter-acting than atracurium or vecuronium and may be the muscle relaxant of choice when the use of anticholinesterases is to be avoided.

The use of a central venous catheter allows not only the measurement of central venous pressure but also permits rapid transfusion to be instituted. Invasive techniques in the presence of anticoagulants must be undertaken with caution and therefore in these circumstances the internal jugular route may be preferred to that of the subclavian vein.

Usually a maintenance infusion of intravenous fluids administered at the rate of 5–7 ml.kg^{-1}.h^{-1} is adequate. If oliguria develops intra- or postoperatively, this is usually due to the release of antidiuretic hormone or to additional fluid losses. Other authorities[23] prefer a maintenance dose of 15 ml.kg^{-1}.h^{-1} Urinary output of 30 ml.h^{-1} appears to be satisfactory but should oliguria develop and fluid losses are corrected, a small dose of diuretic such as bumetanide 0.0075 mg.kg^{-1} intravenously often promotes a diuresis.[24] Alternatively, a small dose of frusemide (20 mg) usually promotes diuresis after a short delay; larger doses are unnecessary as the kidney is often refractory to a high initial dose.[25]

Spinal and extradural analgesia

Although not generally practised in the UK, the exponents of the technique maintain that it provides excellent operating conditions, reduces blood loss and inhibits the endocrine response to surgery, especially postoperative negative nitrogen balance.[26] However, in a series by Worsley et al,[27] some patients had to be transfused postoperatively, presumably for postoperative haemorrhage which might not have been evident during the period of hypotension; nevertheless, the need for transfusion was less than in patients who received general anaesthesia alone. Disadvantages of a spinal technique include hypoventilation in patients breathing spontaneously. Other causes of hypoventilation include the Lloyd-Davies and Trendelenburg positions and the use of intra-operative intravenous sedation.[28]

Surgical procedures in our institutions are often prolonged and the incision is usually extensive. To provide extensive sensory blockade with local analgesia extending from the xiphoid process to the perineum results in marked sympathetic blockade with consequent hypotension and an inability to respond to haemorrhage. However, an infusion of dopamine has been recommended to maintain blood pressure and splanchnic blood flow.[29] The use of anticoagulants, such as heparin, may preclude the use of extradural analgesia; there has been a recent case report of an epidural haematoma, even though the epidural catheter was inserted before the administration of heparin.[30]

An additional problem of spinal analgesia is that by inhibiting sympathetic activity, there is overactivity of the vagus, resulting in a reduction in the calibre of the bowel, especially the small intestine, which might interfere with the technical construction of the anastomosis. Bigler et al[31] reported a case of disruption of the colonic anastomosis, while Carlstedt et al[32] demonstrated that when epidural analgesia was supplemented with general anaesthesia and muscle relaxants, atropine often does not inhibit the increased bowel activity resulting from the use of neostigmine. The disadvantages of spinal and epidural analgesia may be more theoretical than real, but Worsley et al[27] were unable to demonstrate any advantage in terms of the incidence of anastomotic disruption.

Anxiety

It has often been assumed that anxious patients are at a disadvantage and that apprehension of the possible effects of surgery may be detrimental during surgery and in the postoperative period. Mindus[33] recommended the use of benzodiazepines and psychological preparation, but Salmon et al[34] demonstrated that anxious patients had a reduced response to the trauma of major surgery in the peri-operative and postoperative periods. Direct evidence was also provided, indicating that low pre-operative anxiety was associated with a greater endocrine response as assessed by plasma adrenaline and cortisol concentrations.[35] Further work on the influence of patient psychology on postoperative outcome is needed before any clear recommendations can be made concerning this issue.

Intestinal anastomoses

The integrity of intestinal anastomoses may be influenced by surgical technique, local factors, blood supply and anaesthesia.

The rate of anastomotic leak at one of our institutions (St Mark's hospital[36]) is 5% if the anastomosis is above the peritoneal reflection, 19% if it is below the reflection and 50% if there is a peri-anal anastomosis. Worsley et al[27] reported a dehiscence rate of 17%, irrespective of whether the patients had general or spinal analgesia, while Ryan et al[37] found their anastomotic breakdown rate to be 30%, maintaining that the factor responsible for this was epidural opioids administered in the postoperative period.

Infection and trauma increase the activity of collagenase, which might account for the absence of collagen at the site of the anastomosis.[38]

Bell & Lewis[39] and Bell[40] reported the hazards of neostigmine on intestinal anastomoses in patients with inflammatory bowel disease. Whitaker[41] also confirmed that neostigmine increased colonic activity but maintained that this was unlikely to disrupt the anastomosis by direct action, although there was decreased blood flow from contraction of the bowel. Wilkins et al[42] demonstrated that halothane abolished all intestinal activity despite the use of neostigmine, and when halothane was avoided, the increased activity resulting from neostigmine could be alleviated by ensuring that atropine was administered repeatedly to prevent bradycardia following neostigmine; intestinal activity was reflected in pulse rate, with bradycardia being associated with increased colonic activity. Provided that this precaution is taken, the possible hazards of neostigmine can be avoided, while drugs such as atracurium and mivacurium do not necessarily require reversal, thus minimizing the risk of anastomotic disruption. The use of morphine to provide analgesia in the postoperative period is associated with a significantly higher risk of anastomotic disruption than the administration of pethidine.

The danger of anastomotic leak is the occurrence of septic shock leading to peripheral vasodilatation, a reduction in left ventricular performance and damage to the pulmonary endothelial cells. The exact mechanism for the production of septic shock is still obscure, but it is now known that blood monocytes and tissue histiocytes secrete cytokines which result in an increase in tumour necrosis factor or cachectin, which may be responsible for many of the metabolic disturbances.[43] Monoclonal antibodies have been developed to treat gram-negative bacteraemia and septic shock associated with endotoxin but these have proved remarkably unsuccessful.[44,45]

Colonic blood flow

The splanchnic blood flow is of the order of 1500 ml.min^{-1}, which is approximately 25% of the cardiac output, while the blood volume in the splanchnic area is 20–25% of the total blood volume. Haemorrhage of 17% of the blood volume reduces the splanchnic blood flow by 40% without any obvious alteration in systemic blood pressure. Other studies show that a 10% decrease in blood volume, although producing very few changes in blood pressure and cardiac output, reduces colonic blood flow and oxygen delivery by 20%.[46] When the blood pressure falls below 50 mmHg, anastomotic leak rate increases.[47] Foster et al[48] confirmed that oxygen tension in the colon decreased significantly following 10% blood loss, and that tissue perfusion was important, particularly in the elderly.[49] Chou & Gallavan[50] found that an increase in blood flow had little effect on gut motility, but ischaemia and hypoxia produced prolonged paralysis. Increased intra-abdominal pressure also decreases the blood flow to abdominal viscera.[51]

Blood viscosity has been considered to be a factor affecting blood flow to the anastomosis and Tagart[52] reduced the incidence of anastomotic leak by ensuring that the haemoglobin concentration was less than 12.5 g.dl^{-1} before surgery. This was achieved by removing 1–2 units of blood before surgery started. Haemodilution was also thought to be beneficial by Mesh & Gewertz,[53] not only by decreasing the viscosity but also by increasing oxygen consumption. However, there was no compensatory increase in intestinal blood flow in anaemic patients. Hypothermia also decreases oxyen delivery to the intestine.[54] Hypocapnia significantly decreases colonic blood flow;[55] Winso et al[56] confirmed that there was an increase in intestinal vascular resistance associated with hyperventilation. Oxygen tension and pH at the site of the anastomosis are also important in that if tissue oxygen tension in the anastomotic area is above 7.3 kPa (55 mmHg), the leak rate is about 10% whereas if it falls below 3.3 kPa, the rate is almost 100%.[57] Schiedler et al[58] found that if the intramural pH was greater than 7.21 there was little likelihood of ischaemic colitis developing.

Since there are so many variables potentially at work, it is often impossible to pinpoint an exact cause of anastomotic leak. Although morphine increases colonic tone, it also increases splanchnic blood flow by 20%.[59] Andreen[60] concluded that anaesthesia may have some effect on the splanchnic and hepatic circulation, but it may only be of importance when the blood supply to the anastomosis is critical. Studies on blood flow to the colon are confined to total blood flow, whereas the important layer to be considered is the submuscosal layer. The blood flow of the submucosal layer is approximately 20 times that of the muscular layer.[61] Anaesthesia and surgery can cause marked alterations in gut blood flow, but neither surgery nor anaesthesia appears to cause reversal of flow from the submucosal layer.[62] Although many of the inhaled anaesthetic agents do affect mesenteric blood flow, Gelman[63] concluded that surgical procedure and not anaesthesia was the biggest factor in causing the reduction. Halothane increases splanchnic vascular resistance, as does isoflurane[64] but to a lesser extent; enflurane may be the preferred agent.[63] Fentanyl also decreases mesenteric blood flow.

Banks et al[65] summarized many of the factors that affect the mesenteric circulation indicating that H_1- and H_2-receptors are involved, as well as α- and β_2-receptors. Haemorrhage, pain, acidosis and hypothermia increase splanchnic vascular resistance slightly. During hypotension the increase in splanchnic vascular resistance may be 13 times greater than that in the peripheral circulation. Other vasoconstrictors of the mesenteric circulation are vasopressin and angiotensin II. Vasopressin antagonists are being developed but their use is still speculative.[66,67]

Postoperative ileus

Many authorities maintain that paralysis of the gut occurs following most abdominal operations but neither the duration nor the extent of the operation influences the duration of postoperative ileus. Morphine has been implicated but has not been found to affect the duration of ileus.[68] Halothane and enflurane inhibit colonic activity but normal function returns when they are discontinued, while nitrous oxide has little or no effect on contraction of the colon.[69] It has also been maintained that postoperative ileus is a result of increased sympathetic activity; bowel function appears to recover more quickly following epidural analgesia.[70,71] It has been suggested that nitrous oxide may cause intestinal distension; Scheinin et al[72] recommended the use of air instead of nitrous oxide because air not only provided better operating conditions, but also resulted in an earlier resumption of bowel function. Early ambulation is believed to reduce the duration of postoperative ileus, but this has not been confirmed.[73] Catchpole[74] found that lower abdominal operations often resulted in autonomic denervation in the remaining colon and this was another factor which promoted postoperative ileus.

Emergency surgery

In this situation, the anaesthetist may have to deal with a patient who is in circulatory collapse due to dehydration and electrolyte imbalance. The recent Confidential Enquiry into Perioperative Deaths[75] showed that mortality associated with emergency surgery is directly related to inadequate pre-operative correction of fluid and electrolyte imbalances. In addition, abdominal distension may increase abdominal pressure and decrease venous return to the heart. Prolonged vomiting leads to alkalosis, although with inadequate perfusion, metabolic acidosis may ensue. The stomach should be aspirated by nasogastric tube, although this does not always guarantee that the stomach is empty. Pain, morphine and peritoneal irritation are some of the factors involved in delayed emptying of the gastrointestinal tract. In emergency situations with a full stomach, the use of anti-emetics and H_2-antagonists, such as ranitidine, are of little value. If inhalation of gastric contents is suspected, then treatment with tracheal aspiration, bronchial lavage with saline and intravenous administration of hydrocortisone and antibiotics should be instituted immediately. Inhalation of gastric contents results in an immediate fall of Pa_{O_2} and it may be necessary to employ ventilation with a high inspired oxygen concentration.

Care should therefore be taken to prevent regurgitation or vomiting leading to inhalation of gastric contents into the tracheobronchial tract. Techniques favoured include a rapid sequence induction using thiopentone and suxamethonium, with cricoid pressure applied almost as soon as the drugs are given. It must also be remembered that inhalation of gastric contents may occur prior to induction of anaesthesia in debilitated patients. Emergency surgery is often performed for perforated ulcer, acute intestinal obstruction or burst abdomen; burst abdomen is a particularly dangerous situation in that the patient may be relatively well but may have eaten recently.

An alternative technique is to intubate the trachea under local analgesia with 2% lignocaine applied to the piriform fossae; this anaesthetizes the internal laryngeal nerve which supplies the larynx to the level of the vocal cords. Lignocaine may also be applied to the back of the tongue and pharynx, and intubation performed under direct vision.

Postoperative pulmonary function

Respiratory function is often depressed immediately after abdominal surgery as there is a reduction not only in diaphragmatic activity but also in that of the abdominal muscles.[76] Dureuil et al[77] have confirmed that respiratory function is depressed, particularly after upper abdominal surgery, and there was a marked reduction in vital capacity. Scott & Kehlet[78] also confirmed that regional anaesthetic techniques reduced morbidity when the surgical procedure was below the umbilicus but evidence was less convincing for upper abdominal surgery.

Lawrence et al[79] reported that the American Society of Anesthesiologists (ASA) classification failed to identify the risk factors associated with postoperative pulmonary complications. Vodinh et al[80] have stressed the importance of pre-operative spirometry and blood gas analysis. Incentive spirometry has been singularly disappointing in improving diaphragmatic movement postoperatively,[81] but Hall et al[82] reported that incentive spirometry and chest physiotherapy produced comparable results. Roukema et al[83] have found that breathing exercises decrease postoperative complications only in patients with normal lung function. Vodinh et al[80] reported that the only pre-operative risk factors that could be identified were a reduction in the ratio of forced expiratory volume in 1 s to forced vital capacity (FEV_1/FVC) and Pa_{O_2}. Poe et al[84] confirmed that a reduction in FEV_1 was the only indicator of prolonged hospitalization and noted that smoking, old age and obesity did not appear to increase postoperative pulmonary complications. Claims that adequate pain relief reduce pulmonary complications have not been confirmed by Jayr et al,[85] who reported that epidural analgesia with bupivacaine and morphine improved postoperative comfort, but when compared with the control group, the postoperative Pa_{O_2} and spirometric studies were similar.

Upper abdominal surgery reduces functional residual capacity by 30% and this reduction lasts for a week postoperatively. Postoperative hypoxaemia may be due to hypoventilation, intrapulmonary shunt, reduced cardiac output and increased oxygen consumption related to shivering. There may be decreased alveolar ventilation, atelectasis and interstitial lung oedema.[86] Hedenstierna[87] noted that there was a reduction of perfusion of blood through the atelectic zone and this is the major cause of impaired gas exchange. Jones et al[88] confirmed that postoperative hypoxaemia was due to impaired gas exchange during operation and in the postoperative period, and suggested that this might be related to the tone in the bronchi and chest wall as well as vasomotor activity. Patients treated with opioid analgesics suffer episodes of obstructive apnoea during sleep. Prolonged postoperative hypoxaemia may become more apparent with the routine use of continuous monitoring with an oximeter (e.g. see Rosenberg et al[16]).

Chest physiotherapy, as already mentioned, appears to be more successful in patients with normal preoperative lung function and there are limitations to the use of percussion and vibration techniques. Selsby & Jones[89] (see also Hull & Jones[90]) commented favourably on the forced expiratory technique with postural drainage, but one of the disadvantages was that it could also cause bronchospasm and hypoxaemia. Jansen et al[91] have advocated the infusion of doxapram for 6 h postoperatively, repeated if necessary; this led to a reduction in postoperative pulmonary complications and an increase in Pa_{O_2}.

Endocrine response to surgery

Despite recent advances in anaesthesia, most general anaesthetic agents fail to suppress the endocrine response to surgical stimulation. Although it is claimed that these responses are beneficial, there is an increased catecholamine release resulting in increases in cardiac output and oxygen requirements. There is an outpouring of cortisol, adrenocorticotrophic hormone, growth hormone, aldosterone and antidiuretic hormone. There are high levels of blood sugar and the action of insulin is suppressed. Even after an exploratory laparotomy there is protein loss resulting in negative nitrogen balance; up to 500 g of muscle protein may be lost in the process, which Stoner[92] has described as 'autocannabalism'. The outpouring of hormones is well beyond that required to maintain homeostasis; the levels of antidiuretic hormone rise 10-fold, much more than that required to produce a maximum antidiuresis. In addition, the raised levels of antidiuretic hormone result in vasoconstriction, which may affect the splanchnic circulation. Various techniques have been employed to suppress such responses to surgery; these include high-dose opioids and extradural analgesia, the latter being less effective for surgery in the upper abdomen. Another disadvantage of this technique is that, even if the response to surgical stimulation is attenuated, it is effective only during the duration of the extradural blockade.[93]

Metastases

Many factors affect the spread of metastases and the recurrence of carcinoma. It has been suggested that anaesthesia might be implicated, as it suppresses the immune response. However, there are many variables, such as the effect of malignancy on plasminogen activator activity, which may make it easier for secondary tumour cells to lodge in the blood vessels of a particular organ.[94] Blood loss itself has been implicated in the recurrence of carcinoma of the colon. Singh et al[95] also thought that blood loss may affect the growth of established metastases. Stephenson et al[96] found that transfusion of over 11 units of blood carried an unfavourable prognosis, although it is difficult to know whether malignancy was so far advanced that large amounts of blood were required to control massive haemorrhage or that blood itself was a factor. Crowson et al[97] were unable to substantiate the finding that the recurrence rate or the incidence of metastasis was influenced by blood transfusion, but Lawrance et al[98] found that in experimental animals, platelets from the blood that leaks into the peritoneal cavity released growth factors which enhance the recurrence of local malignancy.

Spinal opioids

The use of opioids injected either intrathecally or into the epidural space is particularly useful in the management of patients who have undergone major abdominal surgery. These techniques provide excellent analgesia, including relief of visceral pain, and attenuate the endocrine response to surgery.[13,99]

UPPER ABDOMINAL SURGERY

Gastrectomy

The nature of gastric surgery has changed markedly in recent times with the advent of H_2-receptor blocking drugs and the recognition of the role of *Helicobacter pylori* in the recurrence of peptic ulceration. More emphasis is now paid to the medical management of peptic ulcers, and gastric surgery is more commonly reserved for acute gastric haemorrhage or for gastric carcinoma. Gastrectomy for bleeding gastric ulcer is more common in high-risk, elderly patients, and the procedure carries a high morbidity, and a mortality rate in excess of 20%.[100] Management of patients undergoing gastrectomy for bleeding differs substantially from that of patients who require the procedure for carcinoma.

Gastrectomy for bleeding requires prompt correction of hypovolaemia, as shock is a major risk factor in mortality. Initially, the adequacy of volume replacement can be assessed by pulse rate and blood pressure estimation alone. However, evidence of pre-existing cardiovascular disease necessitates direct measurement of central venous and arterial pressures, since overtransfusion can be as dangerous as untreated shock. Induction of anaesthesia invariably requires preoxygenation and a rapid-sequence induction. During maintenance of anaesthesia, volume replacement must be judged carefully in order to avoid hypotension. Dopamine may be required to preserve renal function and urine output should be monitored closely. The patient's temperature should be measured and the risk of hypothermia reduced by warming intravenous fluids and using a heated mattress. The high peri-operative morbidity and mortality associated with gastrectomy for haemorrhage warrant special care postoperatively, either in an intensive care unit or specialist high-dependency unit.

Patients presenting for gastrectomy for carcinoma are likely to be elderly, may give a history of weight loss and may be in poor physical condition. The nature of the elective surgery permits careful pre-operative assessment, particularly of cardiac and respiratory systems: these patients frequently have a history of heavy smoking. Anaemia, due to chronic blood loss from the tumour, should be corrected and if the patient is particularly cachectic, parenteral feeding may be indicated pre-operatively, via a tunnelled feeding line. The choice of anaesthetic technique is a matter of personal preference; however, a combination of light general anaesthesia and relaxant with regional extradural blockade provides good surgical conditions and effective postoperative analgesia. If a large resection is anticipated, invasive monitoring is required and a careful account must be taken of blood loss. Hypotension may also ensue from traction on the coeliac plexus and is often associated with bradycardia.

Pancreatic surgery

With the exception of drainage of pancreatic cysts, surgery to the pancreas is often major and time-consuming. Drainage of a pancreatic cyst may be required after an attack of pancreatitis and may be performed against a background of sepsis, hyperglycaemia and hypocalcaemia, all of which should be treated adequately prior to surgery. These problems aside, drainage of a pancreatic cyst can be managed like any other upper abdominal procedure.

Carcinoma of the head of pancreas eventually causes a progressive and deepening obstructive jaundice, with weight loss, pain and coagulation abnormalities from lack of vitamin K-dependent clotting factors. Surgical resection by pancreaticoduodenectomy (Whipple's procedure) is a major surgical procedure which requires full invasive monitoring and adequate venous access to allow aggressive correction of blood loss, as well as electrolyte and coagulation abnormalities. Full pre-operative assessment is required with comprehensive assessment of the cardiorespiratory system. Vitamin K may be required to correct coagulation abnormalities. Pain control is particularly important after this procedure. The duration of surgery and the potential severity of pain in the postoperative period render regional analgesia almost obligatory. Extradural blockade with a local anaesthetic followed by opioids — either by bolus or by continuous infusion — provides the most satisfactory management.

Hepatic surgery

Surgical resection of liver abscesses and cysts has been performed for many years. As techniques of liver surgery progress, a number of conditions, formerly considered inoperable, have become amenable to resection of either a lobe or segment of liver (Table 8.1). Included are solitary primary tumours and liver metastases from colorectal cancer, where patients otherwise have a median survival of 10–15 months.[101] Surgical resection of liver metastases can improve survival[102,103] and may be performed if there has been no extra-hepatic spread of tumour. This is a realistic expectation

Table 8.1 Conditions potentially amenable to surgical resection of the liver

Primary tumour
Hepatocellular carcinoma
(80% of primary tumours)

Cholangiocellular carcinoma

Metastases
Colorectal carcinoma

Carcinoid

Infections
Abscesses — protozoal

Hydatid cyst

in the early progress of colorectal tumours only, where seeding is via the portal circulation alone. Improvements in anaesthetic technique and in the understanding of the mechanisms of coagulation have enabled more hazardous procedures, such as resection of tumours in cirrhotic patients, to be performed with greater safety.

Surgical considerations

Scrupulous attention to surgical technique is of paramount importance in limiting blood loss from exposed liver parenchyma. In addition, surgeons may employ various manoeuvres to render the liver safely avascular. These include intermittent clamping of the portal tract, with or without clamping of the supra- and infra hepatic inferior vena cava, or total vascular isolation, with cooling of the liver and venovenous bypass. Veno-venous bypass should be encouraged when inferior vena cava cross-clamping is used, as it permits venous drainage from the portal tract and lower half of the body, preserving renal function and cardiovascular stability, by facilitating return of blood to the heart via the axillary vein.

Even if hepatic vascular isolation is not employed, caval compression from surgical manipulation of the liver can reduce venous return to the heart and thus precipitate wide fluctuations in cardiac output and, hence, changes in blood pressure.

Anaesthetic considerations

While many patients who undergo hepatic resection present for surgery in good health, those with co-existing cirrhosis may present in a poor nutritional condition, with jaundice, coagulopathy, sepsis and renal impairment. Coagulopathy, if present, should be treated aggressively with fresh frozen plasma and platelets as necessary, the aim being to reduce the International Normalized Ratio (prothrombin ratio) to less than 2.0 prior to surgery. Sepsis of any kind must be treated with the utmost vigour, because intra-abdominal sepsis is a frequent postoperative complication of hepatic resection.[104] Renal impairment can be troublesome, particularly if the patient requires blood products for correction of a coagulopathy. Plasma exchange, using plasmapheresis against fresh frozen plasma, can be useful in this situation.[105]

Induction and maintenance of general anaesthesia can, to a large extent, be left to personal preference. However, a number of points should be borne in mind. First, some authorities advocate that nitrous oxide should be avoided if possible; if the surgical procedure is lengthy, prolonged exposure may cause gaseous bowel distension. Second, neuromuscular blockade should preferably be provided by continuous infusion, because acute blood loss accompanied by large transfusions of bank blood may cause fluctuations in the plasma concentration of muscle relaxant administered by bolus dose. Muscle relaxation may therefore prove variable, especially if there are changes in blood pH. Third, the muscle relaxant used should not have to rely upon the hepatic route for clearance; atracurium may be useful in this context. Regional anaesthesia may be useful in hepatic resection, particularly with regard to analgesia in the postoperative period, but care must be exercised in the presence of disturbances of coagulation.

The successful intra-operative anaesthetic management of a patient undergoing hepatic resection rests heavily upon the prompt and appropriate replacement of blood loss. Prompt replacement demands both good venous access and an effective method of rapid infusion. Accurate assessment of blood loss is vital, so frequent estimation should be made of swab and sucker loss together with continuous measurement of intravascular pressures. At the very least, these should include arterial and central venous pressures, and pulmonary capillary wedge pressure if possible. If much blood loss is anticipated, for example if the patient has undergone previous right upper quadrant abdominal surgery, then a 'cell-saver' may be necessary, so that autologous blood may be transfused.[106]

Appropriate blood replacement necessitates the closest possible scrutiny of coagulation status, with aggressive correction of dilutional decreases in platelet and clotting factor concentrations. Hypothermia, liver hypoperfusion and release of necrotic liver-tissue debris into the circulation, following surgical manipulation or de-clamping, may initiate tissue plasminogen activator-mediated disseminated intravascular coagulopathy (DIC) or fibrinolysis. Recognition of DIC may be difficult in the presence of massive blood transfusion, but a rapid decrease in platelet concentration, and laboratory assay of coagulation factors and degradation products, may aid diagnosis. DIC should be treated by platelet transfusion together with administration of cryoprecipitate and fresh frozen plasma as necessary.

Much useful information on coagulation status may be obtained from the thrombo-elastograph,[107] which is small enough to be kept in the operating theatre, and cheap and simple to operate. The device tests the mechanical characteristics of blood coagulum and produces a graphical display over the period of clot formation. From this, an assessment of platelet/coagulation function and fibrinolysis may be made. Aprotinin has been shown to be useful in the management of tissue plasminogen activator-mediated fibrinolysis.[108,109]

Other facets of massive blood transfusion may require careful supervision. Citrate-induced hypocalcaemia should be corrected with calcium chloride, while body temperature should be maintained by use of a warming mattress and limb-swaddling; normal coagulation depends upon the maintenance of body temperature. In general, metabolic acidosis need not be corrected, except in the face of renal impairment, because massive transfusion is invariably followed by a metabolic alkalosis. Renal function should be protected by the administration of mannitol at the start of surgery and a continuous infusion of a renal dose of dopamine.[110,111]

Splenectomy

Splenectomy may be performed in the management of thrombocytopenia or following blunt trauma. Strenuous efforts are often made to preserve the damaged spleen, by repairing tears or performing a partial excision, as evidence has accumulated that resistance to encapsulated organisms, such as *Pneumococcus* or *Haemophilus influenzae*, can decrease following the procedure.

Patients undergoing splenectomy for haematological reasons may have had numerous, sustained spontaneous bleeds and received high-dose corticosteroids. If so, steroids and antibiotics may be required pre-operatively, as may pneumococcal vaccine after surgery. Platelet transfusion will be required to cover surgery if the platelet count has fallen below $40–50 \times 10^9 \, l^{-1}$, although some would advise delaying administration until the splenic artery has been clamped. Naturally, good venous access is mandatory, although this may be difficult via a peripheral vein if the patient has had a prolonged hospital stay. Extreme care should be taken

GALLBLADDER AND BILIARY SURGERY

Cholecystectomy

Cholecystectomy is not only an effective treatment for troublesome gallstones, but also prevents their reformation. If poorly managed, it may be associated with considerable morbidity and a lengthy inpatient stay postoperatively. As a result, a number of alternative treatments for gallstones have been sought. These include various types of dissolution therapy, lithotripsy and laparoscopic cholecystectomy.

The anaesthetic management of cholecystectomy differs little from other upper abdominal surgical procedures and it should present no special problems. Patients are often characterized as being obese, but this is by no means invariable. Surgeons formerly employed Kocher's approach, the incision being below and parallel to the costal margin. However, this was associated with considerable postoperative pain and has fallen into disfavour. Right transverse, median or upper right paramedian incisions are now more common. Surgical access may be improved by introducing a nasogastric tube and emptying the stomach of air. Most surgeons undertake a peroperative cholangiogram to identify the presence of stones in the common bile duct and to confirm the patency of the ampulla of Vater.

Pre- and postoperative analgesia may be difficult in a patient with cholelithiasis, as any opioid which possesses a pure agonist action is capable of inducing spasm in the biliary tract and sphincter of Oddi. Morphine, fentanyl and pethidine are all guilty in this respect but, the effect of pethidine may be less than that of morphine, so it may be used as a premedicant and as a postoperative analgesic. Spasm can be reversed by naloxone, papaverine, nitroglycerine or glucagon. Opioids may prove most useful when given by the epidural route, providing both good operating conditions and effective postoperative analgesia. Plasma concentrations of morphine after epidural administration are low, and unlikely to affect the biliary tract. Naturally, a clotting profile should be checked before using this technique. Some maintain that morphine should be avoided, even in patients who have had a cholecystectomy, as it is still capable of causing spasm of the sphincter of Oddi; this causes an increase in intrabiliary pressure resulting in pain, presumably as a result of stretching of the capsule of the liver.[112]

Lithotripsy

Lithotripsy was originally developed for the treatment of renal calculi, which are shattered by a focused mechancial shockwave. The original technique was painful and required the patient to be anaesthetized, either by epidural or general anaesthesia, and immersed in a water bath for the duration of the procedure. Lithotripsy has been adapted for the treatment of gallstones and technical aspects have been refined almost to the extent that the treatment can be pain-free. While doubt exists as to the long-term efficacy of the treatment in the young, it is undoubtedly of great benefit to the elderly and less fit.

Laparoscopic cholecystectomy

This has become the subject of considerable interest because, in suitable subjects, it allows an appreciable reduction in peri-operative morbidity and postoperative inpatient stay, compared with traditional surgical cholecystectomy. The laparoscope is inserted via a peri-umbilical incision following inflation of the abdominal cavity with carbon dioxide. Three other narrow-bore instruments are then introduced into the peritoneal cavity through the abdominal wall for diathermy, tissue retraction and suction or lavage. In order to obtain good operative access, distension of the abdominal wall must be maintained by continuous insufflation of carbon dioxide and the patient is usually tilted to the left and positioned head-up. These manoeuvres ensure that abdominal contents fall away from the operative site. Video monitors are usually positioned on both sides of the patient to allow both the surgeon and assistants to view the procedure via the laparoscope camera.

From the anaesthetic point of view, the procedure should be confined to patients with an ASA grade of I or II, as a head-up tilt and high intra-abdominal pressure for 2 or more hours require that the patient has a robust cardiovascular system. Good muscle relaxation is required to facilitate surgical access and to permit the gallbladder to be removed via the peri-umbilical wound at the end of the procedure. A nasogastric tube is mandatory, in order that the stomach may be emptied. Monitoring should include non-invasive blood pressure measurement, a peripheral nerve stimulator and pulse oximetry (an ear probe may prove useful, as a finger probe is more likely to be displaced by the surgeon). In addition, end-tidal carbon dioxide concentration should be monitored to ensure that the lungs are adequately ventilated. Hypotension may be avoided by preloading the patient with 500 ml of colloid solution and, if necessary, can be treated with ephedrine.

Biliary reconstruction and drainage

Occasionally, gallbladder surgery can result in damage to the common bile duct, necessitating specialist reconstructive surgery. Biliary reconstruction may also be required in congenital biliary atresia and following pancreatic disease or liver transplantation. Reconstruction is undertaken to allow the biliary tree to drain freely into the gut and the procedure may involve the isolation and mobilization of a loop of small bowel, so that it can be hitched up and sutured to a shortened common bile duct. Invariably, patients have suffered recurrent bouts of cholangitis, sepsis or obstructive jaundice in the past. They may therefore be malnourished and frail. Anaesthetic management centres on the care of a chronically sick patient undergoing a potentially lengthy procedure. Particular attention should be paid to temperature homeostasis, fluid replacement and urine output, and a coagulation profile should be undertaken if there has been a history of jaundice. Monitoring should be invasive and should include arterial and central venous cannulation.

PHAEOCHROMOCYTOMA

Phaeochromocytoma is a rare condition, but is associated with a high mortality rate if the condition is not suspected prior to surgery. The occurrence of hypertension and arrhythmias during surgical operation may suggest the diagnosis. It is said that 10% of tumours are bilateral and 10% are malignant; it must be remembered that other tumours, such as ganglioneuromas and neuroblastomas, are capable of secreting pressor amines.

If the phaeochromocytoma is located in the adrenal gland, then adrenaline and noradrenaline are secreted; tumours in extra-adrenal sites contain mostly noradrenaline. The diagnosis may be made on the basis of a history of syncope, sweating and fainting. The urine may contain excess concentrations of catecholamine metabolites. The diagnosis can now be confirmed using non-invasive techniques. Clonidine, an α_2-agonist, effectively suppresses the plasma concentrations of adrenaline and noraderenaline in essential hypertension, but is ineffective in patients with phaeochromocytoma.[113]

The management of operation is still based on that designed by Ross et al,[114] who advocated the use of pre-operative α-blockade with phenoxybenzamine and the use of β-adrenergic blocking drugs to control tachycardia or persistent ventricular arrhythmias. A number of standard anaesthetic agents have adverse effects at operation and drugs such as atropine and pancuronium, which cause tachycardia, should be avoided. The management of these patients was particularly difficult in a series reported by Ross et al,[114] as in 1967 invasive monitoring was not routine, but now close monitoring is essential and should include electrocardiogram, intra-arterial blood pressure, as well as central venous pressure measurement. During manipulation of the tumour, plasma concentrations of noradrenaline and adrenaline may increase 600-fold.

Other drugs which have been advocated to control blood pressure at operation include prazosin when the tumour is extra-adrenal and also labetalol, although its β-adrenergic action may be a disadvantage. Sodium nitroprusside is also of value in controlling violent fluctuations of blood pressure.

If adequate control of blood pressure has been achieved pre-operatively, there is seldom a need to administer noradrenaline following the removal of tumour. Hypotension may be due to haemorrhage, adrenal failure, inadequate transfusion and the possibility that the adrenergic-blocking agents are still effective. Claims that there is a reduced circulatory blood volume in phaeochromocytoma have not been confirmed.[115-117] Delayed recovery following operation may be due to hypoglycaemia as high concentrations of catecholamines inhibit the action of insulin and, when the tumour is removed, hypoglycaemia may ensue. Care must be taken in the use of intravenous naloxone, which results in an increased level of catecholamines in patients with phaeochromocytoma.[118]

CARCINOID SYNDROME

This syndrome is characterized by vasomotor, gastrointestinal and cardiorespiratory symptoms. The vasomotor symptoms are flushing of the face and neck, while the gastro-intestinal symptoms include diarrhoea and, if there are metastases, pain, hepatomegaly and ascites. Cardiorespiratory symptoms include hypertension, tachycardia, right-sided heart failure, oedema and bronchospasm. Serotonin is said to be responsible for the bronchoconstriction, pulmonary fibrosis and cardiac lesions, while the vasodilatation is due to kinins and prostaglandins. The diagnosis is often made on the basis of increased concentrations of 5-hydroxyindole acetic acid in the urine.

The management of these patients is difficult because it is no longer believed that serotonin is the sole hormone involved and the patient is often asymptomatic unless there are widespread metastases, especially in the liver. Symptomatic treatment is often with methysergide, cyproheptadine and ketanserin. Somatostatin, a growth hormone release-inhibiting factor, can reduce blood concentrations of serotonin and is successful in the management of patients during a crisis at operation.[119,120] Roy et al[121] found that the analogue octreotide reduced plasma concentrations of serotonin and that anaesthesia during resection of the liver was uneventful. Somatostatin appears to control flushing, diarrhoea and wheezing, prevented the release of active substances, and also blocked the peripheral action.[122] Serotonin is usually destroyed in the liver by amine oxidase and symptoms only arise when the liver cannot handle the excess of serotonin. Aprotinin has been advocated to suppress the secretion of bradykinins. At operation, hypertension and bronchospasm may occur. Morphine is avoided because it can release serotonin and most authorities recommend the use of pancuronium.

REFERENCES

1. Kaufman L. Anaesthesia in abdominal surgery. In: Nunn, JF Gray TC, eds. General anaesthesia, 4th edn. London: Butterworths, 1978: pp 1432–1452
2. Kaufman L, Anaesthesia for large bowel surgery: a review. J R Soc Med 1983; 76: 693–696
3. Aitkenhead AR. Anaesthesia and the gastro-intestinal system. Eur J Anaesth 1988; 5: 73–112
4. Heatley RV, Thomas P, Prokipchuk EJ, Gauldie J, Sieniewicz DJ, Bienenstock G. Pulmonary function abnormalities in patients with inflammatory bowel disease. Q J Med 1982; 203: 241–250
5. Bonniere P, Wallaert B, Cortot A et al. Latent pulmonary involvement in Crohn's disease: biological, functional, bronchoalveolar lavage and scintigraphic studies. Gut 1986; 27: 919–925
6. Lemann M, Messing B, D'Agay F, Modigliani R. Crohn's disease with respiratory tract involvement. Gut 1987; 28: 1669–1672
7. Copeland GP, Leinster SJ, Davis JC, Hipkin LJ. Insulin resistance in patients with colorectal cancer. Br J Surg 1987; 74: 1031–1036
8. Painter NS, Truelove SC. Intra-luminal pressure patterns in diverticulosis of the colon. Gut 1964; 5: 201–213, 365–373
9. Parks TG. Rectal and colonic studies after resection of the sigmoid for diverticular disease. Gut 1970; 11: 121–125
10. Sangwan S. Personal communication, 1985
11. Burkitt DS, Donovan IA. Intraluminal pressure adjacent to left colonic anastomoses. Br J Surg 1990; 77: 1288–1290
12. Hatada T, Kusunoki M, Sakiyama T et al. Hemodynamics in the prone jackknife position during surgery. Am J Surg 1991; 162: 55–58
13. Kaufman L. Intraspinal diamorphine: epidural and intrathecal. In: Scott DB, ed. Diamorphine — its chemistry, pharmacology and clinical use. London: Woodhead-Faulkner, 1988: pp 82–96
14. Child C. Glycopyrrolate and the bowel. Anaesthesia 1984; 39: 495
15. Smith DC, Crul JF. Early postoperative hypoxia during transport. Br J Anaesth 1988; 61: 625–627
16. Rosenberg J, Dirkes WE, Kehlet H. Episodic arterial oxygen desaturation and heart rate variations following major abdominal surgery. Br J Anaesth 1989; 63: 651–654
17. Knill RL, Moote CA, Skinner MI, Rose EA. Anesthesia with abdominal surgery leads to intense REM sleep during the first postoperative week. Anesthesiology 1990; 73: 52–61
18. Aitkenhead AR, Robinson S. Influence of morphine and pethidine on the incidence of anastomotic dehiscence after colonic surgery. Br J Anaesth 1989; 63: 230p–231p
19. Martin CS, Asbury A. Sweating and thermoregulation in anaesthesia: a review of the physiology and pharmacology and their relationship to anasthesia. In: Kaufman, L ed. Anaesthesia review 8. London: Churchill Livingstone, 1991: pp 139–158
20. Leading article. Perioperative shivering. Lancet 1991; 338: 547–548
21. Carli F, Emery PW, Freemantle CAJ. Effect of perioperative normothermia on postoperative protein metabolism in elderly patients undergoing hip arthroplasty. Br J Anaesth 1989; 63: 276–282
22. Gelman S. Halothane hepaotoxicity — again? Anesth Analg 1986; 65: 831–834
23. Campbell IT, Baxter JN, Tweedie IE, Taylor GT, Keens SJ. I.V. fluids during surgery. Br J Anaesth 1990; 65: 726–729
24. Kaufman L, Bailey PM. Intravenous bumetanide attenuates the rise in plasma vasopressin concentrations during major surgical operations. Br J Clin Pharmacol 1987; 23: 237–240
25. Noormohamed FH, Lant AF Analysis of the natriuretic action of a loop diuretic, piretanide, in man. Br J Clin Pharmacol 1991; 31: 463–469
26. Vedrinne C, Vedrinne JM Guiraud M et al. Nitrogen-sparing effect of epidural administration of local anesthetics in colon surgery. Anesth Analg 1989; 69: 354–359
27. Worsley MH, Wishart HY, Aitkenhead AR. High spinal nerve block for large bowel anastomosis. Br J Anaesth 1988; 60: 836–840
28. Caplan RA, Ward RJ, Posner K, Chency FW. Unexpected cardiac arrest during spinal anaesthesia: a closed claims analysis of predisposing factors. Anesthesiology 1988; 68: 5–11
29. Lundberg J, Biber B, Delbro D et al. Effects of dopamine on intestinal haemodynamics and motility during epidural analgesia in the cat. Acta Anaesthesiol Scand 1989; 33: 487–493
30. Tekkok IH, Cataltepe O, Tahta K, Bertan V. Extradural haematoma after continuous extradural anaesthesia. Br J Anaesth 1991; 67: 112–115

31 Bigler D, Hjortso NC, Kehlet H. Disruption of colonic anastomosis during continuous epidural analgesia — an early postoperative complication. Anaesthesia 1985; 40: 278–280

32 Carlstedt A, Nordgren S, Fasth S, Appelgren L, Hulten L. Epidural anaesthesia and postoperative colorectal motility — a possible hazard to a colorectal anastomosis. Int J Colorect Dis 1989; 4: 144–149

33 Mindus P. Anxiety, pain and sedation: some psychiatric aspects. Acta Anaesthesiol Scand 1987; 32 (suppl 88): 7–12

34 Salmon P, Pearce S, Smith CCT et al. Anxiety, type A personality and endocrine response to surgery. Br J Clin Psychol 1989; 28: 279–280

35 Salmon P, Kaufman L. Preoperative anxiety and endocrine response to surgery. Lancet 1990; 335: 1340

36 Ritchie J. Personal communication, 1983

37 Ryan P, Scvhweitzer S. Combined epidural and general anesthesia versus general anesthesia in patients having colon and rectal anastomoses. Acta Chir Scand 1989 (suppl 550): 146–151

38 Hawley PR. Infection — the cause of anastomotic breakdown. Proc R Soc Med 1970; 63: 752

39 Bell CM, Lewis CB. Effect of neostigmine on integrity of ileorectal anastomoses. Br Med J 1968; 3: 587–588

40 Bell CM. Neostigmine and anastomotic disruption. Proc R Soc Med 1970; 63: 752

41 Whitaker BL. Observations on the blood flow in the inferior mesenteric arterial system and the healing of colon anastomoses. Ann R Coll Surg 1968; 43: 89–110

42 Wilkins JL, Hardcastle JD, Mann CV, Kaufman L. Effects of neostigmine and atropine on motor activity of ileum, colon and rectum of anaesthetized subjects. Br Med J 1970; 1: 793–794

43 Fong Y, Marano MA, Moldawer LL et al. The acute splanchnic and peripheral tissue metabolic response to endotoxin in humans. J Clin Invest 1990; 85: 1896–1904

44 Ziegler EJ, Fisher CJ Jr, Sprung CL et al. Treatment of Gram-negative bacteremia and septic shock with HA-1A human monoclonal antibody against endotoxin. N Engl J Med 1991; 324: 429–436

45 Wolff SM. Monoclonal antibodies and the treatment of Gram-negative bacteremia and shock. N Engl J Med 1991; 324: 486–487

46 Gilmour DG, Aitkenhead AR et al. The effect of hypovolaemia on colonic blood flow in the dog. Br J Surg 1980; 67: 82–84

47 Schrock TR, Deveney CW, Dunphy JE. Factors contributing to colonic anastomosis. Ann Surg 1973; 177: 513

48 Foster ME, Laycock JRD, Silver IA, Leaper DJ. Hypovolaemia and healing in colonic anastomoses. Br J Surg 1985; 72: 831–834

49 Foster ME, Brennan SS, Morgan A, Leaper DJ. Colonic ischaemia and anastomotic healing. Eur Surg Res 1985; 71: 133–139

50 Chou CC, Gallavan RH. Blood flow and intestinal motility. Fed Proc 1982; 41: 2090–2095

51 Caldwell CB, Ricotta JJ. Changes in visceral blood flow with elevated intraabdominal pressure. J Surg Res 1987; 43: 14–20

52 Tagart REB. Colorectal anastomosis: factors influencing success. J R Soc Med; 1981; 74: 111–118

53 Mesh CL, Gewertz BL. The effect of hemodilution on blood flow regulation in normal and postischemic intestine. J Surg Res 1990; 48: 183–189

54 Mayfield SR, Shaul PW, Oh W, Stonestreet BS. Gastrointestinal blood flow and oxygen delivery during environmental cold stress: effect of anaemia. J Dev Physiol 1989; 12: 219–223

55 Aitkenhead AR, Gilmour DG et al. Effects of halothane and hypocapnia on colon blood flow in the dog. Br J Anaesth 1980; 52: 634–635

56 Winson O, Biber B, Martner J. Effects of hyperventilation and hypoventilation on stress-induced intestinal vasoconstriction. Acta Anaesthesiol Scand 1985; 29: 726–732

57 Shandall A, Lowndes R, Young HI. Colonic anastomotic healing and oxygen tension. Br J Surg 1985; 72: 606–609

58 Schiedler MG, Cutler BS, Fiddian-Green G. Sigmoid intramural pH for prediction of ischemic colitis during aortic surgery. A comparison with risk factors and inferior mesenteric artery stump pressure. Arch Surg 1987; 122: 881–886

59 Leaman LM, Levenson L et al. Effect of morphine on splanchnic blood flow. Br Heart J 1978; 40: 569–571

60 Andreen M. Inhalation versus intravenous anaesthesia. Effect on the hepatic and splanchnic circulation. Acta Anaesthesiol Scand 1982; 26 (suppl 75): 25–31

61 Bond JH, Prentiss RA, Levitt MD, Schoenborn K. The effect of anesthesia and laparotomy on blood flow to the stomach, small bowel and colon of the dog. Surgery 1980; 87: 313–318

62 Kvietys PR, Granger DN. Regulation of colonic blood flow. Fed Proc 1982; 41: 2106–2110

63 Gelman S. General anaesthesia and hepatic circulation. Can J Physiol Pharmacol 1987; 65: 1762–1779

64 Tverskoy M, Gelman S, Fowler KC. Intestinal circulation during inhalation anesthesia. Anesthesiology1985; 62: 462–469

65 Banks RO, Gallavan RH, Zinner MH et al. Vasoactive agents in control of the mesenteric circulation. Fed Proc 1985; 44: 1743–2749

66 Jard S. Mechanisms of action of vasopressin and vasopressin antagonists. Kidney Int 1988; 34 (suppl 26): S38–S42

67 Thibonnier M. Use of vasopressin antagonists in human diseases. Kidney Int 1988; 34 (suppl 26): S48–S51

68 Condon RE, Cowles VE, Schulte WJ, Fantzides CT, Mahoney JL, Sarna SK. Resolution of postoperative ileus in humans. Ann Surg 1986; 203: 574–581

69 Condon RE, Cowles V, Ekbom GA, Schulte WJ, Hess G. Effects of halothane, enflurane, and nitrous oxide on colon motility. Surgery 1987; 101: 81–85

70 Scheinin B, Asantila R, Orko R. The effect of bupivacaine and morphine on pain and bowel function after colonic surgery. Acta Anaesthesiol Scand 1987; 31: 161–164

71 Ahn H, Bronge A, Johansson K, Ygge H, Lindhagen J. Effect of continuous postoperative epidural analgesia on intestinal motility. Br J Surg 1988; 75: 1176–1178

72 Scheinin B, Lindgren I, Scheinin TM. Peroperative nitrous oxide delays bowel function after colonic surgery. Br J Anaesth 1990; 64: 154–158

73 Waldhausen JHT, Schirmer BD. The effect of

ambulation on recovery from postoperative ileus. Ann Surg 1990; 212: 671–677
74 Catchpole BN. Motor pattern of the left colon before and after surgery for rectal cancer: possible implications in other disorders. Gut 1988; 29: 624–630
75 Report of a Confidential Enquiry into Perioperative Deaths. Prepared by Buck N, Devlin HB, Lunn JN. London: The Nuffield Provincial Hospitals Trust and the King's Fund. 1987
76 Duggan JE, Drummond GB. Abdominal muscle activity and intraabdominal pressure after upper abdominal surgery. Anesth Analg 1989; 6: 598–603
77 Dureuil B, Viires N, Cantineua JP et al. Diaphragmatic contractility after upper abdominal surgery. J Appl Physiol 1986; 62: 1775–1780
78 Scott NB, Kehlet H. Regional anaesthesia and surgical morbidity. Br J Surg 1988; 75: 299–304
79 Lawrence VA, Page CP, Harris GD. Preoperative spirometry before abdominal operations. A critical appraisal of its predictive value. Arch Intern Med 1989; 149: 280–285
80 Vodinh J, Bonnet F, Touboul C, Lefloch JP, Becquemin JP, Harf A. Risk factors of postoperative pulmonary complications after vascular surgery. Surgery 1989; 105: 360–365
81 Chuter TAM, Weissman C, Starker PM, Gump FE. Effet of incentive spirometry on diaphragmatic function after surgery. Surgery 1989; 105: 488–493
82 Hall JC, Tarala R, Harris J, Tapper J, Christiansen K. Incentive spirometry versus routine chest physiotherapy for prevention of pulmonary complications after abdominal surgery. Lancet 1991; 337: 953–956
83 Roukema JA, Carol EJ, Prins JG. The prevention of pulmonary complications after upper abdominal surgery in patients with noncompromised pulmonary status. Arch Surg 1988; 123: 30–34
84 Poe RH, Kallay MC, Dass T, Celebic A. Can postoperative pulmonary complications after elective cholecystectomy be predicted? Am J Med Sci 1988; 295: 29–34
85 Jayr C, Mollie A, Bourgain JL et al. Postoperative pulmonary complications: general anesthesia with postoperative parenteral morphine compared with epidural analgesia. Surgery 1988; 1104: 57–63
86 Schwieger I, Gamulin Z, Suter PM. Lung function during anaesthesia and respiratory insufficiency in the postoperative period: physiological and clinical implications. Acta Anaesthesiol Scand 1989; 33: 527–534
87 Hedenstierna G. Gas exchange during anaesthesia. Br J Anaesth 1990; 64: 507–514
88 Jones JG, Sapsford DJ, Wheatley RG. Postoperative hypoxaemia: mechanisms and time course. Anaesthesia 1990; 45: 566–573
89 Selsby D, Jones JG. Some physiological and clinical aspects of chest physiotherapy. Br J Anaesth 1990; 64: 621–631
90 Hull CJ, Jones JG, eds. Symposium on the lung. Br J Anaesth 1990; 65: 1–152
91 Jansen JE, Sorensen AI, Naesh O, Erichsen C, Pedersen A. Effect of doxapram on postoperative pulmonary complications after upper abdominal surgery in high-risk patients. Lancet 1990; 335: 936–938
92 Stoner HB. Metabolism after trauma and in sepsis. Circ Shock 1986; 19: 75–87
93 Bailey PM, Child CS. Endocrine response to surgery. In: Kaufman L. ed. Anaesthesia review 4. London: Churchill Livingstone, 1987: 100–116
94 Harvey SR, Lawrence DD, Madeja JM, Abbey SK, Markus G. Secretion of plasminogen activators by human colorectal and gastric tumor explants. Clin Exp Metast 1988; 6: 431–450
95 Singh SK, Marquet RL, de Bruin RWF, Hop WCJ, Westbroek DL, Jeekel J. Consequences of blood loss on growth of artificial metastases. Br J Surg 1988; 75: 377–379
96 Stephenson KR, Steinberg SM, Hughes KS, Vetto JT, Sugarbaker PH, Chang AE. Perioperative blood transfusions are associated with decreased time to recurrence and decreased survival after resection of colorectal liver metastases. Ann Surg 1988; 208: 679–687
97 Crowson MC, Hallissey MT, Kiff RS, Kingston RD, Fielding JWL. Blood transfusion in colorectal cancer. Br J Surg 1989; 76: 522–523
98 Lawrance RJ, Cooper AJ, Loizidou M, Alexander P, Taylor I. Blood transfusion and recurrence of colorectal cancer: the role of platelet derived growth factors. Br J Surg 1990; 77: 1106–1109
99 Child CS, Kaufman L. Effect of intrathecal diamorphine on the adrenocortical hyperglycaemic and cardiovascular responses to major colonic surgery. Br J Anaesth 1985; 57: 389–393
100 Rogers PN, Murray WR, Shaw R, Brar S. Surgical management of bleeding gastric ulceration. Br J Surg 1988; 75: 16–17
101 Steele G Jr, Ravikumar TS. Resection of hepatic metastases from colorectal cancer. Biological perspectives. Ann Surg 1989; 210: 127–138
102 Allen-Mersh TG. Improving survival after large bowel cancer. Br Med J 1991; 303: 595–596
103 Scheele J, Stangl R, Altendorf-Hofman A. Hepatic metastases from colorectal carcinoma; impact of surgical resection on the natural history. Br J Surg 1990; 77: 1241–1246
104 Pace RF, Blenkharn JI, Edwards WJ, Orloff M, Blumgart LH, Benjamin IS. Intra-abdominal sepsis after hepatic resection. Ann Surg 1989; 209: 302–306
105 Munoz SJ, Ballas SK, Moritz MM et al. Peri-operative management of fulminant and sub-fulminant hepatic failure with therapeutic plasmapheresis. Transplant Proc 1989; 21: 3535–3536
106 Turner DAB. Blood conservation. Br J Anaesth 1991; 66: 281–284
107 Spiess BD, Logas WG, Tuman KJ, Hughes T, Jagmin J, Ivankovich AD. Thromboelastography used for detection of peri-operative fibrinolysis: a report of four cases. J Cardiothorac Anaesth 1988; 2: 666–672
108 Cottam S, Hunt B, Segal H, Ginsburg R, Potter D. Aprotinin inhibits tissue plasminogen activator mediated fibrinolysis during orthotopic liver transplantation. Transplant Proc 1991; 23: 1933
109 Hunt BJ, Cottam S, Segal H, Ginsburg R, Potter D. Inhibition by aprotinin of tPA-mediated fibrinolysis during orthotopic liver transplantation. Lancet 1990; 336: 381
110 Polson PJ, Park GR, Lindop MJ, Calne RY, Williams

R. The prevention of renal impairment in patients undergoing orthotopic liver grafting by infusion of low-dose dopamine. Anaesthesia 1987; 42: 15–19

111 Parker S, Carlon GC, Isaacs M, Howlands WS, Kahn RC. Dopamine administration in oliguria and oliguric renal failure. Crit Care Med 1981; 9: 630–632

112 Parodi JE, Zenilman ME, Becker JM. Characterization of substance P effects on sphincter of Oddi myoelectric activity. J Surg Res 1989; 46: 405–412

113 Bachmann AW, Gordon RD. Clonidine suppression test reliably differentiates phaeochromocytoma from essential hypertension. Clin Exp Pharmacol Physiol 1991; 18: 275–277

114 Ross EJ, Prichard BNC, Kaufman L, Robertson AIG, Harris BJ. Preoperative and operative management of patients with phaeochromocytoma. Br Med J 1967; 1: 191–198

115 Kaufman L. Phaeochromocytoma. In: Kaufman L, ed. Anaesthesia review 1. London: Churchill Livingstone, 1982: pp 21–33

116 Kaufman L. Phaeochromocytoma — update from Anaesthesia Review 1. In: Kaufman L, ed. Anaesthesia review 2. London: Churchill Livingstone, 1984: pp 214–216

117 Hull CJ. Phaeochromocytoma. Diagnosis, preoperative preparation and anaesthetic management. Br J Anaesth 1986; 58: 1453–1468

118 Bouloux PMG, Grossman A, Besser GM. Naloxone provokes catecholamine release in phaeochromocytomas and paragangliomas. Clin Endocrinol 1986; 24: 319–325

119 Kaufman L. Medicine relevant to anaesthesia (1). In Kaufman L, ed. Anaesthesia review 6. London: Churchill Livingstone, 1989: pp 1–20

120 Marsh HM, Martin JK, Kolvs LK et al. Carcinoid crisis during anesthesia: successful treatment with a somatostatin analogue. Anesthesiology 1987; 66: 89–91

121 Roy RC, Carter RF, Wright PD. Somatostatin, anaesthesia, and the carcinoid syndrome. Perioperative administration of a somatostatin analogue to suppress carcinoid tumour activity. Anaesthesia 1987; 42: 627–632

122 Hodgson HJF. Controlling the carcinoid syndrome — simple blocking drugs, somatostatin, and then perhaps embolisation. Br Med J 1988; 297: 1213–1214

9. Anaesthesia for vascular surgery

S. Reiz   P. Coriat

Anaesthetic management, postoperative care and control of acute and chronic pain provide challenging fields for the anaesthetist who devotes interest to vascular surgical patients. These individuals have a high prevalence of concomitant disease related to the heart, the vascular system, the lung and the metabolic system. Their immediate complication rate is therefore high and their medium and long-term survival markedly reduced compared with an age- and sex-matched population without vascular disease. The role of the anaesthetist for vascular patients goes beyond that in most other patient populations since there is a unique opportunity to improve long-term survival and function by applying adequate pre-operative evaluation techniques and refined peri-operative anaesthetic management.

The scope of this chapter is to provide the reader with a comprehensive and clinically relevant insight into the physiological particularities of the vascular surgical patient and how these interact with anaesthetic drugs and techniques as well as with the surgical procedure itself. Pre-operative assessment and risk prediction, monitoring and postoperative care pertinent to the vascular surgical patient will also be discussed.

GENERAL CHARACTERISTICS OF THE VASCULAR SURGICAL PATIENT

Atherosclerosis requiring surgical therapy is most commonly a focal manifestation of a systemic disease with a complex aetiology, dominated by long tobacco use. Multiple organ systems are commonly affected. Coronary artery disease, arterial hypertension, chronic bronchitis and diabetes mellitus are the most frequently encountered diseases complicating the clinical course of the vascular patient. The incidence of these disease varies between populations and with the methods used for their detection (Figs 9.1 and 9.2). Clinical signs of cardiac or pulmonary disease are often absent in patients with decreased functional capacity

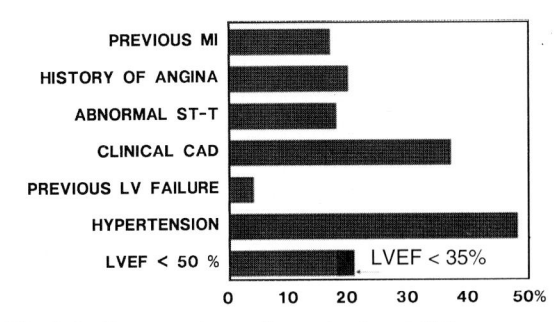

Fig. 9.1 Pre-operative cardiac evaluation of 468 consecutive patients scheduled to undergo abdominal aortic surgery at the Pitié-Salpêtrière unit of vascular surgery, in Paris. Percentage of the population with clinical symptoms. MI = Myocardial infarction; CAD = coronary artery disease; LV = left ventricle; LVEF = pre-operative ejection fraction determined by gated radionuclide angiography. Adapted from Baron et al.[188]

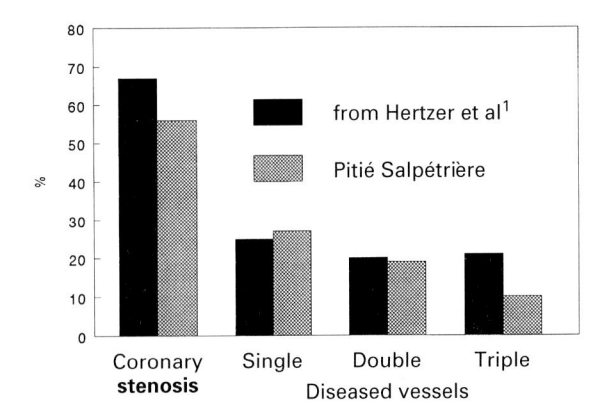

Fig. 9.2 Incidence of coronary artery disease in patients undergoing aortic surgery according to coronary angiographic data. Coronary artery disease was defined as at least one coronary stenosis greater than 50%. From Hertzer et al[1] and unpublished data by Coriat et al.

due to claudication. For instance, clinical evidence of coronary artery disease was found in 36% of patients scheduled for different vascular surgical procedures, whereas coronary angiography revealed significant stenoses in as many as 53–68%[1] (Figs 9.1 and 9.2).

Coronary artery disease

Coronary artery disease is responsible for over 50% of the immediate, medium and long-term mortality and morbidity following vascular surgery.[2–4] Unstable myocardial ischaemia, acute myocardial infarction and ischaemic pulmonary oedema are the most common immediate postoperative cardiac complications. The incidences of these complications vary markedly with the surgical procedure and are highest after aortic reconstruction. For instance, acute myocardial infarction has been reported to occur in approximately 1% of patients subjected to carotid artery surgery,[5] whereas the incidence is 5–15% after abdominal aneurysmectomy.[6] Repetitive myocardial ischaemia, which has been observed in as many as 40% of patients following major vascular procedures, produces myocardial stunning or may lead to infarction with subsequent deterioration of ventricular function[7] and can therefore be expected to shorten long-term survival.[8] Thus, one of the important goals for the peri-operative management of these patients is to avoid myocardial ischaemia. This is achieved mainly by pre-operative anti-anginal therapy, adequate monitoring and accomplishment of peri-operative haemodynamic stability.

Hypertension

Hypertension has been reported in 30–55% of vascular surgical patients (Fig. 9.1, Table 9.1).[9] Baroreflexes are often reset and depressed in hypertensive disease. Advanced age and abnormalities of the cerebral circulation may further depress the baroreceptor-mediated response to increased blood pressure.[10]

Table 9.1 Chronic cardiac medication administered to 468 consecutive patients undergoing abdominal aortic surgery at the Pitié-Salpêtrière unit of vascular surgery (1987–1990)

Long-acting nitrates	13%
ACE inhibitors	14%
Ca^{2+} antagonists	41%
β-Blockers	15%
Vasodilators	12%
Diuretics	11%
Digitalis	1.5%

ACE = angiotensin-converting enzyme.
From Baron et al,[188] with permission.

Morbidity is not increased if blood pressure is adequately controlled pre-operatively.[11] Accordingly, antihypertensive treatment is continued up until the morning of surgery. For instance, β-blockers blunt the stress responses to tracheal intubation and surgical stimulation and decrease the incidence of myocardial ischaemia without increased risk of hypotension following induction of anaesthesia.[12] However, long-acting β-blockers may contribute to decreased cardiac reserve at the time of recovery from anaesthesia.[13] With the introduction of angiotensin-converting enzyme inhibitors, the strategy of maintaining antihypertensive therapy until the morning of surgery may need to be changed. Several recent papers have reported severe hypotension and bradycardia following induction of anaesthesia in patients given these agents.[14]

Left ventricular dysfunction

Patients with chronic hypertensive disease, coronary artery disease and increased impedance to left ventricular (LV) ejection due to atherosclerosis frequently develop impairment of LV function. Those with a history of, or radiological evidence of, congestive heart failure have been shown to have a higher incidence of postoperative pulmonary oedema.[15] Even without clinical or radiological evidence, approximately 17–25% of vascular patients have an LV ejection fraction below 50%, indicating impaired systolic LV function (Fig. 9.1).[16] In addition, diastolic LV function is often depressed by impaired relaxation and compliance. Increased age, aortic atherosclerosis and, most importantly, chronic hypertension contribute to the increased stiffness of the left ventricle. Thus, maintenance of venous return becomes the cornerstone of haemodynamic control in these patients.[17] Finally, myocardial ischaemia may develop in patients with LV hypertrophic cardiomyopathy, even in the absence of coronary artery disease, because coronary vascular reserve is decreased and subendocardial perfusion depends on a high transmural driving pressure.[17]

Diabetes mellitus

The incidence of diabetes mellitus in vascular surgical patients is about 18%. When requiring insulin treatment, diabetes is an independent risk factor for postoperative ischaemic events and congestive heart failure.[18] Those with autonomic neuropathy are often asymptomatic as regards coronary artery disease. The characteristics of the vascular disease tend to lead to repeated peripheral vascular procedures with poor surgical healing. In addition, the coronary arteries are often small in calibre and lesions are of a distal nature. Such patients are most commonly not suited for coronary interventions.

Respiratory disease

Cigarette consumption is the main cause of respiratory dysfunction in vascular disease. Most commonly, a combination of restrictive and obstructive pulmonary disease is present. Smoking has thus been shown as an independent risk factor for postoperative respiratory complications after aortic surgery.[19] Advanced age and obesity, which are associated with decreased values of vital capacity, maximal expiratory flow rate and pulmonary elastic recoil, further increase the risk of pulmonary complications, such as minor and major atelectasis, pneumonia and respiratory insufficiency.[20] Although most common in patients with disabling respiratory disease, these complications are not infrequent in individuals with little or no overt signs of respiratory dysfunction. Thus, a significant number of patients subjected to major vascular surgery may be candidates for prolonged postoperative ventilator therapy.

RISK ASSESSMENT IN VASCULAR SURGERY

The risk of vascular surgery depends on three factors: the patient (with distribution of atherosclerosis and associated diseases), the type of surgery and the peri-operative management of the circulation. The third factor will be discussed in detail in the section on anaesthetic management.

Risk related to patient characteristics

Cardiac risk

A primary goal of the pre-operative cardiac evaluation of the vascular patient is to detect the presence and degree of coronary artery disease. This is important not only to assess operative risk and decide upon the anaesthetic and postoperative management, but also because coronary interventions may improve long-term survival. This latter aspect has attracted increased interest with the rapid development of coronary angioplasty.

Medical history and resting electrocardiogram

A good clinical history is indispensable and provides important information relating to peri-operative management and the risk of cardiac disease. Risk prediction is improved further by adding the information contained in a resting 12-lead electrocardiogram (ECG). For instance, the combination of a history of stable angina pectoris and a pre-operative resting ECG which demonstrates chronic ST segment depression of at least 0.1 mV in two or more leads is associated in vascular patients with a risk of peri-operative ischaemia of over 50%.[21,22] The negative predictive value of a single resting 12-lead ECG in vascular patients with stable coronary artery disease is even more impressive; a normal ECG is associated with an incidence of peri-operative ischaemia in the order of only 8%.

Whenever there are clinical signs of an ongoing evolution of coronary artery disease, patients should be referred to a cardiologist for further evaluation. These signs include recent myocardial infarction and unstable (recent or accelerating) angina pectoris. If the vascular disease requires immediate surgery, it has been suggested that optimization of medical therapy, directed monitoring and aggressive circulatory control over at least the first 3 postoperative days improve outcome.[23]

Most studies of vascular surgical patients have failed to identify stable angina pectoris as an independent cardiac risk factor.[11,24,25] This may be because those patients who had indications for coronary interventions had already been subjected to therapy.[24,25] Our approach to the vascular surgical patient with angina pectoris is not different from that in medical patients: patients are referred for coronary angiography if age and clinical status suggest that coronary intervention might be beneficial. If angioplasty or surgical revascularization is not indicated or possible, optimal anti-anginal therapy is instituted.

A more complex problem in the assessment of cardiac risk of vascular surgery is the lack of adequate functional cardiac history in many patients. For instance, Leppo et al[6]. reported, in a series of 100 aortic surgical patients, that 8 of 15 patients who suffered a peri-operative myocardial infarction had no pre-operative clinical evidence of coronary artery disease. As further shown by Hertzer and colleagues,[1] 14% of vascular patients with triple-vessel disease and 22% of those with double-vessel disease had no angina pectoris or other history of cardiac disease. This illustrates that vascular patients may need to undergo further pre-operative tests to identify the presence and degree of coronary artery disease, and to predict cardiac risk.

Several non-invasive techniques may improve the identification of high-risk patients undergoing vascular surgery. These tests include exercise ECG, ambulatory ECG, dipyridamole-thallium scintigraphy (DTS) and determination of LV ejection fraction by gated radionuclide imaging. At present, the results of some of these tests are also considered to be helpful in selecting patients in whom coronary angiography and subsequent coronary intervention might reduce the risk of the scheduled vascular procedure and improve long-term survival.[26,27]

The ideal pre-operative screening test should be simple, inexpensive, non-invasive and fairly sensitive and specific in respect of the following two questions:

1. Can I identify the patient who will be at risk of peri-operative cardiac events?
2. Can I identify the patient with correctable coronary artery lesions?

Exercise electrocardiography

Exercise ECG has traditionally been recommended for use in vascular surgical patients on the basis that it should reliably identify patients at risk of postoperative cardiac complications. This suggestion has been challenged in several more recent studies in which a positive exercise test was not an independent predictor of cardiac risk. One of these studies even noted that the most severe postoperative cardiac complications occurred in patients who either refused the test or were unable to participate.[25] The present opinion is that maximal exercise testing should be avoided in patients with aortic aneurysm. In addition, it is impossible to perform the test adequately in patients with occlusive disease of the lower extremities. However, submaximal exercise combined with intravenous dipyridamole and subsequent thallium imaging might prove useful for identification of at-risk patients (see below).

Ambulatory ECG

In cardiological practice, the frequency and magnitude of ischaemic ST segment changes on ambulatory ECG monitoring have proved reliable in identifying the severity and long-term prognosis of coronary artery disease.[28] The technique is particularly helpful because of the high incidence of silent ischaemic episodes.[29] Consequently, this technique has also been applied in the pre-operative evaluation of vascular patients.[30–32] Encouraging results have been reported; in one study, the negative predictive power was close to 100%, although it was only 86% in the other (Table 9.2).

Dipyridamole-thallium scintigraphy

Dipyridamole, which dilates non-stenosed coronary vessels, increases flow to normal territories at the expense of flow to jeopardized myocardium as identified by an intravenous injection of thallium-201. This effect may be enhanced by increasing heart rate, either by upright tilting or by submaximal exercise before injection of the isotope. A territory which, on both initial and delayed (3–4 h after thallium injection) imaging lacks perfusion (i.e. a fixed defect), denotes a previous infarct, whereas an initial imaging defect which appears normal on delayed imaging (redistribution) suggests a critically perfused area.[33]

All published studies to date using DTS in vascular surgical patients have applied the resting technique. The ability of DTS to predict postoperative myocardial ischaemia, infarction and cardiac death was first reported by Boucher *et al.*[34] They studied patients subjected to lower-limb revascularization in whom there was a high clinical suspicion of coronary artery disease. Eight of 16 patients with redistribution on pre-operative DTS developed acute postoperative coronary events which were fatal in 4. None of 32 patients with normal DTS or fixed defects had ischaemic complications. In a subsequent study, Leppo *et al.*[6] confirmed that redistribution was the best predictor of postoperative myocardial infarction. In contrast to Boucher *et al*, these investigators also included patients without clinically suspected coronary artery disease. In

Table 9.2 Correlation between pre-operative ischaemia and major cardiac events

	Raby et al[30]*	Mangano et al[62]*	Fleischer et al[32]+
Number of patients studied	176	47ξ	14ξ
Pre-operative ischaemia (%)	18	23	16
Postoperative cardiac events (%)	7	23	17
Positive predictive value (%)	37.5	23	38
Negative predictive value (%)	99	87	86 Vascular patients
			99 Non-vascular patients

* 48 h pre-operative Holter monitoring;
+ at least 12 h pre-operative Holter monitoring;
ξ vascular and non-vascular patients.

addition, they demonstrated that redistribution reliably identified patients with significant coronary artery disease.

Recently, the resting DTS technique has been applied in large-scale studies.[16,35] These have revealed several limitations of the test when applied for risk prediction in vascular surgery. First, DTS shows redistribution in more than 50% of vascular surgical patients,[16,24,35] i.e. also in those with non-significant (less than 50%) coronary artery stenoses. It might be expected that a temporary perfusion defect might appear in a territory distal to an insignificant stenosis, primarily as a result of relative overperfusion of adjacent myocardium supplied by a normal artery. This would explain the low positive predictive value of DTS when applied for risk prediction in patients with suspected coronary artery disease. Thus, several studies have demonstrated that more than 75% of patients with redistribution did not experience postoperative cardiac complications.[16,24,35] Second, recent studies have provided evidence suggesting that resting DTS is not reliable for risk stratification when applied in vascular patients without clinical evidence of coronary artery disease.[35,36] This is of particular concern because non-invasive tests should be preferred in these patients, in whom the incidence of cardiac complications is not negligible. Finally, and most importantly, the sensitivity of resting DTS to predict complications may be less impressive than described initially. Several factors which influence the distribution of thallium may explain this. For instance, the ability to identify a significant stenosis of the left anterior descending coronary artery diminishes if one or two of the other major arteries are critically stenosed.[37,38] This is because dipyridamole-induced coronary vasodilatation produces little or no maldistribution of blood flow in severe multivessel disease. Furthermore, for imaging and anatomical reasons, single-vessel disease involving the circumflex or right coronary artery is poorly detected compared to stenosis of the left anterior descending artery.[38] A technical factor described recently may also explain part of the lack of sensitivity of redistribution in identifying high-risk patients or detecting significant coronary stenoses. Delayed re-injection of thallium has demonstrated that the conventional technique incorrectly identifies a considerable proportion of myocardial segments as being irreversibly injured.[39] This could explain the high incidence of cardiac complications reported by McEnroe et al.[40] in vascular patients with permanent defects on resting DTS.

In order to overcome some of the short-comings of DTS, two techniques aimed at potentiating the degree of inhomogeneous myocardial perfusion produced by dipyridamole have been proposed. These include upright tilting[41] or submaximal exercise.[42] In addition, re-injection of thallium before the delayed imaging is recommended in all patients with initial perfusion defects.[39] There are, as yet, no data to confirm that either of these modifications of the original DTS improves risk prediction in vascular surgical patients. However, preliminary results from studies combining upright tilting and thallium re-injection with DTS do confirm a marked improvement in the ability to identify patients with significant coronary artery disease by this technique (Table 9.3). For all these reasons, resting DTS is progressively being abandoned in favour of the newer modifications of the test.

Angioscintigraphy and echocardiography

LV angioscintigraphy provides objective assessment of systolic function. LV dilatation is one of the common compensatory mechanisms in the face of decreased contractility. Thus, a decline of LV injection is an early and accurate marker of decreased cardiac reserve.[43] In addition, as many as 30% of vascular patients may be unable to give a relevant history of decreased LV function. Patients with clinically suspected coronary

Table 9.3 Ability of dipyridamole-thallium scintigraphy (DTS) to detect coronary artery stenosis in two series of patients from the Pitié-Salpétrière hospital in Paris, scheduled to undergo abdominal aortic surgery. In the first 132 patients a resting DTS was performed; the following 123 patients were tilted after dipyridamole injection but before thallium infusion. In addition, in the latter series, a second injection of thallium was performed prior to the delayed imaging in all patients who demonstrated initial perfusion defects.

	Resting DTS		DTS with tilt and re-injection	
	Initial defect	Redistribution	Initial defect	Redistribution
Sensitivity (%)	51	32	82	64
Specificity (%)	59	74	62	59
Positive predictive value (%)	48	50	66	70
Negative predictive value (%)	62	61	58	51

From unpublished data by Coriat et al.

artery disease and low ejection fraction most commonly have severe triple-vessel disease and poor long-term prognosis.[44] Moreover, these are the patients who benefit most from coronary interventions.[45]

In vascular patients, several studies have documented that a pre-operative ejection fraction lower than 50% is associated with a higher incidence of coronary artery disease, and consequently with an increased cardiac complication rate.[15] In addition, the knowledge of pre-operative ejection fraction could assist the anaesthetist in decision-making as regards choice of anaesthetic technique, level of monitoring and peri-operative use of cardiac medication.

Echocardiography is an excellent technique to provide qualitative information regarding global and segmental LV function. It has the advantage over nuclear techniques of being simple, inexpensive and easily repeatable. The M-mode technique is of limited value for assessment of global ventricular function because many vascular patients have segmental wall motion abnormalities, but it is particularly well-suited to detect ventricular hypertrophy. The two-dimensional image of the short axis of the left ventricle obtained by the transthoracic approach allows the best estimate of LV function. The addition of transmitral Doppler signals provides the opportunity to assess the filling pattern of the left ventricle. Thus, the technique provides combined information relating to LV diastolic function and venous return.

When the ECG is inconclusive, echocardiography further improves the ability to diagnose a previous myocardial infarction, to identify precisely its localization and to appreciate its extent. A short-coming of the technique is its inability to provide information on critically perfused myocardium unless that area is ischaemic. Data in the cardiology literature document that exercise and/or dipyridamole echocardiography provide reliable information on risk territories.[46] No studies evaluating the ability of echocardiography to predict operative risk have been published to date.

Risk related to type of surgery

Cardiac and other adverse outcomes vary greatly with the type of surgery, mainly as a consequence of differences in peri-operative stress, including the consequences of major vessel clamping, amount of bleeding, volume shifts, metabolic changes and postoperative pain.

Carotid artery surgery

The risks of carotid endarterectomy are almost exclusively coronary and/or cerebral.[47-52] This procedure is only moderately stressful for the heart, as illustrated by an incidence of peri-operative myocardial infarction of less than 2% despite an incidence of significant coronary artery disease around 75%.[47] However, data from Ennix et al[50] published over 10 years ago indicate that considerably mortality (18.2%) from peri-operative myocardial infarction occurred in individuals who would now undergo coronary angioplasty prior to coronary bypass surgery in association with their carotid endarterectomy.

Myocardial infarction is also responsible for around 70% of late mortality after carotid endarterectomy.[53] This implies that identification of significant coronary artery disease is important in this patient population despite the low immediate postoperative cardiac morbidity.

Aortic surgery

Mortality within the first 30 days of elective abdominal aortic surgery is in the range of 2-5%[16,54,55]. Cardiac events account for approximately half the deaths.[55] The surgical influence on cardiac and other morbidity following abdominal aortic reconstructive surgery is principally related to the following three factors: elective or emergency operation (two- to five-fold difference), level of clamping (infra- or suprarenal) and aneurysm or occlusive disease of the aorta (two fold difference).[54] Morbidity in survivors of aortic surgery is important principally because it prolongs hospital stay and can be associated with impaired long-term prognosis. Its incidence is not quite clear from the literature. For example, there are large variations in the reported incidence of non-lethal peri-operative myocardial infarction. The incidence of Q-wave and enzyme-verified infarctions varies between 4 and 6% in most retrospective surgical series,[55-57] but in recent prospective studies, specifically aimed at identifying peri-operative transmural and non-Q-wave infarctions, an incidence three to five times higher has been reported.[6,16]

Other morbidity after abdominal vascular surgery affects mainly the lungs and the kidneys (Fig. 9.3).[54] Postoperative respiratory morbidity is important because of weakened respiratory muscle function, impaired lung elasticity and obstructive lung disease, frequently encountered in the vascular patient. Other factors which determine the incidence of respiratory complications are the site of the surgical incision and whether or not emergency surgery was performed. For instance, thoracic aortic repair, which requires a thoracotomy and collapse of the left lung, carries an

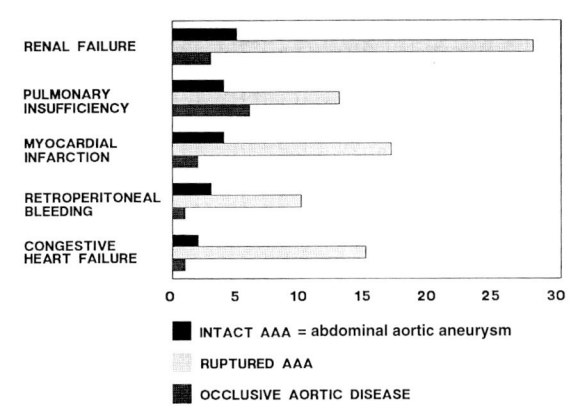

Fig. 9.3 Postoperative complications in 557 patients subjected to abdominal aortic reconstruction reported by Diehl et al.[4] AAA = Abdominal aortic aneurysm.

elevated risk. Likewise, a retroperitoneal approach to the subrenal aorta is the technique preferred over the abdominal incision in patients with pre-existing impairment of respiratory function.

The frequency of pulmonary complications is directly related to the intensity with which they are sought and to the definitions employed, e.g. minor or major atelectasis, pneumonia, etc. However, these complications alone do not usually result in death. In a study by Diehl et al,[54] the overall incidence of postoperative pulmonary insufficiency after elective or acute abdominal aortic aneurysm repair was comparable to that of myocardial infarction or congestive heart failure (Fig. 9.3). However, mortality from respiratory failure was only around 0.2% compared with 65% from cardiac complications. Both respiratory and cardiac complications were approximately doubled after emergency aortic aneurysm repair. Similar results were found in a recent prospective study of morbidity and mortality of patients subjected to elective abdominal aortic surgery.[16] This study also demonstrated an important cross-link between respiratory and cardiac complications. Thus, if combined with a cardiac complication, respiratory dysfunction which, *per se*, was not related to increased mortality carried an increased risk of death compared to a cardiac complication alone.[16]

Pulmonary function tests are often undertaken in the vascular patient because retrospective studies have demonstrated that abnormal pre-operative lung function is associated with increased respiratory failure after upper abdominal surgery.[20] However, unless these tests reflect markedly impaired respiratory function (FEV_1 <1.5 l or Pa_{CO_2} >6 kPa), they carry poor

positive predictive power and have low specificity.[9,54] Nevertheless, there are several reports in the literature demonstrating surprisingly low morbidity when major aortic surgery is performed in patients with incapacitating respiratory function in whom special precautions have been taken. These measures include pre-operative optimization of lung function, incentive spirometry and effective postoperative analgesia continued for several days after surgery in an intensive care unit.

Impairment of renal function is as common (around 6%) as myocardial infarction or major respiratory complications following elective abdominal aortic surgery.[58] However, dialysis is rarely indicated. In contrast, the incidence of renal failure, often requiring aggressive treatment, is high (around 29%) after emergency repair of abdominal aortic aneurysm.[54] Renal complications increase approximately three- to four-fold if the pre-operative serum creatinine concentration exceeds 190 µmol/l (2 mg/dl).[19] Pre-existing causes of decreased renal perfusion and function in vascular patients include atheroma of the renal arteries, hypertension, diabetic nephropathy and inadequate perfusion due to reduced cardiac output (LV dysfunction or hypovolaemia). In addition, pre-operative angiography often contributes to further renal dysfunction by a direct toxic effect of the contrast medium and hypovolaemia due to hyperosmotic polyuria.

Infrarenal aortic surgery may reduce renal perfusion and function by several mechanisms, e.g. changes in intravascular volume distribution, LV dysfunction, adverse consequences of aortic clamping on renal haemodynamics and micro-embolization of atheroma located above the clamp.[59] The incidence of renal dysfunction is higher if the aorta is cross-clamped above the renal arteries. Adequate hydration before and after angiography and maintenance of intravascular volume throughout the peri-operative period have been shown to be effective in reducing the risk of renal dysfunction after abdominal aortic surgery.

Peripheral vascular surgery

Although, intuitively, peripheral arterial revascularization appears to be a minor vascular surgical procedure, it carries a risk which may be as high as that of major vascular procedures.[60] This is because such operations are often subacute or acute and performed in patients of advanced age who are in poor medical condition. There are few good epidemiological studies of outcome related to medical factors following peripheral vascular surgery since the overall result is more a function of successful revascularization than of the anaesthetic management.

A practical approach to cardiac risk assessment prior to vascular surgery

The most crucial aspect of the approach to the cardiac risk assessment of the vascular surgical patient is the clinical suspicion of coronary artery disease based on history and resting ECG. In addition, the type of surgery should be considered, e.g. a more extensive evaluation is justified when high-risk surgery is planned.

In the absence of signs and symptoms suggesting coronary artery disease, the current opinion is to proceed directly to surgery. This attitude ignores the fact that over 10% of such patients will develop peri-operative cardiac complications.[24] However, the positive predictive power and the specificity of additional sophisticated tests are too low to justify their use in such patients. Peri-operative ischaemia monitoring should, nevertheless, be used for the purpose of detecting at-risk patients in this population.

In the patient with symptomatic coronary artery disease, the usual cardiological approach should be followed. This may vary markedly between countries, and among institutions in one country.

In patients with clinically suspected coronary artery disease, additional tests should be used for two reasons: first, because this subgroup of patients is more prone to develop peri-operative complications. Second, these additional tests are particularly helpful for risk stratification. Both ambulatory ECG and DTS have been recommended because they evaluate the functional status of the coronary circulation. The future will decide which of these methods will carry the best cost/benefit ratio as regards referral for coronary angiography. In the literature, it is recommended that coronary angiography is used selectively according to the prior test result.[61] One explanation for this restrictive approach is the relatively high risk of coronary angiography in vascular surgical patients. In addition, there are at present no studies which confirm convincingly an overall decreased mortality if coronary bypass surgery is performed before peripheral vascular surgery. Although it has been demonstrated that the mortality of the peripheral procedure is reduced to approximately one-half, the mortality of a coronary bypass procedure in vascular surgical patients is five to eight times that recorded in a coronary artery bypass population without peripheral vascular disease.[62] It remains to be shown if the use of coronary angioplasty prior to peripheral vascular surgery can provide a more satisfactory overall outcome.

Peri-operative monitoring pertinent to the vascular surgical patient

Cardiovascular monitoring

The main goals of monitoring the cardiovascular system in vascular surgery are to preserve organ perfusion pressure, to maintain adequate oxygen delivery to the periphery, to maintain an adequate preload and to detect myocardial ischaemia. The high level of interest in such monitoring is the result of a need for deeper insights into cardiac physiology among anaesthetists and data suggesting that peri-operative maintenance of haemodynamic stability would reduce the incidence of myocardial ischaemia, and thus improve the cardiac status of the patient with coronary artery disease.[62] In two separate studies, invasive monitoring of the circulation and aggressive treatment of circulatory dysfunction appeared to reduce the risk of re-infarction after non-cardiac surgery.[22,63] However, at present, no controlled studies have reliably documented a reduction in peri-operative morbidity in patients subjected to invasive or non-invasive cardiovascular monitoring.[64]

Detection of myocardial ischaemia

Since myocardial ischaemia is the main morbidity factor in vascular surgery, it appears logical to detect this abnormality before profound cardiac functional disturbances or myocardial injury have developed. This is not always detected by conventional intensive care unit oscilloscope monitoring, as illustrated by a trend printout obtained retrospectively from the first postoperative night in a patient subjected to aortic aneurysm resection in whom an ambulatory ST segment analysis device was used (Fig. 9.4). This patient, who had pre-existing slight ST segment depression in his

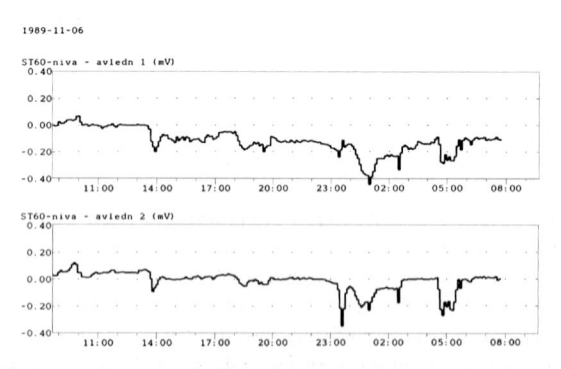

Fig. 9.4 Printout of a Holter electrocardiogram recording (upper panel lead V5; lower panel; lead II) in a patient during (08.30–13.00) and after (13.00–07.30) abdominal aortic surgery. For discussion, see text.

anterior chest leads on the pre-operative ECG, developed further ST segment depression of 0.1–0.4 mV in lead V5 which lasted for approximately 14 of the 18 postoperative hours. He subsequently went on to infarct part of his anterior ventricular wall. The standard intensive care unit monitor had been displaying an uncalibrated lead II, in which the ambulatory monitor revealed that only short periods of new ST changes had occurred.

In the remainder of this section, we will present current opinion on methods used for detection of ischaemia during and after vascular surgery.

The awake patient. Many anaesthetists and surgeons still maintain that the awake patient is the best monitor of myocardial oxygenation and that, if possible, surgery in patients at risk of myocardial ischaemia should be performed under local or regional anaesthesia. However, in addition to the fact that patients under the influence of premedication and adjunct sedatives may fail to report angina pectoris, it appears that the incidence of myocardial ischaemia is higher in conscious patients than during general anaesthesia provided that haemodynamics are carefully controlled. Using two-lead (II and V5) ambulatory ECG recorders, one study performed in vascular and other major abdominal surgical patients demonstrated a 19% incidence of new myocardial ischaemia over the 24 h preceding the operation.[65] All these ischaemic episodes were silent, i.e. unaccompanied by any chest discomfort. In comparison, the overall incidence of ischaemia during general anaesthesia and surgery was 14%. Data from our research group, using 12-lead ECG combined with metabolic sampling of lactate from the myocardium for identification of new ischaemia immediately prior to major vascular surgery, have revealed an incidence of 11%. Despite being specifically questioned, only 1 of 13 ischaemic patients in this study reported cardiac symptoms suggestive of ischaemia. This confirms the high proportion of silent myocardial ischaemia documented in previous studies[66] and coincides with data from ischaemic patterns during daily activities in patients with stable coronary artery disease.[67] All these data suggest that awake patients cannot reliably monitor their own myocardial oxygenation. Furthermore, being awake during surgery may contribute to an increased risk of myocardial ischaemia due to higher myocardial oxygen requirements than under general anaesthesia. The findings also suggest that a pre-induction ECG should be performed and compared to the control ECG from the ward before anaesthesia is induced in a patient at high risk of myocardial ischaemia.

Electrocardiography. Electrocardiography is by far the most commonly employed technique to detect myocardial ischaemia during and after surgery. Depression and pseudonormalization of the ST segment are the most common ECG abnormalities indicating subendocardial ischaemia. ST segment elevation indicating spasm-induced transmural ischaemia or new necrosis is far less commonly reported during anaesthesia.[68] The degree of new ST segment deviation caused by myocardial ischaemia is directly proportional to the size of the ischaemic territory when few ECG leads are utilized[69] and has been shown to have prognostic importance in coronary artery bypass surgery.[70] The criteria used to describe abnormality indicating ischaemia, e.g. a horizontal or down-sloping ST depression of at least 0.1 mV measured 60–80 ms after the J-point or at the J-point respectively in at least one lead, or ST elevation of at least 0.2 mV in at least two leads, have been directly adopted from the exercise laboratory. When used in a Caucasian population with a moderate prevalence of coronary artery disease, the specificity of these criteria is excellent provided that recommended band-widths are used, but they may be too strict when applied in a population at high risk of coronary artery disease, such as those with peripheral vascular disease.

The conventional lower band-width cut-off used in most operating room ECG monitors is 0.5 Hz, compared to 0.05 Hz recommended for diagnostic purposes. The 0.5 Hz level reduces the interference from respiratory movements and therefore stabilizes the baseline of the ECG signal. However, it leads to distortion of the ECG complex including the ST segment, and therefore reduces the specificity for ischaemia.[71] Thus, monitors without diagnostic band-width (0.5–100 Hz) should not be used in patients in whom detection of ischaemia is important.

The sensitivity of ECG monitoring for ischaemia is extremely variable and related to several factors which normally can be easily controlled. The sensitivity increases with the number of leads. For instance, the combined use of leads II, V4 and V5 detected 96% of ischaemic abnormalities displayed by a 12-lead ECG.[72] If lead V5 or II alone had been used, 74 and 32% respectively of the ischaemic episodes would have been detected. If lead I had been displayed, all ischaemic events would have been undetected.

When an operating room monitor is 'eye-balled' for ischaemic events, additional factors contribute to reduced sensitivity; the monitor has often not been calibrated to display 1 mV as 10 mm, or the calibration is changed to increase the R-wave amplitude in order to allow correct calculation of heart rate. This may be of particular concern in hypoperfusion of the interventricular septum where loss of R-wave amplitude may be the only sign of ischaemia. Furthermore, the iso-electric baseline to which the level of the ST segment is compared is not easily identifiable since no reference lines are provided. Finally, a control ECG complex pattern is not easily remembered, particularly when it is pathological.

Most standard operating room and intensive care unit monitors provide only three ECG cables, thus allowing display of only one extremity lead or one modified chest lead at a time. The lead selected for monitoring under these circumstances should preferably display the anterior wall unless pre-operative exercise test or ambulatory ECG monitoring has displayed another risk territory. Most commonly, the CS5 is used, e.g. the negative electrode is placed on the right shoulder and the positive electrode where the fifth intercostal interspace intercepts the anterior axillary line, since this electrode configuration provides both lead II and a modified lead V5.

The arguments outlined above provide reasons for the development of computerized ECG systems for monitoring ischaemia. These systems usually provide continuous display of two to three leads and the respective mean complexes. They have the ability to display a control complex and to set the reference and measurement points for the ST segment analysis. Furthermore, complexes may be superimposed to facilitate comparison. Finally, trend functions and alarms for abnormal ST segment deviation are available. These systems have markedly improved perioperative detection of ischaemia and the understanding of mechanisms of ischaemia, and are invaluable tools in modern care of cardiac risk patients. However, their sensitivity and specificity, as well as the criteria for myocardial ischaemia, remain to be evaluated in various low- and high-risk populations. Although serving as a gold standard for ischaemia in many studies, it is evident that even a 12-lead ECG does not have a 100% sensitivity for myocardial ischaemia. Insufficient blood flow to the free wall of the right ventricle, the interventricular septum or the high posterior wall of the left ventricle does not usually produce typical changes in any of the 12 standard leads. If ischaemia in these regions is to be documented, alternative electrode placements (right chest or oesophageal) or a spatial technique such as vectorcardiography should be employed. Vectorcardiography enables all parts of the heart to be monitored for ischaemia with approximately the same sensitivity.

Mechanical techniques. There is strong experimental evidence that myocardial ischaemia leads to abnormal wall function and stunning of the ischaemic territory.[73]

Such changes usually occur in the absence of, or prior to, other indicators of ischaemia such as the ECG. Similar observations have been made in the cardiac catheterization laboratory when a coronary artery has been occluded during angioplasty.[74] However, these findings do not imply that all new wall motion abnormality is of ischaemic origin. Animal studies have demonstrated that progressive narrowing of a coronary artery first results in some post-systolic shortening. With further reduction of flow, some systolic lengthening occurs, systolic shortening diminishes and post-systolic shortening increases. With profound flow limitation, only systolic lengthening and post-systolic shortening occur. However, there are several mechanisms other than ischaemia which can result in reduction of systolic shortening and appearance of post-systolic shortening. Systolic shortening is reduced by increased afterload, reduction of preload and negative inotropic intervention,[75] events which occur frequently during anaesthesia and surgery, and in the recovery period. Post-systolic shortening may be the consequence of delayed onset of relaxation, e.g. following administration of calcium antagonists.[76] Finally, a territory of the myocardium comprising a previous subendocardial injury which contracts normally at normal afterload, preload, inotropy and heart rate may display profound mechanical dysfunction without being ischaemic if ventricular loading conditions, heart rate or inotropy increase. Thus, although numerous studies in which new wall motion abnormality is interpreted as being of ischaemic origin appear in the literature, there is serious doubt as to the specificity of such changes unless loading conditions, inotropy and heart rate are kept within normal limits.[75,77] This concern is valid for both echocardiographic techniques (M-mode, external and transoesophageal two-dimensional echocardiography) and other mechanical techniques such as cardiokymography.

Transoesophageal echocardiography (TEE) is highly specific for ischaemia, and it has been suggested that it is the most sensitive technique available. This may be true for patients undergoing coronary angioplasty, when transmural ischaemia, frequently affecting a large territory, is produced. However, these data cannot be extrapolated to the surgical patient in whom ischaemia is usually the consequence of distal, mild and subendocardial oxygen imbalance.[78] This results in far less mechanical dysfunction, often confined to areas of the myocardium not sampled by TEE, such as the left ventricular basal or apical regions, or the right ventricular free wall. This may explain why Leung and co-workers found that only 8 of 18 episodes of ECG ischaemia were identified by TEE.[79] In addition, several other factors may limit the sensitivity of TEE for ischaemia. First, TEE allows only a qualitative assessment of wall motion; thus, conservative criteria such as a worsening of wall motion by two or more grades must be chosen.[77] Second, segmental wall function is difficult to interpret in the presence of heart rate above 90–100 beats/min. Finally, comparison of diastolic and systolic frames necessitates that image borders are referred to a specific geographical axis (i.e. fixed versus floating), which is difficult to determine.[75] Preliminary data from our research group collected in patients with severe left anterior descending coronary artery stenoses subjected to atrial pacing and afterload manipulations suggest that TEE is both less specific and less sensitive for ischaemia than electrocardiographic techniques. However, these results do not exclude the use of TEE for other purposes in the operating room, recovery area or intensive care unit. Estimation of global and regional ventricular function of ischaemic or non-ischaemic origin, volaemic state and valvular function (by added Doppler technique) may be of great value in situations where other invasive or non-invasive techniques often fail to provide adequate diagnosis or to guide therapy satisfactorily.

Haemodynamic indicators of ischaemia. The importance of measuring blood pressure continuously and avoiding hypotension in patients with coronary artery disease has been illustrated by Lieberman and co-workers in patients undergoing coronary artery bypass grafting under halothane anaesthesia.[80] They demonstrated that a decline of systolic blood pressure and mean arterial pressure to below 90 and 65 mmHg respectively or by more than 30% had an 84% predictive efficiency for ischaemia. A comparable efficiency was found for heart rate above 80 beats/min or by more than 20%. This study has not been repeated in non-cardiac surgical patients, in whom coronary artery disease might be less severe and limits for abnormality are probably different. Vascular patients often have a systolic blood pressure which may be markedly elevated, whereas diastolic pressure may be in the normal range. Regardless of the pressure preoperatively, the same nadir of systolic blood pressure will be reached during anaesthesia. Thus, a derived method (e.g. percentage decrease) to describe blood pressure levels associated with increased risk of ischaemia is probably not applicable in the vascular population. Since coronary stenoses are dynamic rather than fixed, and myocardial oxygen requirements usually reduced under anaesthesia, it also appears difficult to apply an absolute level of blood pressure below which a significant risk of ischaemia is present in a non-cardiac surgical population.

It has been suggested that more complex haemodynamic indices such as the rate-pressure product (RPP = SAP × HR, where SAP = systolic arterial pressure and HR = heart rate), the triple index (TI = SAP × HR × PCWP, where PCWP = pulmonary or the pressure/rate ratio (P/R = MAP/HR, where MAP = mean arterial pressure) would be of value for prediction of ischaemia in at-risk patients. RPP and TI correlate well with the onset of ischaemia during exercise testing in patients with documented coronary artery disease but repeated attempts have failed to demonstrate a parallel change in myocardial oxygen requirements during anaesthesia.[81] Indeed, the worst possible haemodynamic combination leading to ischaemia (hypotension and tachycardia) is associated with unchanged RPP and TI. In this context, the use of the P/R appears more logical. The data which suggested its usefulness in predicting ischaemia were collected in dogs with a single, fixed coronary artery stenosis.[82,83] Under these conditions, a ratio less than 1 correlated closely with mechanical dysfunction in the territory supplied by the stenosed artery. However, although the negative predictive value for ischaemia of P/R is high (around 99%), clinical studies have failed to document a good positive predictive value.[84] This is probably because most coronary stenoses are distensible and therefore may dilate, constrict or collapse in response to a number of stimuli. In addition, this index does not take into consideration mechanisms of supply-related ischaemia unrelated to haemodynamic changes.

Other studies have suggested that an elevation of the pulmonary arterial occlusion pressure (PAOP) associated with an abnormal wave form (A-C or v-waves) is a more sensitive index of myocardial ischaemia than ST segment depression in lead V5 of the ECG.[85] In the study by Lieberman et al,[85] an isolated elevation of PAOP to above 15 mmHg had an equally poor predictive efficiency as an elevation of the central venous pressure, approximately equal to tossing a coin. The agreement between an elevated PAOP combined with abnormal pulmonary arterial pressure waveform and myocardial ischaemia has been confirmed in studies by Häggmark *et al* in vascular surgical patients.[86] However, this index did not appear to be more sensitive, or to precede ECG abnormalities. Unless accompanied by an abnormal pressure waveform, the predictive efficiency of PAOP increasing from control by more than 8 mmHg was as poor as that described by Lieberman *et al*.[80] However, patients who demonstrated a comparable increase in PAOP *combined* with abnormal waveform did have a 92% likelihood of being ischaemic, as diagnosed by other methods. Unfortunately, only 13% of all PAOP measurements and 21% of all ischaemic events were associated with an abnormal pressure waveform. These results, as well as data comparing PAOP to regional ventricular wall function,[79] illustrate the limited usefulness of data derived from the pulmonary artery catheter for detection of myocardial ischaemia.

Recent data suggest that detection and prevention of myocardial ischaemia by good haemodynamic control are the first steps which might contribute to a reduction in cardiac morbidity following vascular surgery.[87] At present, the most sensitive and specific method which provides real-time diagnosis of ischaemia is computerized ST segment analysis. Further developments in this area will probably include more leads and/or spatial techniques to improve diagnosis of ischaemia in myocardial territories not routinely sampled by present state-of-the-art ECG technology.

Detection of LV dysfunction

In clinical practice, measurements of stroke volume and PAOP have been used for almost 20 years to detect LV dysfunction during and after anaesthesia. LV dysfunction can be described as systolic or diastolic. The former is a result of decreased inotropy or augmented LV impedance. In most instances of systolic dysfunction, end-systolic and end-diastolic volumes increase in parallel, resulting in little change in stroke volume[43] (Fig. 9.5). If the left ventricle is chronically dilated, systolic dysfunction is only rarely accompanied by a rise in PAOP. Diastolic dysfunction is characterized by a stiffness of the left ventricle, resulting in an increased PAOP, not necessarily associated with a reduction of stroke volume. However, such haemodynamic aberrations may also be the result of other circulatory abnormalities such as volume overload or systolic dysfunction, which require completely different forms of treatment. Clearly, determination of haemodynamic profiles using measurements derived from the pulmonary artery catheter has several limitations when trying to assess LV function accurately.

TEE provides important additional information because it allows precise estimation of size.[77] Thus, the factors responsible for low cardiac output states or increased PAOP can be distinguished more easily (Fig. 9.5). Two-dimensional images of the short axis cross-section are ideally suited for monitoring of LV filling and ejection. Global LV function should be assessed using the most spherical view of the ventricle at the mid papillary levels. The papillary muscles also serve as reference points to ensure that identical cross-sections are obtained. One study performed during abdominal aortic surgery confirms that TEE detected LV function more reliably than did the pulmonary artery catheter.[88]

Anterior and posterior LV wall thickness can be measured by transmitting the M-mode beam through the short axis of the left ventricle. Wall thickness is an important consideration because it allows accurate estimation of the degree of hypertrophy in relation to ventricular diameter. Hypertrophic LV cardiomyopathy (which is frequently encountered in the vascular patient even in the absence of systemic hypertension) is often associated with a stiff ventricular wall and decreased LV compliance. In such cases, the left atrium contributes importantly to stroke volume. Thus, a moderate reduction in left atrial pressure could markedly decrease stroke volume.

Doppler technique applied via the TEE permits analysis of transmitral blood flow, which reflects changes in instantaneous pressure difference between the left atrium and ventricle (Fig. 9.6). At present, no Doppler index can quantify either LV compliance or LV end-diastolic pressure. However, the beat-to-beat assessment of the LV filling pattern improves understanding of the changes which occur as a result of volume loading, myocardial ischaemia and inotropic interventions.

Assessment of intravascular volume

Important volume shifts are observed frequently during and after major vascular surgery. Volume status is particularly difficult to assess during the early recovery period, with rewarming of a shivering patient on mechanical ventilation. There are several reasons why conventional haemodynamic monitoring may be a poor indicator of changes in intravascular volume. During anaesthesia, hypovolaemia frequently occurs without being accompanied by tachycardia.[89] This is because baroreflexes are depressed by anaesthetic agents and because the volume receptors in the right atrium are

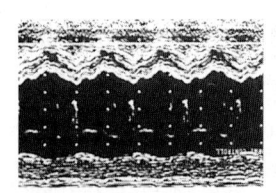

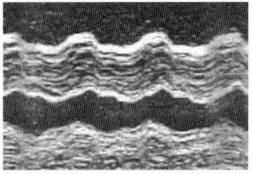

Fig. 9.5 Echocardiograms of the left ventricle from 2 patients obtained peri-operatively using the transoesophageal (two-dimensional and M-mode) approach. Both patients had low blood pressure and in both the pulmonary artery occlusion pressure was 18 mmHg. Echocardiography documented hypovolaemia in a patient with hypertrophic cardiomypathy (left panel) and altered systolic function, with limited left ventricular emptying and enlarged left ventricular cavity in the other patient (right panel).

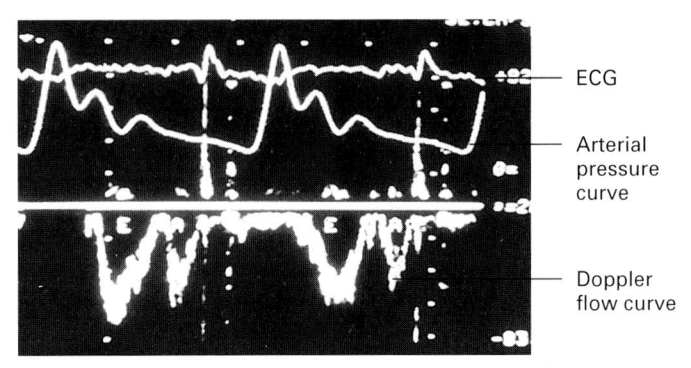

Fig. 9.6 Filling pattern of the left ventricle assessed by the transoesophageal echo–Doppler technique (lower tracing). A normal mitral in-flow velocity profile is shown. The early left ventricular phase (E) is followed by a period of low-velocity flow representing the contribution of atrial contraction (A).

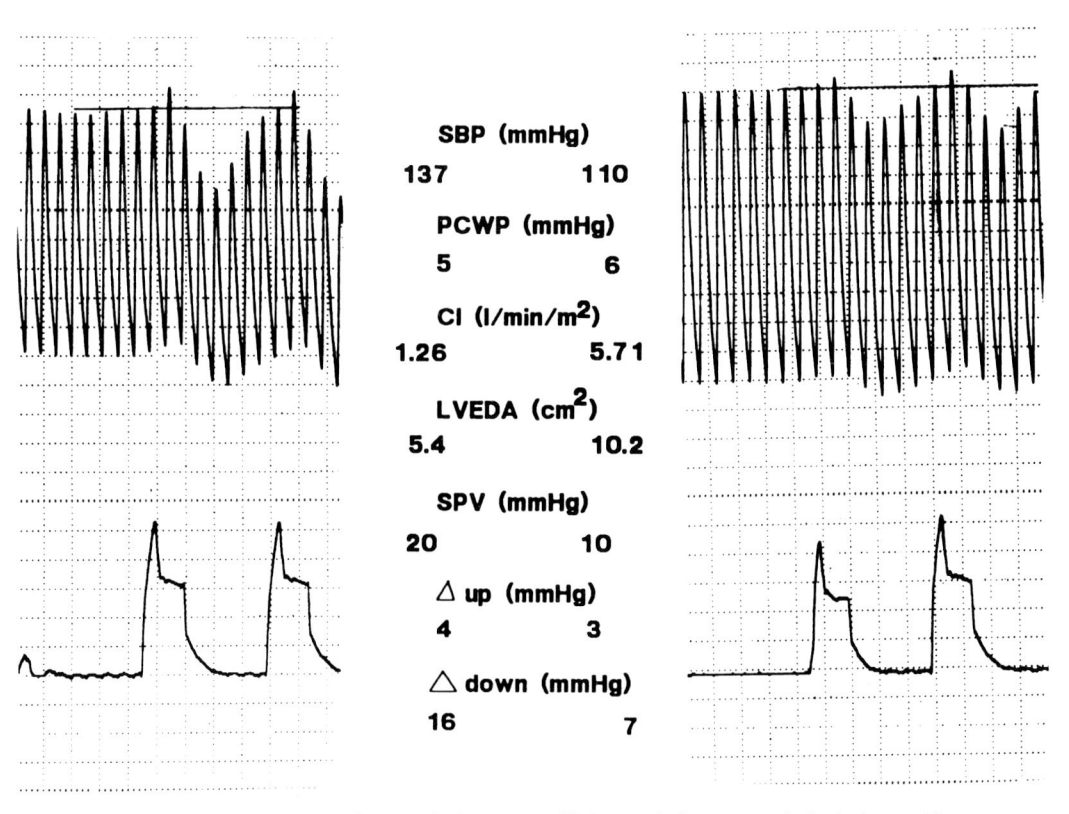

Fig. 9.7 Increased systolic blood pressure (SBP) variation (20 mmHg) recorded postoperatively during positive-pressure ventilation in a patient with hypovolaemia (left panel). After volume loading, SBP variations decreased (right panel). PCWP = Pulmonary capillary wedge pressure; CI- cardiac index; LVEDA = left ventricular end-diastolic area obtained by transoesophageal echocardiographic imaging of the left ventricular cross-sectional area at the insertion of the papillary muscles; SPV = systolic pressure variation.

unloaded by the decreased venous return.[90] Moreover, the main limitation of the pulmonary artery catheter in anaesthesia and surgery is its inability to detect hypovolaemia reliably. Three factors explain why the PAOP overestimates end-diastolic pressure in hypovolaemia. First, hypovolaemia leads to displacement of the pulmonary artery catheter from West zone 3 to zone 2 or 1; consequently, the pressure measured is a reflection of alveolar rather than intravascular pressure. Second, atrial contraction contributes importantly to LV filling during hypovolaemia, and this increases the LV to pulmonary arteriolar pressure gradient. Finally, if tachycardia develops, the premature closure of the mitral valve increases the left atrial to ventricular pressure gradient, while the shortened pressure equilibration time leads to a pressure gradient between the left atrium and the pulmonary artery. In addition, in the presence of a hypertrophic cardiomyopathy which impairs LV compliance, hypovolaemia may be accompanied by an unchanged or even elevated PAOP.

In contrast to the data derived from the pulmonary artery catheter, the analysis of the morphology of the arterial pressure curve is of great clinical interest in the detection of a low preload state during positive-pressure ventilation. The initial phase of lung inflation augments filling of the left ventricle by squeezing the pulmonary veins at the same time as venous return to the right ventricle is reduced. Hypovolaemia augments the resulting influence on systolic blood pressure variations. The magnitude of systolic blood pressure variations observed during positive-pressure ventilation has been shown to correlate closely with preload both experimentally[91] and in patients after aortic surgery[92] (Fig. 9.7). In the clinical study, a systolic blood pressure variation greater than 10 mmHg invariably coincided with an abnormally low preload state detected by TEE (Fig. 9.8). In contrast, PAOP did not reflect preload reliably in animals or in humans.

Detection of cardiogenic pulmonary oedema

The hydrostatic pressure in the pulmonary capillary bed is the principal pressure governing passage of fluid towards the interstitial compartment. In the presence of LV systolic or, more frequently, diastolic dysfunction, pulmonary capillary hydrostatic pressure may exceed the threshold at which acute pulmonary oedema is likely to develop. However, pulmonary oedema is not an inevitable consequence. According to the Starling law, both colloid pressure inside the capillary and hydrostatic pressures outside the capillary counteract the passage of fluid towards the interstitial compartment. In addition, the relationship between pulmonary capillary hydrostatic pressure and PAOP is affected by a number of pathological conditions, such as pulmonary hypertension or increased permeability due to sepsis.

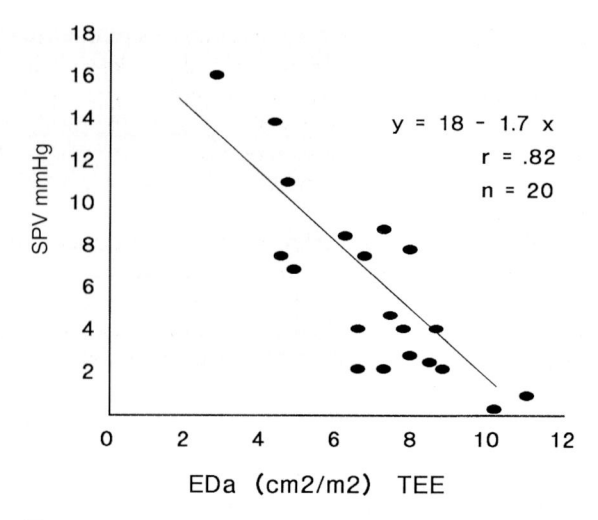

Fig. 9.8 Relationship between systolic pressure variations (mmHg) (SPV) and end-diastolic area (EDa), by transoesophageal echocardiography in patients maintained under fentanyl sedation and mechanical ventilation after abdominal aortic surgery. A close relationship between EDa and SPV was observed, indicating that SPV is preload-dependent.

In clinical practice, pulmonary oedema is an infrequent problem during anaesthesia because most anaesthetic agents or techniques decrease ventricular loading conditions.[8] When pulmonary oedema occurs during vascular surgery, it is usually the result of abrupt or high aortic clamping, severe fluid overload and/or extended myocardial ischaemia. In contrast, patients with limited cardiac reserve are at significant risk of pulmonary oedema in the early postoperative period. Several factors operational at this time contribute to increase both preload and afterload. In particular, the passage from assisted to spontaneous ventilation increases the risk of pulmonary oedema. At the same time, LV function is often depressed by residual anaesthetic agents and myocardial stunning following intra- or postoperative myocardial ischaemia.[7]

Monitoring of organ perfusion pressure

Arterial pressure recorded from a peripheral artery has generally been accepted as a reflection of perfusion pressure governing flow to different central or more distal organs. In vascular surgery, this is probably not always true. Nevertheless, direct arterial pressure monitoring is indicated during aortic and carotid artery surgery. This is principally because meticulous control of blood pressure is needed during surgical manipulations (to avoid myocardial or cerebral ischaemia) and during recovery from anaesthesia (see below).

The assumption that arterial pressure recorded from peripheral vessels truly reflects the levels in the proximal aorta and throughout the arterial system is a simplification, and is probably not valid. Recent studies in humans have clarified the role of arterial distensibility, vascular impedance, pulse-wave velocity and reflection in the generation of the amplitude of the systolic pressure in systemic arteries.[93] Particularly relevant for those who handle vascular surgical patients are the structural changes that occur in peripheral and central arteries due to ageing, atherosclerosis and hypertension,[94] as well as the influence of drugs which alter arterial tone. Ageing, atherosclerosis and hypertension all lead to a similar decrease in vascular distensibility and increased pulse-wave velocity, with premature return of reflected waves from the periphery. Consequently, increased aortic pulse pressure, a late systolic peak and disappearance of diastolic waves in the aortic pressure curve are seen. Peripheral pressure measurements performed in elderly, atherosclerotic and/or hypertensive patients thus underestimate central arterial pressure. In comparison, peripheral vasodilator therapy produces opposite effects on the central to peripheral systolic pressure gradient. Dilatation of small peripheral arteries proximal to the high-resistance vessels, for example, with nitroglycerine, decreases pressure-wave reflection and can therefore reduce aortic systolic pressure by as much as 25 mmHg without altering radial arterial systolic pressure. All these data also indicate that analysis of the arterial pressure waveform to derive indirect estimates of LV systolic function, peripheral vascular resistance or stroke volume is a useless exercise in vascular surgical patients.

Assessment of total body oxygen reserve

Spectrophotometric techniques applied via a pulmonary artery catheter allow continuous monitoring of mixed venous oxygen saturation. This variable indicates the degree to which compensatory mechanisms are activated in order to preserve peripheral oxygenation.[95] Mixed venous oxygen saturation depends principally on total body oxygen consumption and systemic oxygen delivery. In the presence of low total body oxygen consumption, as occurs during general anaesthesia, mixed venous oxygen saturation decreases significantly only if oxygen delivery is severely compromised. Thus, aortic clamping, which reduces total body oxygen consumption by exclusion of areas distal to the clamp, confuses the interpretation of the mixed venous oxygen saturation.

In clinical practice, the main interest in the technique relates to the study of global oxygen balance during stressful situations in which total body oxygen consumption is increased, e.g. after declamping of, particularly, the suprarenal aorta and during recovery from anaesthesia.[96] In these situations, a decrease in mixed venous oxygen saturation is a physiological mechanism designed to ensure peripheral oxygenation. Thus, it does not necessarily indicate that the oxygen needs of the body are not adequately met. However, once the oxygen reserve is used, it is no longer available to compensate for other events which may limit peripheral oxygen delivery. A decrease in mixed venous oxygen saturation to 50% indicates that the oxygen extraction reserve is in the process of being depleted.[97]

At present, the interest in continuous recording of mixed venous oxygen saturation in vascular surgery is limited to major aortic surgery, particularly on the thoraco-abdominal aorta.

Practical guidelines for cardiovascular monitoring of the vascular surgical patient

Extensive invasive monitoring is seldom needed, even in major vascular surgery. When used without precise indications, invasive techniques, particularly pulmonary artery catheterization, may be hazardous to the patient, not only for technical reasons, but also because data derived from the catheter, as described above, may lead to erroneous diagnosis and therapy. This may explain why no benefit of peri-operative use of the pulmonary artery catheter has been found in randomized studies of cardiac surgical patients with normal or impaired LV function. The same argument was put forward to explain the strikingly higher morbidity observed in patients with acute myocardial infarction monitored by a pulmonary artery catheter compared to a matched population cared for without invasive techniques.

We recommend that all vascular patients are monitored for ischaemia using computerized ST segment analysis. In addition, continuous recording of arterial pressure is indicated in all patients undergoing major aortic and neck artery procedures. Patients subjected to peripheral arterial revascularization generally do not need an arterial catheter.

We use pre-operative external two-dimensional echocardiography or radionuclide angiography to determine whether a pulmonary artery or a central venous catheter should be used in abdominal aortic surgery. Central venous access is indicated for transfusion reasons and central venous pressure (CVP) correlates well with PAOP in the majority of vascular patients, regardless of LV function. However, the slope of the CVP/PAOP regression line is low, in the order of 0.2–0.3. This implies that a 10 mmHg rise in PAOP is reflected as only a 2–3 mmHg increase in CVP, a change which would not be detected by standard haemodynamic monitoring system in a patient on positive-pressure ventilation. These data contrast with findings in patients undergoing coronary bypass surgery, in whom a good correlation between CVP and PAOP with a regression line slope around 1 was found, but only in patients whose LV function was preserved.[98] Thus, when pressure data believed to reflect LV end-diastolic pressure are needed, a pulmonary artery catheter should be used. In our long clinical and research experiences from the vascular patient population, we have observed that patients with pre-operative globally depressed LV function or with akinesia or dyskinesia of the anterior and/or septal walls often develop myocardial ischaemia, high PAOP and further deterioration of LV function on TEE during various periods of perioperative stress. In contrast, patients with preserved global and regional LV function rarely display important aberrations of this type unless they have severe coronary stenoses. TEE provides a very useful complement to the pulmonary artery catheter in instances of doubt as to the cause of circulatory dysfunction, and to guide fluid therapy. In our clinical practice, the use of TEE has gradually reduced the need for a pulmonary artery catheter for all indications other than the early detection of cardiogenic pulmonary oedema.

In more complicated aortic surgical procedures, which may include partial bypass or hypothermic cardiac arrest, we may use multiple sites for arterial pressure measurements, pulmonary artery pressure monitoring, continuous display of mixed venous oxygen saturation and TEE. However, no controlled data have indicated that such intense monitoring would improve outcome.

Monitoring of the neurological system

Surgical procedures in which neurological monitoring has been advocated are mainly carotid endarterectomy and thoraco-abdominal aortic resection.

In carotid surgery, some surgeons prefer to operate on conscious patients after performing a deep cervical block.[99] Adequate collateral perfusion is tested by a 1–4 min occlusion of the internal carotid artery. The decision whether or not to use a shunt is based entirely on the clinical appearance of new neurological deficits during this test clamping period. Poor patient cooperation, including involuntary movements during temporary cerebral ischaemia, may make shunt insertion difficult in the awake patient. In addition, late neurological deficits which may occur in the awake patient due to embolization from the shunt can further endanger patient safety.

Other techniques used to monitor the brain when carotid endarterectomy is performed under general anaesthesia include electroencephalography (EEG), measurement of regional cerebral blood flow (r-CBF) and assessment of carotid artery stump pressure, i.e. the pressure distal to the carotid arterial clamp.

The EEG is modified not only by brain ischaemia but also by sedatives and anaesthetic agents, body temperature changes and variations in blood pressure.[100] Both conventional 16-channel raw-signal EEG and more simple EEG devices with fewer leads and fast Fourier analysis for signal processing are highly sensitive for cerebral ischaemia. However, if the EEG is used to assess the need for a shunt, it is possible that its lack of specificity may contribute to increase neurological morbidity by unnecessary shunt insertions. The decision to use EEG monitoring routinely should therefore be based on the neurological morbidity rate of the institution. If this is low (in the order of 1–2%), EEG monitoring will probably not alter neurological outcome. If the neurological deficit rate is higher, and indications and techniques for surgery and anaesthesia are considered to be adequate, EEG monitoring should be considered.

Changes in r-CBF assessed by injection of radioactive xenon directly into the clamped internal carotid artery correlate well with regional cerebral ischaemia. Our opinion is that this rather complicated technique is a research tool rather than a monitoring device with an acceptable cost/benefit ratio.

Measurement of internal carotid artery stump pressure is still used widely to assess whether or not collateral brain perfusion is sufficient. The use of this approach to determine whether a shunt should be inserted has been shown repeatedly to be unreliable.[101] The number of false-positives (i.e. patients with a stump pressure below 60 mmHg and cerebral blood flow above 24 ml/min per 100 g brain tissue) is in the order of 30%. Thus, unnecessary shunting with a potential for neurological complications may occur. However, a stump pressure above 60 mmHg indicates minimal risk of cerebral ischaemia.

Somatosensory evoked potential (SSEP) monitoring has been used in a limited series for surveillance of patients undergoing carotid endarterectomy. It is generally believed that this technique is less reliable than conventional or processed EEG monitoring.[102] More encouraging results of SSEP monitoring have been reported when this technique has been applied in thoraco-abdominal aortic surgery to reduce the risk of paraplegia.[103] However, case reports do indicate that SSEP may be associated with false-negative results.[104] This is basically because SSEPs are mediated via pathways which are anatomically distinctly different from the motor pathways and which have a different blood supply. Limitations of the SSEP also include the interpretation of reversibility of observed defects, and determination of the importance of the length of time that signals have been absent. All these concerns have led to the development of motor evoked potentials (MEP). We cannot at present provide data which reliably document beneficial effects on neurological outcome of this type of monitoring.

PRINCIPLES OF INTRA-OPERATIVE MANAGEMENT

Overall, the anaesthetic management of vascular patients differs little from patients subjected to coronary artery surgery. Specific technical aspects of the various surgical procedures require special attention by the anaesthetist, as they relate to manipulation of the circulation. The overall message is to maintain circulatory stability at or near the patient's normal values. By adopting this approach, the risks of ischaemia and associated cardiovascular complications are minimized.

Premedication and pre-induction management

The high incidence of silent myocardial ischaemia preceding vascular surgery has been referred to above. Ambulatory ECG monitoring has revealed that patients with coronary artery disease admitted to the hospital for vascular or other non-cardiac surgery had approximately a doubling of their ischaemic episodes when monitored on the ward compared to monitoring during their normal daily activities.[30,32] Ischaemia has been documented in 11–30% of patients on arrival in the vascular or cardiac operating suite.[105] This problem is largely overlooked in clinical practice because the anaesthetist seldom takes the time or has the means to perform proper ECG control before inducing anaesthesia. In addition, a significant proportion of ischaemic events are not detected by the ECG. Thus, it is apparent that a significant proportion of vascular patients are anaesthetized in an undiagnosed ischaemic state.

Adequate premedication is the key to avoiding pre-induction ischaemia. We prefer to start premedicating our vascular patients on the night before surgery by giving a sleep dose of a long-acting benzodiazepine. A similar oral dose of this benzodiazepine is given about 1 h before induction of anaesthesia, together with the patient's normal cardiac and antihypertensive medication and intramuscular or subcutaneous morphine, 100–200 µg/kg, combined with scopolamine. Angiotensin-converting enzyme inhibitors are usually discontinued the day before surgery to avoid unexpected hypotension and bradycardia following induction. This format of premedication produces heavy sedation which may be associated with hypoxaemia. Consequently, supplementary oxygen should always be administered during transport of the patient to the operating room. When this regimen is used in patients scheduled for coronary bypass surgery, we have documented a reduction of pre-induction ischaemia to below 1%.

Extensive instrumentation of the patient before induction is seldom necessary. A large-diameter intra-venous cannula and an arterial catheter should be inserted under local anaesthesia, but central venous or pulmonary artery catheterization is best performed after induction, while the patient is being prepared for surgery. For reasons outlined in detail above, pre-operative construction of haemodynamic profiles is a meaningless exercise, particularly because ECG or nuclear techniques provide more reliable estimates of global and segmental LV function.

General anaesthesia

Induction techniques for elective carotid and aortic surgery

The ideal induction technique for elective vascular patients should produce minimal haemodynamic changes, but should blunt the responses to tracheal intubation and other noxious stimuli. This effect cannot be obtained by a single induction agent. With the exception of ketamine and etomidate, all agents used for anaesthetic induction reduce myocardial oxygen requirements. They do this by differential effects on inotropy, heart rate, ventricular loading conditions and wall stress. The haemodynamic changes which occur are principally the results of a direct negative inotropic action and depression of central sympathetic activity leading to decreased venous and arterial tone. In the presence of a hypertrophic cardiomyopathy, reduction in venous tone may lead to severe impairment of LV systolic function (Fig. 9.9).

Numerous studies have demonstrated that short-acting agents such as barbiturates and propofol produce both hypotension and tachycardia in vascular patients and do not offer adequate protection from the stress associated with tracheal intubation.[106–108] A high

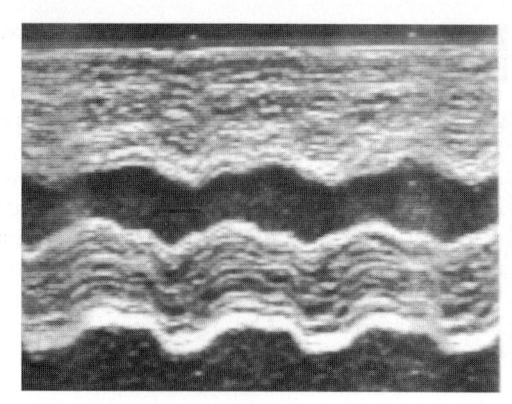

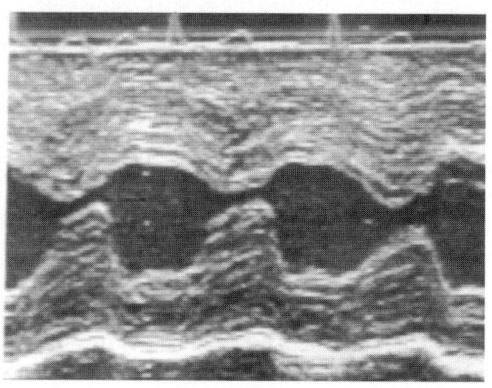

Fig. 9.9 Intra-operative echocardiograms of the left ventricle obtained by the transoeosophageal (M-mode) approach in a patient with left ventricular hypertrophy. At the time when the haemodynamic status was poor (left panel), the echocardiogram documented inadequate preload and impaired contraction pattern. The haemodynamics improved rapidly after administration of intravenous fluids and ephedrine (right panel).

incidence of ischaemia elicited by tracheal intubation after thiopentone induction has been documented in several studies in vascular patients.[107,109,110] To overcome this problem, numerous adjunct techniques have been proposed. These include volatile anaesthetic agents, opioids, intravenous lignocaine, vasodilators, β-blockers and laryngeal nerve block.

High-dose opioid techniques used in cardiac surgery offer the advantage of a very smooth induction and stable conditions for tracheal intubation, but protect the patient poorly from the stress of abdominal surgery.[111] In addition, the elimination half-life of fentanyl is prolonged in patients subjected to aortic surgery,[111] which further extends the respiratory depression associated with this technique. In contrast, a combination of a small dose of midazolam or diazepam (10–25 μg/kg) or thiopentone and fentanyl (5–8 μg/kg) offers the advantage of producing minimal haemodynamic changes while still blunting effectively the response to intubation[112] (see below). Patients with low blood volume and/or increased sympathetic tone may still respond to this induction technique with a marked reduction in venous return. Volume loading and vasoactive amines easily reverse the hypotension.

Non-anaesthetic agents used to smooth out the circulatory responses to induction and intubation in vascular patients comprise mainly β-blockers and intravenous nitroglycerine. A single dose of a long-acting oral β-blocker has been shown to reduce significantly the increase in heart rate and the incidence of ischaemic events in vascular patients with borderline untreated hypertension.[107] Likewise, the use of the ultrashort-acting β-blocker esmolol prior to induction of anaesthesia for carotid artery surgery blunts the response to the noxious stimulus of intubation (Fig. 9.10).[113] Interestingly, this drug also possesses a central effect which reduces the dose of hypnotics needed for induction.[114] When LV function might be chronically depressed, the prophylactic use of intravenous nitroglycerine is a better choice than β-blockers. In a study by Fusciardi and co-workers,[108] an intravenous dose of nitroglycerine 0.9 μg/kg per min started before induction of anaesthesia with thiopentone and fentanyl (3 μg/kg) completely abolished the increases in blood pressure and PAOP, and reduced the

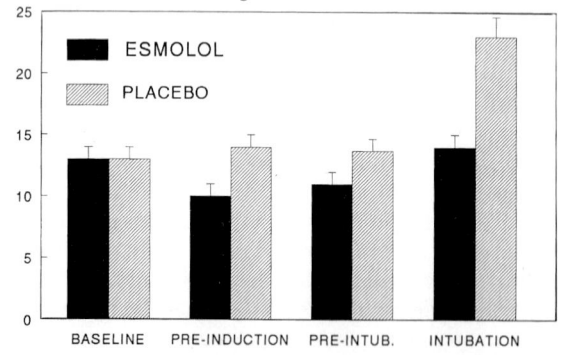

Fig. 9.10 Rate-pressure product changes during induction of anaesthesia and tracheal intubation in patients scheduled for carotid endarterectomy. Five minutes before induction, intravenous administration of esmolol (500 μg/kg per min for 4 min, then 300 μg/kg per min for 8 min) or placebo was started. Anaesthesia was induced with thiopentone at 2–6 mg kg. Adapted from Cucchiara et al.[113] SBP = Systolic blood pressure; HR = heart rate.

incidence of ischaemia compared to patients who did not receive nitroglycerine. Since nitroglycerine decreases preload, volume loading may be necessary with this technique. Similar results to those in the nitroglycerine group were observed if the fentanyl dose (combined with thiopentone) was increased to 8 μg/kg.

The choice of muscle relaxant for induction produces little problem in vascular surgery. Pancuronium, which has been reported to produce tachycardia and increase the risk of ischaemia when used in coronary artery bypass patients, has little haemodynamic effect when administered with benzodiazepines and fentanyl to vascular surgical patients.[115] On the contrary, the combination of a benzodiazepine, fentanyl and vecuronium may sometimes produce profound bradycardia,[45] the mechanism of which is not fully understood.

Emergency aortic surgery. This group of patients comprises those with dissection of the aorta and normal or high blood pressure, and those with retroperitoneal, intra-abdominal, intrathoracic or intrapericardial rupture of an aneurysm associated with more or less profound circulatory shock. In the former group, meticulous control of blood pressure is needed to avoid rupture. A vasodilator may be required, because even a moderate increase in systolic blood pressure may provoke further dissection. Induction techniques are otherwise identical to those described for elective surgery. In patients with a ruptured aneurysm, the haemodynamic state is generally characterized by intense compensatory vasoconstriction. Consequently, all agents which alleviate sympathetic tone are associated with profound hypotension. Induction of anaesthesia is accomplished most commonly with a low dose of fentanyl (2-3 μg/kg) combined with small incremental doses of either etomidate or ketamine, and accompanied by aggressive volume replacement. The essential approach to these patients is to apply the aortic clamp as quickly as possible and then proceed with further placement of monitoring devices, volume replacement and other anaesthetic measures.

Maintenance of anesthesia

The principles of maintenance of anaesthesia for vascular surgery are complicated by the surgical manipulations, which may markedly influence the circulatory status and the homeostasis of the patient. We will describe first the general principles as they relate to choice of primary anesthetic agent and then proceed to discuss more specifically how circulatory control is established in relation to the specific surgical procedure.

As with induction, administration of anesthetic agents for maintenance of anaesthesia should be performed in a fashion that minimizes circulatory changes. The choice of primary anesthetic agent can be left to the discretion of the anesthetist since no published study has reliably identified one agent, inhalational or intravenous, as superior to others. However, it appears evident that techniques involving a single anesthetic agent should be avoided because, inevitably they will have negative side-effects on the circulation or provide insufficient control of noxious stimuli. The actual trend in anaesthesia is therefore to use a basal compound for analgesia, such as fentanyl, and then to add one of the volatile agents to avoid awareness and smooth out the effects of noxious stimuli. In this manner, the side-effects of each agent are minimized.

Several studies performed in cardiac and vascular surgical patients have compared halothane and isoflurane when used to control intra-operative hypertension caused by surgical stimulation under basal fentanyl anaesthesia. Both agents effectively reduced the elevated blood pressure while displaying a different effect on LV function. In one study, performed during sternotomy, halothane decreased stroke index and PAOP remained constant, whereas isoflurane reduced PAOP and improved stroke index.[116] This reduction of wall tension produced by isoflurane will favourably influence subendocardial perfusion, explaining the alleviation of ischaemia observed in some patients. Preliminary results from our group collected in aortic surgical patients have confirmed these systemic haemodynamic differences between the agents. Furthermore, data derived from TEE allowed us to observe improve LV emptying with isoflurane but not with halothane.[117] These results indicate that LV performance is improved when isoflurane is used to control intra-operative hypertension in vascular patients.

The use of isoflurane in patients with coronary artery disease has been controversial despite the obviously beneficial effects on myocardial oxygen balance observed in the treatment of intra-operative hypertension. Under such conditions, ischaemia-induced metabolic coronary vasodilatation will, of course, largely override any direct influence of isoflurane on the coronary vessels. The controversy, which was based on the finding that isoflurane dilated coronary resistance vessels[118,119] and thus had the potential to produce regional and/or transmural flow maldistribution,[120] is now largely resolved. Under certain experimental and clinical conditions, such flow redistribution might cause myocardial ischaemia.[119,120] Several observations explain why ischaemia produced by isoflurane-induced coronary vasodilatation is a rare event in clinical practice. First, isoflurane produces dose-dependent coronary vasodilatation in animals[120] and in patients with vascular and coronary disease.[121] In humans, this vasodilatation is significant only if the inhaled dose is above 1–1.5%, but may occasionally be observed also at lower dose levels. If isoflurane is used as an adjunct to opioids rather than as the sole anaesthetic, as described above, there is consequently no, or negligible, coronary vasodilatation in the majority of patients. Second, the anatomical condition for r-CBF redistribution consists of a territory behind a complete coronary occlusion supplied by collaterals from another, stenosed artery. This anatomical pattern was observed in 23% of patients in the Coronary Artery Surgery Study registry,[122] but is considerably less common in an unselected population of vascular or other non-cardiac surgical patients. A patient with a clinical history of previous myocardial infarction and persistent angina pectoris would have the potential for a steal-prone anatomy. Transmural maldistribution requires a critical stenosis in an epicardial artery, i.e. subendocardial vasodilator reserve should be exhausted. More importantly, and relevant for both transmural and regional flow distribution, are those haemodynamic effects produced by anaesthetic agents which could exhaust subendocardial vasodilator reserve (tachycardia and hypotension), and thereby increase the potential for pharmacologically induced flow maldistribution. However, the negative inotropy produced by isoflurane augments subendocardial vasodilator reserve and thereby counterbalances pharmacological vasodilatation. Finally, although blood flow may be redistributed to some degree by isoflurane, ischaemia would still only develop if oxygen demand exceeds supply in the territory partially deprived of flow.

Simple rules for the use of isoflurane in patients with known or suspected coronary artery disease are therefore to avoid high inspired concentrations of the anaesthetics, to prevent haemodynamic aberrations which increase the potential for flow maldistribution (hypotension and tachycardia) and to monitor the ECG for ischaemia. With this approach, several studies have documented that isoflurane is as safe as other volatile agents or opioids in patients with coronary artery disease.[123]

The influence of nitrous oxide on the cardiovascular system of patients with vascular disease has been the subject of controversy ever since the publication of data demonstrating that this compound was able to produce segmental ventricular wall dysfunction when added to fentanyl or isoflurane in dogs with critical coronary constriction.[124] There is little evidence that this effect is mediated by a direct action on coronary blood vessels because nitrous oxide exerts only mild constriction of epicardial vessels.[125] It appeared in one study[126] as if a low coronary perfusion pressure was a prerequisite for nitrous oxide to produce ischaemia when associated with isoflurane.

Cardiovascular anaesthetists frequently observe that nitrous oxide may produce profound cardiodepression, characterized by progressive falls in blood pressure and cardiac output combined with LV dilatation on TEE, in some rare vascular or cardiac patients with pre-existing LV dysfunction.[127] Nitrous oxide exerts both negative inotropic and sympathetic stimulatory actions.[128] In patients with normal ventricular function, it is therefore conceivable that nitrous oxide does not significantly influence LV function. In contrast, it is possible that the negative inotropy may predominate over the sympathomimetic action in patients with impaired LV function who are already perfused at an elevated sympathetic level. Three studies in patients with normal or decreased LV function scheduled to undergo coronary bypass surgery failed to demonstrate any major influence of nitrous oxide on ventricular function as assessed by TEE.[129-131] However, preliminary data from our group indicate that nitrous oxide administered to patients with coronary artery disease undergoing abdominal aortic surgery was associated with a significantly higher incidence of myocardial ischaemia and greater need for adjunct nitroglycerine during surgical stimulation than in comparable patients randomized to receive a similar anaesthetic without nitrous oxide. These observations were made at identical total minimum alveolar concentration, systemic haemodynamics and inspired oxygen fraction (Table 9.4). It is possible that the contrasting results from these studies could be explained by the fact that the aortic surgical patients were studied at maximal surgical stress and sympathetic levels, whereas the patients scheduled to undergo coronary or carotid surgery were studied in the unstimulated stage, before incision. Consequently, it appears that nitrous oxide, when used in patients with coronary artery disease during major vascular surgery, might be associated with negative circulatory side-effects. If progressive cardiodepression and/or myocardial ischaemia are observed under such conditions, the first step would be to replace nitrous oxide with nitrogen and an equipotent anaesthetic dose of a volatile anaesthetic agent, preferably isoflurane.

Regional anaesthesia

Regional techniques which are applicable for vascular

Table 9.4 Incidence of new 12-lead electrocardiographic, mechanical and metabolic abnormalities recorded in vascular surgical patients not displaying any such aberration while awake. Patients were randomized to receive either isoflurane–fentanyl administered with nitrous oxide/oxygen or with nitrogen/oxygen at $F_{I_{O_2}} = 0.40$

	New intra-operative abnormalities					
	Nitroglycerine treatment	ST segment depression >0.05 mV	ST segment depression >0.1 mV	Type 2 or type 3 CKG	Lactate production	Postop. ST segment depression >0.1 mV
Nitrous oxide/oxygen (%)	18.3	20.5	9.1	23.5	3.5	19.1
Nitrogen/oxygen (%)	0	4.9	0	3.0	1.2	42.9
$P <$	0.001	0.01	0.01	0.01	n.s	n.s

CKG = Cardiokymography.
From unpublished data by Reiz et al.

surgery include central nerve blocks (subarachnoid block, cervical, thoracic and lumbar epidural analgesia) and peripheral nerve blocks (principally deep cervical blocks and upper- and lower-extremity blocks). Only the effects of central blocks are discussed here.

Lumbar epidural and subarachnoid (spinal) analgesia

The main indications for these blocks are to provide anaesthesia for lower-extremity revascularization and/or to afford postoperative analgesia with opioids after major abdominal or thoracic vascular surgery. Graft blood flow is higher if epidural anaesthesia rather than general anaesthesia is employed for peripheral vascular graft surgery.[132] For peripheral revascularization in otherwise healthy, younger patients, we find little difference between the continuous epidural and single-shot subarachnoid techniques, other than the ability to prolong analgesia over many hours by inserting an indwelling epidural catheter. We do not routinely recommend continuous spinal techniques in younger patients because of the high incidence of post-spinal headache in this population when 20-gauge epidural catheters have been inserted intrathecally. The use of ultra-thin catheters may reduce the incidence of headache but has been associated with fragmentation of catheters and other technical problems. However, in older, fragile patients, particularly those with multi-system disease, there is a definite advantage in the continuous spinal technique; the dose of local anaesthetic can be titrated precisely to combine excellent analgesia and rapid onset and offset, with minimal alterations in circulatory status.[133,134]

The main complication of these techniques in relation to vascular surgery is the risk of hypotension with associated myocardial ischaemia. The onset of hypotension is more rapid with spinal analgesia.

Sympathetic block produces regional vasodilatation in blocked areas, with compensatory vasoconstriction in unblocked areas.[135] Dilatation of veins predominates over arterial dilatation because basal sympathetic tone plays an important role, particularly in the adaptation of capacitance vessel tone. The degree of compensatory vasoconstriction is directly proportional to the upper level of a lumbar epidural block and to the change in central venous pressure produced by the block, i.e. the increased vascular tone serves to maintain venous return.[136] These data also explain why patients with elevated sympathetic activity and/or disturbed diastolic LV function, as in hypertrophic cardiomyopathy, are at greater risk of hypotension.

Patients with coronary artery disease respond with maintained or improved global and segmental LV function to the unloading of the left ventricle.[137] However, impairment of segmental LV wall function suggestive of ischaemia has been reported in vascular patients with severe coronary artery disease.[138] For the same reduction in blood pressure, epidural and subarachnoid analgesia decrease myocardial oxygen requirements less than general anaesthesia with volatile anaesthetics.[139] Close control of blood pressure and monitoring for ischaemia are therefore essential when these techniques are applied in vascular patients with coronary artery disease.

Although both epidural and subarachnoid analgesia can reduce the incidence of deep venous thrombosis in patients subjected to hip replacement or plastic surgery, there is no evidence to date of any advantage in this respect in comparison with general anaesthetic techniques in patients undergoing vascular surgery.

With respect to postoperative pain management via indwelling epidural or subarachnoid catheters, we recognize that opioids administered at the lumbar level are also efficient for abdominal or thoracic pain.

However, we believe that it is more practical to place an epidural catheter at the level of the spinal cord which receives afferent impulses from painful areas, because additional treatment with epidural local anaesthetics is often needed to provide adequate pain relief.

Thoracic epidural analgesia

The main indications for thoracic epidural analgesia (TEA) in vascular surgery are to reduce the need for general anaesthetic agents and muscle relaxants during abdominal aortic procedures and to provide optimal conditions for postoperative pain relief.[140] Although TEA for abdominal aortic surgery has been described, we do not recommend its use for thoracic aortic procedures, because surgery itself carries a significant risk of paraplegia.

If an epidural catheter is inserted at a level between T7 and T9, it is possible to titrate the dose of local anaesthetic to provide an adequate block with little or no vasodilatation in the lower extremities. However, it is not always possible to avoid partial blockade of the sympathetic outflow to the heart, which has its principal pathways at the T1–T5 levels. Nevertheless, these effects usually have little influence on cardiovascular status until general anaesthesia is added. Regardless of the agents used, general anaesthesia produces withdrawal of the vasoconstriction which compensates for the regional vasodilatation induced by TEA by depressing central sympathetic outflow. This may result in profound hypotension, sometimes associated with severe bradycardia. In addition to loss of vascular tone and decreased venous return, other mechanisms exist which tend to result in hypotension when TEA is combined with general anaesthesia; these include depressed baroreflexes,[141] negative inotropy produced by the block and by general anaesthetics, and direct vascular effects of the general anaesthetics, in particular opioids and isoflurane. There are also additive negative chronotropic and inotropic effects of high TEA in patients who take chronic β-blocker medication.

This complex interplay between TEA and general anaesthesia may provide difficulties for the anaesthetist in maintaining a stable circulation. This difficulty usually outweighs the benefit of using lower doses of general anaesthetics and the resultant faster recovery. In one study, TEA combined with light general anaesthesia was associated with a stable hypodynamic circulation and little ischaemia in high-risk abdominal vascular patients compared with an equally sick group randomized to receive general balanced anaesthesia, but the incidence of postoperative cardiac complications was the same.[140] A more recent study from our group has confirmed that the intra-operative use of TEA for abdominal aortic procedures does not influence cardiac outcome (Table 9.5).[143] Although the need for postoperative ventilation was significantly reduced by the use of TEA, the pulmonary complication rate was the same as in patients who received general anaesthesia only.[143] However, the intra-operative use of TEA combined with several days of postoperative aggressive pain therapy via the epidural catheter in an intensive care unit may improve the outcome of high-risk patients after abdominal surgery. This suggestion needs further evaluation in a sufficiently large and homogeneous study population before it can be accepted. Presently, there appears to be a trend to insert the thoracic epidural catheter before induction

Table 9.5 Mortality and major postoperative morbidity reported in two studies comparing general anaesthesia (group 1) with thoracic epidural anaesthesia associated with light general anaesthesia (group 2)

	Baron et al[143]		Yeager et al[140]	
	Group 1 ($n = 86$)	Group 2 ($n = 89$)	Group 1 ($n = 25$)	Group 2 ($n = 28$)
Mortality	4	3	4	0*
Cardiac complications	22	19	13	4*
Myocardial infarction	5	5		
Congestive heart failure	7	5		
Prolonged myocardial ischaemia	16	16		
Major infection+	19	10	10	2*
Acute respiratory failure	8	4	8	3
Renal failure	2	4	3	1

*$P < 0.05$ versus group 1.
+General sepsis or pneumonia.

of general anaesthesia, but to use it only to provide analgesia in the recovery period.

Influence and management of surgical manipulations

Aortic surgery

Surgical factors which influence the circulatory stability during aortic resections are principally cross-clamping and unclamping. We shall discuss in detail their respective influence on the heart, the distribution of vascular volume and how these manoeuvres affects other organ systems such as the spinal cord and the brain.

Aortic cross-clamping (AC). AC is characterized by an elevation of impedance to LV ejection, due not only to the mechanical occlusion of the vessel but also to decreased vascular compliance in the region above the clamp. Venous return is reduced less than expected from the large territory excluded from blood flow distal to the clamp because of redistribution of cardiac output towards the territories above the clamp, and significant collateral circulation.[144] AC is associated also with metabolic consequences; there is a reduction in total body oxygen consumption, and it has been suggested that the reduction in cardiac output which accompanies AC is simply due to adaptation to the decreased need for oxygen delivery.[145]

The modification of the circulation produced by AC depends on several factors: the level of clamping (intra-abdominal, suprarenal or thoracic), LV function, the degree of collateral circulation, the agents used for maintenance of anaesthesia and intravascular volume. Before discussing the effects of different levels of AC we will briefly outline the influence of the other mechanisms.

The results of increased afterload and decreased venous return produced by AC depend largely on the degree of pre-existing LV function. The more compromised the heart, the greater is the reduction in LV emptying in response to the elevation of afterload.[43] Even a moderate decrease in venous return may have a pronounced additional negative influence on LV ejection fraction in the face of compromised LV emptying.[43] Haemodynamic studies including estimates of LV volume have demonstrated that AC produces dilatation of the left ventricle which is not necessarily accompanied by an elevation of PAOP.[88] Further deterioration of LV function, which is consistently accompanied by an elevation of PAOP,[146] is observed if myocardial ischaemia is provoked by the increased wall stress.

The presence of a collateral circulation, more developed in patients with chronic atheromatous occlusive disease of the aorta than in those with an aneurysm, would be expected to limit the circulatory consequences of AC. However, several recent studies have documented minimal influence of such collateral circulation.

Two anaesthetic techniques, isoflurane and TEA, have been shown to reduce or eliminate the circulatory consequences of AC. Isoflurane, which reduces arterial tone with little repercussion on LV function, may largely inhibit the rise in afterload following infrarenal cross-clamping, thereby eliminating the need for additional vasodilator therapy. With aortic clamping at higher levels, isoflurane diminishes the need for vasodilator agents to control blood pressure.[147] The splanchnic and thoracic vasodilatation produced by TEA may explain the minimal circulatory effects of infrarenal cross-clamping when this technique is added to a basal fentanyl–nitrous oxide anaesthetic.[142] However, TEA may complicate the management of the circulation following declamping of the aorta and is less easily controlled than a volatile anaesthetic; consequently, isoflurane is the preferred technique.

TEE studies have shown that the repercussions of AC on global and regional LV function is directly related to the level of clamping.[88] The most pronounced circulatory changes are observed with thoracic cross-clamping, a technique with several other implications in respect of anaesthetic management. Access to the thoracic aorta is by a left thoracotomy and collapse of the left lung. Exclusion of the left lung from ventilation is associated with a high risk of hypoxaemia when vasodilators are administered for control of blood pressure; this is because these agents increase the shunt in the right lung and impair pulmonary hypoxic vasoconstriction. Selective high-frequency jet ventilation or continuous positive airway pressure[148] have both been shown to be effective in maintaining normoxia throughout the critical period.

Several experimental studies have demonstrated that thoracic AC produces only marginal decreases in cardiac output if LV function is normal because blood flow is redistributed towards the superior vena cava system.[149] This redistribution, which maintains venous return, can operate only if blood volume is controlled at normal levels. In the absence of partial circulatory assistance devices, the contribution of flow from the inferior vena cava to total venous return is only around 10%. This flow contributes importantly to venous return. Furthermore, it represents the outflow from vital organs distal to the clamp, the perfusion of which depends heavily on the pressure proximal to the clamp.

If this pressure decreases below 120 mmHg, splanchnic perfusion is severely jeopardized. Modern techniques, utilizing partial circulatory assistance devices, have largely eliminated this threat.

Thoracic AC may produce cerebral hypertension by several mechanisms.[150] Because cerebral autoregulation is impaired in patients with atherosclerotic disease, and may be diminished further by volatile anaesthetic agents, the increases in blood pressure and blood volume in the upper part of the body increase cerebral blood flow and favour the development of cerebral oedema. Vasodilators may increase intracranial pressure further. The use of intravenous barbiturates, and meticulous control of systemic blood pressure, diminish the risk of cerebral oedema.

The risk of spinal cord ischaemia is low in abdominal aortic surgery (less than 0.2%).[151] In contrast, there is a high risk in surgery of the thoracic aorta.[152] The risk is directly related to the position of the Adamkiewicz artery. Spinal angiography has demonstrated that patients in whom this artery enters the aorta above or below the aneurysm are at low risk of paraplegia.[153] In contrast, when the Adamkiewicz artery is included in the aneurysm, or cannot be identified on the angiogram, the risk of paraplegia is of the order of 5% if spinal cord revascularization via intercostal arteries is technically possible. If this is not the case, the frequency of paraplegia increases 10-fold.[153] This explains why a shunt does not reduce the risk of paraplegia. Several techniques have been proposed to reduce the risk of spinal cord ischaemia. These include drainage of cerebrospinal fluid to help preserve spinal perfusion pressure[154] and/or administration of intrathecal papaverine with the aim of increasing spinal perfusion.[155] Encouraging results of the latter technique have been obtained both experimentally and clinically. These data await further confirmation from randomized trials before they can be finally accepted.

The kidneys are sensitive to changes in perfusion produced by AC. In addition to the principal factor, which is the level of clamping, two other mechanisms may further impair renal function. These are microembolization of atherosclerotic material and cholesterol from the aortic endothelium, and liberation of circulating myoglobin from rhabdomyolysis in territories distal to the clamp.[156]

Although renal blood flow ceases completely during suprarenal AC, diuresis can be re-established rapidly by adequate hydration following declamping. Renal function usually returns progressively to normal within the first postoperative week.[156] Infrarenal AC also disturbs renal function. A diminution of renal blood flow by almost 40%, and elevation of renal vascular resistance by 75%, have been observed immediately after positioning the clamp.[157] Over 50% of patients subjected to abdominal aortic surgery develop significant elevation of blood urea concentration.[157] If blood pressure and cardiac output are maintained during infrarenal AC, total and intrarenal distribution of blood flow are not affected. Neither sympathectomy by epidural analgesia nor intravenous mannitol infusion influences the consequences of infrarenal AC on renal blood flow.[157] Adequate hydration following declamping is equally effective as mannitol and/or diuretics in limiting renal dysfunction after intrarenal AC.[158]

Aortic declamping. Release of the distal aortic or iliac artery clamps may produce profound haemodynamic disturbances, mainly due to a marked decrease in systemic vascular resistance and diminution of the effective intravascular volume. Diffusion of blood through the aortic graft and vasoplegia with sequestration of blood in the territories distal to the clamp account for the major proportion of the decrease in blood volume. The magnitude of the haemodynamic modifications following unclamping of the aorta is directly proportional to the level of the clamping, i.e. the higher the level, the greater the risk of hypotension. Another factor of importance for hypotension is the release of metabolites with vasodilator and cardiodepressant actions (e.g. adenosine, enosine, inosine, hypoxanthine and plasma purine degradation products) from the territories deprived of flow during clamping. Thus, the longer the clamping period, the greater the risk of high concentrations of such metabolites.

However, the relationship between vascular and intravascular volume is the main determinant of the haemodynamic response to unclamping. Several studies have demonstrated that a fluid challenge aimed at increasing PAOP to well above 12 mmHg is required to ensure haemodynamic stability after the clamp has been removed.[159] The effectiveness of this form of treatment is illustrated by a pronounced increase in cardiac output directly following release of the clamp.

Carotid artery surgery

Patient-related or surgery-related depression of baroreflexes may provoke major hyper- or hypotensive episodes during carotid artery surgery. If untreated, such modifications increase the risk of cardiac and cerebrovascular accidents, and may cause bleeding or rupture of sutures.

As indicated above, the sympathetic depression associated normally with an elevation of systemic blood pressure is blunted in elderly patients, in particular those with cerebral atherosclerosis. This baroreceptor anomaly is observed also in hypertensive patients, who, in addition, have a resetting of their baroreflexes.

Surgery increases the risk of hypertension by two mechanisms. First, clamping of the carotid artery decreases carotid sinus pressure profoundly, leading to increased peripheral sympathetic tone.[160] Second, the partial or complete resection of the nerves to the carotid sinus reduces or completely interrupts the afferent pathways of the baroreflex arch. Consequently, changes in pressure at the level of the baroreceptors are modified less effectively. Animal studies have demonstrated that denervation of afferent pathways to the carotid sinus leads to elevation of systemic blood pressure. Similar results have been observed during carotid artery surgery in humans.[161]

An abrupt reduction of blood pressure is frequently observed after the carotid artery clamp is removed. When surgery is completed and flow re-established, the baroreceptors are exposed to an artificially elevated pressure. The baroreflexes elicit a counter-control, with activation of the parasympathetic system and inhibition of sympathetic tone. The presence of this mechanism has been established indirectly by the finding that local anaesthetics injected around the carotid sinus prevent the fall in blood pressure.[162] However, this method should be used with caution because denervation of the carotid sinus by local anaesthetics deprives the body of an important regulator of systemic blood pressure.

Intra-operative control of haemodynamics

Careful control of systemic haemodynamics is the key to successful outcome after vascular surgery because it reduces the incidence of myocardial ischaemia and diminishes the risk of postoperative ventricular dysfunction in patients with coronary artery disease.

It is common practice to increase anaesthetic depth by administration of volatile anaesthetic agents in response to hypertension and tachycardia during noxious stimuli caused by surgery or by manipulation of the airways. The efficacy of such treatment in vascular patients has been well-established.[163] Vascular hyper-reactivity is a common feature in vascular patients and stress imposed by surgical manipulations may be sudden. Therefore, an anaesthetic agent used to manipulate the circulation should ideally have a rapid onset and offset. At present, the agent used most widely for this purpose is isoflurane. This is mainly because of its peripheral vasodilator action and favourable blood/gas partition coefficient. The potentional role for desflurane or sevoflurane awaits clarification, but their very low blood/gas partition coefficients suggest they may have a useful place in anaesthetic management.

Tachycardia in the presence of normal blood pressure is usually due to hypovolaemia, but, on some occasions, it may not respond adequately to fluid replacement. Under these circumstances, a carefully titrated intravenous dose of a β-blocker has been shown to be effective.[164] In this respect, esmolol has the advantage of being ultra short-acting and cardioselective.[165]

The occurrence of paroxysmal atrial arrhythmias requires rapid treatment with either verapamil or esmolol. Both agents have been shown to be effective and safe, while limiting the increase in heart rate and improving filling of the left ventricle.[166]

Hypotension during vascular surgery is commonly observed prior to surgery, during bleeding and following unclamping of large arteries. Maintenance of effective intravascular volume and control of vascular volume are the cornerstones to avoid profound hypotension. A low blood pressure, which does not respond favourably to reduction or cessation of volatile anaesthetics and fluid loading, should be treated with sympathomimetic agents with predominantly α-adrenergic activity.

Phenylephrine, an α_1-adrenoceptor agonist, is the drug of choice if heart rate is normal or elevated in the presence of hypotension. It increases blood pressure by increasing preload and raising systemic vascular resistance.[167] Simultaneously, heart rate decreases due to activation of the baroreflexes. It has to be noted that this drug may produce substantial pulmonary hypertension due to pulmonary vasoconstriction and increased venous return.

Ephedrine stimulates both α- and β-adrenergic receptors, resulting in increased vascular tone, inotropy and chronotropy. The effect on blood pressure is the consequence of both improved loading conditions and direct cardiac stimulation. Ephedrine is particularly well-suited to treat hypotension in the presence of a low heart rate. There are some well-defined conditions under which acute hypotension is accompanied by a reduction in heart rate. These include activation of the Bezold–Jarisch reflex[168] and reflex cardiac and vasomotor depression elicited by acute and/or severe hypovolaemic hypotension.[169,170] Epidural anaesthesia is associated with an elevated vagal tone, explaining why the decrease in blood pressure is often accompanied by a decrease in heart rate.[171] When combined thoracic epidural analgesia and general anaesthesia are used, even aggressive intravenous fluid administration is often insufficient to maintain adequate systemic blood pressure.[172] Under these circumstances, ephedrine is the agent of choice to treat hypotension. Ephedrine counterbalances the influence of the combined anaesthetic technique on vascular tone, heart rate and inotropy without impairing ventricular emptying (as occurs with phenylephrine; Fig. 9.11).[173]

Treatment of intra-operative myocardial ischaemia

When treatment of myocardial ischaemia is considered, answers to the following questions should be sought first:

1. What haemodynamic changes have precipitated or sustained the ischaemia?
2. Which anaesthetic agent(s) are being, or have been, administered?
3. Does the ischaemia provoke haemodynamic changes which suggest impaired systolic and/or diastolic LV function?

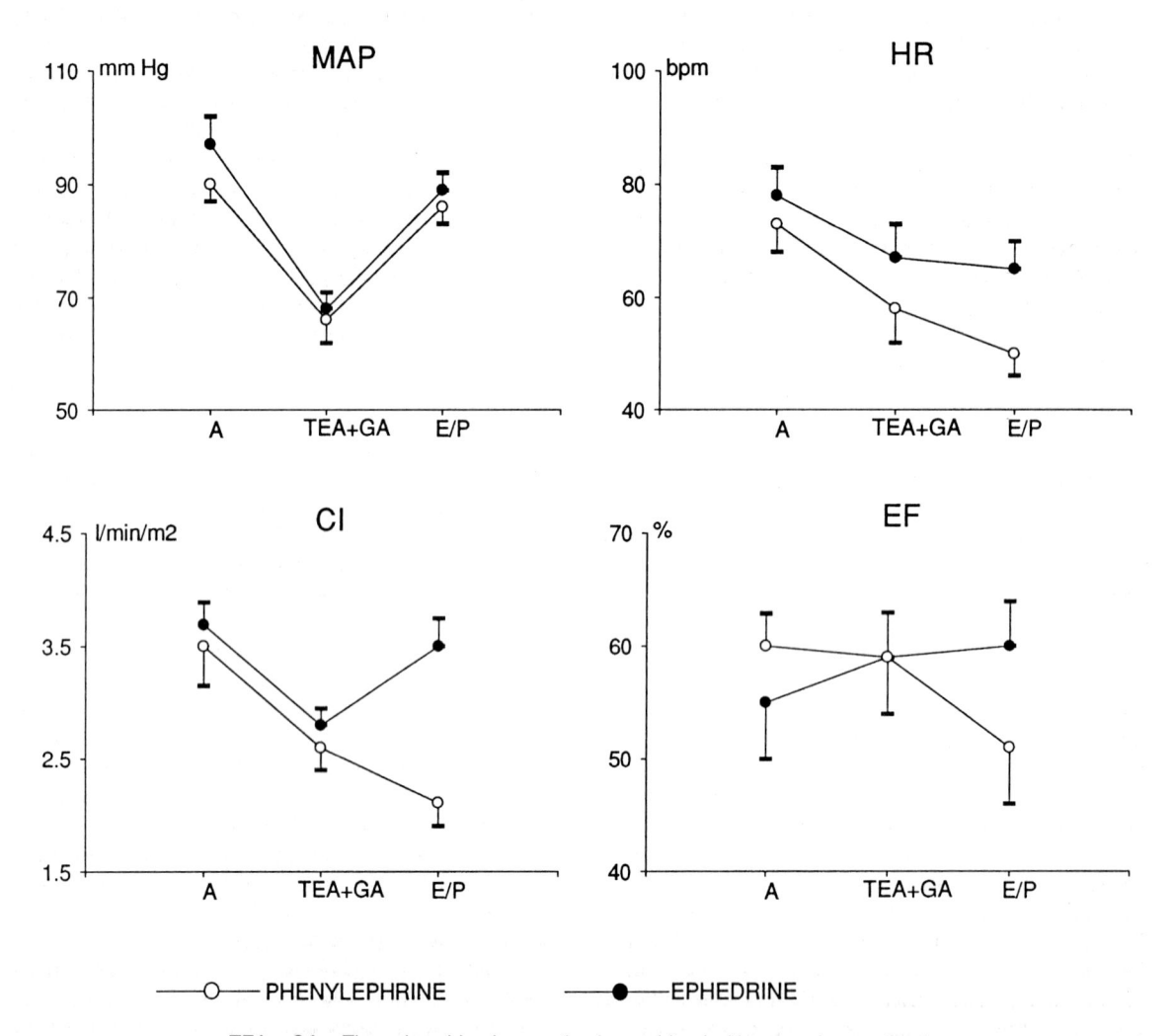

Fig. 9.11 Cardiovascular responses to phyenylephrine or ephedrine used to treat hypotension produced by combined thoracic epidural and light balanced general anesthesia. MAP = Mean arterial pressure; HR = heart rate; CI = cardiac index; EF = ejection fraction area by transoesophageal echocardiography. Three sets of measurements were performed: A = awake; TEA + GA = thoracic epidural anaesthesia combined with general anaesthesia; E/P = after intravenous ephedrine or phenylephrine titrated to obtain a blood pressure comparable to the awake values. Ephedrine improved left ventricular function without modifying heart rate. In contrast, phenylephrine impaired left ventricular systolic emptying, along with a further decrease in heart rate.

Drugs and techniques suitable for treatment of ischaemia due to elevated myocardial oxygen requirements (hypertension, tachycardia and increased inotropy) or decreased supply (hypotension, tachycardia and/or ventricular failure) have been discussed in previous sections of this chapter. Ischaemia which occurs without associated haemodynamic changes indicates an abnormality of coronary vasomotion which is limiting supply (regional or transmural flow maldistribution or coronary vasospasm). The problem of ischaemia related to coronary flow maldistribution has been discussed in depth above, in relation to the use of isoflurane for maintenance of anaesthesia. This section describes the treatment of supply-related ischaemia, thought to be caused by increased tone in dynamic coronary artery stenoses.

Two types of therapy are possible in this situation. Nitroglycerine relieves coronary artery spasm, increases coronary collateral flow and decreases resting tone of dynamic epicardial coronary stenoses.[174] In addition, the drug has a short duration of action, and is easily titrated. However, there is often a reflex increase in heart rate, requiring intravenous fluid administration.

Intravenous calcium antagonists do not decrease preload and can therefore be used to improve myocardial oxygen supply without the risk of increasing demand. The main effects of these drugs are an improvement in subendocardial/subepicardial flow ratio and an increase in coronary collateral blood flow.[175] In addition, when used during opioid-based general anaesthesia, verapamil and diltiazem produce haemodynamic changes which reduce myocardial oxygen requirements.[176,177] Verapamil is effective in relieving ischaemia unrelated to haemodynamic changes and resistant to nitroglycerine infusion.[178] Both verapamil and diltiazem have a rapid onset of action and a relatively short plasma half-life after intravenous administration. When titrated carefully to response, there is little risk of the marked bradycardia which is observed occasionally when acute ischaemia is treated with these drugs. Verapamil is relatively more cardiodepressant than diltiazem[176] and should therefore be avoided in individuals with depressed LV function or those or chronic β-blocker medication. The combined use of intravenous nitroglycerine and a calcium antagonist should be considered if any of these therapies is insufficient by itself in relieving ischaemia thought to be due to coronary artery spasm. This is because these compounds have additive dilator effects on vascular smooth muscle and because further elevation of the dose of a single agent may produce unwanted circulatory effects.[179]

Early postoperative care of vascular patients

Recovery from anaesthesia for major vascular surgery is particularly stressful, with a high incidence of myocardial ischaemic episodes (related mainly to tachycardia), and a significant risk of major cardiac complications. Recent data suggest that ischaemia at this time is the main determinant of adverse cardiac outcome.[180] Therefore, although not yet scientifically proven, all logic dictates that control of haemodynamics which may lead to ischaemia (particularly heart rate) in the early postoperative period is the key to avoiding major cardiac complications.

Low blood volume during rewarming, hypoxaemia, anaemia, the excitation phase associated with emerging from anaesthesia, pain, and the transition from assisted to spontaneous ventilation provoke increases in total body and myocardial oxygen requirements and a decline in myocardial oxygen supply. While the metabolic needs of the body are increased, the following factors may produce a deleterious effect on LV function and thus preclude an adequate total body oxygen delivery. First, a large proportion of vascular patients have pre-existing LV dysfunction, and thus a reduced reserve to handle even limited circulatory alterations. Second, postoperative increases in LV preload, afterload and total body oxygen consumption provoke LV depression in patients with ischaemic heart disease.[181] Third, LV dysfunction is caused by acute myocardial ischaemia. Finally, intra-operative episodes may have caused myocardial stunning which sets the scene for poor ventricular tolerance to circulatory stress.[7]

The main goal in the early postoperative management of vascular surgical patients with documented or suspected coronary artery disease is to decrease metabolic requirements. These are met by an elevation of heart rate, because stroke volume is frequently fixed, and by increased oxygen extraction. Thus, control of heart rate at normal levels by the use of a β-blocker may contribute to inadequate total oxygen delivery and should therefore be undertaken only when the oxygen extraction reserve of the body is sufficient. External heating and intravenous administration of pethidine have both been shown to be effective in reducing the elevated total body oxygen requirements caused by shivering. As discussed in detail in the section on monitoring (see p. 126), evaluation of body oxygen extraction reserve in these instances can be accomplished by measurement of mixed venous oxygen saturation.

Other circulatory aberrations observed frequently in

the early postoperative period after major vascular surgery are mismatching of vascular and intravascular volume, and arterial hypertension. The former problem is particularly evident during rewarming, when blood is diverted from central areas to the periphery because of simultaneous peripheral vasodilatation. Thus, patients who arrive in the recovery room hypothermic and with normal LV filling are at increased risk of hypovolaemia during subsequent rewarming. Similarly, drugs which have central inhibitory effects on sympathetic activity or a direct peripheral vasodilator action, and epidural or subarachnoid local anaesthetics, may produce profound hypotension if administered under these conditions.

Calcium antagonists of the dihydropyridine type are ideally suited to treat early postoperative hypertension.[182] Nifedipine can be given intranasally if the patient is mechanically ventilated; otherwise, the sublingual preparation can be used. Nicardipine has a pharmacokinetic profile which makes repeated intravenous bolus doses appropriate.[183] Several studies have demonstrated the efficacy of these drugs in treating hypertension after vascular surgery without decreasing blood pressure excessively. This is because their arterial dilating effect depends on the level of vascular resistance. Global LV function and cardiac output increase in parallel with the reduction in blood pressure, mainly due to improved LV emptying and the negligible effect on venous return.[183] These effects also favour myocardial oxygen balance by reducing oxygen requirements and increasing oxygen delivery by epicardial coronary vasodilatation. It must be noted, however, that patients with relative hypovolaemia may respond to intravenous dihydropyridine calcium antagonists with an increase in heart rate due to reflex sympathetic activation.

Another drug which can be used to control early postoperative hypertension is labetalol, a combined non-selective β- and α-adrenoceptor blocker. The effectiveness of this drug is controlling postoperative hypertension has been demonstrated in several studies of vascular and cardiac patients (Fig. 9.12).[154,184-186] Although labetalol decreases myocardial oxygen requirements, an 'overshoot' associated with evidence of LV dysfunction is sometimes observed.[187] This is because the β-adrenergic antagonism may predominate over the α-adrenergic vasodilatation, compromising both global ventricular function and total body oxygen extraction reserve.

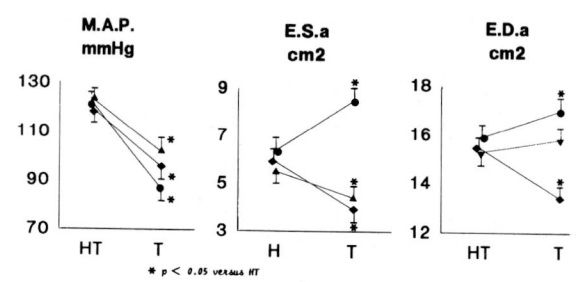

Fig. 9.12 Changes in mean arterial pressure (MAP) and end-systolic (ESa) and end-diastolic areas (EDa) by transoesophageal echocardiography during hypertension and after institution of antihypertensive therapy in patients maintained under fentanyl sedation during mechanical ventilation after abdominal aortic surgery. HT = During hypertension (systolic blood pressure above 170 mmHg); T = after intravenous treatment with labetalol (●), nicardipine (▲) or nitroglycerine (◆) titrated to reduce blood pressure to the pre-anaesthetic levels. All three drugs effectively reduced blood pressure. Labetalol produced normotension by a predominantly cardiodepressant effect, nitroglycerine by reducing preload and afterload and nicardipine by reduction of afterload. Adapted from Le Bret et al[187] and Benammar et al[188] with permission.

ACKNOWLEDGEMENT

This study was supported in part by the Swedish Heart-Lung Foundation.

REFERENCES

1. Hertzer NR, Bevan EG, Young JR et al. Coronary artery disease in peripheral vascular patients. A classification of 1000 coronary angiograms and results of surgical management. Ann Surg 1984; 199: 223–233
2. Reigel MM, Hollier LH, Kazmier FJ et al. Late survival in abdominal aortic aneurysm. World J Surg 1980; 4: 661–667
3. Jamieson WRE, Jancsz TM, Miaygishima RT et al. Influence of ischemic heart disease on early and late mortality after surgery for peripheral occlusive disease. Circulation 1982; 66: 92–99
4. Diehl JT, Cali RF, Hertzer NR et al. Complications of abdominal aortic reconstruction. An analysis of perioperative risk factors in 557 patients. Ann Surg 1983; 197: 49–55
5. Winslow CM, Solomon DH, Chassin MR et al. The appropriateness of carotid endarterectomy. N Engl J Med 1988; 318: 721–726
6. Leppo J, Plaja J, Gionet M et al. Noninvasive evaluation of cardiac risk before elective vascular surgery. J Am Coll Cardiol 1987; 9: 269–276
7. Coriat P, Fauchet M, Bousseau D et al. Left ventricular dysfunction after non cardiac surgical procedures in patients with ischemic heart disease. Acta Anaesthesiol Scand 1985; 29: 804–810
8. Mangano DT. Anesthetics, coronary artery disease and

9. Johnston KW, Scobie TT. Multicenter prospective study on non-ruptured abdominal aortic aneurysms. I. Population and operative management. J Vasc Surg 1988; 7: 69–81
10. Appenzeller O, Descarries S. Loss of baroreceptor reflexes in patient with cerebrovascular disease. Trans Am Neurol Assoc 1971; 89: 177–184
11. Goldman L, Caldera DL, Southwick FS et al. Cardiac risk factors and complications in non-cardiac surgery. Medicine 1978; 57: 357–370
12. Stone JG, Foex P, Sear JW et al. Myocardial ischemia in untreated hypertensive patients: effect of a single small oral dose of a beta-adrenergic blocking agent. Anesthesiology 1988; 68: 495–500
13. Ponten J, Biber B, Bjuro T, Herniksson BA, Hjalmarson A, Lundberg D. β-receptor blockage and spinal anaesthesia. Withdrawal versus continuation of long-term therapy. Acta Anaesthesiol Scand 1982 (suppl); 76: 62–69
14. Mirenda JV, Grissom TE. Anesthetic implications of the renin-angiotensin system and angiotensin-converting enzyme inhibitors (review). Anesth Analg 1991; 72: 667–683
15. Pasternak PF, Imparato AM, Bear G et al. The value of radionuclide angiography as a predictor of perioperative myocardial infarction in patients undergoing abdominal aortic aneurysm resection. J Vasc Surg 1984; 1: 320–325
16. Baron JF, Mundler O, Bertrand M et al. Reexamination of dipyramidamole thallium scintigraphy and gated radionuclide angiography as preoperative screening test prior to abdominal aortic surgery. N Engl J Med 1994; 330: 663–669
17. Nishimura RA, Housmans PR, Hatle LK, Tajik AJ. Assessment of diastolic function of the heart: background and current applications of Doppler echocardiography. Part I: Physiologic and pathophysiologic features. Part II: Clinical studies. Mayo Clin Proc 1989; 64: 71–181
18. Eagle KA, Singer DE, Brewster DC et al. Dipyridamole thallium scanning in patients undergoing vascular surgery. JAMA 1987; 257: 2185–2189
19. Young AE, Sandberg GW, Couch NP. The reduction of mortality of abdominal aortic aneurysm resection. Am J Surg 1977; 134: 585–592
20. Schoonover GA, Olsen GN. Pulmonary function testing in the perioperative period: a review of the literature. J Clin Surg 1982; 1: 125–129
21. Coriat P, Harari A, Daloz M, Viars P. Clinical predictors of intraoperative myocardial ischemia in patients with coronary artery disease undergoing non-cardiac surgery. Acta Anaesthesiol Scand 1982; 26: 287–290
22. Reul CJ Jr, Cooley DA, Duncan JM et al. The effect of coronary bypass on the outcome of peripheral vascular operations in 1093 patients. J Vasc Surg 1986; 3: 788–798
23. Rao TK, Jacobs KH, El-Etr AA. Reinfraction following anaesthesia in patients with myocardial infarction. Anesthesiology 1983; 59: 499–505
24. Cutler BS, Leppo JA. Dipyridamole thallium-201 scintigraphy to detect coronary artery disease before abdominal aortic surgery. J Vasc Surg 1987; 5: 91–100
25. Carliner NH, Fischer L, Plotnick D et al. Routine preoperative exercise testing in patients undergoing major non cardiac surgery. Am J Cardiol 1986; 56: 51–58
26. Hertzer NR, Young JR, Beven EG et al. Late results of coronary bypass in patients with infrarenal aortic aneurysms. The Cleveland Clinical Study. Ann Surg 1987; 205: 360–367
27. Hertzer NR, Young JR, Kramer JR et al. Routine coronary angiography prior to elective aortic reconstruction: results of a selective myocardial revascularisation in patients with peripheral vascular disease. Arch Surg 1979; 114: 1336–1344
28. Hedblad B, Juul-Muller S, Svensson K et al. Increased mortality in men with ST-segment depression during 24 hour ambulatory long-term ECG recording. Eur Heart J 1989; 10: 149–158
29. Rozanski A, Bairey CN, Krantz DS et al. Mental stress and the induction of silent myocardial ischemia in patients with coronary artery disease. N Engl J Med 1988; 318: 1005–1012
30. Raby KE, Goldman L, Creager MA et al. Correlation between preoperative ischemia and major cardiac events after peripheral vascular surgery. N Engl J Med 1989; 321: 1330–1332
31. Pasternak PF, Grossi EA, Baumann FG et al. The value of silent myocardial ischemia monitoring in the prediction of perioperative myocardial infarction in patients undergoing peripheral vascular surgery. J Vasc Surg 1989; 10: 617–625
32. Fleischer LA, Rosenbaum SH, Nelson AH, Barash PG: The predictive value of preoperative silent ischemia for postoperative ischemic cardiac events in vascular and nonvascular surgery patients. Am Heart J 1991; 122: 980–986
33. Albro PC, Gould KL, Westcott RJ, Hamilton GW, Ritchie JL, Williams DL. Non invasive assessment of coronary stenoses by myocardial imaging during pharmacologic coronary vasodilatation. III. Clinical trial. Am J Cardiol 1978; 42: 751–760
34. Boucher CA, Brewster OC, Darling CD, Okada R, Strauss W, Pohost GM. Determination of cardiac risk by dipyridamole. Thallium imaging before peripheral vascular surgery. N Engl J Med 1987 312: 385–394
35. Eagle KA, Coley CM, Newbell JB et al. Combining clinical and thallium data optimizes pre-operative assessment of cardiac risk before major vascular surgery. Ann Intern Med 1989; 110: 859–866
36. Mangano DT, London J, Tubau F et al. Dipyridamole thallium-201 scintigraphy as a preoperative screening test. A reexamination of its predictive potential. Circulation 1991; 84: 493–502
37. Leppo J, Yipintsoi T, Blankstein R et al. Thallium-201 myocardial scintigraphy in patients with triple vessel disease and ischemic exercise stress tests. Circulation 1979; 59: 714–721
38. Gould KLD. Quantitative imaging in nuclear cardiology. Circulation 1982; 66: 1141–1146
39. Dilsizian V, Rocco TP, Freedman NMT et al. Enhanced detection of ischemic but viable myocardium by the reinjection of thallium after stress-redistribution imaging. N Engl J Med 1990; 323: 141–146

40 McEnroe CS, O'Donnell TF, Yeager A, Konstam M, Mackey WC. Comparison of ejection fraction and Goldman risk factor analysis to dipyridamole-thallium 201 studies in the evaluation of cardiac morbidity after aortic aneurysm surgery. J Vasc Surg 1990; 11: 497–504

41 Leppo J, Boucher CA, Okada RD, Newell JB, Strauss HW, Pohost GM. Serial thallium-201 myocardial imaging after dipyridamole infusion: diagnostic utility in detecting coronary stenoses and relationship to regional wall motion. Circulation 1982; 66: 649–657

42 Casake PN, Guiney E, Strauss HW, Boucher CA. Simultaneous low level treadmill exercise and intravenous dipyridamole stress thallium imaging. Am J Cardiol 1988; 62: 799–806

43 Robotham JL, Takada M, Berman M, Harasaura Y. The ejection fraction revisited. Anesthesiology 1991; 74: 172–183

44 Acinapura AJ, Rose DM, Kramer MD et al. Role of coronary angiography and coronary artery bypass surgery prior to abdominal aortic aneurysmectomy. J Cardiovasc Surg 1987; 28: 552–557

45 Cass. Principal investigators. Coronary Artery Surgery Study (CASS): randomized trial of coronary artery bypass surgery: survival data. Circulation 1983; 68: 950

46 McNeer JF, Margolis JR, Lee KL et al. The role of the exercise test in the evaluation of patients for ischemic heart disease. Circulation 1978; 57: 64–71

47 O'Donnel TF, Callow AD, Willet C et al. The impact of coronary artery disease on carotid endarterectomy. Ann Surg 1983; 198: 705–712

48 Sundt TM, Sandok BA, Whisnant JP. Carotid endarterectomy: complications and preoperative assessment of risk. Mayo Clin Proc 1975; 50: 301–309

49 Hertzer NR, Less CD. Fatal myocardial infarction following carotid endarterectomy: 335 patients followed 6–1 years after operations. Ann Surg 1981; 194: 212–218

50 Ennix CL, Lawrie GM, Morris CG et al. Improved results of carotid endarterectomy in patients with symptomatic coronary disease: an analysis of 1546 consecutive carotid operations. Stroke 1979; 10: 122–127

51 Winslow CM, Solomon DH, Chassin MR et al. The appropriateness of carotid endarterectomy. N Engl J Med 1988; 318: 721–727

52 European Carotid Surgery Trialists' Collaborative Group. MRC European Carotid Surgery Trial: interim results for symptomatic patients with severe (70–99%) or with mild (0–29%) carotid stenosis. Lancet 1991; 337: 1235–1243

53 Easton JD, Sherman DG. Stroke and mortality rate in carotid endarterectomy: 288 consecutive operations. Stroke 1977; 8: 565–572

54 Diehl JT, Cali RF, Hertzer NR et al: Complications of abdominal aortic reconstruction. An analysis of perioperative risk factors in 557 patients. Ann Surg 1983; 197: 49–55

55 Freeman WK, Gersh B, Gloviczki P. Abdominal aortic aneurysm and coronary artery disease: frequent companions, but an uneasy relationship. J Vasc Surg 1990; 12: 73–77

56 Crawford ES, Saleh SA, Bobb JW III et al. Infrarenal abdominal aortic aneurysms: factors influencing survival after operation performed over a 25 year period. Ann Surg 1981; 193: 699–704

57 Cappeller WA, Ramirez H, Kortmann H. Abdominal aortic aneurysms. J Cardiovasc Surg 1989; 30: 572–578

58 Tisi GM. Preoperative evaluation of pulmonary function: validity, indications and benefits. Am Rev Respir Dis 1979; 119: 293–298

59 Paul MD, Mazer CD, Byrick RJ, Rose DK, Goldstein MB. Influence of mannitol and dopamine on renal function during elective infrarenal aortic clamping in man. Am J Nephrol 1986; 6: 427–434

60 Dormandy J, Mahir M, Ascady G et al. Fate of the patient with chronic leg ischaemia. J Cardiovasc Surg 1989; 30: 50–57

61 Hertzer NR. Clinical experience with preoperative coronary angiography. J Vasc Surg 1985; 2: 510–514

62 Mangano D, Browner W, Lollenberg M et al. Association of perioperative myocardial ischemia with cardiac morbidity and mortality in men undergoing non cardiac surgery. N Engl J Med 1990; 323: 1781–1788

63 Wells Ph, Kaplan JA. Optimal management of patients with ischemic heart disease for non cardiac surgery by complementary anesthesiologist and cardiologist interaction. Am Heart J 1981; 102: 1929–1037

64 Tuman KJ, McCarthy RJ, Spiess BD et al. Effect of pulmonary artery catheterization on outcome in patients undergoing coronary artery surgery. Anesthesiology 1989; 70: 199–206

65 Fegert G, Hollender M, Browner W et al. Perioperative myocardial ischemia in the non cardiac surgical patient. Anesthesiology 1988; 69: A49

66 Knight AA, Hollenberg M, London MJ et al. Perioperative myocardial ischemia: importance of the perioperative ischemic pattern. Anesthesiology 1988; 68: 681–688

67 Brown FG, Bolson EL, Dodge HT. Dynamic mechanisms in human coronary stenosis. Circulation 1984; 70: 917–922

68 Briard C, Coriat P, Commin P et al. Coronary artery spasm during non cardiac surgical procedure. Anaesthesia 1983, 38: 467–470

69 Miris DM, Ramanathan KB, Wilson JL. Regional blood flow correlates of ST segment depression in tachycardia-induced myocardial ischemia. Circulation 1986; 73: 365–373

70 Thys D, Kaplan JA. Recent advances in electrocardiographic techniques. In: Kaplan JA, ed. Cardiac anesthesia, 2nd, vol 1. Grune Stratton, pp 227–255

71 Griffin RM, Kaplan JA. Myocardial ischemia during non-cardiac surgery. A comparison of different lead systems using computerized ST-segment analysis. Anaesthesia 1987; 42: 155–159

72 London MJ, Hollenberg M, Wong MG et al. Intraoperative myocardial ischemia: localization by continuous 12-lead electrocardiography. Anesthesiology 1988; 69: 232–241

73 Battler A, Froelicher VF, Gallagher KP, Kemper WS, Ross J Jr: Dissociation between regional myocardial dysfunction and ECG changes during ischemia in the conscious dog. Circulation 1980; 62: 735–744

74 Wohlgelernter D, Cleman M, Highman HA et al. Regional myocardial dysfunction during coronary

angioplasty: evaluation by two-dimensional echocardiography and 12-lead electrocardiography. J Am Coll Cardiol 1986; 7: 1245–1254

75 Thys D. The intraoperative assessment of regional myocardial performances: is the cart before the horse? J Cardiothorac Anesth 1987; 1: 273–276

76 Videcoq M, Arvieux CC, Ramsay JG et al. The association isoflurane–verapamil causes regional left ventricular dyssynchrony in the dog. Anesthesiology 1987; 67: 635–641

77 Vandenberg BF, Kerber RE. Transesophageal echocardiography and intra-operative monitoring of left ventricular function. Anesthesiology 1990; 73: 799–801

78 London M, Tubau J, Wrong MG et al. The "natural history' of segmental wall motion abnormalities in patients undergoing non cardiac surgery. Anesthesiology 1990; 73: 644–655

79 Leung JM, O'Kelley B, Browner WS, Tubau J, Hollenberg M, Mangano DT: Prognostic importance of postbypass regional wall-motion abnormalities in patients undergoing coronary artery bypass graft surgery. Anesthesiology 1989; 71: 16–25

80 Lieberman RW, Orkin FK, Jobes DR, Schartz AJ. Hemodynamic predictors of myocardial ischemia during halothane anaesthesia for coronary artery revascularisation. Anesthesiology 1983; 59: 36–41

81 Foex P. Experimental models of myocardial ischemia. Br J Anaesth 1988; 61: 44–55

82 Kotter GS, Kotrly KJ, Kalbfleisch JH et al. Myocardial ischemia during cardiovascular surgery as detected by an ST segment trend monitoring system. J Cardiothorac Anesth 1987; 1: 190–199

83 Buffington C. Hemodynamic determinants of ischemic myocardial dysfunction in the presence of coronary stenosis in dogs. Anesthesiology 1985; 63: 651–662

84 Gordon MA, Urban MK, O'Connor T, Barash PG. Is the pressure rate quotient a predictor or indicator of myocardial ischemia as measured by ST-segment changes in patients undergoing coronary artery bypass surgery? Anesthesiology 1991; 74: 848–853

85 Kaplan JA, Wells PH. Early diagnosis of myocardial ischemia using the pulmonary artery catheter. Anesth Analg 1981; 60: 789–793

86 Häggmark S, Hohner P, Ostman M et al. Comparison of hemodynamic, electrocardiographic, mechanical, and metabolic indicators of intraoperative myocardial ischemia in vascular surgical patients with coronary artery disease. Anesthesiology 1989; 70: 19–25

87 Leung JM, Goehner P, O'Kelly BF et al. Isoflurane anaesthesia and myocardial ischemia: comparative risk versus sufentanil anaesthesia in patients undergoing coronary artery bypass graft surgery. Anesthesiology 1991; 74: 838–847

88 Roizen MF, Beaupre PN, Alpert RA et al. Monitoring with two-dimensional transeosphageal echocardiography: comparison of myocardial function in patients undergoing supraceliac, suprarenal-infraceliac, or infra-renal aortic occlusion. J Vasc Surg 1984; 1: 300–317

89 Leung JM, Chan FW, Mangano DT. Transesophageal echocardiography: prediction of intraoperative hypovolemia. Anesth Analg 1990; 70: S236

90 Baron JF, Decaux-Jacalot A, Edouard A, Berdeaux A, Samii K. Influence of venous return on baroreflex control of heart rate during lumbar epidural anaesthesia in humans. Anesthesiology 1986; 64: 188–193

91 Perel A, Pizov WR, Cotev S. Systolic blood pressure variation is a sensitive indicator of hypovolemia in ventilated dogs subjected to graded hemorrhage. Anesthesiology 1987; 67: 498–502

92 Coriat P, Vrillon M, Perel A, Baron JF et al. A comparison of systolic blood pressure variations and echocardiographic estimates of end-diastolic left ventricular size in patients following aortic surgery. Anesthesia–Analgesia 1994; 78: 46–53

93 O'Rourke MF. The arteries as vascular cushions. In: Arterial function in health and disease. Harlow: Longman, 1982: p67

94 Randall OS, Van Den Bos GC, Westerbof N. Systemic arterial compliance: does it play a role in genesis of essential hypertension? Cardiovasc Res 1984; 18: 455–459

95 Finch CA, Lenfant C. Oxygen transport in man. N Engl J Med 1972; 286: 407–414

96 Reinhart K, Foehring U, Kersting T et al. Effects of thoracic epidural anaesthesia on systemic hemodynamic function and systemic oxygen supply-demand relationship. Anesth Analg 1989; 69: 360–369

97 Matsumura N, Nishijima H, Kojiman S, Hashimoto F, Minami M, Yasuda H. Determination of anaerobic threshold for assessment of functional state in patients with chronic heart failure. Circulation 1983; 68: 360–366

98 Mangano DT. Monitoring pulmonary arterial pressure in coronary artery disease. Anesthesiology 1980; 53: 364–370

99 Cableman CG, Gann DS, Ashworth CJ et al. One hundred consecutive carotid reconstructions: local vs general anesthesia. Am J Surg 1983; 145: 477–483

100 Messick JM, Casement B, Sharbrough FW et al. Correlation of regional cerebral blood flow with EEG changes during isoflurane anaesthesia for carotid endarterectomy: critical rCBF. Anesthesiology 1987; 66: 344–349

101 Shapiro HM. Monitoring in neurological anesthesia. In: Saidman LJ, Smith NT, eds. Monitoring in anesthesia, 2nd edn. Stoneham, MA: Butterworth, 1984: p300

102 Markand ON, Dilley RS, Moorthy SS, Warren C Jr. Monitoring of somato-sensory evoked responses during carotid endarterectomy. Arch Neurol 1984; 41: 376–383

103 Cunningham JN, Laschinger JC, Spencer FC. Monitoring of somatosensory evoked potentials during surgical procedures on the thoraco-abdominal aorta. J Thorac Cardiovasc Surg 1987; 94: 275–285

104 Crawford ES, Mizrahi EM, Hess KR et al. The impact of distal aortic perfusion and somatosensory evoked potential monitoring on prevention of paraplegia after aortic aneurysm operation. J Thorac Cardiovasc Surg 1988; 95: 357–367

105 Furchgott RF. Role of endothelium in responses of vascular smooth muscle. Circ Res 1983; 53: 557–562

106 Martin DE, Rosenberg, Aukburg SJ et al. Low-dose fentanyl blunts circulatory responses to tracheal intubation. Anesth Analg 182; 61: 680–684

107 Stone JG, Foëx P, Sear JW, Johnson LL, Khambatta HJ, Triner L. Myocardial ischemia in untreated hypertensive patients: effect of a single small oral dose

108 Fusciardi J, Godet G, Bernard JM, Bertrand M, Kieffer E, Viars P. Roles of fentanyl and nitroglycerin in prevention of myocardial ischemia associated with laryngoscopy and tracheal intubation in patients undergoing operations of short duration. Anesth Analg 1986; 65: 617–624
109 Stoelting BK. Endotracheal intubation. In: Miller RD, ed. Anesthesia. Churchill Livingstone, 1986, p 523
110 Coriat P, Harari A, Daloz M, Viars P. Clinical predictors of intraoperative myocardial ischemia in patients with coronary artery disease undergoing non-cardiac surgery. Acta Anaesthesiol Scand 1982; 26: 287–290
111 Hudson R, Thomson R, Cannon E et al. Pharmacokinetics of fentanyl in patients undergoing abdominal aortic surgery. Anesthesiology 1986; 64: 334–338
112 Bennet GM, Staley TH. Human cardiovascular responses to endotracheal intubation during morphine N_2O and fentanyl N_2O anesthesia. Anesthesiology 1980; 52: 520–522
113 Cucchiara RF, Benefiel DJ, Matteo RS, DeWood M, Albin MS. Evaluation of esmolol in controlling increases in heart rate and blood pressure during endotracheal intubation in patients undergoing carotid endarterectomy. Anesthesiology 1986; 65: 528–531
114 Geva D, Sagi D, Perel A. Esmolol/N_2O/relaxant: a new effective maintenance technique. Anesthesiology 1990; 73: A320
115 Savarese JJ, Lowenstein E. The name of the game: no anaesthesia by cook book. Anesthesiology 1985; 62: 703–705
116 Hess W, Arnold B, Schulte-Sasse U, Tarnow J. Comparison of isoflurane and halothane when used to control hypertension in patients undergoing coronary bypass surgery. Anesth Analg 1983; 62: 15–20
117 Brusset A, Coriat P, Pazvanska E. Isoflurane vs halothane in control of intraoperative hypertension. Effects on left ventricular function. Anesthesiology 1986; 65: A2
118 Reiz S, Balfors E, Sorensen MB, Ariola S, Friedman A, Truedsson H. Isoflurane — a powerful coronary vasodilator in patients with coronary artery disease. Anesthesiology 1983; 59: 91–97
119 Becker LC. Is isoflurane dangerous for the patients with coronary artery disease? Anesthesiology 1987; 66: 259–269
120 Priebe HJ. Isoflurane and coronary hemodynamics (review article). Anesthesiology 1989; 71: 960–976
121 Becker LC. Is isoflurane dangerous for the patients with coronary artery disease? Anesthesiology 1987; 66: 259–261
122 Buffington CW, Davis KB, Gillispie S, Pettinger M. The prevalence of steal prone coronary anatomy in patients with coronary artery disease: an analysis of the coronary artery surgery study registry. Anesthesiology 1988; 69: 721–727
123 Slogoff S, Keats AS. Randomized trial of primary anesthetic agent on outcome of coronary bypass operations. Anesthesiology 1989; 70: 179–188
124 Philbin DM, Foex P, Drummond G, Lowenstein E, Ryder WA, Jones LA. Postsystolic shortening of canine left ventricle supplied by a stenotic coronary artery when nitrous oxide is added in the presence of narcotics. Anesthesiology 1985; 62: 166–174
125 Wilkowski DA, Still JC, Bonta W, Owen R, Bove AA. Nitrous oxide constricts epicardial coronary arteries without effect on coronary arterioles. Anesthesiology 1987; 66: 659–665
126 Nathan HJN. Control of hemodynamics prevents worsening of myocardial ischemia when nitrous oxide is administered to isoflurane-anesthetized dogs. Anesthesiology 1989; 71: 686–694
127 Balasarawsathi K, Kumar P, Rao TL, El-Etr A. Left ventricular and diastolic pressure as an index for nitrous oxide use during coronary artery surgery. Anesthesiology 1981; 55: 708–709
128 Lunn JK, Stanley TH, Eisele J, Bebster L, Woodward A. High dose fentanyl concentrations and influence of nitrous oxide on cardiovascular responses. Anesth Analg 1979; 58: 390–395
129 Cahalan MK, Prakash O, Rulf ENR et al. Addition of nitrous oxide to fentanyl anaesthesia does not induce myocardial ischemia in patients with ischemic heart disease. Anesthesiology 1987; 67: 925–929
130 Mitchell MM, Prakash O, Rulf NR, Van Daele ERM, Cahalan M, Roelandt JRTC. Nitrous oxide does not induce myocardial ischemia in patients with ischemic heart disease and poor ventricular function. Anesthesiology 1989; 71: 526–534
131 Slavik JR, LaMantia KR, Kopriva CJ et al. Does nitrous oxide cause regional wall motion abnormalities in patients with coronary artery disease? Anesth Analg 1988; 67: 695–700
132 Cousins MJ, Wright CJ. Graft, muscle, and skin blood flow after epidural block in vascular surgical procedures. Surg Gynecol Obstet 1971; 133: 59–67
133 Palas TAR. Continuous spinal anaesthesia versus single shot technique in the elderly. Reg Anesth 1989; 14: 9–14
134 Sutter PA, Gamulin Z, Forster A. Comparison of continuous spinal and continuous epidural anaesthesia for lower limb surgery in elderly patients. A retrospective study. Anaesthesia 1989; 44: 47–50
135 Arndt JO, Höck A, Stanton-Hicks M, Stühmeier K-D. Peridural anaesthesia and the distribution of blood in supine humans. Anesthesiology 1985; 63: 616–623
136 Baron JF, Payen D, Coriat P et al. Forearm vascular tone and reactivity during lumbar anesthesia. Anesth Analg 1988; 67: 1065–1070
137 Baron JF, Coriat P, Mundler O, Fauchet M, Bousseau D, Viars P. Left ventricular global and regional function during lumbar epidural anaesthesia in patients with and without angina pectoris. Influence of volume loading. Anesthesiology 1987; 66: 621–627
138 Saada M, Duval AM, Bonnet F et al. Abnormalities in myocardial segmental wall motion during lumbar epidural anesthesia. Anesthesiology 1985; 71: 26–32
139 Reiz S, Nath S, Rais O. Effects of thoracic epidural block and prenalterol on coronary vascular resistance and myocardial metabolism in patients with coronary artery disease. Acta Anaesthsiol Scand 1980, 24: 11–16
140 Yeager MP, Glass DD, Neff RK, Brink-Johnsen. Epidural anaesthesia and analgesia in high-risk surgical patients. Anesthesiology 1987; 66: 729–735
141 Takeshima R; Dohi S. Circulatory responses to

baroreflexes, Valsalva maneuver, coughing, swallowing and nasal stimulation during acute cadiac sympathectomy by epidural blockade in awake humans. Anesthesiology 1985; 63: 500–508

142 Lunn JK, Dannemiller FJ, Stanley TH. Cardiovascular responses to clamping of the aorta during epidural and general anesthesia. Anesth Analg 1979; 58: 372–378

143 Baron JF, Bertrand M, Barre E et al. Thoracic epidural anaesthesia versus general anaesthesia for high risk surgical patients. Anesthesiology 1991; 75: 611–618

144 Gelman S, Reves JG, Fowler K, Samuelson PN, Lell WA, Smith LR. Regional blood flow during cross-clamping of the thoracic aorta and infusion of sodium nitroprusside. J Thorac Cardiovasc Surg 1983; 85: 287

145 Gelman S, McDowell H, Varner P et al. The reason for cardiac output reduction after aortic cross-clamping. Am J Surg 1988; 155: 578–586

146 Attia RR, Murphy DD, Snider M et al. Myocardial ischemia due to infrarenal aortic cross-clamping during aortic surgery in patients with severe coronary artery disease. Circulation 1976; 53: 961–966

147 Godet G, Bertrand M, Coriat P, Kieffer E, Mouren S, Viars P. Comparison of isoflurane with sodium nitroprusside for controlling hypertension during thoracic aortic cross-clamping. J Cardiothorac Anesth 1990; 4: 177–184

148 Benumof JL. One-lung ventilation. Which lung should be PEEPed? Anesthesiology 1982; 56: 161–162

149 Roberts AJ, Nora JD, Hughes WA et al. Cardiac and renal responses to cross-clamping of the descending thoracic aorta. J Thorac Cardiovasc Surg 1983; 86: 732–755

150 Hantler CB, Knight PR. Intracranial hypertension following cross-clamping of the thoracic aorta. Anesthesiology 1982; 56: 146–147

151 Laschinger JC, Izumoto H, Kouchoukos NT. Evolving concepts in prevention of spinal cord injury during operations on the descending thoracic and thoraco-abdominal aorta. Ann Thorac Surg 1987; 44: 667–674

152 Berendes JN, Bredee JJ, Shipperheyn JJ, Mashhour YAS. Mechanisms of spinal cord injury after cross-clamping of the descending thoracic aorta. Circulation 1982; 66: 1112–1115

153 Kieffer E, Richard T, Chiras J, Godet G, Cormier E. Preoperative spinal cord arteriography in aneurysmal disease of the descending thoracic and thoracoabdominal aorta: preliminary results in 45 patients. An Vasc Surg 1989; 1: 34–46

154 McCullough JL, Hollier LH, Nugen M. Paraplegia after thoracic aortic occlusion: influence of cerebrospinal fluid drainage. J Vasc Surg 1988; 7: 153–160

155 Svensson LG, Von Ritter CM, Groeneveld HT et al. Cross-clamping of the thoracic aorta: influence of aortic shunts, laminectomy, papaverin, calcium channel blocker, allopurinol, and superoxide dismutase on spinal cord blood flow and paraplegia in baboons. Ann Surg 1986; 204: 38–47

156 Mowlan A, McClintock JT, Campbell GS. Effect on renal function of occlusion of the aorta inferior to the renal vessels. Surg Gynecol Obstet 1960; 111: 423–428

157 Gramulin Z, Forster A, Morel D et al. Effects of infrarenal aortic cross-clamping on renal hemodynamics in humans. Anesthesiology 1984; 61: 394–399

158 Bush HL, Huse JB, Johnson WL et al. Prevention of renal insufficiency after abdominal aortic aneurysm resection by optimal volume loading. Arch Surg 1981; 116: 1517–1522

159 Silverstein PR, Caldera DL, Cullen DJ et al. Avoiding the hemodynamic consequences of aortic cross-clamping and unclamping. Anesthesiology 1979; 50: 462–466

160 Bove EL, Fry WY, Gross WS, Stanley JC. Hypotension and hypertension as a consequence of baroreceptor dysfunction following carotid endarterectomy Surgery 1979; 86: 633–637

161 Angell-James JE, Lumley JSP. The effect of carotid endarterectomy on the mechanical properties of the carotid sinus nerve activity in atherosclerotic patients. Br J Surg 1974; 61: 805–811

162 Pine R, Avellone JC, Hoffman M et al. Control of post-carotid endarterectomy hypotension with baroreceptor blockade. Am J Surg 1983; 147: 763–769

163 Roizen MF, Hamilton WK, Sohn YJ. Treatment of stress induced increases in pulmonary capillary wedge pressure using volatile anesthetics. Anesthesiology 1981; 54: 390–398

164 Safwat AM, Reitan JA, Misle GR, Hurley EJ. Use of propranolol to control the rate pressure product during cardiac anesthesia. Anesth Analg 1980; 60: 732–736

165 Kaplan JA. Role of ultrashort acting beta-blockers in the perioperative period J Cardiothorac Anesth 1988; 2: 683–692

166 Michelson EL, Portefield JK, Das G et al. A comparison of esmolol and verapamil in the treatment of atrial fibrillation/flutter. J Am Coll Cardiol 1986; 7: 157A

167 Schwinn DA, Reves JG. Time course and hemodynamic effects of alpha 1 adrenergic bolus administration in anesthetized patients with myocardial disease. Anesth Analg 1989; 68: 571–578

168 Zucker IH. Left ventricular receptors: physiological controllers or pathological curiosities? Basic Res Cardiol 1986; 81: 539–557

169 Sanders JS, Ferguson DW. Profound sympathoinhibition complicating hypovolemia in humans. Ann Intern Med 1989; 111: 439–441

170 Barriot P, Riou B. Hemorrhagic shock with paradoxical bradycardia. Intensive Care Med 1987; 13: 203–207

171 Baron JF, Decaux-Jacolot A, Edouard A, Berdeaux A, Samii K. Influence of venous return on baroreflex control of heart rate during lumbar epidural anaesthesia in humans. Anesthesiology 1986; 64; 188–193

172 Coriat P. Combined thoracic epidural anaesthesia and general anaesthesia: Haemodynamic stability. Acta Anaesthesiol Scand 1991; 96: 35: 95–98

173 Samain E, Coriat P, Le Bret F et al. Ephedrine vs phenylephrine for hypotension due to thoracic epidural anaesthesia associated with light general anesthesia: effects of LV function. Anesthesiology 1990; 73: A82

174 Sorkin EM, Brogden RN, Romankiewicz JA, Intravenous glyceryl trinitrate (nitroglycerin). A review of its pharmacological properties and therapeutic efficacy. Drugs 1984; 27: 45–80

175 Braunwald E. Mechanisms of action of calcium-channel-blocking agents. N Engl J Med 1982; 307: 1618–1627

176 Britt B A. Diltiazem (review). Can Anaesth Soc J 1985; 32: 30–44
177 Godet G, Coriat P, Baron JF et al. Prevention of intraoperative myocardial ischemia during non cardiac surgery with intravenous diltiazem: a randomized trial versus placebo. Anesthesiology, 1987; 66: 241–246
178 Humphrey LS, Black TJ. Intraoperative use of verapamil for nitroglycerin refractory myocardial ischemia. Anesth Analg 1985; 64: 68–71
179 McGregor M. The nitrates and myocardial ischemia. Circulation 1982; 66: 689–692
180 Mangano DT. Hollenberg M, Fegert G et al. Perioperative myocardial ischemia in patients undergoing non cardiac surgery. I: incidence and severity during the 4 day perioperative period. JACC 1991; 17: 843–840
181 Coriat P, Mundler O, Bousseau D et al. Response of left ventricular ejection fraction to recovery from general anesthesia: measurements by gated radionuclide angiography. Anesth Analg 1986; 65: 593–600
182 Godet G, Coriat P, Samama M et al. Treatment of post-carotid endarterectomy hypertension with nifedipine. Effect on hemodynamics and mixed venous oxygen saturation. Anesthesiology 1986; 65: A75
183 Turlapaty P, Vary R, Kaplan JA. Nicardipine, a new intravenous calcium antagonist: a review of its pharmacology, pharmacokinetics and perioperative applications. J Cardiothorac Anesth 1989; 3: 344–355
184 Leslie JB, Kalayjian RW, Sirgo MA et al. Intravenous labetalol for treatment of postoperative hypertension. Anesthesiology 1987; 67: 413–416
185 Sladden RN, Klamerus KJ, Swafford MWG et al. Labetalol for the control of elevated blood pressure following coronary artery bypass grafting. J Cardiothorac Anesth 1990; 4: 210–221
186 Golberg ME, Seltzer J, Azad SS et al. Intravenous labetalol for treatment of hypertension after carotid endarterectomy. J Cardiothorac Anesth 1989; 3: 411–418
187 Le Bret F, Coriat P, Gognach M et al. Transoesophageal echocardiographic assessment of left ventricular function response to labetalol when given to control postoperative hypertension. J Cardiothorac Anesth 1992: 6: 437–443
188 Benammar MS, Coriat P, Houissa M er al. Nicardipine vs trinitrine for treatment of postoperative hypertension: effects on hemodynamics and left ventricular function. Anesthesiology 1987; 67: (Suppl)

10. Thoracic surgery

J. W. W. Gothard

Anaesthesia for thoracic surgery has progressed considerably since the first lung resections were undertaken in the mid-1930s. Gale & Waters introduced single-lumen endobronchial intubation in the USA in 1932 and Magill (1936) refined their techniques with the development of both right- and left-sided endobronchial tubes inserted under direct vision using a rigid intubating bronchoscope.

The control of open pneumothorax by positive-pressure ventilation, as advocated by Waters in the USA and at a later stage by Nosworthy in the UK, was firmly established following the Second World War. This was a direct result of a better understanding of the treatment of open chest wounds, the introduction of muscle relaxants and the development of mechanical ventilators.

Double-lumen endobronchial intubation for thoracic surgery with the Carlen's tube was first reported in 1950. This tube had previously been designed for differential bronchospirometry but subsequently a number of tubes specifically designed for pulmonary surgery were introduced. These included the Bryce-Smith tube (1960) and the Robertshaw right and left tubes (1962). More recently, several manufacturers have introduced plastic disposable double-lumen tubes and as a result there are now only two major manufacturers of rubber re-usable double-lumen endobronchial tubes. Single-lumen endobronchial tubes are no longer produced but fortunately their use is rarely indicated (see sections below on the anaesthetic management of bronchopleural fistula and mediastinal tumours).

Thoracic surgery in the developed countries is now mainly concerned with the diagnosis, staging and resection of neoplastic lung disease, although a number of centres have a major interest in the surgical treatment of both benign and malignant oesophageal disease.

ANAESTHESIA FOR RIGID BRONCHOSCOPY

Diagnostic rigid bronchoscopy

Anaesthesia for rigid bronchoscopy should provide unconsciousness, muscular relaxation, abolition of respiratory tract reflexes, ventilation and a rapid recovery. There are few absolute contra-indications to rigid bronchoscopy but the procedure is hazardous in the presence of hypoxaemia, respiratory tract obstruction and marked superior vena caval obstruction.

Traditionally, sedative premedication combined with an intramuscular vagolytic agent such as atropine or hyoscine is administered prior to rigid bronchoscopy. A vagolytic agent prevents the accumulation of copious salivary secretions during the procedure and may prevent or obtund the bradycardia due to repeated doses of suxamethonium or vagal reflexes. In practice, bradycardia is better treated with intravenous atropine and excess salivation is only a minor problem during recovery from an isolated bronchoscopy or when endobronchial intubation is carried out following the procedure. In low-risk, routine cases many anaesthetists therefore prescribe oral premedication in the form of a short-acting benzodiazepine, such as temazepam. However, sedative premedication should be omitted in patients with poor lung function and respiratory failure, severe superior vena caval obstruction and respiratory tract obstruction. In these patients an intramuscular injection of a non-sedative vagolytic agent such as atropine, given 30–45 min pre-operatively, provides significantly superior operating and recovery conditions.

Cardiovascular instability is common during rigid bronchoscopy (see below) and routine monitoring should include an electrocardiogram, non-invasive blood pressure measurement and pulse oximetry.[1]

Anaesthesia for a routine, isolated bronchoscopy is usually achieved with an intravenous induction agent such as thiopentone, etomidate, methohexitone or propofol. Inhalational induction may be preferred in children and it may be indicated in patients with upper-airway obstruction (see section on laser bronchoscopy, below). Following induction, the depolarizing muscle relaxant suxamethonium is administered so that the rigid bronchoscope can be passed through the fully relaxed vocal cords. Many anaesthetists prefer to spray the cords with plain lignocaine (4 ml of 4%) before bronchoscopy in an attempt to minimize postoperative laryngospasm, although this has only been shown to be beneficial after relatively short procedures.[2] If an operative procedure is to follow the bronchoscopy and there are no contra-indications, such as the anticipation of a difficult intubation, then a non-depolarizing muscle relaxant such as vecuronium or atracurium can be used to provide paralysis from the outset.

The sympatho-adrenal response resulting from instrumentation of the upper respiratory tract during bronchoscopy is similar to that following laryngoscopy and intubation, but may be more marked, with an increase in heart rate and both systemic and pulmonary hypertension. A recent study also suggests that the incidence of myocardial ischaemia may be as high as 10–15% during bronchoscopy, when looked for diligently.[3] In this study, anaesthesia with propofol alone, after pethidine and atropine premedication, provided adequate haemodynamic stability during bronchoscopy and the addition of alfentanil was superfluous. In a comparison group, patients anaesthetized with thiopentone required the addition of alfentanil (18 $\mu g.kg^{-1}$) to obtund the cardiovascular response to bronchoscopy and this caused a decrease in both systolic and diastolic arterial pressures. Propofol would therefore seem an acceptable agent for anaesthetic induction and maintenance during bronchoscopy if administered cautiously in those with diminished cardiovascular reserve. When bronchoscopy is prolonged, increments of an intravenous anaesthetic agent must be given at regular intervals to prevent awareness. Propofol, unlike other agents, can be conveniently given by infusion for a long procedure without the fear of accumulation. Roberts and co-workers have described a simple, manually controlled infusion scheme for the infusion of propofol during surgery which is also suitable for use during bronchoscopy.[4] This is summarized in Table 10.1. Higher infusion rates are required when nitrous oxide is not administered.

Ventilation during bronchoscopy is usually provided by an oxygen-driven Venturi device in adults; alternatively, high-frequency jet ventilation can be used. Oxygen at pipeline pressure (410 kPa) is injected

Table 10.1 Induction and maintenance of propofol anaesthesia

Induction
Propofol 1 mg.kg^{-1}

Maintenance
Propofol 10 mg.kg^{-1}.h^{-1} for 10 min
Propofol 8 mg.kg^{-1}.h^{-1} for 8 min
Propofol 6 mg.kg^{-1}.h^{-1} continuously thereafter

The above regimen, taken from Roberts et al,[4] achieved a mean propofol blood level greater than 3 mg.ml^{-1} with a satisfactory level of anaesthesia, in conjunction with nitrous oxide and fentanyl.

into the open-ended adult bronchoscope via a 16-gauge needle at approximately 12–15 breaths.min^{-1} with the more commonly used Venturi system, allowing adequate time for expiration. Air is entrained into the open-ended adult bronchoscope and ventilation is achieved at inflation pressures not exceeding 30–40 cmH$_2$O. It is important to match the internal diameter of the injector needle to the size of the bronchoscope and to the pressure of the oxygen supply with this technique.[5] Barotrauma to the lungs and airway is always a potential hazard, particularly if the egress of the ventilatory gas is hindered during passive expiration, for example by tumour obstructing the airway or by instrumentation down the bronchoscope. This is particularly likely to occur with small, relatively narrow, paediatric bronchoscopes. It is safer, therefore, to use a conventional manual form of ventilation for children with T-piece circuit attached to the side arm of the bronchoscope and a glass slide occluding the proximal end. This method of ventilation has the added advantage that inhaled anaesthetic agents can be used to ensure lack of awareness during long procedures, such as removal of a foreign body, with the benefit of rapid awakening when required.

Major complications of rigid bronchoscopy under general anaesthesia include the occurrence of arrhythmias, myocardial ischaemia, hypoxaemia, hypercapnia and awareness. The occurrence of arrhythmias during bronchoscopy may be due to pre-existing cardiovascular disease, but can relate to inadequate ventilation and hypercapnia. Arrhythmias frequently resolve if ventilation is increased and anaesthesia deepened.

Awareness, with a reported incidence as high as 4% in some series, can be eliminated if bolus doses of an induction agent are given at regular timed intervals. As discussed previously, an infusion of propofol is more appropriate for long procedures.

At the end of bronchoscopy, it is usual to remove the rigid bronchoscope and maintain ventilation with a mask and airway until spontaneous ventilation is re-established.

During emergence from anaesthesia, upper-airway obstruction is particularly likely to occur as a result of coughing and laryngospasm stimulated by the previous instrumentation and the presence of blood or secretions. Oxygen therapy and all monitoring should therefore be continued until a satisfactory pattern of ventilation has been re-established. If bleeding is significant, for example following biopsy of a tumour, the bronchoscope is left in place until the patient makes spontaneous movements. This allows direct suction in the airway until the last possible moment. The patient can then be turned to the lateral position with the biopsy side down to minimize the possibility of blood soiling the contralateral lung.

Therapeutic rigid bronchoscopy

Laser bronchoscopy

Surgical laser devices can be used in thoracic surgery to resect tracheobronchial tumours. This surgery is usually of a palliative nature and carries a significant mortality. It is often carried out in elderly, debilitated patients with severe bronchial or even tracheal obstruction.[6] The laser is used to resect and cauterize intraluminal tumours within the tracheobronchial tree to relieve breathlessness and haemoptysis. Endobronchial laser therapy can be carried out under local anaesthesia combined with sedation, or under general anaesthesia. Recent experience suggests that general anaesthesia provides superior operating conditions so that palliation can be achieved with fewer treatment sessions and without the problem of bleeding and asphyxiation that has led to death when local anaesthesia has been employed.[7]

A variety of lasers have been used for endobronchial surgery, including the carbon dioxide and neodymium yttrium-aluminium-garnet (Nd-YAG) lasers. The thermal effect of these lasers is the main basis for their efficacy but this also has significant implications for their use during general anaesthesia.[8] There is a considerable fire hazard when lasers are used in the presence of conventional tracheal tubes, particularly in an atmosphere of high oxygen concentration. Foil wrapped, or even metal, tracheal tubes have been used to provide an airway for laser treatment but a simpler approach is to utilize a metal, rigid bronchoscope.[6,7,9] Following induction of anaesthesia, a rigid adult bronchoscope is introduced into the airway and Venturi ventilation commenced (see above). A fibre-optic bronchoscope can then be passed down the lumen of the rigid instrument to reach the area of tumour whilst ventilation continues. An optical fibre is then introduced down the biopsy channel of the fibre-optic instrument in order to transmit the laser beam to the required site. Large biopsy forceps and suction catheters can be passed down the rigid bronchoscope intermittently to remove blood and tumour debris, thus ensuring a relatively clear airway. At times it is necessary to suspend Venturi ventilation whilst smoke particles are sucked from the airway. This does not appear to present an unreasonable hazard when used with appropriate monitoring.

Anaesthesia for laser therapy is carried out using the principles described previously for prolonged bronchoscopy; paralysis is achieved with vecuronium or atracurium and anaesthesia is maintained with propofol. Induction of anaesthesia is particularly hazardous in the presence of upper-airway obstruction and its severity should be assessed before operation clinically and from the chest radiograph and the computed tomographic (CT) scan. The theoretical advantages of an inhalational induction are rarely applicable to this type of palliative surgery carried out in elderly, often debilitated patients but may be considered in extreme circumstances. After pre-oxygenation, intravenous anaesthesia is induced slowly. Intravenous suxamethonium (rather than a non-depolarizing muscle relaxant) is given if there is any doubt about maintenance of the airway. A skilled bronchoscopist should be present from the outset. Once the airway has been secured and ventilation achieved via the rigid bronchoscope, vecuronium or atracurium can be administered.

At the end of laser bronchoscopy, which is often a prolonged procedure, the trachea can be extubated in most patients following the re-establishment of spontaneous ventilation. However, a number of patients require a period of postoperative assisted ventilation for a variety of reasons, including pre-existing muscular weakness residual muscle paralysis and severe stridor.[6,7]

Diathermy resection

Diathermy resection is an alternative and somewhat simpler treatment for intraluminal tumours of the upper tracheobronchial tree. A diathermy resection instrument, incorporating a telescope, is used to remove tumour under direct vision via a rigid bronchoscope. Ventilation is achieved with a Venturi device and the anaesthetic considerations are similar to those discussed for laser bronchoscopy.

Insertion of tracheobronchial stents

Tracheobronchial stents are use to improve airway patency in a variety of pathologies, including tracheal stenosis, narrowing at the site of bronchial anastomoses following sleeve resection and lung transplantation, as well as certain endobronchial tumours.[10] Many different types of stent are available and these continue to proliferate as this is an area of rapid development.

The original Montgomery T-tube is still used to treat proximal tracheal strictures and this allows ventilation through the upright limb of the tube via a tracheostomy. Bifurcating prostheses are available to stent the lower trachea and both main bronchi, and simpler tubular plastic stents can be used in either site. Expanding metal stents are currently in the development phase.

The anaesthetic considerations for the insertion and positioning of intratracheal stents are similar to those for laser bronchoscopy, with ventilation and maintenance of the airway being of most concern. Anaesthesia is maintained intravenously and paralysis provided with suxamethonium initially, followed by vecuronium or atracurium once the airway has been secured bronchoscopically. An inhalational induction may be used, but this is rarely necessary. Maintenance of anaesthesia with spontaneous ventilation for this type of procedure would be very difficult, if not impossible.

In extreme circumstances, partial cardiopulmonary bypass has been instituted to augment oxgenation prior to the insertion of tracheal stents.[11] However, Venturi ventilation can be employed down the standard rigid bronchoscope in most situations, although high frequency jet ventilation is an alternative technique.[11]

As stents are advanced and positioned with grasping forceps placed through the distal end of the bronchoscope, the airway becomes totally blocked and ventilation is impossible. Close co-operation between the anaesthetist and surgeon is essential at this stage and if the stent cannot be positioned before hypoxaemia ensues, it should be rapidly removed and the lungs reventilated. It may take several attempts before the stent is accurately positioned.

If a T-tube is being inserted or replaced it may be possible to use Venturi ventilation via the open limb once the distal T-limb is open. It is essential to ensure that expiration can occur whichever method of ventilation is used, otherwise barotrauma will rapidly ensue, with disastrous consequences.

Once the stent is in place, anaesthesia is discontinued and the patient allowed to breathe spontaneously in a sitting position. Airway patency should be improved by the procedure but there may be short-term problems relating to the presence of blood and secretions, in addition to the general airway trauma. Rarely, stents can move, particularly in the early postoperative period. Acute airway obstruction, which requires immediate re-operation, can result.

ANAESTHESIA FOR MEDIASTINOSCOPY AND MEDIASTINOTOMY

Mediastinoscopy, via a small incision above the suprasternal notch, is carried out to provide a diagnosis in patients with mediastinal lymphadenopathy, and to assess operability in patients with lung cancer.[12] The procedure allows inspection and biopsy, through the mediastinoscope, of paratracheal, superior tracheobronchial and anterior parts of the subcarinal lymph nodes. The great majority of patients with lung cancer are inoperable at presentation. The use of CT scanning and magnetic resonance imaging can identify patients without mediastinal disease who are suitable for surgical resection. However, if enlarged glands are identified by scanning techniques, it is impossible to differentiate between those that contain malignant disease and those that are a result of reactive hyperplasia or old inflammatory disease. Mediastinoscopy should be undertaken in this group of patients to define their operability.

Anterior mediastinotomy allows exploration of tumours and lymph nodes of the anterior mediastinum which are inaccessible by mediastinoscopy. Left anterior mediastinotomy, particularly, is used to assess the lymph node drainage of left upper lobe tumours visually, via the mediastinoscope, and also by digital examination.

Mediastinoscopy and mediastinotomy usually follow on from rigid bronchoscopy. The bronchoscope is removed and tracheal intubation carried out. Muscle relaxation is continued with a short-acting muscle relaxant and anaesthesia is maintained with an inspired gas mixture of oxygen in nitrous oxide (or a suitable air/oxygen mixture) with the addition of volatile agent where appropriate. Postoperative pain is not prominent after mediastinoscopy but may be more evident following mediastinotomy, particularly if a small section of costal cartilage is removed. A relatively small dose of a short-acting opioid, such as fentanyl or alfentanil, can provide adequate analgesia for either procedure.

To aid surgical access during mediastinoscopy, a sand bag is placed under the patient's shoulders and the head is extended as far back as safety permits. A slight head-up tilt prevents venous engorgement, especially in patients whose lymphadenopathy is associated with superior vena caval obstruction. Theoretically, blood pressure should be measured non-invasively on the left arm during mediastinoscopy because unreliable values may be detected on the right if the innominate artery is compressed by the mediastinoscope. In practice, this is rarely a problem.

The most significant complication of either mediastinoscopy or mediastinotomy is major haemorrhage, often related to inadvertent biopsy of a major vascular structure by an inexperienced surgeon. Major bleeding is rare but all patients must have an adequate route for intravenous infusion established prior to surgery.

During mediastinotomy, the pleura may be opened and this is drained during surgical closure. A widebore nasogastric tube is placed in the pleural space through the mediastinotomy wound and the lung is re-expanded manually by the anaesthetist. As the muscle suture line is near completion, a sustained inflation pressure is applied to the lung whilst the tube is withdrawn and the suture line completed by the surgeon to prevent recurrence of the pneumothorax.

At the end of either procedure, muscular relaxation is reversed in the usual manner and spontaneous ventilation is re-established. The tracheal tube is then removed following tracheobronchial suction.

ANAESTHESIA FOR OESOPHAGOSCOPY

Oesophagoscopy is carried out with either a rigid or fibre-optic instrument in order to visualize the lower pharynx and oesophagus and to provide access for biopsy, extraction of foreign bodies, dilatation of strictures and palliative intubation of malignant tumours. Fibre-optic oesophagoscopy can be carried out under intravenous sedation but the rigid oesophagoscope is an extremely bulky instrument which can only be inserted in the anaesthetized patient.

Many patients presenting for oesophagoscopy are cachectic and dehydrated as a result of dysphagia. In this group, anaemia, hypoproteinaemia and electrolyte disturbance are common and should be corrected pre-operatively, where possible. Abnormalities of liver function and blood coagulation are likely to be prominent in patients presenting for injection of oesophageal varices. Hiatus hernia, diverticulum, stricture and achalasia (Fig. 10.1) predispose to reflux of gastric acid or food residues. As a result, bronchopneumonia or even a lung abscess may be present pre-operatively and there is the ever-present risk of further regurgitation peri-operatively.

The lower oesophageal sphincter (LOS), which extends above and below the diaphragm, is now thought to be the major barrier preventing contents regurgitating from the stomach into the lower oesophagus.[13] In the presence of oesophageal disease, the LOS may be less effective, and in some patients with hiatus hernia the LOS is above the diaphragm and therefore unable to adapt to increases in abdominal pressure. Metoclopramide and antacids increase LOS pressure, whereas atropine, glycopyrrolate, opioids and many anaesthetic agents decrease LOS pressure. Despite its effect on the LOS, opioid premedication is often given intramuscularly to fit patients prior to oesophagoscopy. A short-acting oral benzodiazepine may be a better choice in those able to swallow and absorb oral drugs, and it is probably prudent to omit atropine altogether. Premedication should not be given if there is any concern regarding the patient's general physical status.

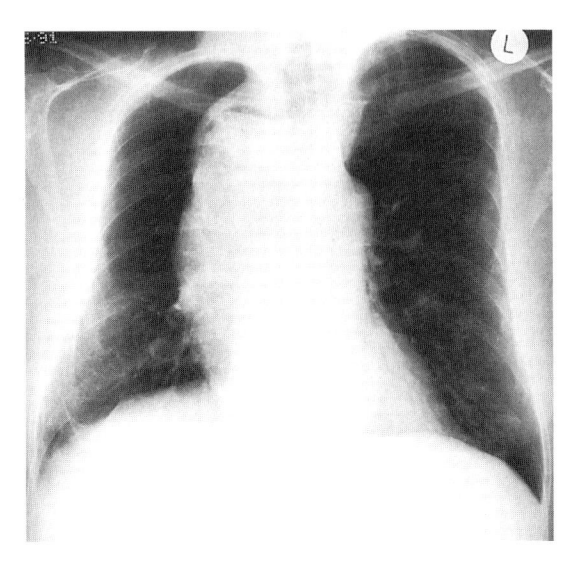

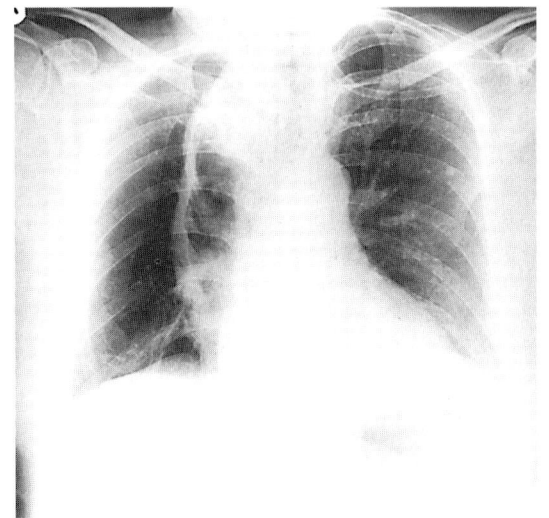

Fig. 10.1 Chest X-ray of a male with achalasia of the oesophagus (a) on presentation and (b) after food residue has been removed at oesophagoscopy.

An H$_2$-antagonist such as ranitidine or cimetidine can be used to raise gastric pH prior to endoscopy. These drugs do not influence LOS pressure and must be given several hours before the procedure to have an effect. Antacid solutions are not usually given prior to oesophagoscopy because they are likely to obscure the operator's view. However, sodium citrate is a suitable clear solution.

Control of reflux during elective oesophagoscopy is usually achieved by physical means. In patients prone to passive regurgitation, particularly the obese with a hiatus hernia, anaesthesia can be induced in a head-up position. Pre-oxygenation is then followed by intravenous induction, using cricoid pressure to occlude the oesophageal lumen when consciousness is lost. Muscle relaxation is then achieved with an adequate dose of suxamethonium, and tracheal intubation carried out with a flexometallic armoured tube, traditionally slightly smaller than would normally be employed.

Anaesthesia can be maintained using inhaled agents, but complete relaxation, with manual ventilation, is essential until the oesophagoscope has been passed through the cricopharyngeal sphincter. Thereafter, full relaxation is still desirable, particularly if biopsy, dilatation or other instrumentation is undertaken via the rigid oesophagoscope. If the procedure is likely to be prolonged, vecuronium or atracurium can be given at this stage, but intermittent administration of suxamethonium is satisfactory for a short procedure.

Recovery of consciousness is supervised with the patient in the lateral position and in a slight head-down tilt. Clinical examination and a chest X-ray are required postoperatively before oral fluid intake is allowed. This is to exclude evidence of oesophageal rupture, including surgical emphysema, pneumo-peritoneum, pneumomediastinum and pneumothorax.

ANAESTHESIA FOR LUNG RESECTION

Lung resection is most commonly undertaken in the developed countries in an attempt to cure lung cancer. Lobectomy and pneumonectomy are the most frequently performed operations but occasionally bi-lobectomy is carried out on the right, and less frequently sleeve resection of a bronchus is combined with lobectomy. The most recently available national figures show a peri-operative mortality of approximately 3% for lobectomy and 6% for pneumonectomy.[14]

Pre-operative assessment

The patient scheduled for lung resection must be fully assessed medically, as for any major surgery. Patients with lung cancer are often lifelong smokers and many are elderly. Cardiorespiratory dysfunction is the major cause of death following lung resection and therefore particular attention must be paid to the patient's pre-operative cardiovascular status and pulmonary function.

A detailed history, clinical examination, chest X-ray and electrocardiogram will reveal many cardiac abnormalities, including ischaemia, cardiac failure and valve disease. Special investigations such as exercise stress testing, echocardiography and angiography may also be indicated. Drug therapy for angina, cardiac failure and arrhythmias should be instituted where appropriate and administered up to the time of surgery; alternatively, existing medical therapy is optimized.

Peri-operative cardiac morbidity for non-cardiac surgery and the assessment of patients with ischaemic heart disease scheduled for non-cardiac surgery have been the subject of two recent authoritative reviews by Mangano and Goldman respectively.[15,16] Outcome studies of intra-operative predictors have shown that prolonged thoracic surgery is associated with an increased risk of cardiac morbidity and Goldman's multifactorial index of cardiac risk in non-cardiac surgery (Tables 10.2 and 10.3) encompasses many of the factors that need to be considered in the pre-operative period. It is worthwhile considering such a scoring system to evaluate risk in the patient presenting for lung resection.

The pulmonary function of patients with carcinoma of the lung is obviously of great importance because their only hope of ultimate cure is surgical resection. Postoperative lung function can be crudely predicted by assuming that each lobe contributes 20% of total

Table 10.2 Multifactorial index of risk in non-cardiac surgery

Risk factor	Points
History	
Myocardial infarction within 6 months	10
Age > 70 years	5
Physical examination	
S3 gallop rhythm or raised jugular venous pressure	11
Important aortic stenosis	3
Electrocardiogram	
Rhythm other than sinus or sinus plus atrial premature beats (APB) on last pre-operative electrocardiogram	7
Ventricular ectopics (> 5 min^{-1})	7
Poor general medical status *	3
Intraperitoneal, intrathoracic or aortic surgery	3
Emergency operation	4

* Includes $P\text{O}_2$ < 8 kPa and $P\text{CO}_2$ > 6.7 kPa.

Table 10.3 Performance of risk index in practice

Points	Life-threatening complications (%)	Cardiac deaths (%)
0–5	0.7	0.2
6–12	5	2
13–25	11	2
26 or more	20	56

function and then deriving post-resection function by simple arithmetic, taking into account the planned operation. Loss of up to 50% of functioning lung tissue (e.g. pneumonectomy) can easily be tolerated in fit patients with good exercise tolerance. Apart from the chest X-ray and CT scans or magnetic resonance imaging carried out to stage the tumour, the only baseline investigation required in these patients is the measurement of forced vital capacity (FVC) and forced expiratory volume in 1 s (FEV_1); these may be performed at the bedside.

Patients with poor lung function often present with a history of dyspnoea and poor exercise tolerance, although this is notoriously difficult to assess objectively. This group, with marginal lung function, is at risk of postoperative respiratory failure particularly if pneumonectomy is planned, and may be chronically disabled if they survive surgery. These patients require formal pulmonary function testing in the laboratory before and after bronchodilator therapy.

Postoperative morbidity and mortality have been related to numerous indices of lung function.[17] Unfortunately, it is impossible to identify any single test which will answer the question: 'Which patient will survive operation with a reasonable quality of life?' The literature on this topic is extensive but much of it dates back 15 or more years, when operative mortality was much higher than currently reported, irrespective of lung function. FEV_1 of 1 l and FVC of 2 l are often quoted as minimal values for pneumonectomy. Additional risk factors include a raised arterial carbon dioxide tension ($Pa\text{CO}_2 > 6.0$ kPa) and increasing age (> 70 years).[18,19] Pulmonary function tests should be interpreted in relation to the size, sex, age and ethnic origin of the patient and some authors quote an FVC of 50% of predicted and an FEV_1 of less than 50% of FVC as values below which mortality rates are likely to rise unacceptably following pneumonectomy.[18,20]

Patients who are at the limit of operability may be further investigated by a variety of sophisticated tests. These include pulmonary artery pressure measurements, to assess unilateral lung function, and exercise testing and radionucleotide techniques, to allow accurate quantification of perfusion and ventilation on a regional basis.[20–22] These techniques are rarely used in clinical practice. A simpler test, that of maximum breathing capacity (MBC),[19,20] appears to correlate well with survival following lung resection. The measurement of MBC is obtained by a period of voluntary hyperventilation through a low-resistance circuit. This is usually for a period of 15 s and minute volume is extrapolated from this. Motivation and sustainable muscle strength contribute to successful performance in this test; as these factors are important in the postoperative recovery period, it is not surprising that the test is reasonably predictive of morbidity and mortality. Patients with an MBC of less than 50% of the predicted value are at increased risk of hospital mortality. A figure of 40 $l.min^{-1}$, or 20 $l.min^{-1}.m^2$ of body surface area, corresponding to an FEV_1 approximately 1 l after resection, is widely regarded as a threshold below which the risks of respiratory failure following pulmonary resection are unacceptable.

Despite the sophistication of currently available specialized tests, it is likely that, in patients with poor lung function, the final decision regarding surgery is made by the surgeon following routine laboratory assessment of pulmonary function and after discussion with the patient and close relatives. A relatively high element of risk may be taken, particularly if there is a good chance of surgical success as ascertained by preoperative staging, because resection currently offers the only chance of long-term survival.[12]

Premedication

Patients scheduled for lung resection tolerate intramuscular premedication with an opioid combined with the sedative anticholinergic hyoscine given 1–2 h before surgery. Atropine or glycopyrronium, (which is less likely to increase heart rate), can be substituted for hyoscine in the elderly.

In patients with poor lung function and upper-airway obstruction scheduled for procedures other than lung resection, it may be wise to omit premedication. Many anaesthetists also prefer to omit opioid drugs from premedication if they intend to use an epidural opioid for postoperative analgesia, using a short-acting oral benzodiazepine in preference.[23]

Induction and maintenance of anaesthesia

Anaesthesia is induced intravenously as for most major surgery. The choice of agent is rarely critical, particularly for a relatively long procedure such as lung resection.

Endobronchial intubation can be performed following

the administration of a non-depolarizing muscle relaxant such as pancuronium for lung resection or a shorter-acting drug for less major procedures, such as lung biopsy. If there is any suspicion that endobronchial intubation may be difficult, suxamethonium is the preferred relaxant provided that there are no indications that manual inflation of the lungs with a mask and airway will be difficult. Suxamethonium provides rapid and profound relaxation in the patient with full dentition and a receding mandible, in whom the placement of a double-lumen endobronchial tube may prove difficult. Musculoskeletal pains following the use of suxamethonium are not a significant problem after thoracotomy.

Positive-pressure ventilation is continued after endobronchial intubation with an inspired gas mixture of 50% oxygen in nitrous oxide or, alternatively, an air/oxygen mixture. A volatile agent such as desflurane, isoflurane or enflurane is used to augment anaesthesia. The choice of agent can be based on standard principles because the effect of these agents on the conduct of one-lung anaesthesia is marginal (see below). It may be necessary to increase the inspired oxygen concentration as high as 100% during one-lung ventilation and the percentage of volatile agent employed must be increased to prevent awareness.

Intravenous opioid analgesics given at the beginning of surgery help to establish analgesia intra-operatively and in the immediate postoperative period. The choice of opioid is not critical but, as the dose is judged empirically on an age and weight basis, many patients require additional increments of the chosen drug at the end of surgery. If epidural opioids are to be used to provide postoperative pain relief, it is best not to use intravenous opioids during surgery. This would certainly be the case if epidural analgesia is established immediately after induction of anaesthesia.

Monitoring

Monitoring for major thoracic surgery should be comprehensive and should include electrocardiography, pulse oximetry, end-tidal gas analysis and invasive, continuous measurement of arterial and central venous pressures. Pulmonary artery catheters can be placed in the lung contralateral to surgery only if radiological screening facilities are available. This is not currently considered justifiable in routine clinical practice.

Endobronchial intubation

Absolute indications for endobronchial intubation during thoracic surgery include:

1. the presence of a bronchopleural fistula
2. gross haemorrhage or infection in the 'surgical' lung
3. bronchoplastic surgery such as sleeve resection and lung transplantation.

Surgery for pleural and cystic lung disease may also be facilitated if endobronchial intubation is employed. Theoretically, lung resection and oesophageal surgery are only relative indications for endobronchial intubation because they can be carried out with standard endotracheal anaesthesia. In practice, however, the ability to collapse the lung on the side of surgery is useful for both types of surgery and the majority of surgeons in the UK would expect to have this facility. A double-lumen endobronchial tube also prevents soiling of the non-surgical lung with blood and pus during lung resection for carcinoma. Although patients with gross infective lung disease uncommonly present for surgery in the UK, many tumours block large bronchi, causing a build-up of infection and even abscess formation distally. Manipulation of the tumour at operation releases this infected material and this can, potentially soil the non-diseased lung, with disastrous consequences.

One-lung anaesthesia is achieved with the use of a double-lumen endobronchial tube inserted immediately following induction of anaesthesia. Single-lumen endobronchial tubes are rarely used and are no longer manufactured.

Double-lumen tubes currently in use fall into two categories: the re-usable red rubber tubes and the disposable designs. The original rubber Robertshaw tube is now made by Phoenix Medical Ltd, with colour-coded bronchial cuffs. A similar, although not identical, tube is manufactured by Rusch (Fig. 10.2). The latter company also produces the rubber Carlen's double-lumen tube and its right-sided version, the White tube; these tubes have a carinal hook. Of the many disposable tubes available, the Bronchocath double-lumen tube (Mallinckrodt, National Catheter Corp.) appears the most widely used (Fig. 10.3), although Rusch also markets a similar product. In addition, Phoenix Medical is about to market a rubber disposable tube made to the original Robertshaw pattern.

The original Robertshaw tubes (Phoenix Medical) are made in right and left forms in three sizes (large, medium and small) with a generous ventilation slot in the bronchial cuff of the right tube to allow ventilation of the right upper lobe. The bronchial cuff and its pilot balloon, along with the ventilation limb, are now conveniently colour-coded in blue rubber. The Rusch Robertshaw tube is made in right and left forms in sizes of 41, 37 and 35 French gauge. The ventilation slot in the bronchial cuff of the right-sided Rusch tube

THORACIC SURGERY 247

is not as large as that of the original Robertshaw tube. The Bronchocath tubes are of similar, but not identical, design to the Robertshaw tubes. These tubes are made of polyvinylchloride in right and left forms in a wide range of sizes — 41, 39, 37 and 35 French gauge. There is also a smaller 28 French gauge tube made only in left form. The configuration of the right bronchial cuff on the Bronchocath (Fig. 10.4) differs from that on the Robertshaw in an attempt to improve efficiency of right upper lobe inflation. However, this design feature has not been wholly successful.

In British practice, a double-lumen tube is placed in the bronchus of the lung contralateral to the side of surgery in order that the diseased lung can be deflated to aid surgery. This also allows the bronchial anastomoses

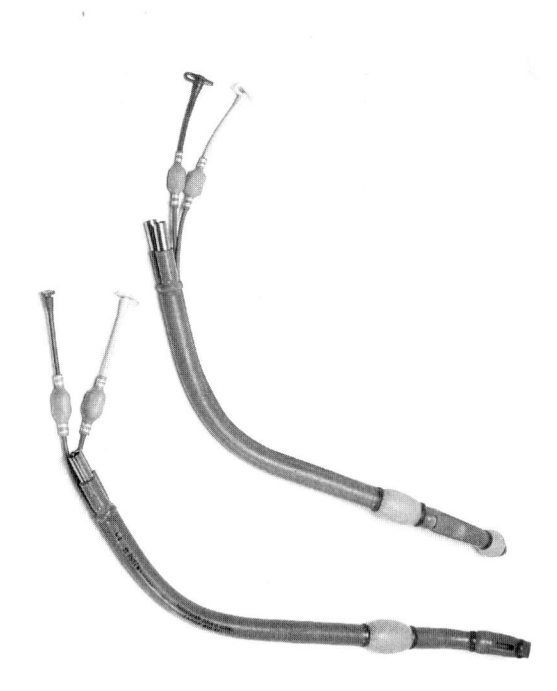

Fig. 10.2 Left and right Robertshaw (Rusch) rubber double-lumen endobronchial tubes.

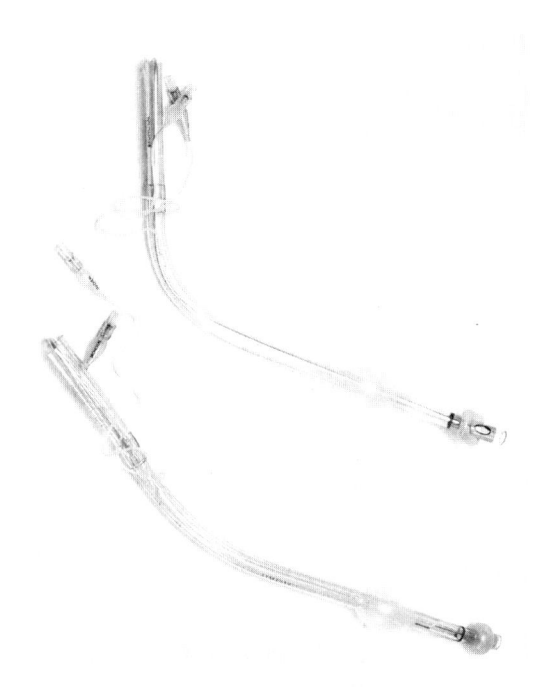

Fig. 10.3 Left and right Bronchocath disposable double-lumen endobronchial tubes.

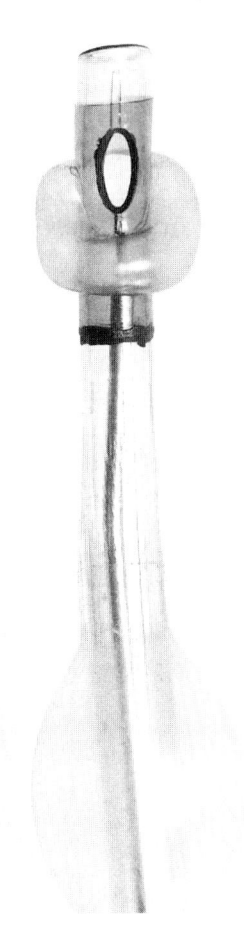

Fig. 10.4 Close-up view showing the bronchial cuff of the right Bronchocath double-lumen tube. Note the ventilation slot.

to be fashioned in an unhurried manner with the tube in place, and creates a division between the two lungs so that there can be no spread of blood or pus from the operative site to the lung. In some centres, left-sided tubes are used exclusively to eliminate the problems associated with right upper lobe ventilation. If this is the case, the tube must be withdrawn into the trachea before left pneumonectomy and left upper lobectomy are completed.

Double-lumen tubes are introduced into the larynx in the normal way. The tube is then advanced blindly (after removing any stilette provided) with a twisting motion towards the side of insertion. Usually the endobronchial portion of the tube is deflected at the carina and passes into the appropriate main bronchus. The position of the tube is checked by alternate auscultation of both lung fields, paying particular attention to the left upper zone with a left tube and the area of the right upper lobe with a right-sided tube. Auscultation is also carried out first with the tracheal limb, and then with the endobronchial limb, occluded to ascertain that isolation of the lungs has been achieved. These checks are repeated after the patient has been positioned for thoracotomy. There is increasing evidence that clinical checks of this nature are inaccurate, and that it is preferable to check the position of endobronchial tubes with a fibre-optic bronchoscope.[24,25] The introduction of slim, relatively inexpensive fibre-optic bronchoscopes/laryngoscopes such as the Olympus LF-1 has made this a practical possibility. The Olympus LF-1 is robust and has a tip of 3.8 mm which can be passed down the lumen of endobronchial tubes as small as the 35 French gauge Bronchocath. The sequence for checking the position of a double-lumen tube is described below.

The bronchoscope (Fig. 10.5) is first passed down the tracheal lumen of the double-lumen tube to check that the bronchial cuff is not obstructing the lower trachea at carinal level or herniating over the main bronchus of the lung to be operated upon. (The bronchial cuff of the Bronchocath is conveniently coloured blue for easy endoscopic identification.) The bronchoscope is then passed down the endobronchial limb to ensure that the upper lobe orifice is not obstructed on the left and that the ventilation slot of a right tube (Fig. 10.6) is directly apposed to the upper lobe orifice, preferably with a clear view of the trifurcation. If any manipulation of the tube is necessary, the tracheal lumen should be re-checked. It is also advisable to repeat the procedure after the patient has been positioned for surgery.[26] The bronchoscope (Fig. 10.7) can be used to place the

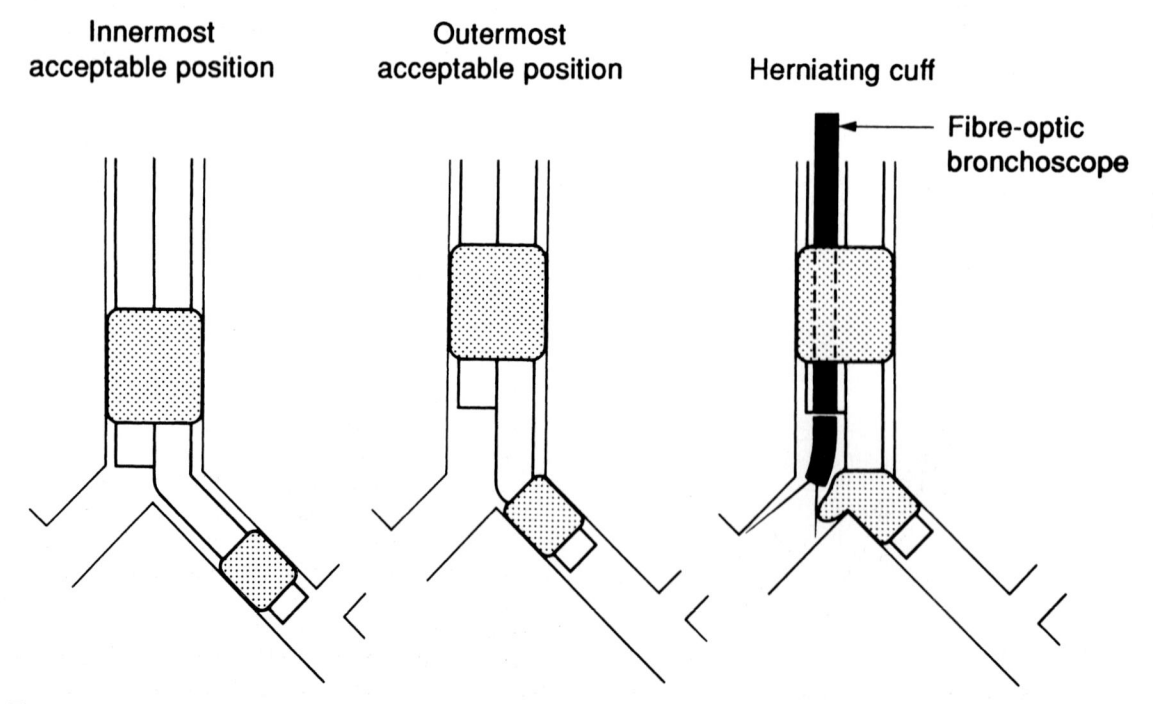

Fig. 10.5 Left-sided double-lumen tube. Checking the position with a fibre-optic bronchoscope.

THORACIC SURGERY 249

endobronchial tube under direct vision from the outset in patients who present with difficult laryngeal intubation, or when the tube cannot be located blindly in the appropriate bronchus. The flexibility of plastic tubes is a distinct advantage when the fibre-optic bronchoscope is used in this way.

Despite accurate initial placement of endobronchial tubes, there is no doubt that movement can occur during surgery.[27] Rubber tubes seem to move less than disposable plastic tubes but in general they are bulkier and less appropriate for small patients. The original pattern right Robertshaw tube (Phoenix Medical) has a large ventilation slot in the bronchial cuff and statistically this is much more likely to be opposite the right upper lobe orifice that that of a similar size Bronchocath.[25] The Rusch Robertshaw tube does not have such a large ventilation slot and any possible advantage of this tube is unproven.

Endobronchial tubes are bulky and may cause laryngeal and mucosal damage. Bronchial rupture can also occur if the distal cuff is overinflated.[28]

Positioning of the patient

Most lung resections are undertaken with the patient in a lateral position. This position can be stabilized with chest and hip supports or, more conveniently, with a mattress which becomes rigid and conforms to the patient's contours once its air is evacuated (Fig. 10.8).

A pillow is placed between the lower leg, which is flexed at the hip and knee, and the upper leg, which lies in a neutral position. The upper arm can be allowed to hang freely above the head, thereby pulling the scapula away from the surgical site; alternatively, it can be placed in an arm support. All potential pressure areas are padded.

One-lung anaesthesia

Distribution of ventilation and perfusion during thoracotomy

In the awake subject in the lateral position, blood flow to the dependent lung increases to approximately 60% of the total because of the effect of gravity on the low-pressure pulmonary system.[29] This is matched by an increase in ventilation as the lower lung is on a steep part of the pressure–volume curve and the lower diaphragm, which is pushed into the chest by the abdominal contents, contracts more effectively from a position of mechanical advantage.

During anaesthesia in spontaneously breathing patients the situation changes. There is a reduction in functional residual capacity (FRC) and both lungs

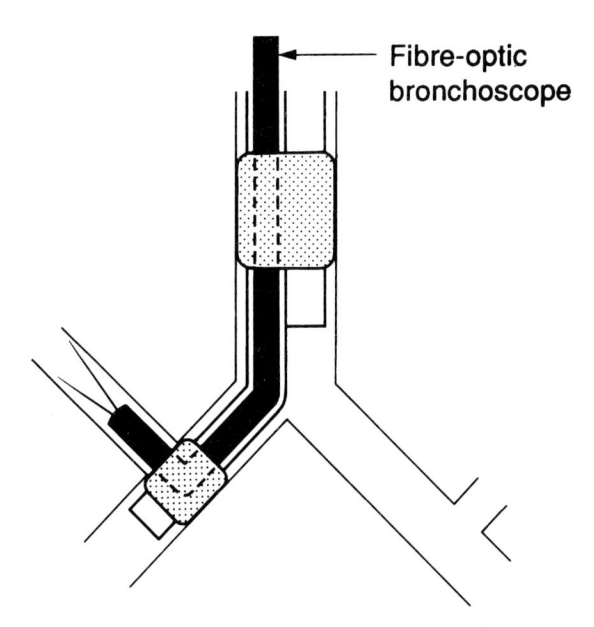

Fig. 10.6 Right-sided double-lumen tube in position.

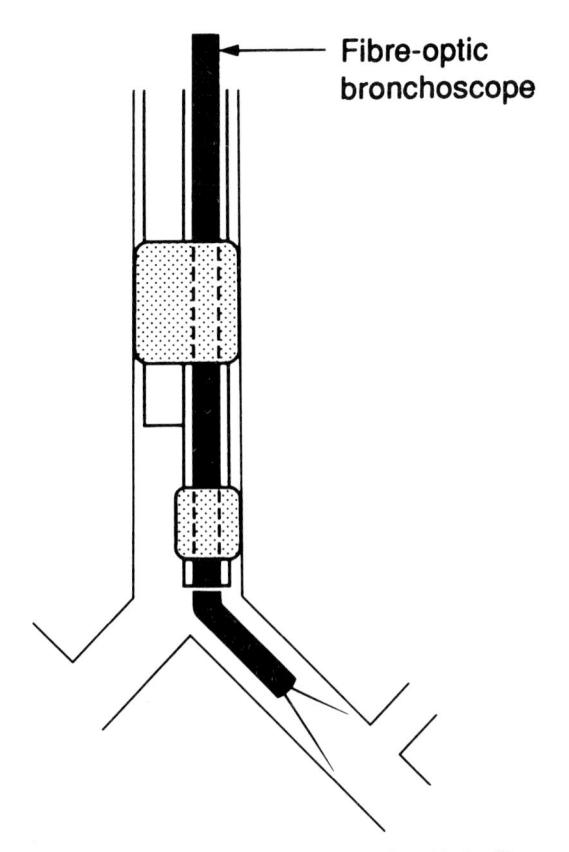

Fig. 10.7 Positioning a double-lumen tube with the fibre-optic bronchoscope.

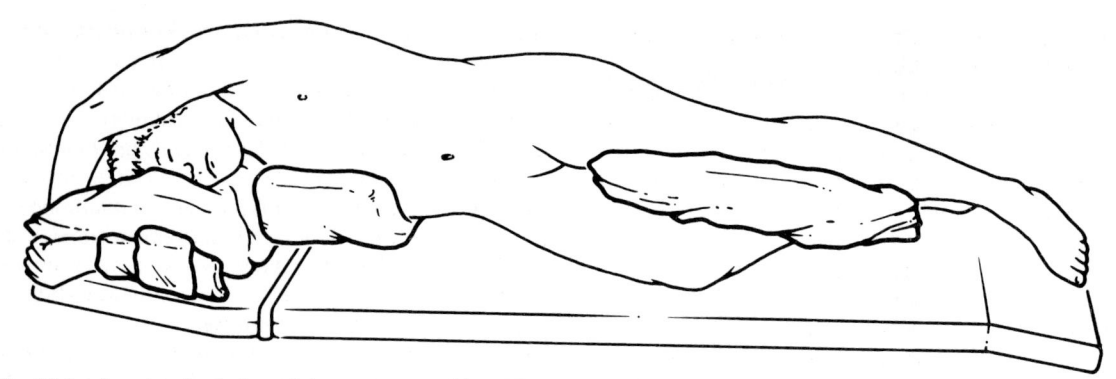

Fig. 10.8 A patient in the lateral thoracotomy position. Note the use of a conformable mattress at chest level to hold the patient in position.

decrease in volume. As a result, the position of the lungs on the pressure–volume curve changes. The non-dependent lung now moves to a steeper part of the curve, and therefore receives more ventilation. Additionally, there is a loss of diaphragmatic tone. The end-result of these changes is that the upper, non-dependent lung, is preferentially ventilated whilst the increased pulmonary blood flow to the lower lung continues.

Paralysis and intermittent positive-pressure ventilation (IPPV) are employed during thoracotomy to overcome the problem of the open pneumothorax. The compliance of the non-dependent lung remains higher than that of the lower lung during positive-pressure ventilation[30] so that preferential ventilation continues to the upper lung, and may be further accentuated when the chest is open.

One-lung anaesthesia is employed at various times during lung resection, primarily to improve surgical access to the non-ventilated lung. This eliminates preferential ventilation to the upper lung but creates a far more serious problem of ventilation/perfusion mismatch.

Physiological aspects of one-lung anaesthesia

Venous admixture. Pulmonary blood flow continues to the upper lung during one-lung anaesthesia, creating a true shunt in a lung where there is blood flow to the alveoli but no ventilation. This shunt is the major cause of hypoxaemia during one-lung ventilation, although the alveoli with low ventilation/perfusion ratios in the dependent lung contribute to some extent. The blood to the upper lung cannot take up oxygen and therefore retains its poorly oxygenated mixed venous composition. This mixes with oxygenated blood in the left atrium causing venous admixture and lowering arterial oxygen tension (PaO_2).

Venous admixture increases from a baseline value of approximately 20% during two-lung ventilation to a level of 30–40% during one-lung ventilation.[31] The PaO_2 can be maintained in the safe range of 9–16 kPa with an inspired oxygen concentration between 50 and 100% in the majority of patients. However, in some individuals, the PaO_2 may fall considerably lower than this, despite a high inspired oxygen concentration.[32–34] This variation is hardly surprising considering the number of interrelated physiological factors that come into play.

Hypoxic pulmonary vasoconstriction. In some clinical and pathological conditions, the phenomenon of hypoxic pulmonary vasoconstriction occurs in the vasculature of poorly oxygenated alveoli, diverting blood flow to better ventilated alveoli and minimizing hypoxaemia.[31,35] The precise mechanism of this effect remains unknown but it may be that endothelial constrictor substance is released at alveolar level in response to hypoxia. Alternatively, hypoxia may inhibit endothelial relaxation substance.

Many factors inhibit hypoxic pulmonary vasoconstriction. These include vasodilator drugs, high or low pulmonary vascular pressures, hypocapnia, volatile anaesthetic agents and handling of the lung. Intravenous anaesthetic agents do not appear to inhibit hypoxic pulmonary vasoconstriction and, in experimental dogs, Lumb et al[36] showed that the shunt during one-lung ventilation was greater during halothane anaesthesia than when ketamine was used. Other workers[37–39] have failed to demonstrate a similar difference in humans, although a recent uncontrolled study showed very low shunt values during one-lung ventilation when propofol and alfentanil were used in a total intravenous anaesthetic technique.[40]

Hypoxic pulmonary vasoconstriction seems, on current evidence, to play little role in reducing hypoxaemia during the time it takes to complete the average lobectomy or pneumonectomy. Volatile anaesthetic agents do not significantly impair arterial oxygenation during one-lung anaesthesia and remain the primary anaesthetic agent of choice for thoracotomy.[35]

Cardiac output. Changes in cardiac output are likely to affect arterial oxygenation during thoracotomy. If oxygen consumption remains steady, a decrease in cardiac output creates a reduced mixed venous oxygen content. Some of this desaturated blood is shunted during one-lung anaesthesia and further exacerbates hypoxaemia. Cardiac output can decrease for a number of reasons during thoracotomy. These include the use of high inflation pressures,[41] the application of positive end-expiratory pressure (PEEP) to the dependent lung[32] and the use of high levels of PEEP to the lower lung combined with continuous positive airways pressure (CPAP) to the upper lung.[42] However, surgical manipulation and retraction around the mediastinum, causing a reduction in venous return, are probably the commonest causes of sudden changes in cardiac output during thoracotomy.

Pre-operative lung function. Diseased lung may have a considerably reduced blood supply as a result of hypoxic pulmonary vasoconstriction or, in some instances, for physical reasons such as collapse/consolidation or infiltration by tumour. Some patients with poor lung function are accepted for lung resection on the basis that their diseased lung is contributing little to gas exchange. If this type of pulmonary disease is largely confined to the side of surgery then one-lung anaesthesia may have little effect on pulmonary gas exchange. Nomoto,[43] using a lung perfusion scanning technique, found that the perfusion partition between the dependent and non-dependent lung correlated significantly with PaO_2 during one-lung ventilation. In patients with empyema, the ratio was as high as 85% and in some the blood flow to the diseased lung was almost immeasurable. In patients with carcinoma, the ratio of perfusion partition was 57% and this group had significantly poorer arterial oxygenation during one-lung ventilation.

Kerr et al[34] reported that patients undergoing lung resection tended to have better arterial oxygenation during one-lung anaesthesia than those undergoing non-resection procedures, such as oesophageal surgery. It was presumed that in the latter group an essentially normal lung was being collapsed to provide surgical access. Katz et al[32] found that patients with a pre-operative FEV_1 nearest the predicted value were more likely to be hypoxic during one-lung anaesthesia. Nomoto[43] also noted an inverse correlation between the pre-operative percentage of predicted vital capacity (VC) and PaO_2 during one-lung ventilation, although other workers have not confirmed this.[44]

Management of ventilation during one-lung anaesthesia

Ventilatory management of the dependent lung is obviously of crucial importance during one-lung anaesthesia. Carbon dioxide elimination is rarely a problem provided that the same minute volume is maintained during one-lung anaesthesia as was employed during the ventilation of two lungs. Ventilator settings are then adjusted to provide adequate alveolar ventilation in the dependent lung without an excessive rise in mean intra-alveolar pressure which directs the low pressure pulmonary blood flow to the non-ventilated lung. It may be necessary to reduce an initial tidal volume of 10–12 ml.kg^{-1} to provide adequate ventilation with a peak inspiratory pressure of 30 cmH$_2$O or less; much depends on the compliance of the lower lung, and occasionally high inflation pressures have to be tolerated for a short period of time. If inflation pressures remain in excess of 30–35 cmH$_2$O despite adjusting the tidal volume to 600 ml or so in the average 70–80 kg adult, the position of the double-lumen tube should be re-assessed. Is a right-sided tube obstructing the right upper lobe orifice, for example? Is a long left-sided tube impinging on the left upper lobe orifice? It may be necessary to reposition the tube and then aspirate secretions from the dependent lung in order to lower peak inflation pressures.

When a satisfactory ventilatory pattern has been established, one-lung anaesthesia can be monitored by continuous pulse oximetry[45] and intermittent arterial blood gas analysis. A PaO_2 of 9 kPa or above, which corresponds to an oxygen saturation of 93.5% with a normal haemoglobin dissociation curve, is tolerable with an inspired oxygen concentration of 50%, even with high inflation pressures. If the PaO_2 remains at or below 8 kPa (91% saturation) then several other measures can be taken to improve oxygenation.

Increasing the inspired oxygen concentration from a baseline of 50% to 100% improves oxygenation because of the increased uptake of oxygen from the alveoli with low ventilation/perfusion ratios in the dependent lung. Many authors advocate the use of 100% oxygen from the beginning of one-lung ventilation and it is difficult to challenge this approach.[31]

Delivery of oxygen to the upper non-ventilated lung by continuous insufflation at a positive pressure of 5–10 cmH$_2$O (analogous to CPAP) improves arterial oxygenation because oxygen is taken up by the pulmonary blood flow to the previously non-ventilated lung.[46] This technique is not commonly used in the UK because it requires ancillary equipment which is unnecessary on a routine basis. Additionally, inflation of the upper lung can impede surgery. However, this technique may be applicable during oesophageal surgery when the left lung is deflated because, as noted previously, this group of patients is more likely to be hypoxaemic. Simple intermittent re-inflation of the upper lung with oxygen has been shown to produce a consistent improvement in oxygenation during one-lung anaesthesia.[47]

PEEP can be applied to the dependent lung with varying results. PEEP does not improve oxygenation in the majority of patients undergoing one-lung ventilation because it tends to decrease cardiac output and, more importantly, it diverts blood flow away from the ventilated lung.[32,48] However, PEEP is beneficial in some patients and may be worthy of trial with careful monitoring by pulse oximetry and blood gas analysis.

PEEP applied to the dependent lung, combined with oxygen delivered to the upper lung to produce CPAP, improves arterial oxygenation during one-lung anaesthesia as the deleterious effect of pulmonary blood flow diversion is negated. However, cardiac output may be substantially reduced by these manoeuvres so that oxygen delivery is not improved significantly.[42] Most anaesthestists find that the disadvantages of this complex technique outweigh any potential short-term advantages unless the need for one-lung anaesthesia is prolonged.

High-frequency jet ventilation

High frequency jet ventilation (HFJV) has been used with some success during thoracotomy via either an endobronchial double-lumen tube or tracheal tube.[49,50] El-Baz et al, using a single-lumen endobronchial tube, demonstrated a reduction in shunt fraction and an improvement in arterial oxygen tension compared with conventional ventilation when HFJV was employed during one-lung ventilation.[51] This improvement was particularly marked when the bronchial cuff was released.

Despite studies showing the HFJV is satisfactory during thoracotomy, it has not been widely accepted. Jenkins et al[49] reported that, although surgical conditions and gas exchange were satisfactory during HFJV, it was difficult to assess adequacy of ventilation. Howland and co-workers found that surgical access was hindered by over-distension of the upper lung during HFJV.[50] Neither group recommended the technique for routine clinical practice.

HFJV may have a role in more specialized circumstances. It has been advocated for the management of patients with a bronchopleural fistula (see below) and for use during a number of operative procedures, including bilateral bullectomy,[52] sleeve resection of the right upper lobe[53] and airway surgery.[11,54]

Termination of anaesthesia

After completion of lung resection and closure of the chest wall, anaesthesia is lightened and spontaneous ventilation re-established in the usual manner. Before removal of the endobronchial tube the patient is placed in a supine position.

Following lobectomy, suction is applied to the bronchi of the intact lung and the remaining lobes of the operated lung. The lungs are manually re-inflated, with the chest drains open to an underwater seal drain. The endobronchial tube is removed when the patient's respiratory effort is satisfactory. A similar sequence is followed after pneumonectomy but the remaining lung is re-inflated until the trachea is approximately central, or slightly towards the side of surgery. The chest drain, if one has been inserted, is then clamped. If a chest drain has not been inserted after pneumonectomy, it may be necessary to aspirate air from the hemithorax on the side of surgery in order to optimize the position of the mediastinum as judged clinically and on an early postoperative chest X-ray.

Patients are placed in the sitting position after removal of the double-lumen tube and allowed to breathe oxygen-enriched air. Further postoperative care is supervised in a high-dependency area or intensive care unit.

Postoperative management

The principles of postoperative management after thoracotomy are similar to those applied after any major operation. Specific areas of concern related to the management of chest drainage, provision of analgesia and the treatment of cardiovascular and respiratory complications.

The management of chest drainage

Chest drains are inserted prior to chest closure after lung resection to drain blood and air from the hemithorax and to allow any remaining lung tissue to expand and fill the cavity. After minor procedures such as open lung biopsy, when the lung is not damaged or bleeding, a temporary chest drain can be inserted and removed immediately after closure of the chest.

Two chest drains (usually wide-bore plastic tubes with end and lateral holes) are inserted following lobectomy. One drain is placed anteriorly in the hemithorax and the other lies in a posterior plane. At least one of the tubes should reach the apex of the cavity. The chest drainage tubes are connected to underwater seal bottles (or drains) which act primarily as a one-way valve but also as a reservoir to collect blood loss. Suction is applied to these drains at a negative pressure of 5 kPa as soon as the chest is closed. It is important to use a suction pump capable of clearing large volumes of air (e.g. modern wall suction units) at this stage. This is because there may be a substantial loss of gas from raw lung surfaces in addition to any air trapped in the chest. A low-volume suction device such as the Robert's pump acts as a plug at the end of the drainage bottle and may result in a tension pneumothorax. Chest drains are removed when they no longer function. Air and fluid loss should have ceased over a 12–24 h period and the loss of 'respiratory swing' on the fluid level is further evidence that the pleural space is obliterated. The drains are removed whilst the patient maintains a positive intra-pleural pressure using a Valsalva manoeuvre. A purse-string suture, placed around the drain site at operation, is then tightened to prevent air entering the chest.

Drainage is not mandatory following pneumonectomy and, as previously discussed, some surgeons close the chest without a drain if they are confident of haemostasis. If drainage is used, a basal drain is inserted as surgery is completed in order to drain blood and manipulate the position of the mediastinum in the early post-operative period. The drainage tube is connected to an underwater seal drainage system, but suction is *never* applied. Following intratracheal suction and removal of the double-lumen tube, with the patient in a supine position breathing spontaneously, the chest drain is clamped when it has been ascertained that the trachea is approximately central. The clamps are only released for 2–3 min in every hour in order to reveal excessive blood loss. The basal drain is usually removed on the day after surgery.

Provision of analgesia

Conacher, in a recent review,[55] has emphasized that thoracotomy causes severe pain and deleterious changes in pulmonary physiology (see below). Despite their respiratory depressant effect, opioid drugs, given intramuscularly or intravenously, are used as the basis of analgesia in most centres. The administration of intramuscular opioids on an 'as required basis' is a poor method of pain control but intravenous opioids, given by continuous infusion, can be effective if managed appropriately by an enthusiastic team.[56] Nurse-controlled and patient-controlled intravenous analgesia has also been used to provide satisfactory pain relief following thoracotomy.[57,58]

The nature of the thoracic cavity allows the use of local anaesthetic and related techniques to provide analgesia after thoracic surgery. A variety of methods have been used.

Intercostal and paravertebral nerve block.
Local anaesthetic intercostal nerve blocks can be established under direct vision before closure of the chest. If several nerves above and below the incision (including those supplying the site of chest drain insertion) are blocked, pain in the immediate post-operative period can be decreased, with a reduction in analgesic requirements.[59] Paravertebral block has been advocated as an alternative to intercostal block because one injection is effective over at least four intercostal spaces and can be conveniently repeated via an indwelling catheter.[60] Additionally, pain from the costovertebral ligaments and posterior spinal muscles, mediated by the posterior primary ramus, is blocked by a paravertebral technique but not by an intercostal one.

Intercostal blocks can be prolonged by cryo-analgesic techniques[61] or by continuous infusion of local anaesthetic agents via an indwelling catheter.[62] Cryo-analgesia of the intercostal nerves has been used successfully for a number of years as an adjunct to other methods of pain relief. However, it cannot be relied upon as the sole method of analgesia following thoracotomy because of the widespread nociceptive input.[63,64] There is also concern that cryo-analgesia may be the cause of long-term dysaesthesia and chronic pain, relating to regeneration of the intercostal nerves.[65,66] However, late chest wall pain is not uncommon following thoracotomy,[67] and this causal relationship is not definitely established.

Epidural analgesia. Local anaesthetic thoracic epidural analgesia can provide excellent pain relief following thoracotomy. The technique is relatively difficult to perform and there is a high incidence of significant adverse effects, including hypotension and urinary retention.[68,70] Thoracic epidural opioids provide adequate analgesia following thoracotomy without hypotension, although respiratory depression is a hazard. The technique of insertion remains difficult, and Bromage has advised against inserting thoracic epidural catheters in the anaesthetized patient because of the risk of neurological damage.[72]

Lumbar epidurals are easier to establish and probably safer than thoracic techniques. Opioids have been used via this route to provide analgesia following thoracotomy. Patrick et al[73] used lumbar epidural diamorphine by infusion and bolus injection to establish analgesia and Badner and co-workers[74] achieved satisfactory pain relief with an infusion of fentanyl. In the former study, there were significant incidences of urinary retention and respiratory depression. In both studies, there was a delay in achieving pain relief so that pain scores were high in the early postoperative period. Badner et al inserted urinary catheters in all patients. There is a significant incidence of urinary retention following thoracotomy irrespective of the method of analgesia used, so it is prudent to catheterize patients in whom epidural analgesia is employed.

Thoracic epidural opioids can be used in combination with local anaesthetic agents to provide analgesia.[75] This may allow a reduction in dosage of both drugs so that the incidence of major side-effects is minimized. This type of technique is probably applicable to lumbar, and certainly high lumbar, epidural analgesia following thoracotomy.

Other methods of analgesia. A variety of other methods of pain relief have been used after thoracotomy. There has been renewed interest in intrapleural regional analgesia,[76,77] and non-steroidal anti-inflammatory agents may have a role to play.[78] The inhalation of 50% nitrous oxide in oxygen (Entonox) is also a simple expedient that can make chest drain removal more comfortable.

Cardiovascular complications

Lung resection imposes considerable strain on the cardiovascular system. After pneumonectomy the entire cardiac output has to pass through one pulmonary vascular bed. This is of little concern in those with a normal pulmonary vascular resistance[21] but can cause right ventricular failure if the pulmonary artery pressure is elevated.

Hypotension in the first 12–24 h following lung resection is often due to vasodilatation as the patient warms peripherally. This usually responds to colloid replacement, monitored by central venous pressure measurements. Active haemorrhage within the chest must also be considered as a cause of hypotension, irrespective of the revealed chest drainage.

In common with other forms of major surgery myocardial infarction can occur in the postoperative period. A high proportion of myocardial infarcts are silent postoperatively[15] and therefore may be difficult to diagnose. If myocardial failure occurs, inotropic therapy, monitored by thermodilution cardiac output and pulmonary capillary wedge pressure measurements, may be required. Measurement of urine output is also essential.

Supraventricular arrhythmias, particularly atrial fibrillation, are common following lung resection. They are more common in the elderly and after extensive surgery. The incidence of atrial arrhythmias is probably lessened by pre-operative digitalization, which also limits the increase in ventricular rate associated with atrial fibrillation. Most centres do not routinely digitalize all patients presenting for thoracotomy. The peak incidence of arrhythmias is delayed until 2–5 days postoperatively; thus, if surgery is extensive, and particularly if there has been dissection within the pericardium, digitalization can be started at operation and continued postoperatively. Verapamil is also effective in reducing the incidence of atrial arrhythmias following thoracotomy if treatment is started in the recovery period.[79] This approach is not followed by all clinicians. Many prefer to diagnose and treat arrhythmias with appropriate drug therapy when they occur, rather than use potentially toxic drugs prophylactically.

Respiratory complications

Pulmonary function changes are considerable following thoracotomy. The extent of these changes depends to a great extent on the nature of surgery but reductions of 50% or more (from pre-operative values) have been widely reported in peak expiratory flow rate, FVC, FEV_1 and MBC.[65,75,80] Adequate analgesia can lead to an improvement in lung function following thoracotomy[80–82] but this is not a universal finding. For example, thoracic epidural analgesia with local anaesthetics may cause a reduction in lung volume,[83] although the analgesic effects of this technique are extremely helpful in allowing effective physiotherapy.[84] In addition, the respiratory depressant effects of conventional intravenous opioid analgesics are well-known and similar problems occur if epidural opioids are used.[85]

The reduction in pulmonary function following thoracotomy often leads to sputum retention which, if inadequately treated, can result in respiratory failure. Once the FEV_1 falls below 1 l, increasing difficulties in sputum clearance are to be expected.[86] Respiratory difficulties are particularly common if the recurrent laryngeal and phrenic nerves have been damaged at operation or if a section of chest wall has been resected. Bronchopleural fistula following lung resection may also precipitate respiratory failure. This is discussed below.

Chest physiotherapy combined with optimal analgesia is the first-line treatment for sputum retention. Appropriate antibiotic therapy is also instituted. If retention of secretions remains a problem, a minitracheotomy can be inserted under local anaesthesia to provide a direct route for suction.[87] Occasionally, these measures are ineffective and mechanical ventilation is necessary.

ANAESTHESIA FOR OTHER SURGICAL PROCEDURES

Repair of bronchopleural fistula

Bronchopleural fistula (BPF) is an abnormal communication between the tracheobronchial tree and the pleural cavity. It is an uncommon condition presenting as a result of trauma, gross infection or, more commonly, when the bronchial stump suture line breaks down following pneumonectomy.

A BPF can occur at any time following pneumonectomy, but commonly presents 2–10 days postoperatively. A small fistula presents as general malaise with a tachycardia and low-grade fever. There may also be episodes of coughing, dyspnoea and wheezing. A large fistula can present dramatically as brownish fluid from the intrathoracic space is coughed up and inhaled into the remaining lung, causing severe bronchoconstriction, dyspnoea and hypoxaemia. Signs of circulatory failure also occur as a result of hypoxia or septicaemia, if the inhaled space contents were infected. This symptomatology is virtually diagnostic of BPF and is usually accompanied by classical X-ray changes;[88] the space fluid decreases dramatically and the remaining lung shows gross evidence of collapse/consolidation (Fig. 10.9). After the sudden occurrence of a large fistula general resuscitative measures are instituted. The patient is supported in the sitting position with the pneumonectomy side dependent. A basal chest drain is then inserted to prevent further spillover of fluid.

Many thoracic surgeons prefer to bronchoscope patients with BPF before surgery in order to confirm the diagnosis, assess the size of the fistula and aspirate infected secretions from the remaining lung. If the fistula proves to be small, it may heal if cauterized with sodium hydroxide or silver nitrate or, alternatively, if an infected pneumonectomy space is chronically drained. A large fistula requires surgical repair.

Anaesthesia for repair of bronchopleural fistula

In the past, endobronchial intubation was carried out under local anaesthesia or after inhalational induction, so that positive-pressure ventilation could be avoided until the fistula was isolated. Both these methods have disadvantages in the ill patient and most experienced thoracic anaesthetists now use a conventional intravenous induction followed by endobronchial intubation facilitated by the use of suxamethonium.

Only atropine premedication is given to the ill patient, who should arrive in the anaesthetic room in the sitting position. This position is maintained on transfer to the operating table and it is then ensured that the chest drain is unclamped and connected to a

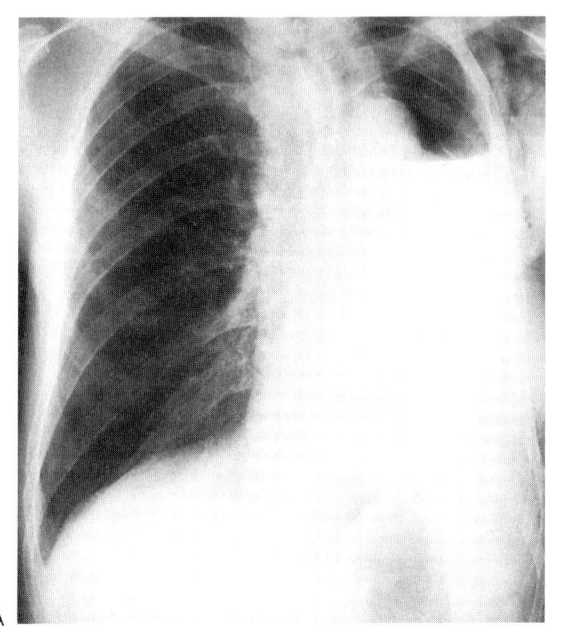

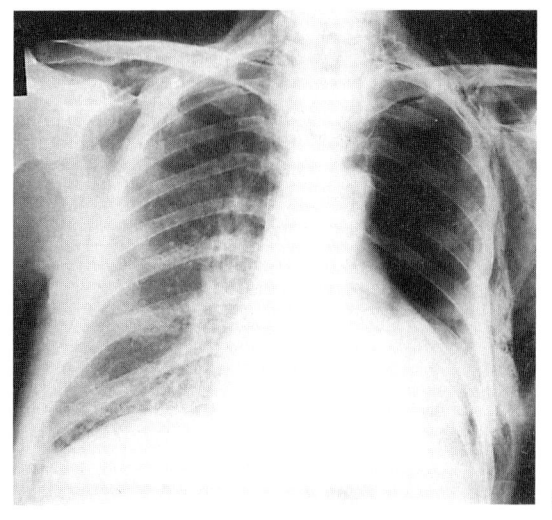

Fig. 10.9 (A) Chest X-ray of a male patient several days after a left pneumonectomy, showing a normal fluid level. (B) Subsequent chest X-ray showing loss of fluid level on the left and soiling of the right lung — radiographic evidence of a bronchopleural fistula.

dependent underwater seal drain. Intravenous access is secured and full monitoring is established. Pre-oxygenation is carried out and then anaesthesia induced with the minimum effective dose of an intravenous agent followed by suxamethonium. Following muscular relaxation the surgeon may undertake bronchoscopy with the rigid instrument to inspect the BPF. Venturi ventilation should be withheld until secretions have been aspirated from the remaining lung. When this has been achieved, ventilation can be commenced. Following bronchoscopy, endobronchial intubation is carried out, if necessary, after an additional dose of suxamethonium.

The type and size of endobronchial tube used for the first operation is usually selected and this can initially be placed blindly in the usual way. However, it is advantageous if a fibre-optic bronchoscope is available so that the endobronchial tube can be positioned accurately using direct vision.[26] If placement of the endobronchial tube proves difficult, the rigid bronchoscope is replaced in the remaining main bronchus to allow Venturi ventilation whilst the situation is re-assessed.

When the fistula has been isolated, a depolarizing muscle relaxant is administered and positive-pressure ventilation started. The patient is then positioned for thoracotomy, taking care not to dislodge the endobronchial tube.

Postoperatively, it is usual to re-establish spontaneous ventilation. This may be inadequate because of the grossly infected remaining lung and the sequelae of a second operation under general anaesthetic. IPPV can be continued conventionally via a disposable plastic double-lumen endobronchial tube or more simply via a tracheal tube. Alternatively, HFJV can be employed.

A number of authors have reported favourably on the use of HFJV in patients with a BPF.[89,90] However, Roth et al[91] found that, despite a reduced peak airway pressure, the air leak through a BPF can increase with HFJV, particularly if chest drain suction is employed. Animal experiments carried out to quantify the effect of HFJV on the air leak through a BPF have produced conflicting results.[92,93] Therefore the role of HFJV in this situation remains to be clarified.

Surgery for cystic lung disease

Surgery for cystic lung disease mainly concerns the excision or obliteration of emphysematous bullae. Excision of large bullae is a relatively major surgical procedure,[94] and therefore less invasive intracavity drainage techniques have been developed to obliterate emphysematous bullae; these latter techniques are particularly useful in relieving symptoms in patients with marginal lung function. Venn et al[95] found that intracavity drainage could be used safely in patients with an FEV_1 as low as 500 ml, with a median improvement in this value of 22% postoperatively. Total lung capacity following drainage was reduced by 11% in the same group of patients. Mortality due to respiratory failure occurred in 2 patients with pre-operative FEV_1 values of 220 and 350 ml respectively; these patients also had high pre-operative $Paco_2$ values of 7.0 kPa or above.

Lung cysts or bullae (Fig. 10.10) are likely to enlarge if nitrous oxide is used during general anaesthesia because the uptake of this gas is faster than the clearance of less soluble nitrogen. Cysts may also be preferentially ventilated during positive-pressure ventilation. These factors may cause lung cysts to enlarge and rupture during surgery, resulting in a tension pneumothorax, particularly if high airway pressures are employed.

Endotracheal anaesthesia can be employed safely for patients undergoing intracavity drainage procedures, provided that an air/oxygen inspired gas mixture is used and ventilation pressures are minimized.

HFJV has been advocated for the intra-operative management of bullectomy.[96] However obligatory end-expiratory pressure is produced by many jet ventilation systems, and pneumothorax remains a complication of their use. A more conventional approach is to separate the two lungs with a double-lumen tube and ventilate the lung contralateral to surgery, omitting nitrous oxide and using low inflation pressures.[97] Bullous lung disease

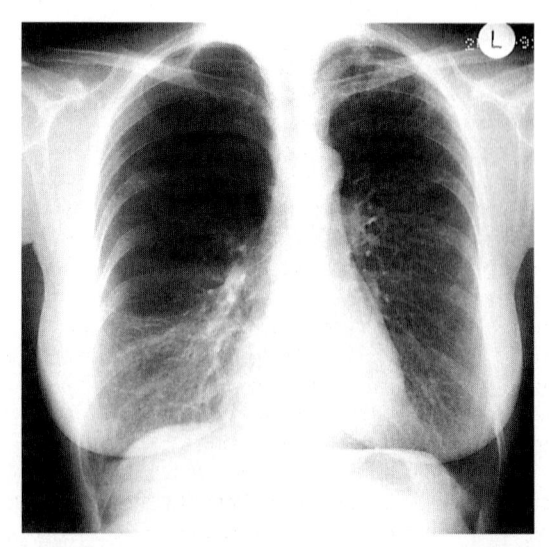

Fig. 10.10 Chest X-ray. Emphysematous bulla in the right lung

is often bilateral and, if so, it is reasonable to ventilate both lungs up to the time that the chest is open; if problems occur with ventilation during this period, the possibility of pneumothorax must be considered. The surgical team should be immediately available to open the chest if a tension pneumothorax occurs.

Adequate postoperative analgesia is essential following bullectomy and intracavity drainage and therefore the use of epidural analgesia should be considered. All patients require careful monitoring of respiratory status in the postoperative period.

Surgery for mediastinal tumours

Mediastinal tumours are rare but patients with these neoplasms frequently present at specialized thoracic surgical units for diagnostic biopsy or resection. The commonest tumours are neural in origin, followed in order of frequency by teratomata and thymic neoplasms. Other lesions found include lymphoma and intrathoracic goitre.

Mediastinal tumours, particularly those in the anterior mediastinum, may cause a variety of difficulties during anaesthesia which are described below.[98-100] Anaesthesia for thymectomy in patients with myasthenia gravis is discussed separately.

Anaesthesia for biopsy and resection of anterior mediastinal tumours

Major anaesthetic problems encountered in association with anterior mediastinal tumours include airways obstruction, compression of intrathoracic vascular structures and the effects of pre-operative radiotherapy and chemotherapy. Intra-operative bleeding may also be severe and adequate central venous access should be established in the systems draining into the superior vena cava and inferior vena cava, in case the former system is damaged or clamped during surgery.

Airways obstruction. Tumour compression of the trachea and main bronchi causes airway obstruction. Patients with an anterior mediastinal tumour commonly present with a cough, dyspnoea and difficulty in breathing, particularly when lying flat. Tracheal compression may be evident on the chest X-ray and this can be evaluated further by CT and magnetic resonance scanning[101] (Fig. 10.11). Pulmonary function tests will confirm airway obstruction.

North American authors have advocated the use of pre-operative radiotherapy or chemotherapy in patients with severe upper airway obstruction given, if necessary, without a firm histological diagnosis.[100] This has not been accepted practice in the UK, where every effort is

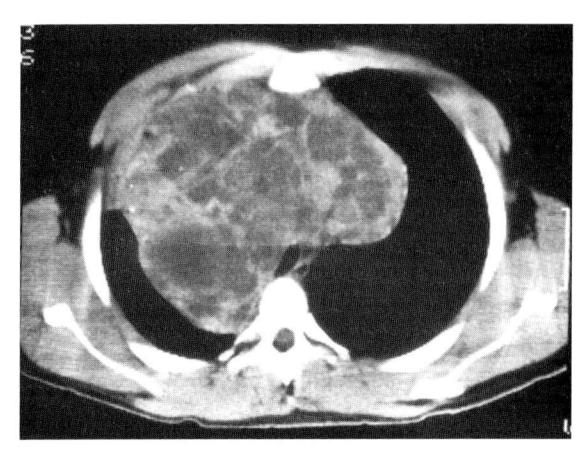

Fig. 10.11 Computed tomographic scan of upper thoracic cavity showing a large mediastinal tumour causing distortion and narrowing of the trachea.

made to establish a tissue diagnosis before beginning any treatment which may mask pathological characteristics of the tumour. There is a risk of severe and even fatal intra-operative respiratory obstruction but this can be minimized by careful planning. This risk is considered justifiable in the context of patients with extremely aggressive tumours whose long-term treatment and survival depend on an accurate histological diagnosis. Ferrari & Bedford (Sloan-Kettering Cancer Center, New York) have recently expressed similar views and reported their experience in 44 children with anterior mediastinal tumours.[102]

Traditionally, it is taught that anaesthesia should be induced by inhalation in the presence of upper airway obstruction. This approach creates a number of problems if the obstruction is due to extrinsic compression by an anterior mediastinal mass.[103] Lung volume is reduced during anaesthesia and bronchial smooth muscle relaxes, thereby increasing the compressibility of the large airways. Partly obstructed ventilation, which is not uncommon during an inhalational induction, generates large negative intrathoracic pressures which tend to flatten an airway already weakened by extrinsic compression. In the majority of patients, intravenous induction can be carried out in the sitting position following pre-oxygenation. After paralysis with suxamethonium, a rigid bronchoscope is passed through the externally compressed trachea and Venturi ventilation started. If compression of the airway is limited to the upper trachea, a tracheal tube can usually be passed through the stricture. Narrowing of the lower trachea or main bronchi may require the use of a longer armoured tracheal tube, or even an endobronchial tube (single- or double-lumen) to negotiate the compression and allow ventilation; these tubes can be placed under direct vision using the fibre-optic or rigid intubating bronchoscope.

Femoral vein to femoral artery cardiopulmonary bypass, established under local anaesthesia, can be used to provide gas exchange during resection of mediastinal tumours in patients with severe airway obstruction.[104] The main disadvantage of this technique is the increased risk of haemorrhage as a result of heparinization.

Following tumour resection, spontaneous ventilation can usually be established despite the presence of an airway weakened by chronic compression. A period of IPPV may be indicated for other reasons such as phrenic nerve section, massive blood loss and prolonged surgery. After biopsy of a mediastinal tumour, spontaneous ventilation may be compromised because of the effects of anaesthesia in a patient with pre-existing respiratory obstruction. Once spontaneous ventilation has been established satisfactorily, a trial of extubation can be carried out with the patient in the sitting position. A few patients require emergency re-intubation followed by a period of mechanical ventilation. Removal of the tracheal tube is possible at a later stage in the majority of these patients once the effects of anaesthesia and surgery have receded. A very small number of patients require treatment of the tumour by radiotherapy, chemotherapy or surgery before they can be weaned from respiratory support; these patients are in a very high-risk category but at least their treatment can be managed with the benefit of accurate histology.

Compression of intrathoracic vascular structures. Obstruction of the superior vena cava is a common presenting feature of anterior mediastinal tumours. Compression of the heart and pulmonary arteries occurs less frequently, as a result of tumour extension, but has been implicated in the death of several patients at induction of anaesthesia.

Pulmonary artery compression is likely if cyanosis is evident in the presence of satisfactory pulmonary function. This is particularly true if the cyanosis is more marked in the supine position or occurs during the straining of defaecation. Cardiac compression presents with the cardiovascular abnormalities associated with pericardial tamponade and is treated using similar principles. Pulmonary artery compression may be alleviated if the patient is anaesthetized in the sitting position. Unfortunately, pulmonary artery occlusion may be most marked on the side on which ventilation is less compromised. In this situation one lung can be inflated easily during anaesthesia but the patient becomes progressively more cyanosed because of poor, or absent, blood flow to that lung. Pulmonary artery compression of this nature may be one of the few indications to use cardiopulmonary bypass before the induction of anaesthesia.

Obstruction of the superior vena cava can present a number of difficulties during anaesthesia. These include a slow induction time if intravenous agents are administered via arm veins, respiratory obstruction and difficulty with tracheal intubation in the presence of oedematous mucosa in the upper airway. None of these factors is an absolute contra-indication to intravenous anaesthesia if the patient is managed in the sitting position and the airway is secured as described above.

Previous chemotherapy and radiotherapy. Pulmonary damage due to bleomycin therapy is of significance in the anaesthetic management of patients with a mediastinal tumour. Bleomycin is used in the treatment of a number of tumours, including primary and secondary teratoma, both of which occur in the mediastinum. Pulmonary damage occurs in 10% or more of patients who receive the drug.[105] It is a dose-related phenomenon which is particularly likely to occur in the elderly, in those with poor lung function and following radiotherapy. Symptoms of pulmonary damage (including shortness of breath, cough and fever) follow a variable time course, but often develop over a period of weeks following treatment. Fine reticular shadows are seen initially on the chest X-ray, but at a later stage more widespread changes may be seen, with linear infiltrates and patchy atelectasis.

There is reasonable evidence that high inspired oxygen concentrations used during and after anaesthesia potentiate the toxic pulmonary effects of bleomycin. The inspired oxygen concentration should therefore be kept at the minimum necessary to provide satisfactory arterial oxygenation. Anaesthesia should be avoided, if at all possible, in those known to have acute bleomycin lung toxicity.

Thymectomy in patients with myasthenia gravis

There are approximately 30–50 cases of myasthenia gravis per million of population. Acquired auto-immune myasthenia gravis is the most common form of the disease and this is more prevalent in females. It is characterized by a weakness and fatigue of voluntary muscles; the initial presentation is often ocular. It is known that there is a marked reduction in acetylcholine receptors at the neuromuscular junction in this disease, and up to 90% of patients have circulating antibodies to these receptors.

Anticholinesterase therapy (usually pyridostigmine) is the first-line treatment for myasthenia but immunosuppressive therapy with corticosteroids and azathioprine may also be used. Plasmapheresis is useful in a proportion of severely ill patients.

The role of the thymus in the aetiology of myasthenia gravis is unclear but up to 75% of patients are improved by thymectomy, and may even achieve complete remission over a variable period of time. A substantial number of the thymus glands removed show evidence of hyperplasia and approximately 15% incorporate a thymoma.

Anaesthetic considerations for thymectomy in myasthenia gravis

Thymectomy can now be undertaken via a transcervical/suprasternal approach. However, a limited, or even complete, median sternotomy is required for an enlarged thymus.

Weakness of the respiratory muscles and inability to cough or swallow are major problems in the management of these patients during and after operation. Peri-operative management of anticholinesterase therapy, induction and maintenance of anaesthesia, the use of muscle relaxants and postoperative ventilation in this context are discussed briefly below. Eisenkraft has reviewed this subject in detail.[106]

Peri-operative anticholinesterase therapy. Anticholinesterase therapy is usually reduced by approximately 20% when the patient is admitted to hospital. This is to prevent overdosage: first, whilst the patient is sedentary in the pre-operative period and second, immediately postoperatively, when the need for anticholinesterases may be substantially reduced. Pyridostigmine is usually withheld on the morning of surgery if respiratory weakness is not a prominent feature symptomatically, and the vital capacity is at least 1 l when a dose of the drug is due. If pyridostigmine is required, an intramuscular injection of 1/30th of the normal oral dose can be given. An oral benzodiazepine is suitable premedication and intramuscular atropine prevents excessive salivation.

When the trachea has been extubated postoperatively, anticholinesterase therapy is recommended. Oral administration of the pre-operative dose regimen is usually satisfactory but, if necessary pyridostigmine can be given intramuscularly in appropriately reduced dosage. Oral administration in the postoperative period is facilitated by passing a nasogastric tube intra-operatively.

Induction and maintenance of anaesthesia. Anaesthesia can be induced intravenously in the usual way and then deepened with an inhaled agent. Myasthenic patients are likely to be more sensitive to the neuromuscular depressant effects of inhaled agents but the extent of this sensitivity varies widely from patient to patient. Isoflurane, which is fairly rapidly eliminated, is a useful agent for use in myasthenics but enflurane and halothane have also been used satisfactorily. In centres where desflurane is available, its rapid elimination may make it the agent of choice.

When the required depth of anaesthesia has been reached, the larynx is sprayed with lignocaine and intubation achieved without the use of muscle relaxants. Mechanical ventilation is continued, controlling the depth of anaesthesia with the chosen inhaled agent.

Use of muscle relaxants. Myasthenics are sometimes resistant to the depolarizing muscle relaxant suxamethonium; however, it can usually be used in relatively normal dosage to produce adequate relaxation for tracheal intubation with a normal recovery time.[106] Suxamethonium may be indicated to facilitate intubation in patients with relatively little muscle weakness or in those at risk of regurgitation.

Patients with myasthenia gravis are sensitive to non-depolarizing muscle relaxants and therefore in the past anaesthetists have avoided their use. However, atracurium, with its unique breakdown properties, has been used successfully to provide muscle relaxation in myasthenics. If neuromuscular transmission is monitored, reduced dosage can be employed, without the need for reversal. Avoiding reversal is advantageous in this group of patients; they may be sensitive to the effects of anticholinesterases in the postoperative period and could therefore develop a cholinergic crisis. Vecuronium has also been used to provide muscle relaxation for thymectomy.[107] Again, monitoring of neuromuscular transmission is an important part of this technique. Mivacurium, a non-depolarizing relaxant with a duration of action less than that of atracurium or vecuronium, may be the agent of choice, although there are no published reports concerning its use in myasthenia at the time of writing.

Post-operative ventilation. It is prudent for IPPV to continue in the initial postoperative period. The effects of anaesthesia are allowed to wear off and then spontaneous ventilation is re-established. Opioids can be used to provide analgesia at a reduced dose during this period. Extubation is performed according to general principles, when the patient is awake and responsive, and able to generate a negative pressure of $-20 \text{ cmH}_2\text{O}$. A few patients require prolonged ventilation, particularly those with severe disease and a previous history of respiratory failure.[106] After surgery, the need for maintenance with anticholinesterases may be decreased or absent. Edrophonium, in doses of 10 mg, can be used to differentiate weakness caused by either too small or too large a dose of anticholinesterase (it will improve the situation in the former and worsen it in the latter).

Tracheal resection

Trauma, tracheostomy and intubation are the usual causes of benign strictures of the trachea. A variety of discrete malignant tumours may also be treated by tracheal resection. Pre-operatively, the site and extent of tracheal narrowing are evaluated after considering clinical history, pulmonary function tests and a penetrated chest X-ray. However, more precise information can be obtained from a CT or magnetic resonance scan (Fig. 10.12).

Surgery on the upper trachea is performed via a cervical incision but right thoracotomy is required for access to the lower trachea and carina. Gas exchange during the resection procedure can be achieved by intubation of the lower trachea or main bronchus through the surgical incision,[108] or by the use of Venturi ventilation[109] or HFJV delivered by a catheter passing beyond the divided trachea.[110,111] Extracorporeal circulation is an alternative for complex resections, particularly those involving the carina, but this carries a high risk of pulmonary haemorrhage associated with heparinization.

Anaesthesia for tracheal resection

Premedication. The majority of patients tolerate light pre-operative sedation with an oral benzodiazepine.

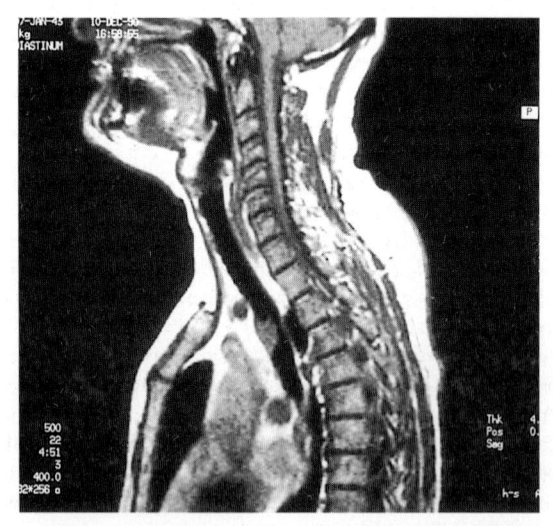

Fig. 10.12 Magnetic resonance scan of the neck and upper thorax. Note the tumour, clearly demonstrated within the trachea at manubrial level.

Respiratory depressant drugs are omitted in those with severe obstruction and it may also be prudent to omit antisialagogues in the same group of patients in case dry secretions lead to further airway narrowing.[108]

Equipment. As with all high-risk airway procedures, all necessary equipment is assembled and checked before induction of anaesthesia. A range of rigid bronchoscopes, including paediatric sizes, must be available. Uncut, cuffed tracheal tubes in a wide range of sizes are laid out in readiness. Several sterile tracheal tubes of suitable size, preferably of the flexometallic type, should also be available for insertion into the distal trachea through the surgical field. A sterile, disposable Bain (co-axial) circuit can be used to connect these tubes to the gas supply on the anaesthetic machine. This type of breathing system is particularly useful for the purpose because it is compact and light in disposable form.

Anaesthetic technique. Pre-oxygenation followed by an intravenous induction and the administration of suxamethonium is a satisfactory technique to allow rigid bronchoscopy in patients with a moderate obstruction, who are dyspnoeic only on exercise. An inhalational induction followed by lignocaine spray to the upper airway can be used in those with more severe obstruction. If manual inflation of the lungs can be achieved easily, a short-acting muscle relaxant may be administered before bronchoscopy. If there is any doubt concerning the ability to ventilate the lungs, muscle relaxants are withheld until the airway has been secured during spontaneous ventilation. A number of patients with severe upper tracheal stenosis may require a tracheostomy distal to the obstuction so that induction of anaesthesia does not pose a problem.

Management of ventilation. The stricture is examined at rigid bronchoscopy. In the majority of cases, some form of tracheal intubation is then possible. With a high tracheal lesion and moderate stenosis, a small tube can usually be passed distally to provide adequate ventilation. Mid to lower tracheal lesions may allow satisfactory inflation via tracheal tube placed above the obstruction, provided the stenosis is not severe. Rarely, it is necessary to pass a paediatric bronchoscope through a severe stenosis in order to dilate the stricture and allow the passage of a small tracheal tube. Occasionally, it may be necessary to continue ventilation via the bronchoscope until a distal airway is established surgically. The use of HFJV via a catheter may also be considered at this stage but it is vitally important that provision is made to allow egress of gas during exhalation.[112]

When the airway is secure, anaesthesia can be maintained with an inhaled agent in oxygen or an air/oxygen mixture. Positive-pressure ventilation can be used following the administration of vecuronium or atracurium in patients whose obstruction has been satisfactorily bypassed.

In mid tracheal lesions, the stricture is identified surgically and the trachea is mobilized above and below. The trachea is then transected below the stricture and a sterile flexometallic or armoured tracheal tube is inserted into the distal segment by the surgeon. Ventilation and anaesthesia are continued via a Bain circuit attached to this second tube. The original tracheal tube is withdrawn proximally but left with its tip through the vocal cords so that it can be advanced at a later stage. The stricture can then be resected and the posterior anastomosis between the upper and lower segments completed whilst the armoured tube is retracted laterally or forwards. The armoured tube is withdrawn after the posterior anastomosis has been reconstructed and then the original tube is advanced into the distal trachea with its tip guided by the surgeon. Ventilation is continued via this tube whilst the anterior part of the trachea is sutured. The tracheal tube can be withdrawn into the upper portion of the trachea after both suture lines have been completed but it may be preferable to leave the tube with its cuff beyond the anastomosis to prevent barotrauma to the suture line.

This technique works well for lesions of the mid or upper trachea and its simplicity has much to commend it over more complex HFJV methods of ventilation. The tracheal tube method of ventilation can be modified for use when the obstruction is in the lower trachea or carinal region but it may be necessary directly to intubate one, or even both, main bronchi. The use of HFJV via relatively fine catheters, which are less likely to obstruct upper lobe bronchi, provides better surgical access in these circumstances, although soiling of the lungs with blood is a potential problem. The relative merits of these techniques have been discussed by Young-Beyer & Wilson.[108]

Postoperative care. In the majority of patients, a concerted effort is made to re-establish spontaneous ventilation to prevent the undesirable effects of prolonged intubation and positive-pressure ventilation on the tracheal suture line. A strong suture is used between the patient's chin and chest wall in order to keep the head flexed, thereby taking tension off the tracheal suture line.

Oesophageal surgery

Surgery is carried out on the oesophagus for repair of hiatus hernia and achalasia. In both these benign conditions, the chief hazards of anaesthesia relate to aspiration of gastric or oesophageal contents into the lungs. The management of these problems is discussed below. Carcinoma of the oesophagus represents a much greater surgical challenge, with operative mortality ranging from approximately 8% for oesophageal resection to 13% for an oesophageal bypass procedure.[113] Long-term surgical results are even more depressing, with 5-year survival being 5% or less in most western series.[114]

Anaesthetic considerations for oesophagectomy

Good pre-operative preparation is essential prior to oesophageal resection. Starvation and nutritional oedema can result from severe dysphagia, and chronic haemorrhage contributes to anaemia and hypoproteinaemia. Every effort should be made to optimize the nutritional state of these patients pre-operatively.[13] A liquid diet may be possible if oesophageal obstruction is not complete but otherwise parenteral nutrition is indicated.

There are few constraints on premedication other than those discussed in relation to oesophagoscopy. The oesophagus is usually approached from a left thoraco-abdominal incision, and the ability to collapse the left lung is useful. Surgery does not involve the lung; thus, a double-lumen tube placed in the left main bronchus is ideal for this purpose because it avoids the problem of right upper lobe ventilation. Hypoxaemia is a potential problem during one-lung ventilation for oesophageal surgery (see above) and therefore oxygen saturation should be monitored continuously.

Blood and fluid loss may be extensive during oesophageal surgery; thus, central venous cannulation is essential. Pulmonary artery catheterization may be indicated in those with myocardial dysfunction. One side of the neck (usually the left) should be kept entirely free from venous lines in case surgical access is required to create an upper anastomosis, when colon is used to replace the oesophagus.

Fit patients may be allowed to breathe spontaneously following a relatively short and uncomplicated operation particularly with the benefit of epidural analgesia. The trachea should not be extubated until the patient is alert and in a sitting position because the conduit of stomach or colon used to replace the oesophagus does not provide a mechanical barrier to prevent aspiration of gastric contents. The majority of patients benefit from a period of mechanical ventilation in the post-operative period. Spontaneous ventilation can be established later in optimal circumstances when heat loss, fluid balance and abnormalities of renal function have been corrected as far as possible.

Chest trauma

Chest trauma requires a multidisciplinary approach to its early management. Blunt chest trauma is relatively common following road traffic accidents. Stabbing and gunshot wounds are major causes of penetrating chest wounds, although the latter remain relatively uncommon in the UK. Blunt chest injuries are rarely isolated events and attention should also be paid to the possibility of neurological damage, abdominal pathology and limb injuries.

Initial emergency care is aimed at the establishment of a satisfactory airway and maintenance of cardiovascular function.[115,118] Immediate chest drainage is indicated for a tension pneumothorax or haemothorax and, if time permits, possible causes of both these conditions should be determined. Thoracotomy in the emergency area is indicated for patients who are apparently dead on arrival in hospital or for patients whose condition deteriorates rapidly despite initial resuscitation.

Possible damage to the lungs and airways include tracheal or bronchial rupture, and pulmonary contusion. Disruption of the diaphragm and the heart and great vessels may also be damaged directly or indirectly. Stab wounds of the chest wall can often be treated conservatively but may require emergency thoracotomy if there are signs of cardiac tamponade or continuing haemorrhage. Damage to the great vessels, particularly closed rupture of the aorta, requires urgent surgical attention in patients who reach hospital alive.

Damage to ribs can cause severe pain and, if extensive, a flail chest wall. In this condition, the thoracic cage is drawn in on inspiration, interfering with ventilation. A minor flail segment can be tolerated in the relatively fit patient if there are no other major injuries. Epidural analgesia can be beneficial in providing optimal analgesia and allowing patients to clear secretions. A number of patients, particularly the elderly and those with multiple injuries, require positive-pressure ventilation to treat respiratory failure and allow adequate analgesia while rib fractures start to heal. Surgical fixation of fractured ribs is now uncommon. This was originally popular in countries where there were inadequate intensive care facilities and prolonged IPPV carried an unacceptably high morbidity and mortality.

REFERENCES

1. Wark KJ, Lyons J, Feneck RO. The haemodynamic effects of bronchoscopy. Effect of pretreatment with fentanyl and alfentanil. Anaesthesia 1986; 41:162–167
2. Augstkalns I, Bradshaw EG. The value of topical lignocaine for bronchoscopy under general anaesthesia. Anaesthesia 1977; 32: 367–370
3. Hill AJ, Feneck RO, Underwood SM, Davis ME, Marsh A, Bromley L. The haemodynamic effects of bronchoscopy. Comparison of propofol and thiopentone with and without alfentanil pretreatment. Anaesthesia 1991; 46: 266–270
4. Roberts FL, Dixon J, Lewis GTR, Tackley RM, Prys-Roberts C. Induction and maintenance of propofol anaesthesia. A manual infusion scheme. Anaesthesia 1988; 43 (suppl): 14–17
5. Bethune DW, Collis JM, Burbridge NJ. Bronchoscope injectors. Anaesthesia 1972; 27: 81–83
6. Hanowell LH, Martin WR, Savelle JE, Foppian LE. Complications of general anaesthesia for Nd: YAG Laser resection of endobronchial tumors. Chest 1991; 99: 72–76
7. George PJM, Garrett CPO, Nixon C, Hetzel MR, Nanson EM, Millard FJC. Laser treatment for tracheobronchial tumours: local or general anaesthesia? Thorax 1987; 42: 656–660
8. Van Der Spek AL, Spargo PM, Norton ML. The physics of lasers and implications for their use during airway surgery. Br J Anaesth 1988; 60: 709–729
9. Conacher ID, Paes ML, Morritt GN. Anaesthesia for carbon dioxide laser surgery in the trachea. Br J Anaesth 1985; 57: 448–450
10. Under M. Tracheobronchial stents and stunts. Chest 1990; 2: 260–261
11. Sherry KM, Keeling PA, Jones HM, Aveling W. Insertion of intratracheal stents. Anaesthetic management using high frequency jet ventilation or cardiopulmonary bypass. Anaesthesia 1987; 42: 61–66
12. Spiro SG. Management of lung cancer. Br Med 1990; 301: 1287–1288
13. Aitkenhead AR. Anaesthesia for oesophageal surgery. In: Gothard JWW, ed. Thoracic anaesthesia. Clinical anaesthesiology, vol 1. London: Baillière Tindall, 1987: pp 181–205
14. United Kingdom Thoracic Surgical Register. 1985–1987. Combined mortality for lobectomy and pneumonectomy.
15. Mangano DT. Perioperative cardiac morbidity. Anesthesiology 1990; 72: 153–184
16. Goldman L. Assessment of the patient with known or suspected ischaemic heart disease for non-cardiac surgery. Br J Anaesth 1988; 6: 38–43
17. Tisi GM. Preoperative identification and evaluation of the patient with lung disease. Med Clin North Am 1987; 71: 399–411
18. Tisi GM. Preoperative evaluation of pulmonary function. Validity, indication and benefits. Am Rev Respir Dis 1979; 119: 293–310
19. Didolkar MS, Moore RH, Takita H. Evaluation of the risk in pulmonary resection for bronchogenic carcinoma. Am J Surg 1974; 127: 700–703
20. Olsen GN, Block AJ, Swenson EW, Castle JR, Wynne JW. Pulmonary function evaluation of the lung resection candidate: a prospective study. Am Rev Respir Dis 1975; 111: 379–386

21. Baier H. Assessment of unilateral lung function. Anesthesiology 1980; 52: 240–247
22. Boysen PG, Clark CA, Block AJ. Graded exercise testing and postthoracotomy complications. J Cardiothorac Anesth 1990; 4: 68–72
23. White PF. Pharmacologic and clinical aspects of preoperative medication. Anesth Analg 1986; 65: 963–974
24. Smith GB, Hirsch NP, Ehrenwerth J. Placement of double-lumen endobronchial tubes — correlation between clinical impressions and bronchoscopic findings. Br J Anaesth 1986; 58: 1317–1320
25. McKenna MJ, Wilson RS, Botelho RJ. Right upper lobe obstruction with right-sided double-lumen endobronchial tubes: a comparison of two tube types. J Cardiothorac Anesth 1988; 2: 734–740
26. Slinger PD. Fiberoptic positioning of double-lumen tubes. J Cardiothorac Anesth 1989; 3: 486–496
27. Saito S, Dohi S, Naito H. Alteration of endobronchial tube position by flexion and extension of the neck. Anesthesiology 1985; 62: 696–697
28. Hannallah M, Gomes M. Bronchial rupture associated with the use of a double-lumen tube in a small adult. Anesthesiology 1989; 71: 457–459
29. Rehder K, Hatch DJ, Sessler AD, Fowler WS. The function of each lung of anesthetized and paralyzed man during mechanical ventilation. Anesthesiology 1972; 37: 16–26
30. Werner O, Malmkvist G, Beckman A, Stahle S, Nordstrom L. Gas exchange and haemodynamics during thoracotomy. Br J Anaesth 1984; 56: 1343–1349
31. Kerr JH. Ventilation and blood flow during thoracic surgery. In: Gothard JWW, ed. Thoracic anaesthesia. Clinical anaesthesiology, vol. 1. London: Baillière Tindall, 1987: pp 61–78
32. Katz JA, Laverne RG, Fairley HB, Thomas AN. Pulmonary oxygen exchange during endobronchial anesthesia. Anesthesiology 1982; 56: 164–171
33. Torda TA, McCulloch CH, O'Brien HD, Wright JS, Horton DA. Pulmonary venous admixture during one-lung anaesthesia. Anaesthesia 1974; 29: 272–279
34. Kerr JH, Crampton Smith A, Prys-Roberts C, Meloche R, Foex P. Observations during endobronchial anaesthesia. II: Oxygenation. Br J Anaesth 1974; 46: 84–92
35. Benumof JL. One lung ventilation and hypoxic pulmonary vasoconstriction: Implications for anesthetic management. Anesth Analg 1985; 64: 821–833
36. Lumb PD, Silvay G, Weinrech AI, Shiang H. A comparison of the effects of continuous ketamine infusion and halothane on oxygenation during one-lung anaesthesia in dogs. Can Anaesth Soc J 1979; 26: 394–401
37. Augustine SD, Benumof JL. Halothane and isoflurane do not impair oxygenation during one-lung anesthesia in patients undergoing thoracotomy. Anesthesiology 1984; 61: A484
38. Rogers SN, Benumof JL. Halothane and isoflurane do not decrease P_aO_2 during one-lung ventilation in intravenously anesthetized patients. Anesth Analg 1985; 64: 946–954
39. Rees DI, Gaines GY. One-lung anesthesia — a comparison of pulmonary gas exchange during anesthesia with ketamine or enflurane. Anesth Analg 1984; 63: 521–525
40. Steegers PA, Backx PJ. Propofol and alfentanil anesthesia during one-lung ventilation. J Cardiothorac Anesth 1990; 4: 194–199
41. Aalto-Setala M, Heinonen J, Salorinne Y. Cardiorespiratory function during thoracic anaesthesia: a comparison of two-lung ventilation and one-lung ventilation with and without $PEEP_5$. Acta Anaesth Scand 1975; 19: 287–295
42. Cohen E, Eisenkraft JB, Thys DM, Kirschner PA, Kaplan JA. Oxygenation and hemodynamic changes during one-lung ventilation: Effects of $CPAP_{10}$, $PEEP_{10}$, and $CPAP_{10}/PEEP_{10}$. J Cardiothorac Anesth 1988; 2: 34–40
43. Nomoto Y. Preoperative pulmonary blood flow and one-lung anaesthesia. Can J Anaesth 1987; 34: 447–449
44. Slinger P, Triolet W, Wilson J. Improving arterial oxygenation during one-lung ventilation. Anesthesiology 1988; 68: 291–295
45. Desiderio DP, Wong G, Shah NK, Liu J, Loughlin CJ, Bedford RF. A clinical evaluation of pulse oximetry during thoracic surgery. J Cardiothorac Anesth 1990; 4: 30–34
46. Rees DI, Wansborough SR. One-lung anesthesia: percent shunt and arterial oxygen tension during continuous insufflation of oxygen to the nonventilated lung. Anesth Analg 1982; 61: 507–512
47. Malmkvist G. Maintenance of oxygenation during one-lung ventilation. Effect of intermittent reinflation of the collapsed lung with oxygen. Anesth Analg 1989; 68: 763–766
48. Capan LM, Turndoff H, Patel C, Ramanathan S, Acinapura A, Chalon J. Optimization of arterial oxygenation during one-lung anesthesia. Anesth Analg 1980; 59: 847–851
49. Jenkins J, Cameron EWJ, Milne AC, Hunter RM. One lung anaesthesia. Cardiovascular and respiratory function compared with conventional and high frequency jet ventilation. Anaesthesia 1987; 42: 938–943
50. Howland WS, Carlon GC, Goldiner PL et al. High-frequency jet ventilation during thoracic surgical procedures. Anesthesiology 1987; 67: 1009–1012
51. El-Baz NM, Kittle CF, Faber LP, Welser W. High-frequency ventilation with an uncuffed endobronchial tube. J Thorac Cardiovasc Surg 1982; 84: 823–828
52. McCarthy G, Coppel DL, Gibbons JR, Cosgrove J. High frequency jet ventilation for bilateral bullectomy. Anaesthesia 1987; 42: 411–414
53. McKinney M, Coppel DL, Gibbons JR, Cosgrove J. A new technique for sleeve resection and major bronchial resection using twin catheters and high frequency jet ventilation. Anaesthesia 1988; 25–26
54. Obara H, Maekawa N, Iwai S, Yamamoto T, Marukawa A. Reconstruction of the trachea in children with tracheal stenosis by using jet ventilation. Anesthesiology 1988; 68: 441–443
55. Conacher ID. Pain relief after thoracotomy. Br J Anaesth 1990; 65: 806–812
56. Church JJ. Continuous narcotic infusions for relief of postoperative pain. Br Med J 1979; 1: 977–979
57. Murphy DF, Opie NJ. Nurse-controlled intravenous

analgesia. Effective control of pain after thoracotomy. Anaesthesia 1991; 46: 772–774
58 White PF. Use of patient-controlled analgesia for postoperative thoracotomy pain. Society of Cardiovascular Anesthesiologists. Proceedings Annual General Meeting 1990; Abstract: 59–60
59 Kaplan JA, Miller ED, Gallagher EG. Postoperative analgesia for thoracotomy patients. Anesth Analg 1975; 54: 773–777
60 Eason MJ, Wyatt R. Paravertebral thoracic block — a reappraisal. Anaesthesia 1979; 34: 638–642
61 Katz J, Nelson W, Forest R, Bruce DL. Cryoanalgesia for post-thoracotomy pain. Lancet 1980; 1: 512–513
62 Safran D, Kuhlman G, Orhant EE, Castelain MH, Journois D. Continuous intercostal blockade with lidocaine after thoracic surgery. Clinical and pharmokinetic study. Anesth Analg 1990; 70: 345–349
63 Keenan DJM, Cave K, Langdon L, Lea RE. Comparative trial of rectal indomethacin and cryoanalgesia for control of early postthoracotomy pain. Br Med J 1983; 287: 1335–1337
64 Roxburgh JC, Markland CG, Ross BA, Kerr WF. Role of cryoanalgesia in the control of pain after thoracotomy. Thorax 1987; 42: 292–295
65 Muller LC, Salzer GM, Ransmayr G, Neiss A. Intraoperative cryoanalgesia for postthoracotomy pain relief. Ann Thorac Surg 1989; 48: 15–18
66 Katz J. Cryoanalgesia for postthoracotomy pain. Ann Thorac Surg 1989; 48: 5
67 Dajczman E, Gordon A, Kreisman H, Wolkove N. Long-term postthoracotomy pain. Chest 1991; 99: 270–274
68 Griffiths DPG, Diamond AW, Cameron JD. Post-operative extradural analgesia following thoracic surgery: a feasibility study. Br J Anaesth 1975; 47: 48–55
69 Conacher ID, Paes ML, Jacobson L, Phillips PD, Heaviside DW. Epidural analgesia following thoracic surgery. A review of 2 years' experience. Anaesthesia 1983; 38: 546–551
70 Matthews PJ, Govenden V. Comparison of continuous paravertebral and extradural infusions of bupivacaine for pain relief after thoracotomy. Br J Anaesth 1989; 62: 204–205
71 Gough JD, Williams AB, Vaughan RS, Khalil JF, Butchart EG. The control of post-thoracotomy pain. A comparative evaluation of thoracic epidural fentanyl infusions and cryo-analgesia. Anaesthesia 1983; 43: 780–783
72 Bromage PR. The control of post-thoracotomy pain. Anaesthesia 1989; 44: 445
73 Patrick JA, Meyer-Witting M, Reynolds F. Lumbar epidural diamorphine following thoracic surgery. A comparison of infusion and bolus administration. Anaesthesia 1991; 46: 85–89
74 Badner NH, Sandler AN, Koren G, Lawson SL, Klein J, Einarson TR. Lumbar epidural fentanyl infusions for post-thoracotomy patients: analgesic, respiratory, and pharmacokinetic effects. J Cardiothorac Anesth 1990; 4: 543–551
75 George KA, Wright PMC, Chisakuta A. Continuous thoracic epidural fentanyl for post-thoracotomy pain relief: with or without bupivacaine? Anaesthesia 1991; 46: 732–736

76 Covino BG. Interpleural regional analgesia. Anesth Analg 1988; 67: 427–429
77 Ferrante FM, Chan VWS, Arthur GR, Rocco AG. Interpleural analgesia after thoracotomy. Anesth Analg 1991; 72: 105–109
78 Cashman JH, Jones RM, Foster JM, Wedley JR, Adams AP. A comparison of infusions of morphine and lysine acetyl salicylate for the relief of pain following thoracic surgery. Br J Anaesth 1985; 57: 255–258
79 Lindgren L, Lepantalo M, Von Knorring J, Rosenberg P, Orko R, Scheinin B. Effect of verapamil on right ventricular pressure and atrial tachyarrhythmia after thoracotomy. Br J Anaesth 1991; 66: 205–211
80 Faust RJ, Nauss LA. Post-thoracotomy intercostal block: comparison of its effects on pulmonary function with those of intramuscular mepeidine. Anesth Analg 1976; 55: 542–546
81 Shulman MS, Brebner J, Sandler A. The effect of epidural morphine on post-operative pain relief and pulmonary function in thoracotomy patients. Anesthesiology 1983; 59: A192
82 Coleman DL. Control of post-operative pain. Nonnarcotic and narcotic alternatives and their effect on pulmonary function. Chest 1987; 92: 520–527
83 Takasaki M, Takahashi T. Respiratory function during cervical and thoracic extradural analgesia in patients with normal lungs. Br J Anaesth 1980; 52: 1271–1276
84 Selsby D, Jones JG. Some physiological and clinical aspects of chest physiotherapy. Br J Anaesth 1990; 64: 621–631
85 Wheatly RG, Somerville ID, Sapsford DJ, Jones JG. Postoperative hypoxaemia: comparisons of extradural, IM and patient-controlled opioid analgesia. Br J Anaesth 1990; 64: 267–275
86 Goldstraw PG. Postoperative management of the thoracic surgical patient. In: Gothard JWW, ed. Thoracic anaesthesia. Clinical anaesthesiology, vol 1. London: Baillière Tindall, 1987: pp 207–231
87 Ryan DW. Minitracheotomy. A new, simple technique for treating patients with retention of sputum. Br Med J 1990; 300: 958–959
88 Lauckner ME, Beggs I, Armstrong RF. The radiological characteristics of bronchopleural fistula following pneumonectomy. Anaesthesia 1983; 38: 452–456
89 Powner DJ, Grenvik A. Ventilatory management of life-threatening bronchopleural fistulae. Crit Care Med 1981; 9: 54–58
90 Feeley TW, Keating D, Nishimura T. Independent lung ventilation using high-frequency ventilation in the management of a bronchopleural fistula. Anesthesiology 1988; 69: 420–422
91 Roth MD, Wright JW, Bellamy PE. Gas flow through a bronchopleural fistula. Measuring the effects of high-frequency jet ventilation and chest-tube suction. Chest 1988; 93: 210–213
92 Spinale FG, Linker RW, Crawford FA, Reines HD. Conventional versus high frequency jet ventilation with a bronchopleural fistula. J Surg Res 1989; 46: 147–151
93 Orlando R, Gluck EH, Cohen M, Mesologites G. Ultra-high-frequency jet ventilation in a bronchopleural fistula model. Arch Surg 1988; 123: 591–593
94 Laros CD, Gelissen HJ, Bergstein JM et al. Bullectomy

for giant bullae in emphysema. J Thorac Cardiovasc Surg 1986; 91: 63–70
95 Venn GE, Williams PR, Goldstraw P. Intracavity drainage for bullous, emphysematous lung disease: experience with the Brompton technique. Thorax 1988; 43: 998–1002
96 McCarthy G, Coppel DL, Gibbons JR, Cosgrove J. High frequency jet ventilation for bilateral bullectomy. Anaesthesia 1987; 42: 411–414
97 Benumof JL. Sequential one-lung ventilation for bilateral bullectomy. Anesthesiology 1987; 67: 268–272
98 Schwartz AJ, Howie M. Case conference — mediastinal mass in a 57-year-old-man. J Cardiothorac Anesth 1987; 1: 71–79
99 Mackie AM, Watson CB. Anaesthesia and mediastinal masses. Anaesthesia 1984; 39: 899–903
100 Neuman GG, Weingarten AE, Abramovitz RM, Kushins LG, Abramson AL, Ladner W. The anesthetic management of the patient with an anterior mediastinal mass. Anesthesiology 1984; 60: 144–147
101 Brown K, Aberle DR, Batra P, Steckel RJ. Current use of imaging in the evaluation of primary mediastinal masses. Chest 1990; 2: 466–473
102 Ferrari LR, Bedford RF. General anesthesia prior to treatment of anterior medistinal masses in pediatric cancer patients. Anesthesiology 1990; 72: 991–995
103 Fletcher R, Nordstrom L. The effects on gas exchange of a large mediastinal tumour. Anaesthesia 1986; 41: 1135–1138
104 Hall DK, Friedman M. Extracorporeal oxygenation for induction of anesthesia in a patient with an intrathoracic tumor. Anesthesiology 1975; 42: 493–495
105 Collis CH. Lung damage from cytotoxic drugs. Cancer Chemother Pharmacol 1980; 4: 17–27
106 Eisenkraft JB. Myasthenia gravis and thymic surgery — anaesthetic considerations. In: Gothard JWW, ed. Thoracic anaesthesia. Clinical Anaesthesiology, vol 1. London: Baillière Tindall, 1987: pp 133–162
107 Nilsson E, Meretoja OA. Vecuronium dose–response and maintenance requirements in patients with myasthenia gravis. Anesthesiology 1990; 73: 28–32
108 Young-Beyer P, Wilson RS. Anesthetic management for tracheal resection and reconstruction. J Cardiothorac Anesth 1988; 2: 821–835
109 Lee P, English ICW. Management of anaesthesia during tracheal resection. Anaesthesia 1974; 29: 305–306
110 Rogers RC, Gibbons J, Cosgrove J, Coppel DL. High frequency jet ventilation for tracheal surgery. Anaesthesia 1985; 40: 32–36
111 Obara H, Maekawa N, Iwai S, Yamamoto T, Marakukawa A. Reconstruction of the trachea in children with tracheal stenosis by using jet ventilation. Anesthesiology 1988; 68: 441–443
112 Larsson S, Nordberg G. Emergency one-lung high-frequency positive-pressure ventilation (HFPPV). Anesth Analg 1987; 66: 471–474
113 United Kingdom Thoracic Surgical Register 1985–1987 Combined operative mortality. Resection and bypass procedures for malignant tumours of the oesophagus
114 Orringer MB. Ten-year survival after esophagectomy for carcinoma. Surgical triumph or biologic variation? Chest 1989; 96: 970–971
115 Alfille PH, Hurford WE. Upper airway injuries. J Clin Anesth 1991; 3: 88–90
116 Cicala RS, Kudsk KA, Butts A, Nguyen H, Fabian TC. Initial evaluation and management of upper airway injuries in trauma patients. J Clin Anesth 1991; 3: 91–98

11. Anaesthesia for pelvic surgery

B. J. Pollard

The pelvis is a shallow bowl formed by the two innominate bones (each comprising ilium, ischium and pubis) on each side and the sacrum posteriorly. The bony pelvis extends upwards posteriorly as the laminae of the iliac bones and in the normal posture tilts forwards as an open-topped bowl.

The principal structures within the pelvis belong to the urinary and genital systems and these will therefore form the main topics for this chapter. A number of major nerves and blood vessels pass through the pelvis, and surgery related to these, and to the bony pelvis, is discussed elsewhere. The other major structure within the confines of the pelvis is the rectum; surgery of the rectum and anus is described in Chapter 8. For the sake of completeness, surgery to the kidney is also included in this chapter.

UROLOGICAL SURGERY

This broad topic describes surgery of the entire urinary system, which includes the kidney, ureters, bladder and urethra. The types of procedure range from the completely non-invasive (e.g. extracorporeal shock-wave lithotripsy; ESWL), through the minimally invasive (e.g. cystoscopy), to major procedures (e.g. nephrectomy). There is an increasing tendency to perform surgery by techniques which are minimally invasive through various endoscopic devices, and much urological surgery lends itself to this approach.[1]

Renal and ureteric surgery

The kidneys and ureters are retroperitoneal structures. Surgical procedures on the lower ureter (e.g. reimplantation or excision) can be performed readily with the patient supine, using an anterior approach through the anterior abdominal wall. However, the surgical approach to the kidney and upper ureter is more logical with a lateral approach, although an anterior incision is possible and is occasionally used.

Positioning of the patient is an important factor in preparation for surgery to the kidney. The patient is usually placed in the lateral position, and the table flexed such that both the trunk and legs are angulated downwards. A 'kidney bridge' may be used to increase lateral flexion in the upper lumbar area to improve surgical access. Great care must be taken in positioning the patient on the table, ensuring that the head, body and legs are supported adequately, and that the degree of lateral flexion is not excessive. Particular care must be taken to prevent undue lateral flexion of the neck.

Pooling of blood in the upper trunk and in the legs is common and it is possible for compression of the vena cava to be produced by the laterally flexed position. The blood pressure must be measured during and immediately after any positional changes, and any cardiovascular instability rectified immediately. The lateral position also leads to considerable mismatch between ventilation and pulmonary perfusion. The upper lung receives preferential ventilation and the lower lung is better perfused (although gas exchange may be better in the lower lung). The pleura may be damaged during surgery, resulting in collapse of the upper lung and further exacerbating the ventilation/perfusion mismatch. Use of the kidney bridge position increases the incidence of postoperative atelectasis of the lower lung.

Many patients who undergo urological operations are elderly and suffer from diseases of the cardiovascular and renal systems. Patients who are scheduled for renal surgery are very likely to have renal insufficiency and this results in a number of additional clinical problems of relevance to the anaesthetist. Pre-existing electrolyte abnormalities are common, and should be corrected by dialysis if appropriate before induction of anaesthesia. Uraemic patients may develop a bleeding diathesis as a result of decreased platelet function. Uraemia may also reduce the requirement for anaesthetic agents, although the cerebral effects of uraemia are uncommon until the blood urea concentration has increased to more than about 20 mmol.l^{-1} (140 mg.dl^{-1}). Suxamethonium is contra-indicated if the serum potassium concentration is elevated. Many patients who suffer from chronic renal failure are chronically anaemic, and a full blood count should be performed as part of the pre-operative preparation. Unless very marked, chronic anaemia should be accepted rather than corrected pre-operatively. Patients who have undergone a period of dialysis within the previous few hours may be relatively dehydrated and careful attention to fluid balance is imperative. Patients with renal disease tend also to suffer from ischaemic heart disease and are often hypertensive; this should be treated if it is significant. There is a considerable potential for blood loss during surgery on the kidney and an intravenous infusion should be established pre-operatively through a cannula of not less than 16-gauge diameter. Blood should be cross-matched and readily available.

General anaesthesia is usually required for these surgical procedures, if only because of the position in which the patient is placed on the table. The procedure may also be lengthy. Muscle relaxation, tracheal intubation and controlled ventilation are required to allow optimum surgical access and because ventilation is impaired by the operating position. A spinal or epidural analgesic block may be performed in order to decrease blood pressure (and thus haemorrhage), and to provide analgesia into the postoperative period. However, the resulting sympathetic blockade may accentuate venous pooling in the legs because the nerve supply to the kidney and ureter arises in the T10–L1 segments and it is necessary to secure a block up to a level of approximately T8. The combination of epidural analgesia and a general anaesthetic is particularly advantageous.

The patient should be returned to the supine position at the end of the procedure and several deep inspirations given in an attempt to improve expansion of the dependent lung. It is possible for the pleura to be opened during surgery (deliberately or inadvertently). The resulting collapse of the upper lung may compromise gas exchange significantly. Under these circumstances, the administration of nitrous oxide should be discontinued before closing the pleura unless a chest drain with underwater seal has been inserted, to prevent the danger of a tension pneumothorax. An increase in airway pressure may provide the first evidence of intraoperative pneumothorax and a chest X-ray should be performed in the recovery room if a pneumothorax is suspected.

When surgery is performed for carcinoma of the kidney, tumour embolus causing sudden collapse and cardiac arrest is an occasional, although uncommon complication.

Extracorporeal shock-wave lithotripsy (ESWL)

The number of open operations for renal stones has decreased dramatically since the introduction of ESWL in the early 1980s. During the course of ESWL, the patient is placed in a tank of water maintained at 36°C and large shock waves are generated in the water by a high-voltage underwater spark discharge, such that their focal point is the centre of the stone. The shock waves result in the disintegration of the stone with negligible trauma to surrounding soft tissues, and the fragments are subsequently passed in the urine.

The awake conscious patient will report that the sensation of a single shock wave is not unpleasant and resembles that of a dull blow. However, sharp pain is produced occasionally, and the upper limit which an awake patient can tolerate is about 100 shock waves, which may not be enough to disintegrate the stone fully. Consequently, sedation, regional anaesthesia or general anaesthesia is required for many patients.

At pre-operative assessment, particular attention should be paid to cardiovascular and respiratory disorders, which should be treated before anaesthesia. Any coagulation disorder must be corrected, and administration of any drugs which affect coagulation (including aspirin) must be discontinued; serious postoperative haematomas may result if clotting is impaired.

If general anaesthesia is the chosen technique, the selection of agents and techniques is determined by the general condition of the patient. However, a technique employing tracheal intubation to secure the airway is strongly recommended because of the relative inaccessibility of the patient during the procedure. Supplementation with an opioid is appropriate in order to obtund increases in blood pressure which might otherwise occur in association with delivery of the shock waves.

Regional blockade may be used for ESWL and the technique of choice is an epidural block. It is necessary to secure a block up to a sensory level of about T6. Epidural blockade is a more flexible method than spinal analgesia. The epidural space must be located using the loss of resistance to saline technique, *not* loss of resistance to air, to prevent the introduction of air bubbles into the epidural space; these may result in spinal cord damage caused by energy dissipation at the air/fluid interface in the epidural space.[2]

A number of patients may tolerate ESWL under the influence of intercostal nerve block from T9 to T12, supplemented if necessary with infiltration of local anaesthetic agent into the skin at the area of shock-wave entry. Care must be taken not to exceed the maximum safe dose of local anaesthetic when such a wide area is to be blocked. Finally, many patients tolerate ESWL under sedation alone, or sedation combined with a lumbar field block at the point of entry of the shock wave, particularly when the more modern lithotripsy machines are used.

There are a number of adverse effects of ESWL, and specific problems related to ESWL.

Cardiac arrhythmias

The shock waves should arrive during the absolute refractory period of the ventricles of the heart.[3] The arrival of a shock wave at any other time may induce atrial or ventricular arrhythmias. The ESWL machine is therefore connected to the electrocardiogram (ECG) monitor, and shocks are triggered by the R wave on the ECG. It is important to apply the electrodes to the patient's chest with great care, and to keep them dry, so that a high-quality signal is produced. If the patient has a cardiac pacemaker, care must be taken to ensure that the shock wave is triggered by the R wave and not by the pacemaker impulses. An additional problem with pacemakers is the potential for physical damage to the pacemaker itself from the shock waves.

Positioning the patient

The patient is placed in a hydraulically operated chair which can be raised or lowered into the bath. Positioning of the patient to ensure that the stone lies in the focus of the shock wave may necessitate various degrees of lateral tilt and bodily contortions. Great care must be taken in the anaesthetized patient to ensure that no damage occurs to joints, nerves, pressure points, etc.

Respiratory movements

The kidneys move with ventilation. During the respiratory cycle, a stone may move in and out of the optimum position in the focus of the wave. Thus, it may be necessary to synchronize the shock wave with the respiratory cycle as well as with the ECG. A possible solution which has been reported is to use high-frequency ventilation, during which the movements of the abdominal viscera, and therefore of the stone, are very small.[4]

Remote monitoring

The position of the patient, partly immersed in a bath of water and surrounded by heavy equipment, makes immediate access very difficult. In addition, X-ray screening may be used intermittently and the anaesthetist may be required to stand behind radio-opaque screens at a distance from the patient. It is therefore imperative that the breathing system, tracheal tube and monitoring probes are attached securely, and that the monitor displays are visible from a distance. A ventilator disconnection alarm is, of course, mandatory.

Haemodynamic effects

The partial immersion of a patient in water produces peripheral compression of the immersed regions. This results in a central shift of blood volume which leads to increases in central venous and pulmonary capillary wedge pressures.[5] The increase in cardiac preload may precipitate cardiac failure in patients with pre-existing heart disease.

On removing the patient from the bath, the blood volume, which had been shifted centrally, is distributed peripherally, and sudden, profound hypotension may result. This effect is exaggerated by the vasodilatation caused by immersion in water at 36°C, and is even more pronounced if epidural block, with its associated sympathetic blockade, has been employed. Vasoconstrictor agents should be readily available at all times. ESWL may induce autonomic hyperreflexia in susceptible patients.

Postoperative problems

There is a relatively high incidence of nausea following ESWL and administration of an anti-emetic during the procedure is desirable. Prolonged shivering may occur during recovery. Urinary retention is common if an epidural block has been employed; insertion of a urinary catheter may be required, particularly as a diuresis is likely to be induced in order to assist in washing out the stone fragments.

Major urinary procedures

Open surgery to the bladder and open (retropubic) prostatectomy are included under this heading. These procedures are major lower abdominal procedures and may last for 1–2 h, or possibly longer in the case of cystectomy or major plastic operations on the bladder. Blood loss may be high and at least one large-diameter intravenous cannula is essential. Blood should be cross-matched and available before starting the procedure. If pre-operative cardiovascular instability exists or prolonged surgery and fluid management are anticipated, then it is wise to consider the use of a central venous line or a pulmonary artery catheter to permit the measurement of central venous pressure and/or pulmonary capillary wedge pressure, and also to act as a second infusion line should it be required.

When total cystectomy is performed, it is usual to fashion an ileal conduit into which the ureters are implanted. It is common for such patients to have undergone pre-operative bowel preparation with evacuant and fluid diet for a number of days. This treatment often renders the patient dehydrated, and cardiovascular instability may appear at induction of anaesthesia unless adequate intravenous fluid replacement is given.

Pre-operative preparation should be directed particularly to the cardiovascular and respiratory systems, because patients scheduled to undergo these procedures are often elderly, and thus may suffer from concurrent disease, related particularly to the cardiovascular and respiratory systems. Renal disease is often present in patients with disorders of the urinary tract and urea and electrolyte concentrations must be measured and, if necessary, brought within the normal range before surgery. It may be wise under these circumstances to avoid agents which rely significantly on the kidney for their excretion (e.g. aminoglycoside antibiotics) or which possess the potential for nephrotoxicity (e.g. enflurane).

The choice of technique depends on the patient's preexisting medical condition, although a technique including tracheal intubation, controlled ventilation, and the use of a neuromuscular blocking agent is appropriate.

Epidural and spinal analgesia are also appropriate techniques, and many anaesthetists combine regional block with light general anaesthesia. This technique also lowers the blood pressure, which may assist in reducing the blood loss. Alternative techniques of induced hypotension may be used for this type of surgery. If induced hypotension is used, meticulous replacement of measured blood loss is essential.

Pain is one of the principal problems associated with major pelvic surgery in the postoperative period. This can be managed in two ways. Conventional opioid preparations may be administered by intermittent bolus dose, infusion or patient-controlled analgesia systems. These techniques are very satisfactory, but some of the side-effects of the opioid drugs, in particular respiratory depression, may be particularly undesirable in the older age group. The second method relies upon regional analgesic techniques. Pelvic surgery lends itself well to the use of an epidural block for postoperative analgesia. A lumbar epidural catheter can be inserted, and analgesic drugs injected. Continuous infusion of bupivacaine (with or without an opioid) through a catheter is the technique of choice. A block encompassing L1–S5 is usually required to ensure adequate analgesia. The ability of a lumbar epidural block to decrease blood pressure may also be of value during surgery. Commonly, the epidural catheter is inserted after induction of anaesthesia and the block maintained throughout anaesthesia and into the postoperative period. The requirement for general anaesthetic agents is also reduced by this technique.

To minimize the incidence of clot retention in the bladder following surgery, a diuretic is often given. Either mannitol or frusemide is suitable, but fluid replacement must be increased at this time in order to compensate for the ensuing diuresis. The risk of intraoperative venous thrombosis is very high during and following pelvic surgery, and appropriate prophylaxis is important.

Transurethral procedures

Many procedures may be performed by this route, including cystoscopy, ureteroscopy, urethroscopy, resection of tumour, resection of prostatic tissue, division of strictures and removal of stones or foreign bodies. The duration of the procedures may range from a few minutes for a diagnostic cystoscopy to more than 1 h for the more complicated procedures. The choice of anaesthetic technique depends upon a number of factors, the most important of which is the patient's general medical condition. Many of the patients who present for these procedures are elderly and may have significant pre-existing medical disorders. Pre-operative assessment is of particular importance. Electrolyte imbalance should be corrected, and the state of hydration reviewed carefully.

Transurethral surgery is performed usually in the lithotomy position and enquiry must be made as to movement or stiffness of hips and knees. It is possible to perform transurethral surgery in other positions if necessary, e.g. by abducting the legs and flexing the knees to a small degree (the Lloyd-Davies position). The use of the lithotomy position is associated with a number of problems. First, ventilation is impaired, principally as a result of the restriction of diaphragmatic movement by compression of the intra-abdominal contents. The Trendelenburg position makes this worse, and leads to a potential reduction in cerebral blood flow due to the increase in intracranial pressure in the head-down position. There is an increased tendency for regurgitation of gastric contents, particularly if the patient has pre-existing symptoms of gastro-oesophageal reflux. In addition, air embolism is possible through any exposed pelvic veins. Many of these problems are exaggerated in the obese patient. It must be remembered also that the lithotomy position produces an autotransfusion of 500–800 ml of blood, which may precipitate left ventricular failure in susceptible patients. At the termination of surgery, if blood loss or fluid has not been replaced adequately, the return of this volume of blood into the legs may cause sudden and marked hypotension.[6] These positional changes may be exaggerated during regional anaesthesia due to the loss of vasomotor tone in the legs. The longer the operation, the greater the leg flexion and the steeper the head-down tilt, the greater is the risk of postoperative atelectasis and hypoxaemia.

The choice of general anaesthetic technique depends principally on the patient's general condition, but a technique involving spontaneous breathing of a volatile agent or an infusion of a short-acting intravenous anaesthetic is suitable for brief operations in the non-obese. The choice of face mask or laryngeal mask should also be considered. For procedures lasting more than 30 min, a technique which includes tracheal intubation and controlled ventilation is more appropriate. In addition, if the surgery involves diathermy close to the obturator nerve pathway, violent movements of the leg may result when diathermy is applied; in these instances, it may also be necessary to use a technique which incorporates a neuromuscular blocking agent. Obese patients do not tolerate the lithotomy position and controlled ventilation is usually indicated in these patients, even for shorter procedures. The use of mivacurium by infusion allows control of ventilation for procedures of duration of 15–30 min and should be considered if assisted ventilation is indicated.

When general anaesthesia is used consideration must be given to the fact that instrumentation of the urethra is particularly stimulating, and an adequate depth of anaesthesia is required to prevent reflex hypertension, tachycardia and possibly laryngeal spasm. A suitable dose of an opioid analgesic, e.g. fentanyl or alfentanil, before induction of anaesthesia, is usually effective. Minor transurethral procedures are often undertaken on an outpatient basis, and consideration should be given to the use of anaesthetic agents from which recovery is rapid (e.g. propofol, desflurane).

There is an increasing tendency in some centres to use a regional technique — either spinal or epidural analgesia. The innervation of the bladder, prostate and lower ureters is from T12 to L3 (sympathetic) and S2 to S4 (parasympathetic). Consequently, a bilateral block to about T10 is necessary. This can usually be achieved using subarachnoid injection of 2.5–3 ml of heavy bupivacaine 0.5%. Cystoscopy may be undertaken after local application of lignocaine gel to the urethra by the surgeon.

These techniques have a number of advantages compared with general anaesthetic techniques; in particular, the patient remains awake and retains control of the airway. A significant proportion of the patients who require this type of procedure have co-existing respiratory disease. In addition, analgesia is continued into the postoperative period. There are a number of contra-indications to spinal or epidural anaesthesia, which include refusal by the patient, infection, septicaemia, disorders of blood clotting and hypovolaemia. However, the majority of contra-indications are relative (e.g. neurological disease, previous surgery to the back). When transurethral resection (TUR) of the prostate or of a bladder tumour is performed, spinal or epidural blockade possesses one further advantage, in that symptoms of the TUR syndrome (see below) may be recognized and treated earlier. Subjective symptoms are usually the first to appear as the TUR syndrome develops. These include nausea, agitation, restlessness and dyspnoea, but these are masked in the anaesthetized patient.

There are, of course, disadvantages of regional techniques, which include the risk of headaches (reduced now that finer needles and pencil-point needles are available) and arterial hypotension if there is pre-existing cardiovascular instability. Management as a day case may not be a contra-indication to spinal anaesthesia provided that the incidence of headache can be made very small by the use of needles with a maximum bore of 26-gauge.[7]

Cysto-urethroscopy can be performed following the topical application of local anaesthetic gel into the urethra. This is particularly effective in females, although the addition of a block of the dorsal nerve of the penis may occasionally be required in men. The technique of sedo-analgesia has been introduced at some centres; the patient receives a small dose of midazolam followed by a local block, and flumazenil is administered at the end of the procedure to reverse the residual effects of midazolam. The success of this technique, of course, hinges on the skill of the surgeon in performing the local block around the perineum.

Dilatation of the bladder is a procedure which is still performed regularly. Direct dilatation of the bladder for 10–15 min during the course of the operation may be required. Fluid is allowed to run into the bladder through the cystoscope or a catheter, and the resulting distension of the bladder allowed to remain for a period of up to 15 min. Distension may result in marked reflex cardiovascular responses; tachycardia, hypertension and cardiac arrhythmias are common during the period of dilatation. It is essential to anticipate these responses and to deepen anaesthesia, or administer an opioid, before dilatation occurs. The surgeon must observe the fluid system continuously, because perforation of the bladder may result from the injudicious use of too high a pressure. If this is not recognized immediately, serious consequences are likely.

The procedure of prolonged balloon dilatation (Helmstein's balloon[8]) for the treatment of bladder tumours is performed occasionally. In this procedure, a distensible balloon is inserted into the bladder and inflated to a pressure of 80–100 mmHg in order to produce pressure necrosis of multiple intravesical tumours. The period of dilatation is prolonged (often up to 8 h), and a continuous regional block, for example an epidural catheter technique, is necessary. Adequate analgesia can usually be produced by a block which extends up to L1.[9]

Transient bacteraemia is common during or immediately after transurethral surgery. In patients with cardiac valvular disease or implanted foreign material, peri-operative antibiotic prophylaxis is essential.[10] Septicaemia leading to septic shock is an occasional end-result. Cysto-urethroscopy, and particularly bladder dilatation, may induce autonomic hyperreflexia in patients with a high spinal cord transection. It is thus important for these patients to receive regional analgesia or general anaesthesia despite the fact that the area of operation is already analgesic.

Transurethral prostatectomy

There are a number of features specific to this procedure in addition to the general considerations pertinent to transurethral surgery. Most notable are blood loss and the transurethral syndrome. Perforation of the bladder is also an occasional complication and the symptoms and signs of this may be masked by general anaesthesia. In addition, a number of surgeons request the administration of a suitable dose of a diuretic agent as the procedure is nearing its end; the resulting diuresis usually maintains flow through the catheter and decreases the likelihood of blockage by a blood clot. An intravenous infusion must always be established before surgery for transurethral prostatectomy starts.

Blood loss. The prostate gland contains numerous large venous sinuses and blood loss during transurethral prostatectomy may be considerable. It is essential to know the pre-operative haemoglobin concentration and for cross-matched blood to be available readily (a minimum of 2 units is recommended). However, the true blood loss may be very difficult to estimate because it is diluted with a large volume of irrigation solution (usually glycine). Consequently, transfusion on empirical grounds is usually performed, using the patient's cardiovascular status and pre-operative haemoglobin concentration as guides. It is possible to assess blood loss more accurately by the use of a colorimeter. A sample of the waste glycine is placed into a previously calibrated colorimeter cell and the haemoglobin concentration of that waste glycine solution determined. From a knowledge of the patient's pre-operative haemoglobin (Hb) concentration and the volume of waste glycine, the blood loss may be calculated using the following formula:

$$\text{Blood loss (ml)} = \frac{V \times 1000 \times C}{\text{Pre-operative Hb}}$$

where V = volume of waste glycine and C = concentration of Hb in waste glycine.

Body temperature decreases if the bladder is irrigated with cold solution and disposable bags of sterile glycine should therefore be warmed to 35°C before use.

The TUR syndrome. TUR of the prostate requires the use of a cystoscope with a movable wire loop, through which is passed the high-frequency current of the cutting diathermy. Continuous irrigation is required through the cystoscope in order to flush away blood and debris and to allow good visibility to be maintained. This continuous irrigation results in distension of the bladder and, because the pressure in the prostatic venous plexuses is low, irrigation fluid tends to pass into the circulation. If the irrigation fluid is physiological saline or an isotonic compound electrolyte solution, e.g. compound sodium lactate, then such absorption is not usually of clinical significance provided that the total volume absorbed is not excessive. However, the irrigation fluid must be a non-electrolyte solution to prevent dissipation of the diathermy current. Water cannot be used because of the danger of haemolysis (water is used for cystoscopy when resection is not required) and the solution of choice in most centres is 1.5% glycine in water. This is slightly hypotonic (2.1% glycine is isotonic) and therefore does not cause haemolysis. It is, nevertheless, absorbed through the prostatic venous plexuses and its excessive absorption may result in the TUR syndrome.[11,12]

The absorption of small volumes of glycine solution is not of any consequence to the patient. However, the greater the duration of surgery, the more extensive the resection and the larger the pressure head of irrigation fluid, the more irrigant solution is likely to be absorbed. Many studies have been undertaken to quantify the volume of irrigating fluid absorbed. In one study, ethanol 2% was added to the glycine irrigating solution; the content of ethanol in the expired breath was related directly to the volume of glycine absorbed.[13] The average rate of fluid absorption is estimated to be between 10 and 30 ml for each minute of resection time.[14] The result of excessive absorption of glycine solution is water overload. All fluid compartments increase in volume, plasma osmotic pressure decreases and tissue oedema develops; of particular importance is the onset of cerebral oedema. Dilutional hyponatraemia occurs, and the serum sodium concentration is the most reliable simple index of absorption. As the plasma sodium concentration decreases from the normal range, there are no clear symptoms or signs until the concentration reaches about 125 mmol.l^{-1}. Below this value, nausea, restlessness, confusion, muscle twitching and hyperreflexia occur. As the concentration decreases still further, the symptoms become more severe, and at values below about 105 mmol.l^{-1}, the patient loses consciousness and irreversible cellular damage is imminent.

The symptoms and signs of the TUR syndrome may be confusing. The patient often presents in the post-operative period with restlessness and agitation. There may be dyspnoea and the patient may complain of nausea, abdominal pains and blurred vision. On examination, the blood pressure is usually raised but there may occasionally be hypotension instead. There is bradycardia, and the ECG shows T wave inversion. If untreated, the syndrome may result in convulsions, pulmonary oedema, cardiovascular collapse and cardiac arrest.[15,16] Because transurethral surgery is more common in older patients, pre-existing cardiovascular disorders and impairment of other body systems may exaggerate the effects and consequences of the TUR syndrome. The degree of hyponatraemia required before the development of symptoms varies markedly, and in some patients, even a modest decrease in the plasma sodium concentration may precipitate the syndrome.

Hyponatraemia is regarded by most authorities as the principal aetiological factor in the transurethral syndrome. However, additional or alternative mechanisms have been proposed. Glycine is an inhibitory transmitter in the central nervous system. It is a polar molecule, but if small quantities do cross into the central nervous system, it is anticipated that unwanted effects would result. Episodes of reversible blindness have been reported in a number of patients who had very high plasma glycine concentrations in the postoperative period.[17] The second possible aetiological factor is ammonia. Ammonia is a metabolite of glycine and in the presence of a high concentration of glycine it is possible that toxic levels of ammonia could be reached.[12,18,19]

The most appropriate management of the TUR syndrome is prevention. The surgeon should be requested to ensure that the reservoir bag of glycine is not placed more than 70–80 cm above the level of the cystoscope and resection should not continue for longer than about 60 min in total. Intravenous replacement fluids should be confined to normal saline and blood loss should be replaced carefully. If there is any suspicion that the TUR syndrome is developing, urgent measurement of plasma sodium concentration should be undertaken. The treatment of an established case of the TUR syndrome remains controversial. Hypertonic sodium chloride solutions have been recommended, and frusemide may have a place. However, administration of hypertonic saline may precipitate fatal cardiovascular collapse,[20] and so it should be used with caution. The author prefers to use isotonic saline alone. Prevention is far better than treatment.

Surgery to the male external genitalia

This subject includes all surgery to the penis and scrotum. Most procedures are not usually lengthy and a technique employing spontaneous breathing through a face mask and airway, or a laryngeal mask airway, is appropriate. Surgery to the penis is very stimulating and a deep level of anaesthesia is required. If anaesthesia is inadequate, hypertension, tachycardia and cardiac arrhythmias result. Laryngeal spasm is also common and can be especially troublesome and even dangerous in small children. An anaesthetic technique which involves simply deep anaesthesia is not the most appropriate, and it is necessary to provide good analgesia before surgery starts. There is also a high requirement for analgesia in the postoperative period. Appropriate analgesia can be provided in one of two ways.

Systemic opioid administration

The effect of a systemic opioid should be maximal before the start of surgery, and to this end, many anaesthetists include an opioid as a premedicant if the patient is to be admitted to hospital. Alternatively, a drug with a rapid onset of action (e.g. alfentanil or fentanyl) may be administered intravenously immediately after induction of anaesthesia. It should be remembered that these drugs also have a short duration of action, and it may be appropriate to administer a suitable dose of a longer-acting opioid during, or immediately after, surgery. A disadvantage of this technique is that respiratory depression may result, and assisted ventilation may be needed on occasions. In addition, opioids tend to increase the arterial carbon dioxide tension in patients who breathe spontaneously.

A high carbon dioxide tension increases the potential for cardiac arrhythmias. In addition, systemic opioids cannot suppress completely sympathetic stimulation resulting from surgery, and endogenous catecholamines are released. Cardiac arrhythmias are therefore not uncommon. A further disadvantage of the use of opioids is the high incidence of postoperative nausea and vomiting.

Local or regional techniques

The combination of general and regional anaesthesia is a better technique for penile surgery. In the presence of a regional block, only a light general anaesthetic is needed — enough to ensure unconsciousness. The regional block is best inserted when the patient is anaesthetized and there are two techniques which are suitable: blockade of the dorsal nerve of the penis, and caudal block. There is little difference in efficacy between the two techniques, although caudal block is associated with a higher incidence of urinary retention. Suitable agents and doses for each block depend, of course, on the age, size and medical background of the patient, but bupivacaine 0.5% is suitable for either, *without* adrenaline for a block of the dorsal nerve of the penis.

Surgical procedures to the penis are usually of a minor nature, e.g. circumcision, but more major procedures, including amputation (partial or total), various plastic procedures and the insertion of Silastic implants are also performed. The use of a combined regional block and general anaesthetic is appropriate for all of these procedures. It must be remembered that the penis is a very vascular structure and there should be an intravenous infusion in situ for all surgery to the penis, with the possible exception of circumcision.

Surgical procedures to the scrotum are generally of a relatively minor nature, for example excision of epididymal cyst or drainage of hydrocoele. General anaesthesia with spontaneous ventilation, or regional anaesthesia, may be employed, the choice being determined by the preferences of the anaesthetist and patient. Some procedures, for example vasectomy, are frequently performed after infiltration of local anaesthetic. Intra-operative stability and postoperative analgesia may be assisted during surgery to the testis if the surgeon infiltrates local anaesthetic solution (without adrenaline) into the spermatic cord at the beginning of surgery.

GYNAECOLOGICAL SURGERY

Perineal surgery

Minor perineal surgery, for example, removal of small skin lesions or repair of an episiotomy, may be performed following simple infiltration with a local anaesthetic agent by the surgeon. If the area is too extensive for the provision of analgesia by local infiltration, then a caudal epidural block is the regional technique of choice. Spinal analgesia is also satisfactory; a saddle block may be produced using hyperbaric local anaesthetic solution injected with the patient in the sitting position. If general anaesthesia is required for these minor procedures, spontaneous ventilation of nitrous oxide and volatile anaesthetic agent is suitable. Patients undergoing perineal surgery are usually placed in the lithotomy position with a 5–10° head-down tilt. It is therefore essential for hip and knee joint mobility to be checked pre-operatively. Obese patients may find difficulty in breathing when placed in this position and patients with gastro-oesophageal reflux may regurgitate. A general anaesthetic with tracheal intubation and controlled ventilation is preferable for these categories of patient and mivacurium is a useful relaxant for shorter procedures.

If more extensive surgery is planned, e.g. vulvectomy (simple or radical), then an intravenous infusion is required. Blood loss may be considerable when radical vulvectomy is performed, and blood must be cross-matched and readily available before the operation starts. Induced hypotension may reduce blood loss and assist the surgeon. A combined general anaesthetic and subarachnoid or continuous epidural block is a suitable technique.

Patients undergoing gynaecological surgery, either minor or major, have a high incidence of postoperative nausea and vomiting and consideration should be given to administering prophylactic anti-emetics in all patients.

Vaginal surgery

Many gynaecological procedures are performed by the vaginal route and include minor procedures (e.g. dilatation of the cervix and curettage, cone biopsy) and major procedures (e.g. vaginal hysterectomy and pelvic floor repair). Colposcopy is usually performed with light sedation alone. General anaesthesia is normally employed for other minor procedures, using a simple technique with spontaneous ventilation. Dilatation of the cervix is stimulating and an adequate depth of anaesthesia is required in order to avoid the reflex hypertension and laryngospasm which would otherwise result. Many of these minor procedures are undertaken on a day-stay basis and appropriate considerations apply (see Chapter 17).

Therapeutic vaginal termination of pregnancy is usually a short procedure. However, the volatile anaesthetic agents cause relaxation of the pregnant uterus and an increased tendency to blood loss. Consequently, they should be used in modest doses, supplemented by an opioid analgesic as well as nitrous oxide; alternatively, a total intravenous anaesthetic technique may be employed. It is common practice to administer a dose of an oxytocic (usually Syntocinon 10 units) during the procedure. Ergometrine has a number of unwanted side-effects which include hypertension, nausea, vomiting and bronchoconstriction, and is now used only rarely.

A similar anaesthetic technique may be employed for surgery to evacuate the retained products of conception, unless the surgery is urgent in an unstarved patient or is required in a patient who is in the immediate postpartum period. In these situations, a rapid-sequence induction technique should be employed, the trachea intubated with a cuffed tracheal tube, and appropriate precautions taken to prevent regurgitation and aspiration of gastric fluid at the end of the procedure.

The major vaginal operations may be performed under general anaesthesia, regional anaesthesia or a combination of the two. When general anaesthesia is considered, the choice of technique depends principally upon the patient's pre-existing medical condition and the anticipated duration of surgery. If a regional block is preferred, a lumbar epidural technique using a catheter is most convenient, although a spinal block is commonly used. The use of a combination of general anaesthesia and a regional block together is attractive as it means that a lighter anaesthetic is possible with a more rapid postoperative recovery; in addition, excellent analgesia is provided in the early postoperative period. An intravenous infusion is essential for the major vaginal procedures whether or not a regional block is employed.

Many gynaecologists infiltrate a local anaesthetic solution with dilute adrenaline around the operation site at the start of surgery. It is important to know the exact quantity which is to be used, the concentration of adrenaline, and the precise time at which it is administered. It is wise to avoid the use of halothane when the surgeon is using adrenaline in this way, because of the increased likelihood of cardiac arrhythmias.

Laparoscopy

This procedure is performed commonly in gynaecology for sterilization, for investigation of infertility and for other diagnostic purposes. During the course of the procedure, the peritoneal cavity is filled with carbon dioxide and the patient placed in the lithotomy position in a steep head-down tilt. The resulting increase in intra-abdominal pressure and elevation of the liver splints the diaphragm and makes spontaneous ventilation very difficult. It also increases the risk of regurgitation of stomach contents. The anaesthetic technique should therefore include the use of a cuffed tracheal tube and controlled ventilation. Hyperventilation is advisable to assist in removing the carbon dioxide absorbed from the peritoneal cavity. Neuromuscular blockade enhances the ability to inflate the abdomen and mivacurium is useful for shorter procedures; otherwise the choice of anaesthetic agent depends upon the patient's general medical condition. Significant haemodynamic changes may occur as a result of the elevated intra-abdominal pressure and the posture of the patient. If the intra-abdominal pressure increases above about 40 cmH$_2$O, compression of the inferior vena cava may reduce venous return profoundly, resulting in a decrease in cardiac output. Uncommon side-effects include gas embolism following the accidental intravenous injection of carbon dioxide, haemorrhage, pneumothorax and perforation of an intra-abdominal viscus.

At the completion of the procedure, the surgeon should remove as much of the carbon dioxide from the abdomen as possible. The patient should be turned to the lateral position before extubation because there is likely still to be a residual increase in intra-abdominal pressure, which increases the risk of regurgitation.

Ectopic pregnancy

Suspected rupture of a tubal pregnancy is an emergency situation. The subjective symptoms may be only of a minor nature, but the patient's condition may deteriorate suddenly and rapidly. The patient must be assessed very carefully before operation, particularly in respect of the cardiovascular status. Acute and continuing intra-abdominal haemorrhage may result in a severely shocked state. These patients are usually young and possess good sympathetic reflexes; consequently, blood loss may be considerable before there are overt signs of hypovolaemia. It is essential to insert at least one large-diameter intravenous cannula before induction of anaesthesia, and, when there is clinical evidence of blood loss, to infuse colloid solutions rapidly; however, if it is clear that massive blood loss is continuing, surgery should not be delayed.

Induction of anaesthesia must be undertaken with great care. A rapid-sequence technique following preoxygenation is appropriate. Following the onset of neuromuscular blockade, intra-abdominal bleeding may accelerate and surgery may be required very quickly. Under these circumstances, it may be necessary to induce anaesthesia in the operating theatre with the surgeon scrubbed and ready to begin. The hypovolaemic patient requires a very much reduced dose of anaesthetic induction agent. If blood pressure is well-maintained after induction of anaesthesia, the surgeon may perform laparoscopy first and then proceed to a laparotomy if the diagnosis is correct. The presence of a grossly shocked, hypovolaemic patient is, however, an indication to proceed directly to laparotomy.

Abdominal gynaecological procedures

Despite the ability of gynaecologists to perform many operations via the transvaginal route, the abdominal approach is necessary for a number of procedures. These operations fall into two principal categories: those on the uterus, and those on the ovaries and fallopian tubes. Operations on the uterus include simple hysterectomy, radical (Wertheim's) hysterectomy, myomectomy and other plastic operations on the uterus. Those on the ovaries and tubes include ovarian cystectomy, oophorectomy, salpinogolysis, sterilization and reversal of sterilization. To these can be added a number of procedures, mostly of a minor nature, to resuspend the uterus and/or ovaries.

All of these operations involve surgery through an incision on the anterior abdominal wall and exposure of the contents of the lower abdomen and pelvis. Consequently, a general anaesthetic technique, which includes a neuromuscular-blocking agent with tracheal intubation and controlled ventilation, is appropriate. The choice of anaesthetic agents depends primarily upon the patient's general medical condition. Hysterectomy is often performed as a treatment for menorrhagia and the patient may be anaemic pre-operatively. A full blood count is therefore essential and pre-operative transfusion should be considered if the haemoglobin concentration is less than 10 g.dl^{-1}.

It is usual to employ an intravenous infusion for all of these operations. The uterus is a very vascular structure, and blood loss may be significant. Blood should therefore be cross-matched and available before operations on the uterus begin. Lower abdominal and pelvic surgery, like perineal surgery, lends itself well to the use of a regional block; either a spinal or epidural block is suitable. If an epidural block is employed, it is wise to insert a catheter in the lumbar region so that adequate local anaesthesia can be given to achieve a block up to a level of about T10. In addition, the presence of a catheter allows the epidural blockade to be continued into the postoperative period in order to obtain good postoperative analgesia.

The more major operations, e.g. radical hysterectomy, may take several hours and blood loss may be considerable. The use of induced hypotension may help to reduce the blood loss. Many anaesthetists find that a combined general anaesthetic and regional block is particularly advantageous for these procedures. The reduction in blood pressure from the epidural assists the surgeon and there is a reduced requirement for general anaesthetic agents; however, excessive reductions in blood pressure should be avoided, particularly in older patients and those with co-existing coronary or cerebral vascular disease. Epidural block is, of course, useful in the management of postoperative pain, which may otherwise be considerable because of the extent of the surgery.

Anterior suspension operations, although of a relatively minor nature, are also associated with a great deal of postoperative pain and discomfort and these patients have a high requirement for postoperative analgesia.

In vitro fertilization

Techniques of in vitro fertilization (IVF) were introduced into clinical practice about 10 years ago. It is common practice to perform a laparoscopy for egg retrieval and, in the technique of gamete intrafallopian transfer (GIFT), the recovered oocyte is then replaced into a fallopian tube together with a quantity of spermatozoa. An alternative method of oocyte recovery is by transvaginal ultrasound, approaching the ovaries via the pouch of Douglas.

It is difficult and uncomfortable to lie motionless for a long time in a head-down position, particularly if the legs are placed in stirrups. The difficulties are exacerbated if the patient is overweight (although such patients are not often accepted into IVF programmes) or if a carbon dioxide pneumoperitoneum is induced for the purposes of laparoscopy. General anaesthesia is used most commonly, and the technique is determined primarily by the surgical approach. However, other techniques have been used, including spinal analgesia, extradural analgesia and sedation.

In addition to the normal considerations appropriate to general or regional anaesthesia (these patients are young and fit), consideration must be given to the effects of the drugs and techniques which are used on the eggs, the fertilization process and the initial development of the embryo. The effects of general anaesthesia on oocyte fertilization and development are still unclear. Present evidence suggests that the success rate of IVF or GIFT may be influenced by the duration of anaesthesia, the use of a carbon dioxide pneumoperitoneum, the order in which the oocytes are retrieved and the stress response to surgery and anaesthesia. A number of anaesthetic agents may also be detrimental and present evidence suggests that halothane should be avoided.[21]

REFERENCES

1. Wickham J. Minimally invasive therapy. Health Trends 1991; 23: 6–9
2. Abbott MA, Samuel JR, Webb DR. Anaesthesia for extracorporeal shock wave lithotripsy. Anaesthesia 1985; 40: 1065–1072
3. Weber W, Madler C, Chaussy C. Anesthesiologische probleme bei der nicht-invasiven zertuemmerung von nierensteinen durch fokussierte stosswellen im ganzkoerperwasserbad. Anesthesist 1983; 32 (suppl): 286–287
4. Carlson CA, Boysen PG, Banner MJ, Gravenstein JS. Conventional vs high frequency jet ventilation for extracorporeal shock wave lithotripsy Anesthesiology 1985; 63: A530
5. Weber W, Chaussy C, Madler C, Peter K, Schueller J. Cardiocirculatory changes during anaesthesia for extracorporeal shock wave lithotripsy (ESWL). J Urol 1984; 131: 246A
6. Little DM. Posture and anaesthesia. Can Anaesth Soc J 1960; 7: 2–15
7. Mudie LL, Cooper GM. Spinal anaesthesia for day case surgery. Curr Anaesth Crit Care 1991; 2: 130–134
8. Helmstein K. Treatment of bladder carcinoma by a hydrostatic pressure technique. Br J Urol 1972; 44: 434–438
9. Lahiri SK, Boys JE. Anaesthesia for bladder inflation therapy. Br J Anaesth 1973; 45: 1162
10. British national formulary, vol 21. London: British Medical Association/Pharmaceutical Press, 1991: p 185
11. Desmond J. Complications of transurethral prostatic surgery. Can Anaesth Soc J 1970; 17: 25–28
12. Ryder KW, Olson JF, Kahnoski RJ, Karn RC, Oel TI. Hyperammonemia after transurethral resection of prostate: a report of two cases. J Urol 1984; 132: 995–996
13. Hahn RG. Ethanol monitoring of irrigating fluid absorption in transurethral prostatic surgery. Anesthesiology 1988; 68: 867–873
14. Hagstrom RS. Studies on fluid absorption during trans-urethral prostatic resection. J Urol 1955; 73: 852–855
15. Henderson DJ, Middleton RC. Coma from hyponatremia following transurethral resection of prostate. Urology 1980; 15: 267–268
16. Reiz S, Dacher M, Kerkoff Y, Olsen B. Non-cardiogenic pulmonary oedema. A serious complication of transurethral prostatectomy. Acta Anaesthesiol Scand 1981; 25: 166–167
17. Ovassapian A, Joshi CW, Brunner EA. Visual disturbance: an unusual symptom of transurethral prostatic resection reaction. Anesthesiology 1982; 57: 332–334
18. Hoekstra PI, Kahnoski RJ, McCamish MA, Bergen W, Heetderks DR. Transurethral resection syndrome — a new perspective: encephalopathy with associated hyperammonemia. J Urol 1983; 130: 704–706
19. Roesch RP, Stoelting RK, Lingeman JE, Kahnoski RJ, Backes DJ, Gephardt SA. Ammonia toxicity resulting from glycine absorption during a transurethral resection of the prostate. Anesthesiology 1983; 58: 577–579
20. Norris TH, Aasheim GM, Sherrand DJD, Trennan JA. Symptomatology, pathophysiology and treatment of transurethral resection of the prostate syndrome. Br J Urol 1973; 45: 420–424
21. Critchlow BM, Ibrahim Z, Pollard BJ. General anaesthesia for gamete intra-fallopian transfer. Eur J Anaesth 1991 8: 381–384

12. Anaesthesia for orthopaedic surgery

L. H. D. J. Booij

Disorders of the musculoskeletal system are among the most frequent diseases in the western world. Their origin may be congenital, traumatic, or the result of disease and/or degeneration. Thus, patients of all ages and with multiple concomitant diseases may require orthopaedic surgery. Consequently, the anaesthetist may be confronted with anaesthetic problems related to age, especially those of the newborn and the elderly, and those related to concomitant diseases and their medication. In the newborn, for example, other congenital abnormalities are frequently present in addition to congenital orthopaedic disorders. Elderly patients have limited cardiorespiratory reserve and may have altered renal and liver function with associated abnormalities of electrolyte and fluid balance. Many patients requiring emergency orthopaedic surgery have sustained multiple trauma, sometimes including visceral, vascular and central nervous system injury, presenting the anaesthetist with additional problems.

Another difficulty for the anaesthetist relates to the fact that the repair of musculoskeletal disorders frequently requires repeated surgery and thus multiple anaesthetics. Corrective operations are, in general, of long duration and problems with temperature maintenance and regulation exist, especially in very young and elderly patients. Infusion of warm fluids, use of heating blankets and the use of a heat–moisture exchanger in the breathing system reduce heat loss.

Many minor orthopaedic procedures (e.g. cast change, joint manipulation, carpal tunnel procedures, fracture reduction, repair of trigger finger, other tendon releases, ganglion resection and arthroscopy) are suitable for day-case surgery, whereas others (e.g. hip replacement, osteotomy, vertebral column surgery) are major operations and require admission to hospital and, in some cases, long-term rehabilitation.

ANTICIPATED PROBLEMS IN ANAESTHESIA FOR ORTHOPAEDIC SURGERY

Co-existing medical disease

If the musculoskeletal disorder is the result of a systemic disease, then this disease may influence the course of the anaesthetic, and is an important determinant in the selection of the technique of anaesthesia and in the choice of individual drugs (see Chapter 2). Systemic disease may also be an important factor in the development of peri-operative complications. For example, pulmonary function is abnormal in many patients with thoracic kyphoscoliosis admitted for surgical correction. Coagulation disorders exist in patients with haemophilia admitted with acute haemarthrosis or for corrective operations after repeated intra-articular bleeding, and the increased risk of acquired immuno-deficiency syndrome (AIDS) must be anticipated because of previous infusions of blood products. There are frequently cardiovascular disorders in patients with Paget's disease (osteitis deformans), and the bones are extremely vascular, often resulting in excessive blood loss during surgery. In patients with advanced rheumatoid arthritis, there may be instability of the cervical vertebral column (usually without compression of the spinal cord), and stiffening of the temporomandibular joint; both conditions have the potential to cause difficulty during tracheal intubation. Frequently, neuromuscular diseases are not restricted to skeletal muscle, causing respiratory dysfunction, but also the myocardium may be involved, leading to haemodynamic disturbances. Careful pre-operative assessment is essential to ensure that possible systemic diseases are detected.

Special problems may also be present if surgery is necessary immediately after trauma (e.g. shock, stress, full stomach, neck injury, neurological damage). Because of other more important injuries, orthopaedic procedures are sometimes delayed, with the possible consequences of infection, aseptic necrosis and contracture formation.

Immobilization and thrombo-embolism

Immobilization and application of a plaster cast are needed after many orthopaedic procedures, with the possible risks of development of deep venous thrombosis and pulmonary embolism, or the occurrence of peripheral neuropathy and decubitus ulcers. Indeed, pulmonary embolism is the main cause of mortality following hip replacement[1]. Polymethylmethacrylic bone cement is used in operations for prosthetic joint replacement. Because these procedures are intramedullary, there is a risk of bone marrow (fat) or air embolus. In addition, the cement itself may embolize or cause an allergic or toxic reaction, resulting in hypotension and hypoxaemia. As the cement hardens, heat is released, and this may cause harmful effects to the bone and bone marrow. Embolism of air, bone marrow, fat or cement may occur during other operations as a result of mechanical manipulation of the bones.[2] Embolism results most commonly in pulmonary and central nervous system complications, but other systems (e.g. kidneys, blood coagulation) may also be involved. Careful positioning during surgery, pre-operative administration of dextran solutions, use of regional anaesthetic techniques, administration of anticoagulation therapy (subcutaneous heparin, oral anticoagulants), early ambulation, early postoperative leg exercises and maintenance of hydration are measures which reduce the risk of thrombo-embolism.

Blood loss and the use of a tourniquet

A number of orthopaedic operations are associated with significant blood loss. Pre-operative autologous blood donation, the use of induced hypotension, intra-operative normovolaemic haemodilution, peroperative salvage and re-infusion of lost blood may be employed to reduce the risk of massive transfusions of homologous blood.

In some orthopaedic procedures, a tourniquet is used to provide a bloodless surgical field or to decrease blood loss. In adults, the recommended inflation pressure for tourniquets is 250–300 mmHg for the upper extremity and 450–500 mmHg for the lower limbs. Before inflation, the limb should be exsanguinated. Inflation of a tourniquet around the lower limb may lead to a significant decrease of the circulatory capacity, resulting in increased afterload, and the risk of heart failure in susceptible patients. The use of a tourniquet imposes the risk of the development of peripheral pressure neuropathy and ischaemic injury to the limb. Haemodynamic instability may occur when acidic products of anaerobic metabolism are released into the systemic circulation when the tourniquet is removed. Unligated vessels will start to bleed after release of the tourniquet. Sickling of erythrocytes may occur when a tourniquet is used with insufficient exsanguination of the limb in patients with sickle-cell disease or trait. Application of a tourniquet may also induce pain, increasing the need for opioids or causing restlessness in the conscious patient if a regional anaesthetic technique is employed. In general, it is accepted that the preferable maximum duration of inflation is 1.5 h, and should not exceed 2 h. In children, the physiological effects of application of a tourniquet are more pronounced than in adults.[3]

Positioning of the patient

Orthopaedic surgery involves all body sites. In many cases, the patient must be placed in other than a supine position. This increases the risk of the development of peripheral pressure and/or stretch neuropathy because anaesthetized patients lack protective reflexes. Most frequently involved is the brachial plexus, followed by the common peroneal, radial and ulnar nerves.[4] Nerves affected by pre-existing neurological disorders such as those associated with diabetes mellitus, herpes zoster, alcoholism and peri-arteritis nodosa are more susceptible to injury. Symptoms of nerve injury may be apparent immediately after surgery, but may not be reported by the patient until 2–3 days later. Although most peripheral nerve injuries recover completely, a residual neurological deficit remains in approximately 10% of affected patients. Careful positioning with prevention of overstretching the joints and padding of possible pressure points reduces the incidence of nerve damage. In the prone position, attention should be paid especially to the eyes and facial nerves. Plaster casts may also contribute to the development of neuropathy. During and after changing the position of the patient, the patency of the airway, the position of the tracheal tube and the patency and connections of the breathing system must be checked.

Tracheal intubation

In a number of orthopaedic patients, problems may occur in association with tracheal intubation either due to aberrant morphology of the face and airways, or because movement of the cervical column may cause spinal cord damage. Hypoplasia of the odontoid process is present in patients with:

1. Morquio syndrome
2. Klippel–Feil syndrome
3. Down's syndrome
4. disproportional dwarfism
5. congenital scoliosis
6. osteogenesis imperfecta
7. neurofibromatosis
8. a number of other rare conditions.

Hypoplasia of the odontoid process may lead to anterior subluxation of the atlas if the neck is hyperextended during tracheal intubation or during positioning of the patient. In Down's syndrome, there is laxity of the transverse ligament which results in atlanto-axial instability with the risk of anterior subluxation on extending the neck. In inflammatory arthropathies (e.g. rheumatoid arthritis, ankylosing spondylitis), the stability of the cervical column may also be impaired.

THE CHOICE OF ANAESTHESIA FOR ORTHOPAEDIC SURGERY

The medical status of the patient admitted for elective orthopaedic surgery should be assessed and made optimal before surgery. The frequency of concomitant systemic medical disorders increases with age, and, as indicated above, many patients who present for orthopaedic surgery have co-existing disease. If patients are admitted for more urgent surgery (e.g. after fracture of the neck of the femur), a balance between delaying surgery and optimizing the patient's general medical status must be sought.

Depending on the site and type of operation, the condition and suitability of the patient and the skills of the anaesthetist, either general or regional anaesthetic techniques can be applied in orthopaedic surgery. In lower limb and pelvic surgery, regional anaesthesia has the advantages of a diminished incidence of thromboembolism, better maintenance of lower limb blood flow, and a decrease in peri-operative blood loss.[5] Local anaesthetics also cause coating of the platelets, thereby decreasing the coagulability of blood. A particular advantage of an epidural technique, either with local anaesthetic or opioid, is its use for treatment of postoperative pain. If intense muscle relaxation is needed (e.g. for reduction of fractures), subarachnoid anaesthesia is more suitable than epidural. A number of blocks (e.g. femoral, sciatic, psoas and ankle blocks) are appropriate for lower limb surgery. Epidural and spinal anaesthetic techniques, both single-shot injection and continuous infusion techniques, have been used for back surgery. For arm surgery, brachial plexus block (by the axillary, supraclavicular or interscalene approach) may be used. For surgery in the lower arm/hand, a more peripheral nerve block (e.g. ulnar, radial and median nerve block) is possible. The blocks can be performed with a variety of local anaesthetics, the choice being determined primarily by the anticipated duration of surgery. The effect of brachial plexus block can be prolonged by repeated administration of local anaesthetic through a catheter placed in the neurovascular sheath.

Intravenous regional anaesthesia (Bier's block) can be used in either the upper or lower limb, and is useful particularly if a bloodless surgical field is necessary. The drug of choice for Bier's block is prilocaine, but the possible occurrence of methaemoglobinaemia after release of the tourniquet must be anticipated. Bupivacaine must not be used for intravenous regional anaesthesia because of its high cardiotoxicity. Local anaesthetic blocks are discussed in more detail in Chapter 23.

One of the advantages of the use of regional anaesthesia in elderly patients is that the deleterious effects of general anaesthesia on mental status and respiratory function are avoided. Combination of a regional technique with sedation or light general anaesthesia may abolish this advantage. However, use of a regional anaesthetic technique does not prevent mental deterioration or confusion in all patients, because factors such as hospitalization, sleep deprivation, alcohol withdrawal and metabolic effects of surgery also contribute.

For prolonged procedures, it is usually necessary to combine a regional technique with sedation or general anaesthesia to prevent discomfort and restlessness.

ANAESTHETIC PROBLEMS IN SPECIFIC ORTHOPAEDIC OPERATIONS

It is impossible to discuss all potential effects of concomitant diseases on the anaesthetic techniques used for all orthopaedic procedures. The following procedures have been selected because of specific difficulties which may arise.

Carpal tunnel release

Carpal tunnel release may occur in association with hyperthyroidism, acromegaly and pregnancy. In these situations, anaesthetic management is influenced by the underlying medical condition.

Congenital dislocation of the hip

This disorder, occurring mostly in girls, is usually recognized shortly after birth, and may be associated with other congenital deformities. The initial therapy should start before the age of 4 years, and entails manipulative reduction and splinting. Skeletal traction or open reduction and osteotomy may be required. Avascular necrosis of the femoral head and cessation of growth of the proximal femoral epiphysis are the major complications. There are no special anaesthetic requirements other than those determined by the age of the patient and any co-existing congenital abnormalities.

Rheumatoid arthritis

Most patients are admitted for prosthetic joint replacement or cervical spinal fusion (anterior or posterior). Although all connective tissue may be involved in this disease, the dominant lesions are found in the joints. Many patients receive long-term corticosteroid therapy, decreasing the ability of the adrenal glands to respond to stress. The cervical vertebrae may be involved in the process, causing instability of the joints and possible dislocation of the altanto-occipital and lower cervical joints.[6] Spinal cord damage may occur in association with movement of the neck during tracheal intubation, and all patients with rheumatoid arthritis should be subjected to evaluation of the cervical vertebral column. Tracheal intubation problems may also occur as a result of involvement of the temporomandibular joint or crico-arytenoid joint.

In 35% of patients, the heart is also involved in the disease process.[7] Pericardial thickening and effusion, valve fibrosis, myocarditis and rheumatoid nodule formation in the cardiac conduction system are the most important abnormalities. Diffuse lung infiltration and pleural effusion may be present, resulting in restrictive pulmonary disease. Twenty-five per cent of patients have a normocytic hypochromic anaemia resistant to iron treatment.

In juvenile rheumatoid arthritis (Still's disease), rash, fever, joint redness, leukocytosis and increased erythrocyte sedimentation rate are dominant symptoms, and polyarthritis, lymphadenitis and splenomegaly are frequently present. Felty's syndrome consists of a triad of rheumatoid arthritis, splenomegaly and neutropenia, sometimes accompanied by anaemia and thrombocytopenia. Frequently, these patients develop a respiratory tract infection following surgery.

Hip surgery

Hip surgery is the most common major orthopaedic procedure performed in the elderly.

Hip fracture

Approximately 80% of patients who sustain hip fracture are female and frail. The fracture may be in the femoral neck (48%), intertrochanteric (48%) or subtrochanteric (4%). The mortality rate following surgery for fractured hip ranges from 6.5 to 31%.[8] Patients with an intertrochanteric fracture have a higher postoperative mortality than those with a fracture of the femoral neck.[9]

The treatment of a fractured hip consists of internal fixation, hip replacement or conservative non-operative therapy. Before fixation of the fracture, patients experience intense pain on movement.

Hip arthroplasty

Most patients admitted for hip replacement are over 65 years of age, and many are overweight, suffer from cardiovascular and/or respiratory disease and take a variety of drugs chronically for co-existing diseases. These factors increase the risk of postoperative complications. The overall mortality rate after hip replacement for arthritis is approximately 2%. The operation is usually performed with the patient in the lateral position.

During arthroplasty, problems may occur due to the fixation of the prosthesis with polymethylmethacrylate cement. Bleeding may be heavy, usually continuing into the early postoperative period, and is made worse by the chronic use of aspirin.

The technique of anaesthesia seems to be of minor importance in relation to the long-term outcome of hip surgery;[10] thus, both regional and general anaesthesia have been recommended. Deep venous thrombosis and pulmonary embolism are the major non-surgical complications of hip surgery; their incidence is diminished when a regional anaesthetic is administered,[11] or if dextran is administered during operation. Use of a regional technique also decreases the need for blood transfusion.

Another problem in this group of elderly patients is impairment of mental function, which is usually transient.[12] Postoperative confusion develops in about 40% of patients. Factors such as hospitalization, sleep deprivation, metabolic effects of surgery and the effect of anaesthetic, analgesic and sedative drugs all contribute to impairment of mental abilities, and it is therefore, in general, independent of the anaesthetic technique.[13] The potential advantage of regional anaesthesia in this respect is lost if sedation or general anaesthesia is employed concurrently.

Knee surgery

Knee joint replacement

This operation is performed mainly in patients with rheumatoid arthritis; thus, other joints and other organ systems are frequently involved in the disease. In many cases, a tourniquet is used to provide a bloodless surgical field. There is a risk of thrombo-embolism in the postoperative period, and brisk blood loss can occur after the tourniquet is released.

Knee arthroscopy

This procedure is frequently performed under local infiltration anaesthesia or under regional anaesthesia. During arthroscopy, surgery (meniscectomy, ligament repair) can be performed within the closed joint.

Spinal column surgery

Surgery on the spinal column is performed for herniated intervertebral disc, correction of scoliosis and spondylosis, resection of neoplasms, spinal fusion or spinal stabilization after trauma.

In some of the patients (e.g. those with cervical vertebral fractures or subluxation of the upper cervical joints), there is a risk of damage to the spinal cord if the neck is moved during tracheal intubation. In others, intubation is difficult because of limited mobility of the neck. Breathing may be compromised by diaphragmatic or intercostal paralysis or kyphoscoliosis, and pre-existing chest diseases are frequently present. Airway management in these patients requires skill and meticulous attention throughout the peri-operative period.

One of the main determinants of the outcome of surgery within the vertebral canal is oxygen delivery to the spinal cord. Blood is delivered to the spinal cord predominantly from a single anterior spinal artery and paired posterior–lateral spinal arteries, which form a long anastomotic channel extending from the upper cervical area to the filum terminale. The blood flow to the grey matter is higher than the blood flow to the white matter. Blood flow to the thoracic cord is 40% lower than that to the cervical and lumbosacral cord. The regulation of blood flow parallels that of the brain. Specifically, hypocapnia decreases and hypoxia increases flow.[14] As in the brain autoregulation occurs when arterial pressure is within the normal range, but is compromised when arterial pressure is below 50 mmHg or above 135 mmHg.[15] The primary route of venous return from the vertebral column and cord is via the vertebral venous plexus, extending from the head to the pelvis, and having extensive connections with the caval system. Because the thin-walled, very compliant venous system does not have valves, its haemodynamics depend upon the pressure gradients within the venous circulation, and on any external pressure applied to the system. Thus, the position of the patient (e.g. abdominal pressure) may cause venous dilatation, with increased venous bleeding during surgery. A variety of positions, using many kinds of support and table frame, have been employed for spinal surgery, but none has proved to be ideal.[16] Accidental kinking of the tracheal tube, pressure damage to eyes and nerves and oozing of the surgical wound have all been described as complications of the patient's position. Blood loss can be heavy, and because most operations are of long duration, hypothermia may develop. Invasive haemodynamic monitoring may be indicated and methods to maintain temperature employed.

Scoliosis

In scoliosis, there is a progressive bony ankylosis of the intervertebral and costovertebral joints, with ribcage deformation. There are various types of scoliosis:[17]

1. idiopathic
2. congenital (e.g. myelomeningocele, spina bifida occulta, hemivertebra, congenital rib fusions)
3. neuromuscular (e.g. poliomyelitis, cerebral palsy, muscular dystrophy, amyotonica congenita)
4. neurofibromatous (von Recklinghausen's disease)
5. mesenchymal (Marfan's syndrome, Morquio's disease, Still's disease, Scheuermann's disease, osteogenesis imperfecta)
6. traumatic (vertebral fracture, irradiation, thoracic surgery).

The most frequent sites of the primary curve are thoracic and lumbar.

In patients with congenital scoliosis, there may be concomitant abnormalities in the central nervous, cardiovascular, pulmonary, gastro-intestinal and urological systems. In idiopathic scoliosis, pulmonary dysfunction (restrictive disease) may be present due to the curvature of the spine, the ribcage deformity and concurrent neuromuscular disease. In these patients, thorough pre-operative evaluation, including pulmonary function testing (total lung volume, vital capacity, residual volume, compliance, diffusion and blood gas analysis), is required.[18] However, in most patients, pulmonary function is not markedly impaired. The primary abnormality in pulmonary gas exchange is ventilation/perfusion maldistribution. In some patients, pulmonary hypertension is present. Disturbances of the mechanism of coughing may occur, and respiratory infection may be present. The anaesthetist must be able to recognize the additional problems related to the original cause of the scoliotic abnormality, especially the neuromuscular diseases.

The operative procedure of spinal fusion and implantation of a Harrington rod, Dwyer device or other support is characterized by extensive blood loss and potential overextension of the cord, which can lead to neurological complications.[19] The incidence of neurological complications is 0.7%. Neurophysiological monitoring (somatosensory evoked potentials) is part of contemporary anaesthesia monitoring during spinal anaesthesia, and has largely replaced perioperative wake-up tests which were performed to exclude possible cord compression.[20] The successful application of neurophysiological monitoring requires expertise, and many factors (e.g. drugs, hypotension, hypothermia, haematocrit and hypoxia) may alter or obliterate the signals, making accurate interpretation impossible.

Severe blood loss occurs frequently during scoliosis surgery, its extent depending on the duration and site of operation, the position of the patient and the anaesthetic technique. The use of autologous blood transfusion, normovolaemic haemodilution, a cell-saver (salvage of blood) and controlled hypotension have all been recommended. If a hypotensive anaesthetic technique is employed, there is a possibility that blood flow to the spinal cord may be compromised. There is an additional damaging effect from direct surgical pressure on the spinal cord,[21] and this is compounded if arterial pressure is low. Somatosensory evoked potential monitoring is particularly valuable in detecting compromised spinal cord perfusion during manipulation of the cord.

General anaesthesia is recommended, avoiding any drug which increases arterial pressure. Tracheal intubation is mandatory, and artificial ventilation should be employed with zero end-expiratory pressure. The standard non-invasive monitors of respiratory and cardiovascular function must be employed, and direct arterial pressure monitoring and central venous pressure monitoring are also required. In the postoperative period, intensive monitoring should be continued, and supplemental oxygen administered. Adequate pain relief is of particular importance. In most institutions, postoperative care is provided in an intensive care or high-dependency unit. In some cases, mechanical ventilation is continued electively in the postoperative period. Meticulous neurological examination should take place repeatedly to detect possible neurological deterioration. In the Dwyer approach, the thorax is opened, leading to additional potential complications.

Patients with scoliosis who require unrelated surgical treatment also present problems to the anaesthetist. Axillary block and epidural or subarachnoid anaesthesia are technically difficult in patients with scoliosis. Airway management problems must be anticipated because of decreased neck mobility. Atlanto-occipital subluxation may also be present. Blind nasotracheal intubation, intubation with the aid of a fibre-optic laryngoscopy, or even tracheostomy, may be necessary. Respiratory and cardiovascular problems may also occur.

Spinal cord injury

Patients with spinal cord injury pose a number of anaesthetic problems.[22] In the acute phase, operations may be performed for associated injuries, and stabilization of the spine or decompression laminectomy may be required. The majority of cases are related to traffic, industrial and sport accidents and involve young patients (15–25 years).

The most frequently involved lesions involve *spinal cord segments* C5–6 or T12–L1. The initiating forces are axial compression, flexion (diving injury), extension (whiplash) and rotation. The mortality rate is higher when the lesion is at the cervical level. The total mortality rate is about 50%, and the cost of treatment of survivors is high because 70% suffer from significant residual neurological deficits. The most common associated injuries in patients with vertebral column trauma are haemo- and pneumothorax, rib fractures and flail chest, pelvic fractures, intra-abdominal blunt injury, fractures of the extremities and head injury.[23] All comatose trauma patients or patients with multiple trauma must be considered to have a spinal cord injury until proved otherwise, and must be transported with the vertebral column immobilized to prevent further injury to the potentially injured cord. When a lesion above C4 is present, assisted ventilation is indicated.

In the acute phase, severe pulmonary oedema is common because blood is shifted from the high-resistance systemic vascular bed to the low-resistance pulmonary vascular bed. Acute spinal cord injury above T5 is characterized by autonomic hypo- or hyperactivity (see below). Initially, there is an immediate hypertensive response with increased systemic vascular resistance, increased myocardial contractility and arrhythmias. This is followed by hypotension and bradycardia (spinal shock). In addition, there is complete loss of visceral and somatic sensation, flaccid paralysis, absent deep tendon and abdominal reflexes and retention of urine and faeces. This state may exist for 3 days to 6 weeks. Stabilization and support of haemodynamics are required during this period. Increasing blood pressure to normal values in order to improve spinal cord perfusion may produce significant improvement in neurological recovery. Although administration of high doses of corticosteroids is still employed in many centres, there is no convincing evidence to support their use.[24]

Pulmonary complications are the most common causes of death during the first 3 months. Respiratory function may improve by 6 months after injury. In chronic spinal cord injury, renal failure as a result of urinary tract infections is the primary cause of death. Rapid and precipitous movements can induce orthostatic hypotension because of the lack of compensatory cardiovascular reflexes. Osteoporosis and pathological fractures are another problem. Poikilothermia may be present. Muscle denervation renders patients prone to hyperkalaemia if suxamethonium is administered.

Autonomic hyperreflexia usually begins 2–3 weeks after trauma, and is characterized by acute generalized autonomic overactivity in response to cutaneous or visceral stimulation below the level of the lesion.[25] It occurs in 65–85% of the patients with a lesion above T7 and is unlikely at a level below T10. It is mediated by the absence of supraspinal inhibitory influences on thoracolumbar sympathetic outflow. The signs and symptoms include hypertension, bradycardia, arrhythmias, headache, nasal congestion, sweating, vasoconstriction and pilo-erection below the spinal cord lesion, vasodilatation above the level of the lesion, convulsions, cerebral haemorrhage, pulmonary oedema and hyperreflexia.[25] Sufficient anaesthetic depth (general, regional or local) can prevent autonomic hyperreflexia. The syndrome may also develop during the recovery period. Treatment consists of elimination of the precipitating stimulus and immediate reduction of blood pressure.

Tracheal intubation of patients with cervical vertebral damage not only poses problems associated with positioning, but may make the application of cricoid pressure, although indicated, hazardous.

Prolapsed intervertebral disc

Intervertebral disc lesions are produced by degeneration and by trauma, and surgery may be performed by an orthopaedic surgeon or neurosurgeon.

Herniation of a disc can occur at any level but occurs most frequently in the lumbosacral area. In uncomplicated cases, there is minimal blood loss, but when more complicated or extended operations are required, blood loss may be heavy. Careful positioning of the patient, avoiding abdominal pressure, is important in minimizing blood loss. Lumbar disc surgery is very painful, particularly when large amounts of bone are removed, and effective postoperative pain relief is important. In a number of hospitals, the procedure is performed under epidural anaesthesia, and the epidural catheter is left in place for postoperative pain management.

In chemonucleolysis, enzymatic dissolution of the nucleus with chymopapain is performed. Anaphylactic reactions and other allergic reactions due to chymopapain, extradural and subarachnoid haemorrhage, infection, nerve root damage and transverse myelitis with paraplegia may occur.[26] They must be treated immediately.

Klippel–Feil syndrome

In this syndrome, congenital fusion of cervical vertebrae, characterized by a short neck with limited motion and a low posterior hairline, exists. Most patients are female, and frequently, additional congenital disorders are present (congenital high scapula, pterygium colli, scoliosis, spina bifida, renal abnormalities, ventricular septal defect, hearing impairment, etc.) In addition, neurological disorders (paraesthesiae and episodic muscle weakness) may be present. Ventilation may be restricted due to deformed costovertebral joints inhibiting chest motion, and to kyphoscoliosis. When anaesthesia is needed, difficulty with tracheal intubation and complications related to the additional abnormalities must be anticipated.

POSTOPERATIVE PAIN MANAGEMENT

Many problems exist with mobilization and rehabilitation after orthopaedic surgery. The experience of pain limits the patient's activities and impairs ambulation. This not only increases the risk of development of deep venous thrombosis, but also may interfere with the technical result of the operation. Pain increases neuro-endocrine activity, alters pulmonary function, causes sleep disturbances, and may increase the risk of myocardial ischaemia in elderly patients and those with cardiovascular disease.

Pain after orthopaedic surgery is frequently severe, although it is generally of short duration and the degree is not always related to the magnitude of the surgery. It must be treated adequately. Conventional parenteral and/or enteral administration of opioid and non-opioid analgesics may be employed, with a varying success rate. Patient-controlled analgesia is now widely accepted as a safe and effective method of postoperative pain management. Regional analgesia with either local anaesthetics or opioids has improved the rate of progress of recovery and rehabilitation after orthopaedic surgery. For this purpose particularly, epidural administration of opioids is valuable, because it retains motor function while blocking the afferent pain systems. However, this technique also has some potential side-effects such as pruritus, nausea and vomiting, sedation, urinary retention and respiratory depression.[27] The use of non-steroidal anti-inflammatory drugs is particularly effective as an adjunct or alternative to opioids after minor or moderate orthopaedic surgery.

Postoperative pain in total hip replacement is usually treated with intermittent intramuscular injections of opioids. However, continuous epidural analgesia or administration of a lateral cutaneous nerve block is much more efficacious.[28,29]

Postoperative pain relief is discussed in detail in Chapter 26.

REFERENCES

1 Johnson R, Green JR, Charnley J. Pulmonary embolism and its prophylaxis following the Charnley total hip replacement. Clin Orthop Rel Res 1977; 127: 123–132
2 Hirsch J. Prevention of deep venous thrombosis. Br J Hosp Med 1981; 26: 143–147
3 Lynn AM, Fischer T, Brandford HG, Pendergrass TW. Systemic responses to tourniquet release in children. Anesth Analg 1986; 65: 865–872
4 Parks BJ. Postoperative peripheral neuropathies. Surgery 1973; 74: 348–357
5 Keith I. Anaesthesia and blood loss in total hip replacement. Anaesthesia 1977; 32: 444–450
6 Crosby ET, Lui A. The adult cervical spine: implications for airway management. Can J Anaesth 1990; 37: 77–93
7 Cathcart ES, Spodick DH. Rheumatoid heart disease: a study of the incidence and nature of cardiac lesions in rheumatoid arthritis. N Engl J Med 1962; 266: 959–964
8 Goucke CR. Mortality following surgery for fractures of the neck of femur. Anaesthesia 1985; 40: 578–583
9 Wickström I, Holmberg I, Stefånsson T. Survival of female geriatric patients after hip fracture surgery. A comparison of 5 anaesthetic methods. Acta Anaesthesiol Scand 1982; 26: 607–614
10 Mckenzie PJ, Wishart HY, Smith G. Long-term outcome after repair of fractured neck of femur. Br J Anaesth 1984; 56: 581–585
11 Modig J, Borg T, Karlström G, Maripuu E, Sahlstedt B. Thromboembolism after total hip replacement: role of epidural and general anesthesia. Anesth Analg 1983; 62: 174–180
12 Millar HR. Psychiatric morbidity in elderly surgical patients. Br J Psychiatry 1981; 138: 17–20
13 Riis J, Lomholt B, Haxholdt O et al. Immediate and long-term mental recovery from general versus epidural anaesthesia in elderly patients. Acta Anaesthesiol Scand 1983; 27: 44–49
14 Marcus ML, Heistad DD, Ehrhardt JC et al. Regulation of total and regional spinal cord blood flow. Circ Res 1977; 41: 128–134
15 Kobrine AI, Doyle TF, Rizolli HV. Spinal cord blood flow as affected by changes in systemic arterial blood pressure. J Neurosurg 1983; 4: 12–15
16 Smith RH, Gramling ZW, Volpitto PP. Problems related to the prone position for surgical operations. Anesthesiology 1961; 22: 189–193
17 Goldstein LA, Waugh TR. Classification and terminology of scoliosis. Clin Orthop 1973; 93: 10–22
18 Kafer ER. Respiratory and cardiovascular functions in scoliosis. Anesthesiology 1980; 52: 339–351
19 MacEwen GD, Bunnell WP, Sriram K. Acute neurologic complications in the treatment of scoliosis: a report of the scoliosis research society. J Bone Joint Surg [Am] 1975; 57A: 404–408
20 Grundy BL, Nash CL, Brown RH. Deliberate hypotension for spinal fusion: prospective randomised study with evoked potential monitoring. Can Anaesth Soc J 1982; 29: 452–462
21 Grundy BL, Nash CL, Brown RE. Arterial pressure manipulation alters spinal cord function during correction of scoliosis. Anesthesiology 1981; 54: 249–253
22 Fraser A, Edmonds-Seal J. Spinal cord injuries. A review of the problems facing the anaesthetist. Anaesthesia 1982; 37: 1084–1098
23 Babinski MF. Anesthetic considerations in the patient with acute spinal cord injury. Crit Care Clin 1987; 3: 619–634
24 Young W, Flamm ES. Effect of high dose corticosteroid therapy in blood flow, evoked potentials, and extracellular calcium in experimental spinal injury. J Neurosurg 1982; 57: 667–673
25 Lambert DH, Deane RS, Mazuzan JE. Anesthesia and the control of blood pressure in patients with spinal cord injury. Anesth Analg 1982; 61: 344–348
26 Reagan JO, Zauder HL. Clinical aspects of chemonucleolysis. Semin Anesth 1987; 4: 51–56
27 Mahoney OM, Noble PC, Davidson J, Tullos HS. The effect of continuous epidural analgesia on postoperative pain, rehabilitation, and duration of hospitalisation in total knee arthroplasty. Clin Orthop Rel Res 1990; 260: 30–37
28 Brands E, Callanan VI. Continuous lumbar plexus block analgesia for femoral neck fractures. Anaesth Intensive Care 1978; 6: 256–258
29 Jones SF, White A. Analgesia following femoral neck surgery. Lateral cutaneous nerve block as an alternative to narcotics in the elderly. Anaesthesia 1985; 40: 682–685

13. Anaesthesia for dental, maxillofacial, thyroid and parathyroid surgery

M.W. Platt

DENTAL PROCEDURES

The incidence of general anaesthesia for dental procedures is declining, from 2 million in 1967 to 371 000 in 1988/89 in England and Wales.[1] This is despite an increase in the number of patients treated in dental schools and hospitals under general anaesthesia. The reduction is due in part to the implementation of recommendations from the Poswillo report advocating that all anaesthetics are given by adequately qualified practitioners, in an appropriate environment and with adequate equipment available. The Poswillo report on *General Anaesthesia, Sedation and Resuscitation in Dentistry*[1] was published in March 1990, and set forth the basic standards acceptable for dental practice, in addition to training requirements for both anaesthetists and dentists. The main recommendations of the report are listed in Appendix A.

Pre-operative considerations

Dental procedures are usually performed on a day-case basis; patients are admitted to hospital on the night before surgery only if it is indicated, for example for management of significant intercurrent disease. Over 70% of dental patients treated under general anaesthesia are children[1] and the majority of procedures comprise dental extraction. The main differences in comparison to other day-case procedures relate to the problem of securing and maintaining an airway for surgery in the mouth, and its protection from blood and debris during the immediate postoperative period.

As for other day-case procedures, patients for outpatient dental treatment should be of American Society of Anesthesiologists (ASA) status 1 or 2.[2-4] There should be no significant cardiac, respiratory, renal or hepatic disease, and no history of bleeding disorders. The surgery intended should be amenable to simple means of postoperative analgesia (that is, by oral medication or, if opioids are needed, this should be for a limited time, e.g. one dose). In addition, as with all outpatient anaesthesia and analgesia, the patient should be discharged accompanied by a responsible adult and should not be left alone for 24 h. Patients who undergo more extensive procedures or require more extensive analgesia should be admitted to hospital for the night following surgery. In addition, adverse social conditions at home may obligate the patient to stay in hospital overnight. Intercurrent disease and bleeding disorders should be adequately assessed and treated pre-operatively. Careful assessment of the mouth and airway should be undertaken during pre-operative assessment, particularly in patients with a dental abscess.

The nature of anaesthesia required in dentistry depends on the type of operation as well as the demeanour of the patient. Dental procedures may be conducted under local or general anaesthesia, or may be performed using relative analgesia with nitrous oxide. Local anaesthesia can also be supplemented by sedation, to reduce anxiety, particularly in very frightened or otherwise anxious patients and those with needle and dental phobias.

Sedative techniques

For adults and older children, an alternative to general anaesthesia is sedation – particularly in those with a phobia of needles in the mouth. Sedation is defined as:[1]

A carefully controlled technique in which a single intravenous drug, or a combination of oxygen and nitrous oxide, is used to reinforce hypnotic suggestion and reassurance in a way which allows dental treatment to be performed with minimal physiological and psychological stress, but which allows verbal contact with the patient to be maintained at all times. The technique must carry a margin of safety wide enough to render unintended loss of consciousness unlikely.

Any other sedative technique is regarded as general anaesthesia.

Intravenous sedation may be achieved with small

intravenous increments of a short-acting benzodiazepine, such as midazolam. Verbal contact should be maintained, and the patient lightly sedated to the point of relief of anxiety, but not loss of consciousness. Midazolam, although short-acting, is more potent at producing loss of consciousness than other benzodiazepines such as diazepam and care should be taken in titrating the total dose required (usually less than 0.1 mg.kg^{-1}). Alternatively, administration of a sedative dose of propofol may be used, either as small boluses (0.3–1.0 mg.kg^{-1}), or as an infusion starting at 3 mg.kg.h^{-1} titrated as necessary, but without inducing anaesthesia.[5-8] Intravenous sedation is not recommended for children, particularly those under 10 years of age, due to its unpredictability.

Inhalational sedation and relative analgesia involve the use of nitrous oxide in concentrations up to 70%, and can be successfully used in both adults and children. Langa first described relative analgesia in 1966, based on the three planes of Guedel's first stage of anaesthesia. The first plane (10–25% nitrous oxide) consists of sedation and some analgesia; the second (25–55% nitrous oxide) is linked with dissociative sedation and greater analgesia, and the third (over 55% nitrous oxide) is associated with total analgesia preceding loss of consciousness.[9] The gases are delivered using apparatus which prevents the administration of less than 30% oxygen (e.g. the Cyprane Quantiflex machine) via a nasal mask (Goldman or Dupaco) with two tubes for the gas flow. From 0% (in oxygen), the concentration of nitrous oxide is slowly increased in increments of 5%. Verbal contact should continue to be maintained throughout the procedure. Above a concentration of 25%, disorientation and confusion, with amnesia, may begin to occur, although a proportion of patients require concentrations of up to 70% for adequate sedation. The term inhalational sedation is therefore limited to the use of nitrous oxide up to a concentration of 30% and is usually used in conjunction with local anaesthesia, whereas relative analgesia allows the use of nitrous oxide up to a concentration of 70% and may not always require the addition of local anaesthesia.[1] Physical contact in the form of a hand on the cheek or stroking the face is often very reassuring to the patient. Recovery from inhalational sedation and relative analgesia is extremely rapid.

General anaesthetic techniques

Any procedure undertaken during general anaesthesia must be performed in an appropriate environment.[1] This includes the use of either a dental chair (with a full range of movements, including the horizontal position and with the ability to be placed rapidly head-down), or a standard theatre trolley or table (with the same ability for the patient to be rapidly placed in the Trendelenburg position). Adequate supplies of tracheal intubation equipment, including appropriate laryngoscopes, tracheal tubes, airways, masks and a breathing system with a reservoir bag allowing positive-pressure ventilation should be the minimum available. Full resuscitation equipment (including a defibrillator) and drugs (including adrenaline) should also be available, in addition to a separate oxygen supply and powerful suction.[1] Appendix B lists the essential drugs and equipment that must be available (from the Department of Health response to the Poswillo report).

Although intermittent-flow anaesthetic machines such as the Walton V, the AE and McKesson machines were developed specifically for dental and maternity use, they are now rarely used. These machines were designed for 'on-demand' gas flow, and some also had the potential for hypoxic mixtures to be given. The Boyle's machine and its derivatives, using only continuous flows of gases and plenum vaporizers, are now more commonly used. Mixer valves, such as the Cyprane Quantiflex, are also popular and prevent the administration of less than 30% oxygen with nitrous oxide, closing off the supply of nitrous oxide if the oxygen supply fails.

There has been much controversy in the past concerning the relative advantages and disadvantages of general anaesthesia in the sitting or supine position for dental surgery.[10] The sitting position was claimed to give better airway maintenance in the unintubated patient, whereas the supine position provided better haemodynamic stability.[11-13] The current consensus is that the supine position is safer, and should be used for induction and maintenance of general anaesthesia for dental surgery, particularly now that the Brain laryngeal mask tends to be favoured in place of nasal or oral airways combined with an oral pack.

Induction and maintenance of anaesthesia for dental surgery may be performed in several different ways. Intravenous induction is standard practice, although children may prefer a gas induction. The use of a eutectic mixture of local anaesthetic (EMLA) cream applied to skin over a suitable vein 2 h pre-operatively makes intravenous induction of anaesthesia in children more acceptable. Propofol is the agent of choice, particularly in outpatients, because of its rapid recovery characteristics, although 1% methohexitone and 2.5% sodium thiopentone remain popular. Etomidate is also used by some dental anaesthetists.

The optimum technique for maintenance of the airway depends on the procedure to be undertaken.

The laryngeal mask is increasingly used in dental outpatient paediatric practice, in preference to the use of a nasal mask for exodontia, and has been shown to reduce the incidence of significant hypoxic episodes.[14-16] Adults who require extensive extractions (especially wisdom teeth extractions) are more safely managed with a nasotracheal tube and throat pack; tracheal intubation should also be used for children who need invasive dental work, such as the removal of palatal teeth, or extensive conservation treatment (including fillings, coatings and crown and bridge work). In children, an orotracheal tube is usually used in preference to a nasal tube to reduce the risk of epistaxis. The preformed RAE tracheal tube is useful for these procedures. Modern plastic tracheal tubes can be soaked in hot water to soften them before nasal insertion. Uncuffed Magill red rubber nasotracheal tubes are still used by some to minimize nasal trauma. Most anaesthetists use a nasal tube of internal diameter 0.5–1 mm less than that which would be used in the mouth, to allow for the narrower nares and to minimize trauma.

Muscle relaxation is usually necessary to pass a tracheal tube (although the use of propofol and alfentanil on induction[17-20] can result in good intubating conditions and is gaining acceptance). Suxamethonium is often used to avoid the necessity of controlled ventilation throughout the procedure. However, the high incidence of postoperative myalgia (despite attempts to minimize this using pre-curarization or other techniques), and the possibility of delayed recovery (in patients with defective or deficient plasma cholinesterase), are significant disadvantages.[20-26] Many anaesthetists use a non-depolarizing relaxant, especially the intermediate-acting agents atracurium[27] and vecuronium, with controlled ventilation.[28] Mivacurium is a shorter-acting non-depolarizing agent which, although metabolized by plasma cholinesterase, does not cause myalgia, and may be particularly useful for procedures lasting less than 30 min.[29-31]

In the absence of paralysis, maintenance of anaesthesia is usually by spontaneous inhalation of a volatile agent. Halothane is more likely to cause arrhythmias, which are common during dental procedures,[32-36] especially when adrenaline is used in local anaesthetic solutions. Enflurane, which is associated with fewer cardiac arrhythmias,[37] is used by many anaesthetists but has the most pronounced respiratory depressant effects of all inhaled agents. Isoflurane has the least effect on the cardiac rhythm, is less of a respiratory depressant than enflurane and is suitable for repeated exposure; consequently, it is regarded by many anaesthetists as the agent of choice. The role of the recently introduced agents, desflurane and sevoflurane, in dental anaesthetic practice awaits clarification, although they have appreciably lower solubilities in blood than the other agents and may be useful for day-case procedures.[38]

Total intravenous anaesthesia with propofol is also commonly used.[39-45] It may be combined with the opioid alfentanil either as a bolus or as an accompanying infusion. Various infusion regimens have been described. All are designed to maintain a plasma steady state at anaesthetic concentrations. The following is an example. After initial doses of propofol (1–2 mg.kg^{-1}) and alfentanil (3.5–10 µg.kg^{-1}), an intravenous infusion of propofol at 12 mg.kg.h^{-1} is continued for 10 min, reduced to 10 mg.kg.h^{-1} for 10 min and then reduced to 8 mg.kg.h^{-1}, from which it can be titrated up or down as necessary. Alfentanil should be administered as an infusion, titrated at a rate of 10–50 µg.kg.h^{-1}.

Opioid supplements are used in most anaesthetic regimens for adults or children undergoing painful procedures such as secondary tooth extraction. If used pre-operatively either in premedication or as part of the induction (i.e. pre-emptively), there is evidence that postoperative analgesia requirements are reduced.[46] Opioid supplementation also smoothes general anaesthesia in an unpremedicated adult day-patient, especially if a tracheal tube is passed. For outpatients, shorter-acting opioids such as fentanyl or alfentanil are preferred, although longer-acting agents such as pethidine and morphine tend to extend analgesia into the postoperative period. The dentist may also provide a regional block which gives analgesia in the early postoperative period, as well as reducing the incidence of intra-operative cardiac arrhythmias (possibly by reducing the requirement for halothane, when it is used, or by reducing the painful stimulus).

It should be remembered that the use of opioids significantly increases the incidence of postoperative nausea and vomiting, and this should be treated prophylactically in the adult outpatient. Metoclopramide 10 mg intramuscularly is a suitable agent. However, propofol is a good anti-emetic;[47,48] as little as 10 mg may significantly reduce the incidence of postoperative nausea and vomiting.[49]

Minimal standards of monitoring should be observed at all times.[50] This includes pulse oximetry, inspired oxygen fraction ($F_{I_{O_2}}$), end-tidal carbon dioxide tension, electrocardiograph (ECG) and blood pressure. It should be remembered that there is a significant lag period before oxygen desaturation is detected by a pulse oximeter and dental anaesthesia is a good example of a situation in which clinical monitoring, and particularly observing the patient's respiration and colour, can forestall impending disaster. The anaesthetist is in a good position to observe these signs, since he or she also aids the dentist by supporting the head and allowing countertraction for the pulling and drilling of teeth.

Postoperative recovery

Adequate postoperative facilities should always be available following any anaesthetic or sedative technique. The patient should be recovered in the lateral position on a trolley, in a 30° head-down position. Oxygen and suction must be available for each patient. Oxygen should be given by face-mask (with either variable or fixed-rate $F_{I_{O_2}}$) until the patient is awake (to avoid diffusion hypoxia). Equipment for resuscitation and tracheal intubation should be available for instant use. Each patient should be continuously supervised while in recovery, until vital signs are stable and consciousness has been recovered.

Patients should be discharged home only when fully recovered and in the care of a responsible adult. Adequate postoperative analgesia can usually be provided by non-steroidal anti-inflammatory agents. The potential side-effects of gastric ulceration and renal suppression should be noted, and the drugs should not be used for prolonged periods, especially in the elderly. Regional nerve blocks are often used in adults for postoperative analgesia, in addition to intravenous dexamethasone to reduce swelling after wisdom teeth extraction and other dental surgery. Children are usually pain-free after exodontia and rarely require more than paracetamol for pain.[51] It behoves a good anaesthetist to monitor postoperative analgesia adequately in all outpatient surgery, and patients should be able to contact somebody at the hospital (either an anaesthetist or a pain nurse), in addition to the dentist, if discomfort or pain arises.

COMPLEX MAXILLOFACIAL PROCEDURES

Advances in modern anaesthesia, intensive care and nursing have enabled the development of increasingly major and complex surgery to the head and neck. During these procedures, the anaesthetist must maintain physiological homeostasis during surgery that may be prolonged and which may be aggravated by major blood loss, fluid and electrolyte changes, heat loss and venous stasis in the lower limbs and pelvis. The development of more comprehensive monitoring of physiological functions has greatly assisted the anaesthetic management of these patients. In addition, improved surgical techniques have reduced the long operating times, resulting in significant decreases in blood loss and in the risks of problems associated with prolonged anaesthesia.

The age of patients varies from the very young to the very old. In addition to surgical correction of facial clefts, surgical correction of major craniofacial abnormalities is performed in ever younger patients, because surgical correction produces better results.[52] Surgical extirpation of malignant tumours of the head and neck has evolved in tandem with the development of free musculocutaneous flaps by plastic surgeons. Often undertaken in the elderly, although also in the middle-aged, these procedures can present major anaesthetic challenges. With constant improvements in major craniofacial surgery, technical demands on the anaesthetist have increased. However, the increasing use of miniplates and screws, providing solid fixation, has reduced the need for jaw wiring, simplifying control of the airway postoperatively.

Adequate oxygenation of the patient is a prime concern, because facial abnormalities are capable of causing airway obstruction and can make control of the airway and tracheal intubation difficult. During surgery, it is necessary to secure the upper airway, while allowing room for the surgeon to manoeuvre.

Anaesthetic aims

The aims of the anaesthetist in maxillofacial surgery include the following:

1. Provision of general anaesthesia for the patient
2. Provision of a secure airway throughout the periods of surgery and recovery
3. Provision of an unobstructed field for the surgeon
4. The management of specific problems, including:
   (a) prolonged surgical and anaesthetic time
   (b) blood loss
   (c) colloid and crystalloid fluid losses
   (d) maintenance of body temperature
   (e) ensuring adequate blood supply to tissue flaps
   (f) postoperative recovery problems.

Pre-operative assessment and premedication

History and examination

Full anaesthetic assessment starts with a complete history and examination. The upper airway needs special attention. Patients with maxillofacial abnormalities often present difficulty with maintenance of the airway and with tracheal intubation. The anatomy of the airway may be grossly displaced due to fracture–dislocation of facial bones and damaged, swollen soft tissues, particularly after major trauma. In 1901, Rene

Le Fort classified fractures of the maxilla after dropping rocks on the faces of cadavers (Fig. 13.1). The evidence for a fracture may be based on the type of accident, the appearance of the face (dish-face appearance, split-open or general facial swelling, or diplopia from upwards movement of the floor of the orbit). High fractures involving the upper part of the nose may include the cribriform plate, resulting in cerebrospinal fluid rhinorrhoea. Injuries to the eye and mandible are present in up to 40% of cases.[53] Radiographs will confirm the type of fracture. The airway should be rapidly assessed and secured as necessary; a tracheostomy may be required.

Other causes of difficult airway management include fixed flexion deformity of the neck due to burn contractures; occluded mouth opening from trauma, scarring or previous surgery (e.g. graft flaps to the lips and cheeks); and trismus due to dental abscess or mandibular or maxillary bone trauma.

Congenital craniomaxillary facial anomalies may present special problems, such as airway obstruction and sleep apnoea, and these should be carefully assessed.[54] The syndromes of Apert and Crouzon are frequently associated with upper-airway obstruction at the nose or palate due to abnormal growth of the maxilla.

Treacher–Collins and Pierre–Robin syndromes are associated with mandibular deformity, which is the commonest cause of tracheal intubation problems in the neonate.

The patient should be carefully assessed for any breathing problems. There may be position-related obstruction, sometimes seen with pharyngeal tumours or thyroid tumours. There may be other difficulties related to breathing, which can be elicited by careful history-taking. In acute trauma, it may be necessary to secure the airway as a matter of urgency. This is usually by tracheal intubation, especially when there is a high risk of aspiration of stomach contents, or when it is impossible to ensure adequate oxygenation by simpler means. In the acute situation, if oxygenation cannot be maintained and tracheal intubation is difficult or impossible, cricothyroidotomy should be performed, and oxygenation maintained via this route until the patient's condition is stabilized.

Investigations

Full baseline haematological, coagulation and biochemical investigations should be performed preoperatively. Blood should be cross-matched, the quantity depending on the surgery; very large volumes may be required for some procedures. Aspirin ingestion

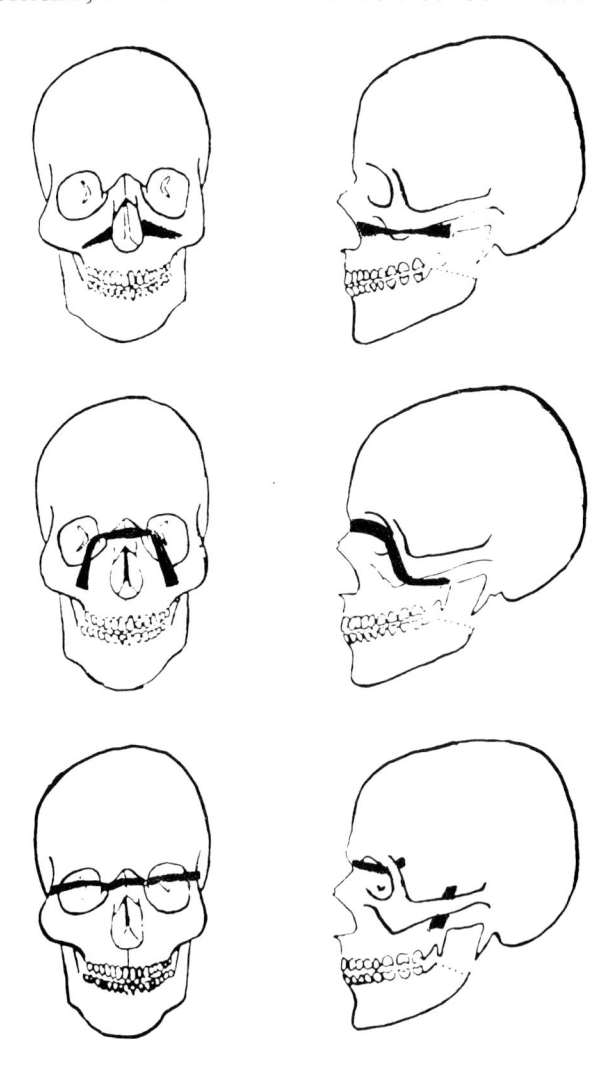

Fig. 13.1 Top: Fracture involving the maxilla only. The fracture line passes through the base of the antrum on either side and across the nasal floor through the septum.
Middle: Posteriorly the fracture line passes up behind the nose in the direction of the malar–maxillary junction, across the posterior wall of the antrum, and across the pterygoid process in the middle and upper third. The anterior fracture line passes into the orbit in the area of the lacrimal bone, and soon emerges again to break across the frontonasal process of the maxilla and the bridge of the nose to meet a similar fracture line on the opposite side. The posterior wall of the orbit is not fractured in this type.
Bottom: There is a craniofacial disjunction, the fracture line passing through both zygomatic arches, both external angular processes of the malar bones, across the back of both orbits, and the back of the nose in the ethmoid area. There is a separation of the nasal bones from the frontal bone. Posteriorly the septum is fractured high up and likewise the pterygoid processes. There is a complete separation of the maxilla, nose and ethmoids and the palatal bones from the base of the skull.

should be stopped at least 2 weeks prior to surgery to allow platelets to resume normal function.[55-58] Although the protease inhibitor and antifibrinolytic agent aprotonin is now routinely used in cardiac surgery to reverse the effects of aspirin on platelet function,[59] it has not yet been shown to be as effective in other forms of surgery; aprotonin is also used to reduce blood loss in repeat heart surgery[59-64] and in liver transplantation surgery.[65,66]

X-rays of the chest, in addition to specific imaging for upper airway and thoracic inlet either by magnetic resonance imaging or computed tomography, should be performed as necessary during the pre-operative assessment. Electrocardiography and other cardiological investigations, in addition to other specific organ function tests such as pulmonary and liver function, should also be undertaken as necessary.

Premedication

Premedication for elective procedures is discretionary. It is desirable to develop a rapport with the patient and to assuage some of the intense anxiety which may, understandably, be present. Sedation should not be used in patients with raised intracranial pressure.

Discuss and plan with the surgeon. After the patient has been assessed and appropriately premedicated, it is important to plan the procedure with the surgeon. This is to ensure safe induction of anaesthesia and airway protection, with the full cooperation of the surgeon. It may be necessary electively to perform tracheostomy at the start of the procedure in order to secure an adequate airway postoperatively, for example, after large deltopectoral flaps used to reconstruct major orofacial defects. Tracheostomy is also considered in cases where pharyngeal oedema is expected to occur, for example as a result of extensive and prolonged surgery involving the pharynx or tongue. The following is a list of possible indications for tracheostomy:

1. Upper airway obstruction:
   (a) marked oedema
   (b) large supraglottic tumours
   (c) laryngeal trauma
   (d) impacted foreign bodies
2. Loss of protective airway reflexes:
   (a) muscle weakness
   (b) unconsciousness
3. Tracheal intubation not feasible:
   (a) limited mouth opening
   (b) massive facial trauma, etc.
4. Loss of airway patency on provision of anaesthesia by mask
5. unstable foreign body present in airway
6. easier airway management after major head and neck surgery.

Induction of anaesthesia

General anaesthesia for maxillofacial surgery may be provided using a variety of techniques.[67] These generally include maintenance with a volatile agent, often supplemented by an opioid such as fentanyl or alfentanil. General anaesthesia may often be combined with regional blockade, particularly for exodontia. Total intravenous anaesthesia using propofol with an opioid such as alfentanil is an alternative. The techniques used are many and varied, the main problems associated with anaesthesia tending to revolve around the provision and securing of the airway, and difficulties associated with prolonged procedures.

Anaesthesia should be induced after a member of the surgical team has arrived. Initial monitoring should include pulse oximetry, ECG and blood pressure cuff; end-tidal carbon dioxide should be monitored immediately after tracheal intubation.[50] Venous access through a large-bore cannula (14- or 13-gauge in adults) should be attained before induction of anaesthesia.

If the airway and tracheal intubation are not expected to be problematic, intravenous induction can be used, and relaxation induced by a long-acting non-depolarizing agent. If problems with tracheal intubation are suspected, fibre-optic-assisted intubation may be indicated. It is an easy art to master, and there are now many published reports of its use in various situations.[68-81]

In patients with acute trauma, in whom rapid-sequence intravenous induction is normally required, any suspected difficulties with tracheal intubation are best managed by awake intubation.

Tracheal intubation equipment

The anaesthetist should be familiar with the equipment and techniques that may be necessary to pass a tracheal tube under difficult circumstances. These techniques should be practised on less difficult patients, and not used for the first time during an acute problem. The following equipment should be available:

1. Laryngeal masks of various sizes
2. Laryngoscopes with straight and curved blades in a range of sizes
3. Fibre-optic laryngoscope (Fig. 13.2)
4. Cricothyrotomy kit (e.g. Portex minitrach)
5. Tuohy needle and epidural catheter

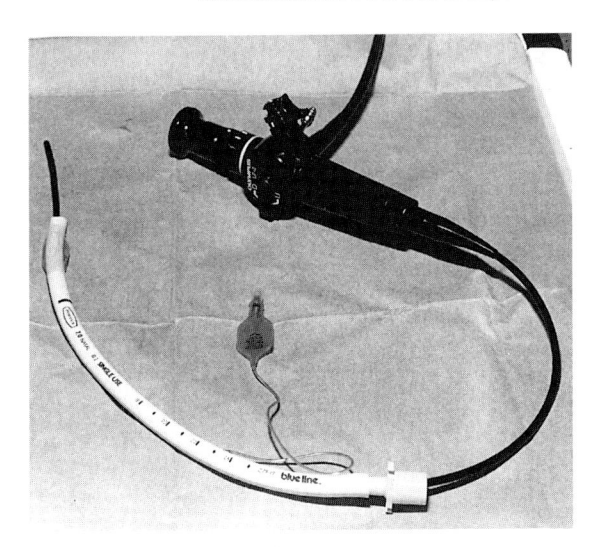

Fig. 13.2 The fibre-optic laryngoscope.

6. Tracheal tubes in a range of sizes
7. Introducers, including an oesophageal bougie.

Details of the use of these items can be found elsewhere, but in skilled hands, a fibre-optic laryngoscope passed orally or nasally under local or general anaesthesia will suffice for many difficult circumstances.

Patients in whom tracheal intubation is impossible by any means may occasionally be managed by the sole use of a laryngeal mask;[82] however, protection of the trachea from oral debris and blood is not guaranteed.

Fibre-optic intubation

For an awake intubation, the airway should be anaesthetized using appropriate agents. A common technique is to use 10% cocaine paste (which also inhibits epistaxis due to its vasoconstrictor properties) for the nostril (applied using three long cotton-wool sticks — at the front, in the middle and at the posterior aspect of the nose, and kept in place for at least 5 min to ensure adequate topical anaesthesia), 2% lignocaine to block the superior laryngeal nerves in the pyriform fossa (via skin injection or using Krause's forceps[83]), and 2% lignocaine applied to the trachea via cricothyroid puncture on deep expiration. If oral intubation is to be performed, the patient can suck a benzocaine lozenge or 10% lignocaine spray may be used topically. After adequate topical anaesthesia is obtained (within the toxic limits of the agents used), phenylephrine drops can be applied to the nose to reduce the risk of bleeding, which may obstruct the lens of the fibre-optic laryngoscope during nasal intubation.

If the patient can be safely anaesthetized before intubation, careful induction is performed, whilst maintaining spontaneous ventilation. This may be achieved by gaseous induction or the judicious use of an intravenous agent such as propofol. The anaesthetic is deepened with the agent of choice; (halothane and sevoflurane are the smoothest agents. It is most helpful for an assistant to support the airway by pulling forward on the angle of the mandible (Fig. 13.3); this also maximizes the pharyngeal space, making it easier to recognize structures with the fibre-optic laryngoscope. Until the trachea is intubated, continuity with the anaesthetic breathing system can be maintained via a nasal airway connected by a 15 mm connector (Fig. 13.3), or via an oral Guedel airway with a 15 mm connector, or even via a laryngeal mask. If the laryngeal mask is slightly withdrawn, the fibre-optic laryngoscope and tracheal tube can pass behind it and into the trachea. Intubation can also be performed through the laryngeal mask itself[84–90] (a size 6.0 mm tracheal tube will pass through a size 3 laryngeal mask airway). A fibre-optic laryngoscope is often used to ensure adequate placement of the tube if blind intubation has been performed through a laryngeal mask.

The best position to pass the fibre-optic laryngoscope at the head of the patient is while standing on a step to gain as much height as possible (Fig. 13.4). This allows positioning of the tip by rotation of the laryngoscope, which is easier when it is as straight as possible.

The tracheal tube is placed over the laryngoscope and positioned as proximally as possible. The laryngoscope may be lubricated along its sides with water-soluble gel to facilitate movement of the tracheal tube over it. Most scopes are designed to take tracheal tubes down to 6.0 mm internal diameter (Fig. 13.2). The

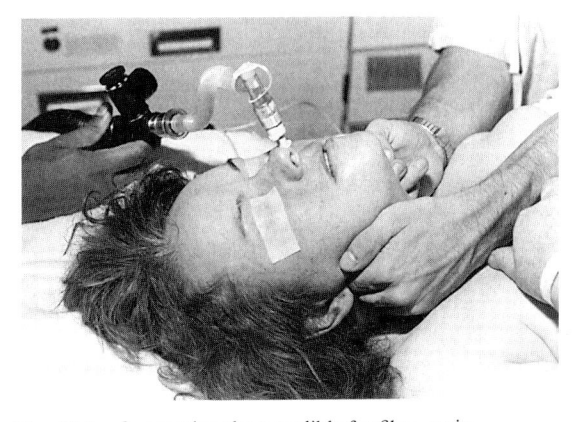

Fig. 13.3 Supporting the mandible for fibre-optic intubation.

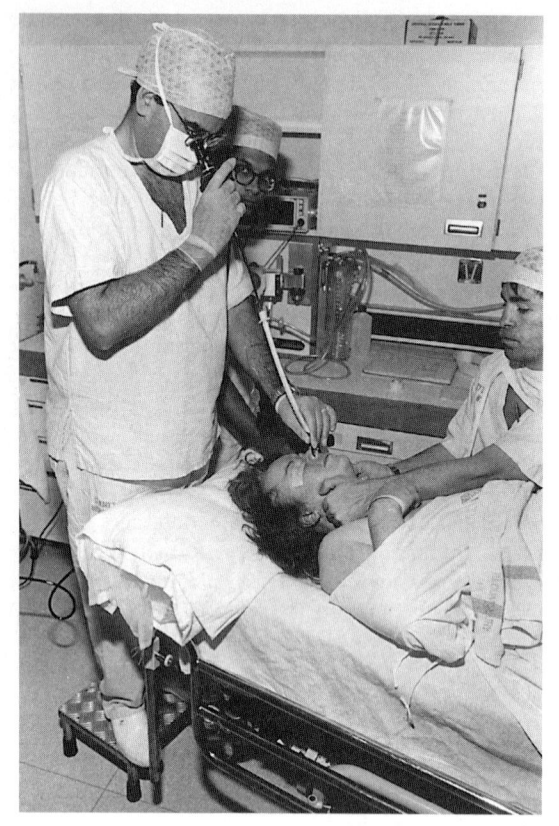

Fig. 13.4 Position for passing the fibre-optic laryngoscope.

distal tip and lens area of the laryngoscope should be cleaned with a proprietary lens cleaner to remove debris and to prevent misting.

The fibre-optic laryngoscope is then passed either nasally or orally. If passed orally in an awake patient, a bite-block will prevent the patient biting the laryngoscope and causing damage. In the nose, structures such as turbinates and the posterior nasal space may be recognized as the laryngoscope is advanced. The tip can be moved in two directions anteroposteriorly on a single plane from a lever on the eyepiece. Turning the whole laryngoscope, keeping it straight, increases the manoeuvrability. As the posterior nasal space is traversed and the laryngoscope tip enters the nasopharynx, or after clearing the mouth in the case of oral intubation, the epiglottis is seen and the hypopharynx comes into view. The laryngoscope is then passed through the vocal cords and into the trachea, which can be recognized by the characteristic appearance of the tracheal rings. Just prior to this, a muscle relaxant can be given intravenously to anaesthetized patients, or more local anaesthetic can be injected through a port of the laryngoscope, to minimize coughing. The tracheal tube is then passed over the laryngoscope, through the vocal cords and into the trachea. The anaesthetic breathing system should then be attached to the tube to enable continuing ventilation (Fig. 13.5). The awake patient is then anaesthetized.

Problems with fibre-optic intubation include inability to see the anatomy clearly. If there is inadequate space between tissues, for example in the presence of severe flexion deformity of the neck or a large tumour of the pharynx or throat, it is difficult to visualize normal structures. Indeed, sometimes until the tracheal rings are visualized, it may be difficult to take bearings and to navigate. Visibility is often improved if an assistant supports the airway, positioning the mandible as far forward as possible. Persistence is the key to success. Provided that the patient has an adequate airway and (in the case of anaesthetized patients) anaesthesia can be successfully maintained, time is not unduly limited. Without technical expertise in this procedure, it is safer not to paralyse the muscles until tracheal intubation is assured.

Tracheal tubes

The selection of design of tracheal tube depends on the site and nature of surgery. RAE tubes are useful, because their shape reduces invasion of the surgical field. An oral RAE tube provides good access for surgery to the upper part of the face. For surgery to the lower half of the face and maxilla, a nasal RAE tube may be used. In circumstances where the tracheal tube is to pass through areas of the surgical field, it is better to use an armoured tube, which can be inserted orally or nasally. Tracheal tubes can be wired to teeth or stitched to the nose to ensure adequate anchorage. If

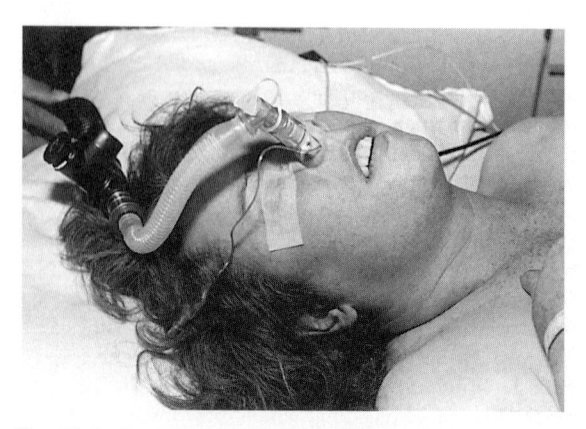

Fig. 13.5 Intubation complete: circuit attached.

the jaws are to be wired together postoperatively, the tube may be changed from oral to nasal during the procedure. However, improved methods of surgical fixation are increasingly used and the jaws may only be wired together while the facial skeleton is being positioned and fixed. A throat pack should be inserted, to prevent accumulation of debris above the tube cuff, but must be removed before long-term wiring of the mandible.

The provision of an adequate unobstructed field for surgery may require some thought and preparation. For extensive surgery of the head involving nose and mouth, a tracheostomy performed at the start of surgery permits an unobstructed field for the surgeon. Nasal intubation makes oral procedures easier, and vice versa. The provision of an adequate field for the surgeon must never conflict with security of the airway. Careful thought in the use of catheter mounts and connectors that do not impinge on the surgeon's field can also help; for example, use of a curved Magill connector, or a preformed oral or nasal RAE tube, can reduce the bulk of equipment extruding from the mouth or nose. Similarly, use of the Rusch tracheostomy tube enables gases to be piped to and from the tracheostomy patient with the minimum of interference with the surgical field.

Maintenance of anaesthesia

Major maxillofacial procedures can last for many hours. The major problems that arise for the anaesthetist then relate to those of prolonged anaesthesia. These include heat loss, blood loss and fluid balance, prolonged exposure to anaesthetic agents and drugs, increased risk of trauma to dependent areas of the body (such as nerve damage and pressure sores), and deep vein thrombosis.

The commonest technique used for maintenance comprises ventilation with a volatile agent supplemented with nitrous oxide and an opioid. The choice of volatile agent depends on individual preference and the characteristics of the patient. Enflurane or isoflurane may be preferred to halothane as these agents are less likely to sensitize the myocardium to endogenous or exogenous catecholamines. Recovery from desflurane anaesthesia, even of prolonged duration, is rapid.[38] In addition, the agent is not arrhythmogenic and, because of its low metabolism, there is little potential for organ toxicity. Its role in this type of surgery awaits evaluation. Sevoflurane is particularly useful for gaseous induction of anaesthesia and this property may make it of value, especially in children. Total intravenous techniques using propofol in conjunction with an opioid such as alfentanil are also used.

The blood pressure is often maintained slightly below normal to reduce surgical bleeding, but not insufficient to maintain good blood flow through tissue transfer or free flaps, if these are constructed. Careful positioning of the patient will optimize venous return, further reducing blood loss. Hypotensive techniques are sometimes used if massive blood loss is anticipated.[91]

The selection of a muscle relaxant depends much on the individual preference of the anaesthetist. Tubocurarine, a long-acting agent, has a greater number of side-effects, particularly histamine release and ganglion blockade. However, some prefer its relative longevity and lack of accumulation of active metabolites, and it is often used as part of a deliberate hypotensive technique. Pancuronium is long-acting and does not release histamine, but it may increase heart rate. The intermediate-acting agents, atracurium and vecuronium, are suitable for use by infusion and, for a given degree of block at the end of surgery, are easier to reverse. As prompt return of muscle power may be an important factor after surgery, their use has much to commend it. Vecuronium accumulates over prolonged periods.[92] Atracurium, because of Hofmann elimination, is not organ-dependent for its elimination, and tends not to accumulate; it may be the drug of choice.

Mechanical ventilation should be employed throughout the procedure, and adjusted to maintain normocapnia or moderate hypocapnia. Profound hypocapnia should be avoided as it may cause vasoconstriction, which can have adverse effects on blood flow to musculocutaneous flaps and other tissue transfers.

Anaesthetic gases should be humidified and warmed to reduce heat and water loss during the procedure and to prevent crusting and tracheal tube obstruction, especially in children. Hypocapnia should be achieved where there is an intracranial component to the surgery. In this instance, isoflurane is preferred to other volatile agents because of its lesser effects on brain blood flow up to 1 minimum alveolar concentration (MAC). Mannitol and cerebrospinal fluid drainage may be required to improve surgical access to the intracranial contents.

Monitoring

In addition to ECG monitoring, pulse oximetry and measurement of inspired and expired gas partial pressures, invasive haemodynamic pressure monitoring is used in the majority of complex maxillofacial procedures. Continuous monitoring of physiological variables allows tighter control of cardiovascular and fluid balance variables during long procedures. Commonly, an intra-arterial cannula, central venous catheter and nasopharyngeal, rectal or aural temperature probes are inserted, as well as a urinary catheter to measure urine output. Some patients with cardiovascular disease may benefit from the use of pulmonary artery pressure monitoring and derived variables such as cardiac index and systemic vascular resistance. The development of intravascular continuous monitoring of oxygen saturation and tension, as well as $P\text{CO}_2$, pH, sodium and potassium sensors will also become increasingly useful, obviating the need for recurrent measurement of arterial blood gases.

Air emboli can be a problem, and these can be assessed by the use of a precordial Doppler detector; end-tidal carbon dioxide monitoring should detect major incidents.

Muscle relaxation should be regularly monitored by train-of-four pattern stimulation. Monitoring is particularly important if an infusion of a neuromuscular blocker is employed.

Homeostasis

Physiological endurance of prolonged complex procedures can be optimized by reducing heat and fluid losses and by paying special attention to pressure areas and deep venous thrombosis (DVT) prophylaxis.[93-96]

Temperature. Normal temperature homeostasis requires the means to detect changes in environmental and core temperatures, and to respond to these changes by behavioural and physiological means. General anaesthesia decreases or ablates these capabilities. All patients undergoing surgery tend to lose heat. Evaporative losses of fluid from surgical sites and the respiratory tract combine with radiant and convective losses to the ambient air to cool the patient. A cold patient is difficult to warm up using external heat sources, mainly because of limited heat transfer with skin vasoconstriction.[92,97] Heat loss can be a significant problem in patients undergoing prolonged and substantial surgery. Surgery for orofacial neoplasia can be especially prolonged, and may involve exposure of large raw areas, exacerbating evaporative heat loss. General anaesthesia promotes heat loss by producing vasodilatation of skin blood vessels (increasing loss by radiation and convection), and inhibits shivering (preventing increased heat production). In addition, many patients who require this type of surgery are of advanced years, with a lower basal metabolic rate and lower body temperature, compounding the effects of heat loss in comparison with younger patients.[98] Postoperatively, shivering increases oxygen consumption, and vasoconstriction increases myocardial workload; both may be particularly stressful to elderly patients.

From the outset, therefore, precautions must be taken to minimize heat losses during prolonged and extensive maxillofacial surgery. These include the use of warming blankets, wrapping limbs in gamgee and foil (or using purpose-made warm air or circulating heated fluid insulating devices,) warming and humidifying inspired gases and warming all infused fluids (especially stored blood) to 37°C. Operating theatre ambient temperature and humidity should also be kept as high as comfortably possible.[99-103]

Avoidance of unintentional trauma and DVT. The patient must be protected from unintentional trauma. All bony protruberances should be well-protected from pressure and knocks. Nerve injuries can be minimized by careful positioning to prevent unnecessary traction on nerve trunks, or pressure on superficial nerves.[104] The eyes must be carefully protected, either by using a protective ointment and covering them carefully with eye-pads and padding, or suturing the eyes closed for the duration of the procedure, especially if the eyes are within the surgical field. The head should be positioned on a soft foam-padded ring. Elastic stockings or calf pump compressors should be used to minimize the risk of DVT. Lithium heparin, given subcutaneously 8-12-hourly, also reduces the incidence of deep venous thrombosis. Both techniques give equivalent results in terms of prophylaxis.[95] Although heparin can cause increased complications from bleeding, these are usually minor.[95]

Fluid balance and blood loss. Fluid balance must be very carefully monitored and maintenance fluids in the form of a crystalloid such as compound sodium lactate should be given early. Many elderly patients tend to be relatively dehydrated when presenting for surgery. Blood loss must be measured continuously. All swabs should be weighed, to give an approximate idea of loss. Total loss may be estimated by adding 25% to the weight of blood measured on swabs, and measuring the volume of blood in suction bottles. Red blood cell replacement should be considered after the first 10% of calculated blood volume has been lost. Plasma expanders in the form of gelatin, starch or albumin are usually used to replace volume in addition to packed red blood cells. Haemodilution may be used to improve blood viscosity in patients who are polycythaemic pre-operatively. This can be particularly important when musculocutaneous or other tissue flaps have been repositioned, as it is important to optimize blood flow through the graft. The haematocrit should be monitored throughout the procedure and maintained above 30% to optimize oxygen delivery.[105,106]

Excessive blood loss requiring massive blood transfusion can cause many complications.[107–116] A disseminated intravascular coagulopathy may occur in addition to simple clotting factor dilution, and appropriate clotting factors and fresh frozen plasma should be available in addition to platelets.

Recovery and postoperative care

At the end of surgery, provided that there is no expectation of significant oedema in the pharynx or upper airway, muscle relaxation can be antagonized and the tracheal tube and throat pack removed when the patient is breathing and has return of pharyngeal reflexes. If the jaws have been wired together, then the patient should pull out the tracheal tube, thus ensuring an adequate return of consciousness with intact pharyngeal reflexes. In this instance, a nasotracheal tube can be withdrawn and cut with its tip in the nasopharynx, allowing its use as a nasal airway and providing access for pharyngeal suction. Wire cutters should be always at hand on the patient's pillow, in case of sudden loss of the airway or vomiting.

Positioning of the patient is important if there has been extensive grafting of musculocutaneous tissue to cover big defects.[117] Pillows can be used to position the patient such that no undue traction or pressure is exerted on the areas concerned.

After very major procedures, when there may have been massive blood loss or where there may be major tissue oedema around the upper airway, the tracheal tube should be left in place and the patient transferred to the intensive care unit. Monitoring should then be continued and tracheal intubation maintained until the patient is normothermic, physiological variables are stable and the adequacy of blood clotting and/or the lack of peripharyngeal oedema confirmed. Extubation may then be performed after 24 h or when the oedema has settled. During this period, mechanical ventilation may be employed, or the patient may breathe spontaneously through the tracheal tube under sedation, as appropriate.

Blood transfusion may be required postoperatively, especially after maxillary surgery. Le Fort fractures of the maxilla and surgical osteotomies of facial bones may cause continued bleeding from open vessels behind the maxilla. Packing of the post-nasal space may be required to stop the blood loss. The upper airway needs careful monitoring in this situation, and may require continued tracheal intubation for its protection, if bleeding is a continuing problem.

Analgesia should initially be provided by intravenous infusion of an opioid. This can be substituted by patient-controlled analgesia when the patient is co-operative. Non-steroidal anti-inflammatory agents may be given with care after blood loss and coagulation defects have been rectified; these drugs inhibit platelets, although diclofenac has been shown not to increase blood loss.[118–124] Long-acting non-steroidal agents such as diclofenac and ketorolac synergize with opioid drugs, reducing the requirement for patient-controlled analgesia. However, non-steroidal anti-inflammatory drugs should not be used in patients with pre-existing peptic ulceration or renal disease, and long-term or high-dose administration may lead to renal failure, especially in the elderly.

Recovery is usually surprisingly rapid and patients generally prosper postoperatively. They may need to return for further surgery, so it is useful to build a rapport, especially with children, to reduce anxiety and tension on future occasions.

THYROIDECTOMY

Physiology and normal function of the thyroid gland

Anatomy and histology

The thyroid gland is a bilobed endocrine gland situated on each side of the trachea and oesophagus behind three strap muscles of the neck. The two pear-shaped lateral lobes, each approximately 5 cm long and extending from the oblique line of the thyroid cartilage to the sixth tracheal ring, are joined by an isthmus which passes over the trachea anteriorly, between the second and fourth tracheal rings. Occasionally a pyramidal lobe is present on the upper border of the isthmus overlying the second and third tracheal rings. The recurrent laryngeal nerve ascends posteriorly between the trachea and oesophagus. The gland is invested by the pretracheal fascia.

Inside the gland, cubical epithelium lines follicles which are filled with colloid containing thyroglobulin. Between the follicles, in connective tissue, are groups of parafollicular cells (C cells) which secrete thyrocalcitonin.

Biochemistry

The thyroid hormones, thyroxine (T_4) and tri-iodothyronine (T_3), are formed in thyroglobulin, an iodinated glycoprotein composed of two protein subunits which are synthesized in the rough endoplasmic reticulum of follicular cells, where mannose is incorporated. Iodine accounts for 65% of the weight of T_4. Being a relatively scarce element on the earth, the thyroid gland has mechanisms to concentrate and store the iodine as the ion, I⁻ (iodide). Iodide is concentrated by active transport from the blood into the follicular cells, where it is rapidly oxidized and incorporated into protein (tyrosine), with little free iodide remaining; this is known as organification of the iodine. After iodination of tyrosine residues of the polypeptide precursors of thyroglobulin to produce mono- and di-iodotyrosine, coupling of these agents by peroxidase[125] within lysosomes produces the hormones T_4 and T_3. There is approximately 15 times as much T_4 as T_3 in thyroglobulin, and slightly less than this in the plasma. The daily intake of iodine from the diet is approximately 150–300 mg, and about 5–30% is taken up by the thyroid gland. Areas of the world that have low amounts of iodine in the environment, causing a depleted iodine intake, are associated with a high incidence of endemic goitre.

Hormone release and circulation

Thyroid-stimulating hormone (thyrotropin, TSH), released from the anterior pituitary gland in response to thyrotropin-releasing hormone (TRH) from the hypothalamus, acts on the thyroid gland to augment the uptake of iodide, in addition to the increased activation of thyroglobulin uptake by follicular cells from colloid stores.[126] Plasma T_4 and T_3 inhibit the release of TRH from the hypothalamus. In the plasma, only 0.02% of total plasma T_4 and 0.3% of plasma T_3 is free. The rest is bound to plasma proteins,[127] of which thyroxine-binding globulin (TBG) is the most important, binding 75% of serum T_4 and T_3. Trans-thyretin (pre-albumin), albumin and haemoglobin[128] are the other main binding proteins. Drugs and other substances such as fatty acids can interfere with protein binding of the thyroid hormones.[129,130] Drugs such as steroids can reduce the amount of circulating TBG, and phenytoin and large doses of salicylates and other non-steroidal anti-inflammatory agents compete for binding to TBG, increasing free serum T_4 and T_3. T_3 is three to four times as potent as T_4 in its metabolic effects. Although the majority of thyroid hormone released from the thyroid gland is thyroxine, 30–40% of T_4 is de-iodinated to T_3 in the liver and kidney.

Target organs and effects

Thyroid hormones affect many biological processes. Intracellular receptors located in the nucleus have now been demonstrated, with a 10-fold greater affinity for T_3 than T_4, and it is via these that their effects are produced.[131–139] It has now also been shown that endogenous ligands (such as the retinoids) and various drugs (such as amiodarone, frusemide and phenytoin) can modulate and influence the activity of thyroid hormones on these receptors.[140–143] Protein-binding sites for T_3 have also been demonstrated in the plasma membrane, the mitochondria, the cytosol and endoplasmic reticulum of cells, although the function of these sites is unclear.[144,145] Thyroid hormones are involved in fetal development of the brain, in addition to other tissues.[146,147]

The first change seen in the cell after exposure to T_3 or T_4 is an increase in the activity of DNA-dependent RNA polymerase in the nucleus of cells. This is followed by an increase in amino acid incorporation into mitochondrial and microsomal proteins. Subsequently, the basal metabolic rate rises in parallel with the activity of cytochrome oxidase. Following physiological doses of T_3, mitochondria of skeletal muscle are seen to be enlarged, denser and more numerous. The basal metabolic rate increases under physiological conditions after a lag period of some 30 h. However, a very large dose of T_4 produces this effect within 2 h. An increasing number of thyroid hormone effects on cell metabolism and genetic regulation in the nucleus are beginning to be unravelled.[148–157] One of the most interesting is the acute effect of thyroid hormone on calcium uptake by the heart,[153] which is thyroid hormone-specific. An additional effect is that of thyroid hormone on sugar uptake by cells in the body, using calcium as a second messenger.[158]

The thyroid hormones are removed from the circulation by the liver, which converts them to less active pyruvic acid derivatives.

Calcitonin

Calcitonin, produced by the C cells of the thyroid, is a peptide hormone which antagonizes the effect of parathyroid hormone on bone and inhibits active bone resorption, resulting in a decrease in plasma calcium concentration. In the kidney, it promotes phosphate excretion.

Regulation of thyroid function

The thyroid gland is controlled by a number of feedback loops involving the hypothalamus and the pituitary. T_4 is the predominant hormone released from the thyroid gland, and it is converted to T_3 in the liver and kidney. Both T_4 and T_3 suppress the release of TSH from the pituitary gland, which also converts T_4 to T_3. TSH stimulates all of the steps to production of thyroid hormone in the thyroid gland via the activation of adenylate cyclase. TRH is released from the hypothalamus probably in response to reduced serum T_3 levels. Somatostatin, other neuropeptides and dopamine also inhibit TSH release from the pituitary.[159] It is likely that peptides such as vaso-active peptide and somatostatin also have a part to play in the intrathyroid regulation of thyroid hormone synthesis.[160,161]

Hyperthyroidism

Thyroid gland dysfunction gives rise to two different problems: hyperfunction of the thyroid gland (hyperthyroidism or thyrotoxicosis) or hypofunction of the thyroid (decreased secretion of thyroid hormone, hypothyroidism or myxoedema). Physical enlargement of the gland (goitre) may cause discomfort or more serious symptoms such as dysphagia or respiratory problems. Goitre usually has no associated functional abnormality (non-toxic goitre), but may be associated with hyperthyroidism (toxic goitre) and occasionally hypothyroidism (seen with Hashimoto's and Reidel's thyroiditis and carcinoma). Simple goitre is usually associated with a smooth, colloidal enlargement of the gland. However, it may become nodular or multinodular, with nodules of gland tissue which may be active (hot) or inactive (cold).

Non-toxic goitre

Enlargement of the thyroid gland may occur physiologically during puberty, pregnancy and the menopause. Pathological non-toxic goitre may occur for the following reasons:

1. Iodine deficiency (a daily intake of less than 100 mg) or relative iodine deficiency (during pregnancy) may cause non-toxic goitre.
2. Substances in the diet such as turnips, swedes, soya beans and drinking water in the Himalayas may be goitrogenic. Fluoride excess and calcium excess have also been implicated. These substances can inhibit the uptake of iodine into the thyroid, or the production of T_4. Drugs may also cause goitre, particularly if hyperthyroidism is overtreated. Goitre and hypothyroidism may occur in the newborn if the mother has been taking antithyroid drugs during pregnancy or lactation.
3. Genetic defects in thyroid function may give rise to goitre. These include the inability to concentrate iodide, to bind iodine or to form iodothyronines.

The lack of iodine, whatever its cause, results in hyperplasia of the gland, which is initially colloidal, but becomes multinodular if it persists.

Simple diffuse goitre usually does not require treatment. The treatment of pathological goitre is to give iodine as iodized salt. For large diffuse goitres, T_4 may be given to reduce activity of the gland and to reduce the size of the goitre.

Toxic goitre (primary hyperthyroidism)

Graves' disease (primary enlargement of the gland associated with hyperthyroidism) is the second commonest endocrine disorder (after diabetes mellitus) and affects 1.9% of the female population. The cause of primary hyperthyroidism remains unknown, but it is likely to be an auto-immune disorder.[162-165] The hyperthyroidism occurs despite suppression of TSH. The thyroid stimulation is thought to be by antibody stimulation of the TSH receptor on the surface of thyroid gland cells. Long-acting thyroid stimulator (LATS) is a family of immunoglobulins that has been found in many patients with hyperthyroidism. It is believed that B lymphocytes produce antibodies to TSH receptors (TRAb; thyroid receptor antibodies). These antibodies are polyclonal and may be stimulatory or inhibitory depending on receptor kinetics.

The clinical features of hyperthyroidism may be summarized as follows:

1. Weight loss, due to raised metabolic rate
2. Preference for cold weather
3. Raised body temperature and increased sweating
4. Fine tremor of the hands
5. Nervousness and irritability
6. Palpitations secondary to effects of thyroid hormones on the heart, in addition to effects of a raised cardiac output
7. Diarrhoea
8. Menorrhagia
9. Loss of hair
10. Muscle weakness
11. Exophthalmos.

Most of these signs and symptoms relate to the increased metabolic rate caused by raised T_3 and T_4 levels. The ophthalmopathy seen in 50% of patients with Graves' disease is rare in other causes of hyperthyroidism. The aetiology is unknown but patients tend to have very high circulating titres of antibodies, suggesting a link with auto-immunity.

Thyroid storm

This is now a rare condition, but may occur in patients

inadequately treated for hyperthyroidism, or with intercurrent infection, or postoperatively following subtotal thyroidectomy and occasionally after radio-iodine therapy. Peri-operatively, it has been confused with malignant hyperthermia and successfully treated with intravenous dantrolene.[166-168] Both syndromes have similar presentations, and treatment is along similar lines.

Thyroid storm is a potentially fatal condition (with a mortality of 20–40%) consisting of marked fever, tachyarrhythmias (which may cause death) and brain irritability. The most effective treatment is by large doses of intravenous propranolol with appropriate antithyroid drugs (e.g. propylthiouracil 400 mg, iodine and hydrocortisone). The patient should also be given oxygen, fluids and electrolytes, and cooled using ice packs, fans and cool intravenous fluids. If the condition occurs under general anaesthesia, it may be difficult to differentiate from malignant hyperthermia and intravenous dantrolene should also be given.

Other causes of hyperthyroidism

In addition to Graves' disease, hyperthyroidism may be due to:

1. toxic multinodular goitre
2. toxic adenoma
3. iodide-induced hyperthyroidism
4. subacute thyroiditis (auto-immune disease such as Hashimoto's disease, and Reidel's thyroiditis, where fibrosis of the gland occurs)
5. factitious (exogenous) thyrotoxicosis
6. neonatal thyrotoxicosis
7. TSH-secreting pituitary tumour
8. pituitary-induced hyperthyroidism
9. choriocarcinoma of uterus or testicle or hydatidiform mole
10. struma ovarii
11. hyperfunctioning thyroid carcinoma (usually metastatic).

Investigation of hyperthyroidism

Laboratory investigations. Virtually all patients with hyperthyroidism have an elevated T_4 free fraction. If this is equivocal, or not raised, an elevated T_3 fraction may indicate T_3 thyrotoxicosis, which occurs in 3–5% of patients. More sophisticated testing of T_4 to T_3 conversion inhibition and tests of thyroid regulation may be required.[169] In the latter instance, serum thyrotropin can be measured using TSH-IMA (TSH immuno-assay), or TRH infusion tests. TSH-IMA testing is also used to monitor patients receiving thyroid hormone replacement therapy.

Other specific tests include antithyroid antibodies (especially thyroid microsomal antibody) in Hashimoto's thyroiditis; thyroglobulin antibodies, also present in Hashimoto's thyroiditis; antibodies against thyroid stimulating hormone receptors in Graves' disease; and serum thyroglobulin determinations, used in follow-up of patients with metastatic thyroid carcinoma following surgery.

Thyroid scan. Iodine isotopes, ^{123}I or ^{131}I, which are trapped in the thyroid gland in the same way as ordinary iodine, are used; ^{123}I, which is less radioactive, is preferred, especially in young patients.

Pertechnetate ($^{99m}TcO_4^-$) may also be used. This substance is trapped, but not organified by the gland, and a scan is performed 30 min after injection.

Ultrasound scan. This can differentiate solid and cystic gland enlargements. It may detect nodules as small as 1–2 mm in size.

Computed tomography and magnetic resonance imaging. These techniques, in addition to giving information about gland size, can also detect compression or invasion of the trachea and the degree of obstruction of the thoracic inlet by large retrosternal goitres.

Chest radiography and barium swallow are also used to assess the degree of gland enlargement.

Treatment of hyperthyroidism

Antithyroid drugs. The first objective, particularly in Graves' disease, is to suppress elevated thyroid hormone secretion rate. The most commonly used drugs are thiourea derivatives. Carbimazole, which is metabolized to the active metabolite methimazole, and propylthiouracil both inhibit the organification of iodine in the thyroid gland. Propylthiouracil also inhibits conversion of T_4 to T_3. Both drugs are concentrated within the hyperactive gland, enabling dosage to be as infrequent as once or twice daily. Reduction of serum T_4 levels precedes a reduction in metabolic effects of T_4, and there may be as much as a 5–10-day lag period for this to occur. Agranulocytosis can occur in 0.2–0.5% of patients taking these drugs, and careful monitoring is essential.

Iodide as potassium iodide, 1 g.ml^{-1}, 3 drops twice a day, or Lugol's solution (125 mg iodide per ml) 10 drops per day, inhibits both thyroid hormone release and thyroid hormone synthesis. This is most effective for short-term treatment for up to 28 days; the thyroid hormone levels start to increase again if treatment is more prolonged. This form of treatment may be given for short periods to patients who are allergic to thiourea drugs. Iodide is also given to reduce thyroid gland vascularity just prior to surgery, but it interferes with the postoperative administration of radio-iodine.

Lithium carbonate may also be used, as it inhibits release of thyroid hormone from the thyroid gland. It is useful for patients who are allergic to thiourea compounds. Patients should be monitored for evidence of lithium toxicity, which can mimic thyrotoxicosis.

β-Adrenergic blocking agents. There is a striking similarity between the effects of hyperthyroidism and catecholamine excess. However, in hyperthyroid patients, excess amounts of catecholamines are not present and the molecular basis for the similarity remains obscure, except that hyperthyroidism is associated with an augmentation of the number of β-adrenergic receptors in the heart. β-Receptor blockade produces a marked reduction in cardiac symptoms, particularly tachycardia and palpitations. However, it should not be used in patients with cardiac failure or bronchospasm. β-Blockade does not reduce the raised metabolic rate of hyperthyroid patients.

Radio-iodine. Radio-active iodine, ^{131}I, has been used since the 1940s. A carefully calculated dose of iodine delivering 6000–7000 rad is associated with a resolution of hyperthyroidism in 6 months in some 80% of patients. It remains a popular treatment with many endocrinologists. The principal complication is hypothyroidism, which occurs in 10% of patients in the first year, and increases at about 5% per year thereafter over 20 years. There is no increased risk of thyroid carcinoma or leukaemia after this treatment. However, there is reluctance to employ radio-iodine in women of child-bearing age, although no increased risk of fetal malformation has been reported.

Surgery. Removal of a portion of the thyroid gland to control hyperthyroidism is traditional, effective and reliable.

Thyroidectomy may be indicated for simple multinodular goitre if only to reduce the incidence of carcinoma. Solitary nodular goitres need to be investigated first to identify whether they are 'hot' or 'cold', i.e. if they are productive or non-productive. Hot nodules may be suppressed by giving T_4, or if not, by surgery, which usually comprises removal of the nodule. Cold nodules are first investigated by needle aspiration under local anaesthetic. They may be cystic or solid. Cytology is important to exclude malignancy, and frozen section is recommended during operation. Large goitres or substernal goitres should be excised to prevent tracheal compression and the onset of respiratory symptoms.[170,171]

Surgery for auto-immune thyroiditis (Hashimoto's disease) or Reidel's thyroiditis (a collagen disorder) is rarely needed unless the goitre becomes large or uncomfortable.

Hypothyroidism

Hypothyroidism is a syndrome of symptoms and signs that results from a deficiency of thyroid hormone. It is classified as *primary* (acquired auto-immune disease,[172] such as Hashimoto's thyroiditis; the consequence of thyroidectomy or radioiodine treatment; congenital, as in thyroid agenesis; or goitre secondary to enzyme deficiency or maternal antithyroid treatment[163]) or *secondary* (due to hypothalamic or pituitary dysfunction).

The common symptoms of hypothyroidism include the following:

1. Weakness and fatigability
2. Dry, coarse skin with hair loss
3. Swelling of the limbs, hands and face
4. Cold intolerance, decreased sweating
5. Husky voice
6. Weight gain
7. Decreased appetite
8. Memory impairment
9. Hearing deficiency
10. Arthralgia and paraesthesiae
11. Constipation
12. Muscle cramps.

These symptoms are caused predominantly by a reduced metabolic rate and the deposition of hygroscopic mucopolysaccharide in the vocal cords, oropharynx and subcutaneous and other tissues, from which the name 'myxoedema' arises.

Treatment of hypothyroidism

Thyroid replacement therapy is the treatment for hypothyroidism. Laevothyroxine is the most commonly used agent, because it provides stable and easily measured serum thyroid hormone levels.

Myxoedema coma

In severe thyroid hormone depletion, the patient may lapse into a coma. This can occur in the myxoedematous patient during times of increased physiological stress such as pregnancy, cold and infection. It may also occur iatrogenically, after the administration of sedatives or anaesthesia[173] to a hypothyroid patient. Treatment of myxoedema coma is with intravenous laevothyroxine 2 μg.kg^{-1} and 100 μg every 24 h thereafter. Hydrocortisone (adrenocortical deficiency also occurs), rehydration and rewarming, sometimes with positive-pressure ventilation, are also required. The precipitating cause should also be treated.

Effects of anaesthesia and surgery on thyroid gland function

The effects of the stress response to anaesthesia and surgery on thyroid hormones are generally a suppression of activity. TSH release is suppressed and TSH is altered, having reduced glycosylation, and becoming less potent in stimulating the release of T_4 from the thyroid gland.[174,175] In addition, T_4 appears to be converted to *reverse* T_3, which is inactive, and lower serum concentrations of T_3 are present.[176] Most of these changes may be the result of high dopamine levels in the circulation,[177] which rise as part of the stress response to surgery. However, despite the reduced levels of thyroid hormones, a hypermetabolic response is still mounted.

The effects of anaesthetic agents differ. An increase of TSH secretion occurs with general anaesthesia (thiopentone/pethidine/pancuronium/nitrous oxide), but is unchanged with epidural anaesthesia.[178] General anaesthesia with volatile agents tends to reduce T_4 levels and increase reverse T_3 levels, and may be the cause of the changes seen generally in anaesthesia and surgery described above.[179-183] High-dose fentanyl anaesthesia for cardiac surgery results in a fall in T_3 and T_4 levels, and an increase in *reverse* T_3 levels.[184]

Although changes occur, it is unclear if they are clinically significant in the context of surgery for thyroid gland disease.

Anaesthetic management for thyroidectomy

Anaesthesia for thyroidectomy can be performed using regional or general anaesthetic techniques. Regional anaesthesia is used in some countries, provided that the surgery required is not too extensive. For subtotal or total excision of a thyroid gland which does not include retrosternal spread, surgery may be performed under a cervical plexus block,[185,186] or local bilateral infiltration. The majority of thyroidectomies in the UK and USA are performed under general anaesthesia.

Pre-operative assessment

The patient should be carefully assessed pre-operatively. In addition to the medical considerations reviewed above, other salient features need to be carefully appraised. Particular attention should be paid to the airway. A large substernal thyroid gland may obstruct the trachea by compression,[171] which may only be apparent to the patient in certain postures or positions. Occasionally, a patient may present acutely with respiratory obstruction requiring immediate intubation of the trachea.[170] A large thyroid gland may also cause obstruction to the thoracic inlet, affecting the oesophagus (dysphagia), or venous drainage (obstructed jugular veins). Long-standing goitre, especially with a very large thyroid gland, may result in tracheomalacia, in which the tracheal cartilage has been invaded by thyroid tissue. This can cause serious problems, particularly postoperatively. An oesophagogram, together with chest radiographs, can be of benefit in identifying potential difficulties. Computed tomography or magnetic resonance imaging of the thoracic inlet and thorax can be of great help in assessing the extent of thyroid tumour, particularly those with retrosternal spread, and its encroachment upon the airways.

Drug treatment

In the uncontrolled thyrotoxic patient, there is a risk of postoperative thyroid storm,[187] and in the hypothyroid patient, there is a risk of postoperative myxoedema coma.[173] In the hyperthyroid patient, control is achieved by the use of antithyroid drugs such as carbimazole, as described above. Patients who have a tachyarrhythmia or other signs and symptoms of increased sympathetic drive should be treated with β-adrenergic blockers.

If radio-iodine is not to be given postoperatively, potassium iodide should be given to reduce gland vascularity prior to surgery. This is usually started 10–20 days before the operation. Even patients who are euthyroid may have a hyperplastic and vascular gland.

Hypothyroid patients controlled on L-thyroxine should continue their treatment up to the day of surgery. If untreated hypothyroid patients present for surgery, then at least 48 h of thyroxine T_4 treatment should be provided before surgery, if possible.[188] This should be allied with steroid replacement therapy, since adrenocortical insufficiency is usually associated with hypothyroidism.

Premedication. The patient should be appropriately premedicated for the attenuation of anxiety (using intramuscular drugs such as opioids, or a sedative hypnotic and anti-emetic; or oral sedatives such as the benzodiazepines, sometimes combined with an anti-emetic drug such as prochlorperazine). The use of antimuscarinic agents such as atropine may produce unwanted tachyarrhythmias in hyperthyroid patients.

Induction and tracheal intubation

It is important to assess the upper airway carefully and to consider specific investigations to rule out any encroachment from tumours causing tracheal compression, invasion of tracheal rings or deviation of the trachea, all of which can make airway management and tracheal intubation difficult.

If difficult tracheal intubation is anticipated, advance consideration must be given to the use of techniques discussed in the previous section on maxillofacial surgery. Fibre-optic techniques of intubation are usually used in these cases.[189]

For surgery on a thyroid gland with extensive retrosternal spread, where thoracotomy is required, a double-lumen endobronchial tube should be passed if possible. This permits deflation of a lung to improve surgical access if necessary.

A large-bore intravenous cannula should be inserted prior to induction of anaesthesia. After awake intubation, induction may proceed intravenously with the induction agent of choice (thiopentone is most commonly used). If intubation is to be performed after induction of anaesthesia in the spontaneously breathing patient, judicious use of intravenous propofol while deepening anaesthesia with a volatile agent such as isoflurane is the preferred method. If no problems are anticipated with airway management or tracheal intubation, induction may proceed intravenously followed by muscle relaxation with short-acting (suxamethonium), intermediate-acting (mivacurium, atracurium or vecuronium) or long-acting (tubocurarine, pancuronium) agents.

Access to the head is limited during the procedure, so the tracheal tube and catheter mount connections should be securely anchored in position. The surgeon may flex and extend the neck during the procedure; consequently, a non-kinking flexometallic tracheal tube is preferable to a simple plastic tube. The eyes should be protected by ointment and eyepads, and taped closed. This is particularly important in patients with ophthalmopathy.

Maintenance of anaesthesia

The patient is positioned slightly head-up to improve venous drainage from the site of operation, with the head extended, sometimes with a roll behind the shoulders, and the head resting on a head-ring. Anaesthesia is generally maintained with nitrous oxide and a volatile agent. Spontaneous ventilation is used by some anaesthetists, but there is a greater risk of air embolus, tachyarrhythmias may be induced by hypercapnia in the hyperthyroid patient and unacceptably deep levels of anaesthesia may be required to control blood pressure. The hypothyroid patient, often relatively hypovolaemic, is also more unstable under these conditions. There are no disadvantages to intermittent positive-pressure ventilation in these patients, and most anaesthetists consider it more appropriate.[188,190]

Isoflurane produces a lower increase in T_4 levels than halothane,[179] and also is less likely to cause ventricular arrhythmias, particularly if the surgeon injects adrenaline.[191] Opioid supplementation is often used to smooth the anaesthetic and reduce the risks of coughing and straining, which have an adverse effect on blood loss and the surgical field.

Hypotensive anaesthetic techniques are used by some anaesthetists to improve the surgical field and reduce blood loss. However, careful positioning of the patient and a smooth general anaesthetic usually obviate the need for this requirement. Volatile agents such as isoflurane and desflurane, which are good vasodilators, tend to reduce arterial and venous blood pressure, leading to an improved surgical field without the need for specific hypotensive agents.

Monitoring. ECG, blood pressure measurement, capnography and pulse oximetry should be used on all patients undergoing general anaesthesia.[50]

In patients who require extensive surgery including thoracotomy, invasive monitoring of blood pressure and central venous pressure is usually required.

Hypotensive anaesthetic techniques, if used, are more safely performed if arterial pressure is monitored continuously.

Recovery

At the end of surgery, neuromuscular blockade is reversed, and when the patient is breathing adequately, the tracheal tube should be removed under direct vision. The vocal cords can then be visualized and any damage to recurrent laryngeal nerves ascertained.

Postoperative problems

Nerve injury. If both recurrent laryngeal nerves have been damaged, the vocal cords are fixed in adduction, and the tracheal tube should be left in place at the end of the operation. A tracheostomy may be required, and if permanent damage has been sustained, further surgery will be required to widen the glottis. If only one nerve has been damaged, the other vocal cord can compensate and intervention is not necessary.

Rarely, the superior laryngeal nerve may be damaged,

and paralysis of the cricothyroid muscle results in a changed voice, in addition to swallowing problems due to sensory loss from the hypopharynx.

Haemorrhage. Primary haemorrhage into the neck can be a dire emergency because tracheal obstruction may occur very rapidly. Stitch-cutters or staple removers should be at hand at all times, so that the tissues can be released if obstruction occurs. This complication usually presents within hours of surgery. The trachea should be re-intubated if obstruction develops.

Oedema. Occasionally, oedema of the larynx and/or pharynx may occur, leading to stridor. If very severe, this may require a temporary tracheostomy.

Tracheomalacia or tracheal collapse. Tracheomalacia is a very rare complication and usually follows thyroidectomy associated with malignancy. Malignant invasion of the tracheal rings renders the trachea liable to collapse after removal of the tumour. Re-intubation is necessary before tracheal stenting and reconstructive surgery at a later date. Tracheal collapse can also occur if it has been necessary to remove tracheal cartilage during the operation.

Thyrotoxic crisis. Similar to a thyroid storm, although less severe, this is a rare occurrence in the patient who has been adequately prepared preoperatively. It is most likely to occur in the uncontrolled thyrotoxic patient. Treatment consists of rehydration and antithyroid therapy (propylthiouracil 400 mg 6-hourly, sodium iodide 250 mg 6-hourly and hydrocortisone 100 mg 6-hourly). Cooling, administration of antipyretic agents such as paracetamol and support of cardiac failure and renal function with adequate oxygenation should also be provided if indicated.

Hypocalcaemic tetany. This tends to occur within a few days of operation when parathyroid glands have also been removed. Treatment is with calcium and vitamin D. Acute tetany can be treated with intravenous calcium.

The parathyroid glands

Anatomy and physiology

There are normally four parathyroid glands, each usually situated behind a pole of the thyroid gland. The parathyroid glands secrete parathyroid hormone (parathormone, PTH) which is part of a complex control system for plasma calcium and phosphate concentrations, also regulated by vitamin D. Vitamin D is produced in the skin by ultraviolet irradiation of 7-dehydroxycholesterol, as well as being absorbed from the diet in the jejunum. Vitamin D is then hydroxylated in the liver from where it is transported to the kidney. Here, it is further metabolized under the regulation of calcium, phosphate and PTH. Low calcium and phosphate concentrations with high PTH cause stimulation of metabolism to produce more $1,25(OH)_2D$, the active form of vitamin D. Prolactin and growth hormone may also stimulate this production.

Target organs for vitamin D and parathormone

Bone, gut and kidney are the principal target organs for vitamin D, but many other tissues such as pituitary, parathyroid glands, pancreas, brain and lymphocytes also contain receptors for $1,25(OH)_2D$. In gut, this compound increases calcium absorption from the intestine. In bone, more re-absorption tends to occur to increase plasma levels of calcium, although bone and cartilage formation can be stimulated under certain conditions. The role of vitamin D in the kidney, independent of PTH, is unclear. PTH acts directly on bone and kidney to increase plasma levels of calcium by mobilizing bone and inhibiting calcium excretion via the kidney. PTH also prevents hyperphosphataemia by increasing phosphate excretion from the kidney via a direct action on the tubules. Calcitonin, released from the C cells of the thyroid gland, can be considered a counter-regulator of PTH, with essentially opposite effects.

Pathology

Hypoparathyroidism occurs most commonly within 1–2 days after thyroidectomy if the parathyroid glands are inadvertently removed. It may also occur temporarily after partial parathyroid excision for adenoma.

The syndrome is characterized by neuromuscular irritability due to a decreased threshold of cell membrane excitation, characterized by paraesthesiae and tetany. Convulsions, spasms and dyspnoea with wheezing and stridor may also occur. Elicited signs of latent hypocalcaemia include Trousseau's sign (tetany of the hand after application of a tourniquet to the upper limb above systolic pressure). Chvostek's sign is elicited by tapping the facial nerve anterior to the ear lobe or just below the zygomatic arch, to induce facial spasms. Other signs include ECG changes, calcification of basal ganglia and papilloedema. Rickets and osteomalacia may also develop. The serum calcium concentration is low, and distinguishes some of the clinical features from metabolic alkalosis. There may also be hypomagnesaemia.

Hyperparathyroidism occurs with uncontrolled excess

release of PTH from one or more parathyroid glands which become adenomatous. Its aetiology is unknown, but the condition is often familial and may be associated with carcinoma (in less than 2% of patients). Symptoms and signs can be remarkably varied and include polyuria, polydipsia, hypertension, uraemia and anorexia. Hypercalcaemia, hypercalciuria (often presenting as nephrolithiasis), and osteitis fibrosa cystica (painful bones) occur.

Treatment

Hypoparathyroidism. Treatment of hypocalcaemia is initially with intravenous calcium (especially in the presence of stridor), followed by regular oral calcium and ergocalciferol (vitamin D_2). Stridor suggests involvement of the larynx and it is important to secure the airway; tracheal intubation may be necessary in severe cases.

Hyperparathyroidism. Treatment of hyperparathyroidism is by excision of adenomatous or extraneous gland tissue. Most parathyroid adenomas can be diagnosed on initial inspection by the surgeon, since they are obviously enlarged, and excision is confirmed by histology. Abnormal glands may also be situated in abnormal places such as the mediastinum (up to 20%). The skill of the surgeon is paramount in the recognition of the gland. Excision of the adenoma is usually curative. Anaesthetic considerations are very similar to those for thyroid surgery.

REFERENCES

1. Poswillo DE. Chairman: General anaesthesia, sedation and resuscitation in dentistry: report of an expert working party. London: Standing Dental Advisory Committee, Department of Health. 1990
2. Reiner SA, Sawyer WP, Clark KF, Wood MW. Safety of outpatient tonsillectomy and adenoidectomy. Otolaryngol Head Neck Surg 1990; 102: 161–168
3. Llewellyn J, Berger B, Glandon GL, Keithley J, Levin D. Postoperative complications in same day admission surgery. QRB 1989; 15: 49–53
4. Scaife JM, Campbell I. A comparison of the outcome of day-care and inpatient treatment of paediatric surgical cases. J Child Psychol Psychiatry 1988; 29: 185–198
5. Valtonen M, Salonen M, Forssell H, Scheinin M, Viinamaki O. Propofol infusion for sedation in outpatient oral surgery. A comparison with diazepam. Anaesthesia 1989; 44: 730–734
6. Skipsey IG, Colvin JR, Mackenzie N, Kenny GN. Sedation with propofol during surgery under local blockade. Assessment of a target-controlled infusion system. Anaesthesia 1993; 48: 210–213
7. Ghouri AF, Taylor E, White PF. Patient-controlled drug administration during local anesthesia: a comparison of midazolam, propofol, and alfentanil. J Clin Anesth 1992; 4: 476–479
8. Oei-Lim LB, Vermeulen-Cranch DM, Bouvy-Berends EC. Conscious sedation with propofol in dentistry. Br Dent J 1991; 170: 340–342
9. Langa H. Relative analgesia in dental practice, 2nd edn. Philadelphia, PA: WB Saunders 1976
10. Sykes P (ed) Drummond-Jackson's dental sedation and anaesthesia. London: SAAD. 1979
11. Al-Khishali T, Padfield A, Perks ER, Thornton JA. Cardiorespiratory effects of nitrous oxide: oxygen: halothane anaesthesia administered to dental outpatients in the upright position. Anaesthesia 1978; 33: 184–188
12. Tomlin PJ. Deaths in out-patient dental anaesthetic practice. Anaesthesia 1974; 29: 551–570
13. Bourne JG. Fainting and cerebral damage: a danger in patients kept upright during dental gas administration and after surgical operations. 1957; 2: 499–505
14. Bailie R, Barnett MB, Fraser JF. The Brain laryngeal mask. A comparative study with the nasal mask in paediatric dental outpatient anaesthesia. Anaesthesia 1991; 46: 358–360
15. Kendall N. The Brain laryngeal mask. An alternative to difficult intubation. Br Dent J 1990; 168: 278
16. Alexander CA. A modified Intavent laryngeal mask for ENT and dental anaesthesia. Anaesthesia 1990; 45: 892–893
17. Davidson JA, Gillespie JA. Tracheal intubation after induction of anaesthesia with propofol, alfentanil and i.v. lignocaine. Br J Anaesth 1993; 70: 163–166
18. Grange CS, Suresh D, Meikle R, Carter JA, Goldhill DR. Intubation with propofol: evaluation of pretreatment with alfentanil or lignocaine. Eur J Anaesthesiol 1993; 10: 9–12
19. Coghlan SF, McDonald PF, Csepregi G. Use of alfentanil with propofol for nasotracheal intubation without neuromuscular block. Br J Anaesth 1993; 70: 89–91
20. Alcock R, Peachey T, Lynch M, McEwan T. Comparison of alfentanil with suxamethonium in facilitating nasotracheal intubation in day case anaesthesia. Br J Anaesth 1993; 70: 34–37
21. Oxorn DC, Whatley GS, Knox JW, Hooper J. The importance of activity and pretreatment in the prevention of suxamethonium myalgias. Br J Anaesth 1992; 69: 200–201
22. McLoughlin C, Elliott P, McCarthy G, Mirakhur RK. Muscle pains and biochemical changes following suxamethonium administration after six pretreatment regimens. Anaesthesia 1992; 47: 202–206
23. Editorial. Suxamethonium myalgia. Lancet 1988; ii: 944–945
24. O'Sullivan EP, Williams NE, Calvey TN. Differential effects of neuromuscular blocking agents on suxamethonium-induced fasciculations and myalgia. Br J Anaesth 1988; 60: 367–371
25. Ostergaard D, Viby Mogensen J, Hanel HK, Skovgaard LT. Pretreatment with pancuronium before

suxamethonium administration in patients heterozygous for the usual and the atypical plasma cholinesterase gene. Acta Anaesthesiol Scand 1991; 35: 502–507
26 Ostergaard D, Engbaek J, Viby Mogensen J. Adverse reactions and interactions of the neuromuscular blocking drugs. Med Toxicol Adverse Drug Exp 1989; 4: 351–368
27 Luyk NH, Weaver JM, Quinn C, Wilson S, Beck FM. Comparative trial of succinylcholine vs low dose atracurium-lidocaine combination for intubation in short outpatient procedures. Anesth Prog 1990; 37: 238–243
28 Harper NJ, Chadwick IS, Linsley A. Suxamethonium and atracurium: sequential and simultaneous administration. Eur J Anaesthesiol 1993; 10: 13–17
29 Wrigley SR, Jones RM, Harrop Griffiths AW, Platt MW. Mivacurium chloride: a study to evaluate its use during propofol–nitrous oxide anaesthesia. Anaesthesia 1992; 47: 653–657
30 Basta SJ. Clinical pharmacology of mivacurium chloride: a review. J Clin Anesth 1992; 4: 153–163
31 Savarese JJ, Ali HH, Basta SJ et al. The clinical neuromuscular pharmacology of mivacurium chloride (BW B1090U). A short-acting nondepolarizing ester neuromuscular blocking drug. Anesthesiology 1988; 68: 723–732
32 Kaufman T. Cardiac arrhythmias in dentistry. Lancet 1965; ii: 287
33 Ryder W. The electrocardiogram in dental anaesthesia. Anaesthesia 1970; 36: 492–497
34 El-Hakim M. Cardiac dysrhythmias during dental surgery. Comparison of hyoscine, glycopyrrolate and placebo premedication. Anaesthesiol Reanim 1991; 16: 393–398
35 Hamilton-Farrell MR, Nightingale JJ. Cardiac dysrhythmias, carbon dioxide tensions and blood halothane concentrations during dental anaesthesia. Eur J Anaesthesiol 1988; 5: 323–329
36 Rodrigo CR. Cardiac dysrhythmias with general anesthesia during dental surgery. Anesth Prog 1988; 35: 102–115
37 Ryder W, Wright CJ. Halothane and enflurane dental anaesthesia. Anaesthesia 1981; 36: 492–497
38 Wrigley SR, Fairfield JE, Jones RM, Black AE. Induction and recovery characteristics of desflurane in day case patients: a comparison with propofol. Anaesthesia 1991; 46: 615–622
39 Lim BL, Low TC. Total intravenous anaesthesia versus inhalational anaesthesia for dental day surgery. Anaesth Intensive Care 1992; 20: 475–478
40 Dachowski MT, Kalayjian R, Angelillo JC, Dolan EA. Continuous infusion of methohexital and alfentanil hydrochloride for general anesthesia in outpatient third molar surgery. J Oral Maxillofac Surg 1989; 47: 233–237
41 van Leeuwen L, Zuurmond WW, Deen L, Helmers HJ. Total intravenous anaesthesia with propofol, alfentanil, and oxygen–air: three different dosage schemes. Can J Anaesth 1990; 37: 282–286
42 Bostek CC, Fiducia DA, Klotz RW, Herman N. Total intravenous anaesthesia with a continuous propofol–alfentanil infusion. CRNA 1992; 3: 124–131
43 Valanne J. Recovery and discharge of patients after long propofol infusion vs isoflurane anaesthesia for ambulatory surgery. Acta Anaesthesiol Scand 1992; 36: 530–533
44 Langley MS, Heel RC. Propofol. A review of its pharmacodynamic and pharmacokinetic properties and use as an intravenous anaesthetic. Drugs 1988; 35: 334–372
45 Sonne NM, Clausen TG, Valentin N, Halck S, Munksgaard A. Total intravenous anaesthesia for direct laryngoscopy: propofol infusion compared to thiopentone combined with midazolam and methohexitone infusion. Acta Anaesthesiol Scand 1992; 36: 250–254
46 Richmond CE, Bromley LM, Woolf CJ. Preoperative morphine pre-empts postoperative pain. Lancet 1993; 342: 73–75
47 Raftery S, Sherry E. Total intravenous anaesthesia with propofol and alfentanil protects against postoperative nausea and vomiting. Can J Anaesth 1992; 39: 37–40
48 Watcha MF, White PF. Postoperative nausea and vomiting. Its etiology, treatment, and prevention. Anesthesiology 1992; 77: 162–184
49 Borgeat A, Wilder Smith OH, Saiah M, Rifat K. Subhypnotic doses of propofol possess direct antiemetic properties. Anesth Analg 1992; 74: 539–541
50 Recommendations for standards of monitoring. London: Association of Anaesthetists of Great Britain and Ireland. 1988
51 Fung DE, Cooper DJ, Barnard KM, Smith PB. Pain reported by children after dental extractions under general anaesthesia: a pilot study. Int J Paediatr Dentistry 1993; 3: 23–28
52 Muhlbauer W, Anderl H, Heeckt P et al. Early operation in craniofacial dysostosis. World J Surg 1989; 13: 366–372
53 Harding Rains AJ, Ritchie HD. Face, lips, palate, facio-maxillary injuries, ear. In: Bailey and Love's short practice of surgery. London: HK Lewis, 1975: p 491
54 Lauritzen C, Lilja J, Jarlstedt J. Airway obstruction and sleep apnea in children with craniofacial anomalies. Plast Reconstr Surg 1986; 77: 1–5
55 Speechley JA, Rugman FP. Some problems with anticoagulants in dental surgery. Dent Update 1992; 19: 204–206
56 Conti CR. Aspirin and elective surgical procedures. Clin Cardiol 1992; 15: 709–710
57 Shirvani R. An evaluation of clinical aspects of post operative autotransfusion, either alone or in conjunction with pre operative aspirin, in cardiac surgery. Br J Clin Pract 1991; 45: 105–108
58 Rawitscher RE, Jones JW, McCoy TA, Lindsley DA. A prospective study of aspirin's effect on red blood cell loss in cardiac surgery. J Cardiovasc Surg Torino 1991; 32: 1–7
59 Bo L, Belboul A, al-Khaja N, Dernevik L, Raberts D, William-Olsson G. High-dose aprotinin (trasylol) in reducing bleeding and protecting lung function in potential bleeders undergoing cardiopulmonary bypass. Chin Med J Engl 1991; 104: 980–985
60 Bidstrup BP, Royston D, Sapsford RN, Taylor KM. Reduction in blood loss and blood use after cardiopulmonary bypass with high dose aprotinin (Trasylol). J Thorac Cardiovasc Surg 1989; 97: 364–372

61. Havel M, Teufelsbauer H, Knobl P et al. Effect of intraoperative aprotinin administration on postoperative bleeding in patients undergoing cardiopulmonary bypass operation. J Thorac Cardiovasc Surg 1991; 101: 968–972
62. Lu H, Soria C, Commin PL et al. Hemostasis in patients undergoing extracorporeal circulation: the effect of aprotinin (Trasylol). Thromb Haemost 1991; 66: 633–637
63. Schonberger JP, van-Zundert A, Bredee JJ et al. Blood loss and use of blood in internal mammary artery and saphenous vein bypass grafting with and without adding a single, low-dose of aprotinin (2 million units) to the pump prime. Acta Anaesthesiol Belg 1992; 43: 187–196
64. Royston D, Bidstrup BP, Taylor KM, Sapsford RM. Reduced blood loss following open heart surgery with aprotinin (Trasylol) is associated with an increase in intraoperative activated clotting time (ACT). J Cardiothorac Anesth 1989; 3(suppl 1): 80
65. Mallett SV, Cox D, Burroughs AK, Rolles K. The intra-operative use of Trasylol (aprotinin) in liver transplantation. Transplant Int 1991; 4: 227–230
66. Mallett S, Rolles K, Cox D, Burroughs A, Hunt B. Intraoperative use of aprotinin (Trasylol) in orthotopic liver transplantation. Transplant Proc 1991; 23: 1931–1932
67. Broennle AM, Teller I. Anaesthesia for craniofacial procedures. Clin Plast Surg 1987; 14: 17–26
68. Williams PJ, Bailey PM. Management of failed oral fibreoptic intubation with laryngeal mask airway insertion under topical anaesthesia. Can J Anaesth 1993; 40: 287
69. Whitley BD, Bell WM. External and internal rigid fixation. Ann R Australas Coll Dent Surg 1991; 11: 199–208
70. Maroof M, Siddique MS, Khan RM. Modified laryngeal mask as an aid to fiberoptic endotracheal intubation. Acta Anaesthesiol Scand 1993; 37: 124
71. Kelly WB, Gupta B. Fibreoptic laryngoscopy after thyroid surgery. Can J Anaesth 1992; 39: 513
72. Cooper DW, Long GT. Difficult fibreoptic intubation in an intellectually handicapped patient. Anaesth Intensive Care 1992; 20: 227–229
73. Smith M, Calder I, Crockard A, Isert P, Nicol ME. Oxygen saturation and cardiovascular changes during fibreoptic intubation under general anaesthesia. Anaesthesia 1992; 47: 158–161
74. Smith JE, King MJ, Yanny HF, Pottinger KA, Pomirska MB. Effect of fentanyl on the circulatory responses to orotracheal fibreoptic intubation. Anaesthesia 1992; 47: 20–23
75. Brimacombe JR. LMA in awake fibreoptic bronchoscopy. Anaesth Intensive Care 1991; 19: 472
76. Smith JE, Sherwood NA. Combined use of laryngeal mask airway and fibreoptic laryngoscope in difficult intubation. Anaesth Intensive Care 1991; 19: 471–472
77. Randell T, Valli H, Lindgren L. Effects of alfentanil on the responses to awake fiberoptic nasotracheal intubation. Acta Anaesthesiol Scand 1990; 34: 59–62
78. Rashid J, Warltier B. Awake fibreoptic intubation for a rare cause of upper airway obstruction — an infected laryngocoele. Anaesthesia 1989; 44: 834–836
79. Ovassapian A, Krejcie TC, Yelich SJ, Dykes MH. Awake fibreoptic intubation in the patient at high risk of aspiration. Br J Anaesth 1989; 62: 13–16
80. Wei WI, Siu KF, Lau WF, Lam KH. Emergency endotracheal intubation under fiberoptic endoscopic guidance for malignant laryngeal obstruction. Otolaryngol Head Neck Surg 1988; 98: 10–13
81. Stool SE. Intubation techniques of the difficult airway. Pediatr Infect Dis J 1988; 7(suppl): S154–S156
82. Allen JG, Flower EA The Brain laryngeal mask. An alternative to difficult intubation. Br Dent J 1990; 168: 202–204
83. Churchill Davidson HC (ed) Thoracic anaesthesia In: A practice of anaesthesia. London: Lloyd-Luke (Medical Books) 1984: p 376
84. Williams PJ, Bailey PM. Management of failed oral fibreoptic intubation with laryngeal mask airway insertion under topical anaesthesia. Can J Anaesth 1993; 40: 287
85. Higgins D, Astley BA, Berg S. Guided intubation via the laryngeal mask. Anaesthesia 1992; 47: 816
86. Chadd GD, Walford AJ, Crane DL. The 3.5/4.5 modification for fiberscope-guided tracheal intubation using the laryngeal mask airway. Anesth Analg 1992; 75: 307–308
87. Iversen AD. [Difficult intubation-helped by a laryngeal mask] Ugeskr Laeger 1992; 154: 1782–1783
88. Silk JM, Hill HM, Calder I. Difficult intubation and the laryngeal mask. Eur J Anaesthesiol 1991; (suppl 4): 47–51
89. Heath ML. Endotracheal intubation through the laryngeal mask — helpful when laryngoscopy is difficult or dangerous. Eur J Anaesthesiol (suppl 4): 41–45
90. Heath ML, Allagain J. Intubation through the laryngeal mask. A technique for unexpected difficult intubation. Anaesthesia 1991; 46: 545–548
91. Bonnet C, Roche B, d'Athis F, du Cailar J. Nicardipine vs trinitrin for controlled hypotension in maxillo-facial surgery. Cah Anesthesiol 1992; 40: 171–175
92. Segredo V, Caldwell JE, Matthay MA, Sharma ML, Gruenke LD, Miller RD. Persistent paralysis in critically ill patients after long-term administration of vecuronium. N Engl J Med 1992; 327: 524–528
93. Comerota AJ, Katz ML, White JV. Why does prophylaxis with external pneumatic compression for deep vein thrombosis fail? Am J Surg 1992; 164: 265–268
94. Dujon DG, Chatzis LA, Hart NB. Thromboembolic prophylaxis in plastic surgery: an appraisal. Br J Plast Surg 1992; 45: 418–420
95. Marshall JC. Prophylaxis of deep venous thrombosis and pulmonary embolism. Can J Surg 1991; 34: 551–554
96. Clagett GP, Reisch S. Prevention of venous thromboembolism in general surgical patients. Results of meta-analysis. Ann Surg 1988; 208: 227–240
97. Ereth MH, Lennon RL, Sessler DI. Limited heat transfer between thermal compartments during rewarming in vasoconstricted patients. Aviat Space Environ Med 1992; 63: 1065–1069
98. Phillips R, Skov P. Rewarming and cardiac surgery: a review. Heart Lung 1988; 17: 511–520
99. Carli F, Emery PW, Freemantle CA. Effect of peroperative normothermia on postoperative protein

metabolism in elderly patients undergoing hip arthroplasty. Br J Anaesth 1989; 63: 276–282
100 Sessler DI, McGuire J, Sessler AM. Perioperative thermal insulation. Anesthesiology 1991; 74: 875–879
101 Deriaz H, Fiez N, Lienhart A. [Effect of hygrophobic filter or heated humidifier on peroperative hypothermia.] Ann Fr Anesth Reanim 1992; 11: 145–149
102 May C. Observations on temperature changes in patients undergoing insertion of a dynamic hip screw. Br J Theatre Nurs 1992; 1: 6–8
103 Bissonnette B. Temperature monitoring in pediatric anesthesia: Int Anesthesiol Clin 1992; 30: 63–76
104 Berwick JE, Lessin ME. Brachial plexus injury occurring during oral and maxillofacial surgery: a case report. J Oral Maxillofac Surg 1989; 47: 643–645
105 Winslow RM. Optimal hematologic variables for oxygen transport, including P50, hemoglobin cooperativity, hematocrit, acid–base status, and cardiac function. Biomater Artif Cells Artif Organs 1988; 16: 149–171
106 Messmer K. Hemodilution — possibilities and safety aspects. Acta Anaesthesiol Scand 1988; (suppl 89): 49–53
107 Donaldson MD, Seaman MJ, Park GR. Massive blood transfusion. Br J Anaesth 1992; 69: 621–630
108 Kulkarni P, Bhattacharya S, Petros AJ. Torsade de pointes and long QT syndrome following major blood transfusion. Anaesthesia 1992; 47: 125–127
109 Reddy SV, Sein K. Potassium and massive blood transfusion. Singapore Med J 1991; 32: 29–30
110 Hewitt PE, Machin SJ. ABC of transfusion. Massive blood transfusion. Br Med J 1990; 300: 107–109
111 Brown KA, Bissonnette B, MacDonald M, Poon AO. Hyperkalaemia during massive blood transfusion in paediatric craniofacial surgery. Can J Anaesth 1990; 37: 401–408
112 Sawyer PR, Harrison CR. Massive transfusion in adults. Diagnoses, survival and blood bank support. Vox Sang 1990; 58: 199–203
113 Macfie A, Goiti J, Hunsley J. The use of fresh blood to control severe haemorrhage associated with massive blood transfusion after cardiopulmonary bypass. Eur J Cardiothorac Surg 1990; 4: 171–173
114 Michelsen T, Salmela L, Tigerstedt I, Makelainen A, Linko K. Massive blood transfusion: is there a limit? Crit Care Med 1989; 17: 699–700
115 Dzik WH, Kirkley SA. Citrate toxicity during massive blood transfusion. Transfus Med Rev 1988; 2: 76–94
116 British Society for Haematology. British Committee for Standardization in Haematology Blood Transfusion Task Force. Guidelines for transfusion for massive blood loss. Clin Lab Haematol 1988; 10: 265–273
117 Chandrasekhar B, Terz JJ, Kokal WA, Beatty JD, Gottlieb ME. The inferior trapezius musculocutaneous flap in head and neck reconstruction. Ann Plast Surg 1988; 21: 201–209
118 Rorarius MG, Baer GA, Metsa Ketela T, Miralles J, Palomaki E, Vapaatalo H. Effects of peri-operatively administered diclofenac and indomethacin on blood loss, bleeding time and plasma prostanoids in man. Eur J Anaesthesiol 1989; 6: 335–342
119 Anderson SK, al-Shaikh BA. Diclofenac in combination with opiate infusion after joint replacement surgery. Anaesth Intensive Care 1991; 19: 535–538
120 Laitinen J, Nuutinen L. Intravenous diclofenac coupled with PCA fentanyl for pain relief after total hip replacement. Anesthesiology 1992; 76: 194–198
121 Laitinen J, Nuutinen LS, Puranen J, Ranta P, Salomaki T. Effect of a non-steroidal anti-inflammatory drug, diclofenac, on haemostasis in patients undergoing total hip replacement. Acta Anaesthesiol Scand 1992; 36: 486–489
122 Perttunen K, Kalso E, Heinonen J, Salo J. IV diclofenac in post-thoracotomy pain. Br J Anaesth 1992; 68: 474–480
123 Baer GA, Rorarius MG, Kolehmainen S, Selin S. The effect of paracetamol or diclofenac administered before operation on postoperative pain and behaviour after adenoidectomy in small children. Anaesthesia 1992; 47: 1078–1080
124 Thiagarajan J, Bates S, Hitchcock M, Morgan-Hughes J. Blood loss following tonsillectomy in children. A blind comparison of diclofenac and papaveretum. Anaesthesia 1993; 48: 132–135
125 Nakamura Y, Ohtaki S, Makino R, Tanaka T, Ishimura Y. Superoxide anion is the initial product in the hydrogen peroxide formation catalyzed by NADPH oxidase in porcine thyroid plasma membrane. J Biol Chem 1989; 264: 4759–4761
126 Gerard CM, Lefort A, Christophe D et al. Distinct transcriptional effects of cAMP on 2 thyroid specific genes: thyroperoxidase and thyroglobulin. Horm Metab Res 1990; (suppl 23): 38–43
127 Byfield PG. Plasma transport of thyroid hormones. Acta Med Australia 1988; 15 (suppl; 1): 10–11
128 Sakata S, Komaki T, Nakamura S et al. Binding of thyroid hormones to human hemoglobin and localization of the binding site. J Protein Chem 1990; 9: 743–750
129 Munro SL, Lim CF, Hall JG et al. Drug competition for thyroxine binding to transthyretin (prealbumin): comparison with effects on thyroxine-binding globulin. J Clin Endocrinol Metab 1989; 68: 1141–1147
130 Lim CF, Bai Y, Topliss DJ, Barlow JW, Stockigt JR. Drug and fatty acid effects on serum thyroid hormone binding. J Clin Endocrinol Metab 1988; 67: 682–688
131 Villa-Verde DM, Defresne MP, Vannier-dos-Santos MA, Dussault JH, Boniver J, Savino W. Identification of nuclear triiodothyronine receptors in the thymic epithelium. Endocrinology 1992; 131: 1313–1320
132 Barakat Walter I, Duc C, Sarlieve LL, Puymirat J, Dussault JH, Droz B. The expression of nuclear 3,5,3' triiodothyronine receptors is induced in Schwann cells by nerve transection. Exp Neurol 1992; 116: 189–197
133 Laudet V, Hanni C, Coll J, Catzeflis F, Stehelin D. Evolution of the nuclear receptor gene superfamily. Embo J 1992; 11: 1003–1013
134 Parker MG. Structure and function of nuclear hormone receptors. Semin Cancer Biol 1990; 1: 81–87
135 Moore DD. Diversity and unity in the nuclear hormone receptors: a terpenoid receptor superfamily. New Biol 1990; 2: 100–105
136 Knopp J, Brtko J. Nuclear binding of thyroid hormones and activity of malic enzyme and ornithine decarboxylase in rat liver during postnatal development. Endocrinol Exp 1990; 24: 429–435

137 Lin KH, Fukuda T, Cheng SY. Hormone and DNA binding activity of a purified human thyroid hormone nuclear receptor expressed in *Escherichia coli.* J Biol Chem 1990; 265: 5161–5165

138 Krieger NS, Stappenbeck TS, Stern PH. Characterization of specific thyroid hormone receptors in bone. J Bone Miner Res 1988; 3: 473–478

139 Ashitaka Y, Maruo M, Takeuchi Y, Nakayama H, Mochizuki M. 3,5,3'-triiodo-L-thyronine binding sites in nuclei of human trophoblastic cells. Endocrinol Jpn 1988; 35: 197–206

140 Paradis P, Lambert C, Rouleau J. Amiodarone antagonizes the effects of T_3 at the receptor level: an additional mechanism for its in vivo hypothyroid-like effects. Can J Physiol Pharmacol 1991; 69: 865–870

141 Smith TJ, Davis FB, Davis PJ. Retinoic acid is a modulator of thyroid hormone activation of Ca^{2+}-ATPase in the human erythrocyte membrane (published erratum appears in J Biol Chem 1989; 264: 10326). J Biol Chem 1989; 264: 687–689

142 Pailler Rodde I, Garcin H, Higueret P. Effect of retinoids on protein kinase C activity and on the binding characteristics of the tri-iodothyronine nuclear receptor. J Endocrinol 1991; 128: 245–251

143 Topliss DJ, Hamblin PS, Kolliniatis E, Lim CF, Stockigt JR. Furosemide, fenclofenac, diclofenac, mefenamic acid and meclofenamic acid inhibit specific T_3 binding in isolated rat hepatic nuclei. J Endocrinol Invest 1988; 11: 355–360

144 Ichikawa K, Hashizume K. Cellular binding proteins of thyroid hormones. Life Sci 1991; 49: 1513–1522

145 Segal J. Action of the thyroid hormone at the level of the plasma membrane. Endocrinol Res 1989; 15: 619–649

146 Ferreiro B, Bernal J, Goodyer CG, Branchard CL. Estimation of nuclear thyroid hormone receptor saturation in human fetal brain and lung during early gestation. J Clin Endocrinol Metab 1988; 67: 853–856

147 Palmero S, Prati M, De Marco P, Trucchi P, Fugassa E. Thyroidal regulation of nuclear tri-iodothyronine receptors in the developing rat testis. J Endocrinol 1993; 136: 277–282

148 Shoshan Barmatz V, Shainberg A. Inhibition of Ca^{2+} accumulation in isolated sarcoplasmic reticulum by thyroid hormones. Biochim Biophys Acta 1991; 1065: 82–88

149 Andersson ML, Nordstrom K, Demczuk S, Harbers M, Vennstrom B. Thyroid hormone alters the DNA binding properties of chicken thyroid hormone receptors alpha and beta. Nucleic Acids Res 1992; 20: 4803–4810

150 Yen PM, Darling DS, Chin WW. Basal and thyroid hormone receptor auxiliary protein-enhanced binding of thyroid hormone receptor isoforms to native thyroid hormone response elements. Endocrinology 1991; 129: 3331–3336

151 Valdermarsson S, Ikomi Kumm J, Monti M. Thyroid hormones and thermogenesis: a microcalorimetric study of overall cell metabolism in lymphocytes from patients with different degrees of thyroid dysfunction. Acta Endocrinol Copenh 1990; 123: 155–160

152 Khawaja Y, Dobnig H, Shapiro LE, Surks MI. Increase in hepatic mitochondrial alpha-glycerophosphate dehydrogenase activity after surgical stress in hyperthyroid rats. Endocrinology 1990; 127: 387–393

153 Segal J. Calcium is the first messenger for the action of thyroid hormone at the level of the plasma membrane: first evidence for an acute effect of thyroid hormone on calcium uptake in the heart. Endocrinology 1990; 126: 2693–2702

154 Rapiejko PJ, Watkins DC, Ros M, Malbon CC. Thyroid hormones regulate G-protein beta-subunit mRNA expression in vivo. J Biol Chem 1989; 264: 16183–16189

155 Depix M, Lavandero S, Sapag-Hagar M. The role of thyroid hormones in the control of beta-adrenergic receptors in rat mammary gland. Res Commun Chem Pathol Pharmacol 1989; 64: 79–86

156 Franklyn JA. The molecular mechanisms of thyroid hormone action. Baillières Clin Endocrinol Metab 1988; 2: 891–909

157 Hoch FL. Lipids and thyroid hormones. Prog Lipid Res 1988; 27: 199–270

158 Segal J. In vivo effect of 3,5,3'-triiodothyronine on calcium uptake in several tissues in the rat: evidence for a physiological role for calcium as the first messenger for the prompt action of thyroid hormone at the level of the plasma membrane. Endocrinology 1990; 127: 17–24

159 Denver RJ, Licht P. Modulation of neuropeptide-stimulated pituitary hormone secretion in hatchling turtles. Gen Comp Endocrinol 1990; 77: 107–115

160 Lewinski A, Wajs R, Karbownik M. Effects of pineal-derived indolic compounds and of certain neuropeptides on the growth processes in the thyroid gland. Thyroidol Clin Exp 1992; 4: 11–15

161 Ahren B. Regulatory peptides in the thyroid gland — a review on their localization and function. Acta Endocrinol Copenh 1991; 124: 225–232

162 Flynn SD, Nishiyama RH, Bigos ST. Autoimmune thyroid disease: immunological, pathological, and clinical aspects. Crit Rev Clin Lab Sci 1988; 26: 43–95

163 McKenzie JM, Zakarija M. Fetal and neonatal hyperthyroidism and hypothyroidism due to maternal TSH receptor antibodies. Thyroid 1992; 2: 155–159

164 Rees Smith B, McLachlan SM, Furmaniak J. Autoantibodies to the thyrotropin receptor. Endocrinol Rev 1988; 9: 106–121

165 Mariotti S, Chiovato L, Vitti P et al. Recent advances in the understanding of humoral and cellular mechanisms implicated in thyroid autoimmune disorders. Clin Immunol Immunopathol 1989; 50: S73–S84

166 Peters KR, Nance P, Wingard DW. Malignant hyperthyroidism or malignant hyperthermia. Anesth Analg 1981; 60: 613–615

167 Bennett MH, Wainwright AP. Acute thyroid crisis on induction of anaesthesia. Anaesthesia 1989; 44: 28–33

168 Christensen PA, Nissen LR. Treatment of thyroid storm in a child with dantrolene. Br J Anaesth 1987; 59: 523

169 Liewendahl K. Assessment of thyroid status by laboratory methods: developments and perspectives. Scand J Clin Lab Invest 1990; (suppl 201): 83–92

170 Maruotti RA, Zannini P, Viani MP, Voci C, Pezzuoli-G. Surgical treatment of substernal goiters. Int Surg 1991; 76: 12–17

171 Melliere-D, Saada F, Etienne G, Becquemin JP,

Bonnet F. Goiter with severe respiratory compromise: evaluation and treatment. Surgery 1988; 103: 367–373

172 Amino N. Autoimmunity and hypothyroidism. Baillières Clin Endocrinol Metab 1988; 2: 591–617

173 Ragaller M, Quintel M, Bender HJ, Albrecht DM. Myxedema coma as a rare postoperative complication. Anaesthetist 1993; 42: 179–183

174 Zaloga GP, Chernow B, Smallridge RC et al. A longitudinal evaluation of thyroid function in critically ill surgical patients. Ann Surg 1985; 201: 456–464

175 McLarty DG, Ratcliffe WA, McColl K, Smyth L. Thyroid hormone levels and prognosis in patients with serious non-thyroidal illness. Lancet 1975; ii: 275–276

176 Burr WA, Black EG, Griffiths RS, Hoffenberg R, Meinhold H, Wenzel KW. Serum triiodothyronine and reverse triiodothyronine concentrations after surgical operation. Lancet 1975; ii: 1277–1279

177 Kaptein EM, Spencer CA, Kamiel MB, Nicoloff JT. Prolonged dopamine administration and thyroid hormone economy in normal and critically ill subjects. J Clin Endocrinol Metab 1980; 51: 387–393

178 Noreng MF, Jensen P, Tjellden NU. Per- and postoperative changes in the concentrations of serum thyrotropin under general anaesthesia, compared to general anaesthesia with epidural analgesia. Acta Anaesthesiol Scand 1987; 31: 292–294

179 Oyama T, Latto P, Holaday DA, Chang H. Effect of isoflurane anaesthesia and surgery on thyroid function in man. Can Anaesth Soc J 1975; 22: 474–477

180 Oyama T, Shibata S, Matsuki A, Kudo T. Serum endogenous thyroxine levels in man during anaesthesia and surgery. Br J Anaesth 1969; 41: 103–108

181 Chikenji T, Mizutani M, Kitsukawa Y. Anaesthesia, not surgical stress, induces increases in serum concentrations of reverse triiodothyronine and thyroxine during surgery. Exp Clin Endocrinol 1990; 95: 217–223

182 Massart C, Le Tellier C, Malledant Y, Leclech G, Nicol M. Modulation of the functional properties of human thyrocytes in monolayer or follicle culture: effects of some anaesthetic drugs. J Mol Endocrinol 1991; 7: 57–62

183 Ho WM, Wang YS, Tsou CT et al. 1989 Thyroid function during isoflurane anesthesia and valvular heart surgery. J Cardiothorac Anesth 1989; 3: 550–557

184 Imberti R, Maira G, Confortinin MC, Preseglio I, Domenegati E. Effect of fentanyl–oxygen anesthesia during cardiac surgery on serum thyroid hormones. Acta Anaesth Belg 1988; 39: 217–222

185 Rudenko MI, Pas'ko VG. A method of cervical plexus anesthesia during surgery of the neck and its organs. Anesteziol Reanimatol 1991; 2: 47–49

186 Saxe AW, Brown E, Hamburger SW. Thyroid and parathyroid surgery performed with patient under regional anesthesia. Surgery 1988; 103: 415–420

187 Murkin JM. Anesthesia and hypothyroidism: a review of thyroxine, physiology, pharmacology and anesthetic implications. Anesth Analg 1982; 61: 371–383

188 Mercer DM, Eltringham RJ. Anaesthesia for thyroid surgery. Ear Nose Throat J 1985; 64: 375–378

189 Younker D, Clark R, Coveler L. Fiberoptic endobronchial intubation for resection of an anterior mediastinal mass. Anesthesiology 1989; 70: 144–146

190 Sebel PS. Thyroid and parathyroid disease. Curr Anaesth Crit Care 1992; 3: 23–29

191 Eger EI. Isoflurane — a review. Anesthesiology 1981; 55: 559–576

Appendix A: Principal recommendations of the Poswillo report

PRINCIPAL RECOMMENDATIONS (GENERAL ANAESTHESIA)

1. The use of general anaesthesia should be avoided wherever possible
2. The same general standards in respect of personnel, premises and equipment must apply irrespective of where the general anaesthetic is administered
3. Dental anaesthesia must be regarded as a postgraduate subject
4. All anaesthetics should be administered by accredited anaesthetists who must recognize their responsibility for providing dental anaesthetic services
5. Anaesthetic training should include specific experience in dental anaesthesia
6. Health authorities should review the provision of consultant dental anaesthetic sessions to ensure they are sufficient to meet local needs
7. Doctors and dentists with knowledge, experience and competence sufficient to satisfy the Royal College of Anaesthetists and the Faculty of Dental Surgery be under no detriment
8. The no-detriment arrangements must have been implemented within 2 years of the publication of the report
9. The administration of general anaesthesia, in dental surgeries and clinics equipped to the recommended standards of monitoring necessary for patient safety, shall continue
10. An electrocardiogram, a pulse oximeter and a non-invasive blood pressure device are essential for the non-invasive monitoring of a patient under general anaesthesia
11. A capnograph should be used where tracheal anaesthesia is practised
12. A defibrillator must be available
13. Equipment conforming to recognized standards should be purchased and installed, regularly serviced and maintained in accordance with manufacturers' instructions
14. General anaesthesia surgeries should be subject to inspection and registration
15. Intravenous agents should be administered via an indwelling needle or cannula which should not be removed until the patient has fully recovered
16. Appropriate training must be provided for those assisting the anaesthetist and the dentist
17. At no time should the recovering patient be left unattended
18. Adequate recovery facilities should be available
19. Good contemporaneous records of all treatments and procedures should be kept
20. Written consent should be obtained on each occasion prior to the administration of a general anaesthetic
21. Consideration should be given to developing a national general anaesthetic/sedation consent form for general dental practitioners
22. Patients should be provided with comprehensive pre- and post-treatment instructions and advice

PRINCIPAL RECOMMENDATIONS (SEDATION)

1. Sedation should be used in preference to general anaesthesia wherever possible
2. For sedation by inhalation the minimum concentration of oxygen should be fixed at 30% by volume
3. A British Standard for relative analgesia machines should be developed
4. Flumazenil should be reserved for emergency use
5. Intravenous sedation should be limited to the use of one drug with a single titrated dose and an endpoint remote from anaesthesia
6. The use of intravenous sedation in all children should be approached with caution
7. Practical training in sedation for dentistry should be provided by dentists

8. More emphasis should be given to undergraduate education in sedation
9. Undergraduates should have had experience of administering inhalational sedation in 10 cases
10. All undergraduates should be proficient in venepuncture
11. Undergraduates should have had experience of managing at least 5 cases involving intravenous sedation
12. Interested dentists should complete a recognized course in intravenous sedation within 2 years of qualification. Refresher training should be sought at appropriate intervals thereafter
13. Guidance should be provided for Postgraduate Dental Deans in the organization of courses
14. Dentists should make themselves conversant with the syllabus for the advanced certificate for dental surgery assistants
15. Dentists must be aware of the significance of pulse oximetry readings
16. All patients treated with the aid of sedative techniques should be accompanied by a responsible person
17. Prior written consent to treatment should be obtained and comprehensive written pre- and post-treatment instructions and advice be provided.

PRINCIPAL RECOMMENDATIONS (RESUSCITATION)

1. Every member of the dental team should be trained in resuscitation. Training should be a team activity
2. Resuscitation procedures should be regularly practised in the surgery under simulated conditions
3. A medical history, including any medication the patient may be receiving, should be obtained prior to every course of treatment
4. Written instructions should include the importance of not consuming food or drink for at least 4 h prior to general anaesthesia or sedation
5. All dental staff must be fully conversant with, and proficient in, the basic life support skills
6. Every member of the dental team should have their proficiency in cardiopulmonary resuscitation tested and certified
7. Dentists must be proficient in the use of airway adjuncts
8. Dental students should be taught basic life support very early in their course. By graduation they must have knowledge of formal airway management and be proficient in the use of airway adjuncts
9. All dental anaesthetists must have advanced life support skills
10. All dentists should look critically at their surgeries to ensure their suitability for resuscitation
11. Every dental surgery should be equipped to enable resuscitation to be performed
12. The drugs listed should be available in every dental surgery
13. All dental practitioners should be proficient in venepuncture
14. Stocks of drugs should be reviewed regularly and out-of-date stock replaced
15. The listed items of equipment as set out in Appendix B should be available in surgeries as appropriate

Appendix B: (Department of Health recommendations from Poswillo report)

LIST OF DRUGS FOR EMERGENCY USE

Drugs to be available in every dental practice

1. Oxygen
2. Adrenaline 1 mg in 1 ml or 10 ml — × 5 ampoules
3. Lignocaine 1% (10 ml) — × 5 ampoules
4. Atropine 0.6 mg (1 ml) — × 5 ampoules
5. Calcium chloride 13.4% (10 ml) — × 2 ampoules
6. Sodium bicarbonate 8.4% (50 ml) — × 3 ampoules
7. Glyceryl trinitrate tabs 300 µg — × 10 tablets
   or Glyceryl trinitrate 400 µg per dose — × 1 sublingual spray
8. Aminophylline 250 mg (10 ml) — × 2 ampoules
9. Salbutamol inhaler 100 µg per dose — × 2 refills
10. Chlorpheniramine maleate 10 mg (1 ml) — × 2 ampoules
11. Dextrose 50% (50 ml) — × 1 vial
12. Hydrocortisone 100 mg (2 ml) — × 5 ampoules
13. Midazolam 10 mg (5 ml) — × 5 ampoules
14. Infusion solutions
    (a) Dextrose 4%/saline 0.18% — 500 ml × 2
    (b) Colloid solution — 500 ml × 2

Drugs to be available in dental practices providing intravenous sedation

1. Flumazenil 500 µg (5 ml) — × 5 ampoules
2. Naloxone 0.4 mg (1 ml) — × 5 ampoules

Drugs to be available in dental practices providing general anaesthesia

1. Suxamethonium 100 mg (2 ml) — × 5 ampoules

LIST OF ESSENTIAL ITEMS OF EQUIPMENT FOR RESUSCITATION WHICH MUST BE AVAILABLE IN EVERY DENTAL PRACTICE

Airway maintenance

1. Suction apparatus — powered and portable (independently powered)
2. Simple airway adjunct (e.g. pocket resuscitator mask with valve)
3. Cricothyroid puncture needle — × 1

Oxygen and artificial ventilation

1. Portable oxygen with appropriate valves, metering and delivery system
2. Self-inflating bag, valve and mask with oxygen enhancement facility

Maintenance of circulation

1. Disposable syringes (sizes 2, 5, 10 ml) — × 5 of each size
2. Disposable needles (sizes 21 and 23 G) — × 10 of each size
3. Disposable intravenous cannulae (sizes 16 and 22 G) — × 5 of each size
4. Disposable intravenous infusion sets — × 2
5. Scissors — × 1
6. Tourniquet, sphygmomanometer and stethoscope — × 1 of each
7. Injection swabs

LIST OF ESSENTIAL ITEMS OF EQUIPMENT REQUIRED IN A DENTAL PRACTICE WHERE DENTAL GENERAL ANAESTHESIA IS ADMINISTERED

1. An electrocardiogram
2. A pulse oximeter

3. A non-invasive blood pressure device
4. A capnograph (where tracheal anaesthesia is practised)
5. A defibrillator

LIST OF ESSENTIAL ITEMS OF ADDITIONAL EQUIPMENT FOR RESUSCITATION IN A SEDATION SURGERY

Airway maintenance

1. Suction tubing and Yankauer sucker × 1 of each
2. Suction catheters — sizes 6, 10 FG × 2 of each
3. Oropharyngeal airways — sizes 1, 2, 3 × 1 of each

LIST OF ESSENTIAL ITEMS OF ADDITIONAL EQUIPMENT FOR RESUSCITATION IN A GENERAL ANAESTHETIC SURGERY

1. Suction tubing and Yankauer sucker × 1 of each
2. Suction catheters — sizes 6, 10 FG × 2 of each
3. Oropharyngeal airways — sizes 1, 2, 3 × 2 of each
4. Nasopharyngeal airways — sizes 6, 7, 8 mm × 1 of each
5. Disposable tracheal tubes — sizes 4.5, 5, 6, 7, 8, 9 mm × 1 of each
6. Macintosh laryngoscope × 1
   Adult blade × 1
   Child blade × 1
   (with batteries and spare bulbs)
7. Catheter mount × 1
8. Mouth gag — with offset jaws × 1
9. Magill intubating forceps × 1
10. 20 ml syringe for tube cuff inflation × 1
11. KY jelly × 1
12. Adhesive tape × 1

14. Anaesthesia for ENT and ophthalmological surgery

A. W. A. Crossley

GENERAL PRINCIPLES

Although the similarities between anaesthesia for ear, nose and throat (ENT) surgery and anaesthesia for eye surgery may not be apparent on superficial inspection, the two areas share much in common. Both require a high degree of co-operation between surgeon and anaesthetist, and a high degree of understanding of both parties of the challenge faced by the other. Both may involve surgery at the extremes of age, and in both areas the anaesthetist is removed from direct access to the airway. In addition, active intervention by the anaesthetist may be required to control blood pressure. A sound understanding of the principles of surgery and physiology is necessary to perform an accurate pre-operative assessment in patients who can be as challenging as any an anaesthetist may face. Little surgery in either field is life-saving, but most brings benefit to the patient in terms of relief of symptoms and improvement in quality of life.

Pre-operative assessment

In both ENT surgery and in ophthalmology, patients may present at the extremes of age. The very young present for examination under anaesthesia. This may be necessary for assessment of hearing, of sight or for diagnosis of congenital abnormality. Children presenting in this way may have multiple handicaps, or other congenital abnormalities. In particular, congenital heart disease is common in this group. Young children also present commonly for strabismus surgery, tonsillectomy and adenoidectomy, and for the insertion of grommets. In procedures that require tracheal intubation, the young child presents a different challenge to the adult patient, because of the differences in the anatomy of the airway.[1] Compared with the adult, the larynx is in a more cephalad position, and the tongue is larger with respect to the size of the oral cavity. In the infant, the epiglottis is relatively larger and less flexible than in the adult, and assumes a greater angle with the anterior pharyngeal wall, making it more prominent. In the child, the cricoid ring forms the narrowest part of the airway, whereas in the adult this is usually the rima glottidis.

Many patients who present for cataract surgery are elderly and suffer from multiple systemic illnesses such as diabetes mellitus, hypertension, ischaemic heart disease and chronic lung disease. They may be receiving multiple drug therapy and they require special care in assessment, more time than younger patients for that assessment, and appropriate pre-operative management. Systemic hypertension is commer with increasing age, and the more elderly patients tend to be treated with less modern therapy regimens.[2] In some areas of the UK, chronic respiratory disease is common in elderly men, who are often surprisingly stoical about their disability. Their ability to hold a conversation with friends whilst walking and their pattern of daily activities outside the home then assume greater importance in the pre-operative assessment. In diabetic patients, control of blood sugar may be less than adequate and the problem of compliance is compounded by poor eyesight and confusion, making the self-administration of insulin difficult, if not impossible. The problems associated with anaesthetizing for the elderly patient have been discussed by Waldmann.[3]

Maintenance of the airway

In both ENT surgery and ophthalmology, the anaesthetist is removed from the operative site and is distanced from the patient. In all but the most simple procedures, this necessitates tracheal intubation in order to provide a secure airway. The act of intubation in itself may introduce difficulties which must be resolved, since in ENT practice many patient have conditions of infective or allergic origin, and consequently may have reactive airways. Intubation in these patients may provoke bronchospasm, and the chances of laryngospasm following extubation are high. In a spontaneously breathing patient at light levels of anaesthesia, the patient may cough as a result of the presence of the tracheal tube. The deep anaesthesia required to overcome this is not consistent with the rapid recovery expected of a patient who may have blood and possibly pus or fragments of tissue in the vicinity of the larynx following extubation. Coughing makes ENT surgery difficult in two respects; first, movement of the patient's head interferes with surgical manipulation, and second, venous congestion caused by coughing increases blood loss from the operative site and further obscures the operative field. In the intra-ocular procedure, coughing and straining upon the tracheal tube raise intra-ocular pressure, and make surgery both difficult and hazardous. A technique of light general anaesthesia combined with muscular paralysis and intermittent positive pressure ventilation overcomes many of these difficulties, but does not necessarily allow a smooth extubation without coughing, which is of equal importance, particularly in eye surgery.[4]

Removal of the anaesthetist from the patient's head necessitates precautions to protect the patient's eyes from injury. The cornea of all patients under general anaesthesia should be protected and kept moist, as must those of other unconscious patients. The tear film maintains the translucency of the cornea, and is important in the nutrition of the cornea in that it permits diffusion of oxygen from the atmosphere, and has bactericidal properties. In order to maintain the tear film in the absence of blinking it is useful to instil artificial tears (hypromellose) or to use an ophthalmic ointment to protect the cornea, and unless surgery dictates that the eyes be left uncovered, the eyelids should be closed and the eyes protected by suitable padding.

Intra-operative control of blood pressure

The advent of the operating microscope in ENT surgery produced a major advance in reconstructive surgery of the middle ear. A primary requirement of this branch of surgery is a relatively bloodless field, and this has led to the use of varying degrees of controlled hypotension for procedures in which the operating microscope is employed.

A variety of techniques have been used to lower systolic blood pressure deliberately for middle-ear surgery. Profound hypotension (to systolic blood pressures less than 50 mmHg) has been employed and reported to be without complication,[5] but it is debatable whether such levels of hypotension are always safe, whether they are required for middle-ear surgery, or indeed whether hypotension is desirable at all. In most instances, a meticulous anaesthetic technique based upon mechanical ventilation to normocapnia, and with the strict avoidance of hypoxaemia, tachycardia or obstruction to venous drainage from the operative site, is sufficient to ensure an adequate surgical field. It has been reported that the blood pressure achieved with a hypotensive technique does not affect the quality of the surgical field.[6] Furthermore, despite apparent safety of the techniques employed, complications are not unknown,[7,8] even though most patients undergoing middle-ear surgery are otherwise healthy adults.

Nevertheless, if otherwise ideal anaesthesia has been obtained, moderate controlled hypotension may be induced as an adjunct to obtaining a good operative field. Artificial ventilation with halothane or isoflurane may be all that is required to lower the blood pressure, particularly with 10–15° of head-up tilt, or if tubocurarine is used to obtain neuromuscular paralysis. The addition of small amounts of the adrenoceptor antagonist labetalol has been used in association with halothane anaesthesia and gives controllable hypotension.[9] Continuous infusion of the ganglion blocker trimetaphan,[10] of mixtures of trimetaphan and sodium nitroprusside,[11,12] or of nitroglycerine[13] has also been used. The use of sodium nitroprusside is associated with a rise in blood pressure when the infusion is discontinued, and with tachyphylaxis. Both phenomena are mediated through the renin–angiotensin system.[14,15] The adenine nucleotides, adenosine and adenosine-5'-triphosphate, have also been investigated for their hypotensive effects.[16]

In ophthalmology, profound hypotension may occasionally be required to provide satisfactory conditions for local resection of choroid tumours.[4]

The requirements for laser surgery

Lasers produce a monochromatic non-divergent beam of intense light and may be used locally to destroy tissue. Medical lasers are of a number of types. The carbon dioxide laser and the neodymium yttrium–aluminium–garnet (Nd-YAG) lasers emit in the infrared spectrum, their emission being absorbed heavily by water. When the water in question is intracellular, the cell contents boil and the cell is destroyed, with little damage to adjacent structures.[17] The Nd-YAG laser emission can be transmitted via a fibre-optic cable directly to the lesion under treatment. The argon laser emits in the blue-green region of the visible spectrum, and its energy is therefore absorbed heavily by red or black pigments. It may be used for the treatment of port wine stains, haemangiomata, and for the removal of tattoos. The ruby laser emits light in the red part of the visible spectrum and is used for photocoagulation of diabetic retinopathy.

The carbon dioxide laser is now established in the treatment of lesions of the oral cavity, larynx and trachea. The advantages of laser surgery over conventional microsurgery lie in the accuracy of the device, and the absence of bleeding and oedema, leading to rapid healing and good functional results. A high degree of co-operation between surgeon and anaesthetist is required in this field because of the shared responsibility for the airway.[18] The problem for the anaesthetist arises from the presence of a high-energy ignition source (the laser beam) in the airway together with oxygen, nitrous oxide and combustible materials such as the wall of a conventional tracheal tube. Nitrous oxide is an oxidizing agent and supports combustion in its own right.[19] The potential for conflagration is clearly high.

The laser beam is most likely to come into contact with combustible material in the form of the tracheal tube, and various tactics have been adopted to allow the co-existence of tube and laser. A standard polyvinylchloride tracheal tube may be protected from contact with the laser beam by wrapping it in wet gauze or reflective aluminium foil or by coating it with dental acrylic.[20-22] None of these approaches is ideal, not least because it is possible for incandescent tissue particles to ignite the tube.[21] Wet gauze dries out rapidly, and aluminium foil does not protect a tube from repeated strikes from the laser beam. The cuff of the tracheal tube must be protected separately, usually by a pledget of wet cotton introduced above the cuff by the surgeon. Attempts to produce laser-proof tracheal tubes by coating them with a fine reflective layer of metal have proved disappointing,[23] but a flexible metal tube[24] is satisfactory and relatively atraumatic in use. The addition of 60% helium to the fresh gas flow is reported to retard laser-induced fires in polyvinylchloride tracheal tubes.[25]

An alternative approach to protecting the tracheal tube is to provide anaesthesia without one. Jet insufflation using the Sanders injector and a foil-wrapped cathether placed through the vocal cords[26] or via the operating laryngoscope or bronchoscope[18] provides satisfactory operating and ventilatory conditions. Alternatively, intravenous anaesthesia in combination with superior laryngeal nerve block and spontaneous ventilation may be used.[27]

In addition to the possibility of fire within the patient's airway, other hazards are associated with the surgical use of lasers. Laser beams reflected from foil-wrapped tracheal tubes may cause burns elsewhere in the pharynx.[28] Misdirected beams have been reported to cause damage distant to the site of surgery, and pneumomediastinum and pneumothorax have resulted.[29,30] Operating room personnel are at risk from stray laser beams or reflected laser light. Visible laser beams may cause retinal damage,[31] whilst the carbon dioxide and Nd-YAG lasers are associated with corneal damage.[32] For this reason, all attendants must wear suitable eye protection.

Autonomic reflexes evoked by surgery

It is well-recognized that surgical stimulation within the facial area and oropharynx may evoke a variety of autonomic reflexes. Oral surgery under general anaesthesia is associated with a high incidence of cardiac arrhythmias,[33] mediated via the fifth cranial nerve in association with volatile agents which sensitize the myocardium to the effects of endogenous catecholamines. Ventricular arrhythmias may also occur under general anaesthesia in association with infiltration of solutions containing catecholamine vasoconstrictors, and with the use of topical cocaine as a vasoconstrictor. In dogs, the arrhythmic threshold for adrenaline is lower under general anaesthesia with halothane than it is in the awake state, but is the same as the awake state when anaesthesia is maintained with isoflurane or fluroxene.[34] In a similar study[35] in patients undergoing transsphenoidal hypophysectomy, the median effective dose (ED_{50}) for the ventricular arrhythmic effects of adrenaline was found to be 2.1 $\mu g.kg^{-1}$ under halothane anaesthesia, 6.7 $\mu g.kg^{-1}$ under isoflurane anaesthesia and 10.9 $\mu g.kg^{-1}$ under enflurane anaesthesia. When lignocaine was administered with the adrenaline, the ED_{50} for arrhythmias under halothane anaesthesia rose to 3.7 $\mu g.kg^{-1}$ suggesting that lignocaine offered some protection from adrenaline. Tucker et al[36] demonstrated in dogs that there are differences between the arrhythmic effects of different catecholamines under anaesthesia. In this study, continuous infusion of adrenaline during halothane anaesthesia produced more ventricular arrhythmias than did metaraminol, and metaraminol more than ephedrine. No arrhythmias were observed in association with phenylephrine infusion except at high dose, and the incidence of arrhythmias with all the drugs was reduced considerably when the animals were anaesthetized with isoflurane. Whilst the commonest rhythm disturbance during ophthalmic surgery is bradycardia associated with the oculocardiac reflex (see below), it is worth noting that supraventricular and ventricular arrhythmias are also common during strabismus surgery, cataract operations, iridectomy and enucleation. Junctional rhythms, which may persist for several minutes and be associated with extrasystolic beats, may occur, as may prolonged ectopic rhythms.[37]

Cocaine is used topically within the nose, primarily for its vasoconstrictor action, and may be used alone or in conjunction with adrenaline. Its vasoconstrictor effects arise from its ability to block uptake$_1$, that is re-uptake of noradrenaline into sympathetic nerve endings. The same mechanism also results in tachyarrhythmias and systemic hypertension. Cocaine is absorbed rapidly when applied to the nasal mucosa, accounting for its popularity by this route as a drug of abuse.[38] Significant arrhythmias may be associated with the absorption of cocaine in this manner[39] and myocardial infarction has been reported.[40]

The oculocardiac reflex

Bradycardia may be induced by stimulation within the facial area. When this occurs in association with stretching of the ocular muscles, often during strabismus surgery, it is known as the oculocardiac reflex. This problem is not confined to strabismus surgery and may also occur during cataract operations under general or local anaesthesia, iridectomy and enucleation.[37] Nor is the problem confined to stimulation of the extra-ocular muscles; severe bradycardia may be induced by stimulation of structures within an empty orbit.[41] A blepharocardiac reflex may also be evoked by traction on the levator aponeurosis or retractors of the lower eyelid in patients undergoing ptosis or entropion surgery.[42] A similar reflex may be evoked during resection of peri-orbital tumours,[43] by trigeminal ganglion injection,[44] by elevation of a fractured zygoma,[45] or by intranasal surgery.[46] During strabismus surgery, the oculocardiac reflex is particularly prevalent; in one study as many as 90% of patients given no anticholinergic premedication exhibited the reflex. This was reduced to an incidence of approximately 50% when glycopyrrolate or atropine was administered intramuscularly as premedication.[47] Glycopyrrolate or atropine given intravenously at the time of induction of anaesthesia is effective in preventing the reflex in the majority of patients;[47,48] there is no difference in incidence between patients breathing spontaneously and those who receive controlled ventilation.[49]

Diffusion of nitrous oxide into gaseous spaces

Nitrous oxide is 30 times more soluble in blood than is nitrogen.[50] As a consequence, when an air-filled space is in contact with plasma equilibrated with nitrous oxide, nitrous oxide diffuses from the plasma into the gaseous cavity faster than nitrogen can diffuse in the opposite direction. In these circumstances, the volume of the gaseous cavity must increase.[51,52]

This process has consequences in ENT surgery, and to a lesser extent in ophthalmology. The middle ear is an air-filled space which increases in volume during anaesthesia with nitrous oxide. Pressure rises in the middle ear until spontaneous escape occurs through the eustachian tube. In the presence of an intact tympanic membrane, the result is increased middle-ear pressure and a bulging, tense tympanic membrane, particularly if the eustachian tube is blocked. The increase in middle-ear pressure may result in barotrauma to the ossicular chain and other structures of the middle ear, particularly when there has been previous reconstructive surgery.[53] Casey & Drake-Lee[54] have shown in children that the increase in middle-ear pressure occurs rapidly on exposure to nitrous oxide, and that it is more rapid in the presence of intermittent positive-pressure ventilation than with spontaneous ventilation. Middle-ear pressure does not increase in patients who receive oxygen or oxygen-enriched air instead of nitrous oxide during anaesthesia.[55] During recovery from anaesthesia, the reverse process occurs, and nitrous oxide diffuses down a steep concentration gradient faster than it is replaced by nitrogen. As a consequence, middle-ear pressure is reduced and the tympanic membrane is pushed inwards by atmospheric pressure. The combination of a high initial rate of pressure increase when nitrous oxide is first introduced and prolonged anaesthesia results in profound subatmospheric pressures in the postoperative period.[56]

A similar problem caused by the diffusion of nitrous oxide occurs in ophthalmology when a bubble of the gas sulphur hexafluoride is introduced into the anterior chamber or vitreous, for example during surgery for retinal detachment. The solubility of nitrous oxide in blood is 117 times greater than that of sulphur hexafluoride and its diffusion coefficient is twice as great. As a consequence, in patients whose lungs are ventilated with gas mixtures containing nitrous oxide, the bubble volume may increase by as much as 96% within 30 min and 240% after 3 h.[57,58] The change in bubble volume can be largely avoided by ventilation with air, and to a lesser extent by ventilation with pure oxygen. If a patient who has undergone intravitreal injection of sulphur hexafluoride requires a further anaesthetic, nitrous oxide should be avoided for a period of at least 10 days, this being the duration of persistence of the sulphur hexafluoride bubble. The increase in intra-ocular pressure occasioned by the increase in volume of the bubble might impair the retinal circulation. Furthermore, discontinuation of nitrous oxide administration at the end of surgery might shrink an intravitreal gas bubble and impair the results of surgery.

It should be remembered that the same process causes the pressure in the cuff of a tracheal tube to increase with time[59] and this may lead to damage to the tracheal mucosa.[60] The same process has been reported to affect the cuff of a laryngeal mask airway.[61]

Principles of postoperative recovery

The provision of an adequate recovery area that is well-equipped and properly staffed with trained personnel is mandatory for both ENT surgery and ophthalmology. The recovery needs of the ENT and eye surgery patient differ somewhat and reflect the nature of the surgery and the population upon which it is being performed. Severe postoperative pain is uncommon following ENT or eye surgery.

In ENT surgery, there is often blood or pus in the oropharynx at the end of surgery, and continued ooze of these fluids postoperatively. Severe blood loss in quantities that require intervention is uncommon, but may occur, particularly from the tonsillar bed. Many patients recover from anaesthesia with nasal packs in situ, and require both reassurance and the support of an oral airway. Many patients are young children, and accordingly may require additional reassurance and comfort.

In ophthalmology, many of the patients are elderly with multiple systemic diseases. Following intra-ocular surgery, coughing, retching or vomiting in the postoperative period raise intra-ocular pressure dramatically and may put the eye at risk.[62]

ANAESTHESIA FOR SPECIFIC ENT PROCEDURES

Tonsillectomy

The aim of anaesthesia for tonsillectomy is to provide deep anaesthesia that obtunds visceral and somatic reflexes, whilst allowing a rapid return to consciousness and the return of protective airway reflexes at a time when there is certain to be blood in the vicinity of the larynx. A technique based upon tracheal intubation under the effect of suxamethonium followed by deep inhalational anaesthesia with spontaneous ventilation is satisfactory. Muscle paralysis with a competitive neuromuscular blocker allows lighter anaesthesia and consequently a more rapid return of protective reflexes. The trachea should not be extubated until the patient is awake and lying on the left side with the shoulders over a pillow and the head dependent. This tonsillar recovery position ensures that the mouth is lower than the larynx and encourages drainage of blood. The use of the left lateral position facilitates re-intubation should it become necessary, since the tongue then falls to the side under the influence of gravity. Close observation during the recovery period is required to exclude continued bleeding.

Post-tonsillectomy bleeding occurs usually within 6 h of surgery.[63] Haemorrhage may be rapid and require resuscitation, although it may go unnoticed initially because the blood is swallowed. The anaesthetist is then faced with (usually) a child with a full stomach, hypotension and a tachycardia. Adequate pre-operative resuscitation is essential before returning to the operating theatre, the degree of tachycardia being a useful sign of the efficacy of fluid replacement. Fluid replacement should be with colloid solutions, or blood, depending upon the estimate of blood loss. In any event, blood should be available before returning to the operating theatre. Induction of anaesthesia should occur only in the presence of a senior anaesthetist, and should be performed on a tipping table with good suction immediately to hand.

A rapid-sequence induction of anaesthesia with pre-oxygenation and cricoid pressure may be followed by maintenance with inhaled anaesthetics, but the author considers that in small children an inhalational induction with halothane, cricoid pressure, and with the child in the left lateral position is safer, since blood from the pharynx then drains freely. This technique avoids the hazards associated with rapid-sequence induction if intubation proves to be difficult. Once the airway is secure, the child can be turned on to his or her back and the stomach emptied with a wide-bore orogastric tube. Maintenance, extubation and recovery are as for the elective case.

Microlaryngoscopy

The requirements for successful microlaryngoscopy are that there should be free access to the pharynx unhindered by anaesthetic apparatus, and an immobile relaxed larynx. A technique based upon mechanical ventilation through a small-diameter orotracheal tube satisfies both requirements. Alternatively, jet ventilation via the laryngoscope has proved popular.[64–67] High-frequency jet ventilation has also been advocated.[68]

Light premedication is desirable, and benzodiazepines are satisfactory. The anaesthetic technique chosen depends in part upon prior knowledge of the pathology involved. Small lesions such as vocal cord polyps require no special precautions, but large lesions that may cause obstruction require careful assessment and handling. Some supraglottic tumours are large and friable, and may cause obstruction. Control of the airway may be lost during an intravenous induction, and in these cases, an inhalational induction is advisable. Direct laryngoscopy under deep inhalational anaesthesia can then form the basis for further management. The management of laser surgery to the larynx has been discussed above.

Middle-ear surgery

As with any surgery conducted with an operating microscope, an immobile field is essential. The second requirement, discussed above, is to provide conditions conducive to a dry operating field. The patient should be adequately sedated before induction. Any factor that may lead to tachycardia should be avoided. For this reason anticholinergic premedication should be omitted, but benzodiazepines, morphine and cyclizine, or papaveretum and hyoscine are suitable alternatives. Intravenous induction followed by paralysis with a competitive neuromuscular blocker allows smooth tracheal intubation. The use of fentanyl or alfentanil at induction reduces the sympathetic response to tracheal intubation.

Intermittent positive-pressure ventilation with an inhaled agent may be used for maintenance of anaesthesia. The vasodilatation associated with isoflurane may be used to advantage in producing moderate hypotension, without recourse to more invasive methods of blood pressure control. The patient's neck should be in a position to allow unimpeded venous drainage, and ventilation to normocapnia established. Light anaesthesia or response to painful stimulus should be avoided. It is useful to start anti-emetic therapy during anaesthesia, since nausea and vomiting are common following middle-ear surgery and may disrupt the surgical repair. Cyclizine is a useful and long-acting anti-emetic in this respect. The problems associated with the use of nitrous oxide in this situation have been discussed above.

Laryngectomy

Careful pre-operative assessment will determine the degree of respiratory obstruction caused by the tumour. If stridor is present, sedative premedication should be omitted. The anaesthetist should anticipate difficult laryngoscopy and intubation, due to the anatomical distortion caused by the tumour, which is often friable and liable to haemorrhage. A range of tracheal tubes should be immediately available, in anticipation of inability to pass a large tube past the tumour. If there is significant obstruction, an inhalational induction is advisable, and the surgeon should be at hand in case emergency tracheostomy is required. If the patient already has a tracheostomy, then all that is required is to change the tracheostomy tube for one that will accept a catheter mount, and to proceed with intravenous induction. Maintenance by mechanical ventilation with an inhaled agent provides satisfactory conditions for what may be a protracted procedure.

In the absence of a previously formed tracheostomy, that procedure is performed during the dissection of the larynx. The tip of the tracheal tube is withdrawn from the trachea into the larynx, and the surgeon cannulates the trachea with a tracheostomy tube. The change-over from one tube to the other must be performed smoothly, and to this end, all tubes and connections should have been checked with the anaesthetist before the change-over becomes irrevocable. The anaesthetist should not withdraw the tracheal tube from the larynx until the tracheostomy tube is secure.

ANAESTHESIA FOR OPHTHALMOLOGY

Factors affecting intra-ocular pressure

The aqueous humour is a clear, colourless aqueous solution that is present in the anterior and posterior chambers of the eye, and was described first by Aristotle. Its composition is similar to that of other extracellular fluids, although it is rich in bicarbonate ion and ascorbic acid.[69] The functions of the aqueous humour are to maintain the intra-ocular pressure and hence the shape of the cornea and anterior chamber, and to carry nutrients to the avascular lens and cornea whilst removing products of metabolism from these structures.

The aqueous humour is formed continuously by the ciliary body in the posterior chamber by a process that involves both active secretion of ions and ultrafiltration of plasma. Of these two processes, active ionic secretion appears to be the more dominant.[70] The fluid formed flows though the pupil into the anterior chamber which it then leaves via the trabecular drainage system in the iridocorneal angle to drain into the canal of Schlemm and ultimately to the episcleral veins on the surface of the eye.

The intra-ocular pressure is determined largely by the rate of formation of the aqueous humour and the ease with which it drains. Pressure from extra-ocular structures may also be transmitted to the contents of the eye, as are pressure changes induced by changes in choroidal volume. Intra-ocular pressure is altered by changes in posture mediated through changes in venous pressure. Similarly, coughing and vomiting increase intra-ocular pressure by increasing central venous pressure. Changes in arterial pressure have little effect upon intra-ocular pressure in the intact eye because of autoregulation. However, changes in intra-ocular pressure may have a marked adverse effect upon choroidal and retinal blood flow, particularly if intra-ocular pressure is increased in the presence of low systemic arterial pressure. The normal intra-ocular pressure is between 10 and 20 mmHg. There is a diurnal variation in pressure of 2–3 mmHg, with the peak pressure usually occurring in the early morning during sleep.

Control of intra-ocular pressure is important to the anaesthetist because of the disruption of the contents of the globe that may ensue if the globe is opened when intra-ocular pressure is raised. Even when the globe is open and intra-ocular pressure is the same as atmospheric, any factor which increases intra-ocular pressure in the intact eye will result in ocular contents moving towards the incision. Furthermore, the sudden release of a high intra-ocular pressure may result in rupture of the short posterior ciliary arteries, leading to expulsive haemorrhage. Massive serous choroidal effusion may also occur in these circumstances, with similar results but a better prognosis.[71] Control of intra-ocular pressure is also of importance in patients with severe angle-closure glaucoma, in whom a rise in intra-ocular pressure may reduce disc perfusion to the point where blindness results.

When assessing the effects of an anaesthetic technique or single agent upon intra-ocular pressure, care must be taken to ensure adequate control of all the experimental variables that may alter intra-ocular pressure. In particular, strict control of ventilatory and circulatory parameters is required. In deciding upon an appropriate anaesthetic technique for a given situation, care must also be taken to view the technique as a whole and avoid fixation upon any one aspect of the intra-operative control of intra-ocular pressure. For example, intramuscular morphine has been shown to reduce intra-ocular pressure and might be used as premedication in combination with an anticholinergic agent.[72] However, it is generally recognized that the use of opioids for premedication for most intra-ocular surgery is at best unnecessary, and may be harmful because of an increased incidence of postoperative nausea and vomiting. Van den Berg and colleagues[73] reported that the incidence of vomiting after eye surgery was highest after squint surgery (41%), but that there was a modest but significant incidence after intra-ocular surgery (13%), when its occurrence is almost certainly of greatest importance. The incidence of nausea and vomiting was higher in females undergoing ocular surgery than in males, but age had no effect upon the incidence. The incidence was raised in those who received opioid premedication compared with those who received a benzodiazepine, but the expected beneficial effects of premedication with an anti-emetic were not demonstrated. The medicolegal implications of vomiting after intra-ocular surgery are clear.[62]

Intravenous anaesthetic agents

Many anaesthetic agents have been shown to reduce intra-ocular pressure. With the exception of ketamine, the induction agents currently available lower intra-ocular pressure.[74] Sodium thiopentone and etomidate lower intra-ocular pressure significantly when used as induction agents. Propofol produces greater depression in intra-ocular pressure than does thiopentone.[75] Benzodiazepines given intravenously for induction of anaesthesia or immediately prior to induction also lower intra-ocular pressure.[76,77] Ketamine may produce a significant rise in intra-ocular pressure.[78]

Neuromuscular blockers

The competitive neuromuscular antagonists lower intra-ocular pressure[74] by decreasing tone in the extra-ocular muscles. In contrast, the use of suxamethonium is associated with increased intra-ocular pressure. The extra-ocular muscles, in common with the striated muscle of the upper oesophagus and the intrinsic laryngeal muscles, are among the few examples of striated muscles in the mammal which receive multiple innervation.[79] Multiply innervated muscle cells receive a dense innervation derived from many neurones over all of their surface, in contrast to the single muscle end-plate derived from a single axon in focally innervated fibres. Such muscles respond to suxamethonium by sustained contraction.

Numerous experimental and clinical studies have confirmed that suxamethonium raises intra-ocular pressure. However, this observation must be kept in perspective. The increase in intra-ocular pressure observed following an intubating dose of suxamethonium is generally of the order of 5–10 mmHg, although Lincoff et al[80] reported a maximum increase of 38 mmHg. This is in comparison to the rise caused by coughing of 40 mmHg,[4] and the rise of 6 mmHg caused by tracheal intubation in the absence of coughing.[81] The act of blinking raises intra-ocular pressure in the intact eye by 10 mmHg.[82] Various attempts have been made to obtund the rise in intra-ocular pressure caused by suxamethonium, including pretreatment with lignocaine, with diazepam, with competitive neuromuscular antagonists and with small 'self-taming' doses of suxamethonium. None of these manoeuvres is fully effective. Administration of acetazolamide to reduce the production of aqueous humour before induction of anaesthesia is effective in preventing the response to suxamethonium.[83] The use of suxamethonium should be avoided in the glaucomatous eye.

Tracheal intubation

The act of tracheal intubation may increase intra-ocular pressure.[84-87] The rise in intra-ocular pressure during extubation may be as great, or greater than, that experienced during intubation.[88] The use of the laryngeal mask airway is associated with less change in intra-ocular pressure, both during insertion and removal,[88,89] than that related to intubation or extubation of the trachea, although other factors such as security of the airway may need to be considered during ophthalmological procedures and may justify tracheal intubation. In one study[90] in which the larynx was examined using a fibre-optic bronchoscope passed via a laryngeal mask, the oesophageal opening could be seen clearly in 9% of patients. This observation is of relevance in any situation in which regurgitation of stomach contents may occur. In one patient in the study, the laryngeal mask airway was partially displaced during draping, and this has relevance in situations in which the anaesthetist does not have ready access to the airway after surgery has started.

Inhaled agents

The inhaled agents decrease intra-ocular pressure through a variety of mechanisms, including alteration in central control of intra-ocular pressure, alteration in aqueous outflow facility and alteration of extra-ocular muscle tone. Conflicting results have been reported for trichloroethylene, which may raise or lower intra-ocular pressure,[74] but the remaining volatile agents usually lower intra-ocular pressure by 20–40%, depending upon anaesthetic depth.

Carbon dioxide tension

Arterial carbon dioxide tension is a major determinant of intra-ocular pressure, and carbon dioxide washout by hyperventilation may be used to decrease intra-ocular pressure rapidly; the fall in intra-ocular pressure parallels that in intracranial pressure under similar circumstances.[91,92] Under general anaesthesia employing controlled ventilation to normocapnia, intra-ocular pressure decreases by approximately 50% when halothane is used and by about 35% with the use of enflurane.[93,94] Ventilation to normocapnia is achieved readily by the use of a single-limb co-axial Bain anaesthetic breathing system in conjunction with a suitable ventilator. The changes in intra-ocular pressure that occur with changes in arterial carbon dioxide tension are thought to be mediated through changes in choroidal blood flow.[95]

While in general it is important to avoid open surgery upon the globe whilst the intra-ocular pressure is high, a profoundly low intra-ocular pressure resulting in an eye which is 'too soft' during cataract surgery may prevent insertion of the lens implant. A similar problem may make corneal grafting difficult, and a soft eye induced by retrobulbar block may also make intra-ocular surgery more difficult under local anaesthesia.[4,96]

Local anaesthesia for ophthalmological procedures

Until recent years, most ophthalmological procedures in the UK were performed under general anaesthesia and, when local anaesthesia was used, the block was usually provided by the surgeon. Consequently, the practice of local anaesthesia for eye surgery by anaesthetists was confined to a few interested individuals. There is a wide range of eye procedures that may be performed under local anaesthesia,[97] and the involvement of anaesthetists in providing local blocks for ophthalmological surgery has increased considerably.

Lid surgery may be performed readily under local anaesthesia. Local infiltration of lignocaine 1 or 2% allows removal of superficial lesions such as papillomata, sebaceous cysts or chalazion. Topical anaesthesia to the conjunctiva, usually with amethocaine 1%, allows removal of foreign bodies from the cornea or minor surgery to the cornea or conjunctiva. Cocaine 4% is also useful in this respect, but causes corneal opacity and cannot therefore be used in situations in which it is necessary to obtain a view through the cornea, as in treatment of retinal detachment. It is also a mydriatic and thus contra-indicated in glaucoma.

Local anaesthesia for intra-ocular surgery, such as extraction of cataract, is more demanding. A combination of retrobulbar block with facial nerve block and topical anaesthesia to conjunctiva and cornea produces both intra-ocular and extra-ocular anaesthesia with paralysis of the facial and extra-ocular muscles.[97] Complications of the technique include retrobulbar haemorrhage, damage to the orbital contents and dural puncture.[98,99] A technique of peri-ocular infiltration that does not require facial nerve block and that appears to be relatively free of complications has been described.[98,100] The use of local anaesthesia for cataract surgery prevents the adverse metabolic and cardiovascular effects that are seen when the procedure is performed under general anaesthesia.[101] Widespread use of local anaesthesia for cataract extraction would allow many more patients to be treated as day cases, as is routine in other countries.[102] Sedation is often provided during eye surgery performed under local anaesthesia. There are risks of airway obstruction and depression of ventilation, particularly in elderly patients, and it is essential that adequate monitoring is undertaken.

General anaesthesia for ophthalmological procedures

Extra-ocular procedures

Examination under anaesthesia. It is important to diagnose and, if possible, correct ocular abnormalities as early in life as possible. Abnormalities of vision that result in failure to produce a focused image on the retina in the first few months of life lead to failure of development of the neural pathways to the visual cortex, and thus to failure of development of binocular vision.[103,104] Restoration of binocular vision requires early correction of strabismus.[105] Children usually require general anaesthesia for examination and indirect ophthalmoscopy, which may involve manipulation of the globe. Other congenital abnormalities are often present. Down's syndrome is common in this group, as is the rubella syndrome, both of which are associated with a high incidence of cataract and with cardiac abnormalities.

It is unusual to require tracheal intubation for these procedures, and anaesthesia can be provided successfully using intravenous induction, or gaseous induction with the inhalational agent of the anaesthetist's choice, and maintenance via a face mask. Halothane is still used frequently in this situation and is preferred for its rapidity of onset and smooth induction, although the author has found enflurane to be equally satisfactory. Premedication is usually unnecessary (apart from application of Emla cream if intravenous induction is planned), and most of these children may be treated successfully as day cases. Children with Down's syndrome may be unusually sensitive to atropine, and if used, the dose should be reduced.[106] Children with Down's syndrome may also have cervical spine abnormalities. It is important to ensure that the neck is supported adequately at all times during the procedure, and that excessive movement of the head upon the neck is avoided.

Strabismus surgery. Surgery for correction of strabismus is the commonest ophthalmological procedure encountered in children. In one paediatric unit, 57% of all children presenting for ophthalmological procedures were scheduled for correction of squint, and of these, 7% were under the age of 1 year.[107] Malignant hyperpyrexia is associated with strabismus and with ptosis,[108–110] and is commoner in the young than in the adult.[110–112] Upper respiratory tract infection is common in children and should be regarded as an absolute contra-indication to anaesthesia, since it greatly increases the incidence of postoperative laryngeal spasm, particularly when tracheal intubation has been employed.

The problems associated with the oculocardiac reflex have been discussed above. Children under 1 year of age should receive intramuscular atropine preoperatively. Older children may be premedicated with a sedative. None is ideal, but trimeprazine tartrate and the benzodiazepines, diazepam and temazepam, have been found to be useful. The application of Emla cream to the dorsum of one or other hand is a useful adjunct to venous cannulation. If not given as premedication, then a muscarinic antagonist should be given i.v. at induction of anaesthesia; glycopyrrolate has been shown to be more effective against the oculocardiac reflex than atropine.[47] Induction of anaesthesia may be by inhalational anaesthesia in the younger child, or by intravenous induction with thiopentone, or with propofol in children over the age of 3 years. Tracheal intubation is required, and may be secured following administration of suxamethonium, alfentanil,[113] or a competitive neuromuscular blocker. Artificial ventilation is obviously required throughout the procedure if a competitive neuromuscular blocker is used, although the author has found a technique using spontaneous ventilation to be satisfactory during strabismus surgery. Extubation is performed under deep inhalational anaesthesia, and the child recovered in a lateral position. There is a high incidence of vomiting after strabismus surgery in children and an anti-emetic should be routinely administered.

Dacrocystorhinostomy. This procedure is performed in cases of obstruction of the nasolacrimal duct. An anastomsis is performed between the medial half of the lacimal sac and the nasal mucosa lining the middle meatus of the nose. A silastic tube may be left in place through this anastomosis to encourage its patency.

Anaesthesia may be provided by a technique which includes tracheal intubation. The aim, as in other head and neck surgery, is to provide an immobile and relatively bloodless surgical field. Intermittent positive-pressure ventilation to normocapnia and the use of a head-up tilt provide satisfactory conditions. Care should be taken to avoid tachycardia and venous congestion caused by malposition of the head. Specific measures to lower arterial blood pressure are usually unnecessary, but may be employed a throat pack should be used.

Radiotherapy in children. Radiotherapy is used in the treatment of retinoblastoma and rhabdomyosarcoma. Children present for repeated treatments which will almost always require general anaesthesia so that the child remains relatively immobile during exposure. The anaesthetist is always remote from the patient for periods of 2–3 min during treatment. Pulse oximetry and electrocardiogram monitoring are mandatory during these periods. Closed-circuit television monitoring and capnography have been found useful.[107] Anaesthesia using ketamine alone provides suitable conditions in these children. It may be given initially by the intramuscular route.[114] Intravenous access may be secured on the first visit under anaesthesia. The cannula may then be secured and flushed with heparinized saline and the parents instructed as to simple hygiene and care of the cannula. In this way, intravenous cannulation may be maintained over a period of weeks, and intravenous induction with ketamine used on subsequent visits. Inhalation induction and maintenance with isoflurane have been shown to be safe and allow for more rapid recovery than ketamine — an important consideration if radiotherapy is taking place on a daily basis.[115]

Intra-ocular procedures

The penetrating eye injury. Trauma is the commonest cause of unilateral blindness.[116] The patient is commonly a child who is frightened and distressed, and who may have eaten immediately prior to the accident. It is often impossible even to examine such a child without general anaesthesia. When associated with other injuries, the ocular injury may often be left safely while more major injuries are treated.

Induction of anaesthesia and tracheal intubation should be smooth and free of coughing. It should be remembered that the injured child will cry and rub the injured eye at the time of the injury, and together these actions will raise intra-ocular pressure and compound the injury, and may be associated with prolapse of the intra-ocular contents. In these circumstances, and in the presence of a full stomach, the use of suxamethonium to achieve tracheal intubation cannot be discouraged. No attempt should be made to empty the stomach by means of a nasogastric tube, as this inevitably leads to further distress and a rapid rise in intra-ocular pressure. Similarly, inhalational induction may be more distressing for the child than a well-conducted intravenous induction.

The use of suxamethonium may be avoided by the use of alfentanil in combination with a competitive neuromusuclar blocker.[113] Pre-oxygenation should be undertaken, and a large dose of competitive neuromuscular blocker given together with the alfentanil. Anaesthesia should then be induced with thiopentone, and cricoid pressure applied. Good intubating conditions are achieved within 1 min of administration of vecuronium. Maintenance of anaesthesia with intermittent positive-pressure ventilation and an inhalational agent provides satisfactory conditions for surgery.

Intracapsular extraction of cataract. This is by far the most commonly performed intra-ocular procedure. If the outcome is to be successful, then the principles concerning the control of intra-ocular pressure outlined above must be adhered to. The anaesthetic technique must be smooth and flawless, with rigid avoidance of respiratory obstruction, coughing, straining or vomiting. Once the eye is open, the intra-ocular pressure is the same as atmospheric pressure, but any disturbance that would previously have led to an increase in intra-ocular pressure will now cause movement of the intra-ocular contents towards the incision, and may result in prolapse of intra-ocular structures. Furthermore, surgery is performed using an operating microscope, and movement of the field of surgery is therefore undesirable.

These conditions dictate that general anaesthesia, when employed, is performed using muscular paralysis and intermittent positive-pressure ventilation. Premedication with a benzodiazepine is satisfactory if required, but opioids should be avoided because of the higher risk of postoperative nausea and vomiting. An anti-emetic should be given at, or shortly after, induction of anaesthesia. Any intravenous induction agent may be employed in combination with fentanyl or alfentanil. Etomidate is useful in these patients, many of whom are elderly with a high incidence of cardiovascular and respiratory disease. The principal means of lowering intra-ocular pressure is through the use of an inhaled agent, and the reduction in pressure that is achieved is proportional to the depth of anaesthesia.[117] A modest head-up tilt should be employed, and positive end-expiratory pressure and excessive peak inflation pressure avoided. Ventilation should be to normocapnia.[93,94] or to moderate hypocapnia, which will aid the decrease in intra-ocular pressure by choroidal vasoconstriction. Extubation should be performed under deep anaesthesia in order to avoid coughing at that time. If opioids are used postoperatively then they should always be given in combination with an antiemetic.

Anaesthesia for the procedure of vitrectomy is similar. It differs in the longer duration of surgery, and the possible use of sulphur hexafluoride within the eye. If the latter is used then nitrous oxide should be discontinued beforehand, and anaesthesia continued using oxygen-enriched air as the carrier gas for the inhalational agent, with additional supplements of intravenous opioid or hypnotic as necessary.[118]

REFERENCES

1 Eckenhoff JE. Some anatomic considerations of the infant larynx influencing endotracheal anesthesia. Anesthesiology 1951; 12: 401–410
2 Knight PR, Hantler CB. Anesthesia and the geriatric patient: hypertension in the elderly. Clin Anesthesiol 1986; 4: 1003–1023
3 Waldmann C. Anaesthesia for the elderly. In: Kaufman L, ed. Anesthesia review 9. Edinburgh: Churchill Livingstone, 1992: pp 194–211
4 Holloway KB. Control of the eye during general anaesthesia for intra-ocular surgery. Br J Anaesth 1980; 52: 671–679
5 Kerr AR. Anaesthesia with profound hypotension for middle ear surgery. Br J Anaesth 1977; 49: 447–452
6 Eltringham RJ, Young PN, Fairburn ML, Robinson JM. Hypotensive anaesthesia for microsurgery of the middle ear. A comparison between enflurane and halothane. Anaesthesia 1982; 37: 1028–1032
7 Condon HA. Deliberate hypotension in ENT surgery. Clin Otolaryngol 1979; 4: 241–246
8 Pasch T, Huk W. Cerebral complications following induced hypotension. Eur J Anaesthesiol 1986; 3: 299–312
9 Scott DB, Buckley FP, Littlewood DG, MacRae WR, Arthur GR, Drummond GB. Circulatory effects of labetalol during halothane anaesthesia. Anaesthesia 1978; 33: 145–156
10 Scott DB, Stephen GW, Marshall RL, Jenkinson JL, MacRae WR. Circulatory effects of controlled arterial hypotension with trimetaphan during nitrous oxide/halothane anaesthesia. Br J Anaesth 1972; 44: 523–527
11 MacRae WR, Wildsmith JAW, Dale BAB. Induced hypotension with a mixture of sodium nitroprusside and trimetaphan camsylate. Anaesthesia 1981; 36: 312–315
12 Wildsmith JAW, Sinclair CJ, Thorn J. MacRae WR, Fagan D, Scott DB. Haemodynamic effects of induced hypotension with a nitroprusside–trimetaphan mixture. Br J Anaesth 1983; 55: 381–389
13 Guggiari M, Dagreou F, Lienhart A et al. Use of nitroglycerine to produce controlled decreases in mean arterial pressure to less than 50 mmHg. Br J Anaesth 1985; 57: 142–147
14 Khambatta HJ, Stone JG, Khan E. Hypertension during anesthesia on discontinuation of sodium nitroprusside-induced hypotension. Anesthesiology 1979; 51: 127–130
15 Fahmy NR, Sunder N, Moss J, Slater E, Lappas DG. Tachyphylaxis to nitroprusside: role of the renin–angiotensin system and catecholamines in its development. Anesthesiology 1979; 51: S72

16 Fukunaga AF, Flacke WE, Bloor BC. Hypotensive effects of adenosine and adenosine triphosphate compared with sodium nitroprusside. Anesth Analg 1982; 61: 273–278
17 Hermens JM, Bennet MJ, Hirshman CA. Anesthesia for laser surgery. Anesth Analg 1983; 62: 218–229
18 Conacher ID, Paes ML, Morritt GN. Anaesthesia for carbon dioxide laser surgery on the trachea. Br J Anaesth 1985; 57: 448–450
19 Leonard PF. The lower limits of flammability of halothane, enflurane and isoflurane. Anesth Analg 1975; 54: 238–240
20 Vourc'h G, Tannieres ML, Freche G. Anaesthesia for microsurgery of the larynx using a carbon dioxide laser. Anaesthesia 1979; 34: 53–57
21 Hirschman CA. Indirect ignition of the endotracheal tube during carbon dioxide laser surgery. Arch Otolaryngol 1980; 106: 639–641
22 Kumar A, Frost E. Prevention of fire hazard during laser microsurgery. Anesthesiology 1981; 54: 350
23 Russell CA. Tracheal tubes for laser surgery. Anaesthesia 1984; 39: 293–294
24 Norton ML, de Vos P. New endotracheal tube for laser surgery of the larynx. Ann Otolaryngol 1978; 87: 554–557
25 Pashayan AG, Gravenstein JS. Helium retards endotracheal tube fires from carbon dioxide lasers. Anesthesiology 1985; 62: 274–277
26 Rontal E, Rontal M, Wenokur ME. Jet insufflation anesthesia for endolaryngeal laser surgery: a review of 318 consecutive cases. Laryngoscope 1985; 95: 990–992
27 Young PN, Robinson JM. Anaesthesia for microsurgery of the larynx. Ann R Coll Surg Engl 1983; 65: 135
28 Gupta B, Lingam RP, McDonald JS, Gage F. Hazards of laser surgery. Anesthesiology 1984; 6`: A146
29 Emery RE. Laser perforation of a main stem bronchus. Anesthesiology 1986; 64: 120–122
30 Ganfield RA, Chapin JW. Pneumothorax with upper airway laser surgery. Anesthesiology 1982; 56: 398–399
31 Wolbarshi M, Fligster KE, Hayes JR. Retinal pathology of neodynium and ruby laser burns. Science 1965; 150: 1453–1454
32 Leibowitz HM, Peacock GR. Corneal injury produced by carbon dioxide laser radiation. Arch Ophthalmol 1969; 81: 713–721
33 Ryder W. Cardiac rhythm during dental anaesthesia. Proc R Soc Med 1971; 64: 82–83
34 Joas TA, Stevens WC. Comparison of the arrhythmic doses of epinephrine during forane, halothane and fluroxene anesthesia in dogs. Anesthesiology 1971; 35: 48–53
35 Johnston RR, Eger EI, Wilson C. A comparative

interaction of epinephrine with enflurane, isoflurane, and halothane in man. Anesth Analg 1976; 55: 709–712
36 Tucker WK, Rackstein AD, Munson ES. Comparison of arrhythmic doses of adrenaline, metaraminol, ephedrine and phenylephrine during isoflurane and halothane anaesthesia in dogs. Br J Anaesth 1974; 46: 392–396
37 Alexander JP. Reflex disturbances of cardiac rhythm during ophthalmic surgery. Br J Anaesth 1975; 59: 518–524
38 Fischman MW, Schuster CR, Resnekon L. Cardiovascular and subjective effects of intravenous cocaine administration in humans. Arch Gen Psychiatry 1976; 33: 983–989
39 Bromley L, Hayward A. Cocaine absorption from the nasal mucosa. Anaesthesia 1988; 43: 356–358
40 Chiu YC, Brecht K, Dasgupta DS, Mhoon E. Myocardial infarction with topical cocaine anesthesia for nasal surgery. Arch Otolaryngol 1986; 112: 988–990
41 Kerr WJ, Vance JP. Oculocardiac reflex from the empty orbit. Anaesthesia 1983; 38: 883–885
42 Andersen RL. The blepharocardiac reflex. Arch Ophthalmol 1978; 96: 1418–1420
43 Khan F, Ankutse MM, Muhja R. Oculocardiac reflex from the empty orbit. Anaesthesia 1986; 41: 441–442
44 Davies A. Bradycardia and asystole associated with trigeminal ganglion injection. Anaesthesia 1988; 43: 895
45 Shearer ES, Wenstone R. Bradycardia during elevation of zygomatic fractures. Anaesthesia 1987; 42: 1207–1208
46 Baxandall ML, Thorn JL. The nasocardiac reflex. Anaesthesia 1988; 43: 480–481
47 Mirakhur RK, Jones CJ, Dundee JW, Archer DB. IM or IV atropine or glycopyrrolate for the prevention of oculocardiac reflex in children undergoing squint surgery. Br J Anaesth 1982; 54: 1059–1063
48 Meyers EF, Tomeldan SA. Glycopyrrolate compared with atropine in prevention of the oculocardiac reflex during eye-muscle surgery. Anesthesiology 1979; 51: 350–352
49 Mirakhur RK, Shepherd WFI, Jones CJ. Ventilation and the oculocardiac reflex. Anaesthesia 1986; 41: 825–828
50 Steward A, Allott PR, Cowles AL, Mapleson WW. Solubility coefficients for inhaled anaesthetics for water, oil and biological media. Br J Anaesth 1973; 45: 282–293
51 Thomsen K, Terkildsen K, Arnfred I. Middle ear pressure variations during anaestheia Arch Otolaryngol 1965; 82: 609
52 Waun JE, Sweitzer RS, Hamilton WK. Effect of nitrous oxide on middle ear mechanics and hearing acuity. Anesthesiology 1967; 28: 846
53 Man A, Segal S, Ezra S. Ear injury caused by elevated intratympanic pressure during general anaesthesia. Acta Anaesthesiol Scand 1980; 24: 224–226
54 Casey WF, Drake-Lee AB. Nitrous oxide and middle ear pressure. Anaesthesia 1982; 37: 896–900
55 Mann MS, Woodsford PV, Jones RM. Anaesthetic carrier gases. Anaesthesia 1985; 40: 8–11
56 O'Neill G. Prediction of post-operative middle ear pressure changes after general anaesthesia with nitrous oxide. Acta Otolaryngol (Stockh) 1985; 100: 51–57

57 Wolf G, Capuano C, Hartung J. Effect of nitrous oxide on gas bubble volume in the anterior chamber. Arch Ophthalmol 1985; 103: 418–419
58 Wolf GL, Capuano C, Harting J. Nitrous oxide increases intra-ocular pressure after intravitreal sulfur hexafluoride injection. Anesthesiology 1983; 59: 547–548
59 Stanley TH. Nitrous oxide and pressures and volumes of high- and low-pressure endotracheal tube cuffs in intubated patients. Anesthesiology 1975; 42: 637–640
60 Klainer AS, Turndorf H, Wu W, Maewal H, Allender P. Surface alterations due to endotracheal intubation. Am J Med 1975; 58: 674–683
61 Lumb AB, Wrigley MW. The effect of nitrous oxide on laryngeal mask cuff pressure. Anaesthesia 1992; 47: 320–323
62 Davies R. Vomiting after removal of cataract. Lancet 1979; ii: 1030
63 Crysdale WS, Russel D. Complications of tonsillectomy and adenoidectomy in 9409 children. Can Med Assoc J 1986; 135: 1139
64 Oulton JL, Donald DM. A ventilating larygoscope. Anesthesiology 1971; 35: 540–542
65 Lee ST. A ventilating laryngoscope for inhalational anaesthesia and augmented ventilation during laryngoscopic procedures. Br J Anaesth 1972; 44: 874–878
66 Smith RB, Babinski M, Petruscak J. A method for ventilating patients during laryngoscopy. Laryngoscope 1974; 84: 553–559
67 Poling HE, Wolfson B, Siker ES. A technique of ventilation during laryngoscopy and bronchoscopy. Br J Anaesth 1975; 47: 328–384
68 Babinski M, Smith RB, Klain M. High-frequency jet ventilation for laryngoscopy. Anethesiology 1980; 52: 178–180
69 Kinsey VE, Reddy DVN. Chemistry and dynamics of aqueous humour. In: Prince JH ed.The rabbit in eye research. Springfield, IL: Charles C. Thomas, 1964: pp 218–319
70 Cole DF. Secretion of the aqueous humour. Exp Eye Res 1977; 25(suppl): 161–176
71 Ruiz RS, Salmonsen PC Expulsive choroidal effusion. Arch Ophthalmol 1976; 94: 69–70
72 Leopold IH, Comroe JH. Effect of intramuscular administration of morphine, atropine, scopolamine and neostigmine on the human eye. Arch Ophthalmol 1948; 40: 285–290
73 van den Berg AA, Lambourne A, Clyburn PA. The oculo-emetic reflex. Anaesthesia 1989; 44: 110–117
74 Murphy DF. Anaesthesia and intra-ocular pressure. Anesth Analg 1985; 64: 520–530
75 Mirakhur RK, Shepherd WFI. Intra-ocular pressure changes with propofol ('Diprivan'): comparison with thiopentone. Postgrad Med J 1985; 61: 41–44
76 Pino-Capote JA. Decrease in intra-ocular pressure produced by i.v. and conjunctival diazepam. Br J Anaesth 1978; 50: 865
77 Fragen RJ, Hauch T. The effect of midazolam maleate and diazepam on intra-ocular pressure in adults. Arzneimittel-Forsch 1981; 31: 2273–2275
78 Adams AK. Ketamine in paediatric ophthalmic practice. Anaesthesia 1973; 28: 212–213

79 Bowman WC. Pharmacology of neuromuscular function. Bristol: John Wright, 1980
80 Lincoff HA, Ellis CH, DeVoe G et al. The effect of succinylcholine on intra-ocular pressure. Am J Ophthalmol 1955; 40: 501–510
81 Joshi C, Bruce DL. Thiopental and succinylcholine: action on intra-ocular pressure. Anesth Analg 1975; 54: 471–475
82 Miller D. Pressure of the lid on the eye. Arch Ophthalmol 1967; 78: 328–330
83 Carballo AS. Succinylcholine and acetazolamide (Diamox) in anesthesia for ocular surgery. Can Anaesth Soc J 1965; 12: 486–498
84 Drenger B, Pe'er J. Attenuation of ocular and systemic responses to tracheal intubation by intravenous lignocaine. Br J Ophthalmol 1987; 71: 546–548
85 Mirakhur RK, Elliott P, Shepherd WFI, Archer DB. Intra-ocular pressure changes during induction of anaesthesia and tracheal intubation. A comparison of thiopentone and propofol followed by vecuronium. Anaesthesia 1988; 43: 54–57
86 Mostafa SM, Wiles JR, Dowd T, Bates R, Bricker S. Effects of nebulized lignocaine on the intra-ocular pressure responses to tracheal intubation. Br J Anaesth 1990; 64: 515–517
87 Robinson R, White M, McCann P, Magner J, Eustace P. Effect of anaesthesia on intra-ocular blood flow. Br J Ophthalmol 1991; 75: 92–94
88 Lamb K, James MFM, Janicki PK. The laryngeal mask airway for intra-ocular surgery: effects on intra-ocular pressure and stress responses. Br J Anaesth 1992; 69: 143–147
89 Holden R, Morsman CDG, Butler J, Clark GS, Hughes DS, Bacon PJ. Intra-ocular pressure changes using the laryngeal mask airway and tracheal tube. Anaesthesia 1991; 46: 922–924
90 John RE, Hill S, Hughes TJ. Airway protection by the laryngeal mask. Anaesthesia 1991; 46: 266–367
91 Smith RB, Aass AA, Nemoto EM. Intra-ocular and intracranial pressure during respiratory alkalosis and acidosis. Br J Anaesth 1981; 53: 967–972
92 Samuel JR, Beaugie A. Effect of carbon dioxide on the intra-ocular pressure in man during general anaesthesia. Br J Anaesth 1974; 58: 62–67
93 Adams AP, Freedman A, Henville JD. Normocapnic anaesthesia for intra-ocular surgery. Br J Ophthalmol 1979; 63: 204–210
94 Rose NM, Adams AP. Normocapnic anaesthesia with enflurane for intra-ocular surgery. Anaesthesia 1980; 35: 569–575
95 McLaren Wilson T, Le May M. Experimental and clinical study of factors influencing choroidal blood flow. Trans Ophthalmol Soc 1974; 94: 378–382
96 Duke-Elder S. The venous pressure of the eye and its relation to the intra-ocular pressure. J Physiol 1962; 61: 409–418
97 Allen ED, Elkington AR. Local anaesthesia and the eye. Br J Anaesth 1980; 52: 689–694
98 Fry RA, Henderson J. Local anaesthesia for eye surgery — the peri-ocular technique. Anaesthesia 1989; 45: 14–17
99 Rubin AP. Editorial — Anaesthesia for cataract surgery- time for change? Anaesthesia 1990; 45: 717–718
100 Davis DB. Posterior peribulbar anaesthesia; an alternative to retrobulbar anaesthesia. J Cataract Refractive Surg 1986; 12: 124–128
101 Barker JP, Vafidis GC, Robinson PN, Hall GM. Plasma catecholamine response to cataract surgery: a comparison between general and local anaesthesia. Anaesthesia 1991; 46: 642–645
102 Hamilton RC, Gimbel HV, Strunin L. Regional anaesthesia for 12 000 cataract extraction and intra-ocular lens implantation procedures. Can J Anaesth 1988; 35: 615–623
103 Hubel DN, Weisel TN. Receptive fields, binocular interaction and functional architecture in the cat's visual cortex. J Physiol 1962; 160: 106–154
104 Wybar K, Taylor D. Sensory aspects of deranged binocular vision. In: Perkins ES, Hill DWH, eds. Scientific foundations of ophthalmology. London: Heinemann Medical, 1977: p 231
105 Taylor DM. Congenital esotropia management and prognosis. New York: Intercontinental Medical Book, 1972
106 Harris WS, Goodman RM. Hyperreactivity to atropine in Down's syndrome. N Engl J Med 1968; 279: 407–410
107 Arthur DS, Dewar KMS. Anaesthesia for eye surgery in children. Br J Anaesth 1980; 52: 681–688
108 Relton JES, Britt BA, Steward DJ. Malignant hyperpyrexia. Br J Anaesth 1973; 45: 269–275
109 Hogg S, Renwick W. Hyperpyrexia during anaesthesia. Can Anaesth Soc J 1966; 13: 429
110 Smith RJ. Preoperative assessment of risk factors. Br J Anaesth 1988; 60: 317–319
111 Britt BA, Kalow W. Malignant hyperthermia: a statistical review. Can Anaesth Soc J 1970; 17: 293
112 Ording H. Incidence of malignant hyperthermia in Denmark. Anesth Analg 1985; 64: 700–704
113 Morton NS, Hamilton WFD. Alfentanil in an anaesthetic technique for penetrating eye injuries. Anaesthesia 1986; 41: 1148–1151
114 Sandford FG, Jones CW. Immobilisation for radiotherapy by ketamine. Anesthesiol Rev 1976; 3: 16
115 Jones RM, Diamond JG, Power SJ, Bajorek PK, Mundai IT. A prospective study of liver function in infants and children exposed to daily isoflurane for several weeks. Anaesthesia 1991; 46: 686–688
116 Editorial. Surgical management of ocular trauma. Br J Ophthalmol 1976; 60: 731
117 Al-Abak HM, Samuel JR. Further observations on the effects of general anaesthesia on intra-ocular pressure in man; halothane in nitrous oxide and oxygen. Br J Anaesth 1974; 46: 756–759
118 Mirakhur RK. Anaesthetic management of vitrectomy. Ann R Coll Surg (Engl) 1985; 67: 34–36

15. Obstetric analgesia and anaesthesia

H. Breivik   D. Bogod

The lives and well-being of two or more individuals are in the hands of the anaesthetist faced with the task of relieving the pain of vaginal delivery or anaesthetizing a patient for instrumental or surgical delivery. Marked alterations of anatomy and physiology that are significant for the anaesthetist, and sometimes dramatic pathophysiology, accompany pregnancy and the progress of labour and delivery. The pharmacodynamics and pharmacokinetics of anaesthetic and analgesic drugs are altered. The effects on the fetus and the newborn of drugs given to the mother may alter significantly the short- and long-term well-being of the child. Maternal and fetal emergencies happen at any time of the day or night; some of the most challenging situations in an anaesthetist's working career may occur in the middle of the night in the delivery room, with trainee or junior staff the most experienced at hand.

Consequently, obstetric anaesthesia and analgesia may cause more trepidation than most other sections of anaesthetic practice. However, the satisfaction obtained from a successful outcome in the delivery room or the obstetric room is tremendously rewarding to the obstetric anaesthetist. For this to occur regularly, a thorough understanding of anatomy, physiology, pharmacology and pathophysiology of pregnancy and delivery is mandatory.

ANATOMY, PHYSIOLOGY AND PHARMACOLOGY

Pain pathways[1]

During the first stage of labour, pain results from dilatation of the cervix and lower uterine segments, and distension of the body of the uterus. The intensity of the pain is related to the strength of the uterine contractions and the pressure generated. Whereas the pain of normal labour and delivery is experienced as moderate to severe, the pain experience is very severe and exhausting during prolonged or complicated labour.

The noxious impulses from the uterus and the cervix are transmitted through afferent sympathetic nerves through the pelvic and hypogastric sympathetic plexuses, to the thoracolumbar sympathetic chain. They pass through the white communicating rami between the sympathetic chain and the spinal nerves, entering the posterior horn of the thoracic spinal cord through the dorsal roots of T11 and T12 (early labour), as well as at T10 and L1 (late first stage).

It is most likely that low back pain during the first stage of labour is referred pain from dorsal rami of somatic spinal nerves T10 to L1. Pressure on nerves and nerve roots of the lumbosacral plexus produces referred pain through segments L1 to S2 and below during the latter part of the first stage when the fetal head descends into the pelvis and causes distension of pelvic structures. This causes low back pain as well as discomfort in the thighs and legs.

During the second stage of labour, noxious impulses from dilatation and trauma of the birth canal are transmitted through branches of the pudendal nerves to segmental levels S2, S3 and S4. The pudendal nerves supply the posterior two-thirds of the labia majora, the vagina, anus and pelvic floor. The anterior third of the labia majora is supplied by genital branches of the genitofemoral nerve. For satisfactory anaesthesia during Caesarean section under spinal or epidural anaesthesia, it is necessary to have an upper sensory level to at least T4, as well as complete sacral anaesthesia. Bonica has reviewed in detail the pain of labour and delivery, the untoward effects of severe labour pain on the mother's respiratory, cardiovascular and metabolic functions, and the undesirable effects on progress of labour and on the fetus.[1]

Pain in the shoulder area after delivery may be referred pain from the diaphragm, irritated by blood or air in the peritoneal cavity. Retrosternal pain and shoulder pain may also be caused by amniotic fluid or air emboli, the latter occurring in approximately 50% of patients who undergo Caesarean section.[2]

Physiological changes

Respiratory system[1,3,4] (Table 15.1)

There is a 20% reduction in the functional residual capacity and its two components, the residual volume and the expiratory reserve volume. Inspiratory capacity increases so that total lung capacity is unchanged. There is no significant change in closing capacity and small airway closure occurs in more than 50% of supine mothers during tidal volume breathing.[4] Tidal volume increases by 40%, but dead space is unchanged. Respiratory rate increases by about 15%, minute ventilation by about 50% and alveolar ventilation by 70%. This causes a decrease of 1.3 kPa (10 mmHg) in arterial $P\text{CO}_2$ and a similar increase in arterial $P\text{O}_2$. Arterial pH is unchanged and there is thus a decrease of 4–5 mmol.l^{-1} in serum bicarbonate concentration and base excess.[3,5]

During the final part of the first stage of labour, and in the second stage, an intermittent increase in maternal minute ventilation up to 300% may occur during painful uterine contractions. This marked maternal hyperventilation causes hypocapnia with arterial $P\text{CO}_2$ decreased to 3 kPa (20 mmHg) or less, and pH above 7.55. Between contractions, these women hypoventilate and are intermittently hypoxaemic, with a 10–50% decrease in arterial $P\text{O}_2$, fetal hypoxaemia and late fetal heart rate decelerations.[1,5] Epidural analgesia eliminates this hyperventilation–hypoventilation sequence.[1]

In spite of capillary engorgement and swelling of the mucous membranes of the respiratory tract, airway resistance decreases by more than 40% during pregnancy. Chest wall compliance is reduced, but lung compliance is unchanged.

Oxygen uptake is increased by 20% because of increased maternal metabolism and work of breathing.[6] The oxyhaemoglobin dissociation curve is shifted to the right at the end of normal (but not in pre-eclamptic) pregnancy; P_{50} is increased from about 3.6 to 4.1 kPa (26.7–30.4 mmHg). This allows a greater volume of oxygen to be released to the tissues at a given $P\text{O}_2$.[7] Oxygen reserve is decreased because of the decrease in functional residual capacity. The increased oxygen consumption results in the rapid development of hypoxaemia during apnoea or hypoventilation.[5]

The decrease in functional residual capacity and the increase in alveolar ventilation increase the rate at which inhalational anaesthesia is induced. The increased cardiac output partly counteracts the effect of increased alveolar ventilation. However, the minimum alveolar concentration (MAC) required to produce loss of movement to surgical stimulation is reduced by about 40%.[8] These changes significantly speed up the rate of inhaled induction of anaesthesia.

Cardiovascular system[1,3] (Table 15.2)

As maternal oxygen uptake increases to meet the increased metabolic demands of the growing fetus, uterus and placenta, the maternal cardiovascular

Table 15.1 Changes at term of pregnancy in respiratory, acid–base and inhalational anaesthetic variables[1,3–5]

Variable	Change
Total lung capacity	No change
Vital capacity	No change
Functional residual capacity	−20%
Residual volume	−20%
Expiratory reserve volume	−20%
Inspiratory reserve volume	+20%
Closing capacity	No change
Tidal volume	+40%
Dead space	No change
Respiratory rate	+15%
Minute ventilation	+50%
Alveolar ventilation	+70%
Airway resistance	−40%
Lung compliance	No change
Chest wall compliance	−45%
FEV$_1$	No change
Arterial $P\text{O}_2$	+1.3 kPa (10 mmHg)
Arterial $P\text{CO}_2$	−1.3 kPa (10 mmHg)
Arterial pH	No change
Serum bicarbonate/base excess	−4–5 mmol.l^{-1}
P_{50}	3.6 → 4.1 kPa (26.7 → 30.4 mmHg)
Oxygen consumption	+20%
Oxygen reserve	Decreased
Inhalational anaesthesia induction	More rapid
MAC for inhalational anaesthetics	−40%

FEV$_1$ = Forced expiratory volume in 1 s; $P\text{O}_2$ = partial pressure of oxygen; $P\text{CO}_2$ = partial pressure of carbon dioxide; = MAC = minimum alveolar concentration.

Table 15.2 Cardiovascular, blood and fluid volume changes in late pregnancy

Variable	Change
Total blood volume	Increase by 1500–2000 ml
Plasma volume	Increase by 1200–1700 ml
Red blood cell volume	Increase by 250–400 ml
Haemoglobin concentration	Decrease to 105–110 g.l^{-1}
Extracellular extravascular fluid	
Without clinical oedema	Increase by about 2000 ml
With slight clinical oedema	Increase by about 5000 ml
Cardiac output	Increase by 2–3 l.min^{-1}
During uterine contractions	Increase up to 14–15 l.min^{-1}

From Hytten & Chamberlain,[3] with permission.

system adapts; vascular resistance decreases (caused at least in part by oestrogen and prostacyclin) and cardiac output increases by 30–50%. Additional increases in cardiac output occur during labour, peaking to 12–14 l.min^{-1} during painful contractions.[1,3] Considerable confusion exists in the literature concerning the magnitude of the circulatory changes during the latter part of pregnancy and the puerperium. However, studies using Doppler and M-mode echocardiography show that cardiac output remains elevated at the end of pregnancy and during delivery and the puerperium, decreasing to non-pregnant values within a few weeks after delivery.[9]

Blood volume and composition[3]

Maternal blood volume increases by about 40% (by 1.5–2.0 l) during pregnancy. Plasma volume increases from about 40 to 60 ml.kg^{-1} (2.6–4.2 l) during late pregnancy, more in multigravidas and patients with multiple pregnancy than in primigravidas. Red blood cell volume increases from about 25 to 30 ml.kg^{-1}. Consequently, haemoglobin concentration decreases to about 105–110 g.l^{-1} (10.5–11.0 g.dl^{-1}). This dilutional anaemia of pregnancy decreases blood viscosity and is one of several factors that promote an increase in cardiac output and oxygen delivery.

Plasma proteins are diluted so that their total concentration declines from about 70 to 60 g.l^{-1}, but the total amount in the circulation increases. The reduction in albumin from 35 to 25 g.l^{-1} has significance for transcapillary extracellular fluid balance; plasma colloid osmotic pressure decreases from 28 to about 22 mmHg (and to about 17 mmHg in pre-eclampsia).[10] For drugs which bind to albumin, the fraction of bound drug decreases, but the total amount of bound drug may not be decreased.[3] The concentrations of most globulins increase during pregnancy.[3] Of particular importance is the fact that α_1-acid glycoprotein concentration decreases significantly during pregnancy from about 1 to 0.4 g.l^{-1}. The basic drug bupivacaine (pKa = 8.1) is bound to this acid plasma protein, and the free fraction of bupivacaine increases from about 5% to more than 8%.[11] This may in part explain the increased toxicity of bupivacaine in pregnancy.

Extracellular extravascular fluid[3]

During normal pregnancy, water is stored in the ground substance of connective tissue, increasing extracellular fluid volume by about 2 l in the absence of obvious oedema. With slight generalized oedema, a pregnant woman may have accumulated about 5 l of additional extracellular extravascular fluid.

The increased extracellular fluid, capillary engorgement and vascular congestion of mucous membranes cause swelling of the upper airways and larynx. Traumatic manipulation with a laryngoscope blade, tracheal tube or suction catheter rapidly increases this swelling and aggravates difficult intubation conditions.

The softening of the ground substance of connective tissues may render the ligamentum flavum so soft that resistance to the advancing epidural needle becomes unrecognizable.

Haemostasis and fibrinolysis[3]

Normal pregnancy is accompanied by major changes in the coagulation system; plasma fibrinogen concentration increases during normal pregnancy by about 50% from 2.5 to 4.0 g.l^{-1}. Similarly, increases in all other coagulation factors, except factors V, IX and XIII, contribute to a hypercoagulable state in the pregnant woman at term. The platelet count is moderately reduced in about 10% of normal pregnancies. There is an ongoing local utilization of coagulation factors in the placenta during pregnancy with an explosion of the coagulation process at placental separation; the immediate formation of a fibrin mesh on the placental site represents about 10% of the total circulating fibrinogen. If this mechanism fails, the placental blood flow of 500–800 ml.min^{-1} rapidly causes catastrophic haemorrhage. The normal average blood loss of about 500 ml during vaginal delivery, and 1000 ml during vaginal delivery of twins or during Caesarean section, is tolerated well because of the increased blood volume.

Fibrinolytic activity is decreased and remains low during labour until about 1 h after placental delivery. Pulmonary thrombo-embolism is a major contributor to maternal mortality; in the most recent national statistics from the UK, thrombosis and thromboembolism were the commonest causes of death in late pregnancy.[12] In spite of the ongoing coagulation process in the placenta, fibrin degradation products are low during normal pregnancy and delivery. In pre-eclampsia, coagulation and fibrin deposition in the intervillous spaces and in the walls of the spiral arteries of the placenta, as well as placental fibrinolysis, are increased, causing decreased placental perfusion and increased circulating fibrin degradation products.

Gastro-intestinal system

Although the generalized relaxation of smooth muscles during pregnancy may influence gastro-intestinal motility, gastric emptying may not be reduced much during normal pregnancy.[13] However, the fact remains that gastric content has a low pH (gastrin is produced by the placenta), and when labour has started, gastric emptying is slowed by pain, anxiety and opioid drugs. Lower oesophageal sphincter pressure is reduced,[14] and intragastric pressure often increases in the parturient. An increased risk of regurgitation and aspiration of acid stomach contents is therefore present during labour and delivery if general anaesthesia is induced or consciousness is impaired from exhaustion, pre-eclampsia or heavy sedation.

Prophylactic regimens with metoclopramide to hasten gastric emptying and increase lower oesophageal sphincter tone, as well as timely administration of H_2-receptor antagonists such as cimetidine or ranitidine, may reduce the risk. Treatment failures and side-effects (neurological dysfunction from dopamine antagonism, multiple drug interactions from H_2-antagonists) reduce their benefits. Prudent measures include administration of non-particulate antacid (30 ml of 0.3 M sodium citrate) immediately before rapid-sequence induction of general anaesthesia. Correct application of cricoid pressure until verified correct placement of a cuffed tracheal tube usually prevents the severe form of acid aspiration pneumonitis. The same precautions should be taken before any general anaesthetic administered during the first 48 h after delivery.

Hepatic and metabolic function[3]

Plasma cholinesterase activity is reduced during pregnancy, but the duration of effect of a single dose of suxamethonium is not prolonged in term-pregnant patients.[15,16] This appears to be due to an increased volume of distribution that offsets the decreased elimination of suxamethonium.[16] There are no reports of clinically significant delays in the metabolism of chloroprocaine.

Pre-existing diabetes mellitus may be unmasked or exacerbated by increased cortisol and human placental lactogen concentrations. The ability to handle a glucose load is decreased and the transplacental passage of glucose may stimulate fetal secretion of insulin. A maternal glucose infusion of 6 g.h^{-1} may cause neonatal hypoglycaemia.

Renal function

Renal plasma flow and glomerular filtration rate increase by approximately 50%. Creatinine clearance increases, reducing upper limits for normal serum creatinine concentration. Tubular re-absorption of glucose is reduced; glycosuria is common, and cannot be used as a screening test for abnormal glucose metabolism in pregnancy.[3]

Nervous system

The anaesthetic requirements for inhalational anaesthetics, as measured by MAC in animals, decrease by up to 40% during pregnancy.[8] This may be related to pregnancy-induced activation of the endogenous pain-inhibiting endorphin system,[17] and there is probably a contribution from the increased plasma concentrations of progesterone, which has been shown to cause sedation or even loss of consciousness in high doses.[18,19]

The onset of local anaesthetic block is significantly faster in nerves excised from pregnant animals than from non-pregnant animals.[20] Epidural or spinal anaesthesia is more rapid and more widespread during the first trimester, even before vertebral venous congestion and decreased cerebrospinal fluid volume can contribute to the spread of the injected local anaesthetic solution.[21]

Aortocaval compression

When pregnant women in the latter half of pregnancy are forced to stay in the supine position, compression of the vena cava and the abdominal aorta by the uterus results in the supine hypotensive syndrome.[22-24] This phenomenon includes hypotension, slowing of the heart rate — sometimes severe — pallor, sweating, nausea, vomiting, slow cerebration, and even loss of consciousness and convulsions. The inferior vena cava is completely compressed in about 90% of the cases, causing a decrease of venous return to the heart and hence a reduction in cardiac output and uteroplacental perfusion. In most women, a compensatory increase in peripheral vascular resistance occurs, maintaining arterial pressure in the upper part of the body.[24] In some women, however, the physiological co-arctation caused by compression of the abdominal aorta causes a temporary increase in arterial pressure in the aortic arch. This may initiate the baroreceptor reflex, causing bradycardia. Bradycardia and the decreased stroke volume from compromised venous return produce a profound decrease in blood pressure.

It is imperative that the anaesthetist recognizes the importance of aortocaval compression. When adaptation by the mother is impaired by drug-induced depression of the cardiovascular system, sympathetic blockade, blood loss or hypoxaemia, a catastrophic situation may develop rapidly. Any such aggravation of the effects of aortocaval compression can cause a precipitous fall in blood pressure and cardiac arrest on induction of spinal, epidural or general anaesthesia.[25,26] Spinal anaesthesia for Caesarean section has in the past had a sinister reputation in many countries because of catastrophic interactions with the supine hypotensive syndrome.[27,28]

Even when the supine position causes minimal maternal symptoms, severe effects on uterine perfusion can occur. The decrease in cardiac output and compression of the abdominal aorta decrease pressure in the uterine arteries even when the mother is able to compensate fully by vasoconstriction to maintain a normal blood pressure in the upper part of her body. The increased venous pressure below the compression of the vena cava increases uterine venous pressure, further decreasing uterine perfusion pressure. Fetal distress may result.[29,30]

Aortocaval compression can be prevented or relieved by left uterine displacement. This can be accomplished by manual displacement of the uterus to the left, by tilting the operating or delivery table laterally to the left, or by placing a small pillow under the patient's right buttock, elevating this part by 10–15 cm.[30,31] If this fails to relieve the problem, it is worth trying right lateral tilt, which may be more effective in 15% of women (Marx GF; personal communication). Wrapping of the lower limbs with elastic bandages has also been used to encourage venous return.[32]

Cerebrospinal fluid and epidural venous congestion

Since the spinal canal is a fairly rigid tube, the volume of cerebrospinal fluid must decrease when epidural veins are distended by increased pressure in the vertebral venous system. A dose of local anaesthetic injected into the subarachnoid space is introduced into a volume of cerebrospinal fluid which is lower than that in the non-pregnant patient (about 70 ml). When the mother is turned from one lateral position through the supine position to the opposite lateral position, the variation in engorgement of the vertebral venous system causes an exaggerated upward movement of the injected local anaesthetic solution. This phenomenon must be recognized by the anaesthetist; taking advantage of the phenomenon adds to the success of a spinal or epidural block, whereas ignorance may cause severe complications.[33,34]

Uterine blood flow

Uterine perfusion pressure and uterine vascular resistance determine uterine blood flow, which is approximately 700 ml.min^{-1} in the pregnant uterus at term.

Aortocaval compression in the supine position decreases uterine perfusion pressure by increasing uterine venous pressure, and by decreasing uterine arterial pressure directly from aortic compression and indirectly from decreased cardiac output. Uterine vascular resistance increases during uterine contractions. Vasopressors with pure α_1-adrenergic action can increase uterine vascular resistance. Ephedrine, the vasopressor of choice in obstetrics, increases venous return, heart rate, cardiac output and systemic arterial pressure indirectly, without increasing peripheral resistance significantly. In numerous clinical studies, ephedrine has been shown to be a safe and effective vasopressor in the obstetric patient with hypotension.[35] However, a minute dose of an α_1-adrenergic agonist, such as phenylephrine 0.1 mg intravenously, produces a similar clinical response as administration of ephedrine without causing tachycardia, which is undesirable in some patients.[35]

Uterine contractile activity and progress of labour

Labour and delivery are traditionally divided into three stages. The *first stage* starts with the initial contractions of the uterus. Initially, there is a *latent phase* with slow dilatation of the cervix, lasting around 8 h in the nulliparous patient, and 4–5 h in the multiparous. The first stage continues with an *active phase*, with uterine contractions lasting about 1 min, occurring every 3 min, and achieving an intra-uterine pressure of between 50 and 70 mmHg (10 mmHg between contractions). During the active phase of the first stage, the cervix is dilated from 2 to 10 cm in the course of 4–6 h in the nulliparous parturient, and in 1-2 h in the multiparous.

The *second stage* of labour starts when cervical dilatation is complete and lasts until delivery of the baby. This takes about 1 h in nullipara and about 30 min in the multiparous woman.

The *third stage* is from delivery of the baby until expulsion of the placenta and the fetal membranes.

Prolongation of the latent phase of the first stage (defined as more than 20 h in the nulliparous, more than 14 h in the multiparous) may be caused by anaesthesia or drugs which decrease uterine activity, e.g adrenaline (see below). The active phase of the first stage can be slowed (less than 1.2 cm dilatation per hour in the nulliparous, less than 1.5 cm.h^{-1} in the multiparous) or arrested by cephalopelvic disproportion malposition and malpresentation of the fetus. These factors may also be responsible for slowing or arrest of descent of the fetus in the second stage. The effects of epidural analgesia on progress of labour are discussed below.

Fetal monitoring[36]

The normal fetal heart rate (FHR) is between 120 and 160 beats.min^{-1}. The short-term variability in beat-to-beat FHR is between 10 and 25 beats.min^{-1}. Slowing of FHR coinciding with an increase in uterine pressure (*early deceleration*), caused by compression of the fetal head and vagal discharge, is normal and benign. *Late deceleration*, occurring 20–30 s after the onset of uterine contractions, indicates uteroplacental perfusion insufficiency.

Umbilical cord compression is the commonest cause of FHR deceleration occurring at *variable* onset in relation to uterine contraction. Maternal hypotension or uterine hypertonicity causing insufficient uteroplacental perfusion are the common causes of *prolonged deceleration* of FHR. If a beat-to-beat FHR variability of more than 5 beats.min^{-1} occurs between decelerations, this indicates sufficient fetal oxygen reserve. FHR *acceleration* indicates fetal well-being, except when it follows variable deceleration and is associated with loss of beat-to-beat FHR variability. If fetal capillary blood can be sampled, a pH below 7.20 suggests significant fetal asphyxia. A fetal scalp capillary pH above 7.25 is satisfactory.

Placental transfer of anaesthetic drugs

The lipid diffusion barrier between the maternal and the fetal circulation within the placenta allows rapid transplacental transfer of small (<500 Dalton) non-ionized lipophilic molecules that are poorly protein-bound. The main driving force is the concentration gradient of free, unbound and un-ionized drug across the placental barrier. Drugs that are highly ionized at normal pH cross the placental barrier slowly. This is true for all the *neuromuscular blocking drugs*, which are also poorly lipid-soluble.[37] Most other drugs used during anaesthesia are of low molecular weight, relatively lipid-soluble, partly ionized and partly protein-bound.

Transfer of drugs across the placenta is determined also by placental blood flow. Thus, the fraction of a drug bolus which crosses the placenta is significantly smaller when intravenous injection is performed during a uterine contraction than during relaxation.

All *inhalational anaesthetics* cross the placental barrier easily. However, the time constant for fetal drug equilibration is around three times as long as that of other maternal tissues. Even for the quickly equilibrating nitrous oxide, studies in sheep have shown that maternal–fetal equilibration takes 40 min.[38] Therefore, inhalational anaesthetics do not reach the fetus in significant amounts during a normal general anaesthetic for Caesarean section, as long as the induction–delivery time is not unduly prolonged. It is also of significance that MAC values for volatile anaesthetics are higher in newborn babies than in older individuals.[39]

Intravenous anaesthetic drugs such as thiopentone cross the placental barrier readily and produce peak concentrations in the fetus after a few minutes. Thereafter, the decline in fetal plasma concentration follows that of the mother; the decisive driving force of placental transfer of a small molecular weight, lipophilic, non-ionized drug such as thiopentone is the concentration gradient, initially determined mainly by the dose administered to the mother. Later, individual maternal distribution and elimination variables determine fetal drug exposure.[40]

All the *opioid drugs*, of which pethidine (meperidine) is still the most commonly used for pain relief in labour, cross the placental barrier easily. Pethidine administered intramuscularly reaches a peak maternal plasma concentration after approximately 45 min, and the terminal elimination phase of the plasma concentration curve starts 1–1.5 h after administration. A high plateau of pethidine concentration occurs in the fetus between 1 and 5 h after intramuscular administration to the mother.[41] Whereas the maternal pethidine half-life is about 3.5 h, the elimination half-life from neonatal blood is around 25 h. The elimination half-life of the opioid receptor antagonist naloxone is much shorter than that of pethidine.[42] Fetal elimination of other opioid analgesics is similarly prolonged.

Ionization and protein binding of local anaesthetic drugs

Transplacental transfer of local anaesthetic drugs illustrates the importance of ionization and protein binding. The amide local anaesthetic drugs are weak bases with pKa values between 7.7 and 8.1. The non-ionized base penetrates diffusion barriers, whereas it is the ionized, cationic form of the local anaesthetic molecule that is pharmacodynamically active, both in blocking nerve conduction and in provoking toxic effects in the myocardium and central nervous system.

Since the pKa values (the pH at which the concentrations of base and cation are equal) are close to physiological pH, changes in maternal and/or fetal acid–base status significantly alter the proportions of the active ionized, non-diffusible form and the non-ionized, diffusible base form of the drugs. When the mother hyperventilates to a pH above 7.5, the diffusible, non-ionized fraction increases, and more drug crosses the placental barrier. In the case of intrauterine asphyxia and fetal acidosis, the transferred local anaesthetic base is ionized inside fetal cells to the active cation form (cation trapping). Local anaesthetic drugs act on the intracellular aspect of the sodium channels, and since pH is lower in the intracellular fluid, this cation trapping phenomenon greatly aggravates and magnifies the toxic effects of local anaesthetics on the fetal heart and nervous tissues.

The local anaesthetic amide with the highest pKa, bupivacaine, binds (about 95%) to the acid α_1-glycoprotein. Protein-bound drugs do not cross the placenta. The concentration of acid α_1-glycoprotein is markedly reduced in maternal plasma, increasing the unbound bupivacaine fraction that is free to diffuse across the placenta from 5 to 8%.[11] This is one reason for the increased action and side-effects of bupivacaine, both in the mother and the fetus/neonate. This should be borne in mind when considering epidural analgesia or anaesthesia where intra-uterine fetal distress has led to fetal acidosis. However, the benefits of a regional technique upon uterine blood flow in both normal[43] and pre-eclamptic[44] women, along with the avoidance of the risks associated with general anaesthesia, may mean that an epidural is the best clinical compromise in these circumstances.

Fetal effects of anaesthetic drugs

Since most anaesthetic drugs that enter the fetal circulation have very prolonged elimination half-lives in the neonate, even tiny amounts may have prolonged effects on the newborn baby. Major effects on vital functions occur after large doses of opioid analgesics and large intravenous maternal injections of local anaesthetics. The prolonged, but clinically less impressive, effects of anaesthetic drugs on the neonate may still have significant and long-lasting behavioural sequelae. Behavioural studies of babies show that consolability may be affected for a long period after normal doses of pethidine to the mother.[45] Other assessments made as long as 5 years after delivery, however, have shown no correlation between anaesthetic or analgesic technique and childhood development.[46,47]

Anaesthetic drugs and uterine activity

Volatile inhalational anaesthetics depress uterine muscle contractions (force and frequency). There are no major differences among the conventional volatile anaesthetics in equipotent doses.[48] Even at 1.5 MAC enflurane, the contractility and the frequency of uterine contractions are reduced only to about 80 and 60% respectively of the control values.[49] Nitrous oxide and most intravenous anaesthetic drugs have insignificant effects. Thus, the depression of uterine muscle activity may be regarded as clinically unimportant with the amount and concentrations of anaesthetic drugs being used in clinical practice today.

Non-anaesthetic drugs and uterine contractility

Oxytocin

An intravenous infusion of oxytocin 5–10 units causes effective uterine constriction in the third stage of labour. Transient vasodilatation and decreases in arterial blood pressure usually result from an intravenous bolus dose of oxytocin.

Ergometrine

This drug causes generalized vasoconstriction in the mother if administered intravenously. The normal increases in blood volume and central venous pressure in the third stage of labour are considerably exaggerated for up to 1 h.[50] A hypertensive crisis, myocardial ischaemia or infarction, or cardiac failure may follow in patients with hypertension or heart disease, or in patients who have recently received a vasopressor.[51] Severe bronchospasm has also been reported.[52] If oxytocin is not available, ergometrine 0.2 mg may be given intramuscularly to treat postpartum haemorrhage. One should be prepared to treat myocardial ischaemia and hypertension with glyceryl trinitrate or a calcium antagonist. Ergometrine-induced bronchoconstriction may be a serotoninergic effect and may require treatment with chlorpromazine or a volatile anaesthetic.[52]

β-Adrenergic drugs

β_2-Adrenergic drugs (salbutamol, terbutaline, orciprenaline, isoprenaline, ritodrine) are used to suppress uterine contractions. Their β_1-agonist activity and β_2-effects outside the uterus cause cardiovascular side-effects and metabolic changes such as tachycardia, pulmonary oedema (especially when corticosteroids are co-administered) and hypokalaemia.[2,53] β-Agonist drugs must be stopped before induction of anaesthesia and fluid overload during anaesthesia must be carefully avoided in patients who have received these drugs.

Prostaglandins

Uterine contractions are stimulated by the prostaglandins $PGF_{2\alpha}$ and PGE_2. They are used primarily for therapeutic termination of pregnancy, e.g. with fetal death in utero, but have been used postpartum when all other agents fail to achieve uterine contractions. $PGF_{2\alpha}$ has positive chronotropic and α-adrenergic effects. PGE_2 causes maternal systemic arterial and pulmonary arterial pressures to decrease.[52]

ANALGESIA FOR VAGINAL DELIVERY

Systemic medication

Tranquillizers/sedatives

Barbiturates, phenothiazines and hydroxyzine can all be used to reduce anxiety. However, neurological and autonomic side-effects as well as prolonged effects on the newborn's neurobehavioural score have reduced the use of these drugs. Benzodiazepines are transferred rapidly to the fetus. Diazepam and its metabolites have prolonged (in some cases, very prolonged) effects on neonatal neurobehaviour, feeding, temperature control, muscle tone and ventilation.[54] This is also true for the more recent benzodiazepines, such as lorazepam and midazolam.[55,56] The anterograde amnesia[57] produced in many patients is another significant drawback for most parturients, who wish to be awake, alert, pain-free and remember the birth of their child. In modern obstetric practice, the father or another relative is allowed to remain with the parturient throughout labour. This has reduced remarkably the need for pharmacological anxiolysis and sedation. When such drugs are necessary, they are now, in recognition of their very potent and prolonged effects on mother and child, administered in minute doses compared to a few years ago.

Opioid analgesics

Opioid analgesics, administered intramuscularly or intravenously, could theoretically provide significant analgesia during labour. Unfortunately, dosage and effect are limited by maternal and neonatal side-effects, so that only moderate pain relief can be obtained with these drugs. Practice varies around the world. However, pethidine (meperidine) seems to be the most common opioid drug administered systemically for obstetric analgesia. Morphine, fentanyl, alfentanil, nalbuphine and butorphanol are all used in some places.

Pethidine (meperidine). The usual intramuscular dose of 50–100 mg gives peak analgesic effects after about 45 min. The analgesic effect of 25–50 mg pethidine by intravenous administration peaks after 5–10 min. The duration of analgesia is approximately 2 h, depending on the dose administered.[58] Pethidine has significant effects on the newborn baby. Infants born less than 1 h or more than 4 h after administration of pethidine 50–100 mg are less depressed than infants born 2–3 h after its administration. As with other opioid analgesics, pethidine causes a dose-related prolongation of time to regular sustained ventilation, reduced Apgar score, decreased oxygen saturation and respiratory acidosis in the newborn. Neurobehavioural effects can be demonstrated.[59–61] Neurobehavioural dysfunction may be caused in part by the very long elimination half-time (more than 60 h) of the active metabolite norpethidine.[61]

Morphine. After administration of intramuscular morphine, analgesia is slower in onset and longer in duration than after pethidine. In equi-analgesic doses, however, morphine produces more respiratory depression of the newborn for a longer time after administration than does pethidine.[62] Morphine is therefore not a favoured drug for obstetric analgesia.

Fentanyl. The peak analgesic effect occurs within 5 min after intravenous injection of fentanyl. The duration of effect is about 30 min. Intravenous fentanyl (1 µg.kg^{-1}) given up to 15 min before Caesarean delivery does not appear to depress the newborn.[63]

Alfentanil. Alfentanil has an even shorter onset time and duration than fentanyl. Alfentanil and fentanyl are indicated only when rapid-onset analgesia of short duration is required, such as during outlet forceps extraction.

Butorphanol and nalbuphine. These two synthetic agonist–antagonist opioid analgesics, in equi-analgesic doses (2 and 10 mg, respectively) produce similar degrees of respiratory depression as morphine 10 mg. Higher doses cause more maternal side-effects and affect neonatal neurobehavioural scores adversely.[64,65] Thus no obvious medical advantages have been shown for these analgesics.

Patient-controlled analgesia

Patient-controlled analgesia with intravenous administration of opioid analgesics is now well-established and widely used for postoperative pain.[66] This method was assessed for obstetric pain as early as 1970.[67] Its main advantage is the psychological benefit from the patient's ability to be in control of analgesic administration. Patient-controlled analgesia has been slow to appear in labour units, in spite of the wide use of opioid analgesics for labour pain. If the reported decrease in total dose and reduced maternal side-effects are confirmed, increased utilization of patient-controlled analgesia for labour pain can be anticipated.[65,66,68]

Ketamine

Low-dose ketamine (<0.5 mg.kg^{-1}) provides adequate analgesia without adverse effects on uterine blood flow, uterine tone or neonatal status.[69,70]

Inhalational analgesia

A majority of parturients are offered pethidine 100 mg intramuscularly early in labour, from which they obtain some relief for about 2 h. Conservative attitudes towards the use of pethidine injections make inhalation of nitrous oxide the mainstay of pain relief in normal labour in many maternity units.[71,72] In some countries, premixed nitrous oxide and oxygen 50%–50% (Entonox) is available. Uncertainties about stability of the mixture at low ambient temperatures have prevented Entonox from becoming more widely available. Various portable machines exist for administration of nitrous oxide blended with oxygen through an on-demand valve. Nitrous oxide concentrations can be varied from 0 up to 75% in oxygen. Face masks must be equipped with scavenging devices in countries where the authorities are concerned about occupational exposure of labour room personnel to nitrous oxide.[73] For self-administration, a concentration above 50% nitrous oxide should not be allowed.

At one time, volatile anaesthetics with analgesic properties were used widely, administered either through simple draw-over vaporizers, or through the precision vaporizer of an anaesthetic machine. *Methoxyflurane* is still used for obstetric analgesia in some countries because of its satisfactory analgesic properties. It is prudent, however, to restrict the total dose to less than 15 ml to prevent inorganic fluoride concentrations rising above 25 µmol.l^{-1} in maternal blood.[74]

The usual concentration of methoxyflurane for self-administration is about 0.3%, for *enflurane* 0.3–1.0% and for *isoflurane* 0.2–0.7%. Such concentrations will not change uterine contractility or responsiveness to oxytocin. The neonate is not affected by these analgesic concentrations of self-administered inhalational agents.

To obtain the optimal effect of inhalational analgesia, it is imperative that midwives understand the kinetics of inhalational anaesthetics and are able to instruct the parturients accordingly. For nitrous oxide, even at 50% concentration, there is a time lag of about 45 s after the start of efficient inhalation with a tightly fitting mask before the mother feels any effects. It is therefore essential that inhalation commences at the start of uterine contraction. Once the active phase of the first stage is well-established, self-administered inhalation is interrupted by the uterine contractions. If inhalation of 50% nitrous oxide goes on for a prolonged period, many mothers become confused, amnesic and unco-operative. Nitrous oxide concentration must then be reduced or the number of inhalations limited between contractions.

Labour and delivery can be made reasonably tolerable in a completely midwife-administered regimen with pethidine for the early part of the first stage, supplemented later in the first stage with properly self-administered nitrous oxide, methoxyflurane, enflurane or isoflurane, and local anaesthetic infiltration of the perineum for the second and third stages. However, if labour is prolonged, or more painful than average, regional analgesia is the only effective way of providing satisfactory and safe pain relief.

REGIONAL ANAESTHESIA

Perineal infiltration and pudendal nerve block

Perineal infiltration with a local anaesthetic solution prior to episiotomy is performed by the obstetrician or the midwife just before delivery.

Pudendal nerve block is performed by the obstetrician or the midwife[72] through the vagina with the patient in the lithotomy position and the delivery table tilted towards the left. The pudendal nerve loops below the ischial spine and sacrospinous ligament. A needle with a guard (Kobak needle — 'Iowa trumpet') is placed on the sacrospinous ligament and a loss of resistance technique used as the needle passes through the ligament, or the needle is passed through the mucosa just below the ischial spine and the ligament. Ten millilitres of local anaesthetic solution (lignocaine or mepivacaine 10 mg.ml^{-1} or chloroprocaine 20 mg.ml^{-1}) containing adrenaline is injected, after appropriate aspiration. This block is adequate for outlet forceps delivery as well as for episiotomy repair.

Paracervical block

All visceral afferent nerve fibres from the uterus, cervix and upper vagina will be anaesthetized by 5–8 ml of local anaesthetic solution injected submucosally at the 4 and 8 o'clock positions of the vaginal fornix lateral to the cervix. Any local anaesthetic solution (without adrenaline) other than bupivacaine may be used. This technique has fallen out of favour because of the high incidence of fetal bradycardia and neonatal depression, although it is still in use by obstetricians in some countries.[72] These complications are related to the close proximity of the injected local anaesthetic to the uterine artery.[75]

Lumbar epidural analgesia

The gold standard for obstetric pain relief is epidural analgesia which, with appropriate timing and optimal combinations of drugs, can render childbirth pain-free without impeding the progress of labour. However, this requires expertise and experience. The technical details of establishing an epidural block are the same as those described under lumbar epidural anaesthesia elsewhere in this book. The 'hanging drop' technique is inappropriate because of positive lumbar epidural pressure.[76] The paramedian approach to the epidural space facilitates catheter placement.[77] In the following sections, the indications for various regimens for epidural drug administration as well as some obstetric complications are discussed.

Indications for lumbar epidural analgesia for vaginal delivery

Indications for lumbar epidural analgesia for vaginal delivery vary with the availability of resources and of alternative analgesic techniques. Cultural differences and local traditions strongly influence indications for epidural analgesia for labour. The following are examples of indications that result in a 15–20% overall epidural rate.[71,72]

1. Ideally, lumbar epidural analgesia should be considered when labour is well-established and the contractions are subjectively so painful that the mother wishes more effective pain relief than that which can be obtained from reassurance, pethidine and properly administered inhalational analgesia.
2. In a painful, prolonged first stage, the parturient becomes exhausted, and the increasing levels of endogenous catecholamines, metabolic acidosis and maternal hyperventilation weaken uterine contractions and impede progress of labour.
3. In pre-eclampsia, the beneficial effects on maternal blood pressure and uteroplacental perfusion, as well as progress of labour, are of value to both mother and fetus.
4. In breech presentation, well-conducted epidural analgesia prevents the urge to bear down before full cervical dilatation and allows the parturient to collaborate with the obstetrician throughout the second stage.
5. In multiple pregnancies, epidural analgesia enables the mother to participate fully and is beneficial to the fetuses.
6. In the presence of intra-uterine dysmaturity, epidural analgesia reduces stress and trauma to the fetus, and maintains uteroplacental perfusion.
7. After intra-uterine fetal death, the parturient should be spared the pain and suffering of labour and delivery.
8. After previous Caesarean section, epidural analgesia often makes vaginal delivery possible, by ensuring optimal analgesia.[78] The probability of uterine rupture is not increased; symptoms of uterine rupture are not concealed by epidural analgesia.[78,79]

Contra-indications to epidural analgesia for vaginal delivery

Proven allergy to local anaesthetic drugs is an absolute contra-indication. The following problems usually preclude epidural catheterization:

1. clinical bleeding tendency of any kind, or a platelet count below 50×10^9/l or bleeding time >10–12 min.[80,81] Low-dose heparin and low-dose acetylsalicylic acid are usually not contra-indications to epidural analgesia (see below)[81]
2. infection in the back or in the skin of the intended puncture site
3. unstable neurological disease
4. hypovolaemic shock
5. proven cephalopelvic disproportion
6. refusal by the patient.

Dosage regimens for lumbar epidural analgesia

A large variety of 'recipes' have been described, with local anaesthetic solutions in varying concentrations and volumes, given intermittently or as a continuous infusion, and with or without addition of an opioid and/or adrenaline. Questions of technique relating to catheter type, approach to the epidural space, test doses and management of complications are discussed later in this chapter.

Intermittent local anaesthetic bolus injections. Bupivacaine, with its beneficial ratio of sensory-to-motor blockade, high protein binding and long duration of effect, is still by far the most frequently used drug for obstetric epidural analgesia. Fear of bupivacaine cardiotoxicity has made chloroprocaine or lignocaine (lidocaine) first choice in some countries (Table 15.3).

A traditional approach has been to administer a volume of 3 ml of bupivacaine 0.25% (2.5 mg.ml^{-1}) as a test dose after the catheter has been inserted, with the parturient in the right lateral position. Thereafter, with the mother turned to the left lateral position, the loading dose of bupivacaine 0.25% is injected in doses of 3 ml + 3 ml. A top-up dose is given as 6–8 ml of

Table 15.3 Suggested regimen for epidural analgesia for vaginal delivery

1. Check equipment, drugs and procedures for *treatment of complications* and for *resuscitation of mother and child*
2. Appropriate *haemodynamic monitoring* from start of block until the block has worn off
   Appropriate fetal monitoring
3. *Epidural catheter*, 18 G, placed with loss of resistance technique and paramedian approach, between L2–3 or 3–4, with the patient in the right lateral position. Advance 4–5 cm
4. It is mandatory that the patient maintains a *lateral position* throughout labour, but shifts from side to side every hour to prevent unilateral block
5. *Epidual test dose:* bupivacaine 0.25% (2.5 mg.ml^{-1}) 3 ml
   Alternatives: Lignocaine 1% (10 mg.ml^{-1}) + adrenaline 5 μg.ml^{-1} 3 ml
   Lignocaine 1% (10 mg.ml^{-1}) + adrenaline 5 μg.ml^{-1} 3 ml + fentanyl 50 μg
6. Activate epidural catheter when cervix is about 5 cm dilated in nulliparas, 3 cm in multiparas
   Epidural loading dose with bupivacaine 0.25%, 3 ml; turn patient to *left lateral* position and inject another 3 ml. Add 50 μg of fentanyl to this loading dose (if not added to the test dose)
   Alternatives: Lignocaine 1% (10 mg.ml^{-1})
   Chloroprocaine 2% (20 mg.ml^{-1}) (not in combination with fentanyl)
7. *Continuous epidural infusion* after appropriate evaluation of the loading dose:
   Bupivacaine 0.0625–1.25% (0.625–1.25 mg.ml^{-1}), 10 ml.h^{-1}
   Alternatives: Lignocaine 0.33–0.5% (3.3–5 mg.ml^{-1}), 10–15 ml.h^{-1}
   Chloroprocaine 0.5% (5 mg.ml^{-1}), 30 ml.h^{-1}
   Add fentanyl 1 μg.ml^{-1} to the most dilute solutions (not to chloroprocaine)
8. Check *sensory level* every hour and adjust infusion rate and/or concentration appropriately
   Rapidly disappearing block may mean migration of catheter into epidural vein
9. *Patient's ability to move legs* should be monitored every 30 min. Increasing motor block indicates subarachnoid migration of catheter
10. Check for *abnormal back pain* (symptom of epidural haematoma) for 12 h after block

bupivacaine 0.25% about every hour or at the earliest sign of pain break-through. This bolus dose should be given in incremental doses of 3 ml, with the usual precautions and observations for subarachnoid or intravascular injection, and appropriate cardiovascular monitoring thereafter.

Continuous-infusion epidural analgesia. *Safety and quality of analgesia* are improved by using a continuous infusion epidural analgesia technique. This increases safety by abolishing the hypotension after bolus injections of more than 30–40 mg bupivacaine.[82] By reducing the concentration of local anaesthetic, and increasing the volume, satisfactory analgesia can be maintained or improved, and side-effects from motor blockade of pelvic muscles are reduced. Bupivacaine concentrations as low as 0.08% (0.8 mg.ml^{-1}), at an infusion rate of 20–25 ml.h^{-1}, have been shown to result in significantly fewer top-up injections for breakthrough pain, compared with bupivacaine 0.25% infused at the same total hourly dose (20 mg.h^{-1}).[82-85]

By using low concentrations and restricting the infusion to provide no more than 20 mg.h^{-1}, a maximum dose of 10 mg would be delivered into the subarachnoid space over 30 min if the catheter migrates through the dura mater. This provides ample time to diagnose this complication, by the appearance of abnormal motor blockade, long before serious hypotension or respiratory muscle paralysis occurs. If the catheter migrates into an epidural vein, the block wears off and the pain of uterine contractions usually increases before central nervous system or cardiotoxic symptoms occur.

Epidural local anaesthetics and opioids. Epidural opioids alone have not been successful for obstetric analgesia.[86] Except during the early part of the first stage of labour, pain relief is insufficient; increasing the dose causes unacceptable side-effects such as nausea, urinary retention, pruritus and respiratory depression.[87] However, a minimal dose of a lipid-soluble opioid, such as fentanyl, definitely increases the rate of satisfactory analgesia when added to very dilute bupivacaine solutions.[88] This makes it possible to reduce further the motor and sympathetic block from bupivacaine and to establish epidural analgesia earlier without impeding progress of the early first stage of labour.[87-91]

Subarachnoid butorphanol and sufentanil (in a high dose) have been shown to be neurotoxic in animals.[92] Sufentanil in a dose of 7.5 μg has been shown to improve onset time and quality of a bupivacaine epidural;[93] this dose is safe when given epidurally but, if accidental subarachnoid injection/infusion occurs, medicolegal difficulties may arise if subsequent neurological problems develop. Alfentanil has not been evaluated for epidural neurotoxicity and appears to have a ceiling effect for spinal analgesia.[87] Epidural administration of morphine causes more severe pruritus than fentanyl.

Thus, *fentanyl* is the opioid of choice for epidural obstetric analgesia. There is now an abundance of clinical experience with fentanyl and the following advice can be given for dosage. A bolus of fentanyl 50 µg can be added to the initial test or loading dose of bupivacaine. Thereafter, a dilute solution of bupivacaine (0.625 mg.ml^{-1} suffices) containing fentanyl 1 µg.ml^{-1} is infused at a rate of 10 ml.h^{-1} initially, and adjusted as needed; a maximum rate of 20 ml.h^{-1} should not be exceeded (Table 15.3).[94]

Whereas a synergism between bupivacaine and fentanyl enhances spinal analgesia, an antagonism appears to exist between chloroprocaine and fentanyl.[95] This has not been observed with any other local anaesthetic. An additional advantage of adding an opioid to the epidural solution is the cessation of shivering that occurs in some parturients.[96]

Epidural infusion of bupivacaine, fentanyl and adrenaline. Opioid drugs cause spinal analgesia by acting on opioid receptors on cells in the substantia gelatinosa of the dorsal horn of the spinal cord. Similarly, activation of post-synaptic α_2-receptors on substantia gelatinosa neurones by adrenaline or clonidine inhibits transmission of pain impulses. Therefore, by adding a small dose of adrenaline to the epidural solution, analgesia is made more dense and the dose of bupivacaine can be reduced further.[87,89,95,97] Adrenaline (1.25 µg.ml^{-1}) also increases the quality of analgesia from dilute bupivacaine 0.125% (1.25 mg.ml^{-1}) solution and sufentanil in a concentration (1 µg.ml^{-1}) definitely below the neurotoxic level.[98]

The following dosing regimen is recommended by Eisenach:[89] a fractional bolus dose of 10 ml containing bupivacaine 0.0625% (0.625 mg.ml^{-1}), fentanyl 1 µg.ml^{-1} and adrenaline 1 µg.ml^{-1} provides pain relief for about 3 h. Continuous infusion rates[87,89,95] should be between 10 and 20 ml.h^{-1}. However, there is an effect of adrenaline on uterine activity, which is discussed below.

Effect of epidural analgesia on progress of labour and rate of instrumental deliveries

Recent reviews of these topics[99–101] can be summarized as follows. Undoubtedly, epidural analgesia (anaesthesia) with heavy-handed dosing of too concentrated a local anaesthetic solution, especially with adrenaline added, may slow or even arrest progress of labour and cause malrotations or malpresentations, increasing the rate of instrumental delivery. However, epidural analgesia, optimally and expertly conducted with dilute solutions of local anaesthetic and opioid, does not impede significantly the progress of labour, either during the first or the second stage. There does not seem to be a limit on how early in labour an epidural block can be started, particularly when such solutions are used. It should be remembered that, although epidural analgesia per se does not reduce uterine contractions, aortocaval compression during epidural analgesia does.[102]

Although a number of publications conclude that there is an increase in the duration of the second stage of labour and higher incidence of instrumental delivery when epidural analgesia is used,[99,100] well-controlled and well-conducted epidural analgesia can lower the forceps rate and is associated with fewer persistent malrotations.[99,103] Epidural analgesia can even help to achieve vaginal delivery as an alternative to Caesarean section in a prolonged, exhausting labour.[104]

If adrenaline in conventional dosage is added to the local anaesthetic solution, uterine contractions definitely decrease.[105] However, epidural analgesia reduces the high levels of endogenous catecholamines in a suffering parturient, thus relieving the endogenous catecholamine inhibition of uterine contractions.[106,107] This is the suggested reason for the beneficial effect on the progress of labour when epidural analgesia is initiated in the prolonged, painful and exhausted first-stage parturient.[104,107,108]

With the abundance of experience that has now accumulated with epidural analgesia, one can state with confidence that the use of a continuous infusion of dilute bupivacaine solution with minimal amounts of fentanyl, optimally tailored to the pain and progress of labour, benefits the parturient as well as the fetus and the neonate. The anaesthetist, the midwife or the patient herself, by using epidural patient-controlled analgesia,[109] can fine-tune epidural pain relief so that pelvic muscle relaxation and bearing-down efforts are not affected adversely.[100] However, there is a fine balance between too little and too much. Complications or unsatisfactory pain relief can occur in the best of hands and it is prudent to have a humble, conservative approach to the practice of epidural analgesia.

Caudal epidural analgesia

Anatomical abnormalities of the sacrum, higher epidural vascularity in the caudal canal and proximity to the rectum and fetal head are among the factors that reduce effectiveness and safety of this approach. Moreover, earlier and more intense perineal anaesthesia and more pronounced pelvic muscle relaxation make tailoring of caudal analgesia to progress of labour difficult. Even when caudal analgesia is used only for the second stage of labour, in combination with lumbar epidural analgesia for the first stage (the double-catheter technique, called the 'Rolls Royce of obstetric analgesia'[110]), the increased complexity and the greater skills required by the anaesthetist often obviate the advantages of the technique.[110,111]

Anaesthesia for vaginal delivery

When anaesthesia is required for vaginal delivery, the same principles apply as for elective or emergency Caesarean delivery. Induction of general anaesthesia requires precautions against aspiration of acid stomach contents into the lungs, and safeguards to ensure adequate anaesthesia and for avoidance of transplacental fetal anaesthetic intoxication. Epidural analgesia can be re-inforced to give satisfactory perineal anaesthesia for forceps delivery or extraction with a dose of concentrated local anaesthetic solution. When rapidity of onset is required and the possibility of intra-uterine fetal acidosis exists, chloroprocaine (or lignocaine) is the best choice. Spinal anaesthesia with a small dose of a hyperbaric solution and the sitting position during and after subarachnoid injection offer the advantages of profound pelvic anaesthesia with minimal fetal effects if maternal haemodynamic stability is maintained.

ANAESTHESIA FOR CAESAREAN SECTION

General considerations

Caesarean sections are performed *electively* because of cephalopelvic disproportion, breech presentation, malpresentation, chronic uteroplacental insufficiency from toxaemia, diabetes mellitus, Rhesus isoimmunization, multiple gestations and fetal abnormalities. *Urgent* Caesarean section is performed because of impending fetal distress or maternal complications such as failure to progress or failure of induction. *Emergency* Caesarean section is performed because of serious maternal complications or serious intra-uterine asphyxia from any cause, e.g. abruptio placentae, placenta praevia, prolapsed umbilical cord, failed forceps or tetanic uterine contrations. *Previous Caesarean section* is no longer an automatic indication for elective Caesarean section. Three out of four patients have a successful trial of vaginal birth after previous transverse uterine incision.[79]

Effects on the mother

Elective Caesarean section should carry only slightly increased risks for the mother, whereas urgent or emergency Caesarean section carries all the added risks of rapid induction of general anaesthesia with a full stomach, increased difficulties with intubation and airway control, exaggerated haemodynamic reactions and postoperative infective, pulmonary and thromboembolic complications. The relative risk of a mother's death is from 2 to 11 times greater with a Caesarean section than with vaginal birth.[79]

Effects on the fetus and newborn

Caesarean section is performed to reduce the fetal risk of a complicated vaginal delivery, or because prompt delivery of the fetus with asphyxia is mandatory. However, compared with normal vaginal delivery, Caesarean section is always associated with a greater perinatal morbidity; all anaesthetic drugs given to the mother, except the neuromuscular blockers, pass to the fetus and have effects on the newborn. Maternal hyperventilation, maternal hypoxaemia or hypercapnia and improperly treated hypotension all have adverse effects on oxygen delivery to the fetus.

Pre-operative preparation for general and for regional anaesthesia

The patient who requires Caesarean section must be assessed and informed by the anaesthetist, and the choice of anaesthetic method discussed. Whenever the patient has an opinion on the choice of anaesthetic technique, this should be accommodated as far as possible. She must be informed of the possibility that an epidural or spinal block may need to be supplemented with systemic analgesia or even general anaesthesia. Evaluation of the airway for possible intubation difficulties and prophylaxis against pulmonary aspiration is just as necessary when a regional technique is anticipated as when general anaesthesia is planned for Caesarean section. Although awareness and wakefulness during general anaesthesia (see below) have been described, modern techniques emphasizing the use of adequate concentrations of volatile agents have made the likelihood of intra-operative recall quite remote. Practice differs as to whether the mother should be warned of the possibility of awareness. In countries where this information is offered it is emphasised that the chance of awareness is low, that it will, in any case, be for a brief period only and that, if it does occur, it is for the benefit of the baby. An explanation of this sort should not cause distress if handled carefully and with sensitivity.

Elective Caesarean section

Regional anaesthesia

Although *infiltration* of the abdominal wall and the uterus with a dilute local anaesthetic solution may enable the obstetrician/surgeon to perform Caesarean section,[110] a central block is commonly far more effective and is to be preferred.

Spinal, epidural or combined spinal and epidural anaesthesia all offer the advantages of decreased risk of gastric acid aspiration, avoidance of depressant anaesthetic drugs on mother and fetus, and a fully conscious mother sharing the joy of a successful delivery. The time required to establish successful spinal or epidural anaesthesia makes them less suitable for emergency Caesarean section. However, in expert hands, induction-to-delivery time can be reduced to about 10 min with spinal anaesthesia[112] and to about 20 min with epidural anaesthesia (with chloroprocaine or lignocaine). If hypotension from aortocaval compression and sympathetic blockade is prevented, the duration of antepartum regional anaesthesia does not affect the outcome of the neonate in elective cases.[113] It is therefore imperative that steps be taken to maintain blood pressure. Prehydration is essential, and volumes as high as 1.5–2.0 l of crystalloid solution are widely recommended. Because sympathetic blockade occurs more rapidly with spinal anaesthesia, it is prudent to give ephedrine 25 mg intramuscularly before induction of spinal anaesthesia, or 10–15 mg intravenously at the induction of spinal anaesthesia.[114]

Haemostasis and lumbar puncture or epidural catheterization. A spinal epidural or subarachnoid haematoma can have devastating effects. It is extremely rare after epidural analgesia.[115,116] However, epidural haematoma can occur spontaneously, on straining (Valsalva manoeuvre) or after minor decelerating trauma.[117,118] It can be expected to be more frequent after traumatic lumbar puncture or epidural catheterization in patients who are taking anticoagulants, patients with thrombocytopenia or patients with prolonged bleeding time from platelet dysfunction or coagulopathy.[119] Due to the increased epidural venous pressure, epidural vein puncture may occur as often as in 18% of obstetric patients during epidural catheterization.[120]

In the treatment of established thrombo-embolic complications, warfarin cannot be used before delivery because it crosses the placenta and causes several fetal haemorrhagic complications. Heparin does not cross the placenta and is the anticoagulant of choice to treat thrombo-embolism occurring during the antenatal period. Lumbar puncture or epidural catheterization should *never* be performed in parturients who are fully anticoagulated or who have obvious platelet dysfunction, thrombocytopenia (platelet count below $50 \times 10^9/l$) and bleeding time longer than 12 min. The situation in parturients who are receiving low-dose heparin thromboprophylaxis or who have been taking low-dose acetylsalicylic acid for pre-eclampsia is more controversial.

Low-dose heparin. Parturients with previous thrombo-embolic complications or with increased risk factors such as age, multiparity, obesity, elective operative delivery or planned oestrogen suppression of lactation, may receive thromboprophylactic treatment. Dextran prophylaxis should not be used antenatally because of the risk of anaphylactoid reactions, even with hapten prophylaxis. Low-dose subcutaneous heparin (or low-molecular-weight heparin) prophylaxis acts primarily by preventing spontaneous conversion of factor X to the activated form Xa. In this low dose, heparin does not interfere with the activation of the normal haemostatic mechanisms at the site of an injury. It does not significantly interfere with platelet function, which is particularly important in achieving a haemostatic seal with small breaks in the vasculature, such as those which occur during epidural catheterization or lumbar puncture.[121] In low-dose heparin prophylaxis, with a normal thrombin time, the level of heparin is so low that it is safe to introduce an epidural catheter.[99] Spinal haematoma in patients on low-dose heparin has been reported, but this was not necessarily related to epidural catheterization.[122] There have been a number of studies using epidural analgesia or epidural anaesthesia in patients on low-dose heparin prophylaxis, as well as in patients on therapeutic heparin doses instituted after an atraumatic placement of an epidural catheter,[123–125] that do not show any increased risk of spinal epidural haematoma. Thus, low-dose heparin prophylaxis in a patient with normal thrombin time and a strong indication for spinal/epidural analgesia should not prohibit an experienced anaesthetist from performing an atraumatic lumbar puncture or epidural catheterization.

Low-dose acetylsalicylic acid therapy. Low-dose acetylsalicylic acid (60–100 mg daily) is now established as a means of preventing pregnancy-induced hypertension with its accompanying placental insufficiency and fetal growth retardation.[126] However, this is true only for those with high risk of developing pregnancy-induced hypertension, especially patients with a history of previous early onset preeclampsia.[127,128] One of the recently published placebo-controlled studies showed that there is no increased risk of low-dose acetylsalicylic acid prophylaxis, especially no increased bleeding or complications to epidural analgesia.[127] The abnormally increased thromboxane production in the placenta of these patients markedly affects the normal thromboxane–prostacyclin balance, increasing platelet aggregation and microvascular occlusion in the placenta. Thromboxane is a potent stimulus for platelet aggregation and vasoconstriction, whereas prostacyclin from vascular endothelial cells is a potent inhibitor of platelet aggregation and causes vasodilatation. Low-dose acetylsalicylic acid (below 100 mg daily) inhibits thromboxane production, whereas high doses (1000– 1500 mg daily) are needed to inhibit endothelial cell production of prostacyclin.[129]

Measurement of the bleeding time is the only practical test of in vivo platelet function. An estimate of bleeding time can be obtained by a technique using a device that is mastered easily by motivated clinicians,[129,130] although reproducibility is poor. The upper limit of normal bleeding time is 10 min. This is generally considered the upper limit for epidural catheterization.[129] However, we agree with those who maintain that even 12 min is acceptable *if* there is a strong indication for a spinal or epidural block.[81] Epidural haematoma secondary to aspirin-induced prolonged bleeding time has been reported in a non-obstetric patient.[131] The bleeding time may return to normal in 72 h after discontinuation of acetylsalicylic acid therapy, but it may take 7 days or more before platelet aggregation tested in vitro returns to normal.[129]

A low-grade thrombocytopenia (97–150 × 10^9/l) occurs in almost 10% of pregnancies without obstetric complications.[132] Thrombocytopenia is more frequent in pre-eclamptic patients and is part of the HELLP syndrome: haemolysis (H), elevated liver enzymes (EL), low platelet count (LP).[133]

Thus, obstetric anaesthetists have an increasingly frequent dilemma — a parturient in whom epidural or subarachnoid block is specifically indicated and a possibility of decreased haemostasis from low platelets and/or platelets inhibited in their function by acetylsalicylic acid therapy. No absolute rules for safe practice can be given.[129] The following seems a reasonable compromise.[81,134]

Platelet numbers below 50 × 10^9/l and/or bleeding time longer than 12 min are *contra-indications* for epidural and subarachnoid blocks. Platelet numbers between 50 and 100 × 10^9/l and bleeding time in the upper-normal range are *relative contra-indications*, e.g. in a patient with suspected difficult intubation and with a fetal indication for urgent Caesarean delivery. With an anaesthetist experienced in the technique, the most prudent method of management is to perform an atraumatic lumbar spinal puncture and to administer a sufficient dose of bupivacaine and opioid to secure good operative anaesthesia and postoperative pain relief.

Symptoms of spinal cord compression. It is mandatory to monitor the postpartum patient who has had epidural or spinal analgesia for signs and symptoms of spinal cord compression or anterior spinal artery syndrome. An epidural, subdural or subarachnoid haematoma usually produces severe *back pain*.[117] As compression ischaemia progresses, paresis and then paralysis of the lower extremities develop, initially with partly intact dorsal column sensations (vibration, proprioceptive sensations). If the cauda equina is compressed, a flaccid paralysis occurs early. It is imperative to respond quickly to any such symptoms and to perform computed tomography, magnetic resonance imaging or myelography. Immediate surgical relief of the compression is needed. Spinal cord ischaemia from compression lasting more than a few hours results in permanent neurological sequelae.[117,118]

Spinal (subarachnoid) anaesthesia. In the USA, spinal anaesthesia is the most commonly used regional anaesthetic technique for Caesarean section and it is undergoing a renaissance in other parts of the world.[135–138] Spinal anaesthesia is established with greater speed than epidural anaesthesia, there is no risk of maternal convulsions and the amount of local anaesthetic that reaches the fetus is minimal. In the hands of an experienced and skilled anaesthetist, spinal anaesthesia can even be chosen as the technique for semi-urgent Caesarean section because of the rapidity with which adequate anaesthesia can be established.[112,113,139]

Spinal needle size and shape. Single-use spinal needles of 25- or 26-gauge are sufficiently stiff to make it relatively easy to perform an atraumatic lumbar puncture for spinal anaesthesia. The cutting edge should be parallel to the long dural fibres. A conical, non-cutting pencil point needle (Whittacre or Sprotte) also reduces post-dural puncture leakage of cerebrospinal fluid.[140] A disposable Whittacre point needle is now available in 27-gauge.

Patient positions. Some anaesthetists prefer to place the patient in a sitting position because the midline of the back is easier to identify, and the cerebrospinal fluid flows more readily through a narrow-gauge spinal needle. However, when the patient is in the right lateral position during puncture and injection, followed by immediate change of position through the supine to the left-tilted position, there is better mixing of local anaesthetic solution with the cerebrospinal fluid and a higher level and improved quality of spinal block.[137]

Recommended doses of the various local anaesthetic solutions for spinal blockade are shown in Table 15.4.

Table 15.4 Dose guide for spinal anaesthesia to T4 for Caesarean section: hyperbaric solutions

	Dosage* according to height (cm)			Onset (min)	Duration (min)
	150–160	160–180	>180		
Bupivacaine	8–10 mg	10–12 mg	12–15 mg	2–4	120–180
Lignocaine	65 mg	70 mg	75 mg	1–3	45–75
Tetracaine	8 mg	9 mg	10 mg	3–5	120–180

*Lower dose in obese, short patients, in multiple gestations.

Bupivacaine is the drug of choice, the hyperbaric solution being more appropriate than the isobaric solution, which causes more pronounced motor blockade and paralysis of the legs and is less predictable in spread. The sensory level should be at least to T4. Even if the sensory level reaches above T1 with bupivacaine, the level for complete motor blockade is several segments lower, minimizing paralysis of the respiratory muscles. A subjective feeling of dyspnoea, which does not imply respiratory inadequacy, may accompany loss of sensation in the thoracic cage and weakness of chest-wall muscles. The appropriate treatment is to warn the patient that this may occur and to provide reassurance. Administration of oxygen by face mask or nasal prongs during spinal or epidural anaesthesia is a prudent precaution which is of value to the fetus and to the mother.[139]

Subarachnoid opioids. The quality of spinal anaesthesia is markedly improved by adding morphine 0.1–0.2 mg to bupivacaine,[138,141,142] although a high incidence of pruritus may be troublesome. Fentanyl also improves and prolongs spinal analgesia with bupivacaine; the optimal dose appears to be between 5 and 10 μg, although the duration of analgesia is less than with morphine.[142,143] The addition of fentanyl 5 μg and morphine 0.1 mg to hyperbaric bupivacaine can give excellent surgical anaesthesia and prolonged pain relief without a significant risk of postoperative respiratory depression.[144]

Postural, post-dural puncture headache. Young female patients have a high incidence of persistent cerebrospinal fluid leakage and postural headache after dural puncture. Parturients are more susceptible to such headaches because of Valsalva manoeuvres and dehydration. Headache severe enough to keep the postpartum patient bed-ridden is especially undesirable as she needs to take care of the neonate and to be mobilized to prevent thrombo-embolic complications.

The magnitude of cerebrospinal fluid leakage is related to the size of the needle hole, as well as the number of needle holes. After an accidental dural puncture with a 16- or 18-gauge epidural needle, crippling headache arises in about 20% and severe headache in about 70–80%.[145] Even with the 26-gauge sharp bevelled (Quincke-point) needle, about 20% of postpartum patients have postural headache, although only 5–6% have headache classified as severe and lasting for more than 1 day.[135] This incidence is reduced to below 2% when a 24- or 25-gauge pencil-point needle is used.[140,146]

In cases of accidental dural puncture with an epidural needle, the incidence of postural headache appears to be reduced by proceeding with successful epidural catheterization and epidural anaesthesia at the same or an adjacent spinous interspace. The use of prophylactic autologous blood patch is controversial.[147,148]

First-line treatment of post-dural puncture headache is by fluid loading and oral paracetamol; caffeine sodium benzoate 500 mg in 500 ml of intravenous glucose[149,150] is favoured by some workers. If headache still persists beyond 2 days, an epidural blood patch is successful in about 95% of cases when using 15–20 ml of the patient's own blood, taken under rigidly aseptic precautions and placed immediately in the epidural space at the site of the previous dural puncture.[151] Some patients experience backache after epidural blood patch, but usually this disappears within a few days.[152] When repeated epidural blood patches fail to relieve post-dural puncture headache, an epidural infusion of saline for 24–48 h is often effective.[153]

Lumbar epidural anaesthesia (Table 15.5). More time is required to establish adequate sensory blockade for Caesarean section with an epidural than with a subarachnoid block. Many anaesthetists prefer epidural to spinal anaesthesia for this reason. Hypotension develops less precipitously than after spinal block. This makes it easier to prevent hypotension, uteroplacental hypoperfusion and catastrophic maternal cardiovascular collapse. The ability to tailor an epidural block and the possibility of continuing with postoperative epidural analgesia are additional advantages. Disadvantages include the higher drug dose (increasing the possibility of local anaesthetic intoxication of mother and child), an inadvertent total spinal block

Table 15.5 Suggested procedure for epidural anaesthesia for Caesarean delivery

1. *Preparations*
   Inform and reassure the patient
   Sodium citrate 0.3 M, 30 ml by mouth < 30 min prior to block
   Position: lateral, right side down (or sitting)
   Oxygen by face mask or nasal prongs
   Electrolyte solution 1000–2000 ml intravenously
   Start cardiovascular monitoring (ECG, pulse oximeter, blood pressure)
   Check resuscitation drugs and equipment:
       Thiopentone/diazepam/midazolam
       Suxamethonium
       Ephedrine, atropine, adrenaline, bretylium
       Ventilation, oxygenation and intubation equipment
       Defibrillator

2. *Localization of epidural space*
   Infiltration (bupivacaine/lignocaine) of skin, subcutaneous tissues, down to lamina
   18-gauge epidural needle
   Paramedian approach L2–3 or L3–4
   Loss of resistance technique

3. *Test dose*
   Bupivacaine 0.5% (5 mg.ml^{-1}) + adrenaline 5 μg.ml^{-1} 3 ml
   Alternatives
   Lignocaine 1–1.5% (10–15 mg.ml^{-1}) + adrenaline 5 μg.ml^{-1} 3 ml
   Chloroprocaine 3% (30 mg.ml^{-1}) 3 ml

4. *Loading dose*
   Bupivacaine 0.5% + adrenaline 5 μg.ml^{-1} 3 ml × 6
   Optional: fentanyl 50–100 μg (1–1.5 μg.kg^{-1})
   Alternatives
   Chloroprocaine 3%, 3 ml × 6
   Lignocaine 2% (20 mg.ml^{-1}) + adrenaline 5 μg.ml^{-1} 3 ml × 6

5. *Epidural catheterization*
   Advanced catheter 4–5 cm, secure well

6. *Extending dose to sensory level > T4*
   Position patient with left lateral tilt
   Bupivacaine 0.5% + adrenaline 5 μg.ml^{-1}, 3 ml increments as needed.
   Maximum total dose 2.5 mg.kg^{-1}
   Chloroprocaine 3%, 3 ml increments as needed
   Maximum total dose 12 mg.kg^{-1}
   Lignocaine 2% + adrenaline 5 μg.ml^{-1}, 3 ml increments as needed
   Maximum total dose 10 mg.kg^{-1}

7. *Cardiovascular monitoring*
   ECG and pulse oximetry continuously, blood pressure every 1–2 min until delivery of baby

8. *Treatment of hypotension < 100 mmHg (or 30% below preblock value)*
   More left lateral tilt, + ephedrine 5–15 mg intravenously, repeat as needed, + increase intravenous infusion rate
   Note: Sudden nausea = hypotension. Give ephedrine first. Check blood pressure

9. *Adrenaline 5–10 μg intravenously*
   If there is severe hypotension and no immediate response to point 8, above

10. *Midazolam*
    0.5–1 mg/diazepam 2.5 mg or intravenously for CNS irritability

ECG = Electrocardiogram; CNS = central nervous system.

and neurotoxic effects from an accidental subarachnoid injection of an epidural dose.

Choice of local anaesthetic. Chloroprocaine 30 mg.ml^{-1} and bupivacaine 5 mg.ml^{-1} are the most commonly used drugs for epidural anaesthesia for Caesarean section. Lignocaine 20 mg.ml^{-1} or mepivacaine 20 mg.ml^{-1}, usually with adrenaline 5 μg.ml^{-1}, are also used.

Chloroprocaine is associated with a minimal risk of systemic toxicity and fetal side-effects, even in the presence of fetal acidosis.[154] Case reports of prolonged neural blockade, and transient or persistent neurological deficits, after inadvertent intrathecal injection of a loading epidural dose of chloroprocaine,[155-157] have been linked to the former formulation of chloroprocaine containing a high concentration of sodium bisulphite in a solution with a low pH[158,159] The preparation of chloroprocaine which is now commercially available for epidural use does not contain bisulphite.

There is an alternative explanation for persistent neurological sequelae after accidental subarachnoid injection of large volumes of local anaesthetic. The increased cerebrospinal fluid pressure and arterial hypotension reduce perfusion pressure in the long anterior spinal artery. This can cause spinal cord ischaemia and the anterior spinal artery syndrome.[160] Chloroprocaine does not seem to be more neurotoxic than lignocaine or bupivacaine when injected in large volumes into the subarachnoid space of animals.[159]

The controversy concerning *bupivacaine* cardiotoxicity[162-165] now seems to be resolved.[166,167] Local anaesthetics block the sodium channels of nerve cell membranes and heart muscle membranes. Sodium channels open briefly during the up-stroke of the action potential and are responsible for fast conduction. Blockade of these sodium channels slows or stops conduction. The effects of blockade of cardiac sodium channels by lignocaine and bupivacaine upon depolarization are similar. Recovery from bupivacaine takes five times longer than recovery from lignocaine. This slow recovery in the presence of bupivacaine causes a frequency-dependent block of the heart at normal heart rates. Whereas lignocaine enters and leaves the sodium channels quickly, bupivacaine enters the sodium channel quickly, but leaves slowly. Thus, cardiotoxic concentrations may accumulate rapidly inside the sodium channels when a large accidental intravenous bolus dose is injected. Re-entry ventricular arrhythmias may arise. The potential of bupivacaine for such electrophysiological cardiotoxicity is about four times that of lignocaine.[167] There is a wide therapeutic ratio even for bupivacaine when administered in a normal mode. The problem arises when bupivacaine is injected accidentally into a vein in a large bolus dose, or with gross overdose.

Bupivacaine is more cardiotoxic in pregnant animals than in non-pregnant animals.[168] This cardiotoxicity is aggravated further by hypercapnic or hypoxic acidosis (which develops rapidly if convulsions occur), probably through intracellular cation trapping of the local anaesthetic molecule.[163,165] Increased acute toxicity from reduced concentration of plasma-binding proteins in parturients has been mentioned above.[11]

Adrenaline 5 µg.ml^{-1} may be added to bupivacaine as well as to chloroprocaine. Adrenaline, by stimulating spinal α_2-receptors, enhances the quality of epidural block,[169] although it does not hasten onset time. Bupivacaine, with adrenaline added for epidural anaesthesia for Caesaren section, should not be used in a dosage above 2.5 mg.kg^{-1}. In non-pregnant patients,[170] the maximum dose of bupivacaine with adrenaline may be as high as 3.5 mg.kg^{-1}.

Choice of epidural opioid. Fentanyl 50–100 µg (1–1.5 µg.kg^{-1} body weight) may be added to bupivacaine for epidural anaesthesia. This significantly improves the quality of the epidural block and does not impair neonatal ventilatory function.[171-173] Morphine 5 mg given epidurally after delivery of the baby provides satisfactory postoperative analgesia for about 23 h with a 0.4% incidence of respiratory depression.[134,175]

Epidural catheter. Local traditions vary with regard to catheter size, end- or side-holes, stiffness and material. An 18-guage catheter of appropriate stiffness and with only an end-hole should theoretically be best. The injected local anaesthetic solution is delivered only to one site, eliminating the possibility of having one hole outside the dura mater and one inside the arachnoid, or one in a vein, or one in the subdural space. An end-hole should also, theoretically, lead to improved detection of intravascular location by the aspiration test, or fluid-column gravitation pull-test, in comparison to a catheter with only side-holes. However, a catheter with an end-hole may be sharper and more easily forced through a thin vein wall, or through the arachnoid membrane if the catheter is in the subdural space.[176]

Midline or paramedian/lateral approach. The midline approach is used traditionally by most anaesthetists. The paramedian approach more often leads to successful and correct catheter placement than the midline approach,[177,178] and a careful technique can eliminate the periosteal trauma which has given rise to the misconception that this approach is more painful than the midline technique.

Test dose for epidural analgesia/anaesthesia. Unfortunately, a negative aspiration test for cerebrospinal fluid or blood is no guarantee that the catheter tip has been positioned correctly. Although the catheter cannot perforate the intact dura mater,[176] a catheter in the subdural, epi-arachnoid space may migrate through the arachnoid membrane. Subdural placement of the epidural needle and catheter is a well-known phenomenon.[179,181] A subdural, epi-arachnoid block may have an onset exactly like that of normal epidural anaesthesia. However, after 20–30 min, the block may increase rapidly to dangerously high levels if a normal epidural loading dose of anaesthetic solution has been injected.

The first epidural test dose must not be larger than the dose that will give a safe level of spinal block if the catheter is in the subarachnoid space; recommended test doses are bupivacaine 10 mg, lignocaine 30 mg or chloroprocaine 90 mg. If injected into the cerebrospinal fluid, these doses will give definite signs of a developing spinal block after 2–3 min.

However, this first test dose will not give any definite symptoms of intravenous injection. This is the reason for the practice of adding adrenaline 15 μg to the first test dose; this dose of adrenaline given intravenously to non-pregnant adult patients creates an increase in heart rate of about 30 beats.min^{-1} and in systolic blood pressure of about 15 mmHg after about 20–25 s, and lasting for about 1 min.[181,182] However, in labouring women, the adrenaline test dose may have poor specificity because of the variation in background maternal heart rate.[183,185]

In the USA, hyperbaric lignocaine (2 ml of lignocaine 15 mg.ml^{-1} in glucose 75 mg.ml^{-1}), with adrenaline 15 μg added, is used extensively as an epidural test dose.[185,186] This is stated to be mandatory (for medicolegal reasons) for epidural anaesthesia for Caesarean section.[186] This test dose gives an objective sensory block at S2 in all cases of subarachnoid injections within 2 min.[185]

As adrenaline also enhances the quality of an epidural block, it should always be used with the test dose if uterine blood flow is not an issue of concern.[187] However, the possibility of a false-negative response to an intravenous adrenaline injection in a parturient must always be kept in mind.

For continuous epidural analgesia, adrenaline is included by those who want to exploit its specific spinal analgesic effect, and omitted by those who are concerned about uterine blood flow,[187,188] or uterine contractions and progress of labour.[100,189]

Incremental epidural loading dose. The first epidural test dose never gives absolute certainty regarding the location of the tip of the epidural catheter. A subarachnoid or intravenous injection of an epidural loading dose can have devastating effects: total spinal block, neurotoxicity, spinal cord ischaemia, cardiovascular collapse or convulsions. Thus, the epidural loading dose of local anaesthetic must always be given in fractional, incremental doses. Doses of 3–5 ml, according to concentration and type of local anaesthetic chosen, with at about 1-min intervals between doses, will provide the vigilant anaesthetist with ample warning of subarachnoid or intravenous injection before a catastrophic dose has been given. However, this requires that the patient is well-informed and that communication, both verbal and visual, is maintained with the patient continuously throughout injection of the loading dose, and for 30 min thereafter. Frequent cardiovascular monitoring during this period is mandatory as well.

Commonly recommended maximal incremental doses[100,136] of bupivacaine are 15 mg every 1–2 min, or 25 mg at intervals of 4–5 min. For lignocaine, a single bolus injection should never exceed 100 mg, and for chloroprocaine, 150 mg.

Incremental extending dose. Epidural injections are additive if repeated at less than 10-min intervals. The level of sensory blockade can be extended one segment[136] by injecting 1.5 ml of bupivacaine 0.5% (5 mg.ml^{-1}), lignocaine 2% (20 mg.ml^{-1}) with adrenaline 5 μg.ml^{-1} or chloroprocaine 30 mg.ml^{-1}.

Prophylaxis and treatment of catastrophic complications of epidural/spinal anaesthesia. It is mandatory that the anaesthetist is mentally prepared for catastrophic events that may strike at any time in the best of hands, and which are always unexpected and inconvenient. All equipment and drugs necessary to treat such complications and to resuscitate mother and child must be immediately available and checked ahead of time.

Using a sensible approach to test-dosing, always using incremental doses for loading and for extending the block, ensuring good patient co-operation, and undertaking vigilant continuous monitoring of the patient's cardiovascular and central nervous system functions, are additional essential precautions.

Convulsions. The vigilant observer is always able to detect warning signs and symptoms. The patient may have subjective sensations of dizziness, tingling, light-headedness, nervousness, apprehension, sudden headache or a metallic taste. Provided that the patient has been warned of these possibilities, she will volunteer the information if any of these symptoms is experienced. Pugnacity, confusion, loquacity or irrationality may become apparent. Twitching of face muscles will be obvious to the anaesthetist in a position to observe the patient's face, before generalized convulsions occur.

Fortunately, such signs of central nervous system irritability occur early after intravenous injection of a local anaesthetic, and *usually before* any cardiovascular signs or symptoms. However, if the patient is heavily sedated, not well-informed or unco-operative, or if the anaesthetist is concentrating on technical details of the block, distracted by other technical difficulties, or absent from the room, a full grand mal seizure, which can develop with surprising rapidity, may occur unexpectedly.

Oxygen administered by mask and bag, simultaneously with diazepam 2.5 mg, midazolam 1 mg or thiopentone 75 mg intravenously, will stop the central nervous system irritability if treatment is started early. However, if grand mal seizures are already present, ventilation becomes compromised. Suxamethonium 1 mg.kg^{-1} followed by tracheal intubation is required if the central nervous system depressant drugs do not stop the seizures immediately. It is mandatory that the patient does not develop hypercapnia, hypoxaemia and acidosis,[163,164] as these aggravate the toxic effects of the local anaesthetic, especially the cardiotoxic effects of bupivacaine. Therefore, administration of suxamethonium and ventilation with 100% oxygen may be life-saving.[163]

Cardiovascular collapse. High epidural, subdural or high subarachnoid anaesthesia with total sympathetic blockade, in a patient under stress with a high vagal tone, decrease venous return, slow the heart and cause a catastrophic drop in cardiac output and arterial blood pressure. If treated immediately with ephedrine 5–25 mg intravenously, atropine 0.5–1 mg or glycopyrrolate 0.25–0.5 mg, simultaneously with head-down tilt, increased intravenous infusion rate, uterine displacement from the vena cava and assisted oxygenation, the situation should be corrected rapidly. However, if delays occur for any reason, the situation deteriorates rapidly and a catastrophe may be unavoidable.[182]

Cardiac arrhythmias. Cardiac arrhythmias occur particularly with intravenous injection or gross overdose of bupivacaine. Ventricular re-entry arrhythmias (ventricular tachycardia or ventricular fibrillation) induced by bupivacaine may be difficult to treat. In animal experiments, bretylium has been shown to be the most effective treatment for bupivacaine-induced ventricular arrhythmias.[190] The dose of bretylium is 5–10 mg.kg^{-1}. Defibrillation, large doses of adrenaline and atropine, correction of acidosis and even extracorporeal assisted circulation have been used in successful resuscitation from severe bupivacaine cardiotoxicity.

Total spinal and high subdural block. When respiratory muscle insufficiency occurs, it is of course mandatory to secure the airway, to ventilate the lungs and to oxygenate the patient appropriately. Cardiovascular support and sedation may be required as well.

Sudden unexpected cardiac arrest during spinal/epidural anaesthesia for Caesarean section. Rarely, incidents of sudden, unexpected cardiac arrest have occurred during spinal or epidural anaesthesia, some for Caesarean section.[25,191] Some of the patients were sedated, so that observation of the central nervous system effects of hypoxia were not recognized.[192] When cardiovascular collapse and cardiac arrest occurred, there was a mean time lag of 8 min from cardiac arrest until administration of the first dose of adrenaline, with a range up to 24 min,[191] indicating suboptimal resuscitation. Prompt administration of adrenaline, in sufficient doses, increases the probability of successful resuscitation.[25] Cardiopulmonary resuscitation in the parturient is unlikely to be successful unless compression of the vena cava is reduced by tilting the patient. If correct resuscitation in the properly positioned patient is not successful after about 5 min, immediate Caesarean delivery must be considered.[100]

Backache after epidural anaesthesia. In a recent study, long-term backache after childbirth occurred in about 18% of women who received epidural analgesia for labour pain and in 10% of those who did not.[193] After elective Caesarean delivery, 14% of those who had epidural anaesthesia and 11% of those who had general anaesthesia had persistent backache. These incidences were derived from a restrospective postal survey with 80% response rate, and may therefore be biased. A Norwegian survey revealed an 11% incidence of backache 1 year after childbirth, irrespective of the method used for relieving labour pain.[194] Thus, the true incidence of long-term backache caused by epidural or spinal analgesia in association with childbirth is probably not significant. Nevertheless, this possibility should be included in the information given to the patient when these techniques of pain relief/anaesthesia are discussed.

An acute, cramping type of severe backache occurring after outpatient chloroprocaine epidural anaesthesia has been ascribed to the ethylenediamine tetra-acetic acid content of the new commercial formulation of chloroprocaine.[195] It has not been observed in obstetric patients. Generous infiltration with a dilute local anaesthetic solution from the skin to the lamina reduces the incidence of post-lumbar puncture or post-epidural backache.[196]

Combined spinal and epidural anaesthesia. The rapidity of induction and the density of a spinal block, combined with the ability to extend the sensory level and to give optimal postoperative analgesia through an epidural catheter, have made the technique of combined spinal and epidural anaesthesia popular in orthopaedic patients,[171,197] and the technique has been introduced into obstetric anaesthesia practice.[198,199] Whereas the epidural catheter can be inserted after the spinal anaesthetic solution has been injected in surgical patients, it is prudent in obstetric patients to position the epidural catheter first, and then to perform the lumbar subarachnoid puncture and spinal anaesthetic injection. This can be undertaken in the same interspace using an epidural needle and a spinal needle, or through the newly devised epidural–spinal needle combination.[173]

Continuous spinal block. Continuous spinal block, achieved by inserting a catheter through a 21-gauge needle, causes unacceptable incidences of post-dural puncture headache in obstetric patients.[200] The new 32-gauge microcatheters[201] appear to cause an unacceptable incidence of permanent neurological deficits.[89,202]

General anaesthesia for Caesarean delivery

Indications. General anaesthesia is necessary when the patient does not want regional anaesthesia, when regional anaesthesia is medically contra-indicated or when rapid induction is required; in the last instance, a spinal technique may still be a feasible alternative for the experienced practitioner.

Evaluation of the airway and intubation. About 40% of maternal deaths directly attributable to anaesthesia are from anoxia, of which aspiration and difficult intubation are the major causes.[203] If the patient cannot extend the neck well or has micrognathia, significant intubation problems must be expected. Oedema of the upper airway in pregnancy, especially after prolonged labour and in pre-eclampsia,[202,203] and breast enlargement interfering with insertion of the laryngoscope,[206] are among factors that make about 1 in 29 obstetric patients difficult to intubate.[207] Added to these problems are the changes in gastro-intestinal physiology, which place every parturient at high risk of regurgitation and acid aspiration. The need for rapid induction when maternal haemorrhage, fetal distress or some other obstetric emergency is present increases the stress load on the anaesthetist with two or more lives in his/her hands.

The degree of visualization of the soft palate, uvula and faucial pillars can be a sensitive prediction of difficult intubation.[208] The oropharynx should be examined with the patient sitting in front of the anaesthetist, with her head in the neutral position, mouth open and tongue maximally protruded. Intubaton will be increasingly difficult from Mallampati class 1 to class 3.

- *Class 1:* faucial pillars, soft palate, and uvula can be visualized; intubation should be easy
- *Class 2:* faucial pillars and soft palate can be visualized, but the uvula is masked by the base of the tongue; visualization of the glottis may be difficult
- *Class 3:* only soft palate can be visualized; intubation will be difficult.

This Mallampati classification, of course, is not foolproof,[209] but the possibility of performing the operation under regional anaesthesia must be considered carefully when intubation problems are obvious.[210]

Difficult airway and obstetric emergencies

Save the mother or save the child? When it is obvious that the patient has a difficult airway, the fetus is in distress, and regional anaesthesia, for whatever reason, is not possible, the difficult choice must be made between putting the mother's life or brain at risk, and trying to save the fetus. In this extreme situation, medical, medicolegal and ethical considerations all favour overlooking the fetus, and performing a maximal effort to save the mother's life.[100] The eventual outcome may otherwise be that both mother and fetus are lost or severely damaged for life.

Techniques to overcome difficult intubation. Six techniques are in use.[100,203] Any unusual technique for difficult intubation must be learned and practised in patients with normal intubation conditions, to be of any help in difficult situations.

1. Direct laryngoscopy is usually not possible when intubation is difficult. However, by having a variety of laryngoscope blades and a short, or 'polio', laryngoscope handle for very obese or large-breasted patients, it may be possible to visualize the tip of the epiglottis sufficiently to introduce a styletted, appropriately curved, tracheal tube through the glottis. Laryngoscope blades of the following types should be available: Macintosh no. 3 and no. 4, Miller no. 3.[211]

2. Fibre-optic endoscopic tracheal intubation is a powerful method.[210] It requires expensive equipment and sufficient experience and skill to be of any help in a difficult intubation for Caesarean section, when time is limited.

3. Retrograde intubation with an epidural catheter introduced through the cricothyroid membrane has a high success rate.[213] However, this method also requires experience and sufficient time, which may not be available in the obstetric patient.

4. The 'lighted stylet' or 'light wand' technique appears to be easily learned, is atraumatic and does not require more time than an ordinary direct laryngoscopic intubation.[214,215] Again, experience with this method is a prerequisite for obstetric anaesthesia.

5. Blind nasal intubation is an alternative in non-emergency situations. However, in the parturient, the mucous membranes are swollen and friable. This exaggerates the normal complication with nasotracheal intubation; epistaxis occurs easily and rapidly complicates the situation.[215]

6. The laryngeal mask has become popular rapidly

since its introduction in 1983.[216,217] Once in place, and with cricoid pressure maintained, it may be possible to pass a tracheal tube through the laryngeal mask, either blindly or using a fibrescope. The laryngeal mask has been incorporated into some failed intubation drill procedures.[218,219] However, although the laryngeal mask has been used in several million patients in the UK, it has not reached universal familiarity among anaesthetists. As with all the above techniques, appropriate skill in using the laryngeal mask must be acquired in non-emergency patients before it is contemplated when difficulty is encountered in intubation in the parturient. It should be remembered that, even when correctly placed, a laryngeal mask is no guarantee that the airway is protected from gastric contents.

Management of failed intubation. When intubation is obviously very difficult, it is vital to make an early decision to abandon the intubation attempt and ventilate the lungs with 100% oxygen while cricoid pressure is maintained. 'These patients do not die from failure to intubate, but from failure to stop trying to intubate'.[220] Prolonged attempts at intubation provoke retching as the patient wakes up from the induction dose of thiopentone, with the risk of vomiting and subsequent aspiration of the acid gastric contents to the lung. Haemoglobin desaturation occurs rapidly in the apnoeic parturient because of the increased oxygen consumption and reduced functional residual capacity. Repeated attempts at intubation cause swelling and oedema, and may lead rapidly to a completely obstructed upper airway. An extra dose of suxamethonium or administration of another neuromuscular blocking drug should not be employed unless it is decided to proceed with general anaesthesia and ventilation by mask.

In any anaesthesia department, a failed intubation, failed mask ventilation protocol must be established, and practised frequently. Many variations have been published, and local traditions vary.[100,136,137,203,218,219,221] The essentials of a failed intubation protocol should include the following.

1. Call for help from the most experienced staff available.
2. Maintain *correct* cricoid pressure.[222]
3. Maintain patient tilted to the left.[100] Use the head-down position only if regurgitation or vomiting occurs.
4. Ventilate the lungs with 100% oxygen using bag and mask.
5. Use the triple airway manoeuvre.[223] Make sure cricoid pressure is correct, and not a suffocating pinch on the larynx. This results in more difficult ventilation and intubation.
6. If the airway is clear, continue inhalational analgesia and instruct the obstetrician to deliver the baby.
7. If the airway cannot be improved beyond partial obstruction, allow the mother to recover from anaesthesia.
8. If the airway is completely obstructed, perform transtracheal oxygenation, with a catheter-over-needle through the cricothyroid membrane. Use oxygen from the fresh gas outlet of the anaesthesia machine or oxygen cylinder. Jet-ventilation or high-frequency ventilation, if available, makes transtracheal catheter ventilation possible.[224] Misplacement of the cricothyroid catheter is an ever-present risk, and care should also be taken to ensure a clear route for expiratory gases.
9. Cricothyrotomy and ventilation through a mini-tracheotomy tube is an alternative if this method is familiar.

Some authorities[135] place the patient in the left lateral, head-down position and use an oesophageal obturator airway device. However, we agree that the left lateral head-down position can make conditions more difficult for both the anaesthetist and the surgeon, increasing the risk of regurgitation without necessarily reducing the risk of aspiration.[100] The oesophageal obturator airway may be a helpful device in deeply comatose patients, but manipulation of the pharynx and oesophagus in the lightly anaesthetized parturient may easily stimulate retching and vomiting, dramatically worsening the airway situation.[100] If airway obstruction is present, introduction of a laryngeal mask airway may enable ventilation to be maintained; however, the risk of regurgitation remains, and cricoid pressure must be sustained. For further guidelines, see Table 15.6.

Antacid therapy and control of gastric content. Aspiration of acid gastric contents is a depressingly common cause of maternal morbidity and mortality,[225] and has been estimated to result in one maternal death per year for every 1 000 000 inhabitants of the USA.[226] Non-particulate antacid therapy, preferably sodium citrate 0.3 M,[227] in a volume of 30 ml, decreases the hydrogen ion concentration of gastric contents for about 30 min. Unfortunately, a single, pre-anaesthetic dose of sodium citrate fails to raise gastric pH above 3.0 in 30% of emergency patients undergoing Caesarean section, and is not much more effective when given at 2-hourly intervals;[228] in contrast, 6-hourly ranitidine 150 mg followed by a single dose of sodium citrate is 100% effective in raising gastric pH to safe levels. Although individual voices have expressed concern over the trend in anti-aspiration prophylaxis,[220] this

Table 15.6 Failed intubation protocol

Airway and mask ventilation satisfactory
Maintain correct cricoid pressure, mask ventilate and oxygenate
1. *If non-emergency situation*, let patient awaken, postpone surgery, deliver later with regional anaesthesia, awake intubation, or tracheostomy
2. *If maternal emergency, or fetal distress and salvageable fetus*, perform surgery with bag-mask ventilation and oxygenation and appropriate anaesthesia (e.g. halothane + ketamine)

Airway and bag-mask ventilation unsatisfactory
Maintain correct cricoid pressure
1. *If non-emergency* situation, allow patient to wake up, postpone surgery, perform under regional anaesthesia, awake intubation or tracheostomy
2. *If maternal emergency*, or fetal distress (salvageable fetus), transtracheal oxygenation and intravenous anaesthesia for appropriate surgery

Bag-mask ventilation impossible
Maintain correct cricoid pressure. Consider laryngeal mask airway
1. *If non-emergency* situation, transtracheal oxygenation until patient is awake, postpone surgery and perform with regional anaesthesia, awake intubation or tracheostomy
2. *If maternal emergency*, transtracheal oxygenation and intravenous anaesthesia for appropriate surgery
3. *If fetal distress/asphyxia and questionable salvageable fetus*, transtracheal oxygenation until mother wakes up, postpone surgery or vaginal delivery of asphyxiated fetus

---

combination of H_2-receptor antagonist and non-particulate antacid has won widespread favour, and is now in use in 87% of obstetric units in the UK.[229] Unlike sodium bicarbonate, sodium citrate does not generate carbon dioxide in the stomach and thus does *not* interfere with capnography as a diagnostic aid to tracheal versus oesophageal intubation.[230]

There is controversy concerning attempts to empty the stomach in non-elective patients who have recently eaten. If the fetus is at risk, an exacerbation of the fetal condition may be precipitated by the stress and breath-holding during attempted gastric emptying. It is also impossible to empty the stomach completely, even with a large-bore gastric irrigation tube.

Pre-oxygenation and psychological preparation of the patient. It is mandatory that the patient inhales at least four vital capacity breaths of 100% oxygen. This washes out a sufficient amount of nitrogen from the residual lung volume, almost to the same extent as 3–5 min of pre-oxygenation at tidal volume.[231] Whenever possible, pre-oxygenation should be of more than usual duration in this situation, to improve the oxygen reserve as much as possible in face of an increased oxygen consumption and an intubation procedure which may be more difficult than in non-pregnant patients. The anaesthetist or a trained assistant should concentrate on holding the face mask, continuously informing and comforting the patient as the remaining pre-induction preparations are completed.

Induction of unconsciousness. A rapid-sequence induction is mandatory. The Sellick manoeuvre,[222] providing anterior-to-posterior pressure on the cricoid cartilage, should be started as the patient loses consciousness and must be maintained until the lungs are protected by inflation of the cuff of the tracheal tube. Unfortunately, insufficiently trained assistants tend to use a firm, two-finger suffocating bilateral squeeze on the larynx, instead of pushing *downwards* on the cricoid cartilage in a straight anterior-to-posterior direction. This pinch manoeuvre on the larynx makes intubation more difficult and obstructs the laryngeal inlet so that face mask ventilation, if required, is critically compromised.

Atropine decreases the lower oesophageal sphincter pressure, and is therefore omitted by many from the rapid-sequence induction. However, the high sympathetic and vagal tone in the psychologically stressed parturient may predispose to sudden bradycardia at induction, when the sympathetic tone suddenly decreases. This is especially so when the cholinergic drug suxamethonium is given to facilitate intubation. If repeated doses of suxamethonium become necessary, atropine, or preferably glycopyrrolate, must be given.

Rapid and pleasant induction of unconsciousness is achieved with thiopentone, in a dose of about 4 mg.kg^{-1} (or up to 300 mg). However, Tunstall,[232] using the isolated forearm technique, has shown that half of the mothers given this dose of thiopentone respond to command 2–3 min after the start of the injection of thiopentone.

If the patient is in hypovolaemic shock, the induction dose of hypnotic drug must be reduced by at least two-thirds. Ketamine 0.5–1 mg.kg^{-1} given with thiopentone 2 mg.kg^{-1} may be a better choice in asthmatic or hypovolaemic patients.

Neuromuscular blockade for intubation of the

trachea. Suxamethonium (succinylcholine) 1.5 mg/kg remains the most rapidly acting muscle relaxant. It should not be preceded by a defasciculating dose of non-depolarizing muscle relaxant, which delays and antagonizes the effect of suxamethonium. In the event of failed tracheal intubation, the short action of suxamethonium permits an early return of spontaneous ventilation. Suxamethonium also increases lower oesophageal sphincter tone.

Verification of correct tracheal tube placement. Unfortunately, all of the clinical signs which are used to indicate correct tracheal intubation can fail.[233] Surprisingly, unrecognized oesophageal intubation occurs again and again. Unless the patient has recently imbibed a carbonated fluid, a capnograph showing an end-tidal carbon dioxide concentration around 5%, with a normal waveform is the most definite objective indication of correct tube placement.[230,233,234] A high level of suspicion for oesophageal intubation after a difficult intubation procedure helps to prevent the catastrophic sequelae of an unsuspected, unidentified, prolonged oesophageal intubation.

Maintenance of muscle relaxation. When the trachea has been intubated successfully, muscle relaxation should be prolonged by administration of a non-depolarizing drug preferably vecuronium 4 mg or atracurium 25 mg. This will ensure sufficient muscle relaxation for the usual duration of a Caesarean operation. The newborn will not be significantly affected by these doses of muscle relaxants. If a second dose of suxamethonium is necessary, an anticholinergic drug must be administered concomitantly.

Maintenance of unconsciousness and avoidance of awareness. The anaesthetist should always bear in mind the possibility of wakefulness and awareness during general anaesthesia for Caesarean section. Awareness refers to the unfortunate situation in which the patient is able to remember being awake, having pain or hearing conversation, and being unable to indicate her state of mind because of the effects of the neuromuscular blocking drugs. Tunstall[235] has made the useful distinction between the state of wakefulness during balanced anaesthesia, and awareness; the patient may be awake and may be able to indicate this by signalling this to the anaesthetist if the neuromuscular blocking drug is prevented from reaching one forearm by an inflated blood pressure cuff (the isolated forearm technique).[235,236] Patients may frequently have episodes of wakefulness after induction, but are usually not able to recall this after surgery.[137]

Episodes of awareness for which the patient was not given proper postanaesthetic support may have disastrous consequences upon psychological well-being; nightmares, sleep phobia and anxiety states can last for years after such an incident.[237] Such unfortunate patient histories are well known to the public from mass media headlines. Patients with sequelae after awareness have been treated successfully by deliberately inducing amnesic wakefulness under isolated-forearm control during a repeat general anaesthetic.[238]

Unfortunately, wakefulness and awareness result from failure to appreciate the short duration of the induction dose of thiopentone,[232] the considerable time needed for uptake of significant inhalational anaesthetics through the lungs, and the need for adequate maintenance anaesthetic gas concentrations. Unfounded fears that volatile anaesthetics may cause uterine hypotonicity and bleeding also contribute to administration of excessively conservative concentrations of anaesthetics.

By the time that the tracheal tube is in the correct position, the induction dose of the hypnotic drug is losing its effect. Unless administration of the inhalational agents is started immediately and unless sufficiently high concentrations are delivered for the first few minutes, the prolonged lag before the anaesthetic partial pressure reaches a plateau in the central nervous system may result in wakefulness.[232]

Whenever nitrous oxide can be used (when maternal or fetal oxygenation is not a critical issue), it increases the speed of uptake of the volatile anaesthetics through the 'second gas' effect.[239]

Guidelines for anaesthetic administration after tracheal intubation for Caesarean section[232]

1. *No maternal or fetal oxygenation problem:* nitrous oxide 66% inspired concentration for *3 min*, thereafter 50%. Isoflurane 0.75% or enflurane 1% from the start.

2. *When nitrous oxide cannot be used:* isoflurane 3% or enflurane 4% for *3 min*, thereafter isoflurane 1.25% or enflurane 1.75%.

At these concentrations, uterine tone, uteroplacental blood flow and the neonate are not affected significantly.[240]

Suppression of hypertensive response to laryngoscopy. The normal hypertensive response to laryngoscopy and tracheal intubation can be exaggerated in mothers who suffer from pregnancy-induced hypertensive disease. Blood pressure above 160/110 mmHg during the preparatory phase before induction of anaesthesia calls for some measure to blunt this response. The hypertensive response can be blocked in part by administration of a small dose of the rapidly acting potent opioid alfentanil 10 µg.kg^{-1} intravenously as the mother is being pre-oxygenated. A double dose is more effective, but causes a high incidence of neonatal respiratory depression.[137] Alternatives are intravenous hydralazine 10–20 mg 5–10 min before intubation. Where trimetaphan is still available, a titrated infusion of a solution containing 1 mg.ml^{-1} can be used effectively to block the hypertensive response during the induction period without causing any effect on the newborn.[137]

Effect of general anaesthesia on the newborn. Appropriately conducted general anaesthesia is no more depressant to the newborn than regional anaesthesia.[241,242] However, if a concentration of 70–75% nitrous oxide is used for induction and maintenance, neonatal depression may be apparent if pre-delivery anaesthesia lasts longer than 10 min.[242] Provided that at least 50% oxygen is given after the first 3 min, and that the above-mentioned volatile anaesthetic concentrations are not exceeded, and that aortocaval compression is avoided, pre-delivery anaesthesia of up to 30 min does not seem to affect the infant adversely.[243,244]

The uterine incision-to-delivery time appears to be more important to neonatal outcome than the pre-delivery anaesthesia interval; if the uterine incision-to-delivery interval exceeds 180 s, the infant may be affected adversely because of interruption of the placental blood flow.[243]

Urgent Caesarean section

If an epidural catheter has been inserted for analgesia before the need for urgent Caesarean section developed, extension of the epidural analgesia up to thoracic segments T3–T4 and down to S5 is possible by using an extending dose of chloroprocaine 3% (30 mg.ml^{-1}; or lignocaine 2% (20 mg.ml^{-1}) with adrenaline 5 µg.ml^{-1}), in a volume of 1.5 ml per segment. This can be performed only if the patient has a satisfactory blood volume and cardiovascular status, and if the fetus is not suffering severe intra-uterine distress. Extension of the block with bupivacaine for an urgent Caesarean section cannot be recommended because of the time required, as well as the possibility of transplacental cation trapping and the increased risk of cardiovascular and central nervous system depression of the neonate. Spinal anaesthesia in expert hands is an excellent alternative, again provided that there is reasonable cardiovascular stability of the mother. If these conditions are not met, rapid-sequence induction of general anaesthesia is necessary.

Emergency Caesarean section

The time available to extend an epidural block or to induce subarachnoid block may *not* be sufficient, and unless serious intubation problems are expected, rapid-sequence induction of general anaesthesia is the method of choice.

COMPLICATED OBSTETRICS

Antepartum haemorrhage

This is caused most commonly by various degrees of placenta praevia and abruptio placentae. *Placenta praevia* occurs in up to 1% of pregnancies, three times more commonly in those aged more than 35 years than in those younger than 25 years, and causes about 1% maternal and about 25% perinatal mortality.[245] The cardinal symptom is painless, bright red bleeding occurring usually after the seventh month of pregnancy. *Abruptio placentae*, usually during the last 2 months of gestation, and more often in hypertensive patients, occurs in up to 2.4% of pregnant women.[245] The maternal mortality rate is about 10% and perinatal mortality in excess of 50%.[245] The cardinal symptoms are vaginal bleeding of dark, clotted blood, with uterine tenderness and hypertonus. However, in some cases there may be a retroplacental, totally concealed haemorrhage. The possibility of *placenta accreta* should be kept in mind if the patient has a diagnosed placenta praevia and has undergone previous Caesarean section. About 5% of patients diagnosed with placenta praevia have placenta accreta. The bleeding from attempts at removing a placenta accreta can be very marked.

The anaesthetist has to face both the challenge of resuscitating the hypovolaemic mother, sometimes with the added problem of coagulation and haemostatic abnormalities, and administering appropriate anaesthesia for emergency Caesarean section, and sometimes hysterectomy. The usual problems of emergency Caesarean section and general anaesthesia are magnified. The rapid-sequence induction may be modified by using ketamine 0.75–1 mg.kg^{-1} instead of thiopentone.

In these situations, at least two large-bore intravenous cannulae should be inserted, preferably in the antecubital fossae. A neck haematoma from failed central venous catheterization complicates rapid-sequence induction dramatically. This emergency situation requires several well-qualified staff to be in attendance.

Postpartum haemorrhage

After Caesarean delivery, 10 units of oxytocin are added to the intravenous infusion. Intravenous ergometrine should not be used because of the severe maternal vasoconstriction which it causes (see above).

Manual removal of the placenta

The anaesthetic management of this emergency does not differ from anaesthesia for operative delivery, except that nitrous oxide and opioid analgesics can be used as required. Fortunately, any form of regional anaesthetic used for the delivery is usually sufficient for painless manual removal of the placenta. However, one should not be tempted to give intravenous analgesics and sedatives in an attempt to avoid full general anaesthesia; an unanticipated loss of consciousness and of airway protection in a hypovolaemic mother can develop into a catastrophe if regurgitation occurs. This procedure, which is usually a brief and minor operation, may occasionally be unexpectedly difficult and prolonged. A low saddle block is also well-suited for this procedure unless the mother has become severely hypovolaemic.

Toxaemia of pregnancy

Pre-eclampsia/eclampsia

The combination of hypertension, proteinuria and/or oedema is diagnosed as pre-eclampsia; when convulsions and coma appear in addition, the diagnosis is eclampsia. Pre-eclampsia develops in 5–10% of pregnancies, predominantly in the young nulliparous patient. The condition accounts for about 20% of maternal deaths and a considerable proportion of perinatal mortality.[136,221]

The aetiology and pathogenesis of pre-eclampsia and eclampsia are unclear. There may be an immunological mechanism, in which fetal tissues are rejected by the mother, causing placental vasculitis and decreased placental perfusion, with increased production of renin, angiotensin, aldosterone and thromboplastin. There is an imbalance between the placental production of prostacyclin and thromboxane. Thromboxane, the vasoconstrictor and stimulator of platelet aggregation, is relatively increased (about seven times) compared with prostacyclin, the potent vasodilator and inhibitor of platelet aggregation.[246,247]

The pathophysiological changes involve every major organ system. There is generalized vasoconstriction, and the intravascular volume and the functioning extracellular fluid volume are decreased, despite retention of sodium and water and generalized oedema. Fibrin deposits are found in most of the small blood vessels of the body. Glomerular filtration rate and urinary output are reduced. Fibrin deposits are present within the glomeruli, constricting glomerular vessels and increasing glomerular permeability to albumin. Significant coagulopathy, with increased platelet adhesiveness and thrombocytopenia, may occur. Fetal growth retardation and eventually fetal distress are common sequelae to the decreased uteroplacental perfusion.

Pre-eclampsia is classified as *severe* if any of the following symptoms are present: systolic blood pressure above 160 mmHg, diastolic blood pressure above 110 mmHg, proteinuria of more than 5 g in 24 h, oliguria below 400 ml in 24 h, cerebral or visual disturbances, pulmonary oedema, cyanosis or epigastric pain.

The cerebral hyperexcitability which occurs in this condition may be related to focal hypoperfusion. Cerebral haemorrhage and cerebral oedema have been leading causes of death from pre-eclampsia and eclampsia.[248] The HELLP syndrome, with haemolysis, elevated liver enzymes and low platelets, is probably an extreme variant of toxaemia of pregnancy.[133] In untreated pre-eclampsia/eclampsia, pulmonary capillary wedge pressure and cardiac output are low, systemic vascular resistance is high and the heart rate is increased.

Because of increased platelet consumption from thromboxane-induced platelet adherence at sites of endothelial damage, about 20% of patients with pre-eclampsia develop thrombocytopenia of a moderate degree ($100-150 \times 10^9$/l). The concentration of fibrin degradation products may be elevated in a few patients, whereas plasma fibrinogen concentration remains normal unless there is a concomitant placental abruption and enormous coagulation factor consumption. Bleeding time appears to be the most reliable test of clotting abnormalities in pre-eclampsia.[249]

Management of pre-eclampsia/eclampsia is symptomatic. Apart from the recently established treatment with low-dose acetylsalicylic acid to correct the thromboxane/prostacyclin ratio and improve placental blood flow,[126,127] the main goals are to prevent or control convulsions, improve organ perfusion, normalize blood pressure and correct clotting abnormalities. Delivery is the ultimate treatment if pregnancy is close to term and symptoms are resistant to standard measures. The treatment should be continued for about 48 h after delivery. In the USA, the mainstay of management of pre-eclampsia/eclampsia is administration of magnesium sulphate by intravenous infusion.[136,221] Magnesium has anticonvulsant effects and causes peripheral arterial dilatation. Therapeutic maternal blood levels are about 2–3 mmol.l^{-1} (normal 0.7–1 mmol.l^{-1}). The patient usually receives an intravenous loading dose of 4 g (16 mmol.l^{-1}) magnesium sulphate over about 5 min, followed by a continuous infusion of 1–2 g.h^{-1} (4–8 mmol.h^{-1}). Electrocardiogram changes appear as plasma magnesium concentration increases above 2.5 mmol.l^{-1} and become severe at a value of around 5 mmol.l^{-1}. Loss of deep tendon reflexes and skeletal muscle relaxation occur at the same concentration. Respiratory arrest occurs if the concentration increases to 7–8 mmol.l^{-1} and cardiac arrest at a plasma concentration of around 12–15 mmol.l^{-1}.

Magnesium potentiates the duration and intensity of both depolarizing and non-depolarizing muscle relaxants by decreasing the amount of acetylcholine liberated from the motor nerve terminals and by diminishing the sensitivity of the receptor to acetylcholine, as well as by reducing excitability of the skeletal muscle membrane.

Intravenous fluid therapy is directed at correction of the functioning extracellular fluid volume by increasing central venous pressure to approximately 5 mmHg and increasing urine output to about 1 ml.kg^{-1}.h^{-1}. This should be achieved primarily by infusion of balanced crystalloid solution, and then 5% albumin solution.

Antihypertensive medical therapy should be started when the patient has been resuscitated with fluid. Hydralazine is the most commonly used vasodilator because it improves uteroplacental and renal blood flows. This drug can be given orally, intramuscularly or intravenously.

Sodium nitroprusside may be used in severe hypertension, but the dose must be less than 5–10 µg.kg^{-1}.h^{-1} to avoid cyanide toxicity in the fetus.[250] If cerebral oedema is suspected or confirmed, trimetaphan is, theoretically, the preferred hypotensive drug. Other drugs that have been used include α-methyldopa, clonidine, nitroglycerine, ketanserin, atenolol and labetalol.[251]

Anaesthetic management. In pre-eclamptic patients who are volume-replenished and have no haemostatic problems, epidural analgesia/anaesthesia is indicated specifically. It reduces blood pressure, improves maternal haemodynamics and leads to a significant improvement in placental perfusion.[44,252,255] If general anaesthesia is required for a pre-eclamptic/eclamptic patient for Caesarean section, vigorous precautions must be taken to reduce the hypertensive response to laryngoscopy and intubation of the trachea (see above). The risks of cerebral haemorrhage and pulmonary oedema, the primary causes of maternal mortality in this condition, are otherwise unacceptably high.[254,256,275] If magnesium sulphate has been administered, muscle relaxants must be titrated carefully and their effect monitored with the aid of a nerve–muscle stimulator. Calcium is an antidote to magnesium-induced neuromuscular blockade, but also to its hypotensive effect.

Embolism

Embolism is a major cause of maternal mortality.[254] Major *amniotic fluid embolism* is unpredictable, fortunately rare (1/8000–80 000)[258] and presents suddenly with all the signs of a catastrophic reduction in cardiac output, including precipitous decreases in end-tidal carbon dioxide concentration and arterial oxygen saturation. Symptomatic treatment comprises ventilation with 100% oxygen and the use of the Trendelenburg position. Cardiac arrest may follow rapidly. If primary resuscitation is successful, major problems may follow from massive coagulation failure. Venous catheterization in the antecubital fossa rather than in the neck or the subclavian veins is recommended. Expert assistance from a haematologist and the blood bank is required.

Air embolism of low magnitude may occur as often as in two-thirds of Caesarean sections under general anaesthesia and in one-third of Caesarean sections under regional anaesthesia.[258] The frequently patent foramen ovale makes any air bubble a potential hazard. Fall in end-tidal carbon dioxide concentration indicates significant embolism. The risk of major air embolism is reduced by avoiding the following: hypovolaemia, low central venous pressure, unnecessary use of the Trendelenburg position and exteriorizing the uterus.

Thrombo-embolism from deep vein thrombosis (2–12/1000 deliveries) remains a major cause of maternal puerperal mortality.[258] Risk factors that indicate the need for active prophylactic measures include age and parity, obesity, Caesarean section, prolonged bed rest and antithrombin III deficiency. Antithrombin III, the major in vivo inhibitor of thrombin and other coagulation system proteases, is deficient in 1/2000–5000 patients (autosomal dominant antithrombin III deficiency). Symptoms of pulmonary thrombo-embolism range from mild pleuritic chest pain to massive cardiopulmonary collapse and haemoptysis. End-tidal carbon dioxide concentration and arterial oxygenation decrease dramatically. Treatment is symptomatic; the patient should be nursed in the intensive care unit. Heparinization is achieved with an intravenous bolus dose of 5000–10 000 units followed by an infusion of 1000 unit.h^{-1}, adjusted to maintain the activated clotting time at 1.5–2.5 times control (or activated partial thromboplastin time at 2–3 times control). The roles of thrombolytic therapy and surgical embolectomy are limited during pregnancy, and risky in the puerperium.[258]

Breech delivery

Breech presentation occurs in 3–4% of term pregnancies, more often in premature deliveries, and in patients with placenta praevia, a uterine tumour, hydramnios, multiple gestation or multiparity. Epidural analgesia is beneficial for both mother and fetus and is the anaesthetic procedure of choice; the mother is able to co-operate and assist in a controlled descent and expulsion of the child.[254,259-261] The condition of the neonate is improved.[259,261] With effective lumbar epidural analgesia, intra-uterine manipulation can usually be performed between contractions. If uterine relaxation is required to complete breech extraction, administration of nitroglycerine 0.1 mg intravenously causes uterine relaxation after 30 s, lasting about 1 min.[261] However, if the mother is severely hypovolaemic, enflurane or isoflurane anaesthesia after rapid tracheal intubation may be necessary.

Twin or multiple delivery

These occur in about 1% of pregnancies in the general population. However, increasing use of drugs to induce ovulation has increased the incidence markedly in recent years. Pregnancy-induced hypertension, excessive blood loss and hypotonic postpartum uterus occur more frequently. Twins may be delivered vaginally, for which epidural analgesia is well-indicated,[261-263] but triplets (or larger numbers) are usually delivered by Caesarean section. Anaesthesia may be required for reversion, extraction, breech delivery, Caesarean section or mid-forceps delivery. Continuous lumbar epidural analgesia, topped up to produce a sufficiently dense block, is usually the anaesthetic technique of choice; neonatal condition, especially of the second twin, is improved after either vaginal or abdominal delivery.[261,262] The large uterus in cases of multiple gestation exaggerates the problem of aortocaval compression, and uterine displacement and adequate prehydration become especially important.

Preterm labour and delivery

The special anaesthetic requirements and risks during delivery of a preterm fetus, i.e. an infant born before the 37th week of gestation, are the same for a fetus classed as small for gestational age, i.e. an infant born at term but with a weight of more than 2 s.d. below the mean. Almost 10% of all births occur preterm, and cause about 80% of early neonatal mortality.[264] Because of the many severe problems which can occur after preterm delivery (including respiratory distress syndrome, intracranial haemorrhage, hypoglycaemia, hyperbilirubinaemia and hypocalcaemia), obstetricians frequently try to inhibit preterm labour and to enhance fetal lung maturity. Administration of glucocorticoids to the mother for at least 24 h accelerates fetal lung maturation, decreasing the incidence of respiratory distress syndrome and probably bronchopulmonary dysplasia, necrotizing enterocolitis and patent ductus arteriosus, without causing significant maternal complications, or neonatal or developmental sequelae in the child.[264] A common regimen is to give betamethasone 12 mg intramuscularly, repeated after 24 h.

Uterine activity is frequently suppressed by β-sympathomimetics, such as ritodrine and terbutaline. Other tocolytic agents used to delay delivery are magnesium sulphate, prostaglandin synthesis inhibitors (indomethacin) and calcium antagonists (nifedipine).[264] The β-adrenergic drugs used for tocolysis predominantly stimulate $β_2$-receptors and thus cause myometrial inhibition. However, they also have effects on $β_1$-receptors and several maternal complications may arise, including tachyarrhythmias, vasodilatation, hypokalaemia, hyperglycaemia, paralytic ileus, restlessness, tremor, chest pain, myocardial ischaemia, pulmonary oedema and sudden maternal death.[264] Many of these maternal effects cause serious interactions with anaesthetic drugs and techniques. β-Adrenergic stimulation increases renin, aldosterone and antidiuretic hormone secretion.[264]

Aggressive hydration may cause pulmonary oedema in these patients. Tachycardia, myocardial ischaemia, vasodilatation and hypokalaemia all increase the normal risks of general anaesthesia. It is usual to avoid halothane (cardiac arrhythmias), atropine and pancuronium (tachycardia). It is prudent to delay general anaesthesia for at least 3 h after discontinuation of tocolytic agents. Potassium supplementation may be indicated.

Anaesthetic drugs which have crossed the placental barrier to the preterm fetus will remain in the neonate for a prolonged period of time because of the decreased metabolic and excretory capacities of the premature infant. In addition, the immature blood–brain barrier allows more depressant drugs to reach the infant's brain. Bilirubin is carried by albumin, and competition for protein-binding sites may occur with diazepam and its metabolites in the neonate if diazepam has been administered to the parturient. Pethidine (meperidine) and the local anaesthetic drugs are carried by acid $α_1$-glycoprotein, and thus will not compete with bilirubin for carrying protein capacity.

Whenever possible, regional anaesthetic techniques should be used. Well-conducted epidural analgesia should be started early in labour to improve uteroplacental perfusion and, by producing appropriate perineal relaxation, it encourages a slow, well-controlled, vaginal delivery with minimal pushing. It also allows a generous episiotomy when needed, and the use of outlet forceps to protect the preterm fetal head. These effects are all advantageous in reducing the handicaps of the preterm or small-for-gestational-age infant. If conversion to anaesthesia for vaginal or abdominal delivery becomes necessary subsequently, this can be accomplished rapidly by administration of chloroprocaine or lignocaine. Otherwise, spinal anaesthesia minimizes the fetal depression from the anaesthetic procedure.

Maternal hyperventilation and optimal maternal blood gases

Placental transfer of oxygen is adversely affected by maternal hyperventilation.[265,266] Reduced uterine and placental blood flow and increased affinity of maternal haemoglobin for oxygen (Bohr effect) contribute to a reduction in oxygen transfer. Maternal hyperoxia improves fetal oxygen stores and acid–base status during Caesarean delivery under epidural anaesthesia.[267] Oxygen tension of blood in the fetal ductus arteriosus does not reach the critical level at which premature closure of the ductus will be induced, even when the mother breathes 100% oxygen.[267]

CONCOMITANT MEDICAL DISORDERS

Heart disease

Congenital cyanotic heart disease with *Eisenmenger's syndrome* (reversal of left-to-right shunts because of pulmonary hypertension) poses some of the most challenging situations for an obstetric anaesthetist. Eisenmenger's syndrome is the pathophysiological end-result of several congenital heart defects (such as atrial septal defect, ventricular septal defect, patent ductus arteriosus, tetralogy of Fallot and others) which have been untreated or treated incompletely. The increased cardiac output which accompanies advancing pregnancy, combined with the gestational decrease in systemic vascular resistance, in the presence of a fixed and high pulmonary vascular resistance, results in a markedly increased right-to-left shunt. Further circulatory disturbances caused by aortocaval compression or hypotension from general or regional anaesthesia lead to even greater degrees of right-to-left shunt, aggravate cyanosis and can result in sudden death from hypoxaemia.[268,269]

Rheumatic heart disease, with haemodynamically significant mitral stenosis, is aggravated by the physiological changes of the cardiovascular system during pregnancy. Atrial fibrillation is a common problem. Maternal cardioversion with up to 100 J appears to be relatively safe for mother and fetus.[269] Corrective heart surgery has been performed during the second and early third trimester with successful results for mother and child.[270]

Patients with congenital *mitral valve prolapse*, which occurs in up to 17% of women of child-bearing age, usually have an uneventful pregnancy. Prophylaxis against endocarditis is indicated if mitral insufficiency complicates mitral valve prolapse. Endocarditis prophylaxis is also indicated before any invasive procedure in patients with other valvular heart conditions, congenital heart disease and idiopathic hypertrophic subaortic stenosis.[269]

Patients with prosthetic heart valves or other valvular disease that requires anticoagulant treatment throughout pregnancy must be changed to heparin treatment during the first trimester to prevent warfarin embryopathy and, during the weeks preceding delivery, to avoid fetal bleeding caused by the trauma of delivery in an anticoagulated fetus.[269]

The challenge of *anaesthetic management* of parturients with cyanotic heart disease or significant valvular disease is to provide high-quality analgesia (with specific spinal opioid analgesia and slowly titrated, carefully monitored epidural analgesia/anaesthesia) without adversely affecting cardiovascular parameters. This can reduce the cardiac stress associated with labour, delivery and the puerperium. By judicious use of intravenous fluid loading and vasopressor therapy, peripheral vascular resistance can be maintained in an optimal range.

Continuous regional anaesthesia is not contraindicated, and may be the anaesthetic technique of choice in pregnant patients with tight aortic stenosis, idiopathic hypertrophic subaortic stenosis, mitral stenosis, Eisenmenger's syndrome and recent myocardial infarction.[269] Light planes of general anaesthesia have been recommended in the past for Caesarean section, but do not confer any cardioprotective effects in the postpartum period when extra loads on the heart are still significant. However, general anaesthesia may be the only choice if it is necessary for the patient to remain anticoagulated throughout the perinatal period.[261] Oxytocin should be titrated very carefully to reduce postpartum haemorrhage, keeping the vasodilating effects of bolus doses in mind. Ergometrine should be avoided because of the increased cardiovascular stress from acute hypertension.

Morbid obesity

All the normal problems of obstetric anaesthesia are exaggerated in the morbidly obese parturient. Epidural analgesia may be possible, but poses unusual technical challenges.[271] Awake tracheal intubation, if at all possible, should be undertaken if general anaesthesia is required.

Severe kyphoscoliosis

When these patients have developed disabling respiratory disease, the risks of delivery and of any anaesthetic intervention are considerable. Technical difficulties often prohibit epidural analgesia.

Diabetes mellitus

The diabetic mother is predisposed to hypertension and uteroplacental insufficiency, and the offspring to prematurity with a perinatal mortality which still is about twice the norm.[272] The normal hypertensive response to laryngoscopy is exaggerated in the diabetic mother and the administration of hydralazine 10 mg intravenously 5–10 min before induction of anaesthesia, or a rapidly acting opioid such as alfentanil in a moderate dose (see above), should be considered. The stiff-joint syndrome of some juvenile-onset diabetics may make intubation unusually difficult.[273] Epidural or spinal blockade are the anaesthetic techniques of choice for diabetic parturients, and should be employed unless specifically contra-indicated.[272]

Close control of blood glucose is necessary throughout pregnancy to reduce maternal and fetal complications. Maternal hyperglycaemia before delivery leads to neonatal hypoglycaemia. Maternal insulin requirements diminish soon after delivery. Careful monitoring of blood glucose in the parturient, administration of glucose and insulin by titrated intravenous infusion, and subsequent neonatal blood glucose control are mandatory if outcome of infants of diabetic mothers is to be optimized. Intensive observation and treatment by the neonatologist are required also, because there are increased incidences of respiratory distress syndrome, hyperbilirubinaemia, hypocalcaemia and a variety of complex congenital abnormalities.[273]

ANAESTHESIA FOR INCIDENTAL SURGERY DURING PREGNANCY

In the anaesthetic management of pregnant patients who need incidental surgery, the primary concerns are potential teratogenicity of drugs, intra-uterine fetal asphyxia and precipitation of preterm labour.

Intra-uterine asphyxia is avoided by maintaining maternal haemodynamics and gas exchange at normal values. Aortocaval compression is a problem even in the second trimester and should be counteracted by left lateral tilt. Fetal heart rate should be monitored during surgery after the 16th week of gestation.

No anaesthetic drug has been proved to be teratogenic in humans.[274,275] However, any surgery that can be postponed until after the first trimester should be deferred. Elective surgery should be postponed until at least 1 month after delivery of the child.

Any emergency operation should be performed under regional block if the type of surgery or maternal condition permits. However, if uterine manipulation is necessary, a halogenated anaesthetic which decreases uterine contractility should be considered in order to minimize the possibility of preterm labour.

Uterine activity should be monitored continuously after surgery because of the risk that premature labour may be precipitated. β-Adrenergic therapy should be started at the earliest sign of increased uterine activity, and may prevent preterm delivery.

In utero manipulations and surgery of the fetus

High-detail ultrasound visualization of fetal anatomy has made intra-uterine manipulations possible. Treatment of hydrocephalus and obstructive uropathies, umbilical vein blood sampling and direct fetal blood transfusion are among the most commonly performed procedures.[276] Local anaesthetic infiltration of the abdominal wall and administration of intravenous alfentanil to the mother, titrated to make the fetus tolerate the surgical stimulation and inhibit fetal movements, provides satisfactory conditions. If the procedure requires complete inhibition of fetal movements, fetal intramuscular or umbilical vein injection of pancuronium 0.5 mg causes fetal paralysis for 2–4 h without affecting the mother.[277]

REFERENCES

1. Bonica JJ. Pain of parturition. Clin Anaesthesiol 1986; 4: 1–31
2. Malinow AM, Ostheimer GW. Anesthesia for the high-risk parturient. Obstet Gynecol 1987; 69: 951–964
3. Hytten F, Chamberlain G. (eds) Clinical physiology in obstetrics. Oxford: Blackwell Scientific. 1980
4. Russell IF, Chambers WA. Closing volume in normal pregnancy. Br J Anaesth 1981; 53: 1043–1047
5. Norris MC, Chan L. Respiratory disease. In: Datta S, ed. Anesthetic and obstetric management of high-risk pregnancy. St Louis, MO: Mosby, 1991: pp 169–209
6. Pernoll ML, Metcalf J, Schlenker TL, Welch JE, Matsumoto JA. Oxygen consumption at rest and during exercise in pregnancy. Respir Physiol 1975; 25: 285–293
7. Kambam JR, Handte RE, Brown WU, Smith BE. Effect of normal and preeclamptic pregnancies on the oxyhemoglobin dissociation curve. Anesthesiology 1986; 65: 426–427

8. Palahniuk RJ, Shnider SM, Eger EI II. Pregnancy decreases the requirements for inhaled anesthetic agents. Anesthesiology 1974; 41: 82–83
9. Robson SC, Hunter S, Moore M, Dunlop W. Haemodynamic changes during the puerperium: a Doppler and M-mode echocardiographic study. Br J Obstet Gynaecol 1987; 94: 1028–1039
10. Cheek TG, Samuels P. Pregnancy-induced hypertension. In: Datta S, ed. Anesthetic and obstetric management of high-risk pregnancy. St Louis, MO: Mosby, 1991: pp 423–456
11. Wulf H, Münstedt P, Maier Ch. Plasma protein binding of bupivacaine in pregnant women at term. Acta Anaesthesiol Scand 1991; 35: 129–133
12. Report on Confidential Enquiries into Maternal Deaths in the United Kingdom, 1985–1987. London: Her Majesty's Stationery Office. 1991
13. Macfie AG, Magides AD, Richmond MN, Reilly CS. Gastric emptying in pregnancy. Br J Anaesth 1991; 67: 54–57
14. Brocke-Utne JG, Downing JW, Dimopoulos GE, Rubin J, Moshal MG. Effect of domperidone on lower esophageal sphincter tone in late pregnancy. Anesthesiology 1980; 52: 321–323
15. Shnider SM. Serum cholinesterase activity during pregnancy, labor and the puerperium. Anesthesiology 1965; 26: 335–339
16. Leighton BL, Cheek TG, Gross JB. Succinylcholine pharmacodynamics in peripartum patients. Anesthesiology 1986; 64: 202–205
17. Gintzler AR. Endorphin-mediated increases in pain threshold during pregnancy. Science 1980; 210: 193–195
18. Selye H. Studies concerning the anaesthetic action of steroid hormones. J Pharmacol Exp Ther 1941; 73: 127–141
19. Merryman W. Progesterone 'anesthesia' in human subjects. J Clin Endocrinol Metab 1954; 14: 1567–1569
20. Datta S, Lambert DH, Gregus J, Gissen JA, Covino BG. Differential sensitivities of mammalian nerve fibres during pregnancy. Anesth Analg 1983; 62: 1070–1072
21. Fagraeus L, Urban BJ, Bromage PR. Spread of epidural analgesia in early pregnancy. Anesthesiology 1983; 58: 184–187
22. Scott DB, Kerr MG. Inferior vena caval pressure in late pregnancy. J Obstet Gynaecol Br Commonwlth 1963; 70: 1044–1049
23. Bieniarz J, Crottogini JJ, Curuchet E et al. Aortocaval compression by the uterus in late human pregnancy. II. An arteriographic study. Am J Obstet Gynecol 1968; 100: 203–217
24. Lees MM, Scott DB, Kerr MG, Taylor SH. The circulatory effects of recumbent postural change in late pregnancy. Clin Sci 1967; 32: 453–465
25. Hetland S, Polak D, Steen PA. Severe hypotension with regional anaesthesia for caesarean section. Tidsskr Nor Lægeforen 1989; 109: 3093–3094
26. Milsom I, Forssman L, Biber B, Dottori O, Rydgren B, Sivertsson R. Maternal haemodynamic changes during caesarean section: a comparison of epidural and general anaesthesia. Acta Anaesthesiol Scand 1985; 29: 161–167
27. Holmes F. Spinal analgesia and caesarean section. Maternal mortality. J Obstet Gynaecol Br Commonwlth 1957; 64: 229–232
28. Flaatten H, Breivik H. Spinal anaesthesia — time for reevaluation? Tidsskr Nor Lægeforen 1989; 109: 3091–3092
29. Humphrey MD, Chang A, Wood EC, Morgan S, Hounslow D. A decrease in fetal pH during the second stage of labour, when conducted in the dorsal position. J Obstet Gynaecol Br Commonwlth 1974; 81: 600–602
30. Crawford JS, Burton M, Davies P. Anaesthesia for Caesarean section: further refinements of a technique. Br J Anaesth 1973; 45: 726–732
31. Eckstein KL, Marx GF. Aortocaval compression and uterine displacement. Anesthesiology 1974; 40: 92–96
32. Gibbs CP, Werber JV, Banner TE, James CF, Hill CR. Epidural anesthesia: leg wrapping prevents hypotension. Anesthesiology 1983; 59: A405
33. Barclay DL, Renegar OJ, Nelson EW. The influence of inferior vena cava compression on the level of spinal anesthesia. Am J Obstet Gynecol 1968; 101: 792–800
34. Carrie LES, O'Sullivan G. Subarachnoid bupivacaine 0.5% for caesarean section. Eur J Anaesthesiol 1984; 1: 275–283
35. Ramanathan S, Grant GJ. Vasopressor therapy for hypotension due to epidural anesthesia for cesarean section. Acta Anaesthesiol Scand 1988; 32: 559–565
36. Martin R. Prepartum and intrapartum fetal monitoring. In: Datta S, ed. Anesthetic and obstetric management of high-risk pregnancy. St Louis, MO: Mosby, 1991: pp 1–26
37. Duvaldestin P, Demetriou M, Henzel D, Desmonts JM. The placental transfer of pancuronium and its pharmacokinetics during caesarean section. Acta Anaesthesiol Scand 1978; 22: 327–333
38. Dawes GS. The distribution and action of drugs on the fetus in utero. Br J Anaesth 1973; 45: 766–769
39. Gregory GA, Eger EI II, Munson ES. The relationship between age and halothane requirement in man. Anesthesiology 1969; 30: 488–491
40. Morgan DJ, Blackman GL, Paull JD, Wolf LJ. Pharmacokinetics and plasma binding of thiopentone. II. Studies at caesarean section. Anesthesiology 1981; 54: 474–480
41. Tomson G, Garle RIM, Thalme B, Nisell H, Nylund L, Rane A. Maternal kinetics and transplacental passage of pethidine during labour. Br J Clin Pharmacol 1982; 13: 653–659
42. Caldwell J, Natrianni LJ, Smith RL. Impaired metabolism of pethidine in human neonates. Br J Clin Pharmacol 1978; 5: 362–363
43. Hollmen AI, Jouppila R, Jouppila P, Koivula A, Vierola H. Effect of extradural analgesia using bupivacaine and 2-chloroprocaine on intervillous blood flow during normal labour. Br J Anaesth 1982; 54: 837–842
44. Jouppila P, Jouppila R, Hollmen A, Koivula A. Lumbar epidural analgesia to improve intervillous blood flow during labor in severe preeclampsia. Obstet Gynecol 1982; 59: 158–161
45. Brackbill Y, Kane J, Manniello RL, Abramson D. Obstetric premedication and infant outcome. Am J Obstet Gynecol 1974; 118: 377–384
46. Van den Berg BJ, Levinson G, Shnider SM, Hughes SC, Stefani SJ. Evaluation of long-term effects of obstetric medication on clinical development. In:

Abstracts of the Society for Obstetric Anesthesia and Perinatology, Boston 1980: p 52.
47. Ounsted M. Pain relief during childbirth and development at 4 years. J R Soc Med 1981; 74: 629–630
48. Munson ES, Embro WJ. Enflurane, isoflurane and halothane and isolated human uterine muscle. Anesthesiology 1977; 46: 11–14
49. Paull J, Ziccone S. Halothane, enflurane, methoxyflurane, and isolated human uterine muscle. Anaesth Intensive Care 1980; 8: 397–401
50. Greenhalf JO, Evans DJE. Effect of ergometrine on the central venous pressure in the third stage of labour. J Obstet Gynaecol Br Commonwlth 1970; 77: 1066–1069
51. Ostheimer GW. Editorial annotation. Clin Anesth 1986; 4: 166
52. Baskett TF, Writer WDR. Postpartum hemorrhage. In: Datta S, ed. Anesthetic and obstetric management of high-risk pregnancy. St Louis, MO: Mosby, 1991: pp 108–134
53. MacLennan FM, Thomsom MAR, Rankin R, Terry PB, Adey GD. Fatal pulmonary oedema associated with the use of ritodrine in pregnancy. Br J Obstet Gynaecol 1985; 92: 703–705
54. Cree IE, Meyer J, Hailey DM. Diazepam in labour: its metabolism and effect on the clinical condition and thermogenesis of the newborn. Br Med J 1973; 4: 251–255
55. Houghton DJ. Use of lorazepam as a premedicant for caesarean section; an evaluation of its effects on the mother and the neonate. Br J Anaesth 1983; 55: 767–771
56. Seidman SF, Marx GF. Midazolam in obstetric anesthesia. Anesthesiology 1987; 67: 443–444
57. Kanto J, Aaltonen L, Erkkola R, Aarimaa L. Pharmacokinetics and sedative effect of midazolam in connection with caesarean section performed under epidural analgesia. Acta Anaesthesiol Scand 1984; 28: 116–118
58. Sheikh A, Tunstall ME. Comparative studies of meptazinol and pethidine for the relief of pain in labour. Br J Obstet Gynaecol 1986; 93: 264–269
59. Shnider SM, Moya F. Effects of meperidine on the newborn infant. Am J Obstet Gynecol 1964; 89: 1009–1015
60. Hodgkinson R, Bhatt M, Wang CN. Double-blind comparison of the neurobehaviour of neonates following the administration of different doses of meperidine to the mother. Can Anaesth Soc J 1978; 25: 405–411
61. Kuhnert BR, Linn PL, Kennard MJ, Kuhnert PM. Effects of low doses of meperidine on neonatal behavior. Anesth Analg 1985; 64: 335–342
62. Way WL, Costley EC, Way EL. Respiratory sensitivity of the newborn infant to meperidine and morphine. Clin Pharmacol Ther 1965; 6: 454–461
63. Eisele JH, Wright R, Rogge P. Newborn and maternal fentanyl levels at cesarean section. Anesth Analg 1982; 61: 179–180
64. Hodgkinson R, Huff RW, Hayashi RH, Husain FJ. Double blind comparison of maternal analgesia and neonatal neurobehaviour following intravenous butorphanol and meperidine. J Int Med Res 1979; 7: 224–230
65. Frank M, McAteer EJ, Cattermole R, Loughnan B, Staffaord LB, Hitchcock AM. Nalbuphine for obstetric analgesia. A comparison of nalbuphine with pethidine for pain relief in labour when administered by patient-controlled analgesia. Anaesthesia 1987; 42: 697–703
66. Ferrante FM, Ostheimer GW, Covino BG (eds) Patient-controlled analgesia. Boston; MA: Blackwell. 1990
67. Scott JS. Obstetric analgesia. A consideration of labor pain and a patient-controlled technique for its relief with meperidine. Am J Obstet Gynecol 1970; 106: 959–978
68. Robinson JO, Rosen M, Evans JM, Revill SI, David H, Ress GA. Self administered intravenous and intramuscular pethidine. A controlled trial in labour. Anaesthesia 1980; 35: 763–770
69. Janeczko GF, El-Etr AA, Younes S. Low-dose ketamine anesthesia for obstetrical delivery. Anesth Analg 1974; 53: 829–831
70. Akamatsu TJ, Bonica JJ, Rehmet R, Eng M, Ueland K. Experiences with the use of ketamine for parturition: I. Primary anesthetic for vaginal delivery. Anesth Analg 1974; 53: 284–287
71. Lind B, Hoel TM. Alleviation of labor pain in Norway: an interview investigation in 1969 and 1986. Acta Obstet Gynecol Scand 1989; 68: 125–129
72. Gerdin E, Cnattingius S. The use of obstetric analgesia in Sweden 1983–1986. Br J Obstet Gynaecol 1990; 97: 789–796
73. Munley AJ, Railton R, Gray WM, Carter KB. Exposure of midwives to nitrous oxide in four hospitals. Br Med J 1986; 293: 1063–1064
74. Clark RB, Beard AG, Thompson DS, Barclay DL. Maternal and neonatal plasma inorganic fluoride levels after methoxyflurane analgesia for labor and delivery. Anesthesiology 1976; 45: 88–91
75. Ralston DH, Shnider SM. The fetal and neonatal effects of regional anesthesia in obstetrics. Anesthesiology 1978; 48: 34–64
76. Shah JL, Baguley I. Extradural pressure during labour. Br J Anaesth 1987; 59: 127P
77. Blomberg RG, Jaanivald A, Walther S. Advantages of the paramedian approach for lumbar epidural analgesia with catheter technique. A clinical comparison of midline and paramedian approaches. Anaesthesia 1989; 44: 742–746
78. Johnson C, Oriol N. The role of epidural anesthesia in trial of labor. Reg Anesth 1990; 15: 304–308
79. Flamm BL, Lim OW, Jones C, Fallon D, Newman LA, Mantis JK. Vaginal birth after cesarean section: results of a multicenter study. Am J Obstet Gynecol 1988; 158: 1079–1084
80. Schindler M, Gart S, Isert P, Morgans D, Cheung A. Thrombocytopenia and platelet functional defects in pre-eclampsia: implications for regional anaesthesia. Anaesth Intensive Care 1990; 18: 169–174
81. Chestnut DH. Anesthesia for the high risk obstetric patient. 1991 Annual refresher course lectures. American Society of Anesthesiologists. 1991 Lecture no 131.
82. Ewen A, McLeod DD, McLeod DM, Campbell A, Tunstall ME. Continuous infusion epidural analgesia in obstetrics. A comparison of 0.08% and 0.25% bupivacaine. Anaesthesia 1986; 41: 143–147

83 Hanson B, Matouskova-Hanson A. Continuous epidural analgesia for vaginal delivery in Sweden. Acta Anaesthesiol Scand 1985; 29: 712–715
84 Tunstall ME, Ramamoorthy C. Continuous epidural infusion with 0.08% bupivacaine. Anaesthesia 1984; 39: 939–940
85 Ewen A, McLeod DD, McLeod DM, Campbell A, Tunstall ME. Continuous infusion epidural analgesia in obstetrics. Anaesthesia 1986; 41: 760–761
86 Husemeyer RP, Davenport HT, Cummings AJ, Rosankiewicz JR. Comparison of epidural and intramuscular pethidine for analgesia in labour. Br J Obstet Gynaecol 1981; 88: 711–717
87 Finster M, Westrich DJ. Newer trends in obstetric pain relief. Anesth Analg 1991; 72 (suppl): 30–34
88 Cohen SE, Tan S, Albright GA, Halpern J. Epidural fentanyl/bupivacaine mixtures for obstetric analgesia. Anesthesiology 1987; 67: 403–407
89 Eisenach JC. Current trends in obstetric analgesia. Audio Digest Anesthesiology 1991; 33:
90 Murphy JD, Henderson K, Bowden MI, Lewis M, Cooper GM. Bupivacaine versus bupivacaine plus fentanyl for epidural analgesia: effect on maternal satisfaction. Br Med J 1991; 302: 564–567
91 Chestnut DH, Owen CL, Bates JN, Ostman LG, Choi WW, Geiger MW. Continuous infusion epidural analgesia during labor: a randomized double-blind comparison of 0.0625% bupivacaine/0.0002% fentanyl versus 0.125% bupivacaine. Anesthesiology 1988; 68: 754–759
92 Rawal N, Nuutinen L, Raj PP et al. Behavioral and histopathologic effects following intrathecal administration of butorphanol, sufentanil, and nalbuphine in sheep. Anesthesiology 1991; 75: 1025–1034
93 Van Steenberge A, Debroux HC, Noorduin H. Extradural bupivacaine with sufentanil for vaginal delivery: a double-blind trial. Br J Anaesth 1987; 59: 1518–1522
94 Chestnut DH, Laszewski LJ, Polack KL, Bates JN, Manago NK, Choi WW. Continuous epidural infusion of 0.0625% bupivacaine–0.0002% fentanyl during the second stage of labor. Anesthesiology 1990; 72: 613–618
95 Grice SC, Eisenach JC, Dewan DM. Labor analgesia with epidural bupivacaine plus fentanyl: enhancement with epinephrine and inhibition with 2-chloroprocaine. Anesthesiology 1990; 72: 623–628
96 Matthews NC, Corser G. Epidural fentanyl for shaking in obstetrics. Anaesthesia 1988; 43: 783–785
97 Eisenach JC, Grice SC, Dewan DM. Epinephrine enhances analgesia produced by epidural bupivacaine during labor. Anesth Analg 1987; 66: 447–451
98 Vertommen JD, Vandermeulen E, Van Aken H et al. The effects of the addition of sufentanil to 0.125% bupivacaine on the quality of analgesia during labor and on the incidence of instrumental deliveries. Anesthesiology 1991; 74: 809–814
99 Morgan B (ed) Controversies in obstetric anaesthesia. London: Arnold. 1990
100 Ostheimer GW. Contemporary issues in obstetric anesthesia. Anesth Analg 1991; 72 (suppl): 102–108
101 Chestnut DH. Epidural anesthesia and instrumental vaginal delivery. Anesthesiology 1991; 74: 805–808
102 Schellenberg JC. Uterine activity during lumbar epidural analgesia with bupivacaine. Am J Obstet Gynecol 1977; 127: 26–31
103 Phillips KC, Thomas TA. Second stage of labour with or without extradural analgesia. Anaesthesia 1983; 38: 972–976
104 Maltau JM, Anderson HT. Epidural anaesthesia as an alternative to caesarean section in the treatment of prolonged, exhaustive labour. Acta Anaesthiol Scand 1975; 19: 349–354
105 Matadial L, Cibils LA. The effect of epidural anesthesia on uterine activity and blood pressure. Am J Obstet Gynecol 1976; 125: 846–854
106 Lederman RP, Lederman E, Work B et al. Anxiety and epinephrine in multiparous women in labor: relationship to duration of labour and fetal heart rate. Am J Obstet Gynecol 1985; 153: 870–877
107 Shnider SM, Abboud TK, Artal R. Maternal catecholamines decrease during labor after lumbar epidural anesthesia. Am J Obstet Gynecol 1983; 147: 13–15
108 Maltau JM, Anderson HT. Continuous epidural anesthesia with a low frequency of instrumental deliveries. Acta Obstet Gynecol Scand 1975; 54: 401–406
109 Gambling DR, Morland GH, Yu P, Laszlo C. Comparison of patient-controlled epidural analgesia and conventional intermittent 'top-up' injections during labor. Anesth Analg 1990; 70: 256–261
110 Bonica JJ. Obstetric analgesia and anesthesia. World Fed Soc Anaesthesiol. Amsterdam 1980.
111 Sinclair JC, Fox HA, Lentz JF, Fuld GL, Murphy J. Intoxication of fetus by a local anesthetic. A newly recognized complication of maternal caudal anesthesia. N Engl J Med 1965; 273: 1173–1177
112 Brørvik K, Larsen RG, Rolfseng OK, Ulseth E. Quality of anaesthesia for emergency caesarean section. NA Forum (Nor Assoc Anaesthesiol) 1991; 4: 40
113 Shnider SM, Levinson G. Anesthesia for caesarean section. In: Shnider SM, Levinson G, eds. Anesthesia for obstetrics, 2nd edn. Baltimore, MD: Williams & Wilkins, 1987: 1 pp 159–180
114 Gutsche BB. Prophylactic ephedrine preceding spinal anesthesia for cesarean section. Anesthesiology 1976; 45: 462–465
115 Usubiaga JE. Neurologic complications following epidural analgesia. Int Anesthesiol Clin 1975; 13: 1–153
116 Kane RE. Neurologic deficits following epidural or spinal anesthesia. Anesth Analg 1981; 60: 150–161
117 Markham JW, Lynge HN, Stahlman GEB. The syndrome of spontaneous spinal epidural hematoma. J Neurosurg 1967; 26: 334–342
118 Costabile G, Husag L, Probst C. Spinal epidural hematoma. Surg Neurol 1984; 21: 489–492
119 Owens EL, Kasten GW, Hessel EA. Spinal subarachnoid hematoma after lumbar puncture and heparinization. Anesth Analg 1986; 65: 1201–1204
120 McNeill MJ, Thornburn J. Cannulation of the epidural space: a comparison of 18- and 16-gauge needles. Anaesthesia 1989; 43: 750–757
121 Shulman AG. Setting the record straight on low-dose heparin. Lancet 1991; 338: 619–620
122 Metzger G, Singbartl G. Spinal epidural haematoma

following epidural anaesthesia versus spontaneous spinal subdural haematoma. Two case reports. Acta Anaesthesiol Scand 1991; 35: 105–107

123 Rao TLK, El-Etr AA. Anticoagulation following placement of epidural and spinal catheters, an evaluation of neurological sequelae. Anesthesiology 1981; 55: 618–620

124 Odoom JA, Sih IL. Epidural analgesia and anticoagulant therapy. Experience with 1000 cases of continuous epidural. Anaesthesia 1983; 38: 254–257

125 Baron HC, La Raja RD, Rossi G, Atkinson D. Continuous epidural analgesia in the heparinized vascular surgical patient — a retrospective review of 912 patients. J Vasc Surg 1987; 6: 144–146

126 Schiff E, Peleg E, Goldenberg M et al. The use of aspirin to prevent pregnancy-induced hypertension and lower the ratio of thromboxane A_2 to prostacyclin in relatively high risk pregnancies. N Engl J Med 1989; 321: 351–356

127 CLASP Collaborative Group, CLASP: a randomized trial of low-dose aspirin for the prevention and treatment of pre-eclampsia among 9364 pregnant women. Lancet 1994; 343: 619–29

128 Collins R. Antiplatelet agents for IUGR and pre-eclampsia, I: Enkin MW, Keirse MJNC, Renfrew MJ, Neilson JP, red. Pregnancy and childbirth module. 'Cochrane Database of Systematic Reviews: Review No. 04000, 4 May 1994, Published through 'Cochrane Updates on Disk'. Oxford: Update Software, 1994. Disk Issue 2.

129 Macdonald R. Aspirin and extradural blocks. Br J Anaesth 1991; 66: 1–3

130 Hindman BJ, Koka BV. Usefulness of the post-aspirin bleeding time. Anesthesiology 1986; 64: 368–370

131 Locke GE, Giorgio AJ, Biggers SL, Johnson AP, Sabur F. Acute spinal epidural hematoma secondary to aspirin induced prolonged bleeding. Surg Neurol 1976; 5: 293–296

132 Burrows RF, Kelton JG. Incidentally detected thrombocytopenia in healthy mothers and their infants. N Engl J Med 1988; 319: 142–145

133 Patterson KW, O'Toole DP. HELLP syndrome: a case report with guidelines for diagnosis and management. Br J Anaesth 1991; 66: 513–515

134 Schindler M, Gatt S, Isert P, Morgans D, Cheung A. Thrombocytopenia and platelet functional defects in pre-eclampsia: implications for regional anaesthesia. Anaesth Intensive Care 1990; 18: 169–174

135 Gibbs CP, Krischer J, Packam BM, Sharp H, Kirschbaum TH. Obstetric anaesthesia: a national survey. Anesthesiology 1986; 65: 298–306

136 Pedersen H, Santos AC, Finster M. Obstetric anaesthesia. In: Barash PG, Cullen BF, Stoelting RK (eds) Clinical anesthesia. London: Lippincott, 1989: pp 1215–1251

137 Tunstall ME, Ostheimer GE. Obstetrics. In: Nunn JF, Utting J, Brown B. Jr: (eds) General anaesthesia. London: Butterworths, 1989: pp 988–1008

138 Kestin IG. Spinal anaesthesia in obstetrics. Br J Anaesth 1991; 66: 596–607

139 Marx GF, Luykx WM, Cohen S. Fetal–neonatal status following caesarean section for fetal distress. Br J Anaesth 1984; 56: 1009–1013

140 Cesarini M, Torrielli F, Lahaye F, Mene JM, Cabirio C. Sprotte needle for intrathecal anaesthesia for Caesarean section: incidence of postdural puncture headache. Anaesthesia 1990; 45: 656–658

141 Abouleish E, Rawal N, Fallon K, Hernandez D. Combined intrathecal morphine and bupivacaine for cesarean section. Anesth Analg 1988; 67: 370–374

142 Abouleish E, Rawal N, Rashad MN. The addition of 0.2 mg subarachnoid morphine to hyperbaric bupivacaine for Cesarean delivery: a prospective study of 856 cases. Reg Anesth 1991; 16: 137–140

143 Hunt CO, Naulty JS, Bader AM. Perioperative analgesia with subarachnoid fentanyl-bupivacaine for cesarean delivery. Anesthesiology 1989; 71: 535–540

144 Naulty JS. Cesarean delivery analgesia with subarachnoid bupivacaine, fentanyl, and morphine. Anesthesiology 1989; 71: A864

145 Bromage PR. Epidural analgesia. Philadelphia, PA: Saunders, 1987: pp 209–210

146 Hurley RJ, Hertwig LM, Johnson MD, Datta S. Personal communication, 1991

147 Ackerman WE, Colclough GW. Prophylactic epidural blood patch: the controversy continues. Anesth Analg 1987; 66: 913

148 Cheek TG, Banner R, Sauter J, Gutsche BB. Prophylactic extradural blood patch is effective. Br J Anaesth 1988; 61: 340–342

149 Sechzer PH, Abel L. Post-spinal anesthesia headache treated with caffeine. I. Evaluation with demand method. Curr Ther Res 1978; 24: 307–312

150 Jarvis AP, Greenwalt JW, Fagraeous L. Intravenous caffeine for postdural puncture headache. Anesth Analg 1986; 65: 316–317

151 Szeinfeld M, Ihmeidan IH, Moser MM, Machado R, Klose J, Serafini AN. Epidural blood patch: evaluation of the volume and spread of blood injected into the epidural space. Anesthesiology 1986; 64: 820–822

152 Abouleish E, de la Vega S, Blendinger I, Tio TO. Long-term follow-up of epidural blood patch. Anesth Analg 1975; 54: 459–463

153 Baysinger CL, Menk EJ, Harte E. The successful treatment of dural puncture headache after failed epidural blood patch. Anesth Analg 1986; 65: 1242–1244

154 Philipson EH, Kuhnert BR, Syracuse CD. Fetal acidosis, 2-chloroprocaine, and epidural anesthesia for cesarean section. Am J Obstet Gynecol 1985; 151: 322–324

155 Ravindran RS, Bond VK, Tasch MD, Gupta CD, Luerssen TG. Prolonged neural blockade following regional analgesia with 2-chloroprocaine. Anesth Analg 1980; 59: 447–451

156 Reisner LS, Hochman BN, Plumer MH. Persistent neurologic deficit and adhesive arachnoiditis following intrathecal 2-chloroprocaine injection. Anesth Analg 1980; 59: 452–454

157 Moore DC, Spierdijk J, van Kleef JD, Coleman RL, Love GF. Chloroprocaine neurotoxicity: four additional cases. Anesth Analg 1982; 61: 155–159

158 Ravindran RS, Turner MS, Muller J. Neurologic effects of subarachnoid administration of 2-chloroprocaine-CE, bupivacaine, and low pH normal saline in dogs. Anesth Analg 1982; 61: 279–283

159 Gissen AJ, Datta S, Lambert D. The chloroprocaine

controversy. II. Is chloroprocaine neurotoxic? Reg Anesth 1984; 9: 135–145
160 Gissen AJ, Datta S, Lambert D. The chloroprocaine controversy. I. A hypothesis to explain the neural complications of epidural chloroprocaine. Reg Anaesth 1984; 9: 124–134
161 Rosen MA, Baysinger CL, Shnider SM et al. Evaluation of neurotoxicity after subarachnoid injection of large volumes of local anesthetic solutions. Anesth Analg 1983; 62: 802–808
162 Albright GA. Cardiac arrest following regional anesthesia with etidocaine or bupivacaine. Anesthesiology 1979; 51: 285–287
163 Moore DC, Crawford RD, Scurlock JE. Severe hypoxia and acidosis following local anesthetic-induced convulsions. Anesthesiology 1980; 53: 259–260
164 Moore DC, Thompson GE, Crawford RD. Long-acting local anesthetic drugs and convulsions with hypoxia and acidosis. Anesthesiology 1982; 56: 230–232
165 Rosen MA, Thigpen JW, Shnider SM, Foutz SE, Levinson G, Koike M. Bupivacaine-induced cardiotoxicity in hypoxic and acidotic sheep. Anesthesiology 1985; 64: 1089–1096
166 Clarkson CW, Hondeghem LM. Mechanism for bupivacaine depression of cardiac conduction: fast block of sodium channels during the action potential with slow recovery from block during diastole. Anesthesiology 1985; 62: 396–405
167 Kotelko DM, Shnider SM, Dailey PA et al. Bupivacaine-induced cardiac arrhythmias in sheep. Anesthesiology 1984; 60: 10–18
168 Morishima HO, Pedersen H, Finster M. Bupivacaine toxicity in pregnant and nonpregnant ewes. Anesthesiology 1985; 63: 134–139
169 Laishley RS. Morgan BM. A single dose epidural technique for Caesarean section. A comparison between 0.5% bupivacaine plain and 0.5% bupivacaine with adrenaline. Anaesthesia 1988; 43: 100–103
170 Ramamurthy S. Anesthesia. In: Green DP, ed. Operative hand surgery, vol I. New York: Churchill Livingstone, 1982: pp 23–54
171 Gaffud MP, Bansal P, Lawton C, Velasquez N, Watson WA. Surgical analgesia for cesarean delivery with epidural bupivacaine and fentanyl. Anesthesiology 1986; 65: 331–334
172 Preston PG, Rosen MA, Hughes SC et al. Epidural anesthesia with fentanyl and lidocaine for cesarean section: maternal effects and neonatal outcome. Anesthesiology 1988; 68: 938–943
173 Carrie LES. Extradural, spinal or combined block for obstetric surgical anaesthesia. Br J Anaesth 1990; 65: 225–233
174 Benlabed M, Dreizzen E, Ecoffey C, Escourrou P, Migdal M, Gaultier C. Neonatal patterns of breathing after cesarean section with or without epidural fentanyl. Anesthesiology 1990; 73: 1110–1113
175 Leicht CH, Hughs SC, Dailey PA, Shnider SM, Rosen MA. Epidural morphine sulfate for analgesia after cesarean section: a prospective report of 1000 patients. Anesthesiology 1986; 65: A366
176 Hardy PAJ. Can epidural catheters penetrate dura mater? An anatomical study. Anaesthesia 1986; 41: 1146–1147
177 Blomberg RG. Technical advantages of the paramedian approach for lumbar epidural puncture and catheter introduction. A study using epiduroscopy in autopsy subjects. Anaesthesia 1988; 43: 837–843
178 Blomberg RG, Jaanivald A, Walther S. Advantages of the paramedian approach for lumbar epidural analgesia with catheter technique. A clinical comparison of midline and paramedian approaches. Anaesthesia 1989; 44: 742–746
179 Abouleish E, Goldstein M. Migration of an extradural catheter into the subdural space. Br J Anaesth 1986; 58: 1194–1197
180 Lee A, Dodd KW. Accidental subdural catheterisation. Anaesthesia 1986; 41: 847–849
181 Moore DC, Batra MS. The components of an effective test dose prior to epidural block. Anesthesiology 1981; 55: 693–696
182 Moore DC. Toxicity of local anaesthetics in obstetrics. IV. Management. Clin Anaesth 1986; 4: 113–124
183 Cartwright PD, McCarroll SM, Antzaka C. Maternal heart rate changes with a plain epidural test dose. Anesthesiology 1986; 65: 226–228
184 Van Zundert AA, Vaes LE, De Wolf AM. ECG monitoring of mother and fetus during epidural anesthesia. Anesthesiology 1987; 66: 584–585
185 Abraham RA, Harris AP, Maxwell LG, Kaplow S. The efficacy of 1.5% lidocaine with 7.5% dextrose and epinephrine as an epidural test dose for obstetrics. Anesthesiology 1986; 64: 116–119
186 Ostheimer GW. Regional anesthesia. In: Ostheimer GW, ed. Manual of obstetric anesthesic. New York: Churchill Livingstone, 1984: pp 165–220
187 Hood DD, Dewan DM, James FM III. Maternal and fetal effects of epinephrine in gravid ewes. Anesthesiology 1986; 64: 610–613
188 Leighton BL, Norris MC, Sosis M, Epstein R, Chayen B, Larijani GE. Limitations of epinephrine as a marker of intravascular injection in laboring women. Anesthesiology 1987; 66: 688–691
189 Matadial L, Cibils LA. The effect of epidural anesthesia on uterine activity and blood pressure. Am J Obstet Gynecol 1976; 125: 846–854
190 Kasten GW, Martin ST. Bupivacaine cardiotoxicity: comparison of treatment with bretylium and lidocaine. Anesth Analg 1985; 64: 911–916
191 Caplan RA, Ward RJ, Posner K, Cheney FW. Unexpected cardiac arrest during spinal anesthesia: a closed claims analysis of predisposing factors. Anesthesiology 1988; 68: 5–11
192 Keats AS. Anesthesia mortality — a new mechanism. Anesthesiology 1988; 68: 2–4
193 MacArthur C, Lewis M, Know EG, Crawford JS. Epidural anaesthesia and long term backache after childbirth. Br Med J 1990; 301: 9–12
194 Kogstad O. Back ache after childbirth. Tidsskr Nor Lægeforen 1988; 108: 1120–1122
195 Hynson JM, Sessler DI, Glosten B. Back pain in volunteers after epidural anesthesia with chloroprocaine. Anesth Analg 1991; 72: 253–256
196 Peng AT, Behar S, Blancato LS. Reduction of postlumbar puncture backache by the use of field block anesthesia prior to lumbar puncture. Anesthesiology 1985; 63: 227–228
197 Coates MB. Combined subarachnoid and epidural techniques. Anaesthesia 1982; 37: 89–90

198 Rawal N, Schollin J, Wesström E. Epidural versus combined spinal epidural block for cesarean section. Acta Anaesthesiol Scand 1988; 32: 61–66

199 Abouleish E, Rawal N, Shaw J, Lorenz T, Rashad MN. Intrathecal morphine 0.2 mg versus epidural bupivacaine 0.125% or their combination: effects on parturients. Anesthesiology 1991; 74: 711–716

200 Giuffrida JG, Bizzarri DV, Masi R, Bondock R. Continuous procaine spinal anesthesia for Cesarean section. Anesth Analg 1972; 51: 117–124

201 Hurley RJ, Lambert DH. Continuous spinal anesthesia with a microcatheter technique: preliminary experience. Anesth Analg 1990; 70: 97–102

202 Ringler ML, Drasner K, Krejcie TC et al. Cauda equina syndrome after continuous spinal anesthesia. Anesth Analg 1991; 72: 275–281

203 King TA, Adams AP. Failed tracheal intubation. Br J Anaesth 1990; 65: 400–414

204 Brock-Utne JG, Downing JW, Seedat F. Laryngeal oedema associated with preeclamptic toxaemia. Anaesthesia 1977; 32: 556–558

205 Jouppila R, Joupilla P, Hollmen A. Laryngeal oedema as an obstetric anaesthesia complication. Acta Anaesthesiol Scand 1980; 24: 97–98

206 Datta S, Briwa J. Modified laryngoscope for endotracheal intubation of obese patients. Anesth Analg 1981; 60: 120–121

207 Gibbs CP. Gastric aspiration: prevention and treatment. Clin Anesthesiol 1986; 4: 47–52

208 Mallampati SR, Gatt SP, Gugino LD et al. A clinical sign to predict difficult intubation: a prospective study. Can Anaesth Soc J 1984; 32: 429–434

209 Wilson ME, John R. Problems with the Mallampati sign. Anaesthesia 1990; 45: 486–487

210 Malan TP, Johnson MD. The difficult airway in obstetric anesthesia: techniques for airway management and the role of regional anesthesia. J Clin Anesth 1988; 1: 104–110

211 Latto IP. Management of difficult intubation. In: Latto IP, Rosen M, eds. Difficulties in tracheal intubation. London: Baillière Tindall, 1985: pp 99–141

212 Ovasappian A, Yelich S, Dykes MHM, Brunner EE. Fiberoptic nasotracheal intubation — incidence and causes of failure. Anesth Analg 1983; 62: 692–695

213 Dhara SS. Guided blind endotracheal intubation. Anaesthesia 1980; 34: 590–592

214 Ellis DG, Jakymec A, Kaplan RM et al. Guided orotracheal intubation on the operating room using a lighted stylet: a comparison with direct laryngoscopic technique. Anesthesiology 1986; 64: 823–826

215 Fox DJ, Castro T, Rastrelli AJ. Comparison of intubation techniques in the awake patient: the Flexi-lum surgical light (lightwand) versus blind nasal approach. Anesthesiology 1987; 66: 69–71

216 Brain AIJ. The development of the laryngeal mask — a brief history of the invention, early clinical studies and experimental work from which the laryngeal mask evolved. Eur J Anaesthesiol 1991; 4: 5–17

217 Leach AB, Alexander CA. The laryngeal mask — an overview. Eur J Anaesthesiol 1991; 4: 19–31

218 Tunstall ME. Failed intubation in the parturient. Can J Anaesth 1989; 36: 611–613

219 Lim W, Wareham C. The LM in failed intubation. Anaesthesia 1990; 45: 689–690

220 Scott D. Endotracheal intubation: friend or foe? Br Med J 1986; 292: 157

221 Shnider SM, Levinson G. Anesthesia for obstetrics. In: Miller RD, ed. Anesthesia, 3rd edn. New York: Churchill Livingstone, 1990: pp 1829–1873

222 Sellick BA. Cricoid pressure to control regurgitation of stomach contents during induction of anaesthesia. Lancet 1961; ii: 404–406

223 Safar P, Bircher NG. Cardiopulmonary cerebral resuscitation, 3rd edn. London: Saunders. 1988

224 Benumof JL, Scheller MS. The importance of transtracheal jet ventilation in the management of the difficult airway. Anesthesiology 1989; 71: 769–778

225 Report on Confidential Enquiries into Maternal Deaths in England and Wales 1973–1975. London: Her Majesty's Stationery Office. 1982

226 Phillips OC, Frazier TM, Davis GH, Nelson AT. The role of anesthesia in obstetric mortality. Anesth Analg 1961; 40: 557–566

227 Lahiri SK, Thomas TA, Hodgson RMH. Single-dose antacid therapy for the prevention of Mendelson's syndrome. Br J Anaesth 1973: 45: 1143–1146

228 Gillett GB, Watson JD, Langford RM. Ranitidine and single-dose antacid therapy as prophylaxis against acid-aspiration syndrome in obstetric practice. Anaesthesia 1984; 39: 638–644

229 Tordoff SG, Sweeney BP. Acid aspiration prophylaxis in 288 obstetric anaesthetic departments in the United Kingdom. Anaesthesia 1990; 45: 776–780

230 Sum-Ping ST, Mehta MP, Symreng T. Reliability of capnography in identifying esophageal intubation with carbonated beverage or antacid in the stomach. Anesth Analg 1991; 73: 333–337

231 Norris MC, Dewan DM. Preoxygenation for ceasarean section: a comparison of two techniques. Anesthesiology 1984; 81: A400

232 Tunstall ME. The reduction of amnesic wakefulness during caesarean section. Anaesthesia 1979; 34: 316–319

233 Birmingham PK, Cheney FW, Ward RJ. Esophageal intubation: a review of detection techniques. Anesth Analg 1986; 65: 886–891

234 Linko K, Paloheimo M, Tammisto T. Capnography for detection of accidental oesophageal intubation. Acta Anaesthesiol Scand 1983; 27: 199–202

235 Tunstall ME. Detecting wakefulness during general anaesthesia for caesarean section. Br Med J 1977; 1: 1321

236 Rosen M, Lunn JN. (eds) Consciousness, awareness and pain in general anaesthesia. London: Butterworths. 1987

237 Jessop J, Jones JG. Conscious awareness during general anaesthesia — what are we attempting to monitor? Br J Anaesth 1991; 66: 635–637

238 Tunstall ME, Lowit IM. Sleep phobia after awareness during general anaesthesia: treatment by induced wakefulness. Br Med J 1982; 285: 865

239 Eger II EI. Uptake and distribution. In: Miller RD, ed. Anesthesia, 3rd edn. New York: Churchill Livingstone, 1990: pp 85–134

240 Moir DD, Thorburn J. Obstetric anaesthesia and analgesia, 3rd edn. London: Baillière Tindall. 1986

241 James FM III, Crawford JS, Hopkinson R, Davies P, Naiem H. A comparison of general anesthesia and

lumbar epidural analgesia for elective cesarean section. Anesth Analg 1977; 56: 228–235
242 Finster M, Poppers PJ. Safety of thiopental used for induction of general anesthesia in elective cesarean section. Anesthesiology 1968; 29: 190–191
243 Datta S, Ostheimer GW, Weiss JB, Brown WU, Alper MH. Neonatal effect of prolonged anesthetic induction for cesarean section. Obstet Gynecol 1981; 58: 331–335
244 Crawford JS, James FM, Crawley M. A further study of general anaesthesia for caesarean setion. Br J Anaesth 1976; 48: 661–667
245 Abdul-Karim RW, Chevli RN. Antepartum hemorrhage and shock. Clin Obstet Gynecol 1976; 19: 533–559
246 Walsh SW. Preeclampsia: an imbalance in placental prostacyclin and thromboxane production. Am J Obstet Gynecol 1985; 152: 335–340
247 Makila U-M, Jouppila P, Kirkinen P, Viinikka L, Ylikorkala O. Placental thromboxane and prostacyclin in the regulation of placental blood flow. Obstet Gynecol 1986; 68: 537–540
248 Hibbard LT. Maternal mortality due to acute toxemia. Obstet Gynecol 1973; 42: 263–270
249 Kelton JG, Hunter DJS, Neame PB. A platelet defect in preeclampsia. Obstet Gynecol 1985; 65: 107–109
250 Shoemaker CT, Meyers M. Sodium nitroprusside for control of severe hypertensive disease of pregnancy: a case report and discussion of potential toxicty. Am J Obstet Gynecol 1984; 149: 171–173
251 Mabie WC, Gonzalez AR, Sibai BM, Amon E. A comparative trial of labetalol and hydralazine in the acute management of severe hypertension complicating pregnancy. Obstet Gynecol 1987; 70: 328–332
252 Newsome LR, Bramwell RS, Curling PE. Severe preeclampsia: hemodynamic effects of lumbar epidural anesthesia. Anesth Analg 1986; 65: 31–36
253 James FM, Davies P. Maternal and fetal effects of lumbar epidural analgesia for labor and delivery in patients with gestational hypertension. Am J Obstet Gynecol 1976; 126: 195–201
254 James FM, Wheeler AS, Dewan DM. Obstetric anesthesia: the complicated patient, 2nd edn. Philadelphia, PA: Davis. 1988
255 Moir DD, Willocks J. Epidural analgesia in British obstetrics. Br J Anaesth 1968; 40: 129–138
256 Connell H, Dalgleish JG, Downing JW. General anaesthesia in mothers with severe pre-eclampsia/eclampsia. Br J Anaesth 1987; 59 1375–1380
257 Hodgkinson R, Husain FJ, Hayashi RH. Systemic and pulmonary blood pressure during caesarean section in parturients with gestational hypertension. Can Anaesth Soc J 1980; 27: 389–394
258 Skerman JH, Huckaby T, Otterson WN. Emboli in pregnancy. In: Datta S, ed. Anesthetic and obstetric management of high-risk pregnancy. St Louis, MO: Mosby Year Book, 1991: pp 495–521
259 Crawford JS. An appraisal of lumbar epidural blockade in patients with singleton fetus presenting by the breech. J Obstet Gynaecol Br Commonwlth 1974; 81: 867–872
260 Bowen-Simpkins P, Fergusson ILC. Lumbar epidural block and the breech presentation. Br J Anaesth 1974: 46: 420–424
261 McMorland GH, Effer SB. Breech presentation, malpresentation, multiple gestation. In: Datta S, ed. Anesthetic and obstetric management of high-risk pregnancy. St Louis, MO: Mosby Year Book, 1991: pp 74–88
262 Crawford JS. An appraisal of lumbar epidural blockade in labour in patients with multiple pregnancy. J Obstet Gynaecol Br Commonwlth 1975; 82: 929–935
263 Crawford JS. A prospective study of 200 consecutive twin deliveries. Anaesthesia 1987; 42: 33–43
264 Malinow AM, Gershon RY, Alger LS. Preterm labor and delivery. In: Datta S, ed. Anesthetic and obstetric management of high-risk pregnancy. St Louis, MO: Mosby Year Book, 1991: pp 457–485
265 Levinson G, Shnider SM, deLorimier AA, Steffenson JL. Effects of maternal hyperventilation on uterine blood flow and fetal oxygenation and acid-base status. Anesthesiology 1974; 40: 340–347
266 Motoyama EK, Rivard G, Acheson F, Cook CD. Adverse effect of maternal hyperventilation on the foetus. Lancet 1966; i: 286–288
267 Ramanatham S, Ghandi S, Arismendy J, Chalon J, Turndorf H. Oxygen transfer from mother to fetus during caesarean section under epidural anesthesia. Anesth Analg 1982; 61: 576–581
268 Jones A, Foster JMG, Jones RM. The anaesthetic management of the Eisenmenger syndrome. Ann R Coll Surg 1984; 66: 353–355
269 Johnson MD, Saltzman DH. Cardiac disease. In: Datta S, ed. Anesthetic and obstetric management of high-risk pregnancy. St Louis, MO: Mosby Year Book, 1991: pp 210–259
270 Becker RM. Intracardiac surgery in pregnant women. Ann Thorac Surg 1983; 36: 453–458
271 Maitra AM, Palmer SK, Bachhuber SR, Abram SE. Continuous epidural analgesia for cesarean section in a patient with morbid obesity. Anesth Analg 1979; 58: 348–349
272 Datta S, Greene MF. The diabetic patient. In: Datta S, ed. Anesthetic and obstetric management of high-risk pregnancy. St Louis, MO: Mosby Year Book, 1991; pp 407–422
273 Hogan K, Rusy D, Springman SR. Difficult laryngoscopy and diabetes mellitus. Anesth Analg 1988; 67: 1162–1169
274 Duncan PG, Pope WDB, Cohen MM, Greer N. Fetal risk of anesthesia and surgery during pregnancy. Anesthesiology 1986; 64: 790–794
275 Konieczko KM, Chapple JC, Nunn JF. Fetotoxic potential of general anaesthesia in relation to pregnancy. Br J Anaesth 1987; 59: 449–454
276 Elias S, Annas GJ. Perspectives on fetal surgery. Am J Obstet Gynecol 1983; 145: 807–812
277 Corke BC, Seeds JW. Intrauterine fetal manipulations. In: Datta S, ed. Anesthetic and obstetric management of high-risk pregnancy. St Louis, MO: Mosby Year Book, 1991: pp 42–53

16. Anaesthesia for cardiac surgery

M. Salmenperä   C. C. Hug Jr

The successful conduct of cardiac anaesthesia is a demanding task. An appropriate degree of anaesthesia and analgesia is needed to block neurally and humorally mediated responses to the noxious stimuli of surgery and cardiopulmonary bypass (CPB). However, circulatory compromise, particularly after CPB, imposes limits on the use of any drug that depresses the cardiovascular system. Furthermore, normal pharmacokinetics and pharmacodynamics of anaesthetic drugs cannot be assumed because of large shifts of body fluids, blood loss and replacement, temperature variations and changes in perfusion of the organs responsible for drug clearance. Cardiac anaesthetists must therefore have a sound understanding of pharmacology and physiology, especially of normal circulatory control, as well as the pathophysiology of cardiovascular diseases.

The number of cardiac operations performed varies widely in different countries, and generally reflects the availability of health care resources rather than differences in demand. In developed countries, the annual incidence of cardiac operations ranges between 0.05 and 0.15% of the population. An increasing proportion of cardiac operations, presently about 80%, is devoted to ischaemic heart disease or its complications. This chapter deals mainly with anaesthesia and life support procedures for coronary artery bypass grafting (CABG) surgery. Other cardiac diseases that pose specific anaesthetic considerations will be reviewed briefly in the text where the information appropriate for CABG patients clearly is not applicable. The conduct of CPB and the immediate post-CPB period is similar for all types of cardiac operations.

PRE-OPERATIVE PREDICTORS OF OUTCOME

Although the nature of the cardiac disease should have been evaluated thoroughly by clinical and laboratory examinations and the surgical plan delineated pre-operatively, the anaesthetist should re-evaluate the patient's functional status by interview and physical examination. This is especially important if the laboratory tests are remote in time. Also, non-cardiac diseases which might affect peri-operative management and outcome should be recognized and controlled so that the patient is in the best overall medical condition possible. The major problems to be addressed in the pre-operative anaesthetic consultation are listed in Tables 16.1–16.3. Rarely, these consultations will add diagnostic information, change the surgical plan or result in postponement of the operation. Usually, the information gathered serves as a database used for risk stratification and formulation of the plans for anaesthesia and life support. Identification of risk factors associated with adverse outcomes underlies the rational development of an anaesthetic care plan, including the selection of monitoring techniques, in an effort to reduce the morbidity and mortality associated with cardiac surgery.

COMPLICATIONS OF CARDIAC SURGERY

Cardiac morbidity and mortality

Hospital mortality rates for CABG operations vary from 1.5 to 9%.[1-3] Mortality rates have been rising within the last decade and reflect the fact that the patients are older, have more advanced cardiac and systemic diseases, and larger numbers are undergoing re-operations and emergency operations. Re-operations have higher operative mortality than primary operations.[4] Primary aortic valve replacement carries about the same operative risk as primary CABG (1–2%) but the risk is distinctly greater in mitral valve replacement (>5%).[5] Multiple valve replacements and concomitant CABG increase the risk further. Emergency operation is clearly a risk factor in all reports.

Some reversible ventricular dysfunction attributable to ischaemia, cardioplegia, ventriculotomy and CPB is to be expected after cardiac surgery.[6,7] More severe and persistent dysfunction usually implies new structural

Table 16.1 History, symptoms and signs in the cardiac surgical patient: items to be addressed in a pre-operative anaesthesia consultation

Symptoms, signs or disease category	Items of particular interest
Coronary artery disease	Stable or unstable angina pectoris, previous MI, CABG or angioplasty, evidence of ischaemic dysfunction with exercise
Heart failure	Dyspnoea, orthopnoea, cyanosis, fatigue, peripheral oedema, jugular venous distension, hepatic engorgement, laterally displaced apical impulse, hepatomegaly, rales, S3 on auscultation
Functional class	Either New York Heart Association (NYHA) class or Canadian Cardiovascular Society Classification
Hypertension and vascular disease	Association with renal disease, diabetes mellitus, transient ischaemic attacks, history of stroke, claudication, carotid bruit
Pulmonary disease	Asthma, COPD, ventilatory rate and pattern, wheezing on auscultation
Heart rate and blood pressure	BP measurement from both arms, range of HR and BP at rest without symptoms (from chart)
Cannulation sites	Allen's test, phlebitis, previous neck surgery
Non-cardiac diseases	Diabetes mellitus, hypo- and hyperthyroidism, bleeding history, renal failure, hepatic failure, history of hepatitis, drug dependence, alcoholism, tobacco smoking
Concurrent medications	Responses to therapy, previous untoward responses to drugs

MI = myocardial infarction; CABG = coronary artery bypass grafting; COPD = chronic obstructive pulmonary disease; BP = blood pressure; HR = heart rate.

Table 16.2 Investigations used to assess cardiovascular function in the pre-operative cardiac surgical patient.

Test	Items of particular interest (implications for anaesthetic management)
ECG	Rhythm, conduction abnormalities (pacing capabilities before CPB?), strain pattern or LBBB (precludes ECG ischaemia detection), ischaemia (leads to be monitored), left ventricular hypertrophy
Chest X-ray	Pulmonary congestion or oedema, cardiothoracic ratio > 1 (avoidance of anaesthetics which depress myocardial function)
Exercise testing	HR and blood pressure at which ischaemia was evident (lower HR should be maintained in the pre-CPB period), localization of ischaemia (ECG leads to be monitored), evidence of ischaemic dysfunction
Coronary angiography	Vascular territories affected (ECG leads to be monitored), left main equivalent (precise haemodynamic control), diffuse obstruction (increased risk of complications after CPB due to incomplete revascularization), collaterals, 'steal-prone anatomy'
Left ventriculography	Ejection fraction < 0.5, LVEDP > 15 mmHg or increasing more than 5mmHg after contrast injection, akinetic and dyskinetic areas (avoidance of anaesthetics which depress myocardial function)
Cardiac catheterization	Pressure gradients across the valves, valve areas: aortic valve < 0.7 cm^2, mitral valve < 1.0 cm^2 (precise haemodynamic control), degree of regurgitation across the valves, pulmonary vascular pressures and resistance (right ventricular failure possible after CPB), shunts and shunt flows (cardiac output measurement?)
Echocardiography	Valvular abnormalities and function, cardiac chamber enlargement, hypertrophy, regional wall motion abnormalities and estimation of ejection fraction, diastolic dysfunction, intracardiac thrombi, shunts
Nuclear imaging	Myocardial perfusion: thallium uptake and redistribution, infarct detection: technetium uptake

ECG = Electrocardiogram; CPB = cardiopulmonary bypass; LBBB = left bundle branch block; HR = heart rate; LVEDP = Left ventricular end-diastolic pressure

Table 16.3 Pre-operative clinical laboratory examinations of the cardiac surgical patient

Test	Clinical implications for anaesthesia
Haemoglobin/haematocrit	Hct < 25%: red cell transfusion may be needed pre-CPB to maintain myocardial oxygen supply Hct 25–35%: homologous red cell transfusions needed during CPB Hct > 40%: removal (isovolaemic haemodilution) of blood and post-CPB re-infusion should be considered
White cell count	Abnormal values (low or high) may indicate ongoing infection and need to postpone surgery
Potassium	Acute hypokalaemia (< 3.0 mmol.l^{-1}) should be corrected pre-operatively
Urea and creatinine	Pre-operative contrast angiograms are significant risk for impairment of renal function intra-operatively
sGOT and sGPT	High values may indicate acute hepatitis, in which case elective surgery should be postponed
PT, PTT	If clear increases are not explained by heparin or coumarin therapy or by congestive liver failure, haematological consultation should be obtained
Platelet count	The reason (consumption, heparin-induced thrombocytopenia) for counts $< 100 \times 10^9.l^{-1}$ should be evaluated
Template bleeding time	Values > 9 min in patients receiving aspirin may predict bleeding diathesis and increased transfusion requirements after CPB and platelets should be made available

Hct = Haematocrit; CPB = cardiopulmonary bypass; sGOT = serum glutamic oxalo-acetic transaminase; sGPT = serum glutamic pyruvic transaminase; PT = prothrombin time; PTT = partial thromboplastin time.

damage and often co-exists with a peri-operative myocardial infarction (PMI). The incidence of PMI in primary CABG surgery is currently 3–11%.[4,8,9] The mortality of PMI in cardiac surgery has been reported to be between 5 and 12%,[9,10] which is lower than the mortality rates of 36–70% reported if PMI is associated with non-cardiac surgery.[11,12] In addition to causing pump failure, new infarction adds to peri-operative morbidity by causing malignant arrhythmias, prolonging the intensive care unit course, and increasing the risks of pulmonary complications, sepsis, renal failure and ultimately multi-organ dysfunction. More than two-thirds of deaths associated with cardiac surgery are related to worsening cardiac function after CPB.[5]

The sharp increase in operative mortality in patients over 70 years of age may be caused by more severe and complicated cardiac disease as well as advanced concurrent disease.[13] The age-adjusted operative mortality in female patients aged over 40 years is more than twice that of male patients.[13] Small body size may be the dominant factor in this gender difference.

Class IV angina (New York Heart Association or Canadian Cardiovascular Society Classification) patients have double the CABG mortality compared to patients with class <IV angina.[13] Unstable angina pectoris, defined as new-onset angina or increasing severity of angina symptoms, is associated with three to five times greater CABG mortality.[13] Silent ischaemia with electrocardiogram (ECG) changes compatible with myocardial ischaemia, but without angina, may present pre-operatively in more than one-third of CABG patients and appears to be a powerful predictor of PMI.[14] Prior history of myocardial infarction, in contrast to that observed in non-cardiac surgical patients, does not seem to increase the incidence of re-infarction during cardiac surgery.[13] Presence of a significant stenosis (> 50% decrease in diameter) in the left main coronary artery places large areas of myocardium at jeopardy, but its ranking as a risk factor for PMI has decreased markedly.[5] Diffuse coronary atherosclerosis is likely to lead to prolonged surgical ischaemia time and incomplete revascularization, both significant predictors of poor outcome.[5,10]

Impaired ventricular function may be the single most powerful predictor of operative mortality in cardiac surgery. Patients with histories of congestive heart failure, digitalis and diuretic therapy and with rales on physical examination have an operative mortality eight times higher than those without congestive heart failure.[13] Poor left ventricular ejection fraction (EF <0.3) is the most robust pre-operative predictor of the need for postoperative inotropic support[15] and of peri-operative morbidity and mortality associated with CABG surgery.[16,17]

Neurological complications

Neurological complications may be the most significant

menace to the expected quality of life of patients after cardiac surgery. Stroke occurs in 2–5% of CABG patients[18–20] and the incidence is higher in patients undergoing valvular operations.[21] Stroke is the leading contributor to operative mortality in patients with valvular operations and there is an incidence of up to 25% of permanent, often subtle, neuropsychiatric deficits.[21]

In patients older than 70 years, or with prior reversible or irreversible neurological symptoms and calcification of the ascending aorta, the risk of peri-operative neurological complication is increased by at least a factor of three.[22,23] These patients, as well as those undergoing open heart operations and those with asymptomatic carotid artery stenosis, may form a subgroup for which a high priority should be given to attempts to protect the brain pharmacologically and by careful control of haemodynamics peri-operatively.

Pulmonary complications

Pulmonary complications, such as postoperative atelectasis and pneumonia, rarely cause mortality after cardiac surgery, but they prolong mechanical ventilation and complicate the intensive care unit course. Smoking history without signs of respiratory disease does not seem to increase operative risk, but with co-existing bronchitis and/or chronic obstructive pulmonary disease (COPD), the risk for pulmonary complications is increased severalfold.[24] Abstinence from smoking for a minimum of 6–8 weeks can substantially reduce the risk. Pulmonary function testing is helpful in the prediction of respiratory complications in all patients undergoing valvular, but not CABG, operations.[25] Impaired ventricular function is a more significant predictor of prolonged ventilatory support since cardiogenic pulmonary oedema is the most frequent cause of compromised gas exchange after CPB.[26] Bronchospasm, whether associated with asthma or COPD, should be controlled to the maximum degree possible. Bronchospasm may be exacerbated when ventilation is re-instituted after CPB.

Bleeding complications

Between 10 and 20% of cardiac surgical patients develop excessive bleeding and require multiple transfusions.[27] In about half of these, a surgical cause is found and in the rest there is an acquired haemostatic defect, often involving platelets.[28] Although bleeding complications are not likely to be the direct cause of mortality, they are associated with haemodynamic instability and prolonged operation time. They can place heavy demands on the transfusion services. Also, the 2–11% incidence of transfusion-related non-A, non-B hepatitis in cardiac surgery is troublesome.[29,30] Pre-operatively, few patients can be identified to be at a high risk of excessive bleeding. The likelihood of diagnosing an inherited haemostatic defect during pre-operative evaluation is remote, but the potentially catastrophic consequences of coagulopathy mandate that careful bleeding history and a basic haemostatic screen (prothrombin time, partial thromboplastin time and platelet count) must be obtained in every cardiac surgical patient. Two pre-operative factors, repeat sternotomy and aspirin use, are identified in most studies as predictors of a bleeding diathesis after CPB.[31,32] In these patients, all strategies, such as prophylactic administration of aprotinin to decrease bleeding and donor blood exposure, should be considered.[33]

PREMEDICATION AND CHRONIC DRUG THERAPY

The obvious goals of premedication in the cardiac surgical patient are to decrease anxiety, produce amnesia and alleviate pain associated with vascular cannulations. The suppression of anxiety and pain should reduce activation of the sympathetic nervous system and limit untoward circulatory responses that may lead to myocardial ischaemia. The benefits of premedication are likely to extend into the operative period and decrease the incidence and severity of hypertension and tachycardia in response to tracheal intubation and surgical stimulation. The risk of intra-operative awareness can also be reduced — albeit not completely abolished — with appropriate premedication.[34]

The choices of drugs and their dosages are usually determined by the age and physical status of the patient, the nature of the cardiac disease and the type of anaesthesia planned. The combination of diazepam 0.1–0.2 mg.kg^{-1} orally 1–2 h before transfer to the operating room, and morphine 50–100 µg.kg^{-1} and scopolamine 2.5–5 µg.kg^{-1} intramuscularly 30 min before transfer, is appropriate for most cardiac surgical patients. Lorazepam 30–60 µg.kg^{-1} orally or intramuscularly 1–2 h before transfer is an alternative to the combination of diazepam and scopolamine for amnesia and sedation.

One hour should be allowed between the administration of oral medications and the intramuscular injection of scopolamine and morphine because the latter delay gastric emptying. Patients with coronary artery disease benefit from heavy premedication provided that their cardiac and pulmonary functions are adequate. Reduced doses of scopolamine should be used in older patients or omitted altogether in patients over 70 years of age since it can cause the central anticholinergic syndrome, manifested as confusion, agitation and hallucinations.[35]

It may be necessary to reduce doses of premedicant drugs in patients with impaired ventricular function at rest, valvular disease or symptomatic pulmonary disease, in order to avoid hypercapnia and hypoxaemia.[36] All patients, regardless of their ventricular function, should receive supplemental oxygen after premedication. It is highly desirable that patients be observed and monitored with ECG and pulse oximetry in the pre-operative holding area, where inadequate premedication can be remedied by additional doses of appropriate drugs.

Oesophageal reflux and peptic ulcer disease are common in cardiac surgical patients. Since a rapid induction-intubation sequence is seldom a good choice in cardiac surgical patients vulnerable to haemodynamic instability, premedication with an H_2-receptor blocker is advisable for patients at risk of aspiration.

Most chronic medications, including drugs used to treat hypertension and angina as well as cardiac glycosides, are continued until the time of surgery. Aspirin is a notable exception. To avoid excessive blood loss associated with irreversible inhibition of cyclo-oxygenase in the circulating platelets, aspirin therapy should be discontinued at least 5 days pre-operatively to allow for the synthesis of new platelets.[31,32] If anticoagulation is desirable in the patient with unstable angina, who is usually hospitalized, an infusion of heparin can be employed.

The need to continue chronic medications should be evaluated as a part of the overall plans for premedication and anaesthesia (Table 16.4). The patient with coronary artery disease has less myocardial ischaemia, tachycardia and arrhythmias if a β-adrenergic receptor blocker is administered before induction of anaesthesia, provided that there is no contra-indication.[37,38] Moderate doses of β-blockers do not complicate discontinuation of CPB. Since β-adrenergic receptor blockers are competitive antagonists, their effects can be overcome with adrenergic agonists if they are needed after CPB.

Considering the frequent occurrence of silent ischaemia pre-operatively in CABG patients and the present understanding that ischaemia may not be related to increased myocardial oxygen demand,[39] it would seem particularly appropriate to continue coronary vasodilators. However, the prospective studies to date have failed to show the benefit of either prophylactic nitroglycerine[40,41] or calcium channel-blocking drugs[37,38] in decreasing ischaemic events in the period preceding CPB. Nevertheless, it is our practice to administer calcium channel-blocking drugs and nitrovasodilators as a part of premedication. Calcium channel-blocking drugs have the potential to modify intra-operative haemodynamics by decreasing systemic vascular resistance and causing atrioventricular block, especially when large doses are administered during an angioplasty complication.

It may be beneficial to haemodynamic stability to

Table 16.4 Chronic drug therapy commonly taken by patients scheduled for cardiac surgery. Advantages and disadvantages of peri-operative use

Drug category	Advantages	Disadvantages
β-Adrenergic receptor blockers	Less tachycardia, hypertension and myocardial ischaemia	Attenuation of inotropic response to $β_1$-agonists, unopposed α-mediated vasoconstriction ($β_2$-antagonist)
Calcium channel blockers	Prevention of coronary artery (+ graft) spasm	Attenuation of the response to inotropes, AV conduction block
Antihypertensives	Less hypertension	Drug interactions
Anti-arrhythmics	Less arrhythmias	Negative inotropic and chronotropic effects (amiodarone, disopyramide)
Diuretics	None	Hypovolaemia, electrolyte abnormalities
Digitalis	Control of rapid ventricular peri-operative rate in atrial tachyarrhythmias	Toxicity (arrhythmias) with hypokalaemia and hypercalcaemia
Heparin, coumarin or aspirin	Reduced risk of thrombosis before CPB	Bleeding complications and increased donor blood requirements after CPB

AV = Atrioventricular; CPB = cardiopulmonary bypass.

administer the usual morning dose of an antihypertensive that has been used chronically to treat hypertension. However, clonidine is the only chronically administered antihypertensive which must be given as a part of the premedication because sudden cessation of clonidine may precipitate acute hypertension peri-operatively.[42] Clonidine as a premedication has been shown to reduce fentanyl requirements and improve haemodynamic stability in patients undergoing CABG under opioid-relaxant anaesthesia.[43,44] Whether this anaesthetic sparing effect is apparent in patients with chronic clonidine therapy is doubtful.

Digoxin administration with premedication is controversial. Owing to low clearance of digoxin and to potential toxicity, especially with wide variation in serum potassium concentration,[45] digoxin administration is appropriately restricted to those patients who need it to control rapid ventricular response in an atrial arrhythmia. It seems unwise to give amiodarone in the immediate pre-operative period since it has been associated with difficulties in discontinuing CPB.[46] Moreover, amiodarone has a very long half-life.

There is no advantage in administering diuretics pre-operatively since they can be injected intravenously if they are needed intra-operatively. Their use in association with pre-operative fasting may cause hypovolaemia and add to peri-operative haemodynamic instability. Angiotensin-converting enzyme inhibitors seem to make patients susceptible to hypotension and bradycardia, particularly during induction of anaesthesia so it may be prudent not to administer these in the immediate pre-operative period.[47]

Asthmatic patients and COPD patients with bronchospasm should receive all their bronchodilators on the morning of the operation. Steroids should be administered if they have been required previously to control asthma. In a patient with severe asthma, it may be necessary to continue theophylline therapy with an aminophylline infusion, but the risk of arrhythmias must be kept in mind.

Rational management of blood glucose concentration in diabetic patients undergoing cardiac surgery requires intermittent measurements of glucose concentration intra-operatively. Hypoglycaemia is particularly of concern because the normal symptoms are completely masked by general anaesthesia. Hyperglycaemia results in a hyperosmolar state with excessive diuresis, and may be deleterious to ischaemic brain.[48] Oral hypoglycaemic agents should not be given on the day of operation as they are long-acting and may cause hypoglycaemia. A continuous intravenous infusion of soluble insulin at a rate of 1–2 unit.h^{-1} promotes glucose entry into cells and limits the development of hyperglycaemia and its side-effects. Because of the sympathetic endocrine responses to CPB, insulin resistance usually develops, and much larger doses of insulin may be required. Blood glucose concentration must be measured regularly and the insulin infusion rate adjusted to keep glucose concentration in the range of 5–6 mmol.l^{-1} (100–300 mg.dl^{-1}). If hypoglycaemia occurs, 10–20 g of glucose can be injected intravenously; the insulin infusion should be continued.

MONITORING

The presence of severe cardiovascular disease, unstable haemodynamics, co-existing multisystem disease and the unphysiological nature of CPB mandates invasive and expensive monitoring methods in cardiac surgical patients. However, their use should be justified in each case by a cost–benefit analysis and the specific indications for their use documented in the anaesthesia and life support plan. The more extensive the monitoring, the more interpretation is required by the anaesthetists. There is a real risk of inappropriate management caused by erroneous or misinterpreted monitoring data. Extensive monitoring technology is no substitute for vigilance, clinical observations and sound clinical judgement.

Pulse oximetry and capnography

Oxygenation and ventilation are assessed intermittently by blood gas analysis during and after cardiac surgery. However, hypoxaemia and hypercapnia may occur between measurements. Both are deleterious to patients with reduced reserves and continuous monitoring by pulse oximetry and capnography can be life-saving and cost-effective in reducing the need for blood gas analysis.[49] Oximetry can be used as a safeguard against excessive premedication and in uncovering hypoxaemia in a draped patient during vascular cannulations. Although the gradient between end-tidal and arterial carbon dioxide tensions is variable in cardiac surgical patients and cannot be assumed to be unchanged by CPB, capnography is an excellent trend-tracking device which warns of the development of hypo- or hypercapnia, both of which can alter cerebral and coronary blood flow.

Electrocardiography

It is customary to monitor two ECG leads in cardiac surgical patients to detect arrhythmias and myocardial ischaemia. Atrial activity is best detected in lead II. While ischaemic repolarization changes may be detected in lead II if the area of distribution of the right coronary artery is in jeopardy, ischaemic changes occur more commonly anterolaterally, and are detected most frequently by an electrode placed in the V5 position on the chest wall.[50] A five-electrode system is useful, with the limb electrodes placed behind each shoulder and on each side of the lower back, and one electrode placed at the anterior axillary line at the fifth intercostal space. This allows monitoring of all standard and augmented limb leads as well as lead V5.

While a combination of leads II and V5 in one study had a sensitivity of 80% in detection of intra-operative ischaemia, the addition of lead V4 increased sensitivity to 96%.[51] The V4 position places the electrode too close to the surgical field of a median sternotomy. However, these data suggest strongly that sensitivity of ischaemia detection should not be compromised by placing the precordial electrode too laterally in an effort to keep it further away from the operative field. Monitors in the cardiac operation rooms should have a capability to display two leads, usually II and V5 simultaneously. The ECG signal should be calibrated, and a strip chart recorder is mandatory to measure reliably the ST segment changes. While ST deviations may be caused by left ventricular strain, digitalis effect or electrolyte abnormalities, new ST segment deviations of greater than 0.2 mV are practically indicative of ischaemia. ST segment depressions may be ascending, horizontal or descending. Ascending depression can be physiological or related to tachycardia, and only depression exceeding 0.2 mV may signify ischaemia. ST deviation should be calculataed 80 ms from the S-wave nadir. With precise and reliable measurement, a 0.05 mV depression increases the sensitivity (without compromising specificity) of ischaemia detection intra-operatively in CABG patients.[52] Episodic ST elevations in the post-CPB period are common. They may indicate transmural ischaemia secondary to air emboli or coronary artery spasm but more commonly are benign, reversible and not associated with myocardial injury.[53]

Ventricular arrhythmias are detected easily with any ECG lead. However, even lead II may be insufficient to confirm atrial activity in arrhythmias with varying degrees of atrioventricular conduction block. Their detection may be facilitated using ECG electrodes incorporated in an oesophageal stethoscope, in the atrial position of a specialized pulmonary artery catheters, or placed on the atrial epicardium by the surgeon. Bipolar leads from these electrode sites produce prominent P waves which are easily related to QRS complexes, and thus the accuracy of atrial arrhythmia diagnosis approaches 100% with these methods.[54]

Arterial pressure

Intra-arterial pressure monitoring is an absolute requirement for every cardiac surgical procedure. A non-invasive blood pressure measurement technique can serve only as a back-up for technical failures but is unsatisfactory for monitoring because of the rapid changes in arterial pressure encountered routinely during cardiac surgery in relation to abrupt changes in blood volume, surgical manipulation and potent drugs affecting the cardiovascular system. An arterial cannula is also required for frequent sampling of arterial blood. The arterial pressure waveform provides clues to changes in contractility, cardiac output and systemic vascular resistance. Since the cardiac surgical patients require minute-to-minute haemodynamic management depends on decisions that are often based on arterial pressure, every effort should be made to ensure the validity of arterial pressure measurements. Transducer drift may be the most frequent cause of technical errors. Thus, the balancing of the transducers against atmospheric pressure is indicated before induction of anaesthesia and before discontinuation of CPB, and whenever the pressures do not fit the clinical picture. Transducer gain and the strip chart recorder should be calibrated before induction. The dynamic characteristics of the pressure-monitoring system affect the accuracy of systolic pressure measurement. The adequate performance of the intravascular catheter tubing can be confirmed visually by observing oscillations after a rapid flush of the tubing with the constant-flush device.[55] Excessive repetitive oscillations (ringing) or absence of any oscillations suggest that the system is underdamped or overdamped, respectively. The usual causes of these dynamic inaccuracies are blood clots, kinked tubing or air bubbles.

The radial artery of the non-dominant hand is usually chosen as the site for arterial access. If asymmetry in blood pressure measurements is found during pre-operative examination (subclavian stenoses are common complications of atherosclerosis in CABG patients), the radial artery of the side showing the higher pressure approximates to aortic pressure more closely and should be chosen. Axillary, brachial and femoral arteries are alternative sites. They probably should not be used routinely because the complication rates may be higher and access to the cannulation sites is more difficult during surgery should technical problems arise.

Radial artery pressure is usually higher than aortic pressure because of the lower elastance of more peripheral arteries and summation of reflected pressure waves. The pressure differences may be temporarily reversed after CPB when directly measured intra-aortic systolic pressure may exceed the radial pressure by a of 30–40 mmHg.[56,57] The mechanism of the pressure difference has not been resolved completely but it may relate to the localized decrease in vascular resistance after full reperfusion of the forearm muscles rendered relatively ischaemic during hypothermic CPB. The dampened appearance of the pressure waveform with a sluggish upstroke, absence of dicrotic notch and hypotension incompatible with the clinical picture are clues to the significant aortic–radial pressure gradients. Pressure in the ascending aorta can be measured directly with a 22-gauge needle and sterile tubing, which is attached to the same transducer for comparison with the radial artery pressure. The pressure gradient usually disappears within 10–60 min;[56] if it persists, the femoral artery can be cannulated by the surgeon for reliable arterial pressure measurements.

Ventricular filling pressures and cardiac output

At least central venous pressure (CVP) should be monitored in each cardiac procedure in order to maintain circulating blood volume at the level appropriate for optimal cardiac performance. CVP measurement is also required to detect obstruction of venous return during CPB.

Ventricular filling pressure is related to ventricular preload (i.e. end-diastolic fibre length or end-diastolic volume) by a curvilinear relationship (Fig. 16.1a). The pressure–volume relationships are different for each ventricle and are changed during surgery by such factors as inotropic state of the heart, myocardial ischaemia and myocardial oedema. Similar degrees of change in end-diastolic volume cause much less change in CVP than in pulmonary artery occlusion pressure (PAOP) and this discrepancy is further accentuated by low compliance due to left ventricular hypertrophy or impaired diastolic relaxation. In a healthy heart, changes in PAOP typically are twice those in CVP with fluid loading; in diseased hearts, this multiplication factor may be three to five and it may be clinically difficult to distinguish small, but important, changes in the CVP from the background noise (Fig. 16.1b). It is prudent to monitor both CVP and PAOP or left atrial pressure (LAP) when left ventricular function is impaired. PAOP is monitored intermittently. In the absence of tachycardia and increased pulmonary vascular resistance, pulmonary artery diastolic pressure (PADP) is close to PAOP, and can be used to monitor trends in left ventricular preload.[58]

Left atrial (LA) catheters can only be inserted intra-operatively and are not available during induction of anaesthesia or the pre-CPB period. They must be

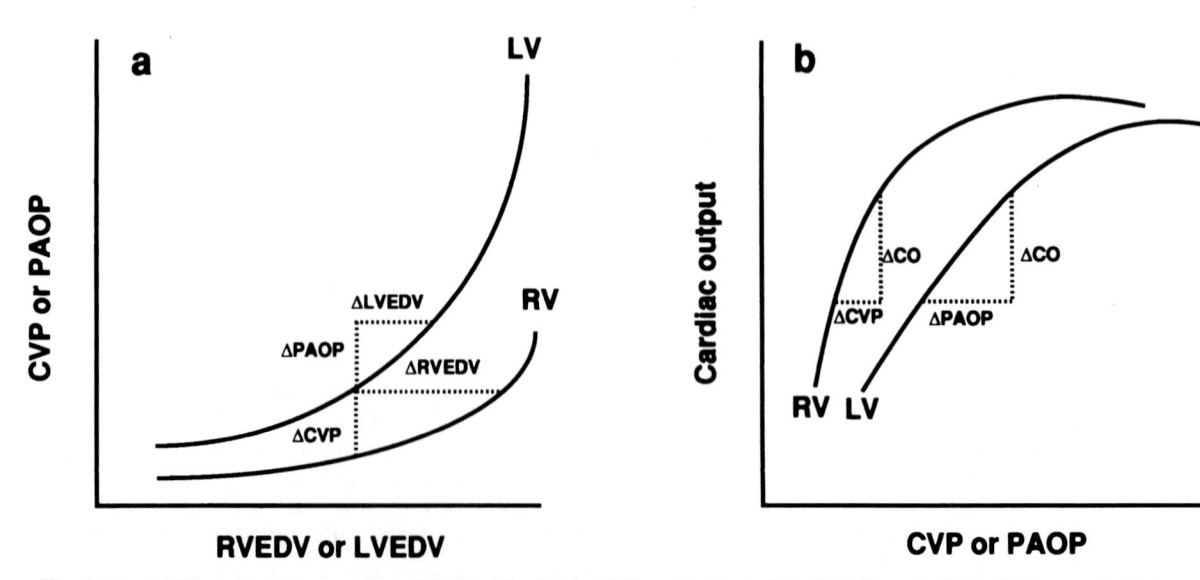

Fig. 16.1 (a) Diastolic pressure–volume relationship of right (RV) and left ventricle (LV). Because RV is thinly muscled it is much more compliant than LV and smaller absolute filling pressures are needed to cause comparable distension than in the thickly muscled LV. Also, equal changes in filling pressure cause greater increases in end-diastolic volume in the right than in the left side. (b) Systolic function (Frank–Starling) curves of RV and LV. Due to the difference in compliance, change in central venous pressure (CVP) is always less than the change in pulmonary artery occlusion pressure (PAOP) for a given change in cardiac output (CO). RVEDV = Right ventricular end-diastolic volume; LVEDV = left ventricular end-diastolic volume.

meticulously maintained to avoid the introduction of air and clot emboli into the systemic circulation. They may be easily dislodged during and after the operation and if the tracing is lost it usually cannot be reinstituted. Removal of LA catheters may cause bleeding. The above drawbacks are not encountered with pulmonary artery (PA) catheters which have their own risks and limitations. However, a PA catheter can be used to measure PA pressures as an indication of right ventricular afterload, and most importantly, cardiac output by thermodilution. There are special types of PA catheters for specific indications, not all of which have been well-delineated (Table 16.5).

The routine use of PA catheters in cardiac surgery remains controversial. A prospective but non-randomized study has failed to show improvement of outcome in patients monitored with PA catheters in comparison to those monitored by CVP alone.[59] PA catheters are monitoring devices, not therapeutic options. Thus, realization of the benefit of PA catheters is use-dependent. Favourable modification of outcome, attributed at least partially to the aggressive haemodynamic management based on the information of PA catheter monitoring, has been suggested in patients with left main coronary artery disease undergoing CABG,[60] and in those undergoing non-cardiac surgery after recent myocardial infarction.[61]

The internal jugular venous approach for insertion of central venous (CV) or PA catheters on either the right or left side is more convenient and reliable in our hands than the use of external jugular veins, although high success rates have been reported for the latter.[62] The subclavian venous access to central circulation has substantially higher complication rates and the steep angles of the catheter often cause damping of the pressure tracings, especially when the sternal retractor is in place. With appropriate pre-anaesthetic medication, CV and PA catheters can be inserted safely, efficiently and with minimal discomfort to the patient before induction of anaesthesia.[63] Haemodynamic instability can occur during and after induction and it is highly desirable that the anaesthetist's attention should not be diverted by the catheterization procedure. Furthermore, the information furnished by a PA catheter already in place can be used to advantage in correcting haemodynamic problems. Central venous access may be important to assure prompt delivery of cardiovascular and anaesthetic drugs. Most of the complications of PA catheters are related to venous cannulation and accidental insertion of a large-bore cannula to the carotid artery.[62] Use of a small-gauge needle on a syringe to identify vessels allows comparison of the colour of the blood with a sample removed from a systemic arterial cannula. When still in doubt, verification of venous pressure levels and fluctuation with respiration or coughing can be accomplished by connecting a sterile tubing to the needle or to an 18–20-gauge venous catheter before inserting larger-

Table 16.5 Use of pulmonary artery catheters (PAC) in adult cardiac surgery

Type of PAC	Monitoring information + clinical utility	Proposed indications
Standard triple-lumen 7-FG thermodilution	Central venous pressure, pulmonary artery pressures, cardiac output, sampling of mixed venous blood	Routine PAC for cardiac surgery
7.5-FG with an additional right ventricular lumen for the introduction of the ventricular pacing probe	As the standard + emergency pacing option	Alternative routine PAC for cardiac surgery
Atrioventricular (AV) pacing PAC with atrial and ventricular pacing electrodes embedded in the catheter body	As the standard + AV pacing capability + AV arrhythmia diagnosis	Left bundle branch block, aortic stenosis, re-operation, combined carotid end-arterectomy and CABG
Oximetry catheter with fibre-optic bundles in the catheter body	As the standard + continuous measurement of saturation of mixed venous blood (measurement of oxygen delivery and/or consumption)	Severe heart failure, patients with mechanical assist devices, ARDS (requirement for PEEP)
Right ventricular volumetric catheter with rapid-response thermistor	As the standard + measurement of right ventricular volumes and ejection fraction	Right heart failure, pulmonary hypertension

CABG = Coronary artery bypass grafting; ARDS = adult respiratory distress syndrome; PEEP = positive end-expiratory pressure.

bore catheters. A Doppler ultrasound probe can be used to identify the jugular vein and guide the insertion of the catheter.[64] Other complications are usually avoidable, inconsequential or rare.[65] The incidence of septic complications is worrying and meticulous attention must be paid to strict sterility during the catheterization procedure and subsequent catheter maintenance.

Since relatively small pressure changes may indicate important changes in preload, careful attention should be paid to the accuracy of the pressure measurements (see above). Continuous display of the pressure waveforms is mandatory to assess the patency of the fluid-filled system and to detect migration of the PA catheter into a permanent wedge position which can lead to misinterpretation of pressures and increased risk of PA rupture by inflation of the balloon.[66] Mean pressures should be read at end-expiration, preferably from a strip chart recorder. Two patterns of venous waveform are common in cardiac surgical patients and are frequently misinterpreted. In atrioventricular dissociation, the atrial systole against closed atrioventricular valves creates large a waves (cannon waves) and regurgitation of blood through incompetent atrioventricular valves causes large v waves during ventricular systole. In both cases, the mean pressures are inaccurate. Instead, end-diastole should be identified using simultaneous recordings of ECG, arterial and PA pressure tracings.[67]

Because of compensatory mechanisms, systemic arterial pressure may not correlate with cardiac output and tissue perfusion. With the measurement of cardiac output and calculation of peripheral vascular resistance, appropriate drug therapy can be instituted early before organ function is compromised. The thermodilution technique is convenient and the only clinically practical method to assess cardiac output repeatedly in cardiac surgical patients. Other techniques (e.g. echo Doppler) make geometric assumptions that often are not valid in cardiac patients. Methods based on the dye dilution or the Fick method are inconvenient and offer no advantages over thermodilution. The thermodilution method is reasonably accurate provided that cardiac output is not extremely low and it can be improved by repeating the injections and averaging the results.[68] Two potential errors in cardiac output measurements should be remembered in cardiac surgery. With tricuspid regurgitation, the indicator is cleared slowly from the right heart and the erroneous results will be associated with a low amplitude and prolonged thermodilution curve. Left-to-right shunts increase the right ventricular rather than systemic cardiac output. Shunts should be suspected when high cardiac output value do not fit with other indicators of tissue perfusion.

Temperature monitoring

Most cardiac operations involve moderate hypothermia during CPB. Temperature gradients usually exist in the patient after CPB because of a significant lag in rewarming of less well-perfused peripheral tissues like muscle and skin. If rewarming is incomplete at the end of CPB, there is 'afterdrop' of the body core temperature as heat moves down its gradient to the periphery. To avoid recooling and its adverse consequences,[69] temperatures should be measured at core sites (e.g. PA catheter thermistor and nasopharynx), and more peripheral sites (e.g. toe or finger, urinary bladder and rectum). The monitoring or bladder temperature may be particularly appropriate during cardiac surgery since a bladder catheter is always inserted; the 'afterdrop' is minimized when temperatures exceeding 36.2°C have been attained before discontinuing CPB.[70]

Urine output

Preservation of renal function is essential to a satisfactory outcome of cardiac surgery. Renal failure is contributory to a prolonged convalescence and high mortality.[71] The volume and quality of urine are indicators of renal function, which is threatened by the injection of radio-opaque contrast agents pre-operatively, low renal perfusion, haemoglobinuria and myoglobinoria during and after CPB. Urine volume alone is not a reliable indicator of cardiac output since it often reflects the large water and osmolar loads of the CPB priming solution, hyperglycaemia and administration of diuretics.

Echocardiography

Transthoracic echocardiography and Doppler flow imaging are useful pre-operatively in defining the anatomy and function of the heart and surrounding structures. This approach is not possible during surgery if the chest wall is the operative site. Lung expansion by intermittent positive-pressure ventilation makes transthoracic echocardiography more difficult to perform. Since the heart lies directly in front of the oesophagus and above the gastro-oesophageal junction, valvular function, chamber filling and contractility can be monitored continuously via crystals incorporated in the tip of the flexible endoscope (transoesophageal echo or TEE). Its close proximity allows the use of high-frequency transducers with improved resolution. Both unidimensional (M-mode), and two-dimensional (2-D mode) imaging is possible with currently available equipment which also permits the colour-coded Doppler images of the blood flow velocity and direction to be superimposed on echo images. TEE technology continues to be developed. Two new features are continuous-wave Doppler, which may allow better analysis of rapid jets and pressure gradient measurements, and biplane transducers, which allow better delineation of anatomy.

An important monitoring application of TEE for cardiac anaesthetists is ventricular wall motion imaging. With the probe at the gastro-oesophageal junction, a short-axis plane of the left ventricle at the papillary muscle level can be imaged. Regional wall motion abnormalities (RWMAs) in this image are more sensitive and earlier indicators of myocardial ischaemia than the ECG.[72,73] Hypokinetic areas may respond to anti-ischaemic drug therapy or revascularization. Akinetic or dyskinetic areas may be more resistant and may signify infarction. Impairment of systolic thickening of myocardium often occurs before RWMAs when ischaemia occurs. Anaesthetists relatively inexperienced at TEE easily learn to interpret wall motion qualitatively.[73] More quantitative evaluation requires planimetry and is presently possible only off-line.

TEE also enables estimation of left ventricular global function and end-diastolic and end-systolic volumes. Fractional shortening and ejection fraction area are calculated from end-diastolic and end-systolic images using M-mode or 2-D views respectively. These calculations may be rendered invalid by the inability to delineate clearly the endocardial border in end-diastolic images. With geometric assumptions, it is possible to calculate ejection fraction.[74] All the echo-indices are unreliable indicators of global cardiac function if RWMAs are present. Monitoring of end-diastolic volume would be very useful in obtaining a more comprehensive picture of preload. There are better correlations between cardiac output and changes in echo-derived estimates of end-diastolic volume than between cardiac output and PAOP after CPB.[75] Although software capable of delineating endocardial borders and providing better estimates of volume and ejection fraction is under development, these can be calculated only off-line at present.

To be useful as a monitoring tool, TEE requires much attention to the image on the screen and the probe needs to be adjusted as surgery proceeds. This may distract the attention of the anaesthetists from the other monitors and duties. The equipment is expensive and few centres are able to provide it for every cardiac operation. These factors and the qualitative nature of the monitoring information have reduced the use of TEE as a monitoring tool. Instead, TEE is usually reserved for those cases in which pre-operative diagnosis requires verification or refinement and the results of surgical intervention need to be assessed intra-operatively.[76] The established indications are evaluation of valvular repair (especially mitral regurgitation) with Doppler colour mapping and identification of aortic dissection sites. There are many new potentially important applications of TEE on the horizon and busy cardiac surgery programmes are likely to benefit from the purchase of the equipment (Table 16.6).

Electroencephalogram monitoring

As cerebral blood flow decreases below normal values, electroencephalogram (EEG) slowing occurs with a reduction of activity at β and α frequencies. EEG slowing is an alerting sign of potential ischaemic injury to the brain. Full multilead EEG monitoring is too cumbersome and requires expert interpretation if the information is needed on-line. In automated real-time EEG analysis, a microprocessor performs a Fourier transformation of the raw EEG signal. EEG activity is then presented as amplitude at discrete frequencies or as a power (amplitude) spectrum at these frequencies at specific sampling intervals or epochs. The changes in power spectra can be assessed visually utilizing any one of a variety of display techniques. The validity and interpretation of the data are enhanced by comparisons of patterns from right and left hemispheres. Shift in the preponderant frequencies can be characterized with numerical descriptors. For example, spectral edge frequency (SEF) is defined as the frequency below which 95% of the EEG power is contained. The SEF appears to be one of the more useful descriptors.

Several factors complicate intra-operative EEG analysis in cardiac surgical patients:

1. Slowing of the EEG is not a specific or sensitive predictor of postoperative neurological disturbances when these are related to focal embolic events, as they often are during cardiac surgery.[77]

2. Anaesthetic drugs and hypothermia cause EEG changes (slowing and increased amplitude) which are difficult or impossible to differentiate from the effects of hypoperfusion.[78,79]

3. Because of the low power of the EEG signal, meticulous preparation of the scalp before application of the electrodes is crucial and the quality of the recording may not remain stable over time. A substantial proportion of EEGs are corrupted by electrical noise during cardiac surgery. This, together with high background variability, suggests that there is very limited value in using the EEG to detect harbingers of

Table 16.6 Intra- and postoperative use of transoesophageal echocardiography

During surgery	Postoperative
Monitoring of regional ventricular function: Hypokinesia, dyskinesia, akinesia Degree of systolic shortening and thickening	*Inadequate imaging through chest wall with suspected* Acute valvular dysfunction Cardiac tamponade Aortic dissection
Monitoring of global LV function Visual assessment of diastolic and systolic areas and calculation of ejection fraction Assessment of preload (ventricular end-diastolic volume)	
Evaluation and detection of: Valvular function before CPB Valvular repair Atrial or ventricular thrombus Intracardiac shunts Intracardiac air Aortic dissection Ventricular aneurysm	

LV = Left ventricular; CPB = cardiopulmonary bypass.

ischaemia.[80] Nevertheless, EEG monitoring may be useful in detecting impaired collateral perfusion in patients with unilateral carotid stenosis and in whom a combined carotid and CABG operation is planned. Misplacement of the aortic cannula can also be detected with EEG monitoring when CPB commences. Pharmacological brain protection with thiopentone or isoflurane requires EEG monitoring to detect the therapeutic end-point of burst suppression; patients are highly variable in terms of their thiopentone dose requirements.[18] Finally, the appearance of activity at higher EEG frequencies suggests emergence from opioid-based anaesthesia and the possibility of becoming aware during the operation.

ANAESTHESIA INDUCTION AND MAINTENANCE

A detailed plan for anaesthetic care and life support should be developed and summarized in the patient's chart in advance of pre-anaesthetic medication, which is often an important part of the plan. It is essential that the equipment and drugs are available as required to implement the plan. The response to pre-anaesthetic medications may indicate that the anaesthetic plan should be altered, and notations on changes should be entered on the anaesthetic record. Calibrated recordings of all ECG leads should be made on the strip chart recorder before induction, for future reference. The baseline haemodynamic profile should also be obtained at this time. Inconsistencies between the pre-operative data and the measurements from the catheterization laboratory may necessitate changes in the management plan. The positioning of the cardiac surgical patient is very important because the operation is lengthy and is likely to involve periods of decreased perfusion which predispose to pressure and stretch injuries.

We routinely perform cannulations of peripheral veins (two 14–16-gauge cannulae), radial artery and jugular vein for PA catheter (through 8.5 F_G introducer) before induction of anaesthesia, with two exceptions. An emergency operation with the requirement to preserve myocardium through expeditious institution of CPB and coronary revascularization may indicate the need to induce anaesthesia with only a single large-bore intravenous cannula in place. The second exception arises in the very anxious patient who is otherwise haemodynamically stable; in such instances, we are willing to induce anaesthesia with ordinary monitoring and a single intravenous cannula, and to complete other vascular cannulations under anaesthesia before skin incision. All cardiac patients should be well oxygenated and the response to added oxygen confirmed by pulse oximetry before induction of anaesthesia. From this point on, a strip chart recorder is run continuously at a low speed throughout the operation to display haemodynamic trends, which are much more valuable guides for management decisions than the momentary oscillographic tracings of absolute values.

No single anaesthetic agent or technique is superior for any or all cardiac surgical patients. The skill of the anaesthetist in using the drugs is undoubtedly more important than the specific technique. The choice of drugs and techniques should be tailored to the individual patient based on pre-operative examination, the experience of the anaesthetists and anticipated time of tracheal extubation after the operation. Cardiac performance and the physiological reserves of the patient are important considerations in developing a rational choice of anaesthetic technique. Most haemodynamic effects of anaesthetics are dose-related. If the circulatory response prohibits high doses needed for induction, the agent may nevertheless be well suited in lower doses as a supplement to other anaesthetic drugs. The haemodynamic effects of anaesthetic agents should not always be viewed as untoward side-effects; rather, these effects may be used to achieve desired haemodynamic goals. Finally, with extensive haemodynamic monitoring, it is usually feasible to detect and correct untoward haemodynamic changes quickly.

Opioids

Are opioids anaesthetics? The answer is a qualified yes; they can render most, although not all, patients unconscious and dose-dependently reduce the requirements of volatile anaesthetics in experimental animals.[81] However, used alone, opioids cannot reliably prevent recall[82] or haemodynamic break through in all patients[83] during noxious stimulation.

The key to effective use of fentanyl-type opioids as anaesthetics is to maintain plasma (and central nervous system) concentrations within a therapeutic range (window). Low-frequency high-amplitude EEG can be maintained[78] with fentanyl plasma concentrations of 10–20 ng.ml^{-1}. The maximum achievable reduction of enflurane minimum alveolar concentration (MAC) by fentanyl in dogs is about 70%, and this corresponds to an average plasma level of 20 ng.ml^{-1} (Fig. 16.2).[84] In cardiac surgical patients, a loading dose and continuous infusion designed to achieve a plasma concentration of 20 ng.ml^{-1} maintained haemodynamics at pre-operative levels and suppressed responses to the noxious stimulation of surgery,[85,86] and vasopressin release.[87] Because of the short distribution half-time of fentanyl, plasma and brain concentrations of fentanyl decline relatively rapidly and administration of a few bolus doses or one large induction dose usually results in fentanyl concentrations that are insufficient to maintain adequate anaesthesia during surgery (Table 16.7). To mediate analgesia opioids must reach μ-opioid receptors within the central nervous system to exert their analgesic and anaesthetic effects. With μ-agonists such as fentanyl and sufentanil, there is a delay of 5–8 min before the maximum concentrations and peak effects of an intravenous dose are achieved.[88]

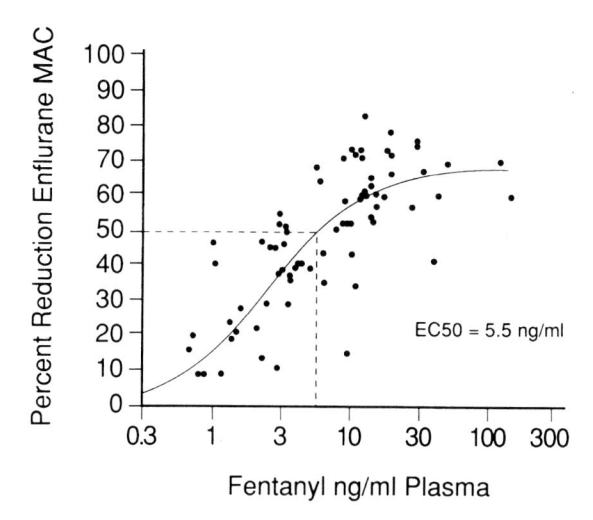

Fig. 16.2 Reduction of enflurane minimum alveolar concentration (MAC) versus plasma concentration of fentanyl in dogs. A ceiling effect is seen and maximum enflurane MAC reduction is evident when plasma concentration exceeds 20–30 ng.ml^{-1}. From Schwieger et al.,[84] with permission.

The clinical implication of this latency is that fentanyl and sufentanil must be administered well in advance of noxious stimuli; after responses to noxious stimuli have occurred, they may be difficult to control with an opioid alone.

The functional status of the sympathetic nervous and cardiovascular systems may modify the haemodynamic course of opioid anaesthesia. Hypertension in response to surgical stimulation is less likely to occur in patients with impaired cardiac function.[89] This does not mean that the quality of anaesthesia is better in these patients, but simply reflects the fact that these patients are unable to maintain stroke volume in the face of increased peripheral resistance produced by sympathetic responses to noxious stimulation. It is important to

Table 16.7 Pharmacokinetics of opioids used in cardiac anaesthesia

Agent	$t_{1/2}\beta$ (h)	Vd (l.kg^{-1})	Cl (ml.kg^{-1}.min^{-1})
Fentanyl	2–4	3–5	10–22*
Sufentanil	2–3	2–3	9–14*
Alfentanil	1–2	0.4–1	3–8

Modified from Hug.[90]
$t_{1/2}\beta$ = Elimination half-time, Vd = volume of distribution, Cl = plasma clearance.
* Equivalent to hepatic blood flow. The clearance of both is flow-dependent.

recognize that the absence of haemodynamic responses to noxious stimulation does not guarantee absence of awareness when an opioid is used as the primary anaesthetic. At present, there is no single reliable guide to confirm the adequacy of opioid anaesthesia in paralysed patients. Complete neuromuscular block should be limited to those periods of the operation in which reflex movements would jeopardize the patient's welfare or the goals of the surgery. Opioids almost invariably should be combined with a hypnotic or inhaled anaesthetic to minimize the risk of awareness. Hypnotics can be administered as premedication and during surgery as supplements at specific times, such as rewarming during CPB, when the possibility of awareness seems to be increased, especially if opioid concentrations are not maintained by an infusion. Benzodiazepines, especially midazolam and diazepam, are usually chosen as supplements for opioid anaesthesia. Their interactions with opioids are still poorly characterized, and vary according to the end-point under investigation. Benzodiazepines may interact in a less-than additive fashion with the opioids in terms of their antinociceptive effect.[84] Their sedative interaction is more likely to be synergistic, and consequently the recovery from opioid anaesthesia may be greatly prolonged if the doses of both the benzodiazepine and opioid are not carefully titrated to the desired effects. The haemodynamic interaction of opioids and benzodiazepines seems to be a low-dose phenomenon. Clinically significant hypotension is often observed when a low dose of either is combined with an induction dose of the other.[91] This hypotension is probably related to abrupt changes in sympathetic tone, and responds well to measures which increase venous return.

The absence of direct depression of the heart by opioids in doses or concentrations many times greater than those used in clinical anaesthesia is the main reason for their popularity in cardiac anaesthesia. Rapid infusions of opioids (e.g. fentanyl >500 µg.min^{-1}) affect cardiac performance by interfering with sympathetic reflexes and causing increased vagal discharge.[92] The resultant decrease in arterial resistance, increase in venous capacitance and bradycardia cause hypotension which responds well to a positional change to augment venous return (Trendelenburg position, leg raising), small doses of a sympathomimetic (ephedrine, phenylephrine) and an anticholinergic (atropine). There are other attractive features of opioids for cardiac patients; these include no interference with autonomic or cardiovascular drugs, preservation of blood flow autoregulation in the central nervous system and coronary circulations, increased toleration of airway manipulation and a tracheal tube, extended postoperative analgesia and no direct organ toxicity. Profound analgesia with opioids may even have anti-ischaemic effects; in one study, their continued administration in the immediate postoperative period decreased the severity of myocardial ischaemic episodes in patients recovering from CABG.[93]

Rigidity occurs frequently during induction of, and sometimes during emergence from, opioid anaesthesia.[83,94] Rigidity occurs typically just before or just after the patient is rendered unconscious. One should withhold attempts to ventilate the lungs at that time because gas is forced into the gastro-intestinal tract and hypotension results from increased intrathoracic pressure, which impedes venous return. The rigidity is typically relieved within 1–2 min by administration of a muscle relaxant. Provided that the patient was breathing 100% oxygen prior to the development of rigidity, apnoeic oxygenation prevents development of hypoxaemia. Hypercapnia can be reversed by mechanical ventilation when the rigidity has been relieved. Pretreatment with subparalysing doses of relaxants before opioid administration may substantially reduce the incidence and intensity of rigidity.[95]

Although morphine anaesthesia, described in 1969 by Lowenstein et al,[96] represents a milestone in the development of cardiac anaesthesia, morphine is no longer used by most anaesthetists who employ an opioid as the primary anaesthetic drug because of histamine release and its vasodilator effect, which limits both the rate of its administration and the maximum dose that is tolerated without the development of excessive oedema. Moderate doses of morphine (1–3 mg.kg^{-1} administered at a rate of 5 mg.min^{-1}) are satisfactory in combination with a benzodiazepine or inhaled anaesthetic. However, most anaesthetists choose either fentanyl or sufentanil.

When used in equipotent doses, fentanyl and sufentanil are virtually indistinguishable. Although better haemodynamic stability during surgery has been claimed after sufentanil,[97] most studies suggest that sufentanil and fentanyl are clinically equivalent in this respect.[98,99] In common with fentanyl, there is a ceiling effect for sufentanil in terms of its reduction of enflurane MAC in dogs,[100] and this observation is compatible with the inability of sufentanil to block sympathetic endocrine–haemodynamic responses to noxious stimuli[101] with doses as high as 40 µg.kg^{-1}, followed by an infusion of 2.0 µg.kg^{-1}.min^{-1}. There is a widely held clinical assumption, supported by at least one study, that the recovery from sufentanil anaesthesia is faster than that from fentanyl.[102] Although this is not readily apparent in terms of the traditionally reported pharmacokinetic variables (Table 16.7), refined pharmacokinetic models suggests that sufentanil is cleared from affected sites in the central nervous system more rapidly than fentanyl if the drug infusions have lasted for more than 3 h.[103] The potential benefits of a more rapid recovery can be realized by titrating sufentanil dose to effect, thereby allowing earlier recovery of spontaneous ventilation, extubation and discharge from the intensive care unit.

Alfentanil anaesthesia for cardiac surgery has been described.[34,86] Rapid equilibration of alfentanil between blood and its receptor sites in the central nervous system allows it to be used as a continuous, variable-rate infusion. Infusion rates between 0.25 and 2.5 µg.kg^{-1}.min^{-1} and plasma alfentanil concentrations of 400–500 ng.ml^{-1} are needed along with 66% nitrous oxide to control somatic and haemodynamic responses during upper abdominal surgery.[104] In cardiac surgery, the incompleteness of anaesthesia with alfentanil is evident. Despite infusion rates as high as 7.8 µg.kg^{-1}.min^{-1} and plasma concentrations exceeding 4600 ng.ml^{-1}, half of the patients in one study were inadequately anaesthetized.[34] Alfentanil is costly and has a relatively long duration of action when its concentrations are sustained at these high levels.

A refined understanding of the pharmacokinetics and dynamics of opioids is emerging.[102] Application of kinetic–dynamic models to computer-controlled infusion devices allows for a calculated concentration in the plasma or at the effect site in the central nervous system to be achieved quickly and varied rapidly according to the patient's needs. Using computer-controlled infusions, opioids and other intravenous anaesthetics can be administered conveniently at variable rates according to the observed responses in a manner similar to the administration of volatile anaesthetics.

Potent inhalational anaesthetics

Halothane, enflurane, isoflurane and desflurane can be used as primary anaesthetics for cardiac surgery in patients with good cardiac performance. The role of sevoflurane remains to be determined. The controlled depression of myocardial contractility and the resulting decrease in myocardial oxygen demand may be used to advantage when coronary flow is limited by proximal stenosis. Indeed, they act favourably on a number of determinants of myocardial oxygen consumption. A controlled decrease in peripheral resistance helps to maintain a normal or slightly decreased systemic arterial pressure, and direct depression of the sino-atrial node and baroreceptor reflex maintains a normal or slightly slow heart rate, except for isoflurane and desflurane at higher inspired rates. Concentrations can be adjusted rapidly to match the changing intensity of surgical nociception, the response to desflurane being especially rapid. Their removal from the body can be hastened by hyperventilation and they can be replaced by intravenous anaesthetics should problems occur. Their principal disadvantage is excessive cardiovascular depression, which limits their use as primary agents in patients with impaired cardiac function.

In humans, neither halothane nor enflurane has been associated with myocardial lactate production, which signifies ischaemia.[105,106] Halothane apparently protects against platelet thrombus formation in stenosed coronary arteries[107] and protects against reperfusion injury after ischaemia in animal experiments.[108] It also has minimal direct effects on coronary vascular resistance, but because of the remote possibility of hepatic injury, halothane is not widely used in adult cardiac surgical patients.

Isoflurane has come under scrutiny because of the claim that it produces myocardial ischaemia, so-called coronary steal, in patients with steal-prone coronary artery disease (CAD),[109,110] and in representative animal models.[111] Steal-prone CAD involves total obstruction in one coronary artery and subtotal obstruction in another; in addition, the coronary beds distal to these stenoses have to be connected via collaterals. Normally, the coronary vasodilatory reserve is used maximally in the bed behind total obstruction, and the flow there is dependent on the pressure gradient across the collaterals. With coronary vasodilators, such as dipyridamole, adenosine and perhaps isoflurane, vasodilatation distal to the partially stenosed vessel decreases pressure; consequently, less flow occurs through the collaterals, and ischaemia may develop in the collateral-dependent zone. This kind of anatomy is not present in the majority of CABG patients. In the CASS study, 'steal-prone' anatomy was identified in 23% of patients.[112] Steal as the mechanism of isoflurane-induced ischaemia remains controversial. First, although isoflurane is a vasodilator, it has not been demonstrated to be a particularly powerful coronary vasodilator and it is not equivalent to adenosine or dipyridamole.[113] Second, hypotension and tachycardia elicited by deep isoflurane anaesthesia complicate interpretation of these studies. The experiments impugning isoflurane do not relate to the manner in which isoflurane is used in clinical practice. When used as an adjunct to opioid anaesthesia, isoflurane effectively controls hypertension associated with surgical stress and even corrects ischaemic myocardial metabolism in that situation.[114] Isoflurane may have direct anti-ischaemic effects on the myocardium. Patients with limited coronary flow reserves were shown to tolerate higher atrial pacing rates without ischaemia under isoflurane anaesthesia than in an awake state.[115]

In the light of the evidence presented above, we feel that isoflurane may be used in patients with established CAD provided that hypotension and tachycardia are avoided. In patients with good left ventricular function, it can also be used as a primary anaesthetic for CABG, as recent controlled clinical studies show that ischaemia is no more frequent with isoflurane, even in patients with steal-prone anatomy, than it is during anaesthesia with halothane, enflurane or sufentanil.[116,117] However, enflurane may be a more reasonable alternative as an inhalational agent for cardiac surgery because isoflurane is prone to cause more tachycardia and vasodilatation, and isoflurane is more expensive than enflurane. If needed for brief periods to control hypertension after sternotomy or vasoconstriction during CPB, isoflurane is a good choice. The role of the newer agent, desflurane, in cardiac anaesthesia, remains to be more clearly defined. Experiments so far suggest that its cardiovascular profile is similar to that of isoflurane,[118] although at greater than 1 MAC concentrations it may cause an even more marked tachycardia than isoflurane. Sevoflurane has been widely used in Japan and may have a role in these patients; its use also remains to be more fully documented.

Nitrous oxide

Nitrous oxide has slight direct cardiac-depressant effects which are usually counteracted by the central sympathomimetic effects of this drug. Background anaesthesia with opioids or volatile anaesthetics interferes with sympathetic outflow from the central nervous system and may uncover myocardial depression.[119] The concerns about the potential of nitrous oxide to cause ischaemia in an area supplied by a critically stenotic coronary artery raised by animal experiments[120] have not been substantiated in humans.[121] Nitrous oxide increases pulmonary vascular resistance, at least in those situations when baseline pulmonary vascular resistance is increased, and this discourages the use of nitrous oxide in patients with valvular heart disease.[122] Nitrous oxide also limits the inspired oxygen concentration. The main case against nitrous oxide in cardiac surgery is its ability to expand and to slow the clearance of air bubbles introduced into the circulation through the extracorporeal circuit and through open chambers in the operative field. These disadvantages do not absolutely contra-indicate the use of nitrous oxide in cardiac surgery, especially before CPB. However, the benefits do not outweigh the potential risks, and most anaesthetists do not use nitrous oxide in their cardiac surgical patients.

Thiopentone

A decrease in sympathetic outflow is primarily responsible for dose-dependent hypotension after an induction dose of thiopentone.[123] This effect is markedly accentuated in patients dependent on sympathetic function to compensate for impaired cardiac performance or hypovolaemia. Withdrawal of sympathetic tone is manifest by increased venous capacitance, decreased arterial resistance and a mild negative inotropic effect. Hypotension during a pure thiopentone induction produces a reflex tachycardia which is accentuated by tracheal intubation. Thus, thiopentone is usually unsuitable as a sole induction agent for cardiac surgery. However, its synergistic hypnotic interaction with opioids can be used to advantage, and very small doses (25–100 mg) can reliably, rapidly and safely induce sleep and control sudden sympathetic responses to noxious stimuli during opioid anaesthesia. The use of thiopentone as a part of brain protection is discussed below.

Propofol

Induction doses of propofol are also associated with sympathetic withdrawal leading to venous and arterial vasodilatation and perhaps negative inotropy.[124] The decrease in blood pressure is comparable or more pronounced than after thiopentone.[125] However, unlike thiopentone, induction with propofol does not usually result in an increase in heart rate because propofol depresses the baroreceptor reflex.[126] Propofol does not attenuate pressor responses to tracheal intubation or surgery. These haemodynamic properties do not make propofol an attractive choice for induction of anaesthesia in most cardiac surgical patients. The haemodynamic course can be attenuated by using staged-infusion regimens of propofol and adding small doses of an opioid to blunt sympathetic responses to noxious stimulation. Propofol has been used successfully to provide postoperative sedation and sleep in the intensive care unit.[127]

Etomidate

Etomidate has minimal effects on the cardiovascular system with the doses required for induction of anaesthesia.[128] Ebert et al demonstrated that etomidate, unlike other intravenous hypnotics, preserves central sympathetic tone and the baroreceptor reflex.[129] This may explain why the addition of fentanyl only minimally augments the cardiovascular depressant effects of etomidate.[130] The suppression of the adrenal cortex after etomidate is not a concern after a single induction dose and the haemodynamic safety of etomidate should be borne in mind if anaesthesia must be induced in a bleeding, hypovolaemic patient after cardiac surgery.

Benzodiazepines

Midazolam and diazepam are the two benzodiazepines used widely peri-operatively in cardiac surgical patients. They differ significantly in their pharmacokinetics; the clearance rate of midazolam is 10–20 times faster, making it suitable for administration as a variable-rate infusion.[131] Midazolam is also two to four times more potent than diazepam. Either drug can be used for induction of anaesthesia, with similar haemodynamic effects.[132,133] The most consistent change produced by benzodiazepine induction is an increase in venous capacitance. Although preload is decreased, cardiac output does not usually decrease proportionally because systemic resistance is also reduced. The overall decrease in mean arterial pressure ranges from 10 to 25%[133] but is much greater in hypovolaemic patients and in those given simultaneous intravenous doses of an opioid.[134] Moderate negative inotropic effects have been reported in the isolated heart but only at concentrations far in excess of those found in plasma after hypnotic doses. Midazolam has a wide margin of safety, with little additional haemodynamic depression when 40 times the standard induction dose is administered to experimental animals.[135]

Benzodiazepines are suitable induction agents for patients with coronary artery disease because myocardial oxygen balance is well maintained.[136] Their biggest disadvantage is that they do not attenuate the haemodynamic responses to tracheal intubation and surgery. Accordingly, concurrent administration of opioids is necessary. However, these combinations do not provide the circulatory stability associated with the use of either agent alone. Pronounced arterial and venous dilation are the primary mechanisms of clinically important hypotension.[89,134]

Although bolus dosing of benzodiazepines to provide the hypnotic component of anaesthesia remains a common practice, the pharmacokinetic profile of midazolam can be used to advantage in producing stable plasma concentrations and effect. Careful titration of small intravenous doses of diazepam (and perhaps midazolam) until consciousness is lost can preserve spontaneous ventilation (in the absence of an opioid).

Ketamine

Ketamine 0.5–1.5 mg.kg^{-1} produces prominent haemodynamic changes, including increases in heart rate, cardiac index and systemic and pulmonary vascular resistance.[137] In normal subjects, the global increases in myocardial oxygen demand are matched by an appropriate increase in coronary blood flow, but in patients with fixed coronary stenosis and reduced coronary flow reserves, the myocardium is put in jeopardy by induction doses of ketamine. Ketamine causes sympathoneuronal release of noradrenaline[137] and also exerts a cocaine-like inhibition of neuronal re-uptake of noradrenaline.[138] The sympathetically mediated haemodynamic changes can be blocked, at least in part, by pretreatment with substantial doses of a benzodiazepine or droperidol.[137,139] An infusion of ketamine after diazepam pretreatment for cardiac procedures is claimed to provide haemodynamic stability comparable to high-dose opioid anaesthesia.[140] Experiments with isolated hearts show that ketamine has a direct negative inotropic effect on the heart, and terminally ill cardiac patients with depleted endogenous catecholamine stores manifest severe additional cardiac decompensation after administration of the drug.[141] After 20 years of clinical use, the precise role of ketamine in cardiac anaesthesia remains unresolved. Presently, we consider ketamine for the induction of anaesthesia in patients dependent on sympathetic activity, such as those with hypovolaemia and severely impaired cardiac contractility. Another advantage of ketamine is its relatively mild depression of spontaneous ventilation. This can be beneficial during induction of anaesthesia in patients in whom intermittent positive-pressure ventilation may seriously compromise cardiac function (e.g. tamponade, pulmonary embolus).

Muscle relaxants

Muscle relaxants are used routinely in cardiac surgical patients to facilitate tracheal intubation, counteract opioid-induced rigidity, limit diaphragmatic and other sudden movements during delicate surgical manoeuvres, suppress body movements to electrical defibrillation, decrease oxygen consumption during CPB, and control shivering after CPB. Usually, prolonged paralysis is not a problem if the plan is to keep the patient deeply sedated and the lungs ventilated mechanically in the postoperative period, at least until normothermia and stabilization of vital functions are achieved. The principal disadvantage of complete paralysis is that purposeful and reflex somatic movements are prevented and these crucial indicators of light anaesthesia are lost. Thus, avoidance of complete neuromuscular block is sound practice to detect intra-operative awareness. Unfortunately, monitoring of neuromuscular blockade by peripheral nerve stimulation is unreliable during hypothermia and low perfusion of the extremities during CPB.

Commonly, suxamethonium (succinylcholine) is omitted in cardiac anaesthesia, and long-acting neuromuscular blockers are used instead for induction and maintenance. This may be a practical choice for lengthy operations but it should be remembered that the circulatory effects of suxamethonium, with modest bradycardia and minimal changes in blood pressure due to transient vagal and ganglionic stimulation, are benign and do not contra-indicate its use in patients (e.g. those at risk of aspiration) in whom rapid development of deep block is desirable.

Pancuronium is vagolytic in paralysing doses, and increases in heart rate are usual after its administration, even in the presence of opioids (all of which increase central vagal activity).[142] Pancuronium may also have sympathomimetic effects which contribute to increases in heart rate and blood pressure which are observed occasionally. The vagolytic effect of pancuronium may be advantageous in a patient with low baseline heart rate due to chronic β-adrenergic blocker therapy and administration of opioid.[143] Vecuronium does not interfere with impulse transmission in the autonomic nervous system. Accordingly, vagotonic effects of many anaesthetic agents are unmasked, with resultant bradycardia. Dangerous bradyarrhythmias may be seen occasionally when vecuronium is combined with high doses of opioids.[143] Atracurium is not widely used in cardiac surgery because of its potential to release histamine when injected in high doses.[144]

Doxacurium and pipecuronium are two new muscle relaxants which, like vecuronium, do not have autonomic nervous system effects. Both are of longer duration than vecuronium. No significant effects have been detected in patients undergoing opioid/benzodiazepine anaesthesia for elective cardiac surgery.[145,146] Both agents are potentially useful as relaxants for cardiac surgery.

MYOCARDIAL PROTECTION BEFORE CPB

A continuous supply of oxygenated blood is essential for normal myocardial function because the heart has a very limited ability to function under anaerobic conditions. During normal resting conditions, the heart uses about 70% of the oxygen contained in the arterial blood delivered to it. Consequently, very little extraction reserve exists to cope with increased oxygen demand. Increased myocardial oxygen demand is met with increased myocardial blood flow by decreasing coronary vascular resistance. The factors which regulate coronary vascular resistance are not completely understood, but there is much evidence to favour the role of adenine nucleotides in matching coronary blood flow to myocardial oxygen demand. With oxygen debt, myocardial adenosine triphosphate and phosphocreatinine concentrations are decreased and the regeneration of adenosine triphosphate is shifted from the tricarboxylic acid cycle to highly inefficient glycolysis. The heart uses glucose delivered by blood as well as that derived from intracellular glycogen stores. Lactic acid is produced, and is not metabolized further in a low-oxygen environment. Contractile dysfunction ensues, and permanent damage results if ischaemia persists for more than 30 min.[147] The clinical consequences depend on the site and size of the ischaemic area. In patients about to undergo CPB and elective ischaemic arrest, adequate energy stores are important and contribute to the success of myocardial preservation during CPB. Despite cardioplegic arrest and hypothermia, there is an obligatory minimum utilization of energy during surgical ischaemic arrest.[148] This continuing metabolic demand can be met with energy stores which existed prior to arrest. The challenge of maintaining these energy stores falls very much on the anaesthetist.

Myocardial oxygen balance

The major determinants of myocardial oxygen demand are ventricular wall tension, contractility and heart rate (Fig. 16.3). Both preload and afterload affect wall

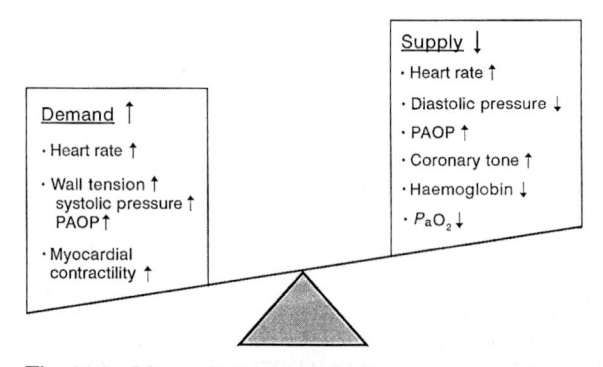

Fig. 16.3 Myocardial oxygen balance: determinants of myocardial oxygen supply and demand.
PAOP = Pulmonary artery occlusion pressure;
Pa_{O_2} = partial pressure of arterial oxygen.

tension. Increases in afterload (aortic pressure and systemic vascular resistance) are particularly detrimental because myocardial energy efficiency is reduced when the greater proportion of myocardial work is devoted to isovolumic work, with its high energy requirements, prior to opening of the aortic or pulmonary valves. Although increases in contractility produced by inotropic agents usually increase oxygen consumption, it may decrease if the failing ventricle empties more efficiently and the wall tension is reduced due to the decrease in chamber size. The increase in myocardial oxygen consumption with heart rate is largely attributable to concomitant increases in myocardial contractility.

The main determinant of myocardial oxygen supply is the coronary perfusion pressure, which varies during the cardiac cycle (Fig. 16.4). This driving pressure is essentially zero in the left ventricular myocardium during systole due to compressive forces exerted on the coronary microvasculature by the high intraventricular systolic pressure. Left ventricular perfusion occurs during diastole and diastolic perfusion time is disproportionately decreased with increases in heart rate.[149] Consequently, tachycardia has the potential to affect both sides of myocardial oxygen balance adversely. Blood supply to the free wall of the right ventricle is continuous throughout the cardiac cycle and, in the presence of pulmonary hypertension, very dependent on adequate aortic pressure. Coronary blood flow is normally autoregulated. Autoregulation is disturbed by coronary vasoconstrictors (e.g. α_1-agonists and hypocapnia) or vasodilators (e.g. nitroglycerine and isoflurane). Decreased oxygen content of blood due to decreased oxygen saturation or low haemoglobin concentration may be a critical factor in the maintenance of myocardial oxygen balance in critically ill patients.

In CAD, the presence of stenoses complicates maintenance of myocardial oxygen balance. The autoregulatory dilation distal to the obstructions helps

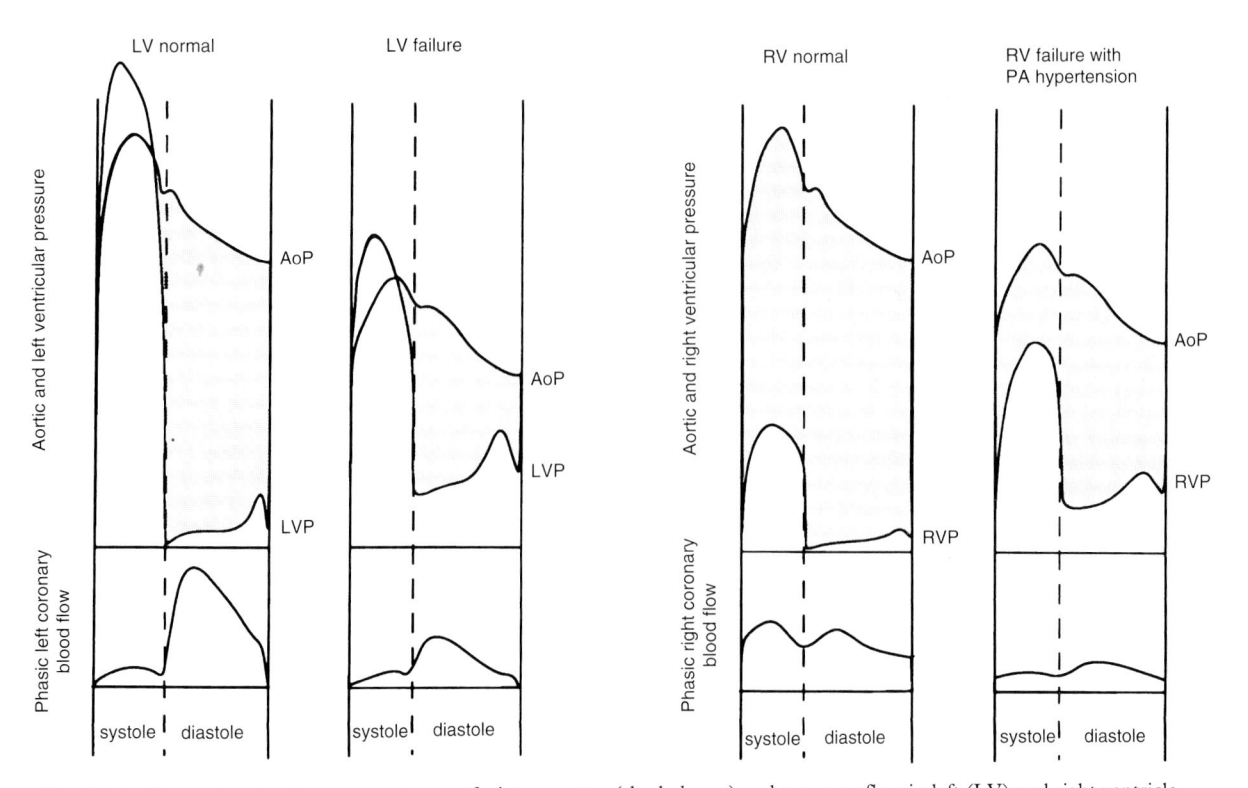

Fig. 16.4 Determinants of coronary artery perfusion pressure (shaded area) and coronary flow in left (LV) and right ventricle (RV). Because of compressive forces during systole, LV coronary blood flow is largely restricted to diastole. LV coronary perfusion is compromised in LV failure because of diastolic arterial hypotension and increased LV diastolic intracavity pressure. Clinically, LV diastolic pressures can be approximated by pulmonary artery occlusion pressure. Increase in heart rate causes disproportionate decrease in the duration of diastole and also decreases perfusion of LV myocardium. RV myocardium receives blood flow throughout the cardiac cycle. RV failure in cardiac surgical patients is usually associated with pulmonary artery (PA) hypertension. In this case, right coronary flow and RV free wall perfusion are compromised by systolic and diastolic arterial hypotension and increased RV intracavity systolic and diastolic pressures. Clinically, RV systolic pressure can be approximated by systolic PA pressure and RV diastolic pressure by central venous pressure. AoP = Aortic pressure; LVP = left ventricular pressure, RVP = right ventricular pressure.

to maintain supply — the so-called vasodilatory coronary vascular reserve. Angina with exertion occurs when the diameter of the lumen has been reduced by about 60%.[147] Practically all the coronary reserve has been exhausted with a luminal narrowing of 70%, and flow distal to the obstruction becomes entirely dependent on the pressure gradients. Since coronary pressures distal to a critical obstruction are typically 55–60 mmHg, diastolic blood pressure considerably above 60 mmHg must be maintained to ensure perfusion. Coronary obstructions are dynamic and may be greatly affected by locally released vasoconstrictors such as serotonin and thromboxane-A_2 from activated platelets. In addition, platelet aggregates and fibrin deposits may rapidly turn a non-significant eccentric atherosclerotic plaque into a significant stenosis.[147]

Detection of myocardial ischaemia

The reported incidence of peri-operative myocardial ischaemia in CABG surgery varies between 10 and 30%.[10,39,150] This variation is probably caused by the different methods used to detect ischaemia. Irrespective of the method used, clinically detected ischaemia represents only the tip of the iceberg of myocardial ischaemia.

Metabolic indicators are very sensitive indicators of ischaemia. Changes in the myocardial content of high-energy phosphates or intracellular pH can now be detected early even in humans, using nuclear magnetic spectroscopy or microelectrodes.[151] Lactic acid spill from ischaemic myocardial areas to the venous effluent can be measured with samples obtained from coronary sinus catheters. Coronary sinus catheterization is only suitable for research applications but has yielded very important information about the effects of anaesthetics on myocardial blood flow and metabolism.[152]

ECG and TEE are two practical methods for monitoring ischaemia in cardiac surgery. The details and their comparison have been discussed previously in the text. Impaired diastolic relaxation is also an early consequence of ischaemia. The increased stiffness results in increased ventricular pressures in order to maintain diastolic filling. Atrial pressure waveforms are accentuated and it is proposed that sudden increases in a and v waves in CVP or PAOP tracings are clinically useful signs of ischaemia.[153]

Prediction of myocardial ischaemia

Measurements of the most important determinants of myocardial oxygen balance have been combined in an effort to develop indices that may offer better prediction of ischaemia. Although there are a number of proposed indices, only two, rate-pressure product (RPP) and pressure/rate quotient, are simple enough to be used clinically. RPP is the product of systolic arterial pressure and heart rate and has been shown to be useful in assessing myocardial oxygen consumption ($M\dot{V}O_2$) and ischaemia during stress testing. Use of RPP to predict ischaemia during anaesthesia and surgery has been disappointing.[154] At least one of the reasons is obvious. Although an increase in heart rate has the potential to cause or worsen ischaemia by increasing oxygen demand and decreasing supply, an increase in arterial pressure may both worsen ischaemia by increasing demand and alleviate it by increasing supply. RPP does not correlate with $M\dot{V}O_2$ in anaesthetized patients.[155] Modification of RPP by the inclusion of PAOP (triple index = RPP × PAOP) does not significantly improve its predictive power for myocardial ischaemia.

Experimental work in animals with critical coronary artery stenosis has demonstrated that ischaemia occurs in the vulnerable areas of myocardium when the ratio of mean arterial pressure to heart rate falls below 1.0.[156] This is in accordance with the time-honoured clinical strategy of keeping normal blood pressure with a low to normal heart rate during anaesthesia in patients with coronary artery disease. Usefulness of this pressure/rate ratio as a clinical tool is in doubt because its power to predict ischaemia has been both confirmed[157] and refuted.[158]

A large proportion of peri-operative ischaemic episodes, perhaps even the majority, seem not to be associated with any haemodynamic changes.[10,39] Consequently, it is unlikely that any index derived from haemodynamic measurements will prove to be a reliable clinical aid to prediction of ischaemia. It may be prudent to maintain haemodynamic variables close to the pre-operative values determined when the patient was free from ischaemic symptoms; however, it is to be expected that ischaemic episodes will occur in some patients, despite careful control of all haemodynamic variables.

Treatment of ischaemia

Anaesthesia may be beneficial to the ischaemic heart and on many occasions haemodynamic aberrations associated with myocardial ischaemia can be controlled by judicious use of anaesthetic agents. If ischaemia is indicated by changes in ECG, TEE or ventricular filling pressures, the treatment strategy depends on whether or not the ischaemia is associated with haemodynamic changes which are potentially detrimental to myocardial oxygen balance.

1. In the absence of haemodynamic changes, acute reductions in coronary blood flow can be presumed to be caused by vasoconstriction in the native coronary arteries, in the stenotic region or in the graft bypassing that region. The mainstays of therapy are nitroglycerine and/or calcium antagonists. Nitroglycerine should be infused initially at a rate of 0.5 µg.kg^{-1}.min^{-1} and the rate increased as necessary; if systemic hypotension occurs, phenylephrine can be used to raise the blood pressure. Nifedipine 10 mg sublingually may also be used, but acute reductions in blood pressure may be problematic.

2. Ischaemia with tachycardia, unresponsive to deepening of anaesthesia, usually responds to intravenous β-blockers. It has been noted[10] that the incidence of PMI is significantly greater when heart rates exceed 110 beats.min^{-1}. Much slower rates are desirable before revascularization, and rates greater than 100 beats.min^{-1} are usually treated in the absence of cardiogenic shock. The ultrashort-acting drug esmolol is an excellent choice if there is concern about ventricular dysfunction or bronchospasm.[159] It is a β$_1$-selective agent with an elimination half-time of 9 min. An initial test dose of 0.15 mg.kg^{-1} can be given and, in the absence of change in heart rate, or any untoward response, this can be doubled every 2–3 min until the desired effect is achieved. Undesirable effects can be expected to dissipate within a few minutes. The favourable response can be maintained with a continuous infusion of esmolol (50–300 µg.kg^{-1}.min^{-1}) or continued with a long-acting β-blocker such as metoprolol (1–2 mg incremental doses).

3. If hypotension is implicated as a cause of, or a contributing factor to, myocardial ischaemia, determination of cardiac output and calculation of systemic vascular resistance are helpful. With low output and low filling pressures, augmentation of preload is logical and an energy-efficient way to increase blood pressure and coronary perfusion. Low values of systemic vascular resistance can be treated with phenylephrine in incremental doses of 50–100 µg. Although adrenergic agonists are coronary vasoconstrictors to some degree, their administration is not usually associated with worsening of myocardial ischaemia. In fact, adrenergic agonists have been shown to increase myocardial perfusion preferentially.[160] If ischaemia is related to hypotension in association with increased filling pressures, therapy with vasopressors should be combined with nitroglycerine.

4. Hypertension, unresponsive to deepening of anaesthesia, should be treated with vasodilators. Titratable and rapidly reversible vasodilators should be used intraoperatively. Sodium nitroprusside is more potent as an arterial vasodilator and its dose–response curve is steeper than that of nitroglycerine.[161] It is the preferred treatment of severe peri-operative hypertension, sometimes in combination with a β-blocker to limit reflex increases in heart rate and renin release. Although nitroprusside has been implicated in the coronary steal phenomenon, worsening of myocardial ischaemia during nitroprusside infusion has not been reported during cardiac surgery.

SPECIFIC VALVULAR DISEASES

Valvular lesions cause pressure or volume overloads which, provided that they are chronic, trigger haemodynamic adaptations that keep patients symptomless at rest for a long time. Ideally, valvular surgery should be performed before the onset of symptoms at rest, as these usually indicate the development of irreversible alterations in the cardiovascular system. Maintenance of haemodynamics close to the pre-operative range is a reasonable goal for the anaesthetic management of patients with valvular disease. Unfortunately, anaesthetists are often faced with patients who have critical valvular lesions and tolerate even minor haemodynamic disturbances poorly. Knowledge of the specific pathophysiology of the different valvular diseases is crucial to the interpretation of monitoring data and to rational therapeutic decision-making (Table 16.8).

Aortic stenosis

Aortic stenosis is a consequence of a degenerative process starting usually on the aortic surface of the valve cusps and exacerbated by high pressure and shear stress imposed by rapid ejection of blood from the left ventricle. The process is much accelerated in congenital bicuspid valves. The severity of aortic stenosis should not be judged from pressure gradients, since the gradient increases as a square of the flow across the valve. A patient with a failing ventricle, unable to maintain cardiac output and with a low flow across the valve, produces a lower gradient than that in a patient with a vigorous ventricle with the same degree of valve obstruction. Calculated valve orifice areas form a better basis for defining the need for surgical correction, which should be performed before the valve area has decreased to less than 0.8 cm^2 (the normal area is 2.6–3.5 cm^2). Thereafter, congestive heart failure usually ensues. A low pulse pressure (< 30 mmHg) usually signifies a critically obstructed aortic valve orifice. EF is usually well-maintained in aortic stenosis until the onset of congestive failure.[162] However, reduced EF may also indicate increased afterload rather than decreased myocardial contractility.

Table 16.8 Goals of haemodynamic management before cardiopulmonary bypass in critical valvular heart disease

Valvular pathology	Heart rate (beats.min^{-1})	Preload	Contractility	Systemic vascular resistance	Pulmonary vascular resistance
Aortic stenosis	⇓, sinus 50–70	⇑	⇔	⇑⇔	⇔
Aortic regurgitation	⇑ ≈ 90	⇑	⇔⇑	⇓	⇔
Mitral stenosis	⇔ 70–90	⇑	⇔	⇔	⇓
Mitral regurgitation	⇑ 80–100	⇓	⇔⇑	⇓	⇓

⇔ = Maintain; ⇑ = increase; ⇓ = decrease.

In aortic stenosis, the left ventricle undergoes adaptive concentric hypertrophy in an attempt to decrease wall stress induced by chronic pressure overload. As a consequence of this compensation (wall stress = intraventricular pressure × ventricular radius/(2 × wall thickness)), systolic function is well-maintained until terminal phases of the disease. However, diastolic function is compromised at an early stage. Low compliance decreases early diastolic filling of the left ventricle and maintenance of preload becomes critically dependent on high filling pressures and preserved atrial systole (i.e. sinus rhythm).[163] The mean PAOP may underestimate left ventricular end-diastolic pressure in ventricles with low compliance. The *a* wave in the PAOP tracing may be a better estimate of left ventricular end-diastolic pressure in this situation. Atrial systole may contribute 30% of left ventricular end-diastolic volume in aortic stenosis compared to 15–20% in a normal patient.

Myocardial oxygen balance is in jeopardy in patients with aortic stenosis. $M\dot{V}o_2$ is increased because of the increased mass of the ventricle and increased workload during the isovolumic contraction before the aortic valve opens. Myocardial oxygen supply is decreased by the elevated end-diastolic pressure and diminished diastolic perfusion time secondary to prolongation of the ejection phase. These factors in combination are responsible for the 30% incidence of symptomatic angina pectoris in patients with critical aortic stenosis despite the absence of coronary artery disease.[164] This pathophysiology sets the goals for anaesthetic management of patients with aortic stenosis (Table 16.8).

Patients with aortic stenosis are liable to malignant arrhythmias. These are due to re-entrant pathways in hypertrophied muscle with patchy ischaemic areas. If ventricular fibrillation develops, it may respond poorly to defibrillation, and closed-chest compression is ineffective in generating blood pressure sufficient to maintain perfusion of the central nervous system and myocardium. The avoidance of a vicious cycle of negative myocardial oxygen balance, decreased cardiac output, hypotension and a further decrease in myocardial perfusion, is a prime concern in the peri-operative management of aortic stenosis patients.

Aortic stenosis often co-exists with significant stenoses in epicardial arteries. This necessitates combined revascularization and valve replacement surgery. These patients cannot be expected to tolerate even moderate peri-operative changes in the determinants of myocardial oxygen balance. Volume overload can result as aortic and mitral regurgitation develop. Although increased systemic vascular resistance and aortic pressure may worsen regurgitation across both valves, therapy is directed at maintaining blood pressure, because of the potentially dire consequences of compromising myocardial oxygen delivery in aortic stenosis.

Aortic regurgitation

Aortic regurgitation (AR) is a volume-overload lesion. Acute and chronic aortic regurgitation have very different presentations. Acute AR, caused commonly by endocarditis or aortic root dissection, increases diastolic volume and causes left ventricular end-diastolic pressure to increase rapidly, sometimes even to a point at which mitral valve closure occurs before end-diastole. Increased left ventricular end-diastolic pressure and functional mitral regurgitation from ventricular dilatation increase pulmonary venous pressures and result in pulmonary oedema. Acute massive AR is incompatible with life and emergency surgical intervention is needed.

Slowly progressing diastolic volume overload in chronic AR results in eccentric ventricular hypertrophy with increased ventricular radius. The diastolic pressure–volume relationship (Fig. 16.1) is shifted down and to the right, and this allows very large end-diastolic volumes to be maintained with low filling pressures. This preload augmentation and the low aortic impedance to ejection are the mechanisms which produce the large stroke volumes needed to maintain adequate forward cardiac output despite significant diastolic regurgitation. Increased ventricular filling pressure is a late feature, but pulmonary congestion and pulmonary hypertension may result from the development of concomitant mitral regurgitation. EF is well maintained initially, but when it begins to decline, there is need for urgent valve replacement.[162]

Forward stroke volume can be augmented in AR by vasodilators. The decrease in aortic pressure also decreases diastolic regurgitation volume by decreasing the aortic to left ventricular pressure gradient. Decreased coronary perfusion subsequent to low diastolic pressure may limit vasodilator therapy in AR. Low heart rates are associated with increased diastolic time and increased regurgitation. Forward cardiac output has been shown to be increased in patients with AR when heart rate is increased, but a ceiling effect has been observed[165] between heart rates of 85–110 beats.min^{-1}. Due to the mechanisms of haemodynamic compensation, patients with chronic AR tolerate the pre-CPB period well. Patients with acute AR need diligent management of haemodynamics to preserve cardiac function and tissue perfusion (Table 16.8).

Mitral stenosis

Mitral stenosis is a consequence of a long-standing degenerative process initiated by rheumatic inflammation. Pure stenosis is observed in about 25% of patients with rheumatic mitral disease; the remainder have varying degrees of mitral regurgitation as well. Significant symptoms are usually observed when the mitral valve area has been reduced to less than 1.5–2.0 cm^2 from the normal 4–6 cm^2. After the valve area has been reduced to <1.1 cm^2, the stenosis is considered to be critical and the LAP to left ventricular end-diastolic pressure gradient increases to more than 20 mmHg, producing pulmonary oedema. LAP greater than 20 mmHg does not appreciably increase transvalvular flow. Persistent high pulmonary venous pressures cause reactive changes in the pulmonary circulation and ultimately a 'second stenosis' develops in the pulmonary vascular bed. Right ventricular failure by this mechanism may be the most significant haemodynamic disturbance before and after valve replacement.

Very little can be done to augment depressed cardiac output before CPB in patients with mitral stenosis. The stenotic orifice limits the effectiveness of preload augmentation, and the infusion of fluids may only increase LAP (not left ventricular end-diastolic pressure) and worsen pulmonary oedema. Correction of bradycardia increases cardiac output, but heart rates in excess of 80–90 beats.min^{-1} increase the transvalvular gradient without much augmentation of flow. Inotropic drugs usually cause tachycardia with little or no change in stroke volume, due to the low preload. Most patients with mitral stenosis are in atrial fibrillation when scheduled for surgery. In this situation, control of ventricular rate by pharmacological blockade of the atrioventricular node with digoxin and/or β-blockers is usually desirable pre- and intra-operatively.

The stenotic mitral valve acts like a waterfall, invalidating assessments of left ventricular preload by measurement of PAOP. In these patients, a thermodilution PA catheter allows measurement of cardiac output and facilitates maintenance of optimal right ventricular loading conditions. Postoperatively, an LAP catheter is needed to assess left ventricular preload in patients who have developed pulmonary vascular hypertension.

Mitral regurgitation

Mitral regurgitation (MR) develops as a consequence of processes that affect the components of the mitral valve apparatus. Valve leaflets may be attacked by rheumatic fever or infective endocarditis. Various connective-tissue diseases may cause weakening and eventually rupture of the chordae tendineae. The posterior papillary muscle often functions abnormally in the presence of posteroseptal ischaemia and may rupture as a complication of myocardial infarction.[166] The left ventricle in MR maintains its high output by preload augmentation, and left ventricular dilatation ultimately increases the mitral valve diameter and the amount of regurgitation. Regurgitation into the low-pressure left atrium serves to unload the left ventricle, and complicates the interpretation of left ventricular EF. A value of EF of less than 0.5 signifies impairment of systolic function, which may become evident after restoration of mitral valve competence by reconstruction or replacement.

The degree of blood regurgitated to the left atrium in patients with MR is dependent on the mitral valve area, the pressure gradient between the left ventricle and atrium, and the duration of systole. Both the mitral area and the pressure gradient are decreased by reduction of left ventricular afterload. Low heart rates increase the duration of systole and the regurgitant fraction. Heart rates between 80 and 100 beats.min^{-1} should be maintained. The upper range may, however, be inappropriate if MR is related to myocardial ischaemia.

In chronic MR, normal compliance of the left ventricle allows efficient filling during early and middle diastole. Atrial systole is not as important, and often is not present because most patients are in atrial fibrillation. In acute MR, the left ventricle fills in the non-compliant part of the pressure–volume curve and depends on atrial augmentation of filling. The pulmonary vascular consequences of chronic and acute MR are different. In chronic MR, distensibility of the left atrium increases over time, along with the increased valvular dysfunction. Chronic subtle elevations of venous pressure produce reactive passive pulmonary arterial hypertension. In acute MR, the lower compliance of the left atrium and pulmonary venous system causes rapidly increasing pulmonary capillary pressures and pulmonary oedema.

OTHER TYPES OF CARDIAC DISEASE AND SURGERY

Re-operations

Up to 15% of cardiac operations are re-operations in many centres. The mortality and morbidity associated with a second heart operation are only moderately greater than for the first operation but the third and subsequent operations have a very high mortality.[167] These patients are very vulnerable in the period before CPB. Scarring and adhesions may bring the anterior wall of the heart into direct contact with the posterior aspect of the sternum and the wall may be torn during sternotomy, with massive blood loss. In addition, functioning grafts are embedded in scar tissue and may be torn when the surgeon tries to expose the usual aortic and vena caval cannulation sites. Rapid transfusions of large volumes of bank blood may be required until emergency CPB is instituted. In haemodynamically unstable patients undergoing re-operation, the option of cannulating the femoral artery for CPB, or at least exposure of the artery, should be considered. Another risk for re-operation is the dislodgement of thrombotic material within old grafts by surgical manipulation, with embolization of the coronaries and sudden ischaemic dysfunction or even cardiac arrest. Both direct pacing and mechanical support of the circulation with internal cardiac massage are difficult or impossible because the epicardium and heart are covered by scar tissue and adherent to surrounding structures. The anaesthetist should be well prepared to treat hypotension, ischaemia and cardiac dysfunction before the circulation fails. Endocardial pacing may be possible using a PA catheter with pacing electrodes on its surface.

End-stage heart failure and cardiac transplantation

Cardiac transplantation is used increasingly as a treatment option for cardiomyopathies of diverse aetiologies not amenable to medical and surgical treatment. In these cases, the challenges of anaesthesia and life support not only include intractable heart failure but also compromised reserves of other organ systems. There are numerous considerations for the anaesthetist, which are described in detail elsewhere.[168]

Three aspects of care are particularly important before CPB in these operations:

1. Communication and co-ordination with all members of the team are of the utmost importance, especially with regard to the timing of premedication, vascular cannulation and induction of anaesthesia. It is imperative that there is no delay between the arrival of the donated organ and its insertion into the recipient because of the need to minimize the organ's ischaemic time.

2. In end-stage heart disease, all of the preload reserves are being used maximally to support pump function. Increasing blood volume may only cause overdistension of the heart and compromise its pumping ability. Afterload reduction with vasodilators is the only medical treatment which can improve the prognosis of these patients. Vasodilator therapy should be continued peri-operatively with due regard to avoiding hypotension during induction of anaesthesia and surgical manipulation. Anaesthetic agents free of significant myocardial depression should be chosen; an appropriate technique comprises the use of an opioid supplemented with small doses of ketamine, and pancuronium for relaxation. Endogenous sympathetic tone is high and supports the circulation; it may be necessary to infuse catecholamines to compensate for sympathetic inhibition induced by anaesthetic drugs. Because of decreased numbers of β-receptors due to down-regulation in response to chronic endogenous adrenergic stimulation, there should be no hesitation in administering higher than normal doses of catecholamines if required.

3. Although some anaesthetists and surgeons do not advocate the use of a PA catheter in heart transplantation, we find them to be very useful. Their main uses are during the discontinuation of CPB, and in the postoperative period. Pulmonary vascular resistance is almost always abnormally high in patients with

cardiomyopathy, and it is important to reduce it to avoid right ventricular failure in the transplanted heart. This can be accomplished only with the information furnished by a PA catheter. Insertion of a PA catheter via the left jugular or subclavian vein is often preferred in order to spare the right internal jugular vein for subsequent endocardial biopsies. A long protective sleeve allows the PA catheter to be withheld in the vena cava or withdrawn from the excised heart and inserted through the donated heart (with the aid of a surgeon from the operation field) before discontinuation of CPB.

Congenital heart disease

Complicated anatomy, functional abnormalities and small body size pose some unique anaesthetic challenges in paediatric surgical patients. The special requirements for equipment, skills and techniques are beyond the scope of the practice of anaesthesia and surgery outside highly specialized centres.[169] Atrial septal defect (ASD) is the only congenital heart disease commonly encountered in the adult cardiac surgical population.

ASD in adolescents or in adults is usually symptomless and discovered incidentally by auscultation or chest X-ray. However, it has the potential for the development of detrimental consequences. Although the shunt in ASD is left-to-right, there is often some bidirectional flow, and the shunt may be reversed transiently when airway manipulations raise right-sided pressures and unload the left side of the heart. Air or any other substance entering the venous circulation may flow into the systemic circulation and produce infarcts in the brain, heart and other organs. High pulmonary blood flow produces chronic pulmonary congestion and reactive pulmonary vascular hypertension. Right heart failure may ensue.

If there is no evidence of increased pulmonary vascular resistance pre-operatively, these patients tolerate anaesthetic techniques that allow early extubation well. It is essential that venous air emboli are avoided. PA catheters are not indicated in ASD. They may interfere with the surgery, and recirculation invalidates cardiac output measurement by thermodilution. If a large left-to-right shunt and increased pulmonary vascular resistance are present, a PA catheter is useful in guiding vasodilator and inotropic therapy used to support right ventricular function after CPB.

Surgery for arrhythmias

Patients with medically intractable arrhythmias are increasingly treated surgically. The condition of patients who present for this type of surgery varies widely. Patients with congenital accessory pathways, such as accessory atrioventricular conduction pathways or Wolff–Parkinson–White syndrome, tend to be young and have good myocardial function. However, patients with arrhythmogenic ventricular foci or intraventricular unidirectional block responsible for ventricular tachycardias by a re-entry mechanism usually have ischaemic cardiomyopathy or a ventricular aneurysm as a complication of myocardial infarction. The expected mortality of arrhythmia surgery varies from 1% for ablation of atrioventricular accessory pathways up to 10% when medically resistant ventricular tachycardia is the indication for surgery.[170] The operative procedure consists of anatomical localization of the arrhythmogenic focus and/or re-entrant pathway by electrophysiological studies and then ablation of the foci and interruption of pathways. Techniques including cryo-ablation, laser coagulation and endocardial resection or encircling ventriculotomy are used. CPB is required for surgical ablation but electrophysiological mapping can be performed before CPB or with the support of normothermic CPB if ventricular tachyarrhythmias are induced. Implantation of an automatic internal cardioverter-defibrillator (AICD) and insertion of the epicardial electrodes do not require CPB, but may be combined with revascularization operations.

Definitive clinical investigations to support current anaesthesia practice for arrhythmia surgery are lacking. The practical guidelines presented below are based on case reports, extrapolation of the results of animal experiments and clinical experience.

1. Doses of anti-arrhythmic drugs may be reduced or discontinued pre-operatively to facilitate identification of abnormal foci and pathways intra-operatively. Nevertheless, the anaesthetist must be prepared to deal with the adverse effects associated with some anti-arrhythmic drugs as well as contending with arrhythmias. Disopyramide and amiodarone have potent negative inotropic properties and cause therapy-resistant hypotension that may complicate the discontinuation of CPB.[146] Small doses of prilocaine or lignocaine can be used for local anaesthesia before insertion of intravascular catheters, but intravenous or intratracheal lignocaine should not be given.

2. Cardioversion or defibrillation is the treatment of choice for arrhythmias should they occur during anaesthesia induction or prior to electrophysiological studies.

3. Thiopentone, benzodiazepines, opioids, volatile agents and nitrous oxide and their combinations can

be used without interference with electrophysiological studies. The desire for early extubation and myocardial function dictates the choice of drugs and their doses. Droperidol should not be used in patients with Wolff–Parkinson–White syndrome because it affects both antero- and retrograde conduction in the atrium in a dose-dependent manner.[171] Drugs with anticholinergic properties (e.g. atropine, pancuronium) and strong sympathomimetic actions (e.g. ketamine) should probably be avoided.

4. If a PA catheter is used, the tip should be introduced initially into the vena cava, and advanced through the right heart into the pulmonary artery after the patient has been cannulated for CPB. Flotation of the PA catheter causes lignocaine-resistant short runs of ventricular tachycardia in up to 65% of patients undergoing CABG.[172] These are likely to be deleterious in patients undergoing arrhythmia surgery because of existing potential re-entrant pathways and compromised ventricular function.

The cardiologist and surgeon seek perfection in the electrophysiological study. This is very important to keep the cure rate high (currently reported as 90% for ventricular tachycardia) and to justify time-consuming procedures which require expensive investment.[170] In some patients, the frequent introduction of ventricular tachycardia and ventricular fibrillation (in AICD insertion) in the presence of normothermia results in slowly recoverable haemodynamic compromise. The anaesthetist continuously monitors the well-being of the patient and should share concerns with cardiologist and surgeon; in some cases, it may be necessary to interrupt the procedure to save the patient.

CARDIOPULMONARY BYPASS

A detailed consideration of the complex subject of CPB is beyond the scope of this chapter. The level of involvement of the anaesthetist in the conduct of CPB varies among cardiac surgical programmes. However, all cardiac anaesthetists must have a thorough understanding of CPB physiology. Maintenance of homeostasis during CPB is tightly coupled with anaesthetic and haemodynamic management, both of which are the responsibility of the anaesthetist. The following sections deal briefly with the basic aspects of extracorporeal systems and those issues of CPB which are particularly important to the anaesthetist.

Extracorporeal systems

Extracorporeal circuits used for CPB vary, depending

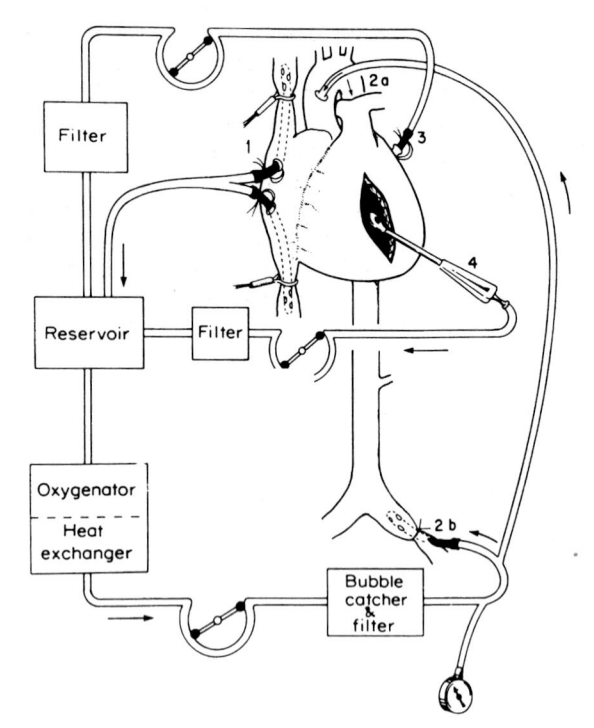

Fig. 16.5 Cardiopulmonary bypass from (1) the vena cava to (2a) the ascending aorta or, alternatively, to (2b) the femoral artery. Blood is also carried to the reservoir from (3) the left ventricular vent cannula and from (4) suction devices to clear the operative field. The arrangement in this diagram is typical for a cardiopulmonary bypass (CPB) circuit with a bubble oxygenator and total CPB tapes are secured around both superior and inferior vena caval cannulae. Modified from Bosé,[151] with permission.

on the patient and the operation. The basic circuit diagram is depicted in Figure 16.5.[173] The tubing and all the components in contact with blood are disposable and consist of various plastics, including polyvinylchloride, polythene, polyurethane, Teflon or polycarbonate. Peristaltic non-occlusive roller pumps generate flow in the CPB tubing. Flow is continuous, but most CPB pumps have an option to vary the instantaneous rate of rotation of roller heads and thus generate pulsatile flow. The benefits, if any, of pulsatile flow during CPB remain unsubstantiated at present.[174] Alternatives to roller pumps have been developed. Vortex centrifugal pumps are thought to produce less blood trauma but they are more complex and expensive, and thus not widely used.

Two basic types of oxygenator are in common use today. In bubble oxygenators, 100% oxygen is broken into microbubbles that percolate through the blood in the reservoir. Gas exchange occurs at the oxygen–blood interfaces and the bubbles are defoamed and vented to the atmosphere. Gas flow is adjusted according to $PaCO_2$ or pH values and PaO_2 and $PaCO_2$ cannot be varied independently without addition of carbon dioxide. In membrane oxygenators, gas exchange occurs through methyl silicone or non-wettable microporous polypropylene membranes. Because no microbubbles are generated, nitrogen can be added during hypothermia, and hyperoxia can be avoided. Hyperoxia during hypothermic CPB is likely to be inconsequential, but during rewarming with high blood flows, oxygen may come out of solution to form microbubbles that enter the systemic circulation. The most important theoretical advantage of membrane oxygenators over bubble oxygenators is reduced direct trauma to the blood elements. Oxygen–blood interfaces in bubble oxygenators cause progressive destruction of platelets and red blood cells.[175] Despite this, most clinical studies which have compared membrane and bubble oxygenators have failed to show differences in blood loss and transfusion requirements.[176,177] Differences between bubble and membrane oxygenators become significant when perfusion times exceed 2–3 h.[178] The claimed advantages of bubble oxygenators, including simplicity of assembly of the circuit and lower priming volume, are now dubious because modern membrane oxygenators share those characteristics and have become much less costly. Most cardiac surgical programmes today use membrane oxygenators exclusively.

The venous blood is collected from the vena cavae and right atrium and drained by gravity (siphon) into the CPB reservoir positioned well below the level of the patient. From this reservoir, the venous blood is pumped through the membrane oxygenator where it is arterialized and returned to the patient through a cannula usually inserted in the ascending aorta; a femoral artery is an alternative site when CPB preparations are to be completed before opening of the mediastinum or in the presence of a contra-indication to cannulation of the ascending aorta. Surgical blood loss is returned to the venous reservoir using cardiotomy suction devices. Screen filters with a pore size of 20–40 μm are required to remove debris from blood suctioned from the operative field. Similar filters are usually placed in the arterial circuit between the oxygenator and the patient to safeguard against accidentally introduced air, microbubbles or debris.

CPB is considered to be *total* when systemic venous return to the heart is totally diverted to the CPB reservoir by placing occlusive tapes around the superior and inferior cava cannulae; blood returning to the left heart is collected by a venting cannula inserted into the left ventricle. *Partial* bypass is used to unload the left ventricle and to support heart function before and after total CPB. CPB using a single combined atrial and vena caval cannula is commonly used for uncomplicated CABG operations and the left ventricle is vented only if ventricular distension begins to occur. The distinction between total and partial CPB is important to the anaesthetist because ventilation must be resumed when there is significant pulmonary blood flow in order to prevent hypoxaemia due to intrapulmonary shunt. Ventilation is unnecessary during total CPB and may be harmful if it causes hypocapnic alkalosis in lung tissue or interferes with the surgery.

The extracorporeal circuit is usually primed with crystalloid or crystalloid–colloid combinations. The addition of hydroxyethyl starch may reduce the immediate postoperative weight gain and limit the increase in shunt fraction after CPB.[179] The haemostatic effects of this colloid, however, limit the dose to be used in the prime and subsequently after CPB. Blood should be added to the prime if the estimated haematocrit after commencement of CPB with 2 l of asanguinous prime is less than 20%.

Haemodynamic management during CPB

Flow rates of 40–60 ml.kg^{-1}.min^{-1} usually maintain adequate systemic oxygen delivery in paralysed adults during moderate or mild hypothermia. Flows as low as 30 ml.kg^{-1}.min^{-1} have been shown not to compromise whole-body oxygenation.[180] Higher flow rates may be necessary in normothermia and if the haematocrit is reduced below 20%. Measurement of oxygen saturation of haemoglobin from the blood returning to the oxygenator is helpful in adjusting the flow rate to the existing need. This measurement can be performed with an oximeter that emits the light beam through a cuvette incorporated in the venous inflow line. The usual target is a venous haemoglobin saturation of at least 60%. Because blood flow is set by the perfusionist, total peripheral resistance is the only physiological determinant of systemic arterial pressure. Peripheral resistance is affected by the viscosity of the blood and arteriolar tone. The initial, often profound, decrease in arterial pressure on commencement of CPB is related to lowered viscosity due to haemodilution by the CPB prime. Viscosity is subsequently increased with hypothermia, and the anaesthetist usually has to deal with increased vascular tone and hypertension, the aetiology of which is obscure. Cerebral blood flow has been shown to be autoregulated when mean arterial pressure is in the range 30–110 mmHg during CPB in patients without cerebrovascular disease or pre-existing hypertension.[181] This contrasts to the corresponding limits of

50–150 mmHg during normal circulation. Since the cerebrovascular status is rarely known for certain, it is prudent to accept blood pressure limits of 50–90 mmHg during CPB. Pressures at the upper range should be adopted in patients with chronic diastolic hypertension, cerebrovascular disease, before aortic cross-clamping in patients with critical coronary stenoses, and after CPB in cases of incomplete myocardial revascularization. Higher pressures are also needed to maintain subendocardial perfusion in hypertrophied myocardium, particularly if that ventricle is fibrillating. Pressures higher than 80 mmHg may increase bleeding and interfere with delicate surgery. High blood flows and systemic pressures increase myocardial perfusion via non-coronary collaterals and lead to warming of the surface-cooled heart and washout of cardioplegic solution. To maintain blood pressure within acceptable limits, an α-adrenergic stimulant (e.g. phenylephrine or noradrenaline) or a vasodilator (e.g. sodium nitroprusside) are the usual drugs of choice.

Venous capacitance is also affected by drugs which interfere with sympathetic nervous discharge or act directly on the venous vasculature. Since arterial inflow and venous return tend to be in balance during stable CPB, a sudden increase in venous capacitance by a vasodilator may sequester up to 1 l of blood and reduce the return to the CPB venous reservoir.[161] Consequently, the perfusionist should be alerted when vasodilator drugs are to be administered so that accidental pumping of air is prevented.

Acid–base management

Decreasing body temperature increases the solubility of carbon dioxide in blood. Thus, $Pa\text{CO}_2$ is decreased, and this increases tissue pH. However, the dissociation constant of water also increases with decreasing temperature, and alkalosis may be optimal for enzyme activity during hypothermia. Blood gas analysers warm samples to 37°C, and normal pH and $Pa\text{CO}_2$ values recorded at 37°C indicate that electrochemical neutrality of water dissociation is maintained. This approach to maintaining $Pa\text{CO}_2$ and pH during hypothermic CPB is known as α-stat regulation. As compared to pH-stat regulation, α-stat regulation during CPB has been shown to maintain cerebral autoregulation closer to normal.[182] Currently, it appears that the majority of cardiac surgical centres utilize the α-stat technique and do not add carbon dioxide to the gas mixture flowing into the CPB oxygenator.

Developments in optical fluorescence chemistry allow for continuous monitoring of blood gases and pH during CPB. They have been shown to perform adequately on the arterial side of the oxygenator.[183] Optical fluorescence measurements of $P\text{O}_2$ have poor accuracy and a significant lag time in the range of values typically found in venous blood, and do not permit reliable determination of venous oxygen tension, which would be useful in assessing the adequacy of oxygen delivery to tissues. However, because the performance of modern oxygenators is very consistent and because significant changes in oxygenation are detected by the less expensive technology of oximetry, the clinical application of continuous blood gas and pH monitoring is limited.

Anticoagulation during CPB

Heparin, a mixture of mucopolysaccharides with a molecular weight ranging from 3 to 30 kDa, causes a 2000–10 000-fold increase in the capacity of the physiological anticoagulant, antithrombin-III, to inactivate thrombin. As a result of this inhibition of the final common pathway of coagulation, nearly complete haemostatic inactivation is obtained with the heparin doses of 300–400 units.kg^{-1} administered before CPB. Failure to produce and maintain anticoagulation leads to massive clotting of blood in the CPB circuit, and death of the patient. Consequently, the importance of a meticulous and consistent approach to heparin anticoagulation during CPB cannot be overemphasized. Heparin should be administered via a central vein after verifying the withdrawal of venous blood into the syringe. All members of the cardiac surgical team should be alert to the administration of heparin. Most importantly, it is imperative to demonstrate heparin effect, usually by prolongation of activated clotting time (ACT), before vascular cannulation for CPB. The ACT should be maintained at greater than 400 s as long as CPB cannulae are in place. A gaussian distribution of heparin dose–ACT response is observed when the standard dose of heparin is given to patients before cannulation for CPB.[184] Some patients fail to reach an ACT of 400 s, despite a dose of 400 units.kg^{-1}. These patients are designated as heparin-resistant, and the reason is usually an acquired deficiency of antithrombin III caused by chronic heparin therapy or a thrombotic process.[185] The resistance can be partly overcome by increasing the dose of heparin, but the initial dose should not exceed 600 units.kg^{-1} as increased postoperative bleeding is likely to result from the antiplatelet effect of heparin. A lower ACT value of 300–350 s may be accepted in these patients provided that the circulating concentration of heparin is > 3 units.l^{-1}; heparin concentration is usually measured by automated titration against known concentrations of protamine (Hepcon). It may be necessary to replenish antithrombin III by an infusion of fresh frozen plasma or with antithrombin III concentrate. Hypothermia slows the elimination of heparin and also potentiates its effects on ACT.[186] Therefore, it is important to repeat ACT at regular intervals, particularly during normothermia and rewarming, and to administer further doses of heparin as needed. Besides its use in the assessment of the adequacy of heparinization, the ACT is used to check the completeness of heparin antagonism by protamine after CPB. It should be borne in mind that ACT is very insensitive to low heparin concentrations and decreased procoagulant activities.[187] Return of ACT to the baseline value registered before anaesthesia does not exclude the presence of coagulopathy or even residual heparin after CPB.

Anaesthesia during CPB

CPB has the potential to alter pharmacokinetics and dynamics. Haemodilution causes rapid declines in plasma drug concentrations. There is a sequestration of some drugs by components of the CPB circuit.[188] Compensation for these effects by administration of supplemental doses of anaesthetic drugs at the start of CPB has been suggested. However, tissues contain substantial stores of anaesthetic drugs, especially those that are lipophilic and known to have a large volume of distribution, and these stores buffer abrupt declines in plasma concentrations of the free drug when CPB is started. Furthermore, because of concomitant dilutional decreases in the concentrations of plasma proteins responsible for drug binding, the concentration of the active moiety, or free drug, changes very little during CPB.[189] The effect of protein binding is often overlooked when considering plasma drug concentration data, which is almost always reported for the total drug in plasma, both free and protein-bound.

Hypothermia decreases brain metabolism and function. Temperatures below 28°C produce unconsciousness. Nevertheless, concern about the adequacy of anaesthetic drug effect remains. Adequate anaesthesia is needed before hypothermia is established, and during rewarming. In some cases, normothermic CPB is used throughout. Although MAC for inhalational anaesthetics is reported to decrease by about 5% per degree Celsius of reduction in body temperature,[190] the dose requirements for anaesthetics acting through receptors rather than physical alterations of membranes may not decrease. Cold may decrease the potency of opioids by decreasing their receptor binding.[191] In the absence of consistent and reliable indicators of anaesthetic depth in patients who are paralysed and undergoing CPB, it may be prudent to continue anaesthetic administration at the rate deemed appropriate before CPB. Moreover, anaesthetics, and opioids in particular, may blunt the stress response induced by hypothermia and CPB. Continuation of opioid infusions at the rate likely to cause the maximum antinociceptive effect before CPB prevents increases in hormones which are under hypothalamic–hypophyseal control (e.g. vasopressin), but activation of the sympatho-adrenal axis still occurs during CPB.[87,192] Blood flow to organs responsible for drug clearance, including lung, liver and kidney, is decreased during CPB.[193] Liver microsomal enzyme activity is decreased by hypothermia and consequently the clearance of anaesthetic drugs which depend largely on hepatic metabolism for their elimination is altered during CPB.[194] Prolongations of elimination half-times have been described for fentanyl and alfentanil in patients undergoing cardiac surgery.[195,196] Reperfusion of the lungs and increased perfusion of skeletal muscles on termination of CPB are at least transiently associated with an increase in plasma concentrations of opioids.[197] These pharmacokinetic changes have the potential to lead to accumulation of opioids if their rate of administration is not reduced after CPB.

Potent inhalational anaesthetics can be added to the gas mixture flowing into the oxygenator and the concentration and anaesthetic depth can be varied rapidly. Haemodilution during CPB decreases the content of volatile agents in blood by virtue of diluting plasma proteins and blood cells; however, hypothermia tends to increase anaesthetic content because of increased solubility of the volatile agents in blood. Overall the wash-in time is somewhat prolonged because tissue capacity is increased by hypothermia.[198] Wash-out in normothermic patients during rewarming is as rapid as from the lungs of a normal patient. The decrease in peripheral vascular resistance produced by inhalational anaesthetics provides the anaesthetist with another therapeutic option to control hypertension during CPB. The disadvantage of volatile anaesthetics is that their administration must be discontinued well in advance of the restoration of spontaneous circulation if their direct negative inotropic effects on the heart are to be avoided. Also, if reliable scavenging of the anaesthetic gases cannot be assured, considerations of the occupational exposure of operating theatre personnel may preclude their use during CPB.

Brain protection during CPB

Global brain ischaemia during CPB is usually of concern

only in patients with cerebrovascular insufficiency. In others, systemic arterial pressures as low as 30 mmHg[181] and systemic flows[180] of 30 ml.kg^{-1}.min^{-1} have been shown to maintain cerebral blood flow and brain oxygenation in hypothermic patients undergoing CPB. In practice, higher values are advocated as a safeguard. Most of the neurological and neuropsychiatric sequelae after CPB are due to focal embolic events. Particulate matter or air may be released to the brain circulation from the heart chambers or the ascending aorta. Emboli are derived from the extracorporeal circuit and most studies suggest that membrane oxygenators and arterial line filtration reduce their occurrence.[199,200] Theoretically, increased brain perfusion may augment central nervous system embolism. pH-stat management increases the brain flow at a given pressure.[182] Prospective clinical studies have shown either no consequences[201] or an increased incidence of neurological dysfunction[202] after luxury perfusion generated by this mechanism.

Thiopentone, in large doses which produce EEG burst suppression, has been shown to reduce neurological morbidity in patients undergoing open cardiac chamber procedures with normothermic bypass.[203] No reduction of neurological complications was found in closed chamber CABG operations with hypothermic CPB.[18] The role of thiopentone loading for brain protection during CPB remains controversial. With some question about its efficacy coupled with an increased need for vasopressor and inotropic support after CPB, the enthusiasm for using high doses of thiopentone for brain protection has waned.

Modification of surgical techniques, such as minimizing manipulation of the ascending aorta, CPB arterial filtration and meticulous removal of air, before allowing blood to be ejected by the ventricle into the arterial system, are probably the most efficacious methods of decreasing the incidence of stroke. Temporary bilateral external compression of the common carotid arteries by the anaesthetist when ventricular ejection begins may divert air and debris to other vascular beds.

Myocardial preservation during CPB

The use of CPB temporarily relieves the heart from its work as a pump. The ability to maintain coronary perfusion pressure and blood oxygenation during CPB creates the best possible situation to rest the heart and allow restoration of myocardial oxygen balance and energy stores before and after application of the aortic cross-clamp. Cardioplegia provides a quiescent heart with minimal oxygen utilization so that coronary perfusion can be interrupted by cross-clamping of the aorta to create a bloodless operative field and to prevent entry of air into the systemic circulation when the left heart chambers are entered. The myocardium does not tolerate total ischaemia beyond 15 min without some irreversible injury to myocytes, and subendocardial necrosis is inevitable after 30–45 min.[147] Ischaemia tolerance is greatly improved with chemical cardioplegia. Cardioplegic solutions have two functions. First, by inducing diastolic arrest, they decrease myocardial oxygen consumption by at least a factor of 5.[204] Second, they provide a milieu that maintains cellular integrity. Failure to provide minimal energy for adenosine triphosphate-dependent membrane ion pumps results in the translocation of calcium to cytoplasm, where it causes sustained interaction of actinomyosin complexes (contracture), and to mitochondria where it uncouples oxidative phosphorylation from the electron transport chain.

The most widely accepted solution is the modification of the solution developed originally at St Thomas's Hospital in London. The ingredients of this solution are shown in Table 16.9. The most important component of this solution is potassium. Perfusion of the heart with a solution containing 15–20 mmol.l^{-1} of potassium elevates the resting membrane potential across the sarcolemma from −90 mV to −60 mV, and this induces asystole. The role of the other components is less clear.

Several experimental and clinical studies have demonstrated the benefit of oxygenating cardioplegic solutions.[205,206] The oxygen content of crystalloid cardioplegia can be doubled from a maximum of 2.2 ml.dl^{-1} at 37°C by decreasing the solution's temperature to 5°C. To increase oxygen delivery with cardioplegia even further, several centres use blood-based cardioplegia. Although the affinity of haemoglobin for oxygen is greatly enhanced by low temperature, oxygen release can be augmented in the myocardium by the development of acidosis due to ischaemia. Superior myocardial preservation with blood over crystalloid cardioplegia has been demonstrated in

Table 16.9 St Thomas's Hospital cardioplegic solution*

Component	Concentration (mmol.l^{-1})
K$^+$	16
Mg^{2+}	16
Ca^{2+}	1.2
Na$^+$	110
Cl$^-$	160
HCO$_3^-$	10

*Unoxygenated pH 7.8; osmolarity 290 mosmol/l.

studies in which the duration of surgical ischaemia has exceeded 2 h.[207] Infusion of cardioplegic solution should be repeated at 20–30-min intervals, not only to maintain cardiac arrest, but also to replenish oxygen and to wash out metabolic end-products. If glycolytic end-products are not washed away, they cause a detrimental feedback inhibition of metabolism.

Usually, cardioplegic solution is infused into the aortic root proximal to the aortic cross-clamp. Typically, asystole is produced by a volume of 200–1000 ml and maintained by volumes of 250–500 ml infused every 20–25 min. To guarantee adequate delivery, the infusion rate must be sufficient to produce an aortic root pressure in the range of normal mean arterial pressure. Roller pumps should be used to infuse cardioplegia. A pressurized bag such as that commonly used for blood transfusion represents a serious compromise that does not guarantee consistent delivery. The presence of an obstructive coronary lesion with poorly developed collaterals causes non-uniform cardioplegic delivery. Retrograde administration of cardioplegia via the coronary sinus offers a significant advantage in these cases and in patients with aortic insufficiency.

Myocardial temperature is decreased by systemic hypothermia, infusion of cold cardioplegic solution, and topical myocardial cooling by an ice-cold saline slush poured or infused into the pericardial space. Hypothermia is an important adjunct to chemical cardioplegia in myocardial preservation because significant additional reductions of $M\dot{V}_{O_2}$ can be achieved with hypothermia after cardioplegia. In addition, temperatures of 15–20°C can maintain asystole and allow for decreased amounts of potassium to maintain cardioplegia. Although myocardial hypothermia is an established part of myocardial preservation protocols, the results of recent experimental and clinical studies have raised doubts regarding the degree of additional protection afforded by hypothermia, and it is not certain that the presumed additional protection justifies the potential detrimental effects of hypothermia. Reperfusion with warm cardioplegic solutions before resumption of contractile activity has been evaluated experimentally and applied clinically, with success,[208] Recently, enhanced myocardial preservation has been claimed using continuous warm blood cardioplegia and omitting hypothermia.[209] It is too early to determine if the results of these studies mandate major revisions in existing myocardial preservation protocols.

Cold potassium cardioplegia with or without blood as a vehicle results in a very low incidence of myocardial injury as assessed by impairment of cardiac function, CK-MB enzyme release or ECG changes. The realization of the full potential of chemical cardioplegia requires consistency in its administration. The anaesthetist should alert the surgeon if redosing is indicated either by the clock or if signs of electrical activity appear in the ECG. Patients with long (>2 h) aortic cross-clamp times could still benefit from improvements in existing methods of myocardial preservation. If energy stores become depleted either because of compromised myocardial oxygen balance before CPB or inadequate protection from ischaemia during aortic cross-clamping, reperfusion injury is likely to occur after CPB. The mechanisms involved are multiple and complex, but presently it is believed that highly reactive superoxide and hydroxyl radicals generated in damaged myocardial mitochondria, endothelial cells or activated leucocytes attack the vital lipid components of the myocardial cell membranes.[210] Recent efforts in the refinement of cardioplegia have been devoted largely to the potential additives that can block the formation of these reactive substances, or can scavenge them.

Discontinuation of CPB

Discontinuation of CPB requires preparations by the anaesthetist. All distractions during the weaning process should be eliminated. Consistent adherence to checklists, such as the one presented in Table 16.10, helps the anaesthetist to make correct decisions in the setting of dynamic physiology and rapidly changing circumstances where the crucial time of decision-making is compressed to a few minutes or less.

The circulatory state and lung function are the key issues to be addressed before attempts are made to transfer the duties of oxygen delivery and carbon dioxide removal from the CPB machine back to the patient's heart and lungs. The lungs should be re-expanded manually to assess their compliance, to detect airway resistance, and to eliminate atelectasis before mechanical ventilation is re-established. Bilateral expansion and resolution of atelectasis should be confirmed visually by observing pleura bulging into the mediastinum and by auscultation laterally, and as posteriorly as possible. If there is evidence of air or a substantial amount of fluid in the pleural space, the surgeon should open the pleura and remove the fluid by aspiration. Wheezing on auscultation using an oesophageal stethoscope helps to differentiate between obstruction and decreased compliance. Obstruction must be relieved before weaning, as it may lead to air-trapping, with increased pulmonary vascular resistance and acute right heart decompensation. In addition, protrusion of the lungs may cause displacement, compression or even detachment of mammary artery

Table 16.10 Checklist for discontinuing cardiopulmonary bypass

1. Patient responsiveness
   - Supplement if needed with an opioid and/or benzodiazepine
   - Deepen neuromuscular block after verifying that patient is anaesthetized (i.e. unconscious)
   - Check that anaesthetic vaporizers are off
2. Monitors
   - Recalibrate pressure transducers
   - Re-activate airway monitors
3. Availability of full-spectrum of vaso-active drugs with the preferred inotrope and vasodilator ready to be infused
4. Laboratory results (<10 min old)
   - Normocapnia, no significant acidaemia
   - K^+ (4.5–5.5 mmol.l^{-1})
   - Hct (18–22%, higher if clinically indicated)
5. Defibrillation/cardioversion and pacing capabilities immediately available
6. Normal body core and peripheral temperatures
7. Ventilation
   - Bilateral lung expansion, resolution of atelectasis
   - Air flow (wheezing, air trapping)
   - Compliance (pulmonary oedema, hydro-, haemo-, pneumothorax)
8. Circulation
   - Venting of intra-arterial air
   - Cardiac rhythm and heart rate
   - Visual impression of right heart filling and contraction
   - ECG (width of QRS, ST changes)
   - Perfusion pressures
   - Blood level in venous CPB reservoir

Hct = Haematocrit; ECG = Electrocardiogram; CPB = Cardiopulmonary bypass.

---

grafts. Increased airway resistance can be treated with the generous use of a nebulized β_2-adrenergic agonist such as albuterol. A T-piece which allows its administration from a metered dose inhaler should always be readily available in the cardiac operating room. In resistant cases, intravenous adrenaline or terbutaline may be needed. Decreased compliance is usually due to extrapulmonary compression. Pneumothorax must be considered, as well as accumulation of blood and irrigation fluids in the chest cavities. Ventilation of the lungs should be initiated before there is significant pulmonary blood flow as evidenced by the appearance of a pulsatile pulmonary artery pressure tracing. Omitting ventilation at this point may result in significant hypoxaemia due to intrapulmonary shunting. When mechanical ventilation has been started, the anaesthetist should check that airway monitors and alarms have been re-activated. After spontaneous pulsatile perfusion has been established, but while still on partial bypass, a pulse oximeter should be functional, and used to assess arterial haemoglobin oxygenation.

Perfusion pressure predicts subsequent mean arterial pressure and should be controlled within a range of 60–80 mmHg with anaesthetics, vasodilators or β-adrenergic agents if necessary, before weaning attempts. Higher pressures increase the pumping work of the heart and may interfere with left ventricular ejection. Lower pressures may provide insufficient coronary perfusion and result in subendocardial ischaemia. There should be at least 500–1000 ml of blood in the venous reservoir of the oxygenator as a preload reserve. Peripheral venous catheters should not be relied upon for large-volume resuscitation during the weaning from CPB. A higher heart rate (between 80 and 100 beats.min^{-1}) than was desirable before CPB is usually required after CPB in order to achieve satisfactory cardiac output. The stroke volume is reduced, and ability to increase stroke volume by augmenting preload is more restricted, because the diastolic function of both right and left ventricles is typically impaired for several hours after CPB, even in patients with excellent pre-operative cardiac function.[6] In addition, provided that revascularization of the heart is complete, myocardial oxygen balance should not be jeopardized by a moderately high heart rate to the same degree as before CPB. Excluding patients with chronic atrial fibrillation, a normal atrioventricular contraction sequence is important and should be established by atrial or atrioventricular sequential pacing if necessary. Pairs of temporary pacing electrodes should be attached on both ventricular and atrial epicardial surfaces. In addition to a stable rhythm, the ECG should show signs of recovery from the hyperkalaemic arrest. Continuation of bypass to rest the heart and allow more time for its recovery of electrolyte and metabolic equilibria should be considered when QRS complexes are wide and ST deviation is large. In anticipation of weaning, calcium (as calcium chloride 1–2 g) is usually administered to correct the mild hypocalcaemia which typically develops during CPB, to produce temporary vasoconstriction and increase contractility, and to antagonize hyperkalaemia persisting from cardioplegia. The routine administration of calcium is controversial. Its inotropic effects are fleeting and it has been shown to attenuate the inotropic action, and to augment the vasoconstrictive effect, of adrenaline.[211] There are also concerns that myocardial reperfusion injury may be worsened and coronary vasospasm exaggerated by increased extracellular ionized calcium. These potentially deleterious effects of calcium have not been substantiated and are probably not important in regard to bolus doses administered during weaning from CPB. Calcium, and other inotropic drugs, should not be administered until the myocardial energy stores have been repleted by allowing sufficient time for coronary perfusion of the heart in the decompressed state on CPB.

The actual weaning starts with gradual occlusion of the venous tubing, thereby diverting more blood to the heart. As less blood returns to the CPB reservoir and the heart increases its pumping, the CPB flow rate is decreased. In essence, as blood enters the heart, it stretches the myocytes to a more optimal length on the length–tension (Frank–Starling) curve (Fig. 16.6). Since quantitative assessment of fibre length or ventricular volume is not available clinically, CVP or PAOP are used as a surrogate of the ventricular preload. Absolute filling pressure values, compatible with weaning, differ from patient to patient, depending on the compliance characteristics of the ventricles. Generally, the lowest filling pressure which results in satisfactory haemodynamics should be sought, because overdistension of the heart chambers is detrimental to their contractile function. If the PAOP reaches 12–15 mmHg and the CVP 8–10 mmHg without satisfactory cardiac performance, it is prudent to begin an infusion of an inotropic agent, even if it is only required for a short period of time, while additional recovery of cardiac function takes place. This approach keeps the heart small, efficient and better perfused than attempts to utilize the extreme upper portion of the Frank–Starling curve. A sluggish upstroke in the systemic arterial pressure tracing and a small difference between systolic and mean arterial pressures suggest poor left ventricular performance. Absence of a step-up between CVP and PA pressure tracings (provided that pulmonary vascular resistance is in the normal range) is typical of significant power failure of the right ventricle and shows that the right ventricle is acting as a conduit, not a pump. A CVP/PAOP ratio exceeding 1 may signify right heart failure and it may be impossible to terminate CPB until right ventricular function is improved. Visual confirmation of cardiac filling and function is important. However, only the right ventricle is readily visible.

With satisfactory systemic, PA and filling pressures, the CPB pump output is gradually reduced to zero and both venous and arterial cannulae are clamped. Thereafter, the pressures should remain stable and the cardiac index should exceed 2.0 l.min^{-1}.m^{-2}. The volume remaining in the CPB reservoir is gradually returned to the patient and the combination of the anti-Trendelenburg position and a venodilator to increase venous capacitance is often used to facilitate emptying the reservoir volume into the patient. It is very important not to allow the heart to distend, since overstretching injures myocytes which regain their function slowly. Hypotension, low cardiac output and high filling pressures cause ischaemic dysfunction rapidly in this situation. It is prudent to resume CPB in order to decompress the ventricle before distension occurs. During a rest period, the beating, nearly empty, heart is supported with partial CPB, while inotropic and vasodilator therapy can be initiated in preparation for another attempt at weaning (Fig. 16.6).

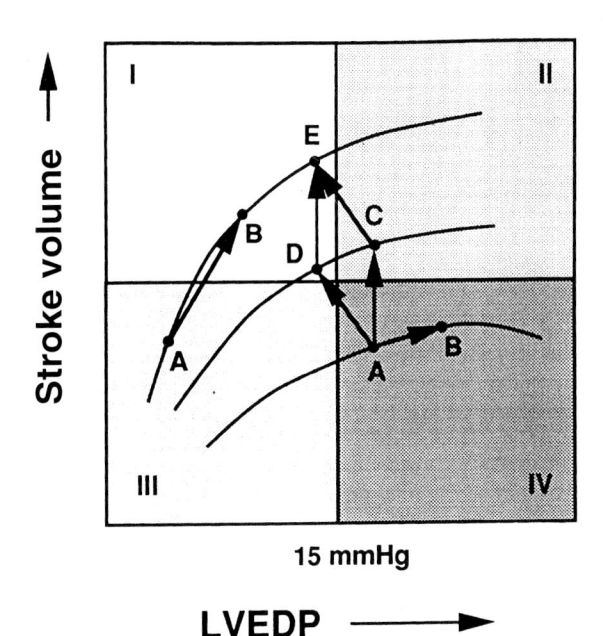

Fig. 16.6 Ventricular function (Frank–Starling) curves after cardiopulmonary bypass. Impaired function indicated by the displacement of the curves downward and to the right. Zone I = normal haemodynamics; II = congestion, III = hypovolaemic low perfusion; IV = congestion and low perfusion. Preload augmentation (A → B) is effective in normalizing haemodynamics if ventricular function is normal. With compromised ventricular function, volume administration only worsens pulmonary oedema. Inotropes (A → C) or afterload reduction with vasodilators (A → D) or their combinations (D → E or C → E) may restore function in those situations. LVEDP = Left ventricular end-diastolic pressure.

Treatment of hypotension and low cardiac output after CPB

After CPB, there is a tendency to slight hypotension, tachycardia, high cardiac output and low systemic vascular resistance.[212] This reflects low blood viscosity (low haematocrit) and perhaps a compensatory response to decrease oxygen-carrying capacity. If myocardial oxygen balance is considered to be in jeopardy, heart rates greater than 110 beats.min^{-1} can be treated cautiously with a β-adrenergic blocker. The ultrashort-acting β-blocker esmolol (5–20 mg intravenously) may be tried first before resorting to longer-acting agents. If hypotension is deemed excessive, adrenergic agonists such as noradrenaline usually increase blood pressure, while stimultaneously providing an inotropic effect to counteract the increased afterload. Although a haematocrit in the range of 18–22% is generally tolerated after CPB, patients with decreased compensatory reserves, such as those with pre-operative heart failure, incomplete revascularization and advanced age, usually require transfusion to raise the haematocrit to 28–30%, which provides a good balance between oxygen-carrying capacity and blood rheology.

The anaesthetist is faced with a demanding therapeutic challenge in a patient with hypotension and low cardiac output after CPB. This is usually due to acute impairment of left heart function. Measurement of factors which determine myocardial performance (heart rate, rhythm, preload, contractility and afterload) and adjustments according to ventricular function curves (Fig. 16.6) should form a rational basis for therapeutic decision-making. Generally, interventions should be made in an escalating manner and the responses confirmed with appropriate haemodynamic measurements (Fig. 16.7).

In heart failure, higher than normal LAP and PAOP may be needed to augment stroke volume. This may indicate systolic heart failure or diastolic heart failure with stiffening of the myocardium.[213] Diastolic failure after CPB can be due to myocardial oedema formation or impaired diastolic relaxation. The latter is an active energy-consuming process, and falls in myocardial ischaemia. An obvious therapeutic intervention is a nitroglycerine infusion. It has been suggested that cyclic adenosine monophosphate-specific phosphodiesterase inhibitors, such as amrinone and milrinone, improve intrinsic diastolic function (lusitropic activity).[214] Usually, diastolic function improves rapidly within the first few hours post CPB. Meanwhile, higher than normal left ventricular filling pressures should be maintained.

Both left and right ventricular contractile function are depressed reversibly after CPB.[6,7] This dysfunction is usually modest and overall cardiac performance can often be maintained at a clinically acceptable level by increased heart rate and slight increases in preload. Reasonable blood pressure is of prime importance for vital organ perfusion after CPB. However, normal blood pressure may be maintained by increased peripheral vasoconstriction. Early detection of low-output

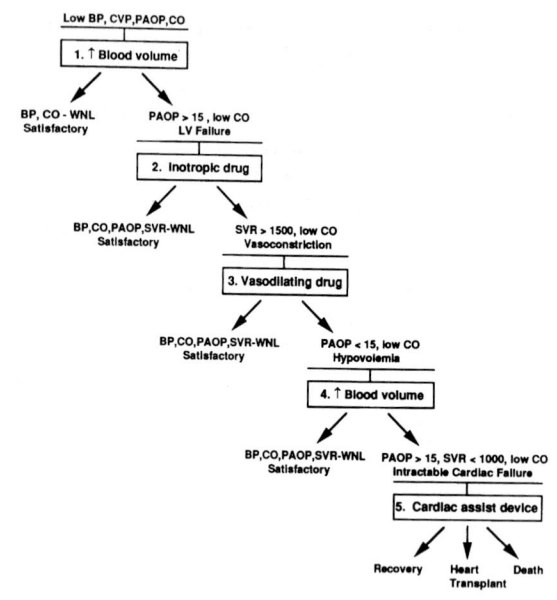

Fig. 16.7 Escalating therapeutic algorithm for low cardiac output and arterial hypotension after cardiopulmonary bypass. Pulmonary artery occlusion pressure (PAOP) is an indirect measure of left ventricular end-diastolic pressure; PAOP greater than 15 mmHg may be necessary in patients with a pressure gradient across the mitral valve and in those with elevated PAOP before surgery as a result of low ventricular compliance. BP = blood pressure; CVP = central venous pressure; CO = cardiac output; SVR = systemic vascular resistance; WNL = within normal limits; ↑= increase. Measurement units are mmHg for pressure, dyn.s.cm^{-5} for SVR, and l.min^{-1} for CO. From Hug,[215] with permission.

syndrome is often impossible without cardiac output monitoring. Reduced total body oxygen consumption, increased lactic acid production and decreased urine output are inevitable consequences. There are no magic numbers which define acceptable haemodynamics in a patient after CPB but systolic blood pressure less than 100 mmHg, cardiac index less than 2 l.min^{-1}.m^{-2} and PAOP exceeding 16 mmHg should raise concern. It is probably better to keep the threshold for initiating inotropic therapy low. In the past, the need for inotropic support after CPB was felt to be an admission of surgical failure and many surgeons were reluctant to see such therapy introduced. This attitude should be discouraged because, when treated aggressively and appropriately, low-output syndrome has an excellent long-term prognosis. The use of inotropic drugs has not been found to be an independent predictor of bad outcome.[15] However, premature prophylactic use of inotropic agents to terminate CPB may be associated with worsening of reperfusion ischaemic injury.[216] The possibility of a surgically treatable cause or institution of mechanical support such as intra-aortic counterpulsation must be considered when faced with high or increasing inotropic requirements after CPB.

Adrenaline or dobutamine are usually the primary choices of inotropic agent for low-output syndrome after cardiac surgery (Table 16.11). Dobutamine may not be as effective as adrenaline or noradrenaline in restoring cardiac output and systemic blood pressure. Dopamine relies for a large part of its action on the release of endogenous catecholamines, which are depleted from the adrenergic nerve terminals in the failing heart and after CPB.[217] These may be the reasons for the attenuation of the effects of dopamine after CPB. In addition, tachycardia and β-receptor-mediated vasoconstriction set the ceiling for the inotropic efficacy of dopamine. For these reasons, adrenaline is preferred to dopamine as the first choice of inotropic drug after CPB. The desired inotropic effect, from modest to maximal, can be achieved rapidly by titration of the adrenaline infusion rate. In contrast to popular belief, adrenaline cause less tachycardia at the equivalent inotropic dose than dopamine[218] or dobutamine[219] in patients after cardiac surgery.

Cyclic adenosine monophosphate-specific phosphodiesterase inhibitors, amrinone, enoximone and milrinone, are the latest additions to the pharmacological armamentarium for treating low-output syndrome after CPB.[220] In addition to their inotropic activity, they are potent vasodilators. The site of action of phosphodiesterase inhibitors downstream from the adrenergic receptor and membrane signal transduction offers a potential for synergistic augmentation of catecholamine inotropic effect. Amrinone is used in patients with pre-existing heart failure, particularly when the first attempt to terminate CPB has been frustrated by poor myocardial performance and high filling pressures. A loading bolus dose of 1.5–2.5 mg.kg^{-1} is administered with a continuous infusion of 5–10 μg.kg^{-1}.min^{-1} to reach therapeutic plasma concentrations.[221]

In a significant proportion of cardiac patients, compromised right ventricular performance is the cause of low-output syndrome. All myocardial preservation techniques are suboptimal with regard to right ventricular preservation and subclinical impairment of right heart function is typical during the first hours after CPB, especially in patients with right coronary artery disease.[222] Overt right heart failure can be precipitated by systemic hypotension and/or pulmonary arterial hypertension. The typical features are an increased CVP, which is disproportionately high compared to left-sided filling pressure, and right ventricular dilatation as observed in the operative field or in the trans-oesophageal echo image. The reversed diastolic pressure gradient shifts the interventricular septum towards the left ventricle and impairs left ventricular filling. The management options for the reversal of right ventricular failure after CPB differ in several respects from those used in left ventricular failure, and are summarized in Table 16.12. The right ventricle

Table 16.11 Inotropic drugs commonly used in cardiac surgery

Drug	Infusion dose	Limitations	Special indications
Adrenaline	2–15 μg.min^{-1}	Tachycardia Vasoconstriction	Difficult weaning from CPB, CPR, anaphylaxis
Noradrenaline	1–20 μg.min^{-1}	Vasoconstriction	Low systemic vascular resistance, right heart failure (support of right coronary perfusion pressure)
Dobutamine	2–15 μg.kg^{-1} per min	Tachycardia Limited efficacy	Congestive heart failure
Dopamine	1–10 μg.kg^{-1} per min	Tachycardia Vasoconstriction Increase in filling pressures Limited efficacy	Renal failure secondary to hypoperfusion, renal effects prominent in a range of 1–2.5 μg.kg^{-1}.min^{-1}
Isoprenaline	1–5 μg.min^{-1}	Tachycardia Arrhythmias	Right heart failure secondary to pulmonary artery hypertension, support of sino-atrial node function after cardiac transplantation
Amrinone	5–10 μg.kg^{-1}.min^{-1} (preceded by bolus of 1.5–2.0 mg.kg^{-1})	Hypotension Limited efficacy as inotrope	To augment β$_1$-agonists during emergence from CPB, congestive heart failure before CPB, right heart failure

CPB = Cardiopulmonary bypass; CPR = cardiopulmonary resuscitation.

Table 16.12 Treatment approaches in postoperative right heart failure

1. Preload augmentation, but avoid cardiac distension injury
   - Volume, or leg elevation (CVP/PAOP < 1!)
   - Establish atrial 'kick' (sinus rhythm, atrial pacing)
2. Afterload reduction (reduction of pulmonary artery pressure)
   - Nitroglycerine, isosorbide dinitrate, sodium nitroprusside
3. Inotropic support
   - Cyclic AMP-specific phosphodiesterase inhibitors, isoprenaline or dobutamine
   - Noradrenaline to maintain systemic blood pressure
4. Ventilatory management
   - Lower intrathoracic pressures (tidal volume < 7 ml.kg^{-1}, low PEEP)
   - Avoidance of respiratory acidosis ($Pa\text{CO}_2$ 4–4.7 kPa; 30–35 mmHg)
5. Mechanical support
   - Intra-aortic balloon counterpulsation to support coronary perfusion pressure
   - Right ventricular assist devices

CVP = central venous pressure; PAOP = pulmonary artery occlusion pressure; AMP = adenosine monophosphate; PEEP = positive end-expiratory pressure; $Pa\text{CO}_2$ = partial pressure of arterial carbon dioxide.

receives oxygen throughout the cardiac cycle, and modest systemic hypotension or pulmonary artery hypertension can result in right ventricular ischaemia (Fig. 16.4). The right ventricle is very sensitive to increased afterload (i.e. pulmonary hypertension or increased pulmonary vascular resistance). In the postoperative cardiac patient, even modest respiratory acidosis can cause significant increases in pulmonary vascular resistance with impairment of right ventricular ejection.[223,224] Maintenance of systemic blood pressure and aggressive treatment and prevention of pulmonary artery hypertension are cornerstones of the treatment of right ventricular failure after cardiac surgery.

Preload augmentation and inotropic drugs are the first treatment options for low-output syndrome after cardiac surgery. If heart failure has a significant congestive component with increased filling pressures, and if systemic vascular resistance is increased, afterload reduction is necessary to relieve congestion, improve myocardial performance at a given level of preload and taper the doses of inotropic drugs needed to support contractility (Fig. 16.6). The introduction of combination therapy with inotropic agents and vasodilators clearly improved the survival of patients with severe left heart failure after cardiac surgery.[225] When properly administered, nitroprusside may improve cardiac output by reducing systemic vascular resistance without significantly lowering systemic arterial pressure. In the presence of ischaemia-induced dysfunction, intravenous nitroglycerine is preferable for reduction of both preload and afterload.

MECHANICAL ASSISTANCE OF THE CIRCULATION AFTER CARDIAC SURGERY

Up to 5% of cardiac surgical patients cannot maintain sufficient oxygen transport despite maximal inotropic support and attempts to maintain optimal loading conditions.[226] In the majority of these patients, the circulation can be supported adequately with intra-aortic counterpulsation. The objective of the treatment is to increase diastolic pressure, coronary perfusion pressure and coronary flow while simultaneously reducing afterload during systole. This is accomplished by cyclically inflating (with helium) and deflating a balloon positioned between the left subclavian and renal arteries in the descending aorta (Fig. 16.8). When positioned and timed properly, diastolic filling of the balloon produces substantial augmentation of coronary perfusion pressure, and rapid deflation at the

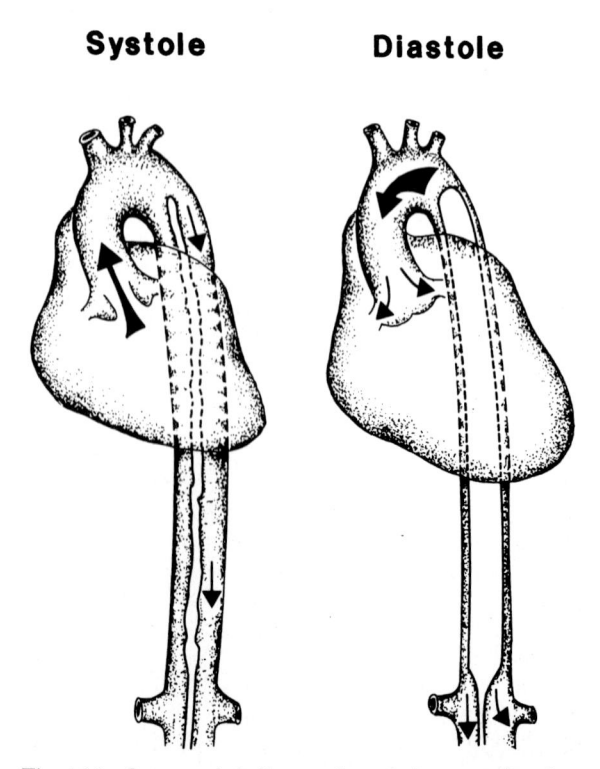

Fig. 16.8 Intra-aortic balloon catheter in its proper location in descending aorta. From Harjula & Salmenperä,[227] with permission.

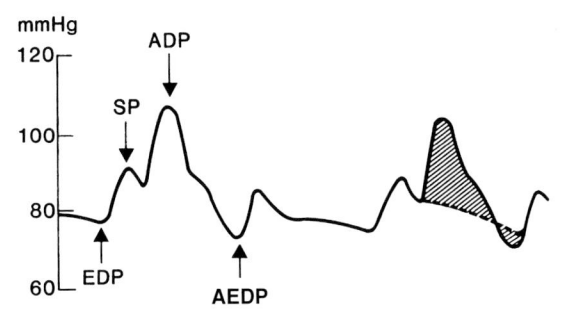

Fig. 16.9 Typical arterial pressure tracing during intra-aortic balloon pumping. In this case, the pulsator assists every other cardiac cycle. The shaded area indicates the pressure change induced by the balloon assist. EDP = End-diastolic pressure; SP = systolic pressure; ADP = augmented peak diastolic pressure; AEDP = augmented end-diastolic pressure. From Harjula & Salmenperä[241], with permission.

end of diastole causes reduced intra-aortic pressure which decreases the isovolumic pressure work of the left ventricle before the aortic valve opens (Fig. 16.9). Myocardial oxygen balance is much improved and intra-aortic balloon pulsation is very effective in reversing ischaemic dysfunction of both right and left ventricles. Increased systemic perfusion pressure allows a decrease in vasopressor administration and thus a trend in cardiac output is the best method to assess the efficacy of, and guide weaning from, intra-aortic counterpulsation. The weaning should occur gradually by decreasing the proportion of assisted cycles. Although intra-aortic balloon pumping should always be considered in the presence of ischaemic dysfunction and increasing inotropic requirements after cardiac surgery, surgical complications at the catheter entry site in the femoral artery, ischaemic complications in the ipsilateral leg and thrombocytopenia are common and serious enough to warrant a conservative attitude towards the use of this treatment modality.[228]

Pumps that can transiently accept the duties of maintaining left and/or right ventricular output remain the only option for the 0.5–1.0% of cardiac surgical patients who cannot be successfully weaned from CPB.[229] When unloaded, both ventricles have the potential to regain function. However, less than 25% of the patients placed on this kind of support survive to be discharged from hospital.[230] Blood pump units consist of three main components: the blood pump, the driving unit and the power supply. All the units may be external but some systems use an intracorporeal pump connected to the other units by a transcutaneous line. Centrifugal and screw pumps are easiest to use but can be employed for short-term assistance only.

Cardiac assistance devices are undergoing constant development and many are experimental. Busy heart surgery programmes should have access to this methodology. Anaesthetists should be familiar with the treatment and monitoring protocols in conjunction with the cardiac assistance devices available in their institution. Because the postoperative care of the patient supported by cardiac assistance devices in the intensive care unit is very time-consuming and expensive, and because the prognosis is dismal, only patients with a reasonable potential for cardiac recovery should be considered for this kind of assisted support. Alternatively, assistance devices can be used as a bridge for heart transplantation if the patient is otherwise eligible for transplantation.

MANAGEMENT OF HAEMOSTASIS AFTER CARDIOPULMONARY BYPASS

Restoration of effective haemostasis after systemic heparinization during CPB is largely the responsibility of the anaesthetist. Reversal of heparin activity is accomplished by administration of protamine, a polycation, which binds to heparin, a poly-anion, forming a non-covalent complex in a dose ratio of 1 mg protamine to 100 units of heparin. The resulting complex cannot bind antithrombin III and the anticoagulant properties of heparin are terminated irreversibly. Complete and sustained reversal is usually accomplished with 1 mg of protamine for each 100 units of heparin administered before CPB. Lower doses may be effective in bringing the ACT to baseline but free heparin activity or heparin rebound is likely with the reduced doses 2–3 h after the initial dose of protamine.[187] If ACT remains higher than baseline, an additional 50–100 mg of protamine can be given safely. If ACT remains elevated, it is probably due to a coagulopathy or to thrombocytopenia.

Infusion of protamine causes hypotension in some patients. This may be a manifestation of classical immunoglobulin E-mediated allergy but various other non-immunological mediators have also been suspected.[231] Occasional patients show a very pronounced increase in pulmonary artery pressure. This catastrophic pulmonary vascular vasoconstriction may lead to circulatory collapse after right heart failure and is mediated by the release of thromboxane A_2.[232] Severe protamine reactions are rare — the incidence is less than 0.1%.[233] Diabetic patients exposed to protamine-containing insulin preparations or those who have previously received protamine for heparin reversal may have a 10–30-fold increased risk of protamine reactions.[234] Several groups have attempted to attenuate protamine reactions by using alternative infusion routes through a left atrial catheter, or directly into the aorta, to allow systemic dilution of protamine before it enters the pulmonary circulation. The results have been inconclusive, and it appears that the site of the infusion is irrelevant as long as the drug is given slowly (< 25 mg.min^{-1}) and in dilute form.

Despite reversal of heparin anticoagulation, a significant proportion of patients continue to bleed excessively. Continuous bleeding into the operative field may significantly prolong chest closure and patients can have excessive chest drainage. The chest drain output should decrease rapidly with time. In the first 3 h after operation, drainage exceeding 3 ml.kg^{-1}.h should cause concern, and after that, values over 1.5 ml.kg^{-1}.h are excessive. The incidence of surgical re-exploration is about 5%[235,236] The putative causes of bleeding after CPB are indicated in Table 16.13. A localized surgical bleeding site is found in most cases. The overwhelming majority of the remainder bleed because of defective primary haemostasis due to acquired platelet dysfunction.[237] It should be remembered that the coagulation cascade is usually functioning well in these patients, and consequently, clots in the operative field, drains or test tubes, do not help to preclude a haemostatic defect. The aetiology of platelet dysfunction is not clear but platelets may be rendered dysfunctional after initial activation in the extracorporeal circuit. Alternatively, mechanical stress or proteolytic activity during CPB may deplete platelets from their constitutional receptor glycoproteins, which are required to mediate platelet adhesion or aggregation.[238] Prophylactic administration of aprotinin, a protease and fibrinolysis inhibitor, has been shown to prevent CPB-induced platelet dysfunction and also seems to cause a dramatic decrease in bleeding and transfusion requirements.[33]

Therapy of ongoing bleeding after CPB should be targeted at the most likely cause. Laboratory diagnosis is likely to be of limited value, partly because of the long time required to obtain the results and partly because of the values, though abnormal, do not often bear a causal relationship to bleeding. However, prolonged template bleeding time (> 12 min) suggests the need for platelet transfusion, irrespective of the platelet count.[237] The starting dose 0.1 units.kg^{-1}. Fresh frozen plasma is often administered, but probably not as often as indicated. Platelet concentrates are actually preparations of platelet-rich plasma, and the plasma component adequately substitutes the coagulation factors, which are rarely decreased beyond critical values. Pharmacological therapy has very limited utility in arresting bleeding once it has been established. Desmopressin acetate causes an increase in the plasma concentration of von Willebrand factor. This plasma factor is needed to bridge the platelets to the site of injury. Available evidence suggests that only occasional bleeding cardiac patients benefit from desmopressin acetate administration.[236]

Table 16.13 Causes of excessive bleeding after cardiopulmonary bypass

Probable
Local surgical bleeding site

Acquired platelet dysfunction

Possible
Pre-operative drug-induced haemostatic dysfunction (aspirin, coumarin)

Pre-operative haemostatic dysfunction attributable to associated disease (uraemia, hepatic failure)

Inherited haemostatic dysfunction (von Willebrand disease, platelet defect)

DIC (sepsis, low-output state)

Primary fibrinolysis

Dilutional coagulopathy and thrombocytopenia

Unlikely
Free heparin (unneutralized and rebound)

Protamine overdose

DIC = Disseminated intravascular coagulation.

VENTILATORY WEANING AFTER CARDIAC SURGERY

Weaning from mechanical ventilation does not usually pose problems in cardiac surgical patients. Extubation in the operating room or during the first hours in the intensive care unit is possible if anaesthesia has been designed to that end. However, this practice is considered by some to be unwise because this is a period of potential instability. Abrupt changes in oxygen consumption due to awakening, residual hypothermia, shivering and pain are more safely treated in ventilated patients. In addition, the stress of re-intubation can be hazardous if the patient has been returned to the operating room for re-exploration because of bleeding. Often, it may be wise to delay extubation until the morning after surgery, when expert help is more readily available if problems arise. Re-intubation of the trachea after the operation may be more difficult than the initial intubation due to soft-tissue oedema around the upper airways after CPB. If the cardiac patient is judged to be clinically ready for extubation, intermittent mandatory ventilation can be reduced fairly rapidly using capnography and pulse oximetry as guides.[49] Blood gas analysis is indicated only at the beginning and end of weaning, and when trend indicators display values which warrant investigation. No T-piece trials are necessary before the removal of the tracheal tube.

The recovery of consciousness and ventilatory drive are prolonged after the use of high doses of opioids with long elimination half-times (Table 16.7). Opioid antagonists have no place in cardiac anaesthesia because they may be hazardous in patients with limited cardiac reserve. It is very important to realize that sleep (natural or drug-induced) has a synergistic effect on ventilatory depression after opioids. Consequently, there is a risk of respiratory depression and arrest if the tracheal tube is removed prematurely; stimulation by the tracheal tube may be the drive that is keeping the patient awake and breathing.

Pulmonary congestion decreases pulmonary compliance and elastic respiratory work, and consequently large negative intrathoracic inspiratory pressures must be developed by the patient to produce adequate lung inflation. These negative swings of intrathoracic pressure increase venous return. Increased diaphragmatic movements may increase intra-abdominal pressure, further increasing pressure gradients or venous return and preload of the heart. Decreased intrathoracic pressure also raises transmural pressure across the ventricular walls and outflow arteries, raising the impedance to ventricular emptying. The increased afterload further increases preload and these changes jeopardize myocardial oxygen balance. Accordingly, myocardial ischaemia and heart failure are well-documented consequences of prematurely discontinued ventilatory support in patients with circulatory compromise.[239,240] Diuretic therapy aimed at reducing hypervolaemia, and vasodilators to reduce wall stress, should be considered before patients with borderline heart failure are exposed to preload and afterload stresses of ventilatory weaning.

LEARNING ABOUT THE POSTOPERATIVE COURSE

Anaesthetists should take time from their busy schedule to review the postoperative course of each cardiac patient. A personal visit and interview are important. This represents a great learning opportunity and helps to improve the public image of the specialty. Many complications, such as awareness, insufficient pain relief and problems related to positioning of the patient during operation may be ignored by members of other specialties, but are often very disturbing to the patient. Clustering of these complications may suggest the need to revise or fine-tune one's practices. Recently, a clear difference in significant morbidity and mortality in CABG procedures, not explicable by the case mix, has been demonstrated among individual cardiac surgeons.[2,3] The causes, as well as the remedies, for these differences are almost certainly multiple. Anaesthetic care does have at least a contributory impact on the outcome of the patient.[241] Learning from complications and recognition that one can do better require courage but are essential for continuous quality improvement.

REFERENCES

1 Cosgrove DM, Loop FD, Lytle BW et al. Determinants of 10-year survival after primary myocardial revascularization. Ann Surg 1985; 202: 480–490
2 Williams SV, Nash DB, Goldfarb N. Differences in mortality from coronary artery bypass graft surgery at five teaching hospitals. JAMA 1991; 266: 810–815
3 O'Connor GT, Plume SK, Olmstead EM et al. A regional prospective study of in-hospital mortality associated with coronary artery bypass grafting. JAMA 1991; 266: 803–809
4 Accola KD, Craver JM, Weintraub WS, Guyton RA, Jones EJ. Multiple reoperative coronary artery bypass grafting. Ann Thorac Surg 1991; 52: 738–744
5 Cosgrove DM. Evaluation of perioperative risk factors. J Cardiac Surg 1990; 5 (suppl): 227–230
6 Breisblatt WM, Stein KL, Wolfe CJ et al. Acute myocardial dysfunction and recovery: a common occurrence after coronary bypass surgery. J Am Coll Cardiol 1990; 15: 1261–1269
7 Mangano DT. Biventricular function after myocardial revascularization in humans: deterioration and recovery patterns during the first 24 hours. Anesthesiology 1985; 62: 571–577
8 Duke PC, Leroux M, Corne R et al. Criteria for the diagnosis of perioperative myocardial infarction in patients undergoing CABG surgery. Can J Anaesth 1990; 37: A150
9 Force T, Hibberd P, Weeks G et al. Perioperative myocardial infarction after coronary artery bypass surgery. Clinical significance and approach to risk stratification. Circulation 1990; 82: 903–912
10 Slogoff S, Keats AS. Does perioperative myocardial ischemia lead to postoperative myocardial infarction? Anesthesiology 1985; 62: 107–114
11 London MJ, Mangano DT. Assessment of perioperative risk. In: Stoelting RK, Barash PG, Gallagher TJ, eds. Advances in anesthesia, vol 5. Chicago, IL: Year Book, 1988: pp 53–87
12 Roberts SL, Tinker JH. Cardiovascular disease, risk and outcome in anesthesia. Edited by Brown DL. Philadelphia, PA: JB Lippincott, 1988: pp 33–49
13 Kennedy JW, Kaiser GC, Fisher LD et al. Clinical and

14 Mangano DT. Pre-operative assessment of the patient with cardiac disease. Baillière's Clin Anaesthesiol 1989; 3: 47–102
15 Royster RL, Butterworth JF, Prough DS et al. Preoperative and intraoperative predictors of inotropic support and long-term outcome in patients having coronary artery bypass grafting. Anesth Analg 1991; 72: 729–736
16 Kuan P, Bernstein SB, Ellestad MH. Coronary artery bypass surgery morbidity. J Am Coll Cardiol 1984; 3: 1391–1397
17 Gersch BJ, Kronmal RA, Frye RL et al. Coronary arteriography and coronary artery bypass surgery: morbidity and mortality in patients aged 65 or older. Circulation 1983; 67: 483–491
18 Zaidan JR, Klochany A, Martin WM, Ziegler JS, Harless DM, Andrews RB. Effect of thiopental on neurologic outcome following coronary artery bypass grafting. Anesthesiology 1991; 74: 406–411
19 Shaw PJ, Bates D, Cartlidge NEF, Heaviside D, Julian DG, Shaw DA. Early neurological complications of coronary artery bypass surgery. Br Med J 1985; 291: 1384–1387
20 Breuer AC, Furlan AJ, Hanson MR et al. Central nervous system complications of coronary artery bypass grafting surgery: prospective analysis of 421 patients. Stroke 1983; 14: 682–687
21 Sotaniemi KA. Brain damage and neurological outcome after open-heart surgery. J Neurol Neurosurg Psychiatry, 1980; 43: 127–135
22 Gardner TJ, Horneffer PJ, Manolio TA, Hoff SJ, Pearson TA. Major stroke after coronary artery bypass surgery: changing magnitude of the problem. J Vasc Surg 1986; 3: 684–687
23 Jones EL, Craver JM, Michalik RA et al. Combined carotid and coronary operations: when are they necessary? J Thorac Cardiovasc Surg 1984; 87: 7–16
24 Warner MA, Divertie MB, Tinker JH. Preoperative cessation of smoking and pulmonary complications in coronary artery bypass patients. Anesthesiology 1984; 60: 380–383
25 Tisi GM. Preoperative evaluation of pulmonary function. Am Rev Respir Dis 1979; 119: 292–310
26 Higgins TL, Yared JP, Paranandi L, Baldyga A, Starr NJ. Risk factors for respiratory complications after cardiac surgery. Anesthesiology 1991; 75: A258
27 Cosgrove DM, Loop FD, Lytle BW et al. Determinants of blood utilization during myocardial revascularization. Ann Thorac Surg 1985; 40: 380–384
28 Woodman RC, Harker LA. Bleeding complications associated with cardiopulmonary bypass. Blood 1990; 76: 1680–1697
29 Ebeling F, Naukkarinen R, Hanhela R et al. Post-transfusion hepatitis after open-heart surgery in Finland — a prospective study. Transfusion Med 1991; 1: 103–108
30 Hoyos M, Sarrión JV, Pérez-Castellanos T et al. Prospective assessment of donor blood screening for antibody to hepatitis B core antigen as a means of preventing posttransfusion non-A, non-B, hepatitis. Hepatology 1989; 9: 449–451
31 Taggart DP, Siddiqui A, Wheatley DJ. Low-dose preoperative aspirin therapy, postoperative blood loss, and transfusion requirements. Ann Thorac Surg 1990; 50: 425–428
32 Ferraris VA, Ferraris SP, Lough FC, Berry WR. Preoperative aspirin ingestion increases operative blood loss after coronary artery bypass grafting. Ann Thorac Surg 1988; 45: 71–74
33 Royston D, Bidstrup BP, Taylor KM, Sapsford RN. Effect of aprotinin on need for blood transfusion after repeat open-heart surgery. Lancet 1987; ii: 1289–1291
34 Hug CC Jr, Hall RI, Angert KC, Reeder DA, Moldenhauer CC. Alfentanil plasma concentration v. effect relationships in cardiac surgical patients. Br J Anaesth 1988; 61: 435–440
35 Flacke WE, Flacke JW. Cholinergic and anticholinergic agents. In: Smith NT, Corbascio AN, eds. Drug interactions in anesthesia. Philadelphia, PA: Lea: & Febiger, 1986: p 160
36 Jones RDM, Kapoor SC, Warren SJ et al. Effect of premedication on arterial blood gases prior to cardiac surgery. Anaesth Intensive Care 1990; 18: 15–21
37 Chung F, Houston PL, Cheng DCH et al. Calcium channel blockade does not offer adequate protection from perioperative myocardial ischemia. Anesthesiology 1988; 69: 343–347
38 Slogoff S, Keats AS. Does chronic treatment with calcium entry blocking drugs reduce perioperative myocardial ischemia? Anesthesiology 1988; 68: 676–680
39 Knight AA, Hollenberg M, London MJ et al. Perioperative myocardial ischemia: importance of the preoperative ischemic pattern. Anesthesiology 1988; 68: 681–688
40 Thomson IR, Mutch WAC, Culligan JD. Failure of intravenous nitroglycerin to prevent intraoperative myocardial ischemia during fentanyl–pancuronium anesthesia. Anesthesiology 1984; 61: 385–393
41 Gallagher JD, Moore RA, Jose AB, Botros SB, Clark DL. Prophylactic nitroglycerin infusions during coronary artery bypass surgery. Anesthesiology 1986; 64: 785–789
42 Brodsky JB, Bravo JJ. Acute postoperative clonidine withdrawal syndrome. Anesthesiology 1976; 44: 517–520
43 Ghignone M, Quintin L, Duke PC, Kehler CH, Calvillo O. Effects of clonidine on narcotic requirements and hemodynamic response during induction of fentanyl anesthesia and endotracheal intubation. Anesthesiology 1986; 63: 36–42
44 Flacke JW, Bloor BC, Flacke WE et al. Reduced narcotic requirement by clonidine with improved hemodynamic and adrenergic stability in patients undergoing coronary bypass surgery. Anesthesiology 1987; 67: 11–19
45 Morrison J, Killip T. Serum digitalis and arrhythmia in patients undergoing cardiopulmonary bypass. Circulation 1973; 47: 341–352
46 Gallagher JD, Lieberman RW, Meranze J, Spielman SR, Ellison N. Amiodarone-induced complications during coronary artery surgery. Anesthesiology 1981; 55: 186–188
47 Colson P, Saussine M, Séguin JR, Cuchet D, Chaptal PA, Roquefeuil B. Hemodynamic effects of anesthesia in patients chronically treated with angiotensin-

converting enzyme inhibitors. Anesth Analg 1992; 74: 805–808
48 Steward DJ, Da Silva CA, Flegel T. Elevated blood glucose levels may increase the danger of neurological deficit following profoundly hypothermic cardiac arrest. Anesthesiology 1988; 68: 653
49 Withington DE, Ramsey JG, Saoud AT, Bilodeau J. Weaning from ventilation after cardiopulmonary bypass: evaluation of a non-invasive technique. Can J Anaesth 1991; 38: 15–19
50 Kaplan JA, King SB. The precordial electrocardiographic lead (V_5) in patients who have coronary-artery disease. Anesthesiology 1976; 45: 570–574
51 London MJ, Hollenberg M, Wong MG et al. Intraoperative myocardial ischemia: localization by continuous 12-lead electrocardiography. Anesthesiology 1988; 69: 232–241
52 Slogoff S, Keats AS, David Y, Igo SR. Incidence of perioperative myocardial ischemia detected by different electrocardiographic systems. Anesthesiology 1990; 73: 1074–1081
53 Leung JM, Hollenberg M, Mangano DT. Prognostic significance of ST-segment elevation in CABG surgery. Anesthesiology 1991; 75: 3A
54 Kates RA, Zaidan JR, Kaplan JA. Esophageal lead for intraoperative electrocardiographic monitoring. Anesth Analg 1982; 61: 781–785
55 Gardner RM. Direct blood pressure measurement — dynamic response requirements. Anesthesiology 1981; 54: 227–236
56 Stern DH, Gerson JI, Allen FB, Parker FB. Can we trust the direct radial artery pressure immediately following cardiopulmonary bypass? Anesthesiology 1985; 62: 557–561
57 Pauca AL, Hudspeth AS, Wallenhaupt SL et al. Radial artery-to-aorta pressure difference after discontinuation of cardiopulmonary bypass. Anesthesiology 1989; 70: 935–941
58 Heinonen J, Salmenperä M, Takkunen O. Increased pulmonary artery diastolic–pulmonary wedge pressure gradient after cardiopulmonary bypass. Can Anaesth Soc J 1985; 32: 165–170
59 Tuman KJ, McCarthy RJ, Spiess BD et al. Effect of pulmonary artery catheterization on outcome in patients undergoing coronary artery surgery. Anesthesiology 1989; 70: 199–206
60 Moore CH, Lombardo TR, Allums JA, Gordon FT. Left main coronary artery stenosis: hemodynamic monitoring to reduce mortality. Ann Thorac Surg 1978; 26: 445–451
61 Rao TLK, Jacobs KH, El-Etr AA. Reinfarction following anesthesia in patients with myocardial infarction. Anesthesiology 1983; 59: 499–505
62 Jobes DR, Schwartz AJ, Greenhow DE, Stephenson LW, Ellison N. Safer jugular cannulation: recognition of arterial puncture and preferential use of the external jugular route. Anesthesiology 1983; 59: 353–355
63 Waller JL, Zaidan JR, Kaplan JA, Bauman DI. Hemodynamic responses to preoperative vascular cannulation in patients with coronary artery disease. Anesthesiology 1982; 56: 219–221
64 Troianos CA, Savino JA. Internal jugular vein cannulation guided by echocardiography. Anesthesiology 1991; 74: 787–789
65 Shah KB, Rao TLK, Laughlin S, El-Etr AA. A review of pulmonary artery catheterization in 6245 patients. Anesthesiology 1984; 61: 271–275
66 Barash PG, Nardi D, Hammond G et al. Catheter-induced pulmonary artery perforation. Mechanism, management, and modifications. J Thorac Cardiovasc Surg 1981; 82: 5–12
67 Moore RA, Neary MJ, Gallagher JD, Clark DL. Determination of the pulmonary capillary wedge position in patients with giant left atrial V waves. J Cardiothorac Anesth 1987; 1: 108–113
68 Levett JM, Repogle RL. Thermodilution cardiac output: a critical analysis and review of the literature. J Surg Res 1979; 27: 392–404
69 Sladen RN. Temperature and ventilation after hypothermic cardiopulmonary bypass. Anesth Analg 1985; 64: 816–820
70 Ramsay JG, Ralley FE, Whalley DG, DelliColli P, Wynands JE. Site of temperature monitoring and prediction of afterdrop during open heart surgery. Can Anesth Soc J 1985; 32: 607–612
71 Gailiunas P, Chawla R, Lazarus JM, Cohn L, Sanders J, Merrill JP. Acute renal failure following cardiac operations. J Thorac Cardiovasc Surg 1980; 79: 241–243
72 Smith JS, Cahalan MK, Benefiel DJ et al. Intraoperative detection of myocardial ischemia in high-risk patients: electrocardiography versus two-dimensional transesophageal echocardiography. Circulation 1985; 72: 1015–1021
73 Abel MD, Nichimura RA, Callahan MJ, Rehder K, Illstrup DM, Tajik AJ. Evaluation of intraoperative transesophageal two-dimensional echocardiography. Anesthesiology 1987; 66: 64–68
74 Teichholz LE, Kreulen T, Herman MV, Gorlin R. Problems in echocardiographic volume determinations: echocardiographic–angiographic correlations in the presence or absence of asynergy. Am J Cardiol 1976; 37: 7–11
75 Thys DM, Hillel Z, Goldman ME, Mindich BP, Kaplan JA. A comparison of hemodynamic indices derived by invasive monitoring and two-dimensional echocardiography. Anesthesiology 1987; 67: 630–634
76 Czer LSC, Maurer G, Bolger AF et al. Intraoperative evaluation of mitral regurgitation by Doppler color flow mapping. Circulation 1987; 76: (suppl. III): 108–111
77 Sainio K, Stenberg D, Keskimäki I, Muuronen A, Kaster M. Visual and spectral EEG analysis in the evaluation of the outcome in patients with ischemic brain infarction. Electroencephalog Clin Neurophysiol 1983; 56: 117–124
78 Sebel PS, Bovill JG, Wauquier, Rog P. Effects of high-dose fentanyl anaesthesia on the electroencephalogram. Anesthesiology 1981; 55: 203–211
79 Russ W, Kling D, Sauerwein G, Hempelmann G. Spectral analysis of the EEG during hypothermic cardiopulmonary bypass. Acta Anesthesiol Scand 1987; 31: 111–116
80 Bashein G, Nessly ML, Bledsoe SW et al. Electroencephalography during surgery with cardiopulmonary bypass and hypothermia. Anesthesiology 1991; 76: 878–891
81 Murphy MR, Hug CC Jr. The anesthetic potency of fentanyl in terms of its reduction of enflurane MAC. Anesthesiology 1982; 57: 485–488

82. Goldman NL, Shah MV, Hebden MW. Memory of cardiac anaesthesia. Physiological sequelae in cardiac patients of intraoperative suggestion and operating room conversation. Anaesthesia 1987; 42: 596–603
83. Waller JL, Hug CC Jr, Nagle DM, Craver JM. Hemodynamic changes during fentanyl–oxygen anesthesia for aortocoronary bypass operation. Anesthesiology 1981; 55: 212–217
84. Schwieger IM, Hall RI, Hug CC Jr. Less than additive antinociceptive interaction between midazolam and fentanyl in enflurane-anesthetized dogs. Anesthesiology 1991; 74: 1060–1066
85. Moldernhauer CC, Hug CC Jr. Continuous infusion of fentanyl for cardiac surgery. Anesth Analg 1982; 61: 206
86. Hynynen M, Takkunen O, Salmenperä M, Haataja H, Heinonen J. Continuous infusion of fentanyl or alfentanil for coronary artery surgery. Plasma opiate concentrations, haemodynamics and postoperative course. Br J Anaesth 1986; 58: 1252–1259
87. Hynynen M, Lehtinen AM, Salmenperä M, Fyhrquist F, Takkunen O, Heinonen J. Continuous infusion of fentanyl or alfentanil in coronary artery surgery. Effects on plasma cortisol concentration, β-endorphin immunoreactivity and arginine vasopressin. Br J Anaesth 1986; 58: 1260–1266
88. Scott JM, Cooke JE, Stanski DR. Electroencephalographic quantitation of opioid effect: comparative pharmacodynamics of fentanyl and sufentanil. Anesthesiology 1991; 74: 34–42
89. Wynands JE, Wong P, Whalley DG, Sprigge JS, Townsend GE, Patel YC. Oxygen–fentanyl anesthesia in patients with poor left ventricular function. Hemodynamics and plasma fentanyl concentrations. Anesth Analg 1983; 62: 476–482
90. Hug CC Jr. Pharmacokinetics and dynamics of narcotic analgesics. In: Prys-Roberts C, Hug CC Jr, eds. Pharmacokinetics in anaesthesia. Oxford: Blackwell, 1984: pp 187–234
91. Tomicheck RC, Roscow CE, Philbin DM, Moss J, Teplick RS, Schneider RC. Diazepam–fentanyl interaction — hemodynamic and hormonal effects in coronary artery surgery. Anesth Analg 1983; 62: 881–884
92. Rosow CE, Philbin DM, Keegan CR, Moss J. Hemodynamics and histamine release during induction with sufentanil or fentanyl. Anesthesiology 1984; 60: 489–491
93. Mangano DT, Siliciano D, Hollenberg M et al. Postoperative myocardial ischemia: therapeutic trials using intensive analgesia following surgery. Anesthesiology 1992; 76: 342–353
94. Christian CM, Waller JL, Moldenhauer CC. Postoperative rigidity following fentanyl anesthesia. Anesthesiology 1983; 58: 275–277
95. Jaffe TB, Ramsey FM. Attenuation of fentanyl-induced truncal rigidity. Anesthesiology 1983; 58: 562–564
96. Lowenstein E, Hallowell P, Levine FH, Daggett WM, Austen G, Laver MB. Cardiovascular response to large doses of intravenous morphine in man. N Engl J Med 1969; 281: 1387–1393
97. de Lange S, Boscoe MJ, Stanley TH, Pace N. Comparison of sufentanil–O_2 and fentanyl–O_2 for coronary artery surgery. Anesthesiology 1982; 56: 112–118
98. Howie MB, McSweeney TD, Lingam RP, Maschke SP. A comparison of fentanyl–O_2 and sufentanil–O_2 for cardiac anesthesia. Anesth Analg 1985; 64: 877–887
99. Thomson RI, Hudson RJ, Rosenbloom M, Meatherall RC. A randomized double-blind comparison of fentanyl and sufentanil anaesthesia for coronary artery surgery. Can J Anaesth 1987; 34: 227–232
100. Hall IR, Murphy MR, Hug CC Jr. The enflurane sparing effect of sufentanil in dogs. Anesthesiology 1987; 67: 518–525
101. Philbin DM, Rosow CE, Schneider RC, Koski G, D'Ambra MN. Fentanyl and sufentanil anesthesia revisited: how much is enough? Anesthesiology 1990; 73: 5–11
102. Sanford TJ, Smith NT, Dec-Silver H, Harrison WK. A comparison of morphine, fentanyl, and sufentanil anesthesia for cardiac surgery: induction, emergence, and extubation. Anesth Analg 1986; 65: 259–266
103. Shafer SL, Varvel JR. Pharmacokinetics, pharmacodynamics, and rational opioid selection. Anesthesiology 1991; 74: 53–63
104. Ausems ME, Hug CC, Jr, Stanski DR, Burm AGL. Plasma concentrations of alfentanil required to supplement nitrous oxide anesthesia for general surgery. Anesthesiology 1986; 65: 362–373
105. Moffitt EA, Sethna DH, Bussell JA, Raymond M, Matloff JM, Gray RJ. Myocardial metabolism and hemodynamic responses to halothane or morphine anesthesia for coronary artery surgery. Anesth Analg 1982; 61: 979–985
106. Moffitt EA, Imrie DD, Scovil JE et al. Myocardial metabolism and haemodynamic responses with enflurane anaesthesia for coronary artery surgery. Can Anaesth Soc J 1984; 31: 604–610
107. Bertha BG, Folts JD, Nugent M, Rusy BF. Halothane, but not isoflurane or enflurane, protects against spontaneous and epinephrine-exacerbated acute thrombus formation in stenosed dog coronary arteries. Anesthesiology 1989; 71: 96–102
108. Marijic J, Stowe DF, Turner LA, Kampine JP, Bosnjak ZJ. Differential protective effects of halothane and isoflurane against hypoxic and reoxygenation injury in the isolated guinea pig heart. Anesthesiology 1990; 73: 976–983
109. Reiz S, Bålfors E, Sørensen MB, Ariola S, Friedman A, Truedsson H. Isoflurane — a powerful coronary vasodilator in patients with coronary artery disease. Anesthesiology 1983; 59: 91–97
110. Moffitt EA, Barker RA, Glenn JJ et al. Myocardial metabolism and hemodynamic responses with isoflurane anesthesia for coronary arterial surgery. Anesth Analg 1986; 65: 53–61
111. Priebe HJ. Isoflurane and coronary hemodynamics. Anesthesiology 1989; 71: 960–976
112. Buffington CW, Davis KB, Gillespie S, Pettinger M. The prevalence of steal-prone coronary anatomy in patients with coronary artery disease: an analysis of the coronary artery surgery study registry. Anesthesiology 1988; 69: 721–727
113. Bollen BA, Tinker JH, Hermsmeyer K. Halothane relaxes previously constricted isolated porcine coronary artery segments more than isoflurane. Anesthesiology 1987; 66: 748–752
114. Sahlman L, Milocco I, Appelgren L, William-Olsson G,

Ricksten SE. Control of intraoperative hypertension with isoflurane in patients with coronary artery disease: effects on regional myocardial blood flow and metabolism. Anesth Analg 1989; 68: 105–111

115 Tarnow J, Markschies-Hornung A, Schulte-Sasse U. Isoflurane improves the tolerance to pacing-induced myocardial ischemia. Anesthesiology 1986; 64: 147–156

116 Leung JM, Goehner P, O'Kelly BF et al. Isoflurane anesthesia and myocardial ischemia: comparative risk versus sufentanil anesthesia in patients undergoing coronary artery bypass graft surgery. Anesthesiology 1991; 74: 838–847

117 Slogoff S, Keats AS, Dear WE et al. Steal-prone coronary anatomy and myocardial ischemia associated with four primary anesthetic agents in humans. Anesth Analg 1991; 72: 22–27

118 Thomson IR, Bowering JB, Hudson RJ, Frais MA, Rosenbloom M. A comparison of desflurane and isoflurane in patients undergoing coronary artery surgery. Anesthesiology 1991; 75: 776–781

119 Moffit EA, Scovil JE, Barker RA et al. The effects of nitrous oxide on myocardial metabolism and hemodynamics during fentanyl or enflurane anesthesia in patients with coronary disease. Anesth Analg 1984; 63: 1071–1075

120 Ramsay JG, Arvieux CC, Foëx P et al. Regional and global myocardial function in the dog when nitrous oxide is added to halothane in the presence of critical coronary artery constriction. Anesth Analg 1986; 65: 431–436

121 Mitchell MM, Prakash O, Rulf ENR, van Daele MERM, Cahalan MK, Roelandt JRTC. Nitrous oxide does not induce myocardial ischemia in patients with ischemic heart disease and poor ventricular function. Anesthesiology 1989; 71: 526–534

122 Schulte-Sasse U, Hess W, Tarnow J. Pulmonary vascular responses to nitrous oxide in patients with normal and high pulmonary vascular resistance. Anesthesiology 1982; 57: 9–13

123 Becker KE, Tonnesen AS. Cardiovascular effects of plasma levels of thiopental necessary for anesthesia. Anesthesiology 1978; 49: 197–200

124 Brüssel T, Theissen JL, Vigfusson G, Lunkenheimer PP, Van Aken H, Lawin P. Hemodynamic and cardiodynamic effects of propofol and etomidate: negative inotropic properties of propofol. Anesth Analg 1989; 69: 35–40

125 Cullen PM, Turtle M, Prys-Roberts C, Way WL, Dye J. Effect of propofol anesthesia on baroreflex activity in humans. Anesth Analg 1987; 66: 1115–1120

126 Patrick MR, Blair IJ, Feneck RO, Sebel PS. A comparison of the haemodynamic effects of propofol (Diprivan) and thiopentone in patients with coronary artery disease. Postgrad Med J 1985; 61: 23–27

127 Russell GN, Wright EL, Fox MA, Douglas EJ, Cockshott ID. Propofol–fentanyl anaesthesia for coronary artery surgery and cardiopulmonary bypass. Anaesthesia 1989; 44: 205–208

128 Colvin MP, Savege TM, Newland PE et al. Cardiorespiratory changes following induction of anaesthesia with etomidate in patients with cardiac disease. Br J Anaesth 1979; 51: 551–556

129 Ebert TJ, Kanitz DD, Berens RJ, Kampine JP. Etomidate induction maintains sympathetic outflow in humans: direct observation from sympathetic recordings. Anesthesiology 1990; 73: A342

130 Lindeburg T, Spotoft H, Sørensen B, Skovsted P. Cardiovascular effects of etomidate used for induction and in combination with fentanyl–pancuronium for maintenance of anaesthesia in patients with valvular heart disease. Acta Anaesthesiol Scand 1982; 26: 205–208

131 Reves JG, Glass P, Jacobs JR. Alfentanil and midazolam: new anesthetic drugs for continuous infusion and an automated method of administration. Mt Sinai J Med 1989; 56: 99–107

132 Samuelson PN, Reves JG, Kouchoukos NT, Smith LR, Dole KM. Hemodynamic responses to anesthetic induction with midazolam or diazepam in patients with ischemic heart disease. Anesth Analg 1981; 60: 802–809

133 Kawar P, Carson IW, Clarke RSJ, Sundee JW, Lyons SM. Haemodynamic changes during induction of anaesthesia with midazolam and diazepam (Valium) in patients undergoing coronary artery bypass surgery. Anaesthesia 1985; 40: 767–771

134 Heikkilä H, Jalonen J, Arola M. Midazolam as adjunct to high-dose fentanyl anaesthesia for coronary artery bypass grafting operation. Acta Anaesthesiol Scand 1984; 28: 683–689

135 Jones DJ, Stehling LC, Zauder HL. Cardiovascular responses to diazepam and midazolam maleate in the dog. Anesthesiology 1979; 51: 430–434

136 Marty J, Nitenberg A, Blachet F, Zouioueche S, Desmonts JM. Effects of midazolam on the coronary circulation in patients with coronary artery disease. Anesthesiology 1986; 64: 206–210

137 Bålfors E, Häggmark S, Nyhman H, Rydvall A, Reiz S. Droperidol inhibits the effects of intravenous ketamine on central hemodynamics and myocardial oxygen consumption in patients with generalized atherosclerotic disease. Anesth Analg 1983; 62: 193–197

138 Hill GE, Wong KC, Shaw CL, Sentker CR, Blatnick RA. Interactions of ketamine with vasoactive amines at normothermia and hypothermia in the isolated rabbit heart. Anesthesiology 1978; 48: 315–319

139 Dhadphale PR, Jackson APF, Alseri S. Comparison of anaesthesia with diazepam and ketamine vs morphine in patients undergoing heart-valve replacement. Anesthesiology 1970; 51: 200–203

140 Hatano S, Keane DM, Boggs RE, El-Naggar MA, Sadove MS. Diazepam–ketamine anaesthesia for open heart surgery: a 'micro-mini' drip administration technique. Can Anaesth Soc J 1976; 23: 648–656

141 Waxman K, Shoemaker WE, Lippman M. Cardiovascular effects of anesthetic induction with ketamine. Anesth Analg 1980; 59: 355–358

142 Thomson IR, Putnins CL. Adverse effects of pancuronium during high-dose fentanyl anesthesia for coronary artery bypass grafting. Anesthesiology 1985; 62: 708–713

143 Salmenperä M, Peltola K, Takkunen O, Heinonen J. Cardiovascular effects of pancuronium and vecuronium during high-dose fentanyl anesthesia. Anesth Analg 1983; 62: 1059–1064

144 Moss J, Rosow CE, Savarese JJ, Philbin DM, Kniffen

KJ. Role of histamine in the hypotensive action of d-tubocurarine in humans. Anesthesiology 1981; 55: 19–25
145 Stoops CM, Curtis CA, Kovach DA et al. Hemodynamic effects of doxacurium chloride in patients receiving oxygen-sufentanil anesthesia for coronary artery bypass grafting or valve replacement. Anesthesiology 1988; 69: 365–370
146 Tassonyi E, Neidhart P, Pittett JF, Morel DR, Gemperle M. Cardiovascular effects of pipecuronium and pancuronium in patients undergoing coronary artery bypass grafting. Anesthesiology 1988; 69: 793–796
147 Norris RM. The pathophysiology of myocardial ischaemia. Baillière's Clin Anaesthesiol 1989; 3: 1–25
148 Buckberg GD, Brazier JR, Nelson RL, Goldstein SM, McConnell DH, Cooper N. Studies of the effects of hypothermia on regional myocardial blood flow and metabolism during cardiopulmonary bypass. I. The adequately perfused beating, fibrillating and arrested heart. J Thorac Cardiovasc Surg 1977; 73: 87–94
149 Boudoulas H, Rittgers SE, Lewis RP, Leier CV, Weissler AM. Changes in diastolic time with various pharmacologic agents. Implication for myocardial perfusion. Circulation 1979; 60: 164–169
150 O'Connor JP, Ramsay JG, Wynands JE et al. The incidence of myocardial ischemia during anesthesia for coronary artery bypass surgery in patients receiving pancuronium or vecuronium. Anesthesiology 1989; 70: 230–236
151 Bosé D. Cellular and mechanical effects of myocardial ischemia. Anesthesiol Clin North Am 1991; 9: 567–472
152 Hall RI, Moffitt EA. The effects of anaesthetics on coronary artery blood flow and myocardial metabolism: a review of studies in animals and man. Baillière's Clin Anaesthesiol 1989; 3: 27–46
153 Kaplan JA, Wells PH. Early diagnosis of myocardial ischemia using the pulmonary arterial catheter. Anesth Analg 1981; 60: 789–793
154 Lieberman RW, Orkin FK, Jobes DR, Schwartz AJ. Hemodynamic predictors of myocardial ischemia during halothane anesthesia for coronary-artery revascularization. Anesthesiology 1983; 59: 36–41
155 Sonntag H, Merin RG, Donath U, Radke J, Schenk HD. Myocardial metabolism and oxygenation in man awake and during halothane anesthesia. Anesthesiology 1979; 51: 204–210
156 Buffington CW. Hemodynamic determinants of ischemic myocardial dysfunction in the presence of coronary stenosis of dogs. Anesthesiology 1985; 63: 651–662
157 Shiraki H, Lee S, Hong J et al Diagnosis of myocardial ischemia by pressure-rate quotient and diastolic time interval during coronary artery bypass surgery. J Cardiothorac Anesth 1989; 3: 592–596
158 Gordon MA, Urban MK, O'Connor T, Barash PG. Is the pressure rate quotient a predictor or indicator of myocardial ischemia as measured by ST-segment changes in patients undergoing coronary artery bypass surgery? Anesthesiology 1991; 74: 848–853
159 Harrison L, Ralley FE, Wynands JE et al. The role of an ultra short-acting adrenergic blocker (esmolol) in patients undergoing coronary artery bypass surgery. Anesthesiology 1987; 66: 413–418
160 Feigl EO. The paradox of adrenergic coronary vasoconstriction. Circulation 1987; 76: 737–745
161 Hynynen M, Palojoki R, Salmenperä M et al. Vasodilator properties of atrial natriuteric factor: a comparison of nitroglycerin, nitroprusside using cardiopulmonary bypass as a study model. J Cardiothorac Anesth 1989; 3: 720–725
162 Ross J Jr. Afterload mismatch in aortic and mitral valve disease: implications for surgical therapy. J Am Coll Cardiol 1985; 5: 811–826
163 Stott DK, Marpole DGF, Bristow JD, Kloster FE, Griswold HE. The role of left atrial transport in aortic and mitral stenosis. Circulation 1970; 41: 1031–1041
164 Hakki AH, Kimbiris D, Iskandrian AS, Segal BL, Mintz GS, Bemis CE. Angina pectoris and coronary artery disease in patients with severe aortic valvular disease. Am Heart J 1980; 100: 441–449
165 Latson TW, Lappas DG. Use of a pacing catheter to control heart rate in a patient with aortic insufficiency and coronary artery disease. Anesthesiology 1985; 63: 712–715
166 Izumi S, Miyatake K, Beppu S et al. Mechanism of mitral regurgitation in patients with myocardial infarction: a study using real-time two-dimensional Doppler flow imaging and echocardiography. Circulation 1987; 76: 777–785
167 Loop FD, Lytle BW, Cosgrove DM. Bilateral internal thoracic artery grafting in reoperations. Ann Thorac Surg 1991; 52: 3–4
168 Curling PE, Kanter KR. Cardiac transplantation: perioperative care. ASA Refresher Course Lectures 1988; 16: 67–80
169 Lake C. Pediatric cardiac anesthesia. Philadelphia, PA: Grune & Stratton. 1988
170 Feinberg BI. Anesthesia and electrophysiologic procedures. In: Kaplan JA, ed. Cardiac anesthesia, 2nd edn. Philadelphia, PA: Grune & Stratton, 1984: pp 751–784
171 Gomexz-Arnau J, Marquez-Montes J, Avello F. Fentanyl and droperidol effects on the refractoriness of the accessory pathway in the Wolff–Parkinson–White syndrome. Anesthesiology 1987; 58: 307–313
172 Salmenperä M, Peltola K, Rosenberg P. Does prophylactic lidocaine control cardiac arrhythmias associated with pulmonary artery catheterization? Anesthesiology 1982; 56: 210–212
173 Nose Y. Manual of artificial organs, vol. 2, The oxygenator. St Louis, MO: CV Mosby. 1973
174 Hickey PR, Buckley MJ, Philbin DM. Pulsatile and nonpulsatile cardiopulmonary bypass: review of a counterproductive controversy. Ann Thorac Surg 1983; 36: 720–737
175 Nilsson L, Bagge L, Nyström SO. Blood cell trauma and postoperative bleeding: comparison of bubble and membrane oxygenators and observations on coronary suction. Scand J Thorac Cardiovas Surg 1990; 24: 65–69
176 Hessel EA, Johnson DD, Ivey TD, Miller DW. Membrane versus bubble oxygenator for cardiac operations. J Thorac Cardiovasc Surg 1980; 80: 111–122
177 Sade RM, Bartles DM, Dearing JP, Campbell LJ, Loadholt CB. A prospective randomized study of membrane versus bubble oxygenators in children. Ann Thorac Surg 1980; 29: 502–511
178 Clark RE, Beauchamp RA, Magrath RA, Brooks JD, Ferguson TB, Welson CS. Comparison of bubble and membrane oxygenators in short and long perfusions. J Thorac Cardiovasc Surg 1979; 78: 655–666

179 Sade RM, Stroud MR, Crawford FA, Kratz JM, Dearing JP, Bartles DM. A prospective randomized study of hydroxyethyl starch, albumin, and lactated Ringer's solution as priming fluid for cardiopulmonary bypass. J Thorac Cardiovasc Surg 1985; 89: 713–722

180 Hickey RF, Hoar PF. Whole-body oxygen consumption during low-flow hypothermic cardiopulmonary bypass. J Thorac Cardiovasc Surg 1983; 86: 903–906

181 Govier AV, Reves JG, McKay RD et al. Factors and their influence on regional cerebral blood flow during nonpulsatile cardiopulmonary bypass. Ann Thorac Surg 1984; 38: 592–600

182 Prough DS, Stump DA, Roy RC et al. Response of cerebral blood flow to changes in carbon dioxide tension during hypothermic cardiopulmonary bypass. Anesthesiology 1986; 64: 576–581

183 Mark JB, FitzGerald D, Fenton T et al. Continuous arterial and venous blood gas monitoring during cardiopulmonary bypass. J Thorac Cardiovasc Surg 1991; 102: 431–439

184 Esposito RA, Culliford AT, Colvin SB, Thomas SJ, Lackner H, Spencer FC. Heparin resistance during cardiopulmonary bypass. The role of heparin pre-treatment. J Thorac Cardiovasc Surg 1983; 85: 346–353

185 Dietrich W, Spannagl M, Schramm W, Vogt W, Barankay A, Richter JA. The influence of preoperative anticoagulation on heparin response during cardiopulmonary bypass. J Thorac Cardiovasc Surg 1991; 102: 505–514

186 Kopriva CJ. The activated coagulation time (ACT), effective hemostasis in cardiac surgery. Ellison N, Jobes DR, eds. Philadelphia, PA: WB Saunders, 1988: pp 155–161

187 Kuitunen AH, Salmenperä MT, Heinonen J, Rasi VP, Myllylä G. Heparin rebound: a comparative study of protamine chloride and protamine sulfate in patients undergoing coronary artery bypass surgery. J Cardiovasc Anesth 1991; 5: 221–226

188 Hynynen M. Binding of fentanyl and alfentanil to the extracorporeal circuit. Acta Anaesthesiol Scand 1987; 31: 706–710

189 Kumar K, Crankshaw DP, Morgan DJ, Beemer GH. The effect of cardiopulmonary bypass on plasma protein binding of alfentanil. Eur J Clin Pharmacol 1988; 35: 47–52

190 Eger EI, Saidman LJ, Brandstater B. Temperature dependence of halothane and cyclopropane anesthesia in dogs. Correlation with some theories of anesthetic action. Anesthesiology 1965; 26: 764–770

191 Puig MM, Warner W, Tang CK, Laorden ML, Turndorf H. Effects of temperature on the interaction of morphine with opioid receptors. Br J Anaesth 1987; 59: 1459–1464

192 Reves JG. Adrenergic response to cardiopulmonary bypass. Mt Sinai J Med 1985; 52: 511–515

193 Koska AJ, Romagnoli A, Kramer WG. Effect of cardiopulmonary bypass on fentanyl distribution and elimination. Clin Pharmacol Ther 1981; 29: 100–110

194 McAllister RG, Tan TG. Effect of hypothermia on drug metabolism. In vitro studies with propranolol and verapamil. Pharmacology 1980; 20: 95–100

195 Bovill JG, Sebel PS. Pharmacokinetics of high-dose fentanyl: a study in patients undergoing cardiac surgery. Br J Anaesth 1980; 52: 795–801

196 Robbins GR, Wynands JE, Whalley DG et al. Pharmacokinetics of alfentanil and clinical responses during cardiac surgery. Can J Anaesth 1990; 37: 52–57

197 Bentley JB, Conahan TJ, Cork RC. Fentanyl sequestration in lung during cardiopulmonary bypass. Clin Pharmacol Ther 1983; 34: 703–706

198 Nussmeier NA, Lambert ML, Moskowitz GJ et al. Washin and washout of isoflurane administered via bubble oxygenators during hypothermic cardiopulmonary bypass. Anesthesiology 1989; 71: 519–525

199 Padayachee TS, Parsons S, Theobold R, Linley J, Gosling RG, Deverall PB. The detection of microemboli in the middle cerebral artery during cardiopulmonary bypass: a transcranial Doppler ultrasound investigation using membrane and bubble oxygenators. Ann Thorac Surg 1987; 44: 298–302

200 Padayachee TS, Parsons S, Theobold R, Gosling RG, Deverall PB. The effect of arterial filtration on reduction of gaseous microemboli in the middle cerebral artery during cardiopulmonary bypass. Ann Thorac Surg 1988; 45: 647–649

201 Murkin JM, Farrar JK, Tweed WA, McKenzie FN, Guiraudon G. Cerebral autoregulation and flow/metabolism coupling during cardiopulmonary bypass: The influence of Pa_{CO_2}. Anesth Analg 1987; 66: 825–832

202 Stephan H, Weyland A, Kazmaier S, Hencke T, Menck S, Sonntag H. Acid–base management during hypothermic cardiopulmonary bypass does not affect cerebral metabolism but does affect blood flow and neurological outcome. Br J Anaesth 1992; 69–51–57

203 Nussmeier NA, Arlund C, Slogoff S. Neuropsychiatric complications after cardiopulmonary bypass: cerebral protection by a barbiturate. Anesthesiology 1986; 64: 165–170

204 Buckberg GD. Myocardial temperature management during aortic clamping for cardiac surgery. Protection, preoccupation and perspective. J Thorac Cardiovasc Surg 1991; 102: 895–903

205 Badenhammer RM, DeBoer LWV, Geffin GA et al. Enhanced myocardial protection during ischemic arrest. Oxygenation of a crystalloid cardioplegic solution. J Thorac Cardiovasc Surg 1983; 85: 769–780

206 Tabayashi K, McKeown PP, Miyamota M et al. Ischemic myocardial protection: comparison of nonoxygenated crystalloid, oxygenated crystalloid, and oxygenated fluorocarbon cardioplegic solutions. J Thorac Cardiovasc Surg 1988; 95: 239–246

207 Feindel CM, Tait GA, Wilson GJ, Klement P, MacGregor DC. Multidose blood versus crystalloid cardioplegia. Comparison by quantitative assessment of irreversible myocardial injury. J Thorac Cardiovasc Surg 1984; 87: 585–595

208 Teoh KH, Christakis GT, Fremes SE et al. Accelerated myocardial metabolic recovery with terminal warm blood cardioplegia (hot shot). Surg Forum 1985; 36: 272–275

209 Lichtenstein SV, Abel JG, Panos A, Slutsky AS, Salerno TA. Warm heart surgery: experience with long cross-clamp times. Ann Thorac Surg 1991; 52: 1009–1013

210 Jennings RB, Steenbergen C Jr. Nucleotide metabolism and cellular damage in myocardial ischemia. Ann Rev Physiol 1985; 47: 727–749

211 Zaloga GP, Strickland RA, Butterworth JF, Mark LJ, Mills SA, Lake CR. Calcium attenuates epinephrine's β-adrenergic effects in postoperative heart surgery patients. Circulation 1990; 81: 196–200

212 Estafanous FG, Urzua J, Yared JP, Zurick AM, Loop FD, Tarazi RC. Pattern of hemodynamic alterations during coronary artery operations. J Thorac Cardiovasc Surg 1984; 87: 175–182

213 Smit VE, Katz AM. Inotropic and lusitropic abnormalities as the basis for heart failure. Heart Failure 1987; 3: 55–56

214 Grayson RF, Marino PN, Kass DA. The effect of amrinone on indices of left ventricular diastolic function assessed by volume (conductance) catheter. Anesthesiology 1988; 69: A103

215 Hug CC Jr. Anaesthesia for adult cardiac surgery. In: Miller RD, ed. Anaesthesia, New York: Churchill Livingstone, 1990; pp 1605–1652

216 Lazar HL, Buckberg GD, Foglia RP, Manganaro AJ, Maloney JV. Detrimental effects of premature use of inotropic drugs to discontinue cardiopulmonary bypass. J Thorac Cardiovasc Surg 1981; 82: 18–25

217 Port JD, Gilbert EM, Larrabee P et al. Neurotransmitter depletion compromises the ability of indirect-acting amines to provide inotropic support in the failing human heart. Circulation 1990; 81: 929–938

218 Stephenson LW, Blackstone EH, Kouchoukus NT. Dopamine vs epinephrine in patients following cardiac surgery: randomized study. Surg Forum 1976; 27: 272–275

219 Butterworth JF, Prielipp RC, Zaloga GP, Royster RL, Robertie PG. Is dobutamine less chronotropic than epinephrine after coronary bypass surgery? Anesthesiology 1990; 73: A61

220 Royster RL, Whiteley JW, Butterworth JF. Amrinone therapy during emergence from cardiopulmonary bypass. J Thorac Cardiovasc Surg 1991; 101: 942–943

221 Bailey JM, Levy JH, Rogers HG, Szlam F, Hug CC Jr. Pharmacokinetics of amrinone during cardiac surgery. Anesthesiology 1991; 75: 961–968

222 Boldt J, Kling D, Thiel A, Scheld HH, Hempleman G. Revascularization of the right coronary artery: influence on thermodilution right ventricular ejection fraction. J Cardiovasc Anesth 1988; 2: 140–146

223 Salmenperä M, Heinonen J. Pulmonary vascular responses to moderate changes in Pa_{CO_2} after cardiopulmonary bypass. Anesthesiology 1986; 64: 311–315

224 Viitanen A, Salmenperä M, Heinonen J. Right ventricular response to hypercarbia after cardiac surgery. Anesthesiology 1990; 73: 393–400

225 Bixler TJ, Gardner TJ, Donahoo JS, Brawley RK, Potter A, Gott VL. Improved myocardial performance in postoperative cardiac surgical patients with sodium nitroprusside. Ann Thorac Surg 1978; 25: 444–448

226 Pennington DG, Swartz M, Codd JE, Merjavy JP, Kaiser GC. Intraaortic balloon pumping in cardiac surgical patients: a nine-year experience. Ann Thorac Surg 1983; 36: 125–131

227 Harjula AJ, Salmenperä M. Surgical management of heart failure. Duodecim 1991; 107: 242–251

228 Isner JM, Cohen SR, Virmani R, Lawrinson W, Roberts WC. Complications of the intraaortic balloon counterpulsation device: clinical and morphologic observations in 45 necroscopy patients. Am J Cardiol 1980; 45: 260–268

229 Zumbro GL, Kitchens WR, Shearer G, Harville G, Bailey L, Galloway RF. Mechanical assistance for cardiogenic shock following cardiac surgery, myocardial infarction and cardiac transplantation. Ann Thorac Surg 1987; 44: 11–13

230 Adamson RM, Dembitsky WP, Reichman RT, Moreno-Cabral RJ, Daily PO. Mechanical support: assist or nemesis? J Thorac Cardiovasc Surg 1989; 98: 915–921

231 Weiss ME, Nyhan D, Peng Z et al. Association of protamine IgE and IgG antibodies with life-threatening reactions to intravenous protamine. N Engl J Med 1989; 320: 886–892

232 Morel DR, Zapol WM, Thomas SJ et al. C5a and thromboxane generation associated with pulmonary vaso- and broncho-constriction during protamine reversal of heparin. Anesthesiology 1987; 66: 597–604

233 Levy JH, Schwieger IM, Zaidan JR, Faraj BA, Weintraub WS. Evaluation of patients at risk for protamine reactions. J Thorac Cardiovasc Surg 1989; 98: 200–204

234 Levy JH, Zaidan JR, Faraj B. Prospective evaluation of risk of protamine reactions in patients with NPH insulin-dependent diabetes. Anesth Analg 1986; 65: 739–742

235 Wasser MNJM, Houbiers JGA, D'Amaro J et al. The effect of fresh versus stored blood on post-operative bleeding after coronary bypass surgery: a prospective randomized study. Br J Haematol 1989; 72: 81–84

236 Czer LSC, Bateman TM, Gray RJ et al. Treatment of severe platelet dysfunction and hemorrhage after cardiopulmonary bypass: reduction in blood product usage with desmopressin. J Am Coll Cardiol 1987; 9: 1139–1147

237 Harker LA, Malpass TW, Branson HE, Hessel EA II, Slichter SJ. Mechanisms of abnormal bleeding in patients undergoing cardiopulmonary bypass: acquired transient platelet dysfunction associated with selective α-granule release. Blood 1980; 56: 824–834

238 Rinder CS, Matthew JP, Rinder HM, Bonan J, Ault KA, Smith BR. Modulation of platelet surface adhesion receptors during cardiopulmonary bypass. Anesthesiology 1991; 75: 563–570

239 Lemaire F, Teboul JL, Cinotti L et al. Acute left ventricular dysfunction during unsuccesful weaning from mechanical ventilation. Anesthesiology 1988; 69: 171–179

240 Hurford WE, Lynch KE, Strauss HW, Lowenstein E, Zapol WM. Myocardial perfusion as assessed by thallium-201 scintigraphy during the discontinuation of mechanical ventilation in ventilator-dependent patients. Anesthesiology 1991; 74: 1007–1016

241 Merry AF, Ramage MC, Whitlock RML et al. First-time coronary artery bypass grafting: the anaesthetist as a risk factor. Br J Anaesth 1992; 68: 6–12

242 Hug CC Jr. Pharmacokinetics and dynamics of narcotic analgesics. In: Prys-Roberts C, Hug CC Jr, eds. Pharmacokinetics in anaesthesia. Oxford: Blackwell, 1984: pp 187–234

243 Hug CC Jr. Anaesthesia for adult cardiac surgery. In: Miller RD, ed. Anesthesia, New York: Churchill Livingstone, 1990; pp 1605–1652

244 Harjula AJ, Salmenperä M. Duodenum 1991; 107: 242–251

17. Day-case surgery

I. Smith   P.F. White

Between 1899 and 1908, Nicoll successfully operated on 8988 children on an outpatient basis in Glasgow and advocated that the practice should be extended to infants and young children.[1] The first free-standing day-case surgical clinic was described by the noted American anaesthesiologist Ralph Waters in 1919.[2] When this anaesthetic practice was started in 1916, it catered primarily to oral surgeons, but later was expanded to include a broader range of surgical procedures. However, it is only in the past two decades that the practice of day-case surgery has begun rapidly to expand. The advantages include decreased costs,[3] increased throughput of patients, leading to increased hospital bed availability and reduced waiting lists, shorter duration of separation of the patient from home and family, and a reduced potential for hospital-acquired infections. Improvements in anaesthetic drugs and techniques have led to more rapid recovery following surgery and have made it possible to perform more extensive procedures on a day-case basis. Typical procedures which are performed as day cases are shown in Table 17.1.

PRE-OPERATIVE ASSESSMENT

For a day-case surgery programme to function safely and efficiently, patient selection is critical. Limiting the choice of patients to those in good general health (i.e. American Society of Anesthesiologists (ASA) class 1–2) can reduce problems, although outpatients with disabling multisystem diseases can be treated without additional complications if they are carefully selected.[4] While studies have shown a greater risk of postoperative complications in patients with pre-existing cardiovascular disease, these risks are considerably reduced if symptoms have been well-controlled for 3 months prior to surgery.[5] Table 17.2 demonstrates the effect of a number of peri-operative factors on the incidence of postoperative complications. The age of the patient may also be a factor in deciding on their acceptability for day-stay surgery. At the one extreme, recovery of fine motor skills may be considerably delayed in the elderly,[6] while at the other, there is a greater risk of postoperative apnoea following surgery in previously premature infants;[7] this effect persists up to about 46 weeks' postconceptual age (gestation plus age from birth).[8] Furthermore, the postoperative care of the very young and the very old may place an excessive burden upon the family. With these possible exceptions, there is no

Table 17.1 Surgical procedures commonly performed as day cases

Dental	Extractions, conservation
Dermatology	Excision of skin lesions
Ear, nose and throat	Tonsillectomy, adenoidectomy, myringotomy, laryngoscopy, polypectomy
Eye	Tonometry, cataracts, strabismus surgery
General surgery	Biopsy and small lesion excision, varicose veins, herniorrhaphy, haemorrhoidectomy
Gynaecology	D&C, Bartholin's cyst, laparoscopic procedures
Orthopaedic	MUA, carpal tunnel, extremity surgery, ganglia
Urology	Cystoscopy, orchidopexy, vasectomy
Paediatric	Circumcision, herniorraphy, EUA
Endoscopy	Endoscopy, colonoscopy, bronchoscopy
Plastic surgery	Cosmetic repairs, septorhinoplasty
Pain management	Chemical sympathectomy, epidural injection, lytic nerve blocks

Modified from Smith & White,[238] with permission.
D&C = Dilatation and curettage; MUA = manipulation under anaesthesia; EUA = examination under anaesthesia.

Table 17.2 Factors influencing the incidence of perioperative complications associated with day-case surgery

Factors	Incidence
Pre-existing disease	
None	1 in 156
Diabetes mellitus	1 in 149
Asthma	1 in 139
Chronic lung disease	1 in 112
Hypertension	1 in 87
Cardiovascular disease	1 in 74
Type of anaesthesia	
Local	1 in 268
Regional	1 in 277
Local/regional with sedation	1 in 106
General	1 in 120
Duration of surgery	
<1 h	1 in 155
1–2 h	1 in 84
2–3 h	1 in 54
>3 h	1 in 35

Modified from White,[237] with permission.

evidence of an overall relationship between postoperative complications and age.[9]

To improve patient safety, reduce cancellations and increase overall efficiency, careful pre-anaesthetic assessment of patients is essential.[10] However, this presents some logistical problems. An interview with the anaesthetist before the day of surgery is theoretically desirable because it allows time to perform selected laboratory investigations and to evaluate any abnormalities. However, it is inconvenient to patients and staff alike and also does not appear significantly to reduce patient anxiety compared with a same-day evaluation.[11,12] Communication by telephone and/or a pre-printed questionnaire can be useful to gather patient information and to convey instructions concerning pre-operative fasting and the appropriate management of co-existing medication. This system is, of course, limited by the patient's access to a telephone, and by postal delays. Once information is collected, it can be used to assist the anaesthetist in requesting appropriate laboratory tests and other special investigations.[13] Patient selection can also be enhanced by closer communication between the anaesthetist and surgeon, so that patient factors, rather than surgical criteria alone, can be used to select patients who are suitable for day-case surgery. General practitioners can also help to select patients, especially with respect to social factors which may be important postoperatively.[10]

Pre-operative evaluation of day-case surgery patients should always include a history and physical examination. Special investigations should be added to confirm or expand clinical findings, but have a limited use in screening for unexpected diseases. Since no laboratory test is 100% specific, there will always be some false-positive results. When such a test is applied to a condition with a low incidence (e.g. when used to screen a healthy population), the majority of positive test results will be false positive.[14] This may result in unnecessary repeat investigations or the performance of other confirmatory tests and will inevitably result in additional costs and delays, while at the same time increasing patient anxiety. Some tests (e.g. chest X-rays) may pose a risk to the patient. Rational use of laboratory tests require that they be applied to a population with a high incidence of the condition being tested for, either as a follow-up to abnormal clinical findings or in selected subpopulations with pre-existing diseases.[15] A computerized patient evaluation (Health Quiz) has been described which can assist in rational selection of tests.[16] Typical guidelines for laboratory testing are shown in Table 17.3.

PREPARATION FOR DAY-CASE SURGERY

Once a proper assessment of the patient has been performed, and any abnormalities that were detected have been corrected, preparation primarily involves the relief of anxiety and a consideration of the need for prophylactic measures to prevent pulmonary contamination by gastric contents.

Patients approaching an operation — even one that medical personnel would consider relatively minor — are frequently anxious. This anxiety may be present for some time before the day of surgery,[17] beginning when the prospect of surgery is first raised, and re-emerging as the patient prepares for the operation. A pre-operative visit with an anaesthetist has been shown to

Table 17.3 Guidelines for pre-operative screening tests in otherwise healthy patients undergoing day-case surgical procedures

Investigation	Population
Full blood count	All adult females Males >50 years
Electrolytes (especially K^+)	Patients >70 years Patients on diuretics, digoxin
Electrocardiogram	Adults >50 years Smokers
Chest X-ray	Patients >70 years
(Pregnancy test)	Females of child-bearing potential

Modified from White,[237] with permission.

reduce anxiety,[18,19] although clearly the timing of this visit (as well as the information conveyed to the patient) is important in achieving the maximum benefit. Reassurance immediately before entering the operating room seems to have the greatest anxiolytic effect.[11] Relaxation exercises have also been shown to reduce anxiety, analgesic requirements and duration of hospital stay.[20] Again, these should be started early for maximum benefit, and could most usefully be taught at the initial surgical visit, especially for patients who were noted to be particularly anxious at that time. Such patients may also benefit from a brief period of treatment with anxiolytic medication (e.g. a sedative–hypnotic on the evening before surgery).

Controversy remains over the relative advantages and disadvantages of treating acute anxiety with pharmacological agents. The greatest fear is that sedative medications will have a prolonged effect and therefore delay recovery and discharge, or impair mental function following discharge. The benzodiazepines are the most appropriate group of agents for day-case premedication. Unlike opioid analgesics, benzodiazepines do not delay gastric emptying.[21] They combine anxiolysis with varying degrees of sedation and amnesia. This anterograde amnesia may frequently be beneficial in blunting memories of unpleasant pre-operative procedures. However, there may also be disadvantages, in that patients may not recall important instructions and recommendations that are given to them by their doctors and nurses.[22] From a medicolegal point of view, informed consent should always be obtained prior to the administration of any centrally active premedicant drug.[23]

Diazepam and lorazepam are both effective anxiolytics; however, they both have a prolonged duration of action and are not really suitable for use in the immediate pre-operative period for sedating day cases. Temazepam has a much shorter half-life and is probably the most commonly used premedicant in the UK. Compared to a placebo, temazepam 20–30 mg administered orally 1 h before surgery resulted in greater sedation and anxiolysis in one study and was associated with fewer induction problems.[24] Furthermore, there was no delay in the time of awakening, the time of walking without assistance or in the degree of postoperative sedation following its use. Triazolam has an even shorter half-life than temazepam and so theoretically should be an excellent choice for premedication in the day-case setting. However, in clinical practice, triazolam results in significant postoperative psychomotor impairment, even when compared to diazepam.[25] Triazolam also has relatively poor anxiolytic properties.[25,26] In the USA, temazepam is not available in the pharmaceutical preparation which is widely used in Europe and as a consequence has a different (and less desirable) onset of action. Therefore, much more interest has been shown in the short-acting, water-soluble agent, midazolam. As commercially supplied, this agent is for intravenous or intramuscular administration. The intravenous route permits the rapid achievement of anxiolysis in patients in whom logistical factors (e.g. transportation delays, rescheduling of cases) prevent the administration of an oral agent. In one study, administration of midazolam 2–3 mg intravenously prior to a sedation technique with propofol enhanced sedation, anxiolysis and amnesia without delaying discharge.[27] When administered prior to general anaesthesia with propofol and nitrous oxide, similar effects were seen. Furthermore, the haemodynamic response to laryngoscopy and tracheal intubation was attenuated.[28] Although midazolam did delay initial awakening in this study, the 1–2 min difference was of little clinical importance and there was no delay in discharge times from the day-case surgery facility. Similarly, the use of intramuscular midazolam 5 mg did not delay recovery in a group of adult day cases.[29]

Although there are advantages to parenteral administration, most patients would prefer an oral premedication. Midazolam liquid can be taken orally and a number of studies have shown this to be effective, although a higher dose is needed compared with intravenous administration. Compared with temazepam 20 mg, midazolam 15 mg by mouth resulted in superior sedation, amnesia and anxiolysis. However, midazolam resulted in a delay in immediate recovery and poorer performance on psychomotor testing.[30] In contrast, another investigation found relatively few differences between the two medications (at the same doses) in terms of effects and recovery, while detecting residual impairment of psychomotor function 4 h postoperatively with either drug.[31] In paediatric patients oral midazolam 0.5–0.7 mg.kg^{-1} was also effective in facilitating separation from parents and resulted in a smoother inhalation induction.[32] One disadvantage of taking the parenteral preparation of midazolam orally is its bitter taste, although this may be masked to some extent by fruit juice. Midazolam may also be administered nasally. This route offers the advantages of a large surface area, good blood supply, a thin barrier to absorption and avoidance of first-pass hepatic metabolism. Midazolam administered nasally has been shown to be effective at a dose of 0.2–0.3 mg.kg^{-1} and to have a rapid onset of action.[33]

Although the benzodiazepines have largely replaced opioid analgesics as premedicant agents, some interest has recently been shown in the use of fentanyl in an oral transmucosal form. Fentanyl can be incorporated into a sucrose matrix (fentanyl ovalette),[34] permitting rapid transmucosal absorption. Dose-ranging studies in children have found the optimal dose to be between 15 and 20 µg.kg^{-1}.[35] Although oral transmucosal fentanyl can reduce agitation, produce sedation and reduce the requirement for postoperative analgesia,[36,37] its use is associated with respiratory depression and high incidences of pruritus and nausea; the latter appear to be dose-independent.[35] Postoperatively, there is also a delay in tolerating oral fluids, resulting in delayed discharge.[36] Although this preparation may have some advantages in patients who are in pain pre-operatively, the high incidence of side-effects would make it unsuitable for routine use. However, the delivery system probably deserves further investigation with other compounds (e.g. benzodiazepines).

The second major area of pre-operative patient preparation relates to the avoidance of pulmonary aspiration of gastric contents. This complication is associated with high morbidity. Furthermore, treatment of established acid aspiration has a very poor success rate. Therefore, prevention of aspiration is considered to be the most effective management. For significant pulmonary damage to occur there must be gastric contents of sufficient volume and acidity to reach and injure the bronchial mucosa. In addition, intragastric pressure must exceed the resistance imposed by the lower oesophageal sphincter, and finally, the protective reflexes of the airway must be markedly reduced or abolished.

By extrapolation from animal experimentation, it is usually assumed that significant pulmonary damage requires the delivery of at least 25 ml of gastric contents at a pH of less than 2.5.[38] This does not necessarily imply that the residual gastric volume should be below 25 ml to prevent aspiration since regurgitation or vomiting is unlikely to result in complete gastric emptying and it is highly improbable that all of the regurgitated stomach contents will enter the bronchial tree. However, it is apparent that the risk to the patient will be reduced if the stomach is as empty as possible and residual contents are at a pH greater than 2.5.

In the early days of anaesthesia, patients were instructed to abstain only from solid food. John Snow advocated administering chloroform at about the time at which patients would be ready for their next meal.[39] This was not, however, because of concern for pulmonary aspiration, but simply to avoid sickness resulting from anaesthetic administration. Indeed, he felt that 'this sickness is not attended with any danger, but it constitutes an unpleasantness and inconvenience'.[39] With the passage of time, guidelines for pre-operative fasting have changed, and many institutions now prohibit all oral intake for a minimum of 6 h pre-operatively, and frequently from midnight of the day before surgery. However, forbidding liquids as well as solids does not follow logically from an understanding of the physiology of normal gastric emptying.

An elegant demonstration of gastric emptying was provided in 1822, when Alexis St Martin, a Canadian fur trader, received a thoraco-abdominal wound from the accidental discharge of a musket. The wound healed, leaving a sinus from his stomach to his anterior abdominal wall, which permitted William Beaumont, an army surgeon, readily to sample the gastric contents and to conduct a series of experiments on the rate of gastric emptying. He discovered that most solids took 4–6 h to be cleared from the stomach, but that 'water, ardent spirits and most other fluids are not affected by the gastric juice and pass from the stomach soon after they have been received'.[40]

Almost 170 years later, Maltby and colleagues[41] administered 150 ml of water to patients 2.5 h pre-operatively and found that gastric volumes at the time of surgery were lower than in patients undergoing a routine 10 h pre-operative fast, presumably because of the peristalsis-inducing effect of water in the stomach. Subsequently, similar observations have been made with other clear fluids, including apple and orange juice, as well as tea and coffee.[42] Milk by itself is not a suitable pre-operative fluid, as it tends to curdle, and then takes several hours to be cleared; however, the small amount present in a cup of tea or coffee is not detrimental.[43] Solutions containing glucose are also rapidly cleared from the stomach, which may be particularly beneficial, as prolonged starvation can increase anxiety and result in hypoglycaemia.[44] In one study children given 3 ml.kg^{-1} of apple juice 3 h before surgery had reduced gastric volume, thirst and hunger compared to children conventionally fasted.[45] Pre-operative oral fluids can also reduce irritability in children.[46] Even a light, low-residue breakfast (buttered toast and tea or coffee) taken 2–4 h pre-operatively has been shown not to increase gastric volume or reduce gastric pH at the time of surgery.[47] Such a regimen may be most appropriate for patients scheduled for afternoon surgery. Most oral medications can be safely taken 1–2 h prior to surgery. Clearly, some of the established practices regarding pre-operative fasting are in need of re-evaluation.[42,48]

Although taking clear fluids can reduce gastric contents compared with fasting, there are still some patients who will not have a completely empty stomach. Therefore, attempts have been made to raise the intragastric pH as well as to decrease the gastric volume. Initially, antacid medications were used to increase gastric pH, but they also increased gastric volume. Omeprazole, a recently introduced proton pump inhibitor, has also been shown to raise intragastric pH. However, it must be taken the evening before outpatient surgery.[49] Therefore, the H_2 receptor antagonists have increasingly been used for this purpose. The dose and timing of drug administration are important in achieving an optimal effect. The addition of metoclopramide 10 mg can assist by reducing residual gastric volume.[50] Ranitidine is slightly more effective than cimetidine.[51] Ranitidine 150 mg, 1–1.5 h pre-operatively has been reported to raise gastric pH to over 2.5 in 80% of patients;[52] however, this still leaves 20% of patients potentially at risk.

Not surprisingly, studies have not shown any reduced morbidity or mortality from routine aspiration prophylaxis with H_2-blocking drugs in healthy day-stay patients. Overall, aspiration pneumonitis is a very rare phenomenon, with an incidence of approximately 5 in 10 000 anaesthetics and a mortality rate close to 0.2 in 10 000.[53] Under such circumstances, it is very difficult to justify the cost and inconvenience of routine prophylaxis with H_2-antagonists, especially as no single agent or combination has been shown to give intragastric conditions indicative of complete protection. The best guidelines would seem to be to permit, and indeed to encourage, one cup of clear fluid 3 h before surgery and to administer H_2-antagonists only to patients with known gastro-oesophageal reflux or others at increased risk of regurgitation.[42]

Further pre-operative preparation involves an explanation to patients of what they are likely to encounter before, during and after anaesthesia. Postoperative instructions are best given prior to pre-medication, as patients are not likely to remember information given after the administration of sedative–amnesic drugs. Important instructions should be reinforced in writing and, where possible, repeated to the patient's escort at the time of discharge.

DAY-CASE ANAESTHESIA TECHNIQUES

The ideal anaesthetic technique would permit a rapid and smooth onset, provide optimum surgical conditions combined with peri-operative analgesia and be followed by rapid recovery without side-effects. Recovery assumes special importance for day cases, because these patients must be able to protect themselves from the challenges of the outside world. Side-effects which would be of limited importance to inpatients assume considerably greater importance in day cases.[54] Although most day-case surgery is performed under general anaesthesia, regional techniques can be effective, especially in urology, gynaecology and orthopaedic surgery. Increasingly, sedative and analgesic drugs are used as supplements for procedures performed under local anaesthesia, referred to in the USA as monitored anaesthetic care.

GENERAL ANAESTHESIA

The ability to provide safe and effective general anaesthesia, with minimal side-effects and rapid recovery, is essential to the smooth functioning of a day-surgery unit.[55] General anaesthesia remains the most common technique because of its popularity with patients, anaesthetists and surgeons alike. Day cases require the same level of basic equipment as inpatients for the delivery of anaesthetic drugs, monitoring and resuscitation. Routine monitoring for day cases should include electrocardiogram and a blood pressure cuff, as well as pulse oximetry and capnography.[56] Monitoring of temperature is desirable for children and adolescents and essential for those at risk of malignant hyperpyrexia.

The conduct of general anaesthesia should follow the same principles as those applied to surgical inpatients. Tracheal intubation is acceptable, although some care may be required in the selection of muscle relaxant drugs. The intermediate-acting agents atracurium and vecuronium are appropriate for many day-case procedures.[57] Their duration of action is sufficiently short that reversal of their effects is usually convenient and postoperative muscle weakness is rarely a problem. Of the two agents, vecuronium may be slightly shorter-acting.[57,58] Suxamethonium can be employed to facilitate intubation, but the myalgia resulting from muscle fasciculations may be distressing to young healthy patients who will be active soon after surgery. Pretreatment with d-tubocurarine 2–3 mg (or a small dose of another non-depolarizing muscle relaxant) can reduce the extent of muscle fasciculation and the associated myalgia. Although rare, suxamethonium is also a potent trigger of malignant hyperpyrexia, and fatal allergic reactions to suxamethonium have been described.[59]

The new non-depolarizing bis-benzylisoquinolinium muscle relaxant mivacurium produces maximum blockade 2–3 min after an intubating dose of 0.2–0.25 mg.kg^{-1} and has a duration of action only two or three times longer than suxamethonium.[60,61] Mivacurium has the potential for histamine release (to a similar degree to that seen with atracurium), which can induce facial flushing and transient decreases in arterial blood pressure.[62] A further disadvantage is that, like suxamethonium, metabolism depends in part on hydrolysis by plasma cholinesterase and prolonged effects have been recorded in patients with atypical plasma cholinesterase.[63] However, the short duration of action and the ability to avoid many of the disadvantages of suxamethonium should make this agent attractive in day cases.[61]

Another alternative to the use of suxamethonium for tracheal intubation is afforded by the laryngeal mask airway,[64] which can be inserted without the use of muscle relaxants. This has reduced the indications for tracheal intubation while maintaining a clear and trouble-free airway. Furthermore, the pressor response to laryngeal mask insertion is no greater than that following insertion of an oral airway[65] and the incidence of postoperative sore throat is similar to that following the use of a face mask and oral airway.[66] The laryngeal mask does not seal the airway against pulmonary aspiration. However, it appears to be well-tolerated at a lighter depth of anaesthesia than is a tracheal tube. Although the value of a tracheal tube in preventing aspiration is often stated, its insertion requires the abolition of protective airway reflexes, which may also be compromised at extubation, thereby providing two periods of risk for aspiration. Indeed, there was an initial doubling of the death rate from pulmonary aspiration following the recommendation that tracheal intubation should be undertaken in all patients undergoing Caesarean section in England and Wales.[67]

Induction of anaesthesia is usually achieved by means of a rapidly acting intravenous agent. Although thiopentone 3–6 mg.kg^{-1} is still the 'gold standard' agent, associated with a rapid induction and minimal side-effects,[68] recovery from its sedative effects can be slow. Methohexitone produces marginally faster awakening and recovery than thiopentone,[68] but recovery of fine motor skills may not return until 6–8 h after an induction dose.[69] Furthermore, it is associated with undesirable effects, such as pain on injection, involuntary muscle activity and hiccuping.

Etomidate produces more rapid and predictable recovery from anaesthesia than the barbiturates, but it also has additional unwanted side-effects.[68] These include pain on injection, irritation of veins, involuntary movements, increased postoperative nausea and vomiting and suppression of adrenal steroidogenesis. Although primarily a problem with prolonged administration, this last effect can occur even after an induction dose of etomidate.[70] Although the clinical implications are unknown, etomidate is probably best reserved for patients in whom its haemodynamic stability confers a definite advantage over other available agents.

Ketamine is not really a suitable agent for day-case anaesthesia. Although the prominent psychomimetic effects during the emergence period can largely be abolished by benzodiazepine pretreatment[71] (e.g. midazolam 0.05–0.1 mg.kg^{-1}), it may not be possible even with subanaesthetic doses to separate analgesia and amnesia from undesirable side-effects, such as dreaming.[72] Furthermore, delays in induction and recovery times impose severe limitations on the use of ketamine for day cases.[73] For similar reasons, benzodiazepines are not suitable induction agents either. Although a specific benzodiazepine antagonist (flumazenil) now exists, induction of anaesthesia with midazolam and subsequent antagonism with flumazenil results in slower recovery times than those achieved with newer induction agents (e.g. propofol).[74] Similar considerations apply to the use of high-dose opioid analgesic drugs for induction, although the shorter-acting opioids (e.g. alfentanil) have been used for maintenance of anaesthesia for brief periods, following induction with other agents.

Propofol has rapidly become the induction agent of choice for day-case surgery.[75] Propofol has the shortest elimination half-life of any of the currently available intravenous induction agents and its use is associated with a low incidence of postoperative side-effects. Its pharmacokinetic profile contributes to a rapid recovery (Fig. 17.1). For example, when compared to methohexitone,[76–78] initial awakening and later recovery were more rapid following induction of anaesthesia with propofol. Propofol also resulted in faster recovery and significantly less mental impairment than etomidate when used in elderly patients.[79] However, the subsequent maintenance technique may affect the rate of recovery. When using halothane and nitrous oxide for maintenance, Sanders and colleagues found that recovery times following induction of anaesthesia with propofol did not differ even from thiopentone.[80] Similarly, Valanne and colleagues[81] found similar recovery following methohexitone and propofol when the combination of enflurane and nitrous oxide was used for maintenance. However, recovery was more rapid and more 'clear-headed' with propofol compared to thiopentone when isoflurane and nitrous oxide were used for maintenance.[82]

Although propofol can produce a greater degree of cardiovascular depression than the barbiturates,[83] it is associated with few peri-operative side-effects. Excitation phenomena occur less frequently than with methohexitone.[81] Pain on injection occurs commonly, although its incidence can be decreased by the use of lignocaine 25–50 mg.[84,85]

The future may see the development of induction

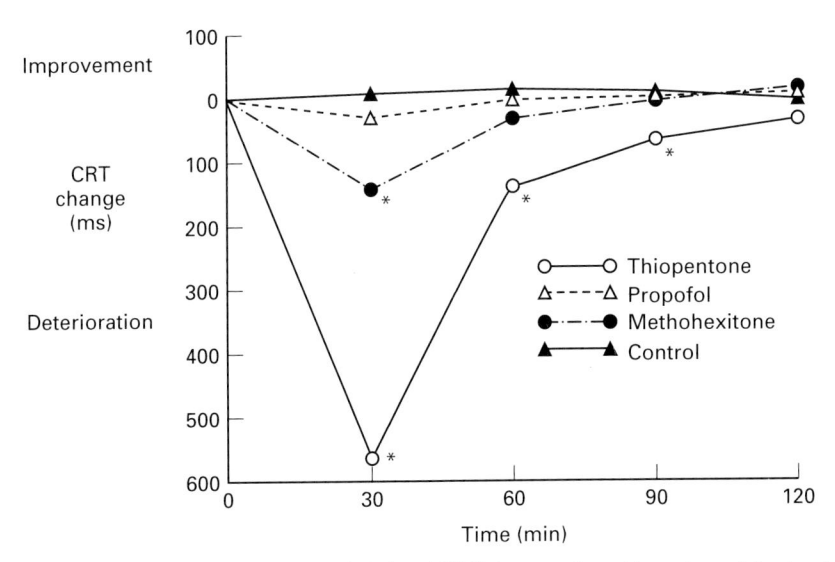

Fig. 17.1 Comparison of mean changes in choice reaction time (CRT) in controls and in patients following induction of anaesthesia with thiopentone, methohexitone or propofol. *P <0.05, from control group. From Mackenzie & Grant,[83] with permission.

agents associated with even more rapid recovery. Preliminary studies with the steroid anaesthetic eltanolone suggest that it possesses excellent haemodynamic stability[86] and an acceptable recovery profile,[87] although less favourable than that of propofol. However, emergence from eltanolone appears to be significantly slower compared to propofol.[88]

In adults, inhalation induction of anaesthesia is uncommon because the intravenous route offers a smoother and more rapid loss of consciousness. The use of a 'single-breath' inhalation technique[89] can increase the speed of induction in a co-operative patient, and would be a highly acceptable alternative, except for the pungency of the available volatile agents. Recovery does not appear to be significantly altered by the use of inhalation induction.[90] In young children, inhalational induction of anaesthesia is frequently preferable to intravenous induction because it avoids 'the needle'. Unfortunately, inhalation induction is often more time-consuming and many children also object to the presence of the face mask and the pungent smell of the volatile agent. The use of inhalation induction has been significantly reduced by the introduction of EMLA cream.

Various distraction techniques can help to reduce these problems. For example, many paediatric anaesthetists introduce the child to the mask at the preoperative visit, so that it is regarded as a toy rather than a piece of medical equipment. A clear plastic mask may be less intimidating than a black rubber one, and is perfectly safe now that explosive agents such as cyclopropane are no longer in use. In many cases, the mask can be avoided altogether; the anaesthetist grips the elbow of the gas delivery circuit and uses cupped hands to channel the anaesthetic vapour over the child's face. As the child begins to succumb to anaesthesia, the face mask can be introduced to complete induction. Permitting the child to sit up during induction may reduce anxiety and increase co-operation. Lying down is associated with bed time, which is unpopular with most children. Allowing the child to stay with the parents during induction may reduce anxiety in the child and result in a smoother induction of anaesthesia.[91] Unfortunately, this technique may well increase anxiety in the parents.[92] The rather pungent smell of the anaesthetic vapour may alarm children; however, this problem can be circumvented by the telling of a story, into which can be woven the presence of a strange smell and a feeling of sleepiness. Fruit-flavoured oils (or lip balm) may also be employed to mask the anaesthetic smell and the child can participate by choosing a favourite flavour.

Halothane is, at present, still the drug of choice for inhalation induction in paediatric patients. Despite the lower blood gas solubilities of isoflurane and enflurane (which should theoretically result in more rapid induction of anaesthesia), clinical comparisons have usually shown halothane to be superior. Kingston compared isoflurane and halothane in unpremedicated children.[93] Children receiving halothane lost consciousness sooner, and were suitable for tracheal intubation earlier than those who receive isoflurane. The children who received halothane also experienced less evidence of airway irritation. There was no discernible difference in emergence times. Other workers have also shown induction with halothane to be both faster[94] and smoother[95] than with isoflurane. Although premedication decreases respiratory irritation during an inhalation induction,[96] there is some evidence that the experience of the anaesthetist has little effect on the incidence of respiratory complications with isoflurane.[97] Using halothane for induction of anaesthesia and then changing to isoflurane for maintenance avoids the problems of induction with isoflurane; however, recovery from isoflurane is associated with more complications than when halothane is used.[98] Indeed, recovery from isoflurane anaesthesia may take longer,[95] despite the apparently more favourable physical properties of isoflurane.[99] Isoflurane may be associated with a higher incidence of minor complications than the other available inhalational agents.[100] Enflurane may be associated with marginally faster emergence from anaesthesia; however, in three-way comparison between enflurane, halothane and isoflurane, halothane was associated with the fastest and smoothest induction and was rated as the best agent overall.[101] When used for dental anaesthesia, Simmons and colleagues found enflurane to be intermediate between halothane and isoflurane in terms of speed of induction, but to result in faster recovery than either of these agents[102] However, a further advantage of halothane is that its cost is markedly lower than all of the alternative agents. Although halothane has become less widely used because of its association with hepatocellular damage, halothane hepatitis is rare in children. In two large series from major children's hospitals (Children's Hospital, Columbus, Ohio and Great Ormond Street, London), the incidence of halothane hepatitis was 1 in 200 311 and 2 in 165 400 respectively.[103,104] However, these were retrospective studies and the possibility of halothane hepatitis in children should not be ignored. In addition, the apparently higher incidence in adults may be related to anaesthesia with halothane in childhood.

Although halothane produces a smooth induction of anaesthesia, more rapid induction would be desirable. Cyclopropane, with a blood:gas partition coefficient of 0.45, can produce rapid inhalational induction in children; however, it is rarely used now, mainly because of its explosive properties. Desflurane, one of the new halogenated ethers with a blood:gas solubility of 0.42, can produce very rapid induction of anaesthesia. Unfortunately, as is the case with isoflurane, it is associated with severe airway irritation in children.[105,106] The other new volatile agent, sevoflurane, also has a low blood:gas solubility (0.69). In contrast to desflurane and isoflurane, this agent possesses minimal airway irritation.[107] Initial studies in children have been encouraging.[108,109] In the former study the authors could detect no difference in the speed of induction or recovery between sevoflurane and halothane, but induction with sevoflurane appeared to be smoother and recovery appeared more complete after sevoflurane at the time of discharge.[108] In the latter study, induction time and duration of anaesthesia were similar in both groups, but significantly more rapid emergence was observed in the sevoflurane group (halothane 9.5 min, sevoflurane 4.3 min mean emergence time).[109]

Further studies with sevoflurane in children are clearly warranted. This agent could well become the future inhalation induction agent of choice for both adults and children.

Irrespective of the method of induction, maintenance of general anaesthesia commonly relies upon a volatile agent in combination with 60–70% nitrous oxide in oxygen. Volatile agents have the advantage of controllability because rapid uptake and elimination through the lungs permit rapid changes in clinical effects. Little difference appears to exist between halothane, enflurane and isoflurane in terms of postoperative recovery times following short procedures.[99,100,110,111] However, minor sequelae (e.g. headache, nausea, dizziness and coughing) are more common following the use of isoflurane than halothane or enflurane.[100] Enflurane has been reported to result in more rapid awakening after brief procedures than halothane.[112] Although it can help to increase throughput in a busy day-case unit, faster awakening by itself is of limited clinical significance. In a small subset of outpatients (e.g. epileptics, patients with a past history of a seizure disorder), enflurane has the added potential disadvantage of possibly causing delayed convulsions.[113]

In the future, the newer and less soluble volatile agents may permit more rapid recovery following their use for maintenance of general anaesthesia. Early recovery following desflurane administration is more rapid than when isoflurane is used, and cognitive function is less depressed in the early postoperative period (Fig. 17.2).[114] Emergence is also more rapid when compared to a maintenance propofol infusion.[115] However, there is no clinically significant decrease in discharge times. Sevoflurane has also been found to result in faster emergence from anaesthesia than isoflurane when used for maintenance of anaesthesia.[108] Although the quality of recovery is allegedly superior with sevoflurane, some workers have failed to detect

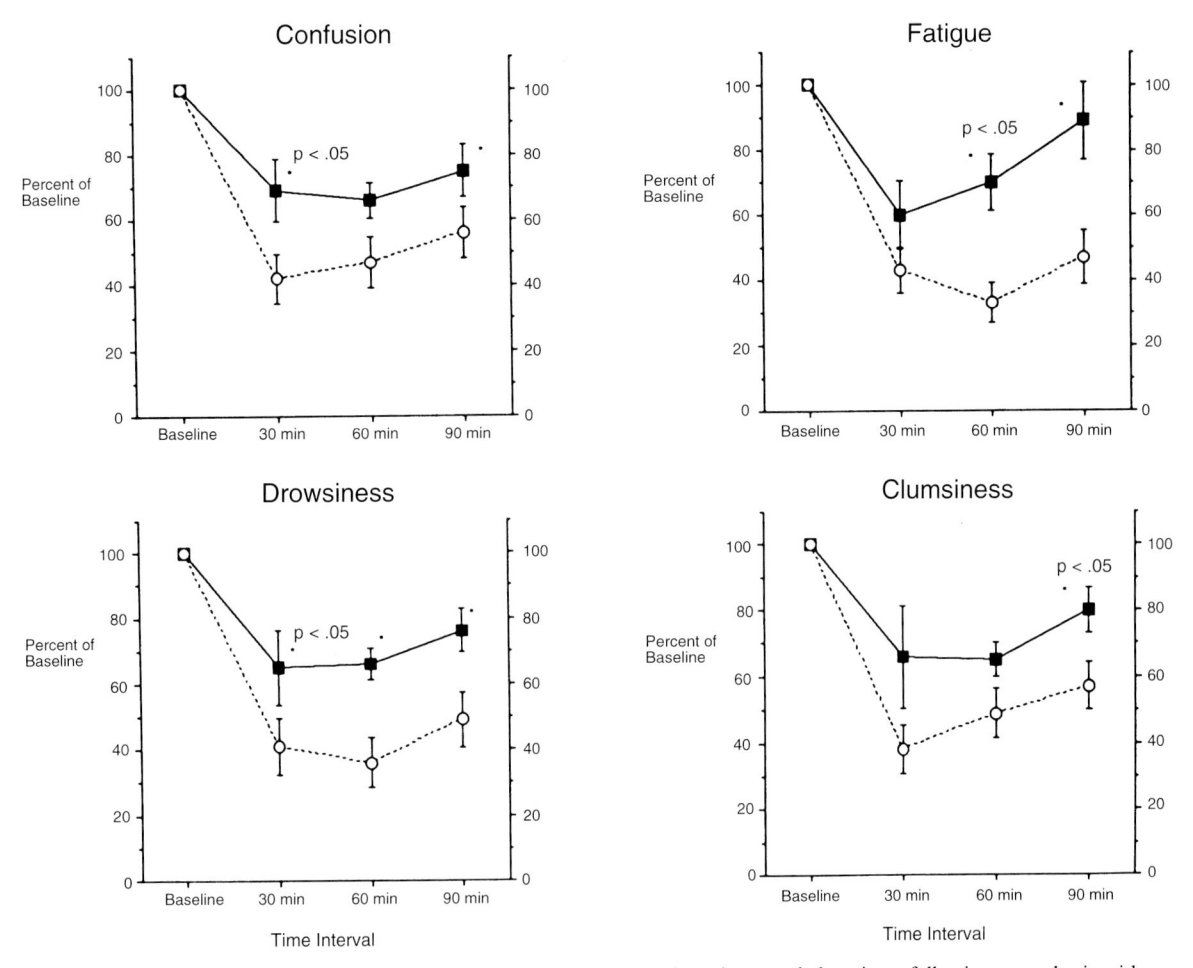

Fig. 17.2 Comparison of visual analogue scales for confusion, fatigue, drowsiness and clumsiness following anaesthesia with desflurane (solid squares) or isoflurane (open circles). From Ghouri et al,[114] with permission. *P <0.05, from isoflurane group.

differences in emergence times when sevoflurane is compared to halothane[108] or enflurane.[116] Emergence and recovery times were similar in women who received either sevoflurane or propofol for induction and maintenance of anaesthesia for day case laparoscopy.[117] Further studies of sevoflurane in day-case anaesthesia are clearly indicated. In addition, some concern has been expressed about the possible nephrotoxicity of sevoflurane. Metabolism of sevoflurane yields free fluoride ions, although the levels reported[107] are comparable to those seen after enflurane anaesthesia (Fig. 17.3). No other signs of toxicity have been reported in clinical practice.

Partly because of the side-effects of the existing volatile anaesthetics, but also because there are situations in which their use is undesirable (e.g. termination of pregnancy), increasing interest is being shown in maintenance of anaesthesia with intravenous agents. In general, the use of an infusion, as opposed to intermittent boluses of drug, has been shown to result in improved intra-operative conditions as a result of improved control of the depth of anaesthesia, lower total drug dosages and faster recovery (Fig. 17.4).[118] To enhance control and decrease recovery times, highly lipid-soluble intravenous agents with short half-life values are desirable. Of the currently available intravenous anaesthetics and analgesics, alfentanil and propofol appear to be the most commonly used. Supplementation of nitrous oxide anaesthesia with alfentanil results in more rapid awakening than when halothane,[119,120] enflurane[121,122] or isoflurane[123] are used. However, alfentanil is associated with a higher incidence of peri-operative apnoea[119,120] although there are no significant differences in later recovery

422 CLINICAL ANAESTHESIA

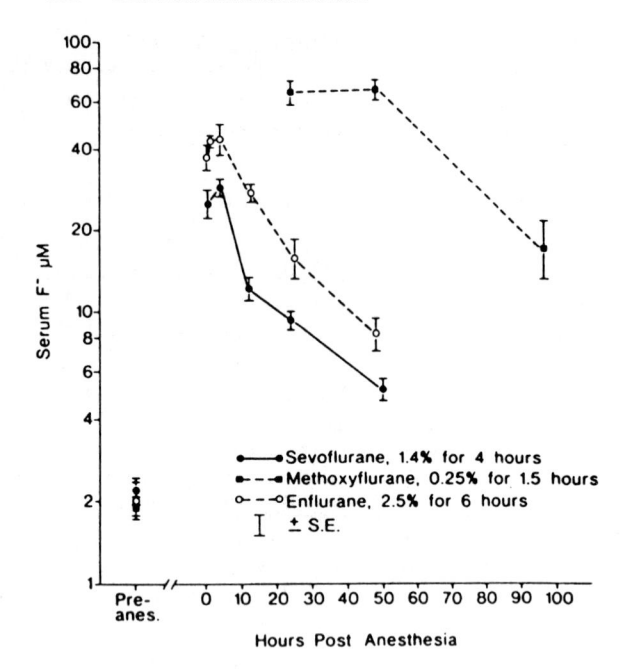

Fig. 17.3 Serum inorganic fluoride ion concentration following anaesthesia with sevoflurane, enflurane or methoxyflurane (in rats). From Cook et al,[242] with permission.

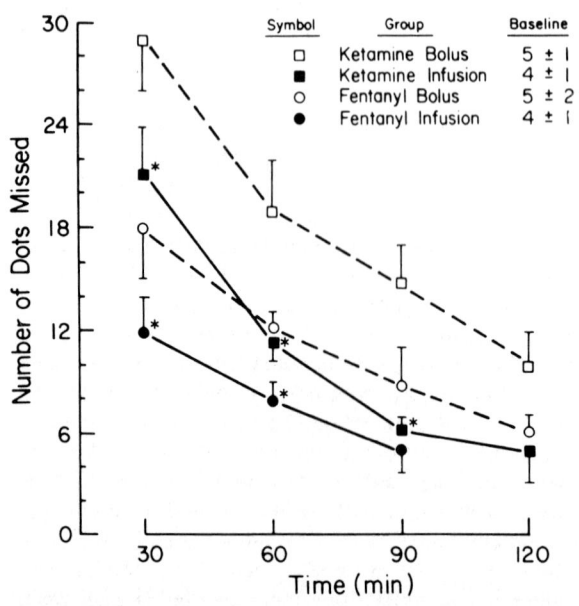

Fig. 17.4 Changes in Trieger scores as a function of time after awakening from anaesthesia maintained by a constant infusion or intermittent boluses of either fentanyl or ketamine. *$P < 0.05$, from respective bolus groups. From White,[118] with permission.

events.[119,123] Similarly, the use of fentanyl results in more rapid awakening than either enflurane or isoflurane, but again without a significant difference in later recovery events.[124] The use of opioid analgesics for anaesthetic maintenance can also result in a significantly increased incidence of postoperative nausea and vomiting.[125] For example, the use of alfentanil or sufentanil for knee arthroscopy resulted in a 45% incidence of nausea, compared to 14–15% with isoflurane.[126,127] Alfentanil has also been shown to impair memory for several hours postoperatively.[128] Opioid analgesics may also be used to supplement maintenance with other agents. For example, the use of fentanyl 1.5 µg.kg^{-1} or alfentanil 8–16 µg.kg^{-1} reduced maintenance requirements of methohexitone, resulted in a smoother peri-operative course and had no adverse effects on awakening or later recovery.[129] Apnoea was seen more frequently with higher doses of alfentanil. When used to supplement enflurane anaesthesia, alfentanil resulted in an improved quality of anaesthesia;[130] surprisingly, alfentanil-treated patients required significantly more postoperative analgesia compared with controls. The authors suggest that this was as the result of decreased volatile anaesthetic uptake in these patients because of opioid-induced ventilatory depression. Alternatively, acute tolerance may have developed in the alfentanil group.[131] As expected, when propofol was used for maintenance of anaesthesia, alfentanil resulted in decreased early postoperative analgesic requirements compared with the use of a β-blocker (esmolol) to supplement propofol and nitrous oxide anaesthesia.[132]

Methohexitone has also been used to provide maintenance anaesthesia for day cases.[78] When used as an alternative to halothane to supplement nitrous oxide, immediate recovery was more rapid following methohexitone; however, later recovery was significantly delayed.[133] Compared with methohexitone, maintenance of nitrous oxide anaesthesia with propofol resulted in more rapid awakening and a shorter time to ambulation.[78] In addition, peri-operative complications (e.g. hiccuping, nausea and vomiting) were decreased in patients who received propofol. Propofol induction and maintenance have also been found to provide more stable anaesthesia, faster recovery and fewer side-effects than etomidate.[134] In comparison with maintenance by inhaled agents, propofol anaesthesia permits faster awakening and discharge than induction with thiopentone and maintenance with halothane,[135] enflurane[136] or isoflurane.[137,138] However, the effects of the induction agent must be considered when making these comparisons. When propofol was used for induction of anaesthesia followed by maintenance with either propofol or isoflurane, propofol maintenance resulted in more rapid awakening but there were no differences in discharge times.[139] Compared with the new volatile anaesthetic desflurane, propofol resulted in slower awakening and longer emergence times; however, later recovery events and discharge times were similar with these two maintenance agents.[115] In this gynaecological day-case population, propofol resulted in a lower incidence of postoperative nausea and vomiting.

ADJUVANTS TO GENERAL ANAESTHESIA

A number of adjunctive medications may be employed to reduce anaesthetic requirements or to modify haemodynamic responses to surgical stimuli. The α_2-agonists can reduce fluctuations in intra-operative arterial blood pressure[140] and can also decrease requirements for both volatile[140] and intravenous[141] anaesthetics. Pre-operative treatment with oral clonidine can enhance sedation; the use of a transdermal clonidine patch prolongs the α_2-agonist effects into the post-operative period, resulting in decreased requirements for opioid analgesics.[142] Dexmedetomidine is a more selective α_2-agonist, which can reduce volatile anaesthetic requirements by up to 90% when administered by a continuous infusion during general anaesthesia.[143] Used as a premedicant before minor gynaecological surgery, dexmedetomidine 0.5–1.0 μg.kg^{-1} resulted in fewer side-effects during the early recovery period, primarily as a result of decreased intra-operative requirements for thiopentone.[144] Used postoperatively, dexmedetomidine 0.4 μg.kg^{-1} reduced opioid analgesic requirements, but at the expense of increased sedation and more frequent episodes of bradycardia.[145] The role of α_2-agonists in anaesthesia, including that for day-case surgery, remains to be clarified.

The autonomic ganglion-blocking drug trimetaphan can effectively attenuate haemodynamic responses during balanced anaesthesia; however, this sympatholytic drug does not control the stress hormone response produced by surgical stimulation as effectively as alfentanil or isoflurane.[146] Esmolol, a cardioselective β-adrenergic antagonist with a very short elimination half-life, can be used to attenuate the haemodynamic response to tracheal intubation. This response is most effectively blunted with a bolus dose of 100–200 mg.[147] The use of esmolol as an alternative to an opioid analgesic offers the potential for more rapid recovery and a lower incidence of postoperative nausea and vomiting in outpatients at risk of opioid-related side-effects. However, when used as an adjunct to propofol and nitrous oxide anaesthesia for outpatient arthroscopy, the use of esmolol resulted in shorter emergence times but without an effect on discharge times or the incidence of postoperative nausea.[132] Furthermore, the use of esmolol (in comparison with alfentanil) resulted in an increase in the severity of early postoperative pain.

REGIONAL ANAESTHESIA

Regional anaesthesia offers the advantage that only that portion of the body which is being operated upon is anaesthetized. Furthermore, the disadvantages of general anaesthesia (e.g. cardiovascular and respiratory depression, impaired mental function and the risks of pulmonary aspiration) are avoided. Regional techniques also provide good analgesia in the early postoperative period. The two most commonly used regional techniques are spinal and epidural anaesthesia. The spinal approach produces a reliable block and also has a faster onset of effect than the epidural route of administration. However, the complications of post-dural puncture headache[148,150] and residual impairment of bladder function have limited its popularity in day cases. Recently, thinner spinal needles have become available; these are reported to reduce the incidence of headache from 37% with 25-gauge to 2% with 27-gauge needles.[151] The use of a pencil-point needle (Sprotte or Whitacre) can also reduce the incidence of headache, even when a larger-gauge needle is used.[152] Using the epidural approach avoids the concern regarding headache (except in the case of accidental dural puncture) and, by using a catheter, permits redosing if the original block is inadequate or of insufficient duration. However, the time required to initiate the block can be a limiting factor when there is a need for rapid patient throughput. Incomplete blocks and 'missed segments' are also troublesome. Fine catheters are now available for continuous spinal blockade. This technique permits greater control and redosing and does not appear to increase the incidence of post-spinal headache.[153] However, there are serious concerns regarding possible neurological complications.

Following surgery performed under spinal or epidural anaesthesia, patients should be kept in the recovery area until they experience return of normal sensation. At that time, autonomic neuropathy and orthostatic hypotension are seldom a problem.[154] Ambulation does not increase the incidence, or prolong the duration, of post-dural puncture headache.[155] The time taken to recover normal sensation varies with the local anaesthetic used. Unfortunately, the choice of available agents is extremely limited (bupivacaine, plain and hyperbaric), such that the duration of action may frequently be inappropriately long for the proposed procedure.

Other regional techniques include caudal blocks, which are particularly useful for anorectal surgery and perineal procedures. For surgery on a single extremity, especially the upper limb, intravenous regional anaesthesia (Bier's block) can be extremely useful. Although there have been concerns about the safety of such a technique, the use of an agent with a high therapeutic index (e.g. prilocaine) and regular testing of the tourniquet can render the procedure safe. Patient comfort is enhanced by the use of a double-cuff technique, inflating the lower (distal) cuff when patients begin to experience discomfort at the proximal cuff.

For upper-extremity surgery, the brachial plexus block is a useful alternative to the intravenous regional technique.[156] Compared with general anaesthesia, this technique results in a decreased postoperative opioid analgesic requirement and normal motor function returns without delaying discharge.[157] Other regional techniques which may have a place in day-case surgery include the three-in-one (femoral obturator and lateral femoral cutaneous nerve) block and the paracervical block. The latter technique resulted in better postoperative analgesia and fewer peri-operative complications (e.g. oxygen desaturation, pain) than propofol when used for termination of pregnancy.[158]

LOCAL ANAESTHESIA

Infiltration of the operative site with local anaesthetic solution is a simple and safe alternative to general or regional anaesthesia. Typical procedures which have been performed under infiltration anaesthesia include vasectomy, hydrocoele repair, hernia repair, eye surgery, arthroscopy and oral surgery procedures. Recently, the use of a local anaesthetic–sedation technique as an alternative to regional or general anaesthesia for day-case laparoscopy has been described.[159] However, the availability of local anaesthetic techniques does not eliminate postanaesthetic side-effects.[160] One of the greatest disadvantages associated with local anaesthesia is the discomfort associated with injection of the medication, both from needle puncture and the initial stinging from the local anaesthetic. A variety of sedative and analgesic drugs can be used to reduce this discomfort. Ketamine can provide good analgesia during the injection of local anaesthetics,[161] but a benzodiazepine should also be administered to decrease ketamine-induced cardiovascular stimulation and to prevent emergence phenomena. The availability of newer preparations of local anaesthetics such as EMLA cream, which can cross intact skin, may expand the range of procedures which can be performed under local anaesthesia. EMLA has been used successfully for skin graft donor sites[162] and recent investigations suggest that it may be a useful adjuvant for extra-corporeal shock-wave lithotripsy.[163,164]

SEDATION-ANALGESIC TECHNIQUES

The operating theatre environment can provoke anxiety in many patients. Sedative–hypnotic medications are frequently employed to allay anxiety during diagnostic procedures which are not particularly painful (e.g. bronchoscopy, endoscopy), or as a supplement to local or regional anaesthesia.[165,166] Benzodiazepines are popular sedative and anxiolytic agents and result in less intra-operative recall than either etomidate or methohexitone.[167] Although decreases in haemoglobin oxygen saturation may occur, the use of a variable-rate infusion with careful titration of dose to the desired clinical effect should ensure that respiratory depression is uncommon. However, the concomitant use of potent, rapidly acting opioid analgesics (e.g. fentanyl) can result in significant ventilatory depression.[168] Residual sedation after higher doses of benzodiazepines may also delay discharge.[167]

The short elimination half-life of propofol suggests that lower (subanaesthetic) doses might be used during local and regional anaesthesia, as well as during diagnostic procedures. An infusion of 4 mg.kg^{-1}.h of propofol provides satisfactory conditions for upper intestinal endoscopy with a rapid and clear-headed recovery.[169] In a dose-ranging study, Smith and colleagues[170] found a loading dose of 0.5 mg.kg^{-1} followed by an infusion of 2 mg.kg^{-1}.h provided optimal sedation and amnesia when used to supplement spinal anaesthesia in elderly patients undergoing urological procedures. In comparison to midazolam, propofol produced less peri-operative amnesia, but resulted in decreased postoperative sedation, clumsiness and confusion.[171] However, propofol did not result in an earlier time to ambulation to discharge.

The availability of the specific benzodiazepine antagonist flumazenil offers the possibility of decreasing the duration of sedative and amnesic effects produced by midazolam. The use of low doses (e.g. 0.01 mg.kg^{-1}) of flumazenil can readily reverse residual sedation, without an increase in anxiety or evidence of an acute stress response.[172] However, the short duration of action of the antagonist (1–3 h) as a result of its rapid elimination ($t_{1/2}\beta$ 0.7–1.3 h) raises the possibility of resedation at a later time during the recovery process. Following sedation with a midazolam infusion, flumazenil improved recovery and permitted discharge more than 20 min earlier compared to a control group.[173] However, sedation with propolol permitted similar recovery times to midazolam–flumazenil and was not associated with recurrence of sedation following discharge, a phenomenon described by several patients who received flumazenil.[173] At present, midazolam appears to offer preferable intra-operative conditions, while propofol has the better recovery profile and the use of a midazolam (2 mg) and propofol (50–75 $\mu g.kg^{-1}.min$) in combination offers advantages over either drug alone.[27]

Sedation with propofol, supplemented with a potent, rapidly acting opioid analgesic (e.g. alfentanil) can provide a satisfactory alternative to other general or regional anaesthetic techniques for many procedures. A combination of fentanyl and propofol sedation provides comparable operative conditions, greater patient acceptability and significantly faster recovery than epidural anaesthesia with lignocaine for extracorporeal shock-wave lithotripsy.[174] A number of other sedation techniques have also been evaluated for this procedure.[175] The availability of ultra-short-acting opioid analgesics (e.g. remifentanil) may permit improved intraoperative analgesia with fewer postoperative side-effects in the future. Experience with postoperative patient-controlled analgesia has led to investigations of both intra-operative patient-controlled analgesia[176] and sedation.[177] Using alfentanil for sedation–analgesia, patients undergoing transvaginal ovum collection preferred to control their own medication and administered similar doses of opioid to those provided when their sedation–analgesia was controlled by the anaesthetist.[176] During epidural anaesthesia, patients allowed to self-administer a sedative mixture containing fentanyl and midazolam rated their level of comfort higher than patients receiving a similar dose of the same medications administered by their anaesthetist.[177]

POSTOPERATIVE PAIN RELIEF

Control of pain is one of the most important postoperative considerations in day-case surgery. The pain is usually most severe in the early postoperative period, at which time the potent, rapidly acting opioid analgesics (e.g. fentanyl, sufentanil) are most appropriate and effective. However, before the patient can be considered fit for discharge, control of pain must be achieved with a simple, safe technique which can easily be managed away from the hospital (e.g. oral analgesics). Although opioid analgesics are associated with sedative and respiratory depressant side-effects, the blood levels required to produce these effects are higher than those required for analgesia. Therefore, these agents are safe if the dose is carefully titrated to achieve the desired analgesic effect. Unfortunately, misconceptions of both medical and nursing staff regarding safety and the potential for addiction mean that patients often receive less medication than is needed to control pain adequately. There is also the concern that aggressive use of opioid analgesics may delay recovery and discharge as a result of opioid-induced nausea, vomiting and sedation. However, this is rarely a problem; indeed, control of pain with opioid analgesics has been shown to reduce postoperative nausea.[178]

The ideal opioid analgesic for postoperative pain relief in the day-case setting is probably yet to be discovered. A rapid onset of action is desirable so that dosage can be easily titrated to effect. However, a very short duration of action (e.g. alfentanil) is undesirable, to avoid the need for frequent redosing. In contrast, drugs that have a long duration of action (e.g. methadone, buprenorphine) may also be inappropriate because any undesirable effects will also be long-lasting. Clearly, the drug must possess adequate analgesic efficacy. This is often a problem with the partial agonist (or agonist–antagonist) drugs, which often have a ceiling with respect to their analgesic effects. Lack of side-effects (e.g. sedation, nausea and vomiting) is also important. Of the currently available agents, fentanyl and sufentanil are the most useful parenteral analgesics in the early postoperative period.

The goal of developing a potent analgesic, devoid of respiratory depressant and emetic effects, has yet to be achieved. In an attempt to overcome deficiencies with existing agents, a number of new synthetic opioids have been developed with differing actions at the opioid receptor subtypes. The hope of maintaining efficacy while at the same time reducing side-effects has not been achieved with some of the newer compounds (e.g. dezocine).[179]

Existing agents may also be administered using alternative delivery systems in an attempt to improve patient acceptability and decrease undesirable effects. Patient-controlled analgesia is becoming increasingly popular for postoperative pain relief in inpatients.[180] Patients generally prefer this technique because it provides an element of control and because they can titrate the analgesic to meet their own personal requirements. Predetermined limits programmed into the infusion pump prevent accidental overdosage and ensure patient safety. Once the unit is set up, analgesia delivery is not dependent on the immediate availability of nursing staff, which benefits the patient as a result of more rapid treatment of pain and could potentially decrease staffing requirements. Recently, investigators have begun to evaluate the possibility of extending the use of patient-controlled analgesia devices into the ambulatory setting.[181] Such a technique would be beneficial when more extensive surgery is performed and adequate analgesia cannot be achieved by oral analgesics. Patient satisfaction was found to be high despite the frequent occurrence of nausea and pruritus. Subcutaneous patient-controlled analgesia might offer an attractive alternative in the outpatient setting.[182–184]

Although parenterally administered opioids produce a rapid onset of analgesic effects, injections can be unpleasant for patients, especially children. Oral opioid analgesics are subject to considerable first-pass hepatic metabolism which decreases their bio-availability. Sublingual, buccal, transnasal and transdermal routes of administration all avoid first-pass clearance and can result in effective analgesic plasma drug levels. Bio-availability is usually lower with non-parenteral administration; however, this can be compensated for by increased dosage. Buprenorphine, a long-acting analgesic, is currently the only commercially available sublingual preparation. Compared with intramuscular administration, sublingual delivery results in similar levels of analgesia.[185] However, buprenorphine is a partial agonist and possesses a ceiling with respect to its analgesic (and ventilatory depressant) effects. It also appears to be associated with a high incidence of nausea. Morphine can also be administered buccally; it produces comparable effects to conventional intramuscular delivery in terms of analgesic effects, and may be associated with fewer adverse effects.[186] The transnasal route has also been employed using butorphanol resulting in analgesia of longer duration than with intravenous administration.[187] The large surface area and excellent blood supply of the nasal mucosa suggest that this route of delivery deserves further evaluation.

Transdermal administration is being employed more frequently for a wide range of compounds (e.g. opioids, vasodilators, α_2-agonists). The lipid-soluble opioid analgesics fentanyl and sufentanil can be absorbed through the skin. However, bio-availability is low and rather unpredictable. In particular, plasma levels can increase considerably following exercise.[188] Additional problems include delayed onset of effects, prolonged duration and the depot effects, resulting in a persistent elevation of plasma concentrations following patch removal. Future developments include the use of iontophoresis to facilitate transfer of larger drug molecules across the skin. This technique may result in a wider range of drugs being delivered transdermally.

Non-steroidal anti-inflammatory drugs (NSAIDs) may be useful when administered as supplements to opioid analgesics. Because oral administration may not be possible in the immediate postoperative period, much attention has focused on NSAIDs which can be administered parenterally. Although parenteral aspirin has little effect on postoperative pain,[189] both diclofenac[190] and ketorolac[191] decrease pain scores and lower requirements for supplemental opioid analgesics. Unlike opioids, the onset of action of NSAIDs is somewhat slower; however, this potential problem can be easily overcome by administering the drug pre-operatively.[192] Pre-operative administration also allows the use of the less expensive oral forms of these agents.

As noted above, the use of regional techniques for intra-operative analgesia can provide a significant degree of postoperative pain relief. Local anaesthetics are increasingly being administered intra-operatively to provide analgesia in the early postoperative period. Caudal nerve block has been performed for this purpose in young children undergoing circumcision and other lower abdominal procedures. Although this technique can be highly effective, it is associated with a significant failure rate and has the potential for troublesome side-effects (e.g. urinary retention and leg weakness).[193] In the case of patients undergoing circumcision, caudal block may delay ambulation and micturition compared with dorsal nerve block. Ilio-inguinal nerve block[194] and block of the dorsal nerve of the penis[195] have been shown to produce levels of analgesia comparable to those achieved with a caudal block following orchidopexy and circumcision, respectively. These nerve blocks are simpler to perform, are inherently safer and are associated with fewer side-effects than caudal analgesia. Simply instilling a long-acting local anaesthetic (e.g. bupivacaine) into the wound is even easier than performing a nerve block. Bupivacaine instillation provides pain relief comparable to that produced by ilio-inguinal nerve block following inguinal hernia repair.[196] Use of a lignocaine aerosol also produces satisfactory analgesia following inguinal herniorrhaphy in adults.[197] For post-circumcision pain, topical application of a lignocaine spray, cream or jelly is as effective as either dorsal nerve block or parenteral morphine, and has fewer side-effects than morphine.[198] Both spray and jelly can be applied painlessly. Furthermore, topical therapy can readily be re-applied by the patient (or parents) at home, thereby ensuring good analgesia during the late recovery period.[199] The effectiveness of these simple methods of pain relief suggests that performing a caudal block (or other major nerve block procedure) for postoperative analgesia may constitute an unnecessary risk for many patients.[200]

Satisfactory postoperative analgesia has also been

reported following wound infiltration with local anaesthetic solution after lower abdominal,[201] gallbladder,[202] sterilization[203,204] and lower-extremity[205] operations. Local anaesthetics can also be injected intra-articularly following arthroscopic surgery. Although most investigators have not demonstrated a significant reduction in postoperative pain using this approach, the injection of 30 ml of bupivacaine 0.5% has recently been shown to decrease postoperative opioid requirements and to improve mobility and discharge times following arthroscopic knee surgery (Fig. 17.5).[206]

Finally, several non-pharmacological methods have been investigated for relief of postoperative pain. An accurate description of the degree of postoperative pain which can be expected by the patient, coupled with reassurance that the pain is normal as well as a description of what measures should be taken to treat it, can result in a significant reduction in the postoperative analgesic requirements compared with patients given no such special care.[207] Transcutaneous nerve stimulation facilitates functional recovery following arthroscopic knee surgery.[208] Cryo-analgesia, a technique involving the freezing of nerves to block pain transmission, was alleged to provide postoperative analgesia for procedures such as herniorrhaphy or cholecystectomy. However, in clinical practice, cryo-analgesia results have been very disappointing.[209]

POSTOPERATIVE NAUSEA AND VOMITING

With the exception of pain, the single most distressing postoperative complication is nausea and vomiting. This side-effect is particularly undesirable in the day-case unit since it interferes with ambulation and discharge. Management should include both attempts at treatment and prevention. Treatment involves the use of one or more of a variety of anti-emetic medications (e.g. metoclopramide, prochlorperazine and droperidol). More recently, antagonists of the 5-hydroxytryptamine type 3 (5-HT$_3$) receptor have been synthesized and these compounds appear to possess potent anti-emetic activity with few side-effects. Of the new 5-HT$_3$ antagonists, ondansetron has been investigated the most extensively. Compared to placebo, ondasetron, 8 mg i.v., was effective as an antiemetic with an incidence of side-effects comparable to the placebo groups.[210] Although formal comparisons with other antiemetics for the treatment of established postoperative nausea have not been performed to date, ondansetron-treated patients with persistent nausea required a smaller number of 'rescue' doses than control patients initially treated with a conventional antiemetic combination consisting of hydroxyzine and metoclopramide.[210] Despite promising initial results with ondansetron, no single agent so far investigated has proved to be effective in all patients.

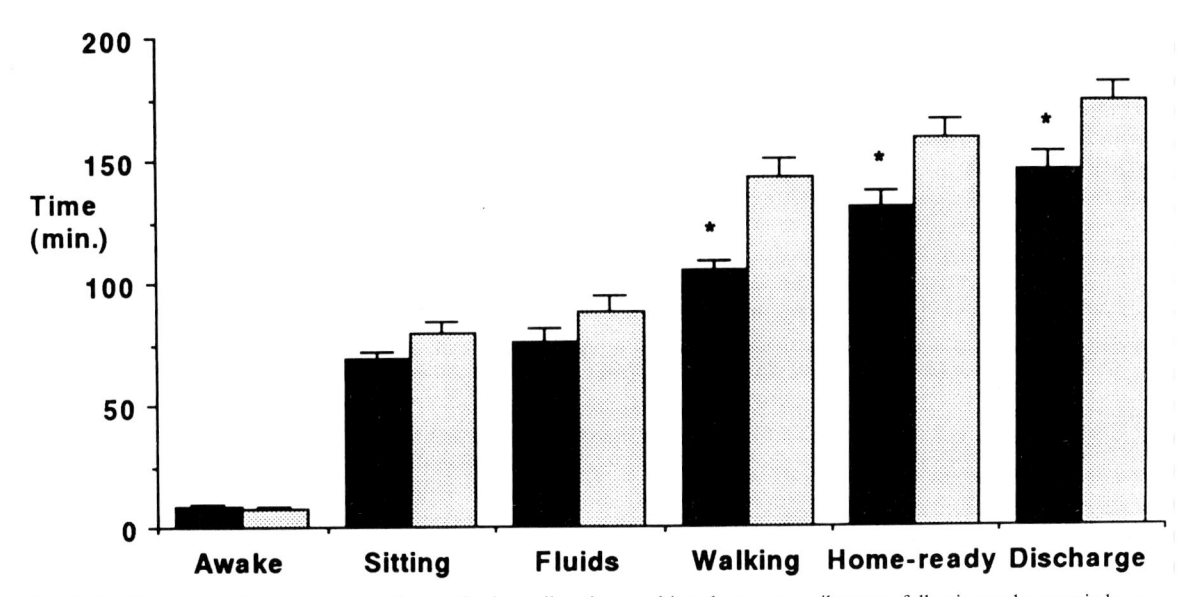

Fig. 17.5 Times from discontinuation of anaesthesia until patients achieved recovery milestones following arthroscopic knee surgery. Filled blocks represent intra-articular instillation of 0.5% bupivacaine; shaded blocks represent saline (control) instillation. *P <0.05, from control group. From Smith et al,[206] with permission.

Anti-emetic agents can also be administered prophylactically, either pre-operatively or during the intra-operative period. These drugs appear to be more effective when administered in this way. Hyoscine (scopolamine) has long been used for treating motion sickness. The transdermal route of delivery has been employed in an attempt to achieve longer-lasting anti-emetic effects. Although in one study nausea was reduced for 24 h compared with placebo, the incidence was still unacceptably high.[211] Furthermore, side-effects such as visual disturbance and drowsiness are common[212] and these may persist for up to 12–24 h.[211] Prophylactic metoclopramide[213,214] and droperidol[215] can both reduce the incidence of postoperative nausea. Droperidol may be more effective than metoclopramide;[216] however, side-effects (e.g. sedation, dysphoria, restlessness, α-blockade) limit its use in the day-case setting. Domperidone appears to be less effective.[214,216] Prophylactic ondansetron in doses of 4 mg or above were significantly more effective than a placebo in preventing nausea and vomiting after day case laparoscopy.[217] Compared to metoclopramide and droperidol, 8 mg of ondansetron was more effective in preventing postoperative emesis (but not nausea) following minor gynaecological operations.[218] Although ondansetron appears to be a useful new antiemetic, droperidol may be a more cost-effective agent for routine prophylactic use.[219] While gastric suctioning has been advocated to reduce postoperative nausea, the results of published studies do not support this recommendation.[220,221] However, when combined with ranitidine 50 mg intravenously[222] or 300 mg orally,[223] gastric suction appeared to decrease postoperative nausea. In view of the potential for trauma associated with the passage of gastric drainage tubes, the anti-emetic effects of ranitidine (and other H_2-blockers) alone warrants further investigation. A multicentre trial is currently underway to investigate the effectiveness of ondansetron 4 mg administered intravenously before induction of anaesthesia in day-case patients.

The treatment and prevention of nausea are still far from satisfactory, and there are several reports describing patients in whom existing anti-emetics were ineffective.[224,225] A number of other factors can influence the incidence of postoperative nausea (Table 17.4), many of which are not under the direct control of the anaesthetist. Nevertheless, avoidance of specific anaesthetic and analgesic medications (e.g. etomidate, opioids, nitrous oxide) may be beneficial in some high-risk individuals. Propofol is associated with a low incidence of emetic sequelae and may possess intrinsic anti-emetic properties.[226,227] Using propofol, esmolol and nitrous oxide for knee arthroscopy, only 6% of patients required anti-emetic medication, compared with a 25% incidence of postoperative nausea using a volatile anaesthetic technique.[206–228] Regional techniques can also help to reduce the incidence of postoperative nausea.[228]

While the future may see the development of more specific and selective anti-emetic agents, other researchers have investigated older non-pharmacological techniques. Interestingly, both acupuncture[229] and acupressure to the flexor surface of the wrist[230] have been shown to reduce nausea after day-case surgery.

Table 17.4 Factors influencing the incidence of postoperative nausea and vomiting

Patient factors	Age (<12 years) Female gender History of motion sickness Morbid obesity Early pregnancy
Gastric factors	Increased gastric volume: 　Anxiety 　Lack of compliance with fasting
Drug effects	Opioid analgesics: 　Pre-operative 　Intra-operative 　Postoperative Volatile anaesthetics Nitrous oxide Etomidate
Surgical factors	Laparoscopy Strabismus surgery Orchidopexy Myringotomy tubes Upper abdominal surgery
Postoperative factors	Hypotension Pain

Based on White & Shafer,[239] with permission.

DISCHARGE CRITERIA

Determining the appropriate time for the safe discharge of a patient following day-case surgery requires and accurate assessment of the patient's recovery from the effects of surgery and anaesthesia.[231] Recovery may be subdivided into three stages: early, intermediate and late. Early recovery, often referred to as the emergence period, involves the initial awakening from anaesthesia and recovery of vital, protective reflexes. Intermediate recovery describes the recovery of cognitive and psychomotor function up to the point at which the patient is fit to be discharged. Late recovery involves a complete return to the pre-operative state and resumption of normal physical and cognitive activities. This process may take several days to weeks.

For the safety of the patient following discharge, it is important that there is a return towards normal levels of physiological functioning prior to discharge. Careful assessment of recovery is becoming more important now that surgery of longer duration is being performed on a day-case basis, and patients with increasingly complex co-existing diseases are considered acceptable candidates. However, important aspects of recovery are difficult to assess using quantitative methodology. There is a wide variety of psychomotor tests (e.g. reaction time, critical flicker fusion time, Maddox wing, p-deletion, Trieger dot and digit-symbol substitution tests)[110] which have been used for research purposes in evaluating new anaesthetic agents and developing discharge criteria. However, most of these tests are too complex and too time-consuming for routine clinical use. In practice, patients should be awake, oriented and able to walk unaided. It is also considered desirable for outpatients to be able to tolerate oral fluids and to pass urine; this recommendation is especially important in the very young and old, in patients having genito-urinary procedures and when large amounts of fluid have been administered during the peri-operative period. Postoperative pain and nausea should not be disabling, and should be easily controlled with non-parenteral medication. Following regional anaesthesia, the ability to walk and to pass urine are probably the most reliable indicators of 'home readiness'. The ability of the patient to run the heel smoothly down the contralateral shin may be a useful indicator of the return of motor and sensory function and is a useful predictor of when ambulation should be attempted.[232] Assessment of recovery following other peripheral nerve blocks is seldom a problem. Residual sensory blockade may be beneficial in decreasing postoperative pain.

Discharge criteria can conveniently be assessed using a simple scoring system[233] or can be recorded by the recovery room staff using a simple check-list (Table 17.5). Anaesthetists and surgeons must be involved in the development of reliable discharge criteria which can be easily interpreted by the nursing staff. These discharge criteria should be tailored to the specific requirements of the centre and may be influenced by the mix of patients and surgical procedures. If such criteria are adequately applied, it is not necessary for medically qualified personnel to be present at the time of discharge. However, a doctor should be available in the day-case facility to advise and assist with any problems or complications which may occur after surgery.

Table 17.5 Discharge criteria following day-case surgery

General
Stable vital signs for at least 30 min
No new postoperative signs or symptoms
No active bleeding
Minimal nausea and vomiting
Oriented to person, place and time
Minimal dizziness after movement or dressing
Pain controlled with oral analgesics
A responsible escort (preferably two for children)

Specific
Ability to pass urine following urological surgery
Normal sensation and circulation after extremity surgery
Return of normal sensation, motor and autonomic function after epidural or spinal anaesthesia

Modified from White,[240] with permission.

Prior to discharge, the patient's dressings should be checked, and verbal and written instructions should be given about dressing care and resumption of normal physical activities. Patients should be encouraged to contact the day-case unit with concerns or postoperative problems. Patients should be accompanied home by a responsible escort, who should also remain with them at home for the first night or arrange for another suitable person to do so. The physical and intellectual capability of the patient's escort should be evaluated by the nursing staff prior to the time of discharge. Some elderly patients may have an escort who is almost equally infirm, while others may be accompanied home by an adult but subsequently left in the care of a child. Small children should ideally be accompanied home by two adults to avoid having the driver distracted by the need to care for their child.

Unfortunately, not all day-case patients pay attention to the advice they are given. A survey performed in the UK in 1972 found that, of all car drivers, 43% drove within 24 h of discharge, 30% drove within 12 h and 9% drove themselves home from the hospital after day-case surgery (one patient even drove a bus full of passengers for 95 miles on the same day as his operation).[234] A more recent American survey conducted in 1990 found that 14% of outpatients drove within 12 h of surgery.[235] Although the newer anaesthetic and analgesic drugs result in less psychomotor impairment than older agents, their use does not ensure sufficiently rapid recovery for driving or the performance of other complex tasks requiring intense concentration and co-ordination on the day of surgery.[69] Unfortunately, the improved recovery after modern anaesthetics may make patients feel that they are capable of performing better than they are able to (secondary to the euphoric effects of these drugs).

Although few sanctions can be used against the patient who deliberately disregards medical advice, it is the responsibility of day-case unit staff to ensure that patients receive appropriate verbal and written instructions for postoperative care and that the patient and escort understand these instructions. Indeed, the medical and nursing staff risk litigation if harm should befall a patient discharged too early, or to whom appropriate advice was not given.[23]

An effective mechanism should exist for the rapid admission of patients to a hospital if unanticipated admission is required. The ability to admit patients is simpler when day-case facilities exist as part of a larger hospital complex rather than as free-standing surgical centres. Overall, approximately 1% of day-case patients require hospital admission for a wide variety of intra-operative and postoperative reasons. This incidence is higher if there is a large percentage of outpatients at the extremes of age (e.g. less than 6 months or over 75 years) or with pre-existing diseases. Unplanned hospital admissions are usually for medical or surgical reasons rather than because of the anaesthetic technique employed. Pain resulting from surgery which has been more extensive than originally envisaged and surgical misadventure (e.g. excessive bleeding or damage to viscera) are the most common surgical problems, while chest pain and arrhythmias are common medical reasons. The commonest anaesthetic-related cause for admission is intractable emesis.[236] Other common reasons for unexpected admission are listed in Table 17.6.

Day-case units should be encouraged to provide follow-up patient care with a telephone call to the patient at home on the first or second postoperative day. Alternatively, the staff may choose to provide the patient with a questionnaire which can be returned in a stamped, addressed envelope. This allows the identification of operative or anaesthetic factors which are associated with a particularly unfavourable (or favourable) postoperative outcome, and can provide important quality assurance data, which may initiate the need to make changes in the policies and procedures of the unit.

SUMMARY

Since its inception in the early 1900s, day-case anaesthesia has expanded considerably, and this growth is continuing today. There is an increasing trend towards performing more lengthy and complicated surgery on an outpatient basis, and the surgical population includes a larger proportion of older and more seriously ill patients. These changes have occurred partly as a result of improvements in anaesthetic techniques, but at the same time, they present new challenges to the anaesthetist.

Improvements in the pharmacological properties of anaesthetic drugs have resulted in agents with more precisely defined effects and with shorter durations of action. The future promises further developments along these lines. However, the incidence of minor, but troublesome, side-effects is still unacceptably high. Pain and postoperative nausea remain areas of concern but active research offers hope for the future.

Anaesthesia for day-case surgery is now regarded as a subspecialty[237] which has encouraged the development of anaesthetic techniques and policies specific to the unique problems presented by ambulatory surgery. Use of rational combinations of drugs and careful selection of technique can provide optimal conditions for surgery, while minimizing recovery times and decreasing side-effects. As increasingly complex surgical cases present for day-case surgery, there must be an expansion of the specialty to include better pre- and postoperative care. In particular, the provision of improved postoperative pain relief and better home health care facilities will be major factors in the continued expansion of day-case surgery. With continuing growth, as Ralph Waters stated in 1919, 'the future for such a venture is bright'.[2]

Table 17.6 Unexpected hospital admission following day-case surgery

Category	Reason for admission

Surgical	Unanticipated extended surgery
	Misadventure
	    Excessive bleeding
	    Uterine perforation
	    Diathermy burn to bowel
	    Perforated bladder or other viscus

Medical	Pre-existing disease (e.g. poorly controlled diabetes)
	Peri-operative complication
	    Chest pain
	    Dyspnoea
	    Arrhythmia

Anaesthetic	Intractable pain Prolonged vomiting Slow recovery/excessive drowsiness Aspiration
Social	Patient/family request General practitioner request Absence of *suitable* escort Nobody available at home

Modified from Korttila,[241] with permission.

REFERENCES

1. Nicoll JH. The surgery of infancy. Br Med J 1909; ii: 753–754
2. Waters RM. The down-town anesthesia clinic. Am J Surg 1919; 33 (suppl): 71–73
3. Kitz DS, Slusarz-Ladden C, Lecky JH. Hospital resources used for inpatient and ambulatory surgery. Anesthesiology 1988; 69: 383–386
4. Natof HE. Pre-existing medical problems. Ambulatory surgery. IMJ 1984; 166: 101–104
5. Federated Ambulatory Surgery Association Special Study 1. 1986. 700 N Fairfax Street, No 520, Alexandria, VA 22314
6. Sear JW, Cooper GM, Kumar V. The effect of age on recovery. Anaesthesia 1983; 38: 1158–1161
7. Steward DJ. Preterm infants are more prone to complications following minor surgery than are term infants. Anesthesiology 1982; 56: 304–306
8. Liu LMP, Coté CJ, Goudsouzian NG et al. Life-threatening apnea in infants recovering from anesthesia. Anesthesiology 1983; 59: 506–510
9. Meridy HW. Criteria for selection of ambulatory surgical patients and guidelines for anesthetic management. Anesth Analg 1982; 61: 921–926
10. Ogg TW. Use of anaesthesia: implications of day-case surgery and anaesthesia. Br Med J 1980; 281: 212–214
11. Arellano R, Cruise C, Chung F. Timing of the anesthetist's outpatient interview. Anesth Analg 1989; 68: 645–648
12. Twersky R, Frank D, Lebovits A. Timing of preoperative evaluation for surgical outpatients — does it matter? Anesthesiology 1990; 73: A1
13. Meyer P, Thisted R, Roizen MF et al. Improving preoperative laboratory test selection. Anesth Analg 1991; 72: S183
14. Roizen MF, Rupani G. Preopreative assessment of adult outpatients. In: White PF, ed. Outpatient anesthesia. New York: Churchill Livingstone, 1990: pp 181–200
15. Charpak Y, Bléry C, Chastang C, Szatan M, Foutgeaux B. Prospective assessment of a protocol for selective ordering of preoperative chest x-rays. Can J Anaesth 1988; 35: 259–264
16. Lutner RE, Roizen MF, Stocking CB et al. The automated interview versus the personal interview. Do patient responses to preoperative health questions differ? Anesthesiology 1991; 75: 394–400
17. Johnston M. Anxiety in surgical patients. Psychol Med 1980; 10: 145–152
18. Egbert LD, Battit GE, Turndorf H, Beecher HK. The value of the preoperative visit by an anesthetist. JAMA 1963; 185: 553–555
19. Leigh JM, Walker J, Janaganathan P. Effect of preoperative anaesthetic visit on anxiety. Br Med J 1977; ii: 987–989
20. Lawlis GF, Selby D, Hinnant D, McCoy CE. Reduction of postoperative pain parameters by presurgical relaxation instructions for spinal pain patients. Spine 1985; 10: 649–651
21. Todd JG, Nimmo WS. Effect of premedication on drug absorption and gastric emptying. Br J Anaesth 1983; 55: 1189–1193
22. Philip BK. Hazards of amnesia after midazolam in ambulatory surgical patients. Anesth Analg 1987; 66: 97–98
23. Wieland JB, Katz LL. Legal considerations in anesthesia for outpatient surgery. In: White PF, ed. Outpatient anesthesia. New York: Churchill Livingstone, 1990: pp 453–472
24. Beechey APG, Eltringham RJ, Studd C. Temazepam as premedication in day surgery. Anaesthesia 1981; 36: 10–15
25. Pinnock CA, Fell D, Hunt PCW, Miller R, Smith G. A comparison of triazolam and diazepam as premedication agents for minor gynaecological surgery. Anaesthesia 1985; 40: 324–328
26. Forrest P, Galletly DC, Yee P. Placebo controlled comparison of midazolam, triazolam and diazepam as oral premedicants for outpatient anaesthesia. Anaesth Intensive Care 1987; 15: 296–304
27. Taylor E, Ghouri AF, White PF. Midazolam in combination with propofol for sedation during local anesthesia. J Clin Anesth 1992; 4: 213–216
28. DeLucia JA, White PF. Effect of midazolam on induction and recovery characteristics of propofol. Anesth Analg 1992; 74: S63
29. Shafer A, White PF, Urquhart ML, Doze VA. Outpatient premedication: use of midazolam and opioid analgesics. Anesthesiology 1989; 71: 495–501
30. Hargreaves J. Benzodiazepine premedication in minor day-case surgery: comparison of oral midazolam and temazepam with placebo. Br J Anaesth 1988; 61: 611–616
31. Nightingale JJ, Norman J. A comparison of midazolam and temazepam for premedication of day case patients. Anaesthesia 1988; 43: 111–113
32. Feld LH, Negus JB, White PF. Oral midazolam preanesthetic medication in pediatric outpatients. Anesthesiology 1990; 73: 831–834
33. Wilton NCT, Leigh J, Rosen DR, Pandit UA. Preanesthetic sedation of preschool children using intranasal midazolam. Anesthesiology 1988; 69: 972–975
34. Stanley TH, Hague B, Mock DL et al. Oral transmucosal fentanyl citrate (lollipop) premedication in human volunteers. Anesth Analg 1989; 69: 21-27
35. Streisand JB, Stanley TH, Hague B, Van Vreeswijk H, Ho GH, Pace NL. Oral transmucosal fentanyl citrate premedication in children. Anesth Analg 1989; 69: 28–34
36. Ashburn MA, Streisand JB, Tarver SD et al. Oral transmucosal fentanyl citrate for premedication in paediatric outpatients. Can J Anaesth 1990; 37: 857–866
37. Feld LH, Champeau MW, Van Steennis CA, Scott JC. Preanesthetic medication in children: a comparison of oral transmucosal fentanyl citrate versus placebo. Anesthesiology 1989; 71: 374–377
38. Roberts RB, Shirley MA. Reducing the risk of acid aspiration during cesarean section. Anesth Analg 1974; 53: 859–868
39. Snow J. On chloroform and other anaesthetics, their action and administration. London: Churchill, 1858: pp 74–75
40. Beaumont W. Experiments and observations on the gastric juice and the physiology of digestion. Plattsburg: Allen, 1833
41. Maltby JR, Sutherland AD, Sale JP, Shaffer EA. Preoperative oral fluids: is a 5 hour fast justified prior to elective surgery? Anesth Analg 1986; 65: 1112–1116

42. Goresky GV, Maltby JR. Fasting guidelines for elective surgical patients. Can J Anaesth 1990; 37: 493–495
43. Scarr M, Maltby JR, Jani K, Sutherland LR. Volume and acidity of residual gastric fluid after oral fluid ingestion before elective ambulatory surgery. Can Med Assoc J 1989; 141: 1151–1154
44. Sutherland AD, Stock JG, Davies JM. Effects of preoperative fasting on morbidity and gastric contents in patients undergoing day-stay surgery. Br J Anaesth 1986; 58: 876–878
45. Splinter WM, Stewart JA, Muir JG. The effect of preoperative apple juice on gastric contents, thirst, and hunger in children. Can J Anaesth 1989; 36: 55–58
46. Schreiner MS, Triebwasser A, Keon TP. Ingestion of liquids compared with preoperative fasting in pediatric outpatients. Anesthesiology 1990; 72: 593–597
47. Miller M, Wishart HY, Nimmo WS. Gastric contents at induction of anaesthesia. Br J Anaesth 1983; 55: 1185–1188
48. Coté CJ. NPO after midnight for children — a reappraisal. Anesthesiology 1990; 72: 589–592
49. Haskins DA, Jahr JS, Ramadyhani U, Texidor M, Kelley D. Does omeprazole, a gastric acid pump inhibitor reduce gastric volume and acidity in outpatients? Anesth Analg 1991; 72: S102
50. Pandit SK, Kothary SP, Pandit UA, Mirakhur RK. Premedication with cimetidine and metoclopramide. Anaesthesia 1986; 41: 486–492
51. Morison DH, Dunn GL, Fargas-Babjak AM, Moudgil GC, Smedstad K, Woo J. A double-blind comparison of cimetidine and ranitidine as prophylaxis against gastric aspiration syndrome. Anesth Analg 1982; 61: 988–992
52. Vinik HR, Covarrubias S. Ranitidine-role of dose and time effect study for prophylaxis of perioperative acid aspiration. Anesthesiology 1990; 73: A13
53. Olsson GL, Hallen B, Hambraeus-Jonzon K. Aspiration during anaesthesia. Acta Anaesth Scand 1986; 30: 84–92
54. Collins KM, Docherty PW, Plantevin OM. Postoperative morbidity following gynaecological outpatient laparoscopy. Anaesthesia 1984; 39: 819–822
55. Shafer A, White PF. New agents and techniques for outpatient anesthesia. Anesthesiol Rep 1990; 3: 82–96
56. Blitt CD. Monitoring during outpatient anesthesia. Int Anesth Clin 1982; 20: 17–25
57. Zuurmond WWA, Van Leeuwen L. Atracurium versus vecuronium: a comparison of recovery in outpatient arthroscopy. Can J Anaesth 1988; 35: 139–142
58. Sengupta P, Skacel M, Plantevin OM. Post-operative morbidity associated with the use of atracurium and vecuronium in day-case laparoscopy. Eur J Anaesth 1987; 4: 93–99
59. Assem ESK, Ling YB. Fatal anaphylactic reaction to suxamethonium: new screening test suggests possible prevention. Anaesthesia 1988; 43: 958–961
60. Goldberg ME, Larijani GE, Azad SS et al. Comparison of tracheal intubating conditions and neuromuscular blocking profiles after intubating doses of mivacurium chloride or succinylcholine in surgical outpatients. Anesth Analg 1989; 69: 93–99
61. Poler S, Watcha MF, White PF. Mivacurium as an alternative to succinylcholine during outpatient laparoscopy. J Clin Anesth 1992; 4: 127–133
62. Savarese JJ, Ali HH, Basta SJ et al. The cardiovascular effects of mivacurium chloride (BW B1090U) in patients receiving nitrous oxide-opiate-barbiturate anesthesia. Anesthesiology 1989; 70: 386–394
63. Østergaard D, Jensen FS, Jensen E, Viby Mogensen J. Mivacurium induced neuromuscular blockade (NBM) in patients heterozygous for the atypical gene for plasma cholinesterase. Anesthesiology 1989; 71: A782
64. Smith I, Joshi G. The laryngeal mask airway for outpatient anesthesia. J Clin Anesth 1993; 5 (supplement 1): 22S–28S
65. Hickey S, Cameron AE, Asbury AJ. Cardiovascular response to insertion of Brain's laryngeal mask. Anaesthesia 1990; 45: 629–633
66. Alexander CA, Leach AB. Incidence of sore throats with the laryngeal mask. Anaesthesia 1989; 44: 791
67. Department of Health and Social security. Report on confidential enquiries into maternal deaths in England and Wales 1964–66. London: HMSO, 1969: pp 68–75
68. White PF. Clinical pharmacology of intravenous induction agents. Int Anesthesiol Clin 1988; 26: 98–104
69. Korttila K, Linnoila M, Ertama P, Häkkinen S. Recovery and simulated driving after intravenous anesthesia with thiopental, methohexital, propanidid, or alphadione. Anesthesiology 1975; 43: 291–299
70. Wagner RL, White PF. Etomidate inhibits adrencortical function in surgical patients. Anesthesiology 1984; 61: 647–651
71. Lilburn JK, Dundee JW, Nair SG, Fee JPH, Johnston HML. Ketamine sequelae. Anaesthesia 1978; 33: 307–311
72. Figallo EM, McKenzie R, Tantisira B, Wadhwa RK, Sinchioco CS. Anaesthesia for dilatation, evacuation and curettage in outpatients: comparison of subanaesthetic doses of ketamine and sodium methohexitone-nitrous oxide anaesthesia. Can Anaesth Soc J 1977; 24: 110–117
73. White PF, Dworsky WA, Horai Y, Trevor AJ. Comparison of continuous infusion fentanyl or ketamine versus thiopental. Anesthesiology 1983; 59: 564–569
74. Forrest P, Galletly DC. Comparison of propofol and antagonised midazolam anaesthesia for day-case surgery. Anaesth Intensive Care 1987; 15: 394–401
75. Smith I, White PF, Nathanson M, Gouldson R. Propofol: an update on its clinical use. Anesthesiology 1994; (in press)
76. O'Toole DP, Milligan KR, Howe JP, McCollum JSC, Dundee JW. A comparison of propofol and methohexitone as induction agents for day case isoflurane anaesthesia. Anaesthesia 1987; 42: 373–376
77. Ræder JC, Misvær G. Comparison of propofol induction with thiopentone or methohexitone in short outpatient general anaesthesia. Acta Anaesthesiol Scand 1988; 32: 607–613
78. Doze VA, Westphal LM, White PF. Comparison of propofol with methohexital for outpatient anesthesia. Anesth Analg 1986; 65: 1189–1195
79. Servin F, Pommereau R, Rowan C, Nimier M, Desmonts JM. Comparison of intraoperative course and recovery following anesthesia with etomidate or propofol in patients over 80 years. Anesthesiology 1990; 73: A318

80 Sanders LD, Isaac PA, Yeomans WA, Clyburn PA, Rosen M, Robinson JO. Propofol-induced anaesthesia. Anaesthesia 1989; 44: 200–204

81 Valanne J, Korttila K. Comparison of methohexitone and propofol ('Diprivan') for induction of enflurane anaesthesia in outpatients. Postgrad Med J 1985; 61 (suppl 3): 138–143

82 Johnston R, Noseworthy T, Anderson B, Konopad E, Grace M. Propofol versus thiopental for outpatient anesthesia. Anesthesiology 1987; 67: 431–433

83 Mackenzie N, Grant IS. Comparison of the new emulsion formulation of propofol with methohexitone and thiopentone for induction of anaesthesia in day cases. Br J Anaesth 1985; 57: 725–731

84 White PF. Propofol: pharmacokinetics and pharmacodynamics. Semin Anesth 1988; 7: 4–20

85 Mirakhur RK. Induction characteristics of propofol in children: comparison with thiopentone. Anaesthesia 1988; 43: 593–598

86 Høgskilde S, Carl P, Sjøntoft E et al. Cardiovascular alterations following iv infusion of pregnanolone emulsion and its vehicle. Acta Anaesth Scand 1991; 35: O89

87 Carl P, Høgskilde S, Nielsen JW et al. Pregnanolone emulsion. Anaesthesia 1990; 45: 189–197

88 Van Hemelnjck J, Muller P, Van Allen H, White PF. Relative potency of eltanolone, propofol and thiopental for induction of anesthesia. Anesthesiology 1994; 80: 36–41

89 Wilton NCT, Thomas VL. Single breath induction of anaesthesia, using a vital capacity breath of halothane, nitrous oxide and oxygen. Anaesthesia 1986; 41: 472–476

90 Nightingale JJ, Stock JGL, McKiernan EP, Wilton NCT. Recovery after single-breath induction of anaesthesia in daycase patients. Anaesthesia 1988; 43: 554–556

91 Hannallah RS, Rosales JK. Experience with parents' presence during anaesthesia induction in children. Can Anaesth Soc J 1983; 30: 286–289

92 Braude N, Ridley SA, Sumner E. Parents and paediatric anaesthesia: a prospective survey of parental attitudes to their presence at induction. Ann R Coll Surg Engl 1990; 72: 41–44

93 Kingston HGG. Halothane and isoflurane anesthesia in pediatric outpatients. Anesth Analg 1986; 65: 181–184

94 Cattermole RW, Verghese C, Blair IJ, Jones CJH, Flynn PJ, Sebel PS. Isoflurane and halothane for outpatient dental anaesthesia in children. Br J Anaesth 1986; 58: 385–389

95 McAteer PM, Carter JA, Cooper GM, Prys-Roberts C. Comparison of isoflurane and halothane in outpatient paediatric dental anaesthesia. Br J Anaesth 1986; 58: 390–393

96 Raftery S, Warde D. Oxygen saturation during inhalation induction with halothane and isoflurane in children. Br J Anaesth 1990; 64: 167–169

97 Phillips AJ, Brimacombe JR, Simpson DL. Anaesthetic induction with isoflurane or halothane. Anaesthesia 1988; 43: 927–929

98 Pandit UA, Steude GM, Leach AB. Induction and recovery characteristics of isoflurane and halothane anaesthesia for short outpatient operations in children. Anaesthesia 1985; 40: 1126–1130

99 Carter JA, Dye AM, Cooper GM. Recovery from day-case anaesthesia. Anaesthesia 1985; 40: 545–548

100 Tracey JA, Holland AJC, Unger L. Morbidity in minor gynaecological surgery: a comparison of halothane, enflurane and isoflurane. Br J Anaesth 1982; 54: 1213–1215

101 Fisher DM, Robinson S, Brett CM, Perin G, Gregory GA. Comparison of enflurane, halothane, and isoflurane for diagnostic and therapeutic procedures in children with malignancies. Anesthesiology 1985; 63: 647–650

102 Simmons M, Miller CD, Cummings GC, Todd JG. Outpatient paediatric dental anaesthesia. Anaesthesia 1989; 44: 735–738

103 Warner LO, Beach TP, Garvin JP, Warner EJ. Halothane and children: the first quarter century. Anesth Analg 1984; 63: 838–840

104 Wark HJ. Postoperative jaundice in children: the influence of halothane. Anaesthesia 1983; 38: 237–242

105 Taylor R, Lerman J, Sikich N, Shandling B. Induction and recovery characteristics of desflurane in infants and children. Anesthesiology 1990; 73: A1246

106 Welborn L, Zwass M, Coté C et al. Comparison of desflurane and halothane anesthesia in pediatric ambulatory patients. Anesth Analg 1991; 72: S320

107 Smith I, Ding Y, White PF. Comparison of induction, maintenance and recovery characteristics of sevoflurane-N_2O and propofol-seroflurane-N_2O with propofol-isoflurane-N_2O. Anesth Analg 1992; 74: 253–259

108 Morisaki H, Suzuki G, Miyazawa N, Kiichi Y, Misaki T, Suzuki A. A clinical trial of sevoflurane in children for herniorrhaphy. J Anesth 1988; 2: 94–97

109 Naito Y, Tamai K, Shingu R, Fujimori R, Mori K. Comparison between sevoflurane and halothane for paediatric ambulatory anaesthesia. Br J Anaesth 1991; 67: 387–389

110 Cooper GM. Recovery from anaesthesia. Clin Anaesth 1984; 2: 145–162

111 Milligan KR, Howe JP, Dundee JW. Halothane and isoflurane in outpatient anaesthesia. Anaesthesia 1988; 43: 2–4

112 Stanford BJ, Plantevin OM, Gilbert JR. Morbidity after day-case gynaecological surgery. Br J Anaesth 1979; 51: 1143–1145

113 Fahy LT. Delayed convulsions after day case anaesthesia with enflurane. Anaesthesia 1987; 42: 1327–1328

114 Ghouri AF, Bodner M, White PF. Recovery profile after desflurane-nitrous oxide versus isoflurane-nitrous oxide in outpatients. Anesthesiology 1991; 74: 419–424

115 Van Hemelrijck J, Smith I, White PF. Use of desflurane for outpatient anesthesia: a comparison with propofol and nitrous oxide. Anesthesiology 1991; 75: 197–203

116 Fredman BD, Nathanson MH, Wang J, Klein K, White PF. Use of sevoflurane vs propofol for outpatient anesthesia: recovery profiles. Anesth Analg 1994; 78: S121

117 Mazze RI, Calverley RK, Smith NT. Inorganic fluoride nephrotoxicity. Anesthesiology 1977; 46: 265–271

118 White PF. Use of continuous infusion versus intermittent bolus administration of fentanyl or ketamine during outpatient anesthesia. Anesthesiology 1983; 59: 294–300

119 Moss E, Hindmarch I, Pain AJ, Edmondson RS. Comparison of recovery after halothane or alfentanil for minor surgery. Br J Anaesth 1987; 59: 970–977
120 Cartwright DP. Recovery after anaesthesia with alfentanil or halothane. Can Anaesth Soc J 1985; 32: 479–483
121 Howie MB, Hoffer LJ, Kryc J et al. TD. A comparison of enflurane with alfentanil anaesthesia for gynaecological surgery. Eur J Anaesth 1989; 6: 281–294
122 Biswas TK, Hatch PD. A comparison of alfentanil, halothane and enflurane as supplements for outpatient urological surgery. Anaesth Intensive Care 1989; 17: 275–279
123 Short SM, Rutherfoord CF, Sebel PS. A comparison between isoflurane and alfentanil supplemented anaesthesia for short procedures. Anaesthesia 1985; 40: 1160–1164
124 Azar I, Karambelkar DJ, Lear E. Neurologic state and psychomotor function following anesthesia for ambulatory surgery. Anesthesiology 1984; 60: 347–349
125 White PF, Coe V, Shafer A, Sung ML. Comparison of alfentanil with fentanyl for outpatient anesthesia. Anesthesiology 1986; 64: 99–106
126 Zuurmond WWA, Van Leeuwen L. Alfentanil v. isoflurane for outpatient arthroscopy. Acta Anaesth Scand 1986; 30: 329–331
127 Zuurmond WWA, Van Leeuwen L. Recovery from sufentanil anaesthesia for outpatient arthroscopy: a comparison with isoflurane. Acta Anaesth Scand 1987; 31: 154–156
128 Kennedy DJ, Ogg TW. Alfentanil and memory function. Anaesthesia 1985; 40: 537–540
129 Cooper GM, O'Connor M, Mark J, Harvey J. Effect of alfentanil and fentanyl on recovery from brief anaesthesia. Br J Anaesth 1983; 55: 179S–182S
130 Collin RIW, Drummond GB, Spence AA. Alfentanil supplemented anaesthesia for short procedures. Anaesthesia 1986; 41: 477–481
131 Koskinen R, Tigerstedt I, Tammisto T. The effect of peroperative alfentanil on the need of immediate postoperative pain relief. Acta Anaesth Scand 1991; 35: 21
132 Smith I, Van Hemelrijck J, White PF. Efficacy of esmolol versus alfentanil as a supplement to propofol-N_2O anaesthesia. Anesth Analg 1991; 73: 540–546
133 Yee P, Galletly DC. Recovery from day-stay anaesthesia — a comparison of an intravenous and inhalational technique of maintenance. Anaesth Intensive Care 1985; 13: 380–382
134 DeGrood PMRM, Harbers JBM, Van Egmond J, Crul JF. Anaesthesia for laparoscopy. Anaesthesia 1987; 42: 815–823
135 Puttick N, Rosen M. Propofol induction and maintenance with nitrous oxide in paediatric outpatient dental anaesthesia. Anaesthesia 1988; 43: 646–649
136 Millar JM, Jewkes CF. Recovery and morbidity after daycase anaesthesia. Anaesthesia 1988; 43: 738–743
137 Gold MI, Sacks DJ, Grosnoff DB, Herrington CA. Comparison of propofol with thiopental and isoflurane for induction and maintenance of general anaesthesia. J Clin Anesth 1989; 1: 272–276
138 Doze VA, Shafer A, White PF. Propofol-nitrous oxide versus thiopental-isoflurane-nitrous oxide for general anaesthesia. Anesthesiology 1988; 69: 63–71

139 Milligan KR, O'Toole DP, Howe JP, Cooper JC, Dundee JW. Recovery from outpatient anaesthesia: a comparison of incremental propofol and propofol-isoflurane. Br J Anaesth 1987; 59: 1111–1114
140 Ghignone M, Quintin L, Duke PC, Kehler CH, Calvillo O. Effects of clonidine on narcotic requirements and hemodynamic response during induction of fentanyl anesthesia and endotracheal intubation. Anesthesiology 1986; 64: 36–42
141 Flacke JW, Bloor BC, Flacke WE et al. Reduced narcotic requirement by clonidine with improved hemodynamic and adrenergic stability in patients undergoing coronary bypass surgery. Anesthesiology 1987; 67: 11–19
142 Segal IS, Jarvis DA, Duncan SR, White PF, Maze M. Perioperative use of transdermal clonidine as an adjunctive agent. Anesth Analg 1989; 68: S250
143 Erkola O, Aho M, Kallio A, Scheinin H, Korttila K. Dexmedetomidine infusion as anaesthetic adjuvant. Acta Anaesth Scand 1991; 35: O80
144 Aantaa R, Kanto J, Scheinin M, Kallio A, Scheinin H. Dexmedetomidine, an α_2-adrenoceptor agonist, reduces anesthetic requirements for patients undergoing minor gynecologic surgery. Anesthesiology 1990; 73: 230–235
145 Aho MS, Erkola OA, Scheinin H, Lehtinen A-M, Korttila KT. Effect of intravenously administered dexmedetomidine on pain after laparoscopic tubal ligation. Anesth Analg 1991; 73: 112–118
146 Monk TG, Mueller M, White PF. Treatment of stress response during balanced anesthesia. Anesthesiology 1992; 76: 39–45
147 Parnass SM, Rothenberg DM, Kerchberger JP, Ivankovich AD. A single bolus dose of esmolol in the prevention of intubation-induced tachycardia and hypertension in an ambulatory surgery unit. J Clin Anesth 1990; 2: 232–237
148 Flaatten H, Raeder J. Spinal anaesthesia for outpatient surgery. Anaesthesia 1985; 40: 1108–1111
149 Flaatten H, Rodt S, Rosland J, Vamnes J. Postoperative headache in young patients after spinal anaesthesia. Anaesthesia 1987; 42: 202–205
150 Clarke GA, Power KJ. Spinal anaesthesia for day case surgery. Ann R Coll Surg Engl 1988; 70: 144–146
151 Kang SB, Goodnough DE, Lee YK, Olsen RA, Krueger LS. Spinal anesthesia with 27-gauge needles for ambulatory surgery patients. Anesthesiology 1990; 73: A2
152 Flanagan JF, Kumatta D, Black D. Comparison of 24 gauge Sprotte and 27 gauge Quincke needle on the incidence of post dural puncture headache. Anesth Analg 1991; 72: S75
153 Moote CA, Varkey GP, Komar WE. Similar incidence of post-dural puncture headache after conventional vs continuous spinal anesthesia. Anesth Analg 1991; 72: S190
154 Farhie SE. Postoperative care after regional anesthesia. Int Anesth Clin 1983; 21: 157–171
155 Carbaat PAT, Van Crevel H. Lumbar puncture headache: controlled study on the preventive effect of 24 hours' bed rest. Lancet 1981: ii: 1133–1135
156 Davis WJ, Lennon RL, Wedel DJ. Outpatient brachial plexus anesthesia. Anesthesiology 1990; 73: A26

157 Baysinger CL, Bowe EA, Bowe LS, Sykes LA. Brachial plexus blockade versus general anesthesia for orthopedic operations on the upper extremity in outpatients. Anesthesiology 1990; 73: A43

158 Ræder JC, Børdahl P, Nordentoft J, Kirste U. Local anaesthesia versus general anaesthesia (TIVA) for outpatient laparoscopic sterilisation. Acta Anaesth Scand 1991; 35: O1

160 O'Sullivan G, Kerr-Muir M, Lim M, Davies W, Campbell N. Day-case ophthalmic surgery: general or local anaesthesia? Anaesthesia 1990; 45: 885–886

161 White PF, Vasconez LO, Mathes SA, Way WL, Wender LA. Comparison of midazolam and diazepam for sedation during plastic surgery. J Plast Reconst Surg 1988; 81: 703–710

162 Goodacre TEE, Sanders R, Watts DA, Stoker M. Split skin grafting using topical local anaesthetia (EMLA): a comparison with infiltrated anaesthesia. Br J Plast Surg 1988; 41: 533–538

163 Monk TG, Ding Y, White PF. Analgesic efficacy of EMLA during outpatient shock-wave lithotripsy. Anesth Analg 1992; 74: S213

164 Pettersson B, Tiselius HG, Andersson A, Eriksson I. Evaluation of extracorporeal shock wave lithotripsy without anaesthesia using a Dornier HM3 lithotriptor without technical modifications. J Urol 1989; 142: 1189–1192

165 Philip BK. Supplemental medication for ambulatory procedures under regional anesthesia. Anesth Analg 1985; 64: 1117–1125

166 Smith I, White PF. Use of intravenous adjuvants during local and regional anesthesia. Curr Rev Clin Anesth 1992; 12: 146–151

167 Urquhart ML, White PF. Comparison of sedative infusions during regional anesthesia — methohexital, etomidate, and midazolam. Anesth Analg 1989; 68: 249–254

168 Bailey PL, Pace NL, Ashburn MA, Moll JWB, East KA, Stanley TH. Frequent hypoxemia and apnea after sedation with midazolam and fentanyl. Anesthesiology 1990; 73: 826–830

169 Dubois A, Balatoni E, Peeters JP, Baudoux M. Use of propofol for sedation during gastrointestinal endoscopies. Anaesthesia 1988; 43 (suppl): 75–80

170 Smith I, Monk TG, White PF, Ding Y. Propofol infusion during regional anesthesia: sedative, amnestic and anxiolytic properties. Anesth Analg 1994; 79: 313–319

171 White PF, Negus JB. Sedative infusions during local and regional anesthesia: a comparison of midazolam and propofol. J Clin Anesth 1991; 3: 32–39

172 White PF, Shafer A, Boyle III WA, Doze VA, Duncan S. Benzodiazepine antagonism does not provoke a stress response. Anesthesiology 1989; 70: 636–639

173 Ghouri AF, Ruiz R, MA, White PF. Effect of flumazenil on recovery after midazolam and propofol sedation. Anesthesiology 1994; 81: 333–339

174 Monk TG, Bouré B, White PF, Meretyk S, Clayman RV. Comparison of intravenous sedative-analgesic techniques for outpatient immersion lithotripsy. Anesth Analg 1991; 72: 616–621

175 Monk TG, Rater JM, White PF. Comparison of alfentanil and ketamine infusions in combination with midazolam for outpatient lithotripsy. Anesthesiology 1991; 74: 1023–1028

176 Zelcer J, White PF, Chester S, Paull JD, Molnar R. Intraoperative patient-controlled analgesia: an alternative to physicians administration during outpatient monitored anesthesia care. Anesth Analg 1992; 75: 41–44

177 Park WY, Watkins PA. Patient-controlled sedation during epidural anaesthesia. Anesth Analg 1991; 72: 304–307

178 Andersen R, Krohg K. Pain as a major cause of postoperative nausea. Can Anaesth Soc J 1976; 23: 366–369

179 Ding Y, White PF. Comparative effects of ketorolac, dezocine and fentanyl as adjuvant, during outpatient anesthesia. Anesth Analg 1992; 75: 566–571

180 White PF. Use of patient-controlled analgesia for management of acute pain. JAMA 1988; 259: 243–247

181 Chandler LH, White PF. Ambulatory PCA — a new approach to postoperative pain management. Anesth Analg 1991; 72: S33

182 Taylor E, White PF. Does the anesthetic technique influence the postoperative analgesic requirement? Clin J Pain 1991; 7: 139–142

183 Urquhart ML, Klapp K, White PF. Patient-controlled analgesia: a comparison of intravenous versus subcutaneous hydromorphone. Anesthesiology 1988; 69: 428–432

184 White PF. Subcutaneous-PCA: an alternative to iv-PCA for postoperative pain management. Clin J Pain 1990; 6: 297–300

185 Shah MV, Jones DI, Rosen M. "Patient demand" postoperative analgesia with buprenorphine. Br J Anaesth 1986; 58: 508–511

186 Bell MDD, Mishra P, Weldon BD, Murray GR, Calvey TN, Williams NE. Buccal morphine — a new route for analgesia? Lancet 1985; 1: 71–73

187 Abboud TK, Zhu J, Gangolly J et al. Transnasal analgesics: a new method for pain relief in post-cesarean section patients. Anesthesiology 1988; 69: A657

188 Sebel PS, Barrett CW, Kirk CJC, Heykants J. Transdermal absorption of fentanyl and sufentanil in man. Eur J Clin Pharmacol 1987; 32: 529–531

189 Foster JMG, Cashman JN, Jones RM. Parenteral aspirin for pain relief in day-case dental anaesthesia. Anaesthesia 1985; 40: 576–578

190 McLoughlin C, McKinney MS, Fee JPH, Boules Z. Diclofenac for day-care arthroscopy surgery: comparison with a standard opioid therapy. Br J Anaesth 1990; 65: 620–623

191 Gillies GWA, Kenny GNC, Bullingham RES, McArdle CS. The morphine sparing effect of ketorolac tromethamine. Anaesthesia 1987; 42: 727–731

192 Campbell WI, Kendrick R. Intravenous diclofenac sodium. Anaesthesia 1990; 45: 763–766

193 Dalens B, Hasnaoui A. Caudal anesthesia in pediatric surgery: success rate and adverse effects in 750 consecutive patients. Anesth Analg 1989; 68: 83–89

194 Hannallah RS, Broadman LM, Belman AB, Abramowitz MD, Epstein BS. Comparion of caudal and ilioinguinal/iliohypogastric nerve blocks for control of post-orchidopexy pain in pediatric ambulatory surgery. Anesthesiology 1987; 66: 832–834

195 Vater M, Wandless J. Caudal or dorsal nerve block? Acta Anaesthesiol Scand 1985; 29: 175–179
196 Casey WF, Rice LJ, Hannallah RS, Broadman L, Norden JM, Guzzetta P. A comparison between bupivacaine instillation versus ilioinguinal/iliohypogastric nerve block for postoperative analgesia folowing inguinal herniorrhaphy in children. Anesthesiology 1990; 72: 637–639
197 Sinclair R, Cassuto J, Högström S et al. Topical anesthesia with lidocaine aerosol in the control of postoperative pain. Anesthesiology 1988; 68: 895–901
198 Tree-Trakarn T, Pirayavaraporn S. Postoperative pain relief for circumcision in children: comparison among morphine, nerve block and topical analgesia. Anesthesiology 1985; 62: 519–522
199 Tree-Trakarn T, Pirayavaraporn S, Lertakyamanee J. Topical analgesia for relief of post-circumcision pain. Anesthesiology 1987; 67: 395–399
200 Anonymous. Analgesia in children after day-case surgery. Lancet 1988; i: 1084–1085
201 Partridge BL, Stabile BE. The effects of incisional bupivacaine on postoperative narcotic requirements, oxygen saturation and length of stay in the post-anesthesia care unit. Acta Anaesthesiol Scand 1990; 34: 486–491
202 Moss G. Discharge within 24 hours of elective cholecystectomy. Arch Surg 1986; 121: 1159–1161
203 McKenzie R, Phitayakorn P, Uy NTL et al. Topical bupivacaine and etidocaine analgesia following fallopian tube banding. Can J Anaesth 1989; 36: 510–514
204 Kaplan P, Freund R, Squires J, Herz M. Control of immediate postoperative pain with topical bupivacaine hydrochloride for laparoscopic fallope ring tubal ligation. Obstet Gynecol 1990; 76: 798–802
205 Bourne MH, Johnson KA. Postoperative pain relief using local anesthetic instillation. Foot Ankle 1988; 8: 350–351
206 Smith I, Van Hemelrijck J, White PF, Shively R. Effects of local anesthesia on recovery after outpatient arthroscopy. Anesth Analg 1991; 73: 536–539
207 Egbert LD, Battit GE, Welch CE, Bartlett MK. Reduction of postoperative pain by encouragement and instruction of patients. N Engl J Med 1964; 270: 825–827
208 Jensen JE, Conn RR, Hazelrigg G, Hewett JE. The use of transcutaneous neural stimulation and isokinetic testing in arthroscopic knee surgery. Am J Sports Med 1985; 13: 27–33
209 Khiroya RC, Davenport HT, Jones JG. Cryoanalgesia for pain after herniorrhaphy. Anaesthesia 1986; 41: 73–76
210 Bodner M, White PF. Antiemetic efficacy of ondansetron after outpatient laparoscopy. Anesth Analg 1991; 73: 250–254
211 Uppington J, Dunnet J, Blogg CE. Transdermal hyoscine and postoperative nausea and vomiting. Anaesthesia 1986; 41: 16–20
212 Tigerstedt I, Salmela L, Aromaa U. Double-blind comparison of transdermal scopolamine, droperidol and placebo against postoperative nausea and vomiting. Acta Anaesth Scand 1988; 32: 454–457
213 Diamond MJ, Keeri-Szanto M. Reduction of postoperative vomiting by preoperative administration of oral metoclopramide. Can Anaesth Soc J 1980; 27: 36–39
214 Madej TH, Simpson KH. Comparison of the use of domperidone, droperidol and metoclopramide in the prevention of nausea and vomiting following gynaecological surgery in day cases. Br J Anaesth 1986; 58: 879–883
215 Lerman J, Eustis S, Smith DR. Effect of droperidol pretreatment on postanesthetic vomiting in children undergoing strabismus surgery. Anesthesiology 1986; 65: 322–325
216 Korttila K, Kauste A, Auvinen J. Comparison of domperidone, droperidol, and metoclopramide in the prevention and treatment of nausea and vomiting after balanced general anesthesia. Anesth Analg 1979; 58: 396–400
217 McKenzie R, Kovac A, O'Connor T et al. Comparison of ondansetron versus placebo to prevent postoperative nausea and vomiting in women undergoing ambulatory gynecologic surgery. Anesthesiology 1993; 78: 21–28
218 Alon E, Himmelseher S. Ondansetron in the treatment of postoperative vomiting: a randomized, double-blind comparison with droperidol and metoclopramide. Anesth Analg 1992; 75: 561–565
219 Watcha MF, Smith I. Cost effectiveness analysis of antiemetic therapy for ambulatory surgery. J Clin Anesth 1994; 6: 370–377
220 Artuso JD, Panico FG. Effects of mechanical evacuation of gastric contents on postoperative nausea and vomiting. Anesthesiology 1990; 73: A1068
221 Schulman SR. The effect of gastric suction on postoperative nausea and vomiting in children. Anesth Analg 1991; 72: S240
222 Kraynack BJ, Bates MF. IV ranitidine reduces nausea and vomiting after propofol-isoflurane anesthesia. Anesth Analg 1991; 72: S145
223 Kraynack BJ, Bates MF. Ranitidine reduces nausea and vomiting after thiopental-isoflurane anesthesia. Anesthesiology 1990; 73: A42
224 Cohen SE, Woods WA, Wyner J. Antiemetic efficacy of droperidol and metoclopramide. Anesthesiology 1984; 60: 67–69
225 O'Donovan N, Shaw J. Nausea and vomiting in day-case dental anaesthesia. Anaesthesia 1984; 39: 1172–1176
226 McCollum JSC, Milligan KR, Dundee JW. The antiemetic action of propofol. Anaesthesia 1988; 43: 239–240
227 Watcha MF, Simeon RM, White PF, Steven JL. Effect of propofol on the incidence of postoperative vomiting after strabismus surgery in pediatric outpatients. Anesthesiology 1991; 75: 204–209
228 Bowe EA, Baysinger CL, Sykes LA, Bowe LS. Subarachnoid blockade versus general anesthesia for knee arthroscopy in out-patients. Anesthesiology 1990; 73: A45
229 Dundee JW, Chestnutt WN, Ghaly RG, Lynas AGA. Traditional Chinese acupuncture: a potentially useful antiemetic? Br Med J 1986; 293: 583–584
230 Fry ENS. Acupressure and postoperative vomiting. Anaesthesia 1986; 41: 661–662
231 Kitz DS, Robinson DM, Schiavone PA, Walsh PR, Conahan TJ. Discharging outpatients. AORN J 1988; 48: 87–91

232 Moore DC. Spinal anesthesia: bupivacaine compared with tetracaine. Anesth Analg 1980; 59: 743–750
233 Chung F. Are discharge criteria changing? J Clin Anesth 1993; 5 (suppl 1): 64S–68S
234 Ogg TW. An assessment of postoperative outpatient cases. Br Med J 1972; 4: 573–576
235 Lichtor JI, Sah J, Apfelbaum J, Zacny J, Coalson D. Some patients may drink or drive after ambulatory surgery. Anesthesiology 1990; 73: A1083
236 Gold BS, Kitz DS, Lecky JH, Neuhaus JM. Unanticipated admission to the hospital following ambulatory surgery. JAMA 1989; 262: 3008–3010
237 White PF. Outpatient anesthesia — an overview: In: White PF, ed. Outpatient anaesthesia. New York: Churchill Livingstone, 1990: pp 1–48
238 Smith I, White PF. Outpatient anaesthesia. In: Nimmo WS, Rowbotham DJ, Smith G (eds) Anaesthesia, 2nd edn. Oxford: Blackwell; 1994: pp 956–981
239 White PF, Shafer A. Nausea and vomiting: causes and prophylaxis. Sem Anesth 1987; 6: 300–308
240 White PF. Outpatient anesthesia. In: Miller RD, ed. Anesthesia. New York: Churchill Livingstone, 1990: pp 2025–2060
241 Korttila K. Recovery period and discharge. In: White PF, ed. Outpatient anaesthesia. New York: Churchill Livingstone, 1990: pp 369–395
242 Cook TL, Beppu WJ, Hitt BA, Kosek JC, Mazze RI. Renal effects and metabolism of sevoflurane in Fischer 344 rats. Anesthesiology 1975; 43: 70–77

18. Anaesthesia for non-surgical interventions

A. W. Harrop-Griffiths

A review of anaesthetic care for individual non-surgical interventions forms the major part of this chapter but the general principles underlying the safe management of patients undergoing these procedures is first reviewed. These will be addressed in four sections: personnel, equipment, patient factors and physical environment.

PERSONNEL

Ideally, all anaesthetic care is provided by a senior anaesthetist experienced in the procedure to be undertaken or by a trainee supervised by such an individual. As the majority of procedures requiring anaesthetic involvement consist of operations performed in operating theatres, either in scheduled sessions or as emergencies, senior anaesthetic staff are rostered to be available to manage these procedures. However, non-surgical interventions are often not afforded such arrangements. Procedures such as computed tomography (CT) and cardiac catheterization do not necessarily require the involvement of an anaesthetist unless the hospital is a specialist paediatric facility. Frequently, the provision of an experienced anaesthetist for patients undergoing these procedures is not made, and if an anaesthetist is required, the task is often delegated to an unsupervised trainee. Similarly, in the ideal situation, the anaesthetist should be accompanied by a trained assistant. The supply of such trained assistants is often matched to regular operating theatre workload and they may not be available when required for occasional employment in non-operating theatre locations.

Therefore, it is important to the safe provision of anaesthetic care for non-surgical procedures that the same standards of supply of senior anaesthetists and anaesthetic assistance be met for both surgical and non-surgical interventions. Indeed, it may be argued that anaesthesia at these 'remote locations' requires a greater level of training and competence than that in large operating theatre suites where a number of anaesthetists are usually available to assist with an emergency.

EQUIPMENT

It is not unusual for equipment from the main operating theatres to be passed on to other locations, such as the X-ray department, radiotherapy unit and cardiovascular laboratory — the sites of non-surgical interventions. Moreover, these sites are sometimes lacking some equipment that might be considered part of standard monitoring in the main operating theatres. It is an important principle that whatever level of anaesthetic and monitoring equipment is deemed appropriate for the anaesthetic care of patients within an institution, it is provided at all locations where anaesthetics are liable to be given. The regular servicing and maintenance of equipment at remote locations must also be ensured to assist safe management.

PATIENT FACTORS

The patient presenting for a non-surgical intervention may have had inadequate pre-operative assessment and investigation. This may occur for a number of reasons:

1. ineffective communication between the physicians managing the patient and the anaesthetic department
2. patient admission only shortly before the procedure to be undertaken
3. lack of appreciation of the physiological impact of the intervention and of anaesthesia if required
4. low prioritization of the procedure.

It is important that patients presenting for non-surgical procedures should receive the same quality of investigation and preparation as any patient undergoing a surgical procedure.

PHYSICAL ENVIRONMENT

It is reasonable to suggest that the ideal environment for the administration of anaesthesia would be a large well-lit room free from obstructions and containing a table capable of being placed in the Trendelenburg position on which is lying a patient to whom the anaesthetist has unrestricted access. In contrast to this ideal is the average CT or magnetic resonance imaging (MRI) scanner room. Although many of the constraints placed upon the anaesthetist by the physical environment of the non-surgical intervention are unavoidable, some of them occur because of inadequate consultation with anaesthetists in the planning stage of new facilities. As far as is reasonably possible, the environment must be made conducive to safe anaesthetic management.

The department should review arrangements for its personnel, equipment, patient preparation and facilities on a regular basis. Audit systems need to be developed and extended to the non-surgical procedure environment so that the provision of suitable anaesthetic care can be monitored, preventable morbidity identified and action taken to prevent recurrence. It is the adoption of such a pro-active approach that underlies the continuing safe anaesthetic care for non-surgical interventions. It appears likely that the frequency of such interventions will increase as new investigational techniques and therapeutic manoeuvres not requiring surgery are developed. Anaesthetists must be involved in the development and planning for the safe conduct of such techniques within an institution in order to minimize risk.

RADIOLOGY

Computed tomography

The primary requirement for a successful CT scan is that the patient should lie motionless in order to minimize movement artefacts and so attain the best possible image. The procedure is not painful and therefore the vast majority of patients can fulfil this requirement without the assistance of an anaesthetist. However, there are specific groups of patients for whom this is not possible. They include the very young, the confused or disoriented, those with movement disorders and the restless, whether through pain or anxiety. Patients in these groups may require an anaesthetist to provide general anaesthesia or sedation with monitored anaesthetic care. An anaesthetist may also be needed when very ill patients, or those requiring controlled ventilation in an intensive care facility, are subjected to CT scanning.

Pre-operative assessment

Although CT scanning can be used to assess a wide variety of pathological conditions, it is often used to provide information about intracranial pathology, or neoplastic disease within the thorax or abdomen. The potential for these disease processes to affect the conduct of the anaesthetic must be evaluated. For instance, if the scan is directed towards the detection of intracranial pathology, the possibility of raised intracranial pressure must be considered and managed appropriately. In addition to a full standard pre-operative assessment, these specific areas of interest must also be addressed.

Communication with the radiologist should be made with regard to the likely duration of the scan and the desirability of ventilatory control. The quality of scans of the thorax and upper abdomen[1] can be affected by movement artefacts and if artificial breath-holding is required, the anaesthetist may have to plan to use neuromuscular-blocking agents. The use of premedicant drugs should be based on the assessment of the patient and consideration of the planned anaesthetic technique. It is not uncommon that well-judged premedication, if appropriate, is all that is necessary to provide a calm and adequately immobile subject for CT scanning.

Preparation

CT scanning rooms are often poorly lit and may be cramped. The anaesthetist should ensure that all anaesthetic and resuscitative equipment is available and functioning in the CT scan room before anaesthesia begins. Trained assistance should be available. Breathing systems and monitoring equipment should have sufficiently long attachments to the patient to allow movement of the scan platform without disconnection. A tipping trolley should be available in the scan room for induction of anaesthesia before the patient is transferred to the scan platform.

Anaesthesia

As the scan is conducted with the patient in a small, dark tunnel, access to the head is often difficult and airway management presents a major point of consideration to anaesthetists. Sedation, whether given in the form of premedication, or intravenously just prior to scanning, is occasionally needed for children or anxious adult patients. If heavy sedation is used, the movements associated with even a modest degree of airway obstruction can result in the production of poor images.[2] Many units successfully use ketamine anaesthesia for children undergoing CT scans, although caution must be exercised in its use in those with suspected raised intracranial pressure.[3] If tracheal intubation is employed to secure and maintain the airway, great care must be exercised in ensuring that kinking of the tracheal tube or disconnection of the breathing system does not occur. Intubation of infants and children may give rise to a significant incidence of post-extubation stridor.[2] The laryngeal mask airway is achieving greater popularity for the maintenance of airway integrity during a CT scan, but a high degree of vigilance should be maintained as kinking has been reported.[4] If tracheal intubation is employed, the use of controlled ventilation should be guided by the requirements of the scan and the likely pathology being investigated — it would be wise to produce modest hyperventilation in those with suspected raised intracranial pressure. Similarly, the choice of inhaled anaesthetic agent should be guided not only by the anaesthetist's preference but also by the patient's likely pathology. Total intravenous anaesthesia has been used successfully in the CT scanner room, although one report on the use of etomidate in this respect noted a high incidence of involuntary movements.[5] Propofol has been investigated as the sole anaesthetic agent for children undergoing CT scanning.[6] It was found to be similar in most respects to thiopentone (with which it was compared), except that recovery time was significantly shorter after propofol. Rectal midazolam has also received attention for this application, but with variable results.[7] On balance, there is no ideal anaesthetic for patients undergoing CT scanning.

Other factors worthy of consideration in relation to CT scanning are the radiation hazards and the use of intravenous contrast media. Radiation exposure during a CT brain scan is similar to that of a skull X-ray,[8] and although this does not represent a large radiation hazard, all personnel should wear appropriate lead protection during scanning and carry film badges to assess longer-term radiation exposure. Intravenous contrast media are commonly used during CT scanning in order to enhance image quality. Such media carry with them a significant incidence of adverse reactions and the anaesthetist must be alert to this possibility. On occasions, radiologists may request that contrast be swallowed by the patient shortly before scanning. This requires an alteration in anaesthetic technique because of the risk of regurgitation.

Multiply traumatized patients must be fully evaluated and their condition stabilized before transfer to the CT scanning facility as there is rarely the space, equipment or personnel in a CT scanner room to manage a patient who suffers acute physiological decompensation.

Before considering the transfer of patients from an intensive therapy unit careful consideration must be given to the patient's suitability for physical transfer.

CT scanning is rarely a life-saving procedure, and the transfer of a patient dependent on positive end-expiratory pressure or inotropic agents is often complicated by technical difficulties in maintaining such therapeutic modalities continuously on the journey to and from the scanning table. Continuous invasive monitoring, although facilitated by the introduction of portable devices, may be difficult during transfer. Appropriate portable ventilation, monitoring and infusion systems must be available before transfer is contemplated.

Magnetic resonance imaging

The development of new therapeutic and diagnostic techniques in medicine presents an ever-increasing challenge to the ingenuity of anaesthetists intent on providing safe care for their patients. Of the recent developments in imaging techniques, none has provided a greater challenge than MRI. While CT scanning has demanded that the patient be immobile in a short dark tunnel at a remote location, MRI has made this demand in a long, dark, noisy tunnel with the added inconvenience of strong and varying magnetic fields.

Many of the general and organizational considerations discussed in previous sections are pertinent to a discussion of anaesthesia for MRI. As with CT scanning, it is usually the young, the sick, the confused and the restless who require anaesthesia. However, to these can be added the claustrophobic. The incidence of claustrophobia sufficiently severe to necessitate general anaesthesia for MRI is up to 7%.[9] The physical and biophysical principles involved in MRI have been reviewed by Nixon and colleagues.[9] There are three physical components of interest to the anaesthetist — static magnetic field, changing magnetic fields and radiofrequency radiation.

Static magnetic field

A static magnetic field of up to 2 T (the earth's magnetic field is 0.00005 T) is used in MRI. This provides a powerful attraction for any ferromagnetic object within the immediate environment of the magnet. Metal objects such as scissors, pens and keys may therefore become fast-moving projectiles and must be excluded from the scanning environment. Ferromagnetic elements contained within the patient may also be displaced, including potential for dislodgement of metal vascular clips on an intracranial aneurysm.[10] Cardiac pacemakers are also at risk, not only from inactivation or conversion to an inappropriate mode by closure of the reed switch, but also from movement causing displacement of the pacemaker box or wire.[11] Other implanted materials are also potentially at risk, although heart valves and cochlear or stapedial implants seldom include ferromagnetic material. Make-ups and tattoos which include metallic dyes have been associated with local irritation.[12]

Changing magnetic fields

Rapidly changing magnetic fields are also utilized in the scanning process. These have the capacity for creating internal electrical currents which, although insufficient to damage biological tissues, may disturb the functioning of pacemaker microcircuitry.[11] A theoretical possibility also exists that these microcurrents may induce seizures in epileptics. However, such an occurrence has not yet been reported.

Radiofrequency radiation

The use of radiofrequency radiation in the scanning process may give rise to the heating of metal implants.[13] Although the degree of heating likely to occur is insufficient to present a risk to patients, caution should be exercised in the scanning of patients with large metal implants.

Occupational risks

Ionizing radiation is not utilized in MRI. Magnetic fields have not been shown to harm tissues and no oncological or genotoxic effects have been found. However, caution has been advised in the use of MRI in the first trimester of pregnancy.[14]

Anaesthetic problems

The problems encountered in providing anaesthetic care for patients undergoing MRI may be divided into two areas: problems with anaesthetic equipment and problems with monitoring.

Equipment

Any loose ferromagnetic object taken close to the magnet is likely to fly towards it and lodge in its midst; the routine practice of anaesthesia is based to a significant extent on the use of loose ferromagnetic objects. In addition, large ferromagnetic objects placed close to the magnet can cause image distortion.

Anaesthetic machines are now constructed mostly of stainless steel which, although ferrous, is not magnetic. However, in many machines, support structures, castors and portions of the cylinder supports are ferromagnetic while gas cylinders almost always are. One solution that has been described has been a modification of a standard anaesthetic machine in which all ferromagnetic elements are replaced with equivalents made from stainless steel or aluminium.[15] The expense of this approach may not appeal to some clinicians, but the logic behind it is sound. An alternative approach which allows the machine to stay close to the magnet is to bolt it securely to the wall of the scanner room, although the possibility that this may cause image distortion should be anticipated.

Most anaesthetic ventilators are incompatible with proximity to an MRI scanner. There exist some pneumatically driven, fluidic-controlled, volume-cycled ventilators which are MRI-compatible.[14] A Servo 900C ventilator has been used in close proximity to the magnet, but great caution must be exercised as the positive end-expiratory pressure valve is controlled by a solenoid.

Assessments of the magnetic attractiveness of items of anaesthetic equipment have been made.[9] Items such as metal tracheal tube connectors, intravenous needles and ballpoint pens contain ferromagnetic material but cannot compare with the attractiveness of a standard laryngoscope. Attempts to overcome this problem include the manufacture of plastic laryngoscopes, but as the batteries of a laryngoscope experience a far greater magnetic force than the laryngoscope itself, a more successful approach has been the development of remote direct current power sources for laryngoscopes.[16]

Although it is possible to modify almost all anaesthetic equipment to contain a safe minimum of ferromagnetic material, the solution most often preferred is the removal of anaesthetic machine, equipment and associated paraphernalia from the scanner room. This cost-effective and pragmatic approach necessitates the provision of an area close to the scanner where anaesthesia can be induced, the placement of the patient on a table or scanning platform which can be rapidly moved during a scan should the need for urgent anaesthetic intervention arise, and the use of an extended anaesthetic breathing system to link the patient safely to the machine.

Monitoring

As the patient undergoing MRI is often hidden in the bore of the magnet during the procedure, adequate monitoring becomes an imperative, and it is an important principle that appropriate monitoring of the patient should not, if at all possible, be compromised by the physical limitations of the scanning environment.

The static magnetic field distorts the cathode ray display of many monitors used in the anaesthetic setting, and the achievement of an adequate picture may require the removal of the display from the scanning room or its orientation so as to minimize the distortion. Electrical wire connections between patient and monitor can act as radiofrequency antennae and can cause distortion of the MRI image.

Electrocardiogram (ECG) systems that include non-ferrous fasteners and electrodes along with signal conduction by telemetry or fibre-optic cables have been used to achieve satisfactory traces, but some form of signal gating is necessary to produce useful results due to radiofrequency interference. T-wave abnormalities of the ECG may be noted in fields greater than 0.3 T.[17] Although striking in their nature, they are free from any association with blood pressure changes, arrhythmias or changes in heart rate.[18]

Pulse oximeters have been found to function adequately, but may suffer periods of interrupted function if placed less that 2 m from the magnet. The probe should be placed on an extremity as far as possible from the scan site and the probe lead conducted some distance to the monitor. A case of burn injury to a finger has been reported in association with the use of a pulse oximeter during MRI when loops of wire were allowed to form.[19]

Automated non-invasive blood pressure monitoring using an oscillometric method is effective in the MRI setting. The use of plastic cuff connectors and extended tubing is necessary. The monitor itself should be placed as far from the magnet as possible. Invasive monitoring systems using either long manometer lines or fibre-optic conduction have been used successfully.

Respiratory gas analysis is an effective method for monitoring ventilation and breathing system integrity. Long sampling lines are required if the monitor itself is to be kept remote from the magnet. Mixing of gas within long lines may give rise to some inaccuracy of carbon dioxide measurements and difficulty in interpretation of waveforms.

Practical application

The vast majority of patients undergoing MRI need no assistance from an anaesthetist. Simple premedication and sedation techniques suffice for most of those who require pharmacological help to stay still and calm in the magnet. The anaesthetist may be involved in monitoring these patients.

A small number of patients need general anaesthesia for MRI. Pre-operative assessment, investigation and preparation should follow standard procedures. Although there is no evidence that the choice of anaesthetic agent affects image quality, it has been reported[9] that controlled ventilation provides superior images when compared with spontaneous ventilation. In a situation where instant access to the patient may not be possible, the patient's airway should, of course, be secured. Tracheal intubation must be considered to be the standard technique at present, although the use of a laryngeal mask airway has recently been described.[20]

If a wall-mounted, well-secured or non-ferromagnetic anaesthetic machine is available close to the magnet, the choice of anaesthetic breathing system should not present a problem. However, the anaesthetic machine is often kept some distance from the magnet. It is then necessary to use an anaesthetic breathing system which can be extended, often to a length of some metres. The Bain system has achieved popularity for this use[14] as it is light, flexible and can be used for either controlled or spontaneous ventilation. Its successful use in paediatric patients undergoing MRI has been described.[21]

When the patient has been anaesthetized and placed on the MRI scanner platform, the breathing tubes and monitoring leads or lines should be secured in such a way that movement of the platform will not give rise to their disconnection. In recently established units, purpose-built ducts are often available through which tubes, lines and leads can be led to the anaesthetic machine and monitors. If problems arise during the conduct of the anaesthetic that require the intervention of the anaesthetist, the patient should be moved into the area of the anaesthetic machine.

A well-designed MRI unit should have adequate recovery facilities. In addition to this, a trained recovery nurse or the continuing presence of the anaesthetist will be necessary until the patient is stable and fully awake.

Arteriography

The advent of digital subtraction angiography (DSA) techniques has substantially reduced the demands upon anaesthetic departments for general anaesthesia for arteriographic investigations. Some centres still practise direct arteriographic techniques, particularly for intracranial lesions, as vascular structures along the base of the skull may be poorly visualized by DSA. In the UK, some centres still conduct the majority of cerebral angiographic procedures under general anaesthesia.[22] Moderate hyperventilation during such procedures produces vasoconstriction in vascular beds where reactivity is preserved and, by slowing transit time through the vessels under investigation, may improve image quality for small lesions.[23] Angio-embolization procedures on the brain or spinal cord are often performed under general anaesthesia as the high incidence of potentially life-threatening complications may be managed more effectively. Anaesthetic considerations for cerebral angiography are necessarily a fusion of those for neuro-anaesthesia and for procedures conducted within the confines of a radiology department in terms of personnel, equipment and environment.

CARDIOLOGY

Cardiac catheterization

In spite of the growth in non-invasive cardiological investigative procedures, cardiac catheterization remains the only way of measuring pressures and saturations within the chambers of the heart and the great vessels. It is also important in the evaluation of the anatomy of the coronary vasculature in preparation for bypass surgery. It is important that the circulation is stable and as near normal as possible for accurate measurements to be made.

A stable and immobile adult patient is usually readily achieved with little or no sedation. However, sedation or anaesthesia will be necessary for paediatric patients, in whom this investigation continues to be common. Well-judged premedication may be all that is necessary for the conduct of the procedure. Different institutions have preferences for different premedicant drugs or combinations of drugs, and local experience should prevail. Cocktails such as pethidine/promethazine/chlopromazine[24] enjoy continuing popularity, but close supervision of the child must be instituted after its administration as respiratory depression can be substantial. Trimeprazine is frequently used and benzodiazepines such as diazepam or midazolam in appropriate doses can also be effective[25] by the oral or rectal route. Very young patients or those with severe hypoxaemia or heart failure may be given no premedication or only a small dose of atropine.

Monitoring should include ECG, pulse oximetry, temperature, blood glucose and arterial blood gas analysis (for acid–base balance disturbances). The use of added inspired oxygen in infants undergoing cardiac catheterization is potentially hazardous. Constriction of the ductus arteriosus in infants with aortic stenosis, aortic arch interruption or co-arctation has been blamed on increased F_{IO_2}.[26] Monitoring with a pulse oximeter facilitates the administration of modestly increased oxygen concentrations when clinically necessary.

If premedication is successful, catheterization can be conducted under local anaesthesia. Caution should be exercised in local anaesthetic dosage as overdose is easy in small children. If lignocaine is used, the dose should be limited to 3 mg.kg^{-1}. Further sedation may be necessary, for which small doses of a benzodiazepine such as diazepam might be appropriate.

In patients for whom general anaesthesia is selected, tracheal intubation with a muscle relaxant and controlled ventilation is commonly used,[27] although different institutions pursue their standard practice for paediatric cardiac anaesthesia.

Cardioversion

Patients presenting for direct current cardioversion vary greatly in age and general fitness for anaesthesia. The procedure may be conducted on an elective basis in an attempt to convert a stable but undesirable rhythm (such as atrial fibrillation without haemodynamic impact) or as an emergency for tachyarrhythmias which jeopardize haemodynamic sufficiency (such as ventricular tachycardia). As careful and thorough a pre-operative assessment as possible within the available time must be made, with particular attention to co-existing conditions (such as hypertension and diabetes) and the presence of concurrent drug therapy (e.g. anticoagulants, digoxin). If the clinical situation allows, patients should undergo an appropriate period of starvation before direct current cardioversion.

The discomfort is such that anaesthesia, or at least amnesia, is desirable. Two general approaches have been used, both having their foundations in the early days of cardioversion as a therapeutic manoeuvre.[28,29] The first is to provide general anaesthesia, using an intravenous induction agent and maintenance of anaesthesia with nitrous oxide and an inhaled agent. This technique has evolved into a simpler but similar technique — intravenous induction after no premedication and maintenance of anaesthesia by continued injections of intravenous agent. Although drugs such as thiopentone and methohexitone do not have an ideal pharmacokinetic profile for repeated injection over a period of time, they continue to be popular because of the extent of experience with their use. Propofol is achieving an increasing degree of popularity for direct current cardioversion because its use is characterized by smooth induction and rapid emergence. Whatever induction agent is used, its administration should be cautious and incremental so as to minimize the cardiovascular side-effects of the drug in a situation of potentially significant pre-existing cardiovascular compromise. The other technique for direct current cardioversion relies on the administration of incremental doses of a benzodiazepine, previously diazepam, but increasingly midazolam, to produce a state of heavy sedation. This technique has a good safety record but suffers from the theoretical disadvantage that drugs of long duration are being administered for a procedure that has only a short duration. The use of midazolam rather than diazepam minimizes this objection.

Whichever technique is used, a comprehensive range of equipment for tracheal intubation, airway management and resuscitation should be immediately to hand. If the patient does not have an empty stomach, rapid-sequence induction with cricoid pressure and the administration of suxamethonium followed by tracheal intubation should be undertaken to provide airway protection. Even if the patient is adequately starved, pre-oxygenation is advisable, followed by continued oxygen administration during anaesthesia as the development of malignant arrhythmias during direct current cardioversion is a potential complication. The occasionally violent and always instantaneous contraction of thoracic and abdominal muscles during the passage of the current may pose a risk to those with severe osteoporosis. It may be wise in this rare instance to ensure some degree of neuromuscular blockade with suxamethonium.

Invasive therapeutic procedures

Invasive paediatric procedures such as balloon atrial septostomy, transluminal angioplasty of aortic coarctation and stenotic pulmonary arteries and occlusion of collaterals may be performed at cardiac catheterization. The procedures tend to last longer than simple catheterization and attention must be paid to temperature maintenance and fluid balance management. The anaesthetist must be prepared to deal with periods of low cardiac output and arrhythmia; thus, monitoring of arterial pressure is usually direct and access to the central venous circulation is desirable, and can often be achieved through the catheter.

Procedures such as coronary angioplasty and balloon valvuloplasty are increasing in popularity. They are most commonly performed on adults and anaesthesia is rarely needed. For this reason, there is a dearth of literature on the subject of anaesthesia for these procedures. The principles of anaesthesia for patients undergoing these procedures differ little from those applicable to any patient suffering from ischaemic or valvular heart disease.

The use of a standard general anaesthetic technique (fentanyl, etomidate, suxamethonium, vecuronium, nitrous oxide, enflurane) for coronary angioplasty has been reported.[30] The paper by Kates et al is interesting for a number of reasons, notably that the anaesthetic technique was reported as successful in this situation and also that the number of authors of the paper exceeded the number of patients in the trial. The same group reported again some 3 years later in relation to a trial comparing general anaesthesia and intravenous sedation for the same procedure. Their conclusions were that general anaesthesia was feasible and that patients preferred it.[31] Although the number of authors had grown from seven to 14, the number of patients had also grown, so that they exceeded the number of authors!

Patients undergoing cardiological electrophysiological testing also rarely require anaesthesia.[32] Procedures beyond simple electrophysiological testing such as closed-chest catheter ablation of conduction pathways or arrhythmogenic foci may involve direct current shocks in the range of 200–400 J. Tachyarrhythmias resulting in cardiovascular decompensation may be caused inadvertently during such procedures and may require direct current cardioversion. As this is known to cause marked discomfort, general anaesthesia may be required briefly.[33] If repeated shocks are likely to be required, or become necessary, continued general anaesthesia may become a rational management option. Inhalational anaesthesia has the theoretical disadvantage that volatile agents may interfere with normal cardiac conduction; consequently, intravenous anaesthesia is often used. Excitatory phenomena and myoclonus associated with the use of etomidate can interfere with accurate intracardiac catheter placement. In the author's experience, the use of a propofol infusion has proved successful whether with controlled or spontaneous ventilation.

RADIOTHERAPY

Radiotherapeutic procedures share common ground with other techniques occasionally requiring anaesthetic involvement: remote location, the presence of bulky equipment in facilities not primarily designed for the administration of anaesthetics and, if the institution is not well-geared towards the regular provision of such anaesthetic services, the consequent logistic and personnel problems. To these can be added an almost exclusively paediatric clientèle, the requirement for repeated anaesthetics within a short period and a biophysical hazard that excludes the anaesthetist from the same room as the patient.

Children presenting for radiotherapy fall largely into one of three groups: those requiring cranial or craniospinal irradiation for leukaemia whether on a therapeutic or prophylactic basis, those with primary intracranial tumours and those needing radiotherapy for primary or metastatic tumours outside the brain.[34] The frequency of such treatments may be up to five times a week for 7 consecutive weeks. Such frequent intervention needs careful and continuing psychological support that is best provided in a specialist centre.

General anaesthesia is usually required for children under the age of 5 years, particularly if the prone position is necessary. Most, though not all, children over this age may be amenable to treatment with or without sedation or appropriate support and bribery.

All radiotherapy, but particularly that administered to the head and neck, requires great accuracy to avoid the irradiation of areas susceptible to and not requiring it. A shell or cast is made for radiotherapy to the head, neck or spinal areas to ensure immobility in a reproducible position.[35] General anaesthesia may therefore be needed for three separate phases — mould production, planning of treatment and treatments.

Mould production

Quick-setting materials such as dental alginate or plaster of Paris are pasted over the child's head to aid in the production of a Perspex mould. Holes are left in the mould for the child's nostrils and mouth, the latter hole being big enough to allow the insertion of an oral airway should this become necessary at a later date.

Planning of treatment

Between one and five planning sessions may be necessary to ensure the correct alignment of treatment regimens.

Treatments

Once the child is accurately positioned with the help of the mould and securing straps to prevent sudden movement, treatment sessions lasting between 10 and 45 min are conducted.

Pre-operative preparation

A standard assessment as for all general anaesthesia should be made. Particular attention must be paid to haemoglobin concentration and white cell and platelet counts, and the possibility of intercurrent infection should be excluded.

In selected children it may be possible to avoid general anaesthesia with judiciously chosen premedication. Unfortunately, as is well-known to anaesthetists everywhere, paediatric premedication is unpredictable and unreliable. There has been a continuing search for the best premedication for children in this, or any other, situation and this search is likely to continue for some time. Agents described have included: chloral, trimeprazine, nepenthe, diazepam, chlorpromazine, pethidine, pentobarbitone, droperidol and methadone.[34] The agents used, as for any paediatric anaesthesia, should be according to the anaesthetist's personal preference or local guidelines and protocols. Repeated radiotherapy sessions within a short space of time do, however, give the anaesthetist an opportunity to discover the agent and dose that suit that particular child. If ketamine forms part of the anaesthetic plan, the inclusion of an anticholinergic in the premedication is recommended.

Anaesthesia

The principal requirement is that the patient should be absolutely still during the treatments. Management of the airway is the most important issue as access is limited not only by the anaesthetist's intermittent exclusion from the immediate environs of the patient but also by the Perspex mould which surrounds the head of many of the patients. Tracheal intubation as part of routine anaesthetic management in this context may appear tempting, but the hazards of the trauma of daily intubation in this age group are best avoided. The aim is therefore to provide light general anaesthesia (the procedure is painless) with spontaneous ventilation with an airway that needs no external support or is amenable to simple adjuncts such as an oropharyngeal tube.

Many anaesthetic agents have been used. Cyclopropane[36] has its proponents, although the accompanying explosion risk would rule it out for many anaesthetists and its availability is declining in many countries. The choice appears therefore to lie between halothane, enflurane and isoflurane with or without nitrous oxide. Halothane is commonly considered to be the easiest agent to use for inhalational induction, but recent reports of 'halothane hepatitis' in children may make anaesthetists more wary of its repeated use.[37,38] This consideration has led to the description of the use of isoflurane for radiotherapy.[38,39]

If inhalational anaesthesia is to be avoided, there is still a wide choice of intravenous or intramuscular agents. After over 40 years' clinical use there are still papers being published on the use of barbiturates for paediatric radiotherapy, e.g. intramuscular methohexitone[40] and intravenous infusions of thiopentone[41] or ketamine.[34] Brett and her colleagues have discussed the anaesthetic requirements of infants undergoing repeated radiotherapy[42] and, like other authors,[38] conclude that appropriately administered general anaesthesia is preferable to sedation using drugs such as benzodiazepines or ketamine.

However, others have advocated the use of ketamine. Its water solubility, suitability for repeated administration, minimal organ toxicity, analgesic properties and its use by the intravenous or intramuscular routes make it attractive and its use is supported by a number of publications.[43–46] Anticholinergic premedication should be considered to reduce the severity of salivation during its use and diazepam administration prior to giving ketamine has been advocated to reduce the incidence of unpleasant emergence phenomena.[34] Caution should be exercised in patients with raised intracranial pressure.

Monitoring

Immediate proximity to the patient during treatment periods is not feasible so appropriate monitoring should be employed. ECG, automated blood pressure measurement and pulse oximetry are commonly employed along with observation either through a window or, if this is not possible, with closed-circuit television.[38] Between treatment periods, the anaesthetist should re-establish direct contact with the patient to ensure that the airway is unobstructed.

ELECTROCONVULSIVE THERAPY

Based on the erroneous premise that schizophrenia and epilepsy could not co-exist and the correct premise that schizophrenic symptoms might be improved after a grand mal convulsion, induced convulsions were first employed as a therapeutic intervention in 1934. Initially, seizures were induced pharmacologically, but since the introduction of electrically induced seizures in 1937, this has become the only method of delivering this treatment. The popularity of electroconvulsive therapy (ECT) waned in the 1950s and 1960s because of the introduction of effective psychopharmacological agents to control the symptoms of schizophrenia and the major affective disorders. A further decrease in its use occurred in the 1970s when public opinion was directed towards its occasional misuses. Although there may now seem to be a slight resurgence of interest in its use, recent anaesthetic literature on the subject is scant and largely restricted to reports of unusual cases and the application of new drugs to the anaesthetic techniques used for ECT. However, two review articles on the subject have been published in the last 10 years, and the interested reader is directed towards these for a detailed bibliography.[47,48]

The treatment

The detailed biological reasons for the undoubted success of ECT in appropriate clinical situations remain largely a mystery. Although several biochemical changes caused by ECT have been determined, the link between these and clinical improvement has not been clearly elucidated.

The aim of the treatment is to produce a seizure; without the seizure there is no therapeutic benefit. Indeed, the duration of the seizure appears to be the primary determinant of success.[49–51] Seizure durations of less than 30 s are probably not effective, while extended seizures may substantially increase post-ictal memory loss and confusion.[52] It may be that there is a duration window of maximum effect; it has been reported that below a seizure aggregate of 210 s within one course, benefits were unlikely to accrue, while if the aggregate exceeded 1000 s, no further improvement would be seen.[53] It has been proposed that a single seizure of between 25 and 60 s is ideal.[54]

A variety of proprietary ECT machines are available which produce a range of stimulus waveforms, durations and intensities. Some also allow the display and recording of electroencephalogram and ECG. What is important is that a stimulus of sufficient magnitude is generated to overcome the patient's variable head resistance and seizure threshold. After preparation of the skin, plate or sponge electrodes are used to minimize impedance. Although psychiatrists debate the merits of unilateral or bilateral ECT, the difference matters little to the anaesthetist. In the former, both electrodes are placed over one temple; in the latter, an electrode is placed on each temple.

There is initially a very brief period of muscular spasm caused by direct muscular and neuromuscular stimulation. This is followed by a tonic phase of between 10 and 20 s which is replaced by a clonic phase of up to 60 s duration. After a brief period of post-ictal coma impossible to separate from the continuing effects of anaesthesia, the patient should awake to consciousness.

Physiological impact of ECT

The cardiovascular changes associated with ECT are characteristic, although rarely reproducible even in the same patient in a single course of treatment. In general, the tonic phase is associated with parasympathetic nervous system stimulation. This may be associated with the development of ectopic pacemakers, bradycardia, extrasystoles, ventricular escape rhythms and even asystole. Hypotension and excess salivation may accompany this phase. During the clonic phase, the sympathetic nervous system predominates. Tachycardia, hypertension, multifocal extrasystoles and bigeminy have all been recorded.

The cardiovascular changes associated with ECT are well tolerated by patients in good health but may pose a substantial threat to patients with ischaemic heart disease, cerebrovascular disease or intracranial pathology. Contra-indications to ECT have been listed[48] but the concept of any absolute contra-indication to ECT has been argued against[55] on the traditional basis that risk/benefit analysis should be considered for each individual patient and that all contra-indications should be considered relative. Listed contra-indications include phaeochromocytoma, raised intracranial pressure, recent myocardial infarction and high-risk pregnancy (although the avoidance of drug therapy that ECT allows may be considered a positive indication for its use in low-risk pregnancy).

The patient

The patient presenting for ECT is often elderly, an unreliable historian and poorly prepared. In addition to this, he or she is likely to be the subject of polypharmacy with drugs that can have a significant impact on anaesthetic management. A study in 1975[55] of 425 patients undergoing ECT showed, not surprisingly, that all patients were receiving some sort of psychotropic therapy, tricyclic antidepressants and benzodiazepines being the most commonly encountered. Both tricyclic antidepressants and monoamine oxidase inhibitors may be associated with hypertensive crises and an increased incidence of arrhythmias. The interaction between these two groups of drugs has been shown to increase duration of anaesthesia and mortality. The temptation, common in anaesthetic practice in other areas, to cease medication with these drugs for a period prior to anaesthesia is unlikely to be a feasible option with regard to ECT. Lithium carbonate may potentiate the effects of neuromuscular blockers. Benzodiazepines can increase convulsion threshold.

Anaesthetic management

Pre-operative evaluation. The patient presenting for ECT should receive the same thorough preparation as that afforded to any patient undergoing anaesthesia. Difficulties may arise when an anaesthetist new to the patient is requested to provide anaesthesia for, say, the fourth treatment in a course of ECT, only to find that the patient has not been investigated to a standard that he or she feels acceptable. It is a great temptation in this situation simply to give the anaesthetic and thereby avoid the delay that further investigation would create. To do this would continue and extend the chain of errors which has already been established. It is found helpful by some anaesthetic departments to establish protocols for the investigation of patients undergoing ECT. Such protocols should assist in the answering of questions such as: 'Is it worth performing coronary angiography for someone about to undergo ECT?'

The standard period of pre-operative starvation within any department should be carried out. This may not be easy, as the patients may be unreliable and unco-operative. Careful supervision by nursing staff is valuable in this situation.

There is some debate concerning the most appropriate premedication. Most are agreed that sedative premedication is undesirable in that it can prolong recovery from anaesthesia. Occasionally, very anxious patients in whom careful explanation and reassurance have failed to allay fears may be considered appropriate for a sedative premedication. In this instance, the use of benzodiazepines is probably most appropriate. The use of anticholinergic agents has stimulated some research and debate. The logic behind the administration of pre-operative anticholinergics lies in the possibility of preventing the bradycardia and excessive secretions theoretically associated with the initial parasympathetic response to ECT. Against this is the possibility of harm deriving from induced tachycardia and confusion and delirium if the anticholinergic has the capacity for crossing the blood–brain barrier. Evidence against the benefit of anticholinergic premedication lies in papers by Vereecke & Troche[56] and Wyant & MacDonald.[57] The first reported no problems with airway secretions or bradycardia in 6000 ECT treatments performed without the benefit of atropine pretreatment. The second reported a controlled study purporting to demonstrate no benefit from atropine pretreatment. Nevertheless, many anaesthetists choose to give an anticholinergic to patients undergoing ECT. Which one should be given? There is probably little to choose between atropine and glycopyrronium; however, the latter, while associated with equivalent protection against vagal bradycardias and excess salivation, is less likely to cause a tachycardia.[58]

Anaesthetic preparation. ECT is often conducted in a facility within the mental health portion of a hospital. The equipment is often remaindered from the main operating theatre suite and may not receive the appropriate maintenance attention. It is vital that all monitoring and resuscitation equipment that the anaesthetist might require is present, adequately maintained and regularly checked. Locally agreed minimum standard monitoring, to include at least continuous ECG, automated blood pressure and oxygen saturation, should be used. A trained anaesthetic assistant should be present along with trained recovery personnel.

Management of the procedure. Reliable intravenous access should be established. Pre-oxygenation need not be considered mandatory,[59] but cannot be argued against unless the individual patient finds the application of a mask particularly distressing. The standard practice of the anaesthetist or the institution should be followed in this respect.

The requirements for ECT include:

1. provision of a sufficient degree of anaesthesia to render the patient unaware of the initial application of current
2. muscle relaxation so that the motor effects of the convulsion are attenuated but not completely eliminated.
3. the use of anaesthetic agents which do not substantially affect seizure threshold.
4. a rapid recovery.

The barbiturate anaesthetics thiopentone and methohexitone have enjoyed the greatest use historically, methohexitone continuing to be the most popular agent for ECT. Although thiopentone is an effective anticonvulsant, current evidence suggests that there may be little to choose between these agents in the ECT setting,[55] although this is not uncontested.[59,60] The use of diazepam has its proponents,[61] but may shorten seizure duration[62] and may be associated with slower induction and recovery.[55] Ketamine has not fared well in comparison with methohexitone for ECT in terms of a slower induction and recover, but appears not to be associated with emergence phenomena in this setting.[63] Reports of the use of etomidate appear favourable,[64,65] but it has not enjoyed direct comparison with methohexitone.

Prior to the introduction of propofol, induction agents such as diazepam, ketamine and etomidate were considered as alternatives to methohexitone when contra-indications to its use existed. Propofol offered potential advantages over methohexitone in terms of its rapid and clear-headed recovery. This application was readily appreciated and reports of its use appeared in the literature. It was soon realized that the use of propofol, when compared with methohexitone, was associated with reduced seizure duration.[66-68] One identifiable benefit, however, is that propofol appears to be better than methohexitone at obtunding the hypertensive response to ECT.

The current status is that methohexitone is still largely unchallenged as the induction agent of choice for ECT. On the rare occasions that methohexitone may not be given to a patient, the second choice lies between propofol and etomidate. The increasing popularity of propofol at the time of writing suggests that it will nudge etomidate into third place in this respect.

Before the advent of neuromuscular blockers, the threat of fractures sustained as a result of the violence of induced convulsions was very real. Suxamethonium is now in almost universal use in order to modify the physical convulsions associated with ECT. The dose should be selected to be one that still leaves some neuromuscular function intact so that the presence and duration of a seizure can be assessed. The use of simultaneous electroencephalogram monitoring or the isolation of an arm from the general circulation with a tourniquet may be used for seizure assessment, but as there appears to be little benefit to be derived from complete neuromuscular blockade at the risk of significantly prolonging apnoea time, the majority of anaesthetists adhere to a low-dose suxamethonium technique. A dose of 0.5 mg.kg^{-1} has been recommended.[69] The well-recognized complications of suxamethonium are pertinent to its use for ECT except that the incidence of muscle pains appears to be low (around 2%).[70] The use of a small dose of a non-depolarizing neuromuscular blocker to attenuate some of the side-effects of suxamethonium has not been investigated in detail with respect to ECT management, and it would seem reasonable for those who practise this technique to continue.

In situations such as pseudocholinesterase deficiency where the use of suxamethonium may be considered to be undesirable, a non-depolarizing neuromuscular blocker may be used. The successful use of gallamine[71] and atracurium[72] has been reported in this context.

Routine tracheal intubation is seldom performed, except where circumstances demand. Although it is claimed that some centres practise routine intubation, the possibility of a greater anaesthetic requirement and an augmentation of the pressor response seem to argue against this practice.

If it is deemed highly desirable to attenuate the sympathetic response to ECT in specific patients, standard measures may be employed. Reports of the use of lignocaine, propranolol, clonidine, sodium nitroprusside and nitroglycerine[73,74] to achieve this end exist.

Postanaesthesia care. The immediate post-ECT period is not without risk.[75] Close supervision and appropriate monitoring are therefore recommended until the patient has regained full consciousness. This should be conducted in an adequately staffed recovery area. Periods of confusion or aggressive behaviour are not uncommon in the recovery period and steps should be taken to ensure the patients' safety in this situation.

REFERENCES

1. Stark DD, Moss AA, Goldberg HI, Davis PL, Federle MP. Magnetic resonance and CT of the normal and diseased pancreas: a comparative study. Radiology 1984; 150: 153–161
2. Ferrer-Brechner T, Winter J. Anesthetic considerations for cerebral computer tomography. Anesth Analg 1977; 56: 344–347
3. Welldorm SG. Anaesthesia for EMI scanning in infants and small children. South Med J 1976; 69: 1294–1295
4. Goldberg PL, Evans PF, Filshie J. Kinking of the laryngeal mask airway in two children. Anaesthesia 1990; 45: 487–488
5. Patel A, Dallas SH. A trial of etomidate infusion anaesthesia for computerised axial tomography. Anaesthesia 1981; 36: 639
6. Valtonen M. Anaesthesia for computerised tomography of the brain in children: a comparison of propofol and thiopentone. Acta Anaesthesiol Scand 1989; 33: 170–173
7. Coventry DM, Martin CS, Burke AM. Sedation for paediatric computerized tomography — a double blind assessment of rectal midazolam. Eur J Anaesthesiol 1991; 8: 29–32
8. Weston G, Strunin L, Amundson GM. Imaging for anaesthetists: a review of the methods and anaesthetic implications of diagnostic imaging techniques. Can Anaesth Soc J 1985; 32: 552–561
9. Nixon C, Hirsch NP, Ormerod IEC, Johnson G. Nuclear magnetic resonance. Anaesthesia 1986; 41: 131–137
10. New PFJ, Rosen BR, Brady TJ et al. Potential hazards and artifacts of ferromagnetic and nonferromagnetic surgical and dental materials and devices in nuclear magnetic resonance imaging. Radiology 1983; 147: 139–148
11. Pavlicek W, Geisinger M, Castle L et al. The effects of nuclear magnetic resonance on patients with cardiac pacemakers. Radiology 1983; 147: 149–153
12. Gangarosa RE, Minnis JE, Nobbe J, Praschan D, Genberg RW. Operational safety issues in MRI. Magnetic Res Imaging 1987; 6: 287–292
13. Davis PL, Crooks L, Arakawa M, McRee R, Kaufman L, Margulis AR. Potential hazards in NMR imaging: heating effects of changing magnetic fields and RF fields on small metallic implants. Am J Roentgenol 1981; 137: 857–860
14. Patteson SK, Chesney JT. Anesthetic management for magnetic resonance imaging: problems and solutions. Anesth Analg 1992; 74: 121–128
15. Rao CC, McNiece WL, Emhardt J, Krishna G, Westcott R. Modification of an anesthesia machine for use during magnetic resonance imaging. Anesthesiology 1988; 68: 640–641
16. Karlik SJ, Heatherley T, Pavan F, Stein J, Lebron F Rutt B. Patient anesthesia and monitoring at a 1.5 T MRI installation. Magnetic Res Med 1988; 7: 210–221
17. Gaffey CT, Tenforde TS, Dean EE. Alterations in the electrocardiogram of baboons exposed to DC magnetic fields. Bioelectromagnetics 1980; 1: 209–212
18. Tenforde TS, Gaffey CT, Mayer BR, Budinger TF. Cardiovascular alterations in Macaca monkeys exposed to stationary magnetic fields; experimental observations and theoretical analysis. Bioelectromagnetics 1983; 4: 1–9
19. Shellock FG, Slimp GL. Severe burn of the finger caused by using a pulse oximeter during MR imaging. Am J Roentgenol 1989; 153: 1105
20. Rafferty C, Burke AM, Cossar DF, Farling PA. Laryngeal mask and magnetic resonance imaging. Anaesthesia 1990; 45: 590–591
21. Boutros A, Pavlicek W. Anesthesia for magnetic resonance imaging. Anesth Analg 1987; 66: 367
22. Walters FJM. Anaesthesia for neuroradiology. Br J Hosp Med 1987; 10: 351–356
23. Du Boulay G, Edmonds-Seal J, Bostick T. The effect of intermittent positive pressure ventilation upon the calibre of cerebral arteries in spasm following subarachnoid haemorrhage — a preliminary communication. Br J Radiol 1968; 41: 46–48
24. Smith C, Rowe RD, Vlad P. Sedation of children for cardiac catheterisation with an ataractic mixture. Can Anaesth Soc J 1958; 5: 35–40
25. Saint-Maurice C, Meistelman C, Rey E, Esteve C, De Lauture D, Olive G. The pharmacokinetics of rectal midazolam for premedication in children. Anesthesiology 1986; 65: 536–538
26. Moffitt EA, McGoon DC, Ritter DG. The diagnosis and correction of congenital cardiac defects. Anesthesiology 1970; 33: 144–160
27. Sumner E. Anaesthesia for patients with cardiac disease. In: Hatch DJ, Sumner E, eds. Neonatal anaesthesia and perioperative care. London: Edward Arnold. 1988
28. Gilston A, Fordham R, Resenkov L. Anaesthesia for direct current shock in the treatment of cardiac arrhythmias. Br J Anaesth 1965; 37: 533–539
29. Nutter DO, Massumi RA. Diazepam in cardioversion. N Engl J Med 1965; 273: 650–651
30. Kates RA, Stack RS, Hill RF et al. General anesthesia for patients undergoing percutaneous transluminal coronary angioplasty during acute myocardial infarction. Anesth Analg 1986; 65: 815–818
31. De Bruijn NP, Hlatky MA, Jacobs JR et al. General anesthesia during percutaneous transluminary coronary angioplasty for acute myocardial infarction. Anesth Analg 1989; 68: 201–207
32. Oliver WC, White RD. Anesthesia: electrophysiologic testing, arrhythmia surgery and aneurysm resection. In: Tarkan S. ed. Cardiovascular anesthesia and postoperative care. Chicago, IL: Yearbook. 1989
33. Davis J, Scheinman MM, Ruder MA et al. Ablation of cardiac tissues by an electrode catheter technique for

34. Filshie J, Harrison CA. Paediatric radiotherapy. In: Filshie J, Robbie DS, eds. Anaesthesia and malignant disease. London: Edward Arnold 1989
35. Dobbs J, Barrett A. Practical radiotherapy planning. In: Practical radiotherapy planning. London: Edward Arnold. 1985
36. Casey WF, Price V, Smith HS. Anaesthesia and monitoring for paediatric radiotherapy. JR Soc Med 1986; 79: 454–456
37. Kenna JG, Neuberger J, Mieli-Vergani G, Mowat AP, Williams R. Halothane hepatatis in children. Bri Med J 1987; 294: 1209–1211
38. Jones RM, Diamond JG, Power SJ, Bajorek PK, Munday I. A prospective study of liver function in infants and children exposed to daily isoflurane for several weeks. Anaesthesia 1991; 46: 686–688
39. Goudsouzian NG, Alifimoff JK, Cote CJ. Isoflurane for radiotherapy in children? Anesthesiology 1988; 68: 648
40. Jeffries G. Radiotherapy and children's anaesthesia. Anaesthesia 1988; 43: 416–417
41. Menache L, Eifel PJ, Kennamer DL, Belli JA. Twice daily anesthesia in infants receiving hyperfractionated irradiation. Int J Radiat Oncol Biol Phys 1990; 18: 625–629
42. Brett CM, Wara WM, Hamilton WK. Anesthesia for infants during radiotherapy: an insufflation technique. Anesthesiology 1986; 64: 402–405
43. Amberg HL, Gordon G. Low-dose intramuscular ketamine for pediatric radiotherapy: a case report. Anesth Analg 1976; 55: 92–94
44. Edge WG, Morgan M. Ketamine and paediatric radiotherapy. Anaesth Intensive Care 1977; 5: 153–156
45. Cronin MM, Bousfield JD, Hewitt EB, McLellan I, Boulton TB. Ketamine anaesthesia for radiotherapy in small children. Anaesthesia 1972; 27: 135–142
46. Piwoz S, Goldstein B. The use of ketamine anesthesia in radiation therapy. Radiology 1973; 109: 725–726
47. Gaines GY, Rees DI. Electroconvulsive therapy and anaesthetic considerations. Anesth Analg 1986; 65: 1345–1356
48. Selvin BL. Electroconvulsive therapy — 1987. Anesthesiology 1987; 67: 367–385
49. Hurwitz TD. Electroconvulsive therapy: a review. Comp Psychiatry 1974; 15: 303–314
50. Kenedell RE. The present status of electroconvulsive therapy. Br J Psychiatry 1981; 139: 265–283
51. Ottosson JO. Experimental studies in the mode of action of electroconvulsive therapy. Acta Psychiatr Scand 1960; 35: 1–141
52. O'Connell RA. A review of the use of electroconvulsive therapy. Hosp Commun Psychiatry 1982; 33: 469–473
53. Maletzky BM. Seizure duration and clinical effect in electroconvulsive therapy. Compr Psychiatry 1978; 19: 541–550
54. Weiner RD. The psychiatric use of electrically induced seizures. Am J Psychiatry 1979; 136: 1507–1517
55. McCleave DJ, Blakemore WB. Anaesthesia for electroconvulsive therapy. Anaesth Intensive Care 1975; 3: 250–256
56. Verheecke G, Troche E. Atropine in ECT. Anaesth Intensive Care 1982; 10: 166
57. Wyant GM, MacDonald WB. The role of atropine in electroconvulsive therapy. Anaesth Intensive Care 1980; 8: 445–450
58. Greenan J, Dewar M, Jones CJ. Intravenous glycopyrrolate and atropine at induction of anaesthesia: a comparison. J R Soc Med 1983; 76: 369–371
59. Woodruff RA, Pitts FN, McClure JN. The drug modification of ECT. 1 Methohexital, thiopental and preoxygenation. Arch Gen Psychiatry 1968; 18: 605–611
60. Pitts FN, Desmaris GM, Stewart W, Schaberg K. Induction of anaesthesia with methohexital and thiopental in electroconvulsive therapy. N Engl J Med 1965; 273: 353–359
61. Martin DJ, Kaelbling R. Diazepam-modified electroconvulsive therapy. Biol Psychiatry 1971; 3: 129–139
62. Stromgren LS, Dahl J, Fieldborg N. Factors affecting seizure duration and number of seizures applied in unilateral electroconvulsive therapy — anaesthetics and benzodiazepines. Acta Psychiatr Scand 1980; 62: 158–165
63. MacInnes EC, James NM. A comparison of ketamine and methohexital in electroconvulsive therapy. Med J Aust 1972; 1: 1031–1032
64. Crispin A, Crommem AM. A progress in electroconvulsive therapy — the non-barbiturate drug etomidate. Acta Psychiatr (Belg) 1977; 76: 678–687
65. O'Carroll TM, Blogg CE, Hoinville EA, Savege TM. Etomidate in electroconvulsive therapy: a within-patient comparison with alphaxalone/alphadalone. Anaesthesia 1977; 32: 868–872
66. Simpson KH, Halsall PJ, Carr CME, Stewart KG. Seizure duration after methohexitone or propofol for induction of anaesthesia for electroconvulsive therapy (ECT). Br J Anaesth 1987; 59: 1323–1324
67. Rouse EC. Propofol for electroconvulsive therapy: a comparison with methohexitone. Preliminary report. Anaesthesia 1988; 43 (suppl); 61–64
68. Dwyer R, McCaughey W, Lavery J, McCarthy G, Dundee JW. Comparison of propofol and methohexitone as anaesthetic agents for electroconvulsive therapy. Anaesthesia 1988; 43: 459–462
69. Pitts FN, Woodruff RA, Craig AG, Rich CL. The drug modification of ECT. 2: succinylcholine dosage. Arch Gen Psychiatry 1968; 19: 595–598
70. Kerr RA, McGrath JJ, O'Kearney RT, Price J. ECT: misconceptions and attitudes. Aust NZ J Psychiatry 1982; 16: 43–49
71. Simpson KH, Halsall PJ. The use of propofol for anaesthesia for electroconvulsive therapy. Anaesthesia 1988; 43: 812–813
72. Brunton CT, Free CW. ECT without suxamethonium. Anaesth Intensive Care 1983; 11: 177–178
73. Dodson ME. Short acting neuromuscular blockers and ECT. Br J Anaesth 1985; 57: 933–934
74. Liu WS, Petty WC, Jeppsen A, Wade EJ, Pace NL. Attenuation of hemodynamic and hormonal responses to ECT with propranolol, xylocaine, sodium nitroprusside or clonidine. Anesth Analg 1984; 63: 244
75. Barker JC, Baker AA. Deaths associated with electropexy. J Ment Sci 1959; 105: 339–348

19. Anaesthesia for plastic, microvascular and burns surgery

D.W. Green

ANAESTHESIA FOR PLASTIC SURGERY

In no other field of specialized surgery has the anaesthetic contribution been so crucial to the development of surgical practice and scope. Indeed, close co-operation between the surgeon and the anaesthetist is considered crucial to the success of surgery, particularly with the use of deliberate arterial hypotension.[1]

Historical review of anaesthetic practice

In a review of the development of anaesthesia for plastic surgery, the recollections of Surgeon-Major Furnell in 1871 of operations before anaesthesia make harrowing reading.[2] The spectre of a young girl with a burn injury of the neck being operated upon with no anaesthesia was considered worse than a 'man being flogged for subordination'; indeed, 'his sufferings were light as air as compared with the agonies this poor girl must have undergone'.

New surgical techniques in plastic and reconstructive surgery have required the development of additional skills in anaesthesia. It is the anaesthetist's responsibility to apply these wisely and safely for maximum benefit to the patient. The requirement in many plastic surgery operations for both surgeon and anaesthetist to have access to the surgical field (the former to operate and the latter for airway protection and control) necessitated advances in anaesthetic techniques which had implications well beyond the boundaries of plastic surgery itself.

Monitoring and blood pressure measurement

In the early 1900s, Harvey Cushing, in Massachusetts, introduced the first anaesthetic record on which were charted observations of pulse and respiration, later adding blood pressure using the Riva-Rocci method. Monitoring is obviously important during any anaesthetic, but became particularly relevant following the introduction of hypotensive techniques. The necessity to have accurate readings at low arterial pressures, which was not possible during deliberate hypotension with the sphygmomanometer, led to the introduction of the oscillotonometer into anaesthetic practice in East Grinstead in the 1950s.[3] Accurate measurement of blood pressure was crucial to the safety of the technique and its applicability to other fields of anaesthesia.

Mouth gags

The fact that ether was still given by insufflation prompted the development of the combined tongue depressor and insufflation tube holder by Crowe and Davis (the latter was Cushing's anaesthetist). This was brought to the UK by Boyle (Boyle–Davis gag) and later converted for use in cleft palate and tonsillar surgery by Dott.

Tracheal intubation and anaesthetic circuits

William Macewen of Glasgow pioneered the use of endotracheal intubation (awake) for oral surgery as an alternative to tracheostomy. Undoubtedly, the most significant event in plastic surgical anaesthesia was the establishment of the unit at the Queen's Hospital in Sidcup under Gillies, Kilner and Newlands in 1917.[2] No specialized anaesthesia was available until the transfer of Magill and Rowbotham in 1919. The initial use of a two-tube (in–out) insufflation endotracheal technique for long periods was considered uneconomical and unphysiological. This led to the development of the single, wide-bore endotracheal tube which was wide enough to allow to-and-fro breathing. The additional developments of laryngoscopes, breathing systems and other tubes by these men advanced anaesthesia in other specialties and in other countries.

Paediatric anaesthesia

Significant developments relevant to plastic surgery

have been the introduction of the T-piece for cleft palate surgery by Philip Ayre of Newcastle-upon-Tyne in 1937, and its subsequent modification by Jackson-Rees to allow controlled ventilation.[4] The interposition of a solenoid 'mechanical thumb' occluder to the expiratory limb of this circuit forms the basis of many paediatric ventilators.

Hypotensive anaesthesia

Apart from airway problems with plastic surgery of the head and neck (which still encompasses a large proportion of plastic surgical operations), the spectre of troublesome bleeding was still evident, despite excellent airway control which had been obtained with tracheal intubation. To overcome this problem, postural ischaemia (head-up-tilt) and hypotensive drugs to 'control the circulation' and reduce operative blood loss were introduced, primarily by Enderby and his colleagues at East Grinstead in the early 1950s. Despite early setbacks, these pioneers established the safety of hypotensive techniques which were subsequently modified and refined for use in other branches of surgery. The use of hypotensive techniques also spawned wide-ranging research into cerebral blood flow and autoregulation which has significantly enhanced our understanding of these systems.[3]

ANAESTHETIC TECHNIQUES

The scope of plastic surgery is wide, with overlap into craniofacial, maxillofacial, oral, head and neck, ear, nose and throat, ophthalmic, burns and neurosurgery.

Deliberate arterial hypotension

The realization that the sympathetic ganglion-blocking drugs penta- and hexamethonium were capable of producing postural hypotension led to their use in plastic surgery in an attempt to lower blood pressure and reduce bleeding.[3] Although the initial drugs had limited success, refinements occurred over the years with the addition of pentolinium, halothane, intermittent positive-pressure ventilation (IPPV), β-blockade and potent direct-acting vasodilators such as sodium nitroprusside (SNP) and glyceryl trinitrate (GTN).[5,6]

Indications for arterial hypotension

There is one simple criterion by which the need for deliberate hypotension should be judged: its application shall be only for the ultimate benefit of the patient.[7]

There are several potential advantages. Blood loss may be reduced so that transfusion becomes unnecessary, or at the very least limited. This has obvious benefits. The duration of the operation is curtailed because less time is required for haemostasis and the surgeon has a much improved view of the operative field. The accuracy of the surgical operation is enhanced. Anatomical structures are more easily delineated so that there is less risk of accidental trauma to vital tissues.

All these effects are laudable, but only if they can be achieved safely and reliably. There have been many reviews of the safety of hypotensive anaesthesia, and controlled studies have been unable to identify any difference in morbidity and mortality provided that the anaesthetist is experienced in the technique and obvious risk factors are taken into account (e.g. cerebrovascular and cardiovascular disease[8]).

Should deliberate hypotension be used?

There are three absolute requirements which must be met before the use of hypotensive anaesthesia is considered:

1. The patient must, in the joint opinion of the surgeon and anaesthetist, derive positive benefit from the application of the technique to that particular operation.

2. The anaesthetist must have been properly trained and be competent, not only to administer a safe and skilled general anaesthetic, but to supplement it with deliberate hypotension, effectively maintained and safely controlled.

3. The surgeon must be sufficiently skilled and experienced to take positive advantage of the improved conditions of the field of operation so that he or she may carry out the operation more swiftly, more accurately and with reduced blood loss.[7]

If these criteria are met, complications are no greater than with conventional techniques.

Technique of hypotension and circulatory control

In the original technique of balanced anaesthesia a triad of narcosis, analgesia and muscle relaxation was stressed. Nowadays, a fourth is added — autonomic control. Techniques of circulatory control are necessary to prevent excessive variation in blood pressure during surgery. Similar techniques are used to produce hypotension. Most anaesthetic agents produce hypotension, e.g. the inhaled agents via cardiac output reduction (halothane) or peripheral vasodilatation (isoflurane).[9] Thus, hypotension is often easily achieved, particularly with the combination of head-up tilt and IPPV. Circulatory control can be difficult to maintain during changes in surgical stimulation, particularly during skin incision. There are three ways to deal with this problem:

1. A large dose of a specific hypotensive drug may be administered before incision to obtund the response; however, there is the possibility of severe hypotension during periods of surgical inactivity (especially with longer-acting agents).

2. A bolus dose of an ultrashort-acting analgesic (such as alfentanil) or anaesthetic (such as propofol) may be given immediately prior to skin incision.

3. The surgeon can infiltrate the operative site with local anaesthetic. In combination with small doses of specific hypotensive drugs, this produces admirable conditions in most patients.

The last option seems to be the most sensible compromise, allowing controlled circulation, but with little danger of profound hypotension. The use of labetalol in combination with the potent inhaled agents has found great favour.[9] Increments of 5 mg intravenously up to a maximum of about 25 mg produce adequate control (systolic blood pressure 60–80 mmHg). Minimal doses are required in older patients (over 50 years). Excessive decreases in blood pressure may be treated by judicious use of intravenous fluids, and reductions in tilt and anaesthetic concentration. Excessive bradycardia, with or without hypotension, is usually effectively reversed by atropine or glycopyrronium, although it may be difficult thereafter to re-establish hypotension.

Cleft lip and palate

The anaesthetic management of paediatric patients for plastic surgical procedures requires close co-operation and understanding between the surgeon and anaesthetist. Success depends upon avoidance of psychological trauma, establishment and maintenance of a secure airway and adequate access to the vascular system.[10]

Correction of cleft lip is usually undertaken in the first 3 months of life for cosmetic reasons as well as for facilitation of feeding. However, the commonly applied rule of 10s (patient greater than 10 weeks of age, 10 lb (4.5 kg) in weight and haemoglobin of 10 g.dl^{-1} or more) is no longer strictly applicable. Lip repair is now undertaken in some centres in the neonatal period in an effort to improve family acceptability and parental bonding. Difficulties experienced mainly relate to the age of the child for those inexperienced in infant procedures, and problems with tracheal intubation.

Normal considerations of anaesthesia for the neonate and infant apply, such as adequate fluid input, intravenous access and maintenance of body temperature. Cleft lip and palate can be associated with the Pierre Robin syndrome and thus the infant may pose problems of intubation and respiratory obstruction due to the presence of a hypertrophic tongue. Intubation may also be difficult if the laryngoscope enters the cleft in the maxilla, but this can usually be avoided.

Blood loss during surgery is usually slight, but intravenous fluids (such as compound sodium lactate in 5% dextrose, or Plasma-Lyte in 5% dextrose) should be administered at a rate of 5–7.5 ml.kg^{-1}.h. Complications specific to cleft lip repair include tracheal tube displacement, either complete or partial. Use of preformed tubes, such as the RAE pattern, have probably not reduced this possibility due to their fixed length and poor shape. The newer Portex Polar and Sheridan tubes may be more suitable. Anaesthesia need only be light, particularly if the surgeon uses local anaesthetic infiltration combined with adrenaline.

Cleft palate repair is usually undertaken at the age of about 6 months to 1 year. Tracheal intubation may prove difficult in inexperienced hands. Blood loss is often significant; it should be measured carefully and replaced if necessary.[11,12]

Facial surgery

This includes anaesthesia for rhytidectomy (face lift), blepharoplasty (eyelid reduction), excision of squamous cell carcinoma and flap repair and rhinoplasty. It is interesting to note the absence of reports of specialized anaesthetic techniques (hypotension apart) in the UK literature. Reports of general anaesthetic and regional/local techniques have mainly emanated from the USA and Canada.

Selection of technique: general versus local anaesthesia and sedation

There is much dispute in the literature about suitability for either technique. Obviously, old and frail patients benefit from a local anaesthetic technique with minimal sedation.[13] Whether there is less morbidity and mortality from this approach is uncertain. As will be seen, the distinction between general and local anaesthesia has become blurred, particularly in relation to techniques involving intravenous sedation.

General anaesthesia. Important considerations include:

1. assessment of the patient

2. selection of a tracheal tube for adequate airway control and surgical access
3. minimizing the risk of postoperative haematoma formation by:
   (a) prevention of coughing and straining on head movement and extubation
   (b) smooth emergence
   (c) prevention of nausea and vomiting postoperatively.

The technique itself is unimportant if these considerations are met. Nasal intubation is preferred by some surgeons as it avoids distortion of facial features, which may occur with a poorly positioned oral tube. If the latter route is chosen, an oral, south-facing Portex Polar tube, with a double bend (unlike the RAE) allows a better seating of the tube on the lower jaw. Anaesthesia is maintained with the patient in the head-up position. For nasal operations the throat is packed. Hypotensive techniques with head-up tilt may be employed to reduce bleeding (see below). If intermediate-acting relaxants such as atracurium are used, evoked reversal of neuromuscular blockade may be formal if appropriate monitoring is used routinely. This allows spontaneous ventilation to be established towards the end of the procedure and extubation of the trachea under reasonably deep levels of anaesthesia to avoid coughing.

In an effort to avoid tracheal intubation, Katz and colleagues used an inhalational technique (for rhytidectomy) using bilateral nasopharyngeal airways combined with local anaesthesia.[14] Intra-operative tracheal intubation was necessary in 7% of cases; most British anaesthetists (and surgeons) would find this requirement unacceptable. The laryngeal mask airway is rapidly finding a place for this type of surgery, as a safe airway can be achieved without the necessity for tracheal intubation.[15]

Kaye & Kruse recognized the problems with procedures performed under heavy sedation, and turned to general anaesthesia for apprehensive, unco-operative or poor physical status patients. The technique included fixation of the orotracheal tube using a strong suture placed round the lower teeth![16]

Local anaesthetic/sedation techniques. The use of office facilities for plastic surgery, particularly in the USA, is becoming more widespread because of rapidly escalating hospital costs, elimination of insurance benefits for cosmetic surgery in hospitals and scheduling difficulties in hospital operating rooms.[17] New techniques have had to be developed in intravenous analgesia and anaesthesia to allow such procedures to proceed in unfamiliar surroundings.[18]

Apart from the injection of diazepam to produce a calm and tranquil patient, followed by local anaesthetic infiltration or regional nerve block,[13] some more ambitious techniques have been described. It should be noted that the distinction between some of these techniques and general anaesthesia is somewhat blurred and indistinct.

Vinnick described his experience of 2000 cases of his office-based dissociative technique using diazepam and ketamine.[17] The technique is described here in detail to emphasize the inexorable progression to general anaesthesia. It consists of premedication 1 h before surgery with lorazepam 4 mg orally together with butorphanol 0.5 mg (an agonist–antagonist opioid similar in activity to pentazocine) and promazine 25 mg intramuscularly. On arrival in the operating room, a 21 G Butterfly needle is inserted into the external jugular vein. This enables the operator to administer additional sedation during the procedure whilst maintaining a sterile environment. Diazepam is administered intravenously in 5 mg increments up to 20 mg until the patient is deeply asleep (i.e. unrousable). A loading dose of ketamine 75 mg is then given intravenously. (The patient is now effectively anaesthetized.) Additional doses of ketamine 25 mg are given as necessary together with glycopyrronium if salivary secretions are a problem.

A somewhat similar technique is described by Buffington et al.[19] Lignocaine infiltration was also used in their cases, which not only included facial surgery but also breast surgery and abdominoplasty. They concluded that it was possible to perform virtually any superficial plastic surgical operation using this technique. There were few complications.

Desnoyers and colleagues from Quebec have also described a pseudosedative technique involving various neuroleptic drugs such as perphenazine, chlorpromazine and pethidine (lytic cocktail). The patient is then sedated with thiopentone/diazepam plus ketamine 25–50 mg intravenously as necessary.[20]

Safety aspects. The use of any of these dissociative techniques should not be attempted unless the office surgical facility is equipped for cardiac and respiratory emergencies with separate personnel, fully qualified in cardiopulmonary resuscitative techniques. Ventilation, pulse, blood pressure, electrocardiogram and oxygen saturation should be monitored.

McNabb & Goldwyn examined the blood gas and haemodynamic effects of sedatives and analgesic techniques when used as a supplement to local anaesthesia in plastic surgery. Blood gas changes revealed a fall of Pa_{O_2} to 9.3 kPa (70 mmHg) in some cases, with a rise in Pa_{CO_2} and a consequent respiratory acidosis. They now recommend the use of supplemental oxygen during these procedures, together with advice to the patient to take regular deep breaths.[21]

Flumazenil and agents for reversible sedation. Flumazenil, a 1,4-imidazobenzodiazepine derivative, is a highly effective, centrally acting, competitive benzodiazepine antagonist with low intrinsic activity. Given the widespread use of benzodiazepines such as diazepam and midazolam in sedative techniques in the office or outpatient setting, it is useful for hastening awakening. Due to rapid hepatic elimination, its half-life is short (about 1 h); nevertheless, a single dose of 0.05–0.1 mg.kg^{-1} intravenously is normally sufficient to attain and maintain the desired level of consciousness. The only consistent side-effect is nausea and vomiting.[22]

With the increasing demands for day surgery, flumazenil is certain to increase the applicability and usefulness of sedative techniques involving benzodiazepines. It is important that anaesthetists become fully involved in the implementation of reversible sedation (which would also involve the administration of naloxone and physostigmine).

Breast reconstruction

The mutilation of the female body by general surgical mastectomy represents one of the most serious psychological problems that patients with breast cancer face. Up to 40% are unable to accept serious, life-threatening disease with the uncertain success of treatment in addition to the disfigurement produced by mastectomy. As a result, many are turning to plastic surgeons for some kind of cosmetic salvage operation.[23] The difficulties encountered in breast reconstruction are substantially increased by previous radical surgery (e.g. pectoralis major removal) or irradiation. In these cases, a transposition flap (e.g. latissimus dorsi or rectus abdomini) is required to fill the defect. Where surgery has been less radical, tissue expanders may be inserted which are filled percutaneously over a period of weeks or months to achieve a suitable skin expansion.

Surgery for breast reconstruction involving flap transposition is long and complex. If the latissimus dorsi flap is chosen, the patient is initially placed on the side opposite to the previous mastectomy. The myocutaneous flap is then raised and tunnelled subcutaneously anteriorly to emerge through the old mastectomy incision. The patient is then carefully turned on to her back, the old incision is extensively undermined and the myocutaneous flap inserted into the margins of the old scar. A prosthesis is inserted under the transposed muscle and the wound closed. The other breast may also require adjustment at the same operation.

A normal general anaesthetic technique is employed and if a number of simple guidelines are followed, surgery is facilitated and blood loss minimized. This involves circulatory control with labetalol and isoflurane. Accurate blood pressure measurement is often hindered by surgical interference, and a blood pressure cuff should be placed on each arm.

Some surgeons feel that breast symmetry can be created optimally when the patient is brought to a totally upright position with the trunk vertical and perpendicular to the floor. Safety is well-documented but depends on planning with the surgeon pre-operatively and allowing time to move the patient.[24]

Surgery may take 2–3 h, with blood loss being replaced with Hartmann's solution and colloid solutions. In a personal series of 75 cases, blood transfusion was rarely necessary.

Conclusion

The major emphasis of plastic surgical anaesthesia is close co-operation between the surgeon and the anaesthetist. Specialized techniques of airway maintenance and circulatory control are major contributions which have been made by plastic surgical anaesthetists to anaesthetic practice in general.

ANAESTHESIA FOR MICROVASCULAR SURGERY

Following the first successful microvascular tissue transfer at East Grinstead, microvascular free transfer surgery has become increasingly common. Units such as Canniesburn in Glasgow and the Royal Marsden in London each undertake between 50 and 100 of these operations each year.[25]

In principle, the technique involves raising a donor tissue flap (which may consist of skin, muscle or bone, or a combination) complete with its own arterial supply and venous drainage. Following preparation of the recipient site (often involving extensive resection of tumour) and identification of a suitable artery and vein for anastomosis, the donor blood supply is divided and quickly attached to the recipient vessels using microvascular surgical techniques. This allows for a one-stage excision and repair of large tumours without the necessity for multistage operations involving pedicle flaps. As a result, these are becoming increasingly less common with a concomitant decrease in multiple-procedure repairs and in the time the patient is required to stay in hospital. In addition, digits can be transferred (e.g. toe to thumb) or emergency operations carried out for re-implantation following traumatic amputation.

Macdonald has summarized the basic anaesthetic requirements for these procedures.[26] The anaesthetist must possess a sound knowledge of circulatory physiology and pharmacology, particularly of the peripheral circulation. Adequate cardiac output and perfusion pressure must be maintained and normocapnia and adequate analgesia provided. Heat loss should be minimized by maintenance of a warm operating environment (22–23°C), use of warming blankets, warmed fluids and humidification of the inspired gas. In general terms, adequate tissue oxygenation must be maintained by optimization of blood flow and oxygen content.

Theoretical considerations

Circulatory control

This has been the subject of a number of useful reviews.[27-29]

Pressure, flow and resistance. The Poiseuille–Hagen equation describes the factors which determine flow of a homogeneous fluid through a non-distensible cylindrical tube:

$$\text{Blood flow} = \frac{\Delta P \pi r^4}{8 \eta l}$$

where ΔP is pressure gradient, r is radius of the tube, l is length of the tube and η is viscosity of the fluid.

Flow to a tissue is equal to the pressure gradient divided by resistance. The resistive component is determined by the radius of the blood vessel and viscosity of the blood. However, because flow is inversely proportional to the fourth power of the radius, changes in radius have a dramatic effect on resistance. In the sections that follow, the importance of this relationship is stressed.

Cardiac output, blood pressure and vascular resistance: principles of peripheral circulatory control. Factors which are relevant to this discussion include those which are likely to activate compensatory mechanisms to maintain blood pressure. Because there is no central control of cardiac output as such, blood pressure is maintained by a sympathetically (α_1-receptor) mediated increase in peripheral vascular resistance at the expense of reductions in cardiac output and oxygen delivery. During microvascular surgery, a decrease in cardiac output is usually due to decreased cardiac preload from hypovolaemia (absolute, due to blood loss or relative, from vasodilatation due to anaesthetic agents). Because maintenance of cardiac output (and oxygen delivery) is of such crucial importance, newer techniques of non-invasive measurement will assume increasing relevance during microvascular surgery. Such methods include oesophageal and transtracheal Doppler ultrasound, and thoracic bioimpedance techniques. These methods have a good correlation with more invasive (and inappropriate) techniques such as thermodilution.[30] Blood pressure must be maintained by volume replacement to restore cardiac output.

Neural control of blood pressure and vascular resistance. The reflex response to hypovolaemia and a falling venous pressure is mediated by the low-pressure cardiopulmonary baroreceptors situated in the vicinity of the superior vena cava and right atrial junction. Hypovolaemia results in an increase in sympathetic tone and peripheral vascular resistance with arteriolar and venular constriction (cardiac output is actually less than normal). The main site of vascular resistance is the arterioles and to some extent the small arteries and the precapillary sphincters. Although this may not be marked in some organ beds (e.g. cerebral), it is significant in skin and muscle. In excess, it is likely to prejudice flap survival.

During anaesthesia, this reflex may be effectively blocked by inhaled agents (halothane > enflurane > isoflurane) and intravenous induction agents (propofol > thiopentone > etomidate), all of which attenuate neural reflexes that stabilize blood pressure. Nitrous oxide, benzodiazepines and opioids such as fentanyl (not morphine and pethidine) have less effect. In addition, because halothane depresses cardiac output more than isoflurane,[31] a maintenance technique with the latter (which also decreases peripheral vascular resistance) is preferable.

The high-pressure baroreceptor reflexes are activated by sensors located in the arch of the aorta and respond to a falling arterial pressure (from any cause) by increased sympathetic activity. Again, although this reflex is partly blocked during anaesthesia, particularly by halothane, thiopentone and propofol, high doses are needed to produce profound hypotension during anaesthesia in the young, normovolaemic patient who is surgically stressed.[22] However, due to alteration in β-receptor affinity and numbers in the elderly, older patients are much more sensitive to the haemodynamic depressant effects of anaesthesia.[32]

Humoral control of blood pressure and vascular resistance. Longer-term effects on blood pressure and peripheral vascular resistance are humorally mediated through release of agents with marked vasoactive properties, such as adrenaline, noradrenaline, vasopressin, prostaglandins, kinins and angiotensin II. Again, excessive activation of humoral compensatory mechanisms due to hypovolaemia or in response to vasodilator agents, such as sodium nitroprusside (see below), may lead to prejudiced graft survival in the postoperative period.

The metabolic responses to anaesthesia and surgery also include increased output of catecholamines, growth hormone, renin–angiotensin–aldosterone, antidiuretic hormone, adrenocorticotrophic hormone and cortisol, and a resultant varying degree of insulin resistance. These result in the common accompaniments of surgery: hypertension, tachycardia, sodium and water retention, and immune depression. Although these responses are neurally mediated and can be blocked by regional anaesthetic techniques, blockade is usually only partial, suggesting an additional local response from the injured tissue. This local wound factor is thought to be the cytokine interleukin-1.[33]

In general, the larger arterioles (first- and second-order) are under predominantly neural influence whilst the smaller arterioles (third- and fourth-order) respond mainly to humoral (and direct vasodilator) influences.[5]

Local control of blood flow. Regulation of blood flow through capillary beds is intended mainly to optimize the supply of adequate oxygen and nutrients to cells requiring them. At any one time, only small sections of the capillary bed are perfused. As metabolism continues to proceed, hypoxia and hypercapnia supervene, together with the production of metabolic products such as adenine, hydrogen ions, potassium and lactic acid. These substances tend to cause relaxation of the precapillary sphincters to allow blood flow to be re-established. Thus, given an adequate supply to the tissue bed (dependent also on remote factors), blood can then be appropriately distributed by local factors.

The role of the endothelium. A recent review of endothelial factors involved in peripheral vascular control suggests that much greater importance should be attached to these factors when considering anaesthetic techniques and use of agents which might improve blood flow and/or rheology.[32] The role of the intact endothelium in the production of vasodilator substances such as endothelium-derived relaxing factor (EDRF, now known to be nitric oxide) and prostacyclin (PGI_2), is substantial. These are produced in response to potentially vasoconstricting factors, such as thromboxane (TxA_2) and adenosine diphosphate (ADP) produced from platelets following vascular damage and endothelial injury. These vasodilator factors, together with fibrinolytic agents such as tissue plasminogen activator (TPA), limit stasis and thrombosis following endothelial damage. In their absence, coagulation and thrombosis occur, the endothelium and distal tissues become hypoxic and events are set in motion which can lead to irreversible damage (Table 19.1).

To complicate the issue still further, intact endothelium also produces vasoconstrictor substances such as endothelium-derived contracting factors (EDCF) and endothelin. The latter is a 21-amino-acid peptide which has greater vasoconstricting activity than any other known hormone. It is also responsible for the metabolism of renin and angiotensin I to produce angiotensin II, another potent vasoconstrictor.

Additional factors of relevance during anaesthesia include the effect on the endothelium of smoking, ageing and arteriosclerosis, and endothelial changes due to hypertension and hyperlipidaemia. In the presence of these factors, the endothelium is much more sensitive to contracting substances as well as being less able to prevent the formation of thrombus due to tissue damage. The effectiveness of vasodilators, such as isoflurane, is also limited. Consequently, the success rate of microvascular surgery is likely to be prejudiced in this group of patients.

It can be seen from Table 19.1 that the situation during anaesthesia and surgery is extremely complex. Agents such as isoflurane and halothane have profound effects on the vascular smooth muscle which can vary according to the concentration and the arteriolar bed studied.

Blood vessel distensibility and critical closing pressure

From the law of Laplace, the tension (T) in a vessel is equal to the product of pressure (P) and radius (R):

$$P = T/R$$
$$\text{or } P = \frac{T\text{ (elastic)} + T\text{ (active)}}{R}$$

T (elastic) is the tension due to elastic recoil of the stretched elastic tissue in the vessel and this decreases as P and R are reduced. T (active) is the tension caused by smooth-muscle contraction from external causes, particularly increased sympathetic activity (see above). For a given pressure, equilibrium is maintained by changes in R and T. If pressure is reduced, there is reduction of R and thus T (elastic). At low levels of pressure, tension is chiefly due to T (active), as T (elastic) cannot fall any further when R is at a minimum. Below this critical level of P, the vessel becomes unstable and closes; this is known as the critical closing pressure (CCP).

Table 19.1 Effect of selected agents on peripheral arteriolar smooth muscle in the presence and absence of intact endothelium

Agent	Effect on smooth muscle with intact epithelium	Mechanism of action	Effect on smooth muscle in absence of epithelium	Mechanism
Acetylcholine (Ach)	Relaxation	Release of NO from intact endothelium which increases cyclic GMP in smooth muscle cells, causing protein kinase activation and relaxation	Constriction	Direct effect
Bradykinin, histamine	Relaxation	As above	?	
Sodium nitroprusside and nitroglycerine	Relaxation	Direct smooth-muscle relaxation by release of NO activation of guanylate cyclase and production of cyclic GMP, as above	Relaxation	Direct smooth-muscle activation of cyclic GMP
Prostacyclin	Relaxation	Stimulates cyclic AMP in smooth muscle	Relaxation if administered exogenously	
Isoflurane (high concentrations)	Relaxation	Release of NO	?	
Halothane	Relaxation	Inhibition of contraction caused by KCl and phenylephrine	Relaxation	Greater effect at higher concentrations
Methylene blue	Contraction	Inhibition of NO	No effect	
Isoflurane and enflurane (low concentration)	Contraction	Inhibition of NO and stimulation of release of EDCF	?	
Phenylephrine and noradrenaline	Contraction	Direct α_1-effect on muscle, inhibited by isoflurane and halothane	Contraction	
Hypoxia	Contraction	Generation of superoxide anions which inactivate NO. Also inhibits relaxation caused by Ach. Inhibits release of NO and stimulates release of EDCF. These effects *may* be prevented by superoxide dismutase		
Thrombin	Contraction	Release of endothelin-1 and thence increase in ITP and calcium-mediated contraction (inhibited by calcium antagonists)	No effect	
Renin	Contraction	Conversion to AT1 and AT2 in the endothelium. Direct effect	No effect	
Angiotensin II	Contraction	Direct effect	Contraction	Direct effect
Endothelin	Contraction	See above. Endothelin is the most potent vasoconstrictor known		

From Hall,[33] with permission.
NO = Nitric Oxide; GMP = guanosine monophosphate; AMP = adenosine monophosphate; KCl = potassium chloride; EDCF = endothelium-derived contracting factor; ITP = intrathoracic pressure; AT1, AT2 = angiotensin I, II.

The value of CCP is thus mainly determined by the value of T (active) or the level of overall tonic influences on the blood vessel. Thus, low pressures which are associated with vasodilatation decrease the value of CCP. As a corollary, in the presence of vasoconstriction the vessel may close at quite high pressures. The implications of avoiding vasoconstrictors which increase T (active) in microvascular surgery are therefore obvious. As stated earlier, blood pressure *must* be maintained by influencing factors which maintain (or increase) cardiac output rather than peripheral resistance. As a corollary, hypotension, if due to vasodilatation with a low T (active) is not, of itself, detrimental.

When considering oxygen delivery to the flap, it is the *local* control of circulation which is paramount. Thus, systemic measures to improve microcirculatory flow may actually divert or 'steal' blood away from the flap. It is likely that local vasodilator influences within the flap will be at a maximum, but systemic humoral influences may override these factors, to cause a reduction in flow. Neural control of the blood vessels of the flap is lost following transfer, but feeding and drainage vessels are still affected.

Viscosity, haematocrit and oxygen delivery

Blood is a non-Newtonian fluid, which means that viscosity is not constant and is determined by flow. Although it has a viscosity which is four to five times that of water, this is substantially reduced when blood is flowing. Rapid laminar flow results in axial streaming of cells so that the shearing stresses at the periphery are reduced along with the effective viscosity. In contradistinction, when flow rates are reduced, viscosity is markedly increased, especially at high haematocrit. This is due to attraction between slow-moving red cells enhanced by fibrinogen and globulins. Consequently, it is important to maintain high flows and a moderate haematocrit during microvascular surgery. In addition, the Fahraeus–Lindqvist effect means that viscosity is low even in very small vessels.

Conclusion

The overall effect of anaesthesia and surgery is to produce a profound alteration in haemodynamics and peripheral circulatory control, to which may be added the additional effects of agents used deliberately to lower blood pressure during tumour removal, such as sodium nitroprusside and labetalol. Although central venous pressure (CVP) is often measured in these patients, it does not provide unequivocal evidence of the state of the peripheral circulation, particularly under general anaesthesia. In the absence of major blood loss (easily measurable in most circumstances), hypotension is likely to be due to the vasodilatory effects of drugs. This can be overcome by a combination of reducing the concentration of inhaled anaesthetic agent and the dose of vasodilator (if used), reducing the postural stress, and finally by judicious fluid replacement until a satisfactory blood pressure is achieved.

In practice, discerning use of inhaled agents provides the anaesthetist with a pharmacological CVP. As homeostatic mechanisms are blocked, arterial blood pressure assumes a proportional relationship to blood volume.

Haematocrit and haemodilution

The effects of haematocrit changes on viscosity, flow and tissue oxygen delivery following haemodilution have been reviewed by Fahmy.[28] In general, a reduction in haematocrit is followed by a marked decrease in viscosity, which would tend to reduce pressure by reducing resistance (see Poiseuille–Hagen equation, above). However, probably as a result of reduced afterload consequent on reduced viscosity, cardiac output increases and there is thus little pressure change. Although oxygen content of blood is reduced by a decrease in haematocrit, oxygen delivery (the product of content and flow) is maintained due to the increase in cardiac output. Local blood flow also increases, thereby maintaining tissue oxygen delivery during normovolaemic haemodilution, and is probably maximal at a haematocrit of about 30–35%. Obviously, in the patient with cardiac decompensation, an increase in cardiac output may not be possible and haemodilution should be avoided.

Normovolaemic haemodilution, particularly if blood is collected following induction of anaesthesia but prior to surgery, is likely to be beneficial by improving local blood flow and thus oxygen delivery, provided that the haematocrit does not decrease below 30%.[28] However, no controlled trials have been reported to recommend its use routinely in microvascular surgery.

Practical considerations

The subject has been comprehensively reviewed.[25,26,34–38] It is important to note that there is little scientific backing for most of the statements made in these articles, or for the techniques used.[39] However, there seems to be a consensus on some factors. The prolonged duration of many of these operations[34] means that care of the patient must be meticulous, rather like the intensive unit (ITU) patient, particularly in respect of the following factors.

Pressure areas

Liberal use of gamgee and padding must be employed. Nerve and muscle damage has occurred during these operations.[34] Bird & Strunin[36] recommend the use of a ripple mattress and frequent limb movement to prevent this complication.

Humidification of inspired gases

This should be routine, but is of particular importance during prolonged surgery.[40,41] Use of a Pall bacterial filter achieves both humidification and decontamination of inspired gases. However, in protracted surgery, an active heated humidifier (such as a Bennett cascade) can be used to warm the patient actively by maintaining inspired gas temperature at 38°C.[42]

Temperature control

Theoretical factors. Neurones in the pre-optic hypothalamic nuclei (POH) are essential for activation of responses to thermal stress. In addition, they control the distribution of blood between the warm internal core and the body shell, which is usually 2°C cooler. Following induction of anaesthesia, these neurones are inhibited. This results in warmer core blood redistributing to the shell due to opening of arteriovenous fistulae.[43] This rapid redistribution of warm blood accounts for the pronounced fall in core temperature which occurs during the first hour or so of anaesthesia. The body then comes into equilibrium and there is a period during which heat loss to the exterior is balanced by internal heat production. This is aided by a proposed return of thermoregulation by the POH.[44] At this stage, the measures alluded to below should prove effective in maintaining body temperature, although at a lower core temperature than normal. No techniques are available to prevent the initial redistributive decline in core temperature.

General anaesthetics such as halothane, and opioids such as fentanyl, depress the threshold for peripheral vasoconstriction under anaesthesia by 2–3°C.[44] Also, by promoting peripheral vasodilatation, inhaled anaesthetics increase heat loss by radiation, conduction and evaporation. Neuromuscular blockers decrease heat production by impeding muscle activity.[44]

On awakening from anaesthesia, activity in the POH returns to levels above normal and shows greater sensitivity to thermal change. This is said to account for the excessive shivering activity which is frequently seen in the immediate postoperative period. Following this, a period of reduced sensitivity of POH is seen and this may result in a delayed return to normal body temperature. There is a compensatory increase in oxygen requirements in the postoperative period due to shivering.[45,46] This may prejudice graft survival and can be reduced by scrupulous attention to minimization of heat loss.

Practical considerations. The patient's temperature must be maintained as near normal as possible. Apart from humidification of gases, this can best be achieved by a warm operating theatre (21–22°C) and covering the patient with plastic or aluminized sheets over all areas which are not needed for surgery. Warming blankets in adults probably make little contribution to maintenance of body temperature.[47] The newer forced-air exchange blankets (e.g. Bair hugger) may prove to be more effective at conserving heat. If blood loss is expected to be excessive (e.g. emergency replantation), an in-line warmer should be employed. The cold stress of 1 unit of bank blood at 4–8°C is equivalent to that of 1 litre of colloid or crystalloid at 16–20°C: body temperature decreases by about 0.25°C.[48] In general, it is advisable to warm all i.v. fluids. If these factors are taken into consideration the anaesthetic technique in itself is not crucially important.

Personnel

Frequent breaks for coffee and other refreshments are necessary during some of the lengthier procedures to prevent excessive fatigue.[49] However, as the procedures become more of a routine, duration in skilled surgical hands is not excessive (average 4 h or less).

Fluid balance and blood loss

Meticulous fluid balance is necessary in the more protracted operations. Although fluids are often titrated to maintain CVP at some predetermined level, as noted previously, there is not much evidence that this has any direct relationship to circulating volume and cardiac output. The use of fluids to improve rheology is discussed later. Excessive administration of crystalloid is generally deprecated, although evidence that it produces oedema is scanty. Blood loss in some of the more prolonged cases can be excessive, and adequate amounts of blood should be cross-matched, and haematocrit checked at frequent intervals.[38]

Blood pressure

This should be maintained at near normal values, particularly if vasodilators are used. However, deliberate hypotension may be used during dissection and removal of the tumour, prior to the taking of the flap.[38] It is preferable to use a short-acting agent during this time so that hypotension may be easily reversed when it is time to reperfuse the flap. Once this has occurred, the aim is to maintain blood flow, which is difficult to predict from measurement of blood pressure alone. Hypovolaemia should be avoided at all costs.

Normoxia and normocapnia

There is a consensus that hypoxaemia should be avoided and that arterial carbon dioxide tension should be maintained at normal levels to prevent the deleterious effects of lowered levels on peripheral perfusion. This is best monitored by measuring end-tidal carbon dioxide tension and by arterial blood gas analysis.[38]

Selection of anaesthetic technique

The diversity of patients who may present for microvascular surgery precludes a detailed discussion of precise anaesthetic techniques. Many of the cases performed for head and neck cancer present problems with respect to previous chemotherapy, poor nutritional state, difficult intubation and poor venous access.[25] The emergency revascularization procedure obviously requires close attention to pre-operative blood loss and repletion, and the need to perform rapid-sequence anaesthetic induction and intubation in a patient with a full stomach.

In general, a balanced technique is used with muscle relaxants and adequate analgesic supplementation. The aim is to reduce stress and the attendant catecholamine secretion which may tend to reduce peripheral blood flow. The use of nitrous oxide could be questioned for any procedure which exceeds 5 h. Air and oxygen is a better solution, in combination with an inhaled agent. Isoflurane is theoretically preferable to halothane or enflurane because of the relative effects on cardiac output.

Local anaesthetic techniques are rarely used, and certainly not in isolation. Epidural anaesthesia supplementation has been advocated for lower abdominal and limb surgery, and brachial plexus block for the upper limb.[38] Systemic heparinization is advocated by some to reduce thrombosis of the graft. Although this might be thought to preclude the use of epidural or intrathecal blocks,[25] these have been successfully used to improve blood flow in microvascular surgery[50] without complication, even in a large series of 912 patients who received systemic heparin.[51]

If a tracheostomy is thought necessary, due to the site and extent of the surgical procedure, it is best performed at the beginning, thus allowing the anaesthetic breathing system to be removed from the surgical field. If this sequence is adhered to, it avoids the necessity for sophisticated oral or nasal tracheal tubes, as these will be replaced by a tracheostomy tube very early in the procedure.

Following anaesthetic induction and tracheal intubation, a wide-bore intravenous cannula is inserted, paying attention to the requirement of the surgeons for free flaps. An arterial cannula is used for continuous blood pressure monitoring and intermittent blood gas analysis, although the frequency of analysis is reduced by continuous measurement of end-tidal carbon dioxide tension and oxygen saturation. To avoid unnecessary trauma to the radial artery, a dorsalis pedis arterial cannula is frequently employed.

It is not generally necessary to insert a central venous catheter unless normovolaemic haemodilution techniques are to be employed. In head and neck surgery, direct access to central veins is often difficult or impossible. Catheters inserted from more peripheral veins (e.g. in the antecubital fossa) have a high failure rate in terms of correct positioning of the tip, and their use is not recommended unless the position is confirmed by X-ray. Accurate measurement of blood loss by swab weighing together with appropriate fluid repletion should ensure normovolaemia and adequate oxygen delivery.

Adjuvant techniques

Graft survival may be enhanced by a number of techniques, including the use of vasodilators, alterations in rheology and hypothermia.

Animal work provides evidence supporting the use of regional and systemic vasodilatation to enhance flap survival in microvascular surgery.

Local vasodilators. Vasodilatation is maximal in the flap itself due to hypoxia, hypercapnia and accumulation of metabolites following devascularization. However, feeding vessels are still subject to systemically induced vasoconstriction which could reduce flow. It seems rational to prevent this effect by the use of *regional* sympathetic block. *Intra-arterial* guanethidine has been used to produce prolonged (>3 days) and localized vasodilatation in experimental studies of flaps in the rabbit ear.[52] Application in humans could include an *intravenous* regional sympathetic block with guanethidine[53,54] when using the radial forearm free flap. Elsewhere, it would be difficult to limit the spread of guanethidine.

Systemic vasodilators. Although systemic vasodilatation with phenoxybenzamine, phentolamine and isoxsuprine is beneficial experimentally, no controlled trial has been carried out in humans. Indeed, *systemic vasodilators may be harmful* as they could produce steal of blood away from the maximally vasodilated flap. In addition, use of SNP causes a reflex increase in plasma renin activity (PRA) and angiotensin II secretion unless the patient is profoundly β-blocked.[6,9] This may cause problematical vasoconstriction when SNP is discontinued in the postoperative period. Nevertheless, systemic vasodilatation has been advocated using SNP or thymoxamine.[35,38]

Altered rheology: hypervolaemic haemodilution. Manipulations in haematocrit by hypervolaemic haemodilution to a haematocrit of 30–35% have been advocated by some.[26] This is rational, based on the evidence presented above.

Altered rheology: dextran administration. Alterations in blood viscosity by administration of dextran 40 is more controversial, but has been recommended.[26,37] Certainly, dextran has useful properties of reducing viscosity, preventing red blood cell rouleaux formation and minimizing platelet adhesion and sludging.

Hypothermia. Although rarely required in elective surgery, hypothermia and tissue perfusion, as is used for maintenance of graft viability for extended periods during transplant surgery, may be useful in emergency surgery for re-implantation. It extends the duration of experimental graft survival.[55]

Coagulation changes in microvascular surgery

One of the main reasons for graft failure is coagulation in the vessels of the transferred flap. The adverse influence of endothelial damage on protection of vessel smooth muscle from constrictor influences has been discussed above and is illustrated in Table 19.1. Virchow's triad suggests that the likelihood of intravascular coagulation is increased by stasis, trauma to the vessel wall and a hypercoagulable state. It is seldom appreciated that it is at least as important to maintain circulating concentrations of factors which reduce abnormal coagulation in major surgery as it is to replace coagulation factors themselves.

Much remains to be learned about the precise role of antithrombin III (AT-III) in thrombosis of transferred flaps and replanted limbs. AT-III binds to thrombin and thus inhibits (abnormal) coagulation. This reaction is greatly enhanced by heparin, which is ineffective in the presence of low AT-III concentrations. Seyfer et al studied the effects of elective, moderate and major trauma surgery on AT-III.[56] Although concentrations were reduced in the former two categories, the third caused a massive decrease, which was related to duration of surgery and the volume of blood transfused. Levels of AT-III were directly related inversely to graft survival. They advocated exogenous repletion of AT-III at an early stage during major surgery (e.g. with fresh frozen plasma or AT-III) and enhancement of its effect by addition of low-dose heparin.

Postoperative care

Intensive peroperative monitoring is futile if it is not continued well into the postoperative period. It is difficult to be precise about the period of vulnerability of the flap. Some quote a period of 48 h.[26] Certainly, the patient should remain well-perfused, warm and painfree during this time. Frequent examinations of the graft should be undertaken.

Reasons for graft failure

Despite all the anaesthetic manoeuvres described above, the main reason for graft failure is surgical. This may be due to poor vessels, poor technique or both. In traumatic amputation, the state of vessels and ischaemic time may be so great as to preclude a successful outcome, however skilled the surgery (and anaesthesia). The anaesthetic technique plays a small, albeit important part in determining graft survival.

The future

A perusal of the literature suggests that we have not discovered the optimal monitoring techniques for either the patient or the graft during these procedures. Since the principal factor on which graft survival depends is adequate oxygenation, it would seem reasonable to monitor oxygenation in the grafted area as well as the patient as a whole. This can easily be achieved in the patient by the use of tissue (conjunctival) oxygen monitoring.[57] This is a very sensitive index of tissue oxygenation and circulatory status and may prove useful as a global monitor during these procedures. Similarly, micro-oxygen electrodes could be inserted under the flap to monitor local oxygenation. Manipulations of blood volume, pressure, rheology and flow could then be scientifically assessed with regard to their effects on these parameters.

Conclusion

Anaesthesia for microvascular surgery is still at the infant stage. Much more scientific evidence is required before rigid advice can be given regarding anaesthetic techniques. Success or failure of the graft is predominantly determined by the surgeon.

ANAESTHESIA FOR BURNS SURGERY

Burn injury may involve skin, muscle or respiratory tract, or any combination. The skin is the largest organ of the body and is most often involved in extensive thermal injury. Because it has a primary commitment to water and heat balance, as well a providing a barrier to infection, it is not surprising that a major burn can produce detrimental effects in these areas. There is now improved understanding of the systemic effects resulting from major thermal injury, particularly in terms of fluid fluxes, stress response, hypermetabolism and immunomodulation. Advances in fluid resuscitation, treatment of infection, maintenance of adequate nutrition and surgical, anaesthetic and nursing techniques have all contributed to a continuing reduction in mortality.[58] In moderate to severe injury, the complexity of treatment necessitates admission to a specialized burns unit.[59-62]

Pathophysiology of major thermal injury

Surface burns may be due to heat, electrical injury or chemicals. In the first, three concentric zones exist in the area of the burn. The central area of coagulation necrosis, representing that part with the greatest exposure to heat, is surrounded by a zone of stasis which is a potentially viable area, and this is surrounded by an area of hyperaemia. Burn involving skin is classified as superficial partial thickness, deep partial thickness and full thickness. Destruction of the protective epidermal layers is described as superficial partial thickness and leads to dysfunction in water and thermal balance, and an increased risk of infection. As more dermal elements are destroyed (deep partial thickness), loss of skin function and delays in healing occur, especially if the wound becomes infected.

Electrical burns pose special problems because the extent of damage is often much greater than suspected. Both the voltage (pressure) and amperage (flow) of electricity are important determinants of injury. The superficial injury is characterized by an entry point of the electric current and an exit point at some distance away, representing the earth point. Between these points, the current takes the line of least resistance, usually muscle, causing extensive myonecrosis. Although there may be few systemic effects of fluid loss, extensive muscle damage and rhabdomyolysis can lead to the later complication of acute renal failure unless extensive debridement takes place immediately.

Chemical burns cause necrosis with similar problems to thermal burns.[63]

Metabolic effects

The metabolic response to burn injury follows two distinct phases. In the first phase, as a result of increased endothelial permeability and loss of protein and fluid, there is stasis in the burn wound, metabolic rate is decreased and this is accompanied by hypovolaemia, hypotension and a reduction in cardiac output. Following resuscitation, there is a second phase which is characterized by a massive increase in flow to the burn wound, hypermetabolism, raised cardiac output and increased oxygen consumption. The metabolic effects have both locally and systemically mediated components (Fig. 19.1). Locally, activation of phospholipase A_2 by heat leads to release of arachidonic acid from phospholipids by a process of lipoperoxidation. Arachidonic acid is then broken down by cyclo-oxygenase and lipoxygenase to prostaglandins and leukotrienes. These eicosanoids, together with autocoids such as histamine and bradykinin and cytokines such as interleukin-1, may be responsible for both the local and systemic increase in endothelial permeability which is characteristic of large burns (> 30% of body surface area or BSA). Although the systemic increase in permeability may be short-lived (<48 h) permeability continues to increase in the burned area itself. This, together with an increased blood flow (following resuscitation), is maintained until healing has taken place. This is worsened by activation of xanthine oxidase, which is an electron donor to oxygen, facilitating the formation of superoxide which can cause longer-term capillary endothelial damage and dysfunction.

Thus, one of the main initial effects of the burn is to produce profound hypovolaemia by a massive internal fluid shift from circulating volume to the interstitial fluid compartment. External fluid losses through the burn wound itself are relatively small in the early stages, but assume greater prominence after the first 48 h. Recent work has concentrated on alterations in the blood–lymph barrier and interstitial fluid and oncotic pressures to account for these losses. The normal slight negativity of interstitial fluid pressure increases dramatically in thermally damaged tissue. This, together with an increase in interstitial oncotic

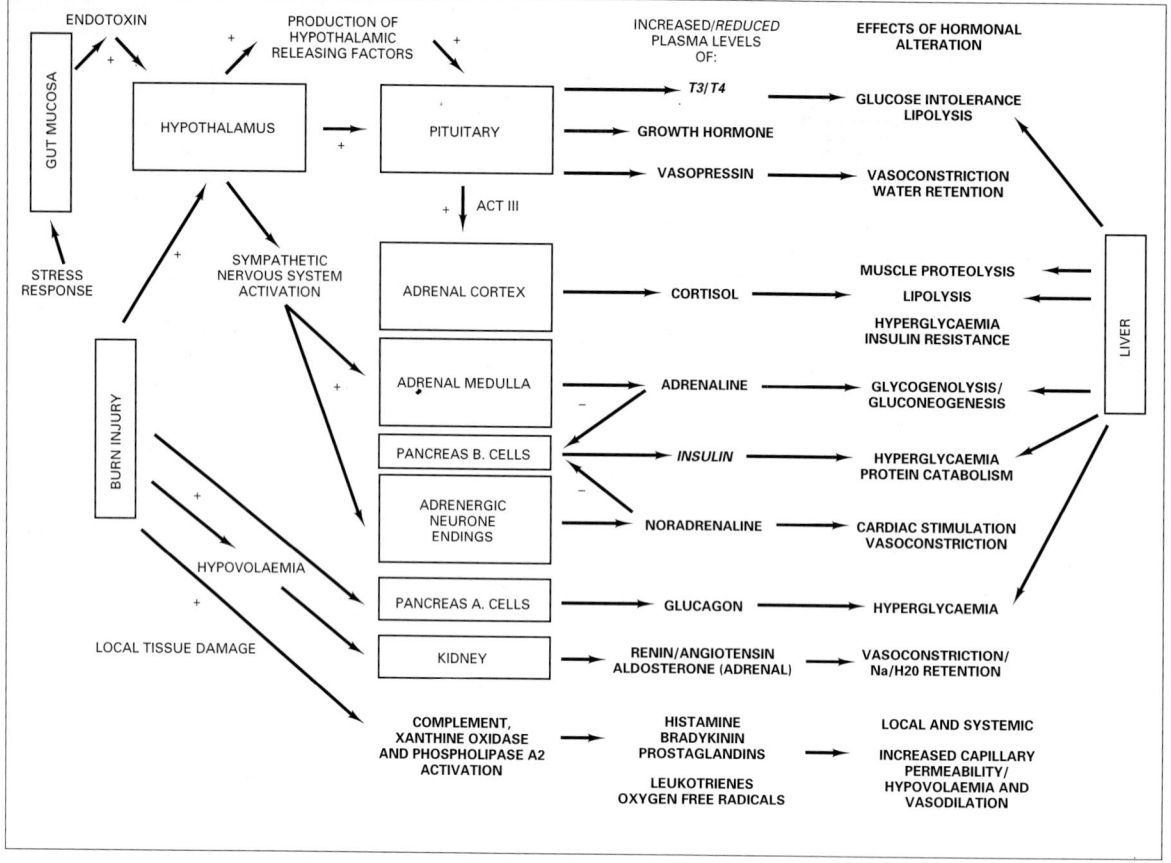

Fig. 19.1 Local and systemic metabolic responses to major thermal injury. ACTH = Adrenocorticotrophic hormone; T3 = tri-iodothyronine; T4 = thyroxine

pressure due to thermally mediated degradation of collagen, leads to a pronounced increase in fluid leakage from the circulating volume into the burn wound, as predicted by the Starling equation.[64] This loss is worsened by destruction of the stratum corneum which results in increased evaporative and heat loss. All these losses are proportional to the size of the affected area.

The systemic component is caused by tissue damage initiating a stress response which is mediated by the hypothalamus via the sympathetic and sensory nerves. This results in an outpouring of many hormones and mediators, as outlined in Figure 19.1. Catecholamines play an important role in sustaining hypermetabolism, the net result being an overall increase in metabolic rate, cardiac stimulation and hyperglycaemia. Decreased concentrations of tri-iodothyronine, thyroxine and insulin occur.[65] These changes produce a marked catabolic state and result in immune suppression. This increases the likelihood of infection at a later stage.

Although oxygen consumption returns to normal following burn excision and grafting in animals,[66] this does not occur in humans, where the excision of large areas of burned tissue does not appear to attenuate the increase fully. This is probably due to the difficulty in excising burn eschar completely in humans. In addition, damage to normal areas used for skin grafting may contribute to raised metabolic rate and oxygen consumption. It seems that this metabolic response cannot be 'switched off' until complete healing has taken place.[67] The data also suggest that elevated blood flow in the burn wound does not play a significant role in the pathogenesis of the hyperdynamic state.[68]

It is pertinent to note that inhalation anaesthesia with either enflurane or isoflurane markedly decreases tissue oxygen requirements in the hyperdynamic burned patient. The reductions in oxygen consumption, cardiac index and oxygen delivery occur in parallel, thus maintaining whole-body oxygen supply–demand balance. The changes are promptly reversed when

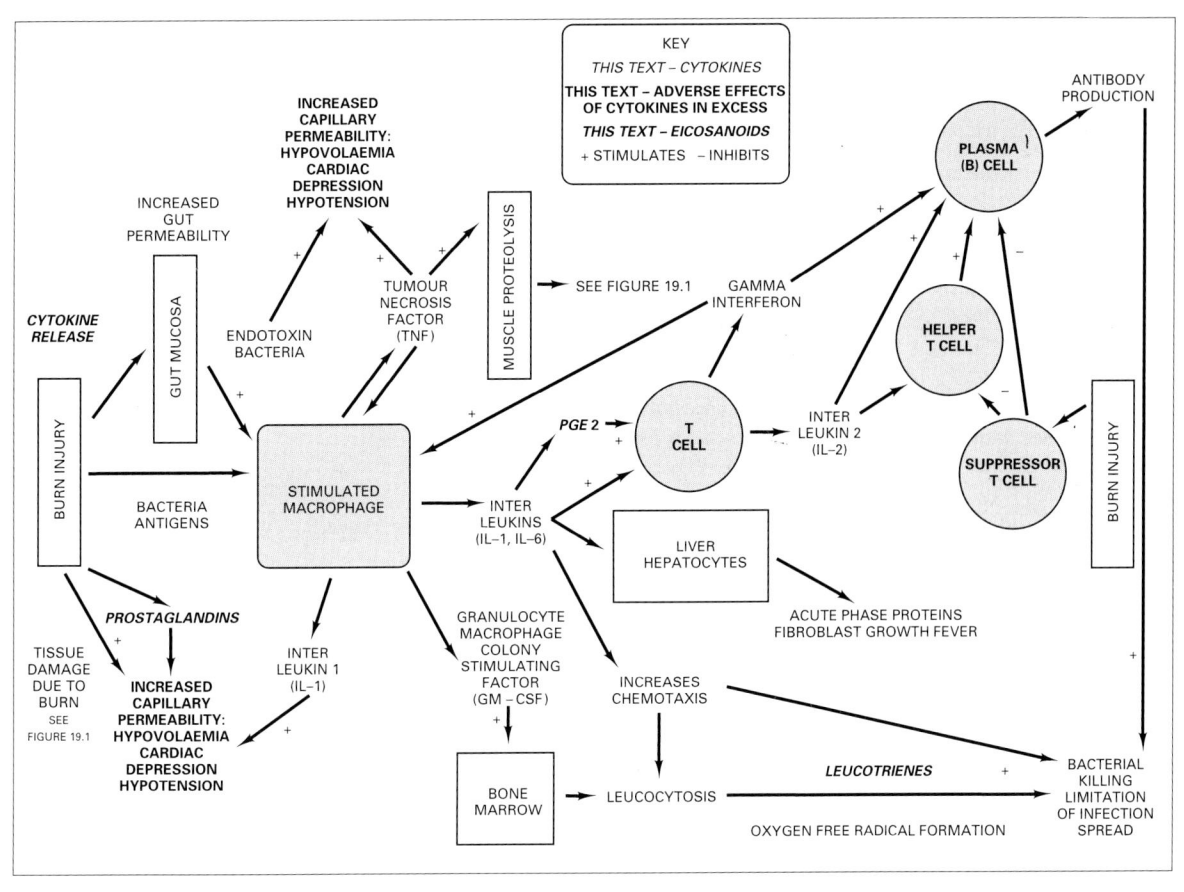

Fig. 19.2 Role of the immune system and cytokines in major thermal injury, including some interactions with the prostaglandins and leukotrienes. PGE_2 = Prostaglandin E_2.

anaesthesia is discontinued.[69,70] The possibility of pharmacologically reducing the metabolic response to the burn injury is being explored.

The increase in metabolic rate in a 50% burn often exceeds 100% of normal, necessitating administration of large quantities of calories, preferably by the enteral route (see below). This increase may be limited by nursing the patient in a thermally neutral environment at about 32°C.[71]

Immunological effects

The interaction between the metabolic and immune response to major thermal injury is extremely complex[65,72] (Fig. 19.2). Increased endothelial permeability, hypovolaemia, hypotension and cardiac depression result in decreased oxygen delivery and consumption. Endotoxaemia, splanchnic ischaemia and hypoxaemia lead to an increase in gut permeability and translocation of bacteria to infect mesenteric lymph nodes and systemic organs.[73,74] This, together with bacterial contamination from the wound itself, leads to activation of macrophages to produce the cytokines, interleukin, tumour necrosis factor and granulocyte macrophage colony-stimulating factors (GM-CSF).[75–78] The net result is to activate helper T cells and B cells so that immunoglobulin antibodies are produced. These, together with circulating opsonins such as fibronectin, bind with the specific bacterial antigens and facilitate bacterial ingestion and killing by polymorphonuclear leukocytes and macrophages. Stimulation of the bone marrow by GM-CSF ensures adequate supplies of leukocytes and chemotaxis is enhanced by interleukin-1 and leukotrienes.

In major thermal injury, exposure of collagen causes activation of Hageman factor (XII) which in turn leads to initiation of coagulation, complement, kinin, prostaglandin/leukotriene and fibrinolytic cascades. Although these are necessary for a favourable outcome, they must be kept in check by inhibitors. For example, local coagulation is desirable to stop bleeding, but disseminated intravascular coagulation is undesirable, as it may result in severe organ dysfunction. Complement activation is necessary at the site of injury to provide a 'homing beacon' for polymorphs and macrophages. Activation is localized to the site of injury by the action of complement inhibitors. In severe trauma, activation and production of complement overwhelm these inhibitory systems and lead to systemic release of the anaphylotoxins, C3a and C5a, both of which exacerbate tissue fluid loss causing widespread activation and margination of polymorphs. This leads to endothelial damage, particularly in the lung. In addition, local factors are produced by the burn wound itself, which can lead to immunosuppression.[79] This may involve increased production of suppressor T cells[80] which inhibit the activity of helper T cells and B lymphocytes.

Adequate initial resuscitation with maintenance of oxygen delivery, together with early excision of the burn wound, is essential to limit these adverse effects and to prevent sepsis.

Haemodynamic effects

Profound haemodynamic changes occur following severe burn injury prior to resuscitation. Fluid loss results in hypovolaemia and a reduction in cardiac output, blood pressure being initially maintained by increased sympathetic tone. The reduction in cardiac output precedes large fluid shifts and may be due to an as yet unidentified myocardial-depressant factor released from the burn wound. Systemic vascular resistance is increased by a combination of haemoconcentration, fluid loss and increased sympathetic tone. In the initial stages, the reduction in blood flow to relatively non-essential areas such as skin, kidney and muscle helps to maintain cerebral, cardiac and hepatic arterial blood flow. In the longer term, failure to reverse these changes by adequate fluid resuscitation leads inexorably to cardiovascular and renal failure, which invariably prove fatal. The realization that burn injury caused massive losses of fluid from the circulating volume was crucial for the introduction of appropriate fluid resuscitation regimens and a reduction in the high mortality which had previously existed (see below).

Loss of functioning red cells may occur in the burned area but this does not usually result in sufficient loss to require transfusion. However, escharotomy may lead to massive blood loss necessitating urgent replacement.

Respiratory effects

The respiratory tract may be involved locally due to thermal injury, inhalation of smoke-containing toxic gases and carbon monoxide, and by the systemic effects of burn injury. With the reduction in mortality of cutaneous burns, smoke inhalation is becoming an increasing cause of morbidity and mortality. Pulmonary pathology, primarily as a result of inhalation injury, now accounts for 20–84% of mortality associated with burns.[81] The presence of an inhalation injury is a strong determinant of mortality.[82] This topic has been the subject of recent reviews.[83-86]

Pulmonary changes from cutaneous burns

Circulating cytokines, prostanoids and autocoids released from burn tissue, together with the fall in plasma oncotic pressure in the early resuscitation phase, particularly when crystalloid regimens are employed sets the scene for alteration in pulmonary endothelial hydrostatic balance.

Starling's law states that the net fluid outflow from plasma to the interstitial space is related to the difference between hydrostatic pressures in the pulmonary capillaries and the interstitium minus the net difference between oncotic pressures in plasma and interstitial fluid, i.e.:

$$\text{Net fluid flow} = K(P_c - P_i) - \sigma(\pi_c - \pi_i)$$

where K is a constant which determines the net flow for any pressure difference which exists, σ is the reflection coefficient and describes how closely the capillary endothelium in the lung approximates to a true semipermeable membrane. For the latter, the value of σ would be 1 and such a membrane would permit the difference in oncotic pressure between the plasma in the capillary (π_c) and the interstitial fluid (π_i) to be fully expressed. The normal value in the lung is about 0.7. However, although the systemic effects of surface burn injury do not appear to increase capillary endothelial permeability to protein, in cases where there is inhalation injury, σ is reduced. As σ approaches zero, fluid movement will be determined solely by the hydrostatic pressure gradient between the capillary (P_c) and interstitial fluid (P_i). Fluid overload, in combination with myocardial depression (a frequent accompaniment of severe burn injury) is likely to lead to an increase in net fluid flow. However, the pulmonary lymphatics have a great capacity to increase lymphatic flow, which drains excess fluid from the interstitium until its capacity is exceeded. Thus, an increase in extravascular lung water with concomitant deterioration in lung function is not an inevitable accompaniment of these changes.

Although a decrease in dynamic lung compliance is seen early after severe burn injury, this is likely to be due to mediator-induced bronchoconstriction (attenuated by ibuprofen) rather than to increased lung water. The mediator may be either thromboxane or a byproduct of oxygen radicals, as evidenced by increased lipid peroxide production in lung tissue.[87] An increase in chest-wall oedema results in an additional decrease in static lung compliance.[88] Marked changes in pulmonary function may occur during burn excision, again due to release of thromboxane from the eschar. This is associated with increased lung lipoperoxidation and decreases in compliance and the Pao_2/Fio_2 ratio, which may be exacerbated by concomitant burn wound infection.[89]

Pulmonary damage due to direct thermal injury and inhalation of toxic gases and carbon monoxide

Effective heat dissipation in the upper airway means that heat damage to the major airways below the carina is unlikely. However, upper airway obstruction due to massive oedema following thermal injury can occur. Direct heat from superheated steam or the inhalation of smoke can cause pulmonary damage, including mucosal oedema and terminal airway collapse due to reduction of surfactant. Reduction in closing volume leads to maldistribution of ventilation and perfusion, with resultant hypoxaemia. Toxic gases in smoke, such as carbon monoxide, hydrogen cyanide, phosgene and acrolein, may also cause pulmonary damage and compromise lung function and gas exchange. This is manifest by increasing hypoxaemia despite a high inspired concentration of oxygen. Histotoxic hypoxia is caused by a direct effect of cyanide on cellular oxygen utilization (see below).

Carbon monoxide. Carbon monoxide, a colourless and odourless gas, is produced from incomplete combustion of carbon-containing materials. Carbon monoxide binds to the haemoglobin molecule 200 times more strongly than oxygen; thus, as little as 0.1% carbon monoxide can reduce oxyhaemoglobin to 50% of normal. The resultant marked decrease in oxygen transport is responsible for the majority of damage due to carbon monoxide. In addition, there is evidence of direct tissue toxicity caused by unbound carbon monoxide found in the plasma.[90] Acute exposure to carbon monoxide presents with symptoms and signs ranging from nausea and headache to coma, convulsions and myocardial infarction, even in patients with normal coronary arteries.[91] Delayed neurological problems are an additional feature in patients recovering from severe carbon monoxide poisoning.

It is important to realize that Pao_2 (and thus calculated oxygen saturation) may be normal or raised (if additional oxygen is being administered) in patients with carbon monoxide poisoning, as is apparent in oxygen saturation measured by a pulse oximeter. Most pulse oximeters are unable to distinguish between oxyhaemoglobin, methaemoglobin and carboxyhaemoglobin. Levels of carbon monoxide may be measured in the expired gas using a carbon monoxide meter or measured in a blood sample using an in vitro spectrophotometric oximeter.

Cyanide. As mentioned earlier, fumes from smouldering plastic can produce toxic gases; hydrogen cyanide is the most important because it can cause histotoxic hypoxia if inhaled. 'Normal' amounts of cyanide are combined with thiosulphate in the liver under the influence of the enzyme rhodanase, forming thiocyanate, which is excreted by the kidney. This system of elimination is relatively inefficient, and excess cyanide becomes a chemical asphyxiant, paralysing mitochondrial respiration and oxidative phosphorylation by combining with cytochrome oxidase.[6,86]

The brain and the heart are most sensitive to the hypoxia produced, with resultant tachycardia, tachypnoea, dizziness and lactic acidosis progressing to stupor, cardiac arrhythmias, apnoea, seizures and death.[92]

Oxygen transport

These changes in cardiovascular, respiratory and cellular function lead to deficiencies in oxygen transport and cellular oxygenation (Fig. 19.3).

Global oxygen transport (oxygen delivery; $\dot{D}o_2$) is equal to cardiac output ($\dot{Q}$) multiplied by the arterial oxygen content. Normally,

$$\dot{D}o_2 = \dot{Q} \text{ (l.min}^{-1}) \times (\text{Hb(g.l}^{-1}) \times 1.34 \times Sao_2(\%)/100)$$
$$= 5 \times (140 \times 1.34 \times 0.97)$$
$$= 1000 \text{ ml.min}^{-1} \text{ (ignoring oxygen in solution)}$$

The intimate associations between the cardiovascular haematopoietic and respiratory systems are clearly seen. Reduction of each to 75% of normal reduces oxygen delivery by over 60%. Recent studies have suggested that critical illness may be associated with inadequate oxygen delivery, with a resultant tissue oxygen debt which is difficult to define by normal clinical criteria. This may be related either to increased oxygen demand or to an inability to extract oxygen from the blood due to a metabolic defect, as occurs in sepsis. To this should be added the extensive oedema

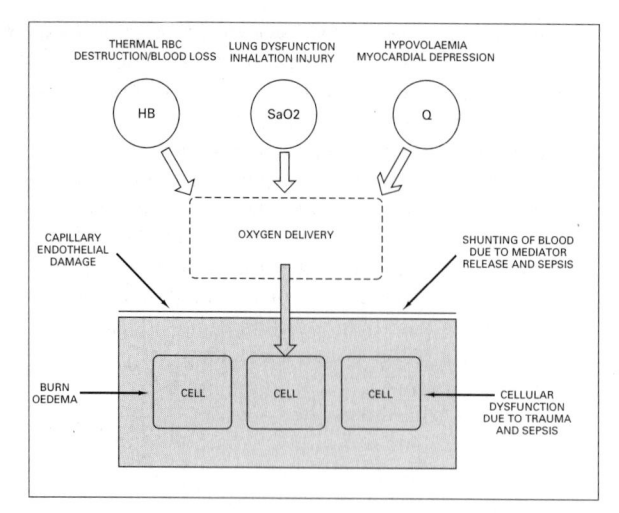

Fig. 19.3 Factors affecting cellular oxygen delivery and utilization. See text for details. QRBC = Red blood cell; HB = Haemoglobin; SaO_2 = saturation arterial oxygen; $\dot{Q}$ = cardiac output.

that occurs in the burn injury, which increases the distance that oxygen has to travel from haemoglobin to cell mitochondria.

Release of inflammatory mediators may result in shunting of blood away from essential capillary beds as well as depressing cellular oxygen uptake (Fig. 19.3). A protracted period of deficient oxygen delivery or utilization sets the scene for eventual organ failure. However, since thermal trauma is associated with activation of xanthine oxidase, increased oxidant release and lipoperoxidation, it would be detrimental to increase oxygen delivery unnecessarily to burned tissues lest this process be exacerbated. Work in sheep has suggested that present methods of measuring effectiveness of resuscitation in thermal injury are inadequate and result in a significant oxygen debt. Increasing oxygen delivery (which could be achieved by transfusion and/or inotropes) restores adequate oxygen delivery without further increasing release of oxidants from the burn wound.[93] This work demands a re-evaluation of present resuscitation regimens in thermal injury.[94]

Early assessment and treatment in major thermal injury

Anaesthetists may be involved in the initial management of burn victims, who should be dealt with and assessed methodically. Associated problems such as fractures, head injury, internal bleeding and drug overdose are common accompaniments and must be noted and treated. The major priority is assessment of the airway and breathing, particularly if there is a possibility of smoke inhalation. Circulatory status is assessed and appropriate fluid resuscitation started. A bladder catheter must be inserted for urine output monitoring. Burn wound care includes cleansing and removal of devitalized tissue, using a strict aseptic technique, application of topical antibiotics and coverings, and administration of tetanus toxoid.

Particular note should be made of circumferential burns. In the peripheries, these may cause circulatory obstruction whilst, in the chest and neck, impede ventilation. Clinical assessment of circulatory adequacy is unreliable so Doppler techniques and measurement of compartment tissue pressures should be undertaken. If in doubt, surgical escharotomy should be performed to relieve pressure; this involves making an incision throughout the length of the eschar to just beyond its boundary. Although this may be accomplished without anaesthetic (because it is usually performed in areas of full-thickness burn), it may be associated with rapid and heavy blood loss necessitating urgent replacement.

Fluid resuscitation

In minor burns of less than 10–15% BSA, aggressive intravenous fluid resuscitation may not be necessary. As larger burns lead to severe depletion of circulating volume, a careful assessment of fluid requirements and adequacy of replacement is mandatory. Given the amounts needed, a reliable, peripheral, wide-bore (14–16 SwG) intravenous cannula is required, preferably inserted through unburnt skin so as to avoid risk of infection.

Unfortunately, controversy exists over the type of fluid to use, the amount required and the end-point of adequate fluid resuscitation following burn injury.[94] Because there are both local and remote changes in vascular endothelial permeability, massive and unpredictable loss of circulating volume and protein may occur. Fluid therapy is directed towards correcting this deficit, thereby maintaining oxygen delivery to the tissues by restoration of cardiac output, whilst at the same time ensuring adequate haemoglobin and pulmonary gas exchange. Indeed, the goal of burned patient fluid resuscitation is the maintenance of organ function at the least immediate or delayed physiological cost.[95]

Following successful resuscitation, there are increases in cardiac output and oxygen consumption — the so-called hyperdynamic phase. This has implications for future management of the patient in terms of anaesthesia, nutrition and drug therapy (see below).

Assessment of the burn area. As fluid therapy is inextricably linked with the percentage of the BSA which is burned, accurate assessment of this area is crucial. It is important to distinguish between hyperaemia (erythema) and the burn itself. The former, though painful, does not contribute to fluid loss and will heal spontaneously provided that it does not become infected. Full-thickness burns have, by definition, no surviving dermis and are anaesthetic. Paradoxically, water and heat loss may be less than through partial-thickness burns due to the destruction of the blood supply.

Assessment of the burn area can be surprisingly difficult. The rule of nines is useful in the adult: there are 11 areas of 9% each and one of 1% (Fig. 19.4). Since a burn injury does not necessarily follow artificial boundaries, an assessment of 1% of the BSA based on the area of the patient's hand, laid flat with fingers together is a better method of estimation. In children, the Lund and Browder charts are more useful due to the difference in BSA of the various parts of the body in the infant and child.[96] For instance, the head represents 20% of BSA in the infant but only 9% in the adult (Fig. 19.5).

Time course of fluid loss. The greatest loss of fluid occurs immediately following the burn injury and gradually subsides over the next 24–48 h. Fluid regimens should reflect this reduction in fluid requirements.

Calculating the requirement. The fluid requirement of the patient is determined by:

1. the percentage of BSA burned (as above)
2. the time of injury, because fluid loss occurs from this time. A considerable deficit may already have arisen by the time the patient has reached a medical facility.
3. the weight (in kilograms) of the patient.

Various fluid regimens have been advocated. In general, the main controversy is whether to give any colloid (dextran, gelatin or albumin) during the initial resuscitation phase.[64,97,98] Some workers have suggested that, because the loss of protein which exists after a burn injury continues for a period of 48 h, it is pointless to give albumin-containing solutions during this phase as the exogenously administered colloid would simply leak out of the circulation into the interstitial fluid. Other workers feel that the evidence suggesting protein leakage is more transient and that solutions that contain colloid (albumin) provide a better resuscitation regimen.[99]

There is little evidence of an increase in remote capillary endothelial permeability to protein in the periphery or in the lung. Thus, thermally mediated systemic oedema and interstitial space expansion are caused and exacerbated by large quantities of crystalloid, which dilute plasma proteins and reduce oncotic pressure. These facts favour the use of colloid solutions in resuscitation. Unfortunately, the burn wound itself does show increased permeability to protein, so excess colloid might exacerbate wound oedema following restoration of endothelial integrity,[100] and delay healing by increasing oxygen diffusion distance as mentioned earlier. In the USA, albumin solutions are becoming scarce and increasing use is being made of synthetic colloids such as Pentastarch which seem equally efficacious.[101] A recombinant albumin preparation is about to undergo clinical trials.

In an effort to limit tissue oedema consequent on infusion of such large quantities of isotonic solutions, hypertonic solutions have been used. Although there is often a useful reduction in the volume of solution required, very few benefits have been observed when compared with other regimens.[102,103] The use of

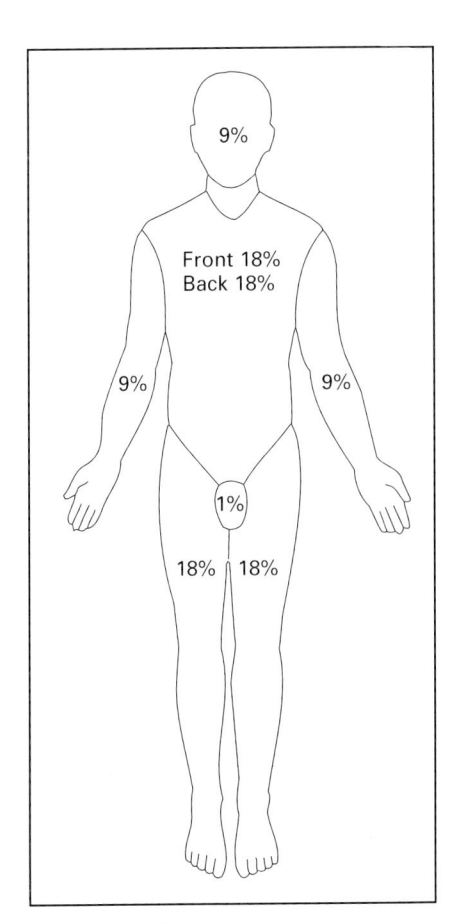

Fig. 19.4 The rule of nines.

CHART FOR ESTIMATING SEVERITY OF BURN WOUND

NAME _____ WARD _____ NUMBER _____ DATE _____
AGE _____ ADMISSION WEIGHT _____

LUND AND BROWDER CHARTS

IGNORE SIMPLE ERYTHEMA

Partial thickness loss (PTL)
Full thickness loss (FTL)

REGION	% PTL	FTL
HEAD		
NECK		
ANT. TRUNK		
POST. TRUNK		
RIGHT ARM		
LEFT ARM		
BUTTOCKS		
GENITALIA		
RIGHT LEG		
LEFT LEG		
TOTAL BURN		

RELATIVE PERCENTAGE OF BODY SURFACE AREA AFFECTED BY GROWTH

AREA	AGE 0	1	5	10	15	ADULT
A = 1/2 OF HEAD	9 1/2	8 1/2	6 1/2	5 1/2	4 1/2	3 1/2
B = 1/2 OF ONE THIGH	2 3/4	3 1/4	4	4 1/2	4 1/2	4 3/4
C = 1/2 OF ONE LEG	2 1/2	2 1/2	2 3/4	3	3 1/4	3 1/2

*Trade mark

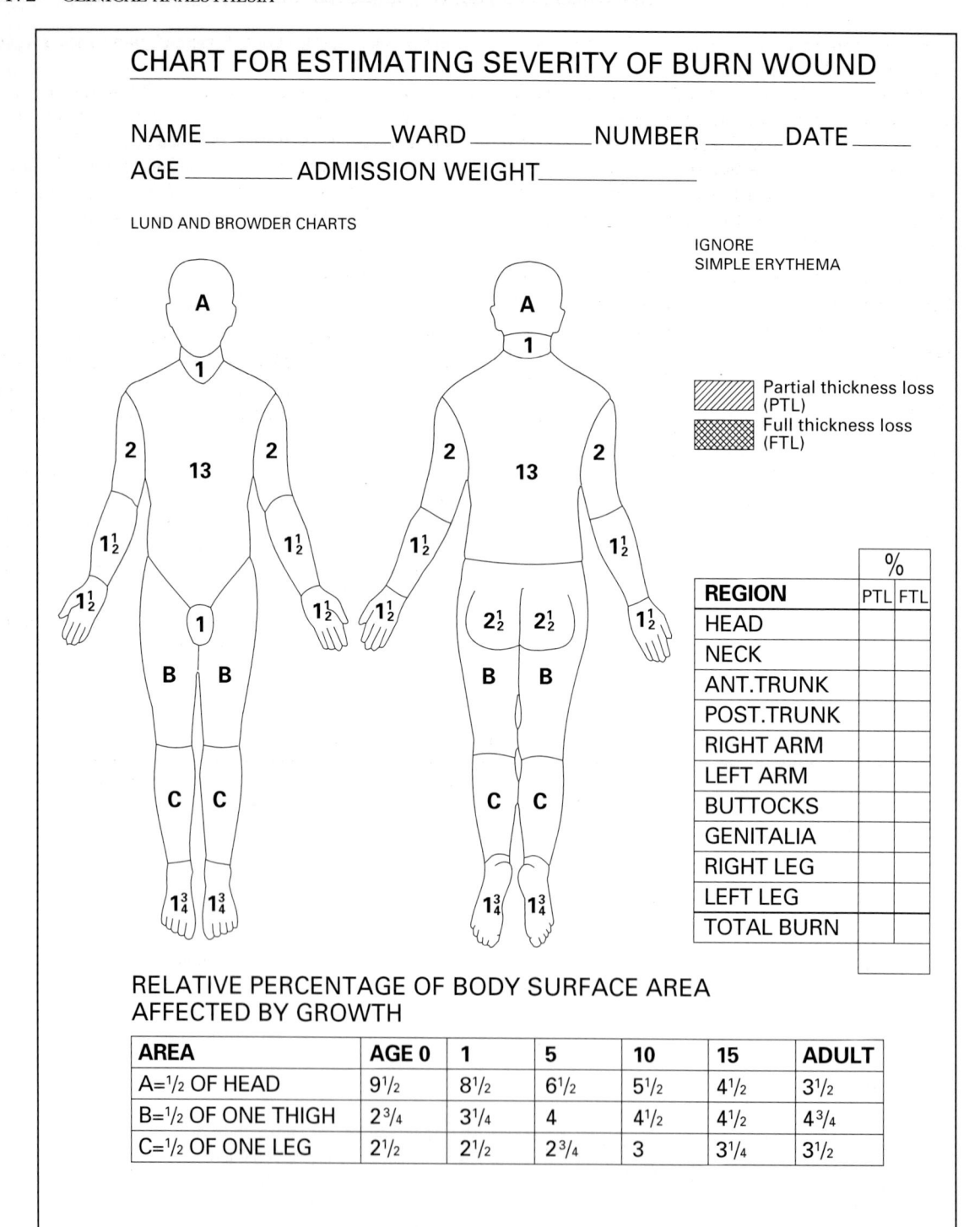

Fig. 19.5 Chart for estimating severity of burn wounds. Courtesy of Smith & Nephew Pharmaceutical.

hypertonic crystalloid combined with dextrans is controversial.[104,105]

For all regimens, a careful check on plasma sodium concentration should be made to avoid excessive hypo- or hypernatraemia. The former can cause severe neurological problems, particularly in children.[106]

Two regimens are illustrated below but as yet, no conclusive evidence exists to suggest that one regimen is preferable to another (Table 19.2).

1. A regimen based initially on lactated Ringer's (Hartmann's; compound sodium lactate) solution at a rate of 2.5–4 ml.kg^{-1} per % BSA burned (plus maintenance fluids) is recommended in the first 24 h by the National Institutes of Health in the USA (Parkland formula).[95]

Example: A 60 kg patient with a 40% BSA burn received at 1400 h. Fluid regimen commencing at 1800 h (using 4 ml.kg^{-1} per % BSA).

In the first 24 h (to 1400 h) the patient will need:

4 × weight × % BSA burned
   = 4 × 60 × 40
   = 9600 ml of Ringer's lactate

50% is given in the first 8 h, 25% in the next 8 h and 25% thereafter.

Thus, 4800 ml must be given by 2200 h (8 h after injury), 2400 ml by 0600 h the following day, and so on.

2. In the UK, the Mount Vernon (Muir and Barclay) formula is often used. This is a regimen which emphasizes the role of plasma protein fraction (PPF).[107]

Here the regimen relies on a 36 h period, with fluid requirements based on six time units of 4, 4, 4, 6, 6 and 12 h. The fluid requirement during each unit is:

0.5 × weight × % BSA burned
   = 0.5 × 60 × 40
   = 1200 ml of PPF in each time unit

Thus, 6000 ml would be infused in the first 24 h. Additional free water in the form of dextrose 5% is also given at a basic maintenance rate of 2000 ml per 60 kg in 24 h. Suitable adjustments are made for infants and children.

These regimens are diametrically opposite to each other in their use (or abuse) of PPF, and many units now administer a regimen based on a compromise between the two extremes. More fluid is necessary in the patient with inhaled pulmonary injury (up to 2 ml.kg^{-1} per % BSA).[85]

Evaporative losses. These are calculated on an hourly basis as 2 ml.m^{-2} BSA for each % BSA burn, e.g. for a 40% burn in a man of 2 m^2 BSA, this would

Table 19.2 Formulae used for estimating adult burn patient resuscitation fluid needs: first 24 h

Formula	Electrolyte	Colloid	Glucose in H$_2$O
Burn budget of F.D. Moore	Lactated Ringer's 1000–4000 ml 0.5 N Saline 1200 ml	7.5% of body weight	1500–5000 ml
Evans	Normal saline 1 ml.kg^{-1} per % burn	1 ml.kg^{-1} per % burn	2000 ml
Brooke	Lactated Ringer's 1.5 ml.kg^{-1} per % burn	0.5 ml.kg^{-1} per % burn	2000 ml
Modified Brooke	Lactated Ringer's 2 ml.kg^{-1} per % burn		
Parkland	Lactated Ringer's 4 ml.kg^{-1} per % burn		
Hypertonic sodium solution (250 mmol.l^{-1})	Volume to maintain urine output at 30 ml.h^{-1}		
Muir and Barclay		0.5 ml.kg^{-1} per % burn in 4, 4, 4, 6, 6 h periods	2000 ml

see Pruitt.[95]

amount to 160 ml.h^{-1}. The sodium content of this fluid should be about 70 mmol.l^{-1}.

Assessment of adequacy of fluid replacement.
The fluid regimens alluded to above can only be guidelines to therapy in the seriously ill patient. Continuous evaluation is needed to assess adequacy so that fluid therapy is titrated to maintain circulating volume, cardiac output and oxygen delivery during the immediate phase when the greatest losses are happening. At the same time, excessive input must be avoided so as to reduce the risk of circulatory overload, excessive weight gain and unnecessary increases in wound oedema.

The best *clinical* sign of adequate fluid intake is urine output. Providing this exceeds 0.5 ml.kg^{-1}.h^{-1} in adults (1 ml.kg^{-1}.h^{-1} in children), fluid input is probably sufficient.[108] A decrease in urine output with a concomitant increase in urine osmolality (>700 mosmol.l^{-1}) together with a low urine sodium (<20 mmol.l^{-1}) is strongly suggestive of inadequate fluid input. Following extensive burns, particularly if associated with muscle damage, urine output must be maintained at supranormal levels (with the use of mannitol if necessary) in order to avoid renal failure from acute tubular necrosis. Low output of iso-osmolar (280–310 mosmol.l^{-1}) urine, with a sodium content of 20–40 mmol.l^{-1}, is strongly indicative of this serious complication. Other indices, such as systemic blood pressure and pulse rate, are less reliable. A rising haematocrit is good evidence that fluid replacement is inadequate.

Aggressive *invasive* haemodynamic monitoring, using a thermal dilution pulmonary artery catheter, is employed in patients with large areas of burns to individualize therapy. Based on measurement of pulmonary artery pressure, cardiac output and left ventricular stroke work index, therapy can be optimized. Infusion of an inotropic agent such as dopamine may be necessary if the patient fails to respond to volume load as a result of myocardial depression. Using these indices, large variations are found in the amount of fluid needed to achieve predefined haemodynamic goals (Table 19.3). Values ranging from 1.42 to 5.34 ml.kg^{-1} per % BSA in the first 24 h, have been reported; less fluid was required in patients who received PPF.[109,110]

Measurement of oxygen delivery, consumption and extraction ratio may reveal occult tissue hypoxia, as mentioned earlier. An increasing metabolic acidosis together with a rising serum lactate concentration provides strong supporting evidence of inadequate resuscitation. Deterioration in pulmonary function limits respiratory compensation in these circumstances and makes overall acidaemia worse.

Table 19.3 Optimal ranges of haemodynamic parameters in adult burned patients

Variable	Value
Mean blood pressure	> 80 mmHg
Pulse pressure	> 40 mmHg
Pulse rate	< 120 beats.min^{-1}
Urine volume	> 0.5 ml.kg^{-1}.h^{-1}
Haematocrit	40–50%
Plasma protein	> 30 g.l^{-1}
Cardiac index	> 2.5 l.min^{-1}
Pulmonary capillary wedge pressure	2–7 mmHg
Central venous pressure	2–7 mmHg
Left ventricular stroke work index	> 25 g.m.m^{-2}
Systemic vascular resistance	1000–1750 dyn.s.cm^{-5}

Data from Aikawa et al.[110]

Assessment and treatment of inhalational injury

Treatment begins with the removal of the victim from the scene of the fire and administration of a high concentration of oxygen; this prevents further exposure and ameliorates other causes of hypoxia.

Careful assessment of the patient with potential upper-airway thermal damage and smoke inhalation is required. Many modalities have been used in the diagnosis of patients likely to develop serious respiratory problems as a result of inhalational injury, and include the following:

1. history (e.g. toxic fume inhalation, smoke-filled room)
2. the presence of facial and nasal burns
3. hypoxia
4. neurological signs due to cerebral hypoxia
5. carbonaceous sputum with auscultatory signs of wheezing and rales
6. elevation of carboxyhaemoglobin concentration to greater than 15% is suggestive of smoke inhalation: >40% causes coma, >60% collapse.
7. appearances on chest X-ray
8. airway mucosal erythema as visualized by fibre-optic bronchoscopy.

None of these is highly predictive. Although hypoxia in the early stages is highly suggestive of pulmonary damage, absence of hypoxia does not preclude the development of problems later on. In recent years assessment of respiratory mucosal damage in the upper and lower airway by the fibre-optic bronchoscope has become the standard technique for assessing these patients with the greatest accuracy.[111,112] Administration of a high concentration of oxygen displaces carbon monoxide from haemoglobin and optimizes oxygen delivery. In exceptional cases of carbon monoxide poisoning (over 30% carboxyhaemoglobin), the patient should be transferred to a hyperbaric oxygen facility.[113] If the patient is unconscious or there is evidence of severe thermal injury (see above) the airway should be immediately secured with a tracheal tube and ventilation commenced with 100% oxygen. Arterial blood gases should be measured, together with carboxyhaemoglobin and cyanide concentrations.

A high index of suspicion of cyanide poisoning is needed in such cases. An unremitting metabolic acidosis in the presence of carboxyhaemoglobin level greater than 15%, despite treatment, is highly suggestive of cyanide toxicity. Some studies have shown a correlation between carboxyhaemoglobin and cyanide levels.[92] Lethal concentrations of cyanide have varied between 0.5 and 3 mg.l^{-1} due to variation in the activity of liver rhodanase, worsened by burn shock, and low levels of thiosulphate (see below). Specific treatment is aimed at detaching cyanide from cytochrome oxidase and thus restoring normal aerobic metabolism.

As in poisoning with sodium nitroprusside, cyanide radicals may be scavenged by binding to:

1. exogenously administered hydroxocobalamin (4 g intravenously over 20 min) to form cyanocobalamin. This is non-toxic and can achieve dramatic reductions in blood cyanide concentrations
2. exogenously administered thiosulphate (12.5 g over 20 min). This forms thiocyanate, which is then excreted via the kidneys
3. an increased level of methaemoglobin, thus forming cyanmethaemoglobin. Methaemoglobin is formed from normal haemoglobin by the inhalation of amyl nitrite (0.2–0.4 ml via rebreathing) or by infusion of sodium nitrite (300 mg over 20 min). Both may cause hypotension, especially the latter
4. exogenously administered cobalt edetate (300 mg intravenously over 1 min) to form the inert complex cobalticyanide. Although this is the recommended treatment for *severe* poisoning, the other treatments are less toxic and should be used in the conscious patient.[86]

(N.B. Doses are for an average 60 kg patient. Suitable adjustments must be made for patients of different weight.)

Nutritional support

Aggressive enteral nutrition by early, continuous tube feeding has become standard practice in burn units over the last 20 years.[62,58] The role of the gut in thermal injury, both as a source of endotoxaemia and bacteraemia and also as the optimum route of nutrition, has been elucidated.[114] The incidence of gastric erosion and ulceration in the burned patient remains high.[115] The mainstay of therapy consists of early enteral nutrition as well as the use of antacids and H$_2$-antagonists such as cimetidine and ranitidine.[58]

Effect of thermal injury on gut endothelial permeability and function

Following major thermal injury, the gut is an innocent bystander in the midst of vast changes in metabolism and haemodynamics. A vital function of the intestinal mucosa is to act as a barrier in preventing the invasion and systemic spread of indigenous bacteria and endotoxin normally contained within the gut lumen. Although during simple starvation there may be a slight increase in gut permeability, in the presence of inflammatory mediators and a reduction in splanchnic blood flow permeability to fluids, bacteria and endotoxin is increased.[73,74,116] This occurs at a time of moderate to severe hepatic dysfunction due to shock and results in the gut being a major source of systemic bacteraemia and endotoxaemia, equivalent to the burn wound itself. In such circumstances, as in many other critical care settings, it is tempting to infer that the gut is incapable of normal function and either to withhold nutritional support or provide it by the parenteral route (total parenteral nutrition; TPN). In the burn setting this move would be disastrous for three reasons.

First, good evidence exists to support the view that adequate gut function can only be restored by oral feeding.[117,118] Although isotopic studies have shown that villous structure is restored by amino acids derived from the blood, TPN is ineffective in prevention or cure of this problem as it appears that luminal nutrients are required for release of hormones trophic to the gut. Table 19.4 shows the effects in the experimental animal of immediate versus delayed full-strength enteral nutrition on jejunal size and function following thermal injury.[117] Many burn units are therefore reviewing their policy of withholding enteral nutrition until after the resuscitation phase. However, there is still debate concerning whether enteral nutrition can be fully utilized at such an early stage in these patients.[114] Second, TPN regimens are associated with infectious complications such as septicaemia and endocarditis, as they usually require central venous catheterization. Third, TPN impairs the body's response to gut-derived endotoxin.[119]

Table 19.4 Effect of enteral nutrition with a high-protein (20–25%) versus traditional nutritional regimen in the burned guinea pig model (30% body surface area burn)

Anatomical and pathophysiological studies	Regimen 1 (high-protein)	Regimen 2 (traditional)
Jejunal mucosal weight (at day 1)	No change	50% reduction
Jejunal mucosal thickness and DNA content	No change	50% reduction
Cortisol levels (24 h to 14 days)	No change	150% increase
Glucagon increase	No change	Significant

Feed administered via gastrostomy tube, immediately post-burn.

Regimen 1: Pumpfeed of milk whey protein (Promix, 15% non-protein calories) and a complex carbohydrate (Polycose, 85% non-protein calories) + added vitamins and minerals.

Regimen 2: Day 1, lactated Ringer's only; day 2, one-third strength formula; day 3, two-third strength; day 4 onwards, full strength.

Data from Alexander & Gottschlich.[117]

A high-protein diet rich in arginine and low in linoleic acid has been found to be effective.[117] Additional glutamine and methionine are also recommended.[114] High glucose concentrations, with a calorie to nitrogen ratio of between 100 : 1 and 150 : 1, are necessary and help to switch off hepatic glycogenolysis and gluconeogensis. Depending on the size of the burn, 1.5–2 times the estimated calorie intake is required. Although thermal injury results in gut ileus, restoration of gut function is definitely impaired by delays in starting enteral nutrition. Recent work suggests that early enteral nutrition can reduce or even prevent the hypermetabolism and immunosuppression of thermal injury, thus reducing morbidity and mortality (Table 19.5).[117,118] As stated above, efforts must be made to limit hypermetabolism by maintaining a high ambient environmental temperature and limiting heat loss.

Effects of the burn injury on drug use in anaesthesia

The profound changes in hepatic, cardiovascular, respiratory and immune function which occur in thermal injury have profound implications for the use of drugs in these patients.[115,120]

Pharmacokinetic changes

Pharmacokinetics describe how the body handles the drug in terms of absorption, distribution, binding, metabolism and excretion. During the early hypodynamic phase, drug absorption from all sites is diminished due to reduced blood flow, thus necessitating administration by the intravenous route in small, divided doses. During the hyperdynamic phase, drug absorption is facilitated. A decrease in albumin concentration leads to increased free fraction of drugs normally bound to this moiety, such as diazepam, whilst an increase in acute-phase proteins results in a decrease in levels of free fraction of basic drugs such as the neuromuscular blockers. Changes in plasma binding on free drug levels are difficult to assess as most laboratories report total drug levels (bound and unbound).

Burn injury results in complex changes in hepatic drug metabolism. A reduction in hepatic blood flow results in decreased clearance of those drugs which have high hepatic clearance (such as the majority of opioids), whilst depressed hepatic enzyme activity, particularly in the septic patient, decreases the clearance of drugs with low to moderate clearance such as diazepam. This may be exacerbated by the administration of drugs such as cimetidine, omeprazole, erythromycin, ketoconazole and metronidazole, which inhibit hepatic metabolism.

However, an increase in glomerular blood flow leads to increased elimination and requirements for drugs excreted unchanged, such as the aminoglycoside antibiotics.

Table 19.5 Nutritional constituents and requirements and their role in thermally injured patients

Dietary constituent	Nutritional and metabolic effects
Amino acids	
Branched-chain amino acids, leucine, isoleucine and valine	Stimulation of protein synthesis, but a major clinical effect on patient outcome yet to be demonstrated
Glutamine	High loss from muscle in injury or sepsis needs increased intake for adequate replacement
Arginine	Essential amino acid during stress. Stimulation of immune system and increased wound healing. Stimulates growth hormone which *may* be beneficial
Methionine	Reduces negative nitrogen balance but full effect remains to be elucidated
Carbohydrate	Necessary for anaerobic glycolysis in the brain and kidney, although the former may adapt to use ketone bodies. Limited to maximum of 30 kcal.kg^{-1}.day^{-1} from glucose before increased incidence of fatty liver and increase in respiratory quotient with excess carbon dioxide production
Fat	Polyunsaturated fatty acids, long- and medium-chain triglycerides provide high-energy source in iso-osmolar solution. Also provide essential fatty acids and phosphate. Medium-chain have easier absorption and utilization than long-chain triglycerides. Can provide up to one-half of energy needs
Trace elements and vitamins	Trace elements, such as zinc, iron and copper are recommended but convincing evidence in favour is scanty. Increased requirement for B complex and C vitamins widely accepted

Data from Henley.[114]

Pharmacodynamic changes

The response of the burned patient to the majority of drugs is not profoundly altered. In general, increased doses are necessary to maintain clinical effect due to pharmacokinetic changes.

Neuromuscular blockers. Changes associated with the use of neuromuscular-blocking drugs can be explained by an effect of the burn injury producing a proliferation of nicotinic acetylcholine receptors over the muscle surface rather than their normal position at discrete end-plate junctions.[115]

Thus, following major thermal injury the depolarizing blocker suxamethonium causes widespread release of potassium from the entire muscle membrane rather than at these distinct sites. The excessive potassium release associated with administration of suxamethonium begins within days after thermal injury and may last up to 2 years. The systemic hyperkalaemia may cause severe arrhthymias, potentially necessitating the use of calcium, bicarbonate and/or glucose/insulin. Suxamethonium should generally be avoided in the burned patient, although it is probably safe if emergency tracheal intubation is required in the immediate phase following burn injury.[121]

Similarly, the increase in receptor sites renders competitive blockers less effective, with many studies showing increased dose requirements for the traditional relaxants, d-tubocurarine and metocurine.[115] The newer agents, atracurium and vecuronium, show similar effects. In adults, there is resistance to atracurium in patients with burns over 33% BSA from about 6 to 300 days (maximum at 15–40), the resistance being proportional to the size of the burned area.[122] Similar results were found in children, the maximum resistance occurring after the first week and being proportional to the burn size. There was no difference in comparison with controls up to the first week or in children who received the drug more than 3 years after the burn.[123] Depending on the size of the burn, the dose of vecuronium needed to produce a 50% reduction in twitch height in paediatric patients was increased by a factor of 2 in burns of less than 40% BSA and fourfold in 60% burns.[124] Thus, major burn injury (>30%) induces a resistance to the effects of competitive neuromuscular blockers which is evident about a week after injury, lasts for up to a year and is proportional to the size of the burn.

An increase in acute-phase proteins, especially α_1-acid glycoproteins, may also increase dose requirements of relaxants by increasing protein binding and thus decreasing the active, unbound fraction.[125]

Intravenous anaesthetics. Few pharmacokinetic and pharmacodynamic data exist for these drugs in the burned patient. Ketamine remains a most useful agent for the following reasons:

1. excellent cardiovascular stability, as its inherent cardiac-depressant effects are offset by its ability to facilitate sympathetic activity.

2. intense intra- and postoperative analgesic effect, available even at subanaesthetic doses
3. effective analgesia (1–2 mg.kg^{-1}) and anaesthesia (5–8 mg.kg^{-1}) by the intramuscular route
4. well-maintained airway reflexes and pharyngeal tone, resulting in excellent airway maintenance without the necessity to intubate the trachea.

This makes the drug particularly appropriate for procedures ranging from minor dressing changes and debridements to major escharotomies.[115] Despite its ideal properties, use of ketamine can result in loss of airway control, and facilities for tracheal intubation and administration of oxygen must be immediately to hand. In addition, arterial hypotension may still occur in the critically ill patient despite use of ketamine; patients must be optimally resuscitated before induction of anaesthesia. The hallucinogenic properties of ketamine during recovery can be diminished by administration of a benzodiazepine, but may still be problematical.[126]

Propofol has been compared with ketamine for induction and maintenance in burned patients. Despite an increased incidence of apnoea and moderate cardiovascular depression on induction, propofol was found to be a satisfactory agent with more reliable duration of action, shorter and more complete recovery and absence of deleterious psychological effects.[127]

Both ketamine[125] and thiopentone show evidence of tolerance in repeated use. Thus, the dose must be carefully titrated to effect; in the author's experience, massive doses of ketamine are sometimes necessary. Requirements for thiopentone are increased in children even 1 year or more after burn injury.[128]

Inhaled anaesthetics. Some authorities believe that halothane remains a useful agent for burn anaesthesia, because of its lack of pungency and ease of use for induction by the inhalational route — a pertinent consideration where venous access may be difficult. Although there is some controversy concerning the use of halothane for repeated anaesthetics in the burns patient,[115,129] medicolegal considerations probably dictate that, unless there is a good indication for its repeated use, multiple exposures to this agent — especially within a short time interval — should be avoided. All potent inhaled agents reduce oxygen consumption in these patients.

Analgesics. Pain management in burned patients is a topic frequently discussed but rarely considered in a scientific manner.[130] The mechanisms of pain production in both the acute and chronic phases remain to be elucidated. In some experimental situations, an acute burn to the hand may result in hyperalgesia (increased pain sensitivity) to subsequent thermal stimuli in other areas.[131] In addition, pain is described as an 'unpleasant sensory and emotional experience'; the latter component should not be underestimated.[132]

Pain relief is required immediately following the burn injury and can be achieved with incremental doses of an intravenous opioid such as morphine. This avoids problems with absorption from poorly perfused skin or muscle at a time when gastric absorption is also impaired. Following resuscitation, analgesia is required both for procedures and for background pain control. Although opioids can be employed for both, the acute, intense analgesia required for debridement and minor escharotomy is best achieved with ketamine. To avoid the necessity for repeated intramuscular injections, opioids may be administered orally or sublingually (e.g. morphine sulphate 20 mg 4-hourly, or buprenorphine 0.4 mg 8-hourly) and the dose adjusted accordingly. Alternatively, if the patient is able to manipulate the controls of an on-demand analgesia apparatus, this may provide a better and more controllable solution,[130] and also facilitates the administration of additional boluses of opioid which may be required for more intense periods of analgesia such as physiotherapy and dressing changes. Using a two-stage infusion regimen, excellent pain relief can be achieved with intravenous methadone.[133,134] The first-stage loading infusion is set at 0.1 mg.kg^{-1}.h^{-1} for 2 h followed by a 10-fold reduction to a maintenance infusion rate of 0.01 mg.kg^{-1}.h^{-1}.

Sedatives. Although the effects of a single dose of a benzodiazepine are unlikely to be modified in the burned patient, repeated doses may result in cumulative effects from agents which have active metabolites and long elimination half-lives. This particularly applies to diazepam; agents such as lorazepam or midazolam are more suitable in the burn/critical care setting.[115]

Antibiotics. From the time of the burn injury until closure has been achieved and the patient discharged from the burn unit, sepsis remains one of the most daunting problems faced by the patient as a result of:

1. the presence of a large devitalized area on the skin acting as a culture medium for exogenous micro-organisms
2. increased permeability of the gut endothelium to endogenous bacteria and endotoxin
3. systemic immunosuppression and modulation resulting from the burn injury and from failure to provide adequate nutrition
4. inappropriate use of antibiotics, resulting in further immunosuppression.

Treatment in the burn unit is obviously directed

towards minimizing these problems. Excision and grafting of the burned area remain the most important facet of treatment, but this takes time, during which the factors listed above must be considered. Although tetanus prophylaxis is still given on admission to the burn unit, routine antistreptococcal therapy has been all but abandoned.[63] Parenteral antibiotics are administered only when there is clear indication of systemic infection. Diagnosis of localized infection in the burn wound is best demonstrated by repeated biopsies of the burn eschar; a count exceeding 10^6 organisms per gram of tissue is deemed significant. As they penetrate burn eschar very poorly, topical antibiotics are used more frequently than in other situations and are applied to the wound following debridement and hydrotherapy. A commonly used agent is silver sulphadiazine, although mafenide acetate, povidone-iodine and silver nitrate are also used. Systemic absorption of these drugs can result in toxicity.[115]

If parenteral antibiotics are required, then higher doses than normal should be administered because of an enhanced rate of drug elimination through the kidney and loss of drug through the burn wound. Particular difficulties are encountered in those drugs such as aminoglycosides (frequently employed to treat systemic *Pseudomonas* infections), which have both increased elimination potential and a very low therapeutic ratio. Careful individualized titration of dose is required with frequent measurement of peak and trough plasma concentrations in order to achieve therapeutic concentrations without inducing nephro- and auditory toxicity. Newer, less toxic agents such as aztreonam may be preferable. As is common in other intensive care settings, the combination of major injury and broad-spectrum antibiotics frequently leads to systemic candidiasis and other fungal infections.[135]

Anaesthetic problems associated with burn excision and grafting

Following resuscitation, attention is directed by the burn team to obtaining skin closure as rapidly as possible in order to minimize the risk of infection, which delays healing and prejudices recovery. Rapid skin closure requires tangential excision of burn eschar and cover of the excised area with autograft under general anaesthesia. The ability to do this depends on the initial size of the burn wound and the availability of donor areas. In addition, burn excision is associated with massive bleeding and this limits the extent of closure that can be achieved during a single session. Use of cutting diathermy, tourniquets where appropriate and even hypotensive anaesthesia limit blood loss and allow more aggressive therapy.

The anaesthetic techniques for burn excision must be meticulously planned and executed.[136] Prior to anaesthesia, the patient's condition must be optimized, particularly with respect to fluid balance and haemoglobin concentration. Adequate amounts of blood should be cross-matched. Enteral feeds are stopped for the minimal time pre-operatively. Facial and neck burns must be assessed to determine whether there will be untoward problems with tracheal intubation.[137] A fibre-optic bronchoscope should be available in case of difficulties, and awake intubation used if necessary.

The patient is at serious risk of profound hypothermia and measures to preserve heat should be adopted. Theatre temperature is maintained around 30°C and surgery limited to 1–2 h. Suxamethonium is avoided and increased dose requirements for competitive neuromuscular blockers anticipated. A peripheral nerve stimulator is useful if a suitable site is available (ulnar or facial nerve).

During surgery, blood is replaced as it is lost, recognizing the difficulties of accurate assessment in these circumstances. The effects of rapid replacement of blood on plasma ionized calcium concentration must be taken into account as hypocalcaemia results in cardiac depression and hypotension. A number of cardiac arrests and severe hypotensive episodes have been witnessed in association with intravenous infusion of fresh frozen plasma, which has been shown in children to cause marked reductions in ionized calcium.[138] Excessive zeal on the part of the surgical team must be avoided so that burn excision is limited, to confine the insult to a manageable level. In a large burn, this means that multiple procedures must be performed before skin closure is achieved.

Conclusion

Thermal trauma produces severe derangements in homeostasis which are proportional to the extent of the injury. Concomitant inhalational damage increases the intensity of the problem and places severe demands on both the patient and the attending staff. A satisfactory outcome cannot be achieved unless there is a sound understanding of these problems. The anaesthetist has a crucial role to play in all aspects of management.

REFERENCES

1. Koopmann CF Jr. Anesthetic considerations in facial plastic surgery: the surgeon's viewpoint. Contemp Anesth Pract 1987; 9: 117–125
2. Bodley P. Development of anaesthesia for plastic surgery. J R Soc Med 1978; 71: 839–843
3. Enderby GEH. Historical review of the practice of deliberate hypotension. In: Enderby GEH, ed. Hypotensive anaesthesia. London: Churchill Livingstone, 1985: pp 75–91
4. Smith RM. Design and function of pediatric anesthesia systems. In: Smith RM, ed. Anesthesia for infants and children. St Louis, MO: Mosby, 1980: pp 128–151
5. Hester JB. The use of sodium nitroprusside as a hypotensive agent in plastic surgery. Postgrad Med J 1974; 50: 582–583
6. Verner I. Techniques for deliberate hypotension: Direct acting vasodilators. In: Enderby GEH, ed. Hypotensive anaesthesia. London: Churchill Livingstone, 1985: pp 164–183
7. Beare RL. Indications for hypotensive anaesthesia. In: Enderby GEH, ed. Hypotensive anaesthesia. London: Churchill Livingstone, 1985; 99–108
8. Green DW. Cardiac and cerebral complications of deliberate hypotension. In: Enderby GEH, ed. Hypotensive anaesthesia. London: Churchill Livingstone, 1985; pp 236–261
9. Green DW. Techniques for deliberate hypotension: pharmacological blockade. In: Enderby GEH, ed. Hypotensive anaesthesia. London: Churchill Livingstone, 1985: pp 109–137
10. Wallace CT. Anesthesia for plastic surgery in the pediatric patient. Clin Plast Surg 1985; 12: 43–50
11. Smith RM. Anesthesia for general, urologic and plastic surgery. In: Smith RM, ed. Anesthesia for infants and children. St Louis, MO: CV Mosby, 1980; pp 408–412
12. Watson JD, Pigott RW. Management of cleft lip and palate. Hosp Update 1991; 17: 306–312
13. Neil RS. Regional analgesia combined with intravenous sedation in major eyelid surgery: an alternative to induced hypotension. Br J Plast Surg 1983; 36: 29–35
14. Katz H, Machida RC, Wooton DG, Amonic R. A technic of general anaesthesia for blepharoplasty and rhytidectomy. Anesth Analg 1976; 55: 165–167
15. Brain AIJ. The laryngeal mask — a new concept in airway management. Br J Anaesth 1983; 55: 801–805
16. Kaye BL, Kruse JC. General anesthesia for rhytidectomy: a review of 100 consecutive cases. Plast Reconstr Surg 1977; 60: 747–751
17. Vinnick CA. An intravenous dissociation technique for outpatient plastic surgery: tranquility in the office surgical facility. Plast Reconstr Surg 1981; 67: 799–806
18. Pratt JM Jr. Analgesics and sedation in plastic surgery. Clin Plast Surg 1985; 12: 73–81
19. Buffington CW, Buehler PK, Glauber DT, Hornbein TF, Hamacher EN. A new system of infiltration anesthesia and sedation for plastic surgery. Plast Reconstr Surg 1984; 74: 671–682
20. Desnoyers Y, Custeau P, Berthiaume J, Dagenais G. Anaesthesia for facial rhytidectomy. Can Anaesth Soc J 1979; 26: 222–224
21. McNabb TG, Goldwyn RM. Blood gas and hemodynamic effects of sedatives and analgesics when used as a supplement to local anesthesia in plastic surgery. Plast Reconstr Surg 1976; 58: 37–43
22. Brogden RN, Goa KL. Flumazenil. A preliminary review of its benzodiazepine antagonist properties, intrinsic activity and therapeutic use. Drugs 1988; 35: 448–467
23. Ward DJ. Breast reconstruction. Hosp Update 1987; 9: 725–734
24. Smooth EC, Ross D, Silverberg B, Ruttle M, Newman LM. The sit-up position for beast reconstruction. Plast Reconstr Surg 1986; 77: 60–65
25. Inglis MS, Edwards JM, Robbie DS, Breach NM. The anaesthetic management of patients undergoing free flap reconstructive surgery following resection of head and neck neoplasms — a review of 64 patients. Ann R Coll Surg Engl 1988; 70: 235–238
26. Macdonald DJF. Anaesthesia for microvascular surgery: a physiological approach. Br J Anaesth 1985; 57: 904–912
27. Hainsworth R. Arterial blood pressure. In: Enderby GEH, ed. Hypotensive anaesthesia. London: Churchill Livingstone, 1985: pp 3–29
28. Fahmy N. Techniques for deliberate hypotension; haemodilution and hypotension. In: Enderby GEH; ed. Hypotensive anaesthesia. London: Churchill Livingstone, 1985: pp 164–183
29. Longnecker D. The microvascular response to hypotensive drugs. In: Enderby GEH, ed. Hypotensive anaesthesia. London: Churchill Livingstone, 1985: pp 54–65
30. Peruzzi WT, Vender JS. Haemodynamic monitoring. Curr Opin Anesth 1991; 4: 47–52
31. Wolf WJ, Neal MB, Peterson MD. The hemodynamic and cardiovascular effects of isoflurane and halothane anesthesia in children. Anesthesiology 1986; 64: 328–333
32. Ebert TJ, Stowe DF. Peripheral circulation: recent insights into autonomic nervous control and endothelial factors relevant to cardiovascular disease and anaesthesia. Curr Opin Anaesth 1991; 4: 3–11
33. Hall GM. Endocrine and metabolic responses to surgery and anaesthesia. In: Nimmo WS, Smith G, eds. Anaesthesia. Oxford: Blackwell Scientific Publications, 1989: pp 396–406
34. Hynynen M, Eklund P, Rosenberg PH. Anaesthesia for patients undergoing prolonged reconstructive and microvascular plastic surgery. Scand J Plast and Reconstr Surg 1982; 16: 201–206
35. Robins DW. The anaesthetic management of patients undergoing free flap transfer. Br J Anaesth 1983; 36: 231–234
36. Bird TM, Strunin L. Anaesthetic considerations for microsurgical repair of limbs. Can Anaesth Soc J 1984; 31: 51–60
37. Jakubowski M, Lamont A, Murray WB, de Wit SL. Anaesthesia for microsurgery. S Afr Med J 1985; 67: 581–584
38. Aps C, Cox RG, Mayou BJ, Sengupta P. The role of anaesthetic management in enhancing peripheral blood flow in patients undergoing free flap transfer. Ann R Coll Surg Engl 1985; 67: 177–179
39. Rylah LT. Does anaesthesia affect free flap survival? Br J Anaesth 1986; 58: 939–940
40. Chalon J, Loew DAY, Malebronch J. Effects of dry

anesthetic gases on tracheobronchial ciliated epithelium. Anesthesiology 1972; 37: 338–343
41 Chalon J, Ali M, Ramanathan S, Turndorf M. The humidification of anaesthetic gases: its importance and control. Can Anaesth Soc J 1979; 26: 361–366
42 Tausk HC, Miller I, Roberts RB. Maintenance of body temperature by heated humidification. Anesth Analg 1976; 55: 719–723
43 Hammel HT. Anesthetics and body temperature regulation. Anesthesiology 1988; 68: 833–835
44 Sessler DI, Olofsson DI, Rubinstein EH, Beebe JJ. The thermoregulatory threshold in humans during halothane anaesthesia. Anesthesiology 1988; 68: 836–842
45 Bay J, Nunn JF, Prys-Roberts C. Factors influencing arterial Po_2 during recovery from anaesthesia. Br J Anaesth 1968; 40: 398–406
46 Jones HD, McClaren CAB. Postoperative shivering and hypoxaemia after halothane, nitrous oxide and oxygen anaesthesia. Br J Anaesth 1965; 37: 35–41
47 Morris RH, Kumar A. The effect of warming blankets on maintenance of body temperature of the anesthetised paralysed adult patient. Anesthesiology 1972; 36: 408–411
48 Sladen RN. Temperature regulation and anesthesia. In: 1990 Annual Refresher Course Lectures. 1990 ASA 243. 1–7
49 Paget NS, Lambert TF, Sridnar K. Factors affecting an anaesthetist's work: some findings on vigilance and performance. Anaesth Intensive Care 1981; 9: 359–365
50 Weber S, Bennett CR, Jones NF. Improvement in blood flow during lower extremity microsurgical free tissue transfer associated with epidural anaesthesia. Anesth Analg 1988; 67: 703–705
51 Baron HC, LaRaja RD, Rossi G, Atkinson D. Continuous epidural analgesia in the heparinized vascular surgical patient: a retrospective review of 912 patients. J Vasc Surg 1987; 6: 144–146
52 Aarts HF. Regional intravascular sympathetic blockade for better results in flap surgery: an experimental study of free flaps, island flaps and pedicle flaps in the rabbit ear. Plast Reconstr Surg 1980; 66: 690–698
53 Hannington-Kiff JG. Intravenous regional sympathetic block with guanethidine. Lancet 1974; i: 1019–1021
54 Holland AJC, Davies KH, Wallace DH. Sympathetic blockade of isolated limbs by intravenous guanethidine. Can Anaesth Soc J 1977; 24: 597–602
55 Tsai TM, Jupiter JB, Serratoni F, Seki T, Okubo K. The effect of hypothermia and tissue perfusion on extended myocutaneous flap viability. Plast Reconstr Surg 1982; 70: 444–454
56 Seyfer AE, Seaber AV, Dombrose FA, Urbaniak JR. Coagulation changes in elective surgery and trauma. Ann Surg 1981; 193: 210–213
57 Abraham E. Conjunctival oxygen tension monitoring. Int Anesth Clin 1987; 25: 97–112
58 Deitch EA. The management of burns. N Engl J Med 1990; 323: 1249–1253
59 Snelling CF. The comprehensive burn unit. Can J Surg 1985; 28: 478–481
60 Feller I, Tholen D, Cornell RG: Improvements in burn care, 1965 to 1979. JAMA 1980; 244: 2074–2078
61 Sevitt S. A review of the complications of burns, their origin and importance for illness and death. J Trauma 1979; 19: 358–369
62 Demling RH. Burns. N Engl J Med 1985; 313: 1389–1398
63 Achauer BM, Martinez SE. Burn wound pathophysiology and care. Crit Care Clin 1985; 1: 47–58
64 Arturson G. Fluid resuscitation in burns and inhalation injury. Curr Opin Anaesth 1990; 3: 275–278
65 Weissman C. The metabolic response to stress: an overview and update. Anesthesiology 1990; 73: 308–327
66 Lalonde C, Demling RH. The effect of complete burn wound excision and closure on postburn oxygen consumption. Surgery 1987; 102: 862–868
67 Demling RH, Frye E, Read T. Effect of sequential early burn wound excision and closure on postburn oxygen consumption. Crit Care Med 1991; 19: 861–866
68 Gregoretti S, Gelman S, Dimick AR. Lack of immediate effects of wound excision on the hyperdynamic circulation of burned patients. J Burn Care Rehabil 1988; 9: 180–183
69 Gregoretti S, Gelman S, Dimick A, Proctor J. Total body oxygen supply–demand balance in burned patients under enflurane anesthesia. J Trauma 1987; 27: 158–160
70 Gregoretti S, Gelman S, Dimick A, Bradley EL Jr. Hemodynamic changes and oxygen consumption in burned patients during enflurane or isoflurane anesthesia. Anesth Analg 1989; 69: 431–436
71 Wilmore DW, Mason AD, Johnson D, Pruitt BA. Effect of ambient temperature on heat production and heat loss in burn patients. J Appl Phys 1975; 39: 593–598
72 Abraham E. Host defense abnormalities after hemorrhage, trauma and burns. Crit Care Med 1989; 17: 934–939
73 Deitch EA. Intestinal permeability is increased in burn patients shortly after injury. Surgery 1990; 107: 411–416
74 Deitch EA, Specian RD, Berg RD. Endotoxin-induced bacterial translocation and mucosal permeability: role of xanthine oxidase, complement activation, and macrophage products. Crit Care Med 1991; 19: 785–791
75 Riley-Paull KL, Munster AM. The role of cytokines in thermal injury. Crit Care Rep 1990; 2: 4–8
76 Marano MA, Fong Y, Moldawer LL et al. Serum cachectin/tumor necrosis factor in critically ill patients with burns correlates with infection and mortality. Surg Gynecol Obstet 1990; 170: 32–38
77 Guo Y, Dickerson C, Chrest FJ, Adler WH, Munster AM, Winchurch RA. Increased levels of circulating interleukin 6 in burn patients. Clin Immunol Immunopathol 1990; 54: 361–371
78 Silver GM, Gamelli RL, O'Reilly ME, Hebert JC. The effect of interleukin-1alpha on survival in a murine model of burn wound sepsis. Arch Surg 1990; 125: 922–925
79 Ferrara JJ, Dyess DL, Luterman A, Curreri PW. Transportation of immunosuppressive substances produced at the site of burn injury into the systemic circulation: the role of lymphatics. J Burn Care Rehabil 1990; 11: 281–286

80 McIrvine AJ, O'Mahony JB, Saporoschetz I, Memmick JA. Depressed immune response in burn patients: use of monoclonal antibodies and functional assays to define the role of suppressor cells. Ann Surg 1982; 196: 297–301

81 Herndon DN, Thompson PB, Trabner DL. Pulmonary injury in burned patients. Crit Care Clin 1985; 1: 79–96

82 Clark CJ, Reid WH, Gilmour WH, Campbell D. Mortality probability in victims of fire trauma: revised equation to include inhalation injury. Br Med J 1986; 292: 1303–1305

83 Zellner PR. The 1990 Everett Idris Evans memorial lecture: the inhalation injury. J Burn Care Rehabil 1990; 11: 487–495

84 Vanacker B, Boeckx W, Van Aken H, Gruwez JA. Current concepts of inhalation injury in burns victims. Acta Anaesthesiol Belg 1989; 40: 107–112

85 Herndon DN, Barrow RE, Linares HA et al. Inhalation injury in burned patients effects and treatment. Burns 1988; 14: 349–356

86 Langford RM, Armstrong RF. Algorithm for managing injury from smoke inhalation. Br Med J 1989; 299: 902–904

87 Jin LJ, Lalonde C, Demling RH. Lung dysfunction after thermal injury in relation to prostanoid and oxygen radical release. J Appl Physiol 1986; 61: 103–112

88 Jin LJ, Lalonde C, Demling RH. Effect of anesthesia and positive pressure ventilation on early postburn hemodynamic instability. J Trauma 1986; 26: 26–33

89 Demling RH, Katz A, Lalonde C, Ryan P, Jin IJ. The immediate effect of burn wound excision on pulmonary function in sheep: the role of prostanoids, oxygen radicals, and chemoattractants. Surgery 1987; 101: 44–55

90 Goldbaum LR, Orellano T, Degal E. Mechanisms of the toxic action of carbon monoxide. Ann Clin Lab Sci 1986; 6: 372–376

91 Mariusnunez AL. Myocardial infarction with normal coronary arteries after acute exposure to carbon monoxide. Chest 1990; 97: 491–494

92 Silverman SH, Purdue GH, Hunt JL, Bost RO. Cyanide toxicity in burned patients. J Trauma 1988; 28: 171–176

93 Demling RH, Lalonde C, Fogt F, Zhu D, Liu Y. Effect of increasing oxygen delivery postburn on oxygen consumption and oxidant-induced lipid peroxidation in the adult sheep. Crit Care Med 1989; 17: 1025–1030

94 Waxman K. Toward a re-evaluation of burn resuscitation. Crit Care Med 1989; 17: 1077

95 Pruitt B. Fluid resuscitation for extensively burned patients. J Trauma 1981; 21: 690–692

96 Lund CC, Browder NC. Estimation of area of burns. Surg Gynecol Obstet 1944; 79: 352–358

97 Hall KVN, Sorenson B. The treatment of burn shock: results of a five year randomised controlled clinical trial of dextran 70 vs. Ringer's lactate solution. Burns 1978; 5: 107

98 Hughes KR, Armstrong RF, Brough MD, Parkhouse N. Fluid requirements of patients with burns and inhalation injuries in an intensive care unit. Intens Care Med 1989; 15: 464–466

99 Carvajal HF, Parks DH. Optimal composition of burn resuscitation fluids. Crit Care Med 1988; 16: 695–700

100 Baxter CR, Shires GT. Physiological response to crystalloid resuscitation in severe burns. Ann NY Acad Sci 1968; 150: 874–894

101 Waxman K, Holness R, Tominaga G, Chela P, Grimes J. Hemodynamic and oxygen transport effects of pentastarch in burn resuscitation. Ann Surg 1989; 209: 341–345

102 Monafo WW, Chuntrasakaul C, Ayvazian VH. Hypertonic sodium solutions in the treatment of burn shock. Am J Surg 1973; 126: 778–783

103 Gunn ML, Hansborough JF, Davis JW, Furst SR, Field TO. Prospective, randomized trial of hypertonic sodium lactate versus lactated Ringer's solution for burn shock resuscitation. J Trauma 1989; 29: 1261–1267

104 Onarheim H, Missavage AE, Kramer GC, Bunther RA. Effectiveness of hypertonic saline–Dextran 70 for initial fluid resuscitation of major burns. J Trauma 1990; 30: 597–603

105 Horton JW, White DJ, Baxter CR. Hypertonic saline dextran resuscitation of thermal injury. Ann Surg 1990; 211: 301–311

106 Sarnaik AP, Meert K, Hackbarth R, Fleischmann L. Management of hyponatraemic seizures in children with hypertonic saline: a safe and effective strategy. Crit Care Med 1991; 19: 758–762

107 Muir IFK, Barclay TL, Settle JAD. The practical management of burns shock. In: Muir IFK, Barclay TL, Settle JAD (eds) Burns and their management, 3rd edn. London: Butterworths, 1987: pp 30–35

108 Settle JAD. Urine output following severe burns. Burns 1974; 1: 23–42

109 Aikawa N, Martyn JAJ, Burke JF. Pulmonary artery catheterisation and thermodilution cardiac output determination in the management of critically ill burned patients. Am J Surg 1978; 135: 811–819

110 Aikawa N, Ishibiki K, Naito O, Abe O. Individualised fluid resuscitation based on haemodynamic monitoring in the management of extensive burns. Burns 1982; 8: 249–255

111 Moylan JA, Adib K, Birnbaum M. Fiberoptic bronchoscopy following thermal injury. Surg Gynecol Obstet 1975; 140: 541–543

112 Hara KS, Prakash UBS. Fiberoptic bronchoscopy in the evaluation of acute chest and upper airway trauma. Chest 1989; 96: 627–630

113 Wiseman DH, Grossman AR. Hyperbaric oxygen in the treatment of burns. Crit Care Clin 1985; 1: 129–145

114 Henley M. Feed that burn. Burns 1989; 15: 351–361

115 Martyn J. Clinical pharmacology and drug therapy in the burned patient. Anesthesiology 1986; 65: 67–75

116 Grimble G, Payne-James JJ, Rees R, Silk DBA. Enteral nutrition: novel substrates. Int Care and Clin Mon 1989; 10: 51–57

117 Alexander JW, Gottschlich MM: Nutritional immunomodulation in burn patients. Crit Care Med 1990; 18: S149–S153

118 Mochizuki H, Trocki O, Dominioni L, Brackett KA, Joffe SN, Alexander JW. Mechanism of prevention of post-burn hypermetabolism and catabolism by early enteral feeding. Ann Surg 1984; 200: 297–310

119 Fong Y, Marano MA, Barber A et al. Total parenteral

nutrition and bowel rest modify the metabolic response to endotoxin in humans. Ann Surg 1989; 210: 449–457
120 Bonate PL. Pathophysiology and pharmacokinetics following burn injury. Clin Pharmacokinet 1990; 18: 118–130
121 Gronert GA, Theye RA. Pathophysiology of succinylcholine hyperkalaemia. Anesthesiology 1975; 43: 89–99
122 Dwersteg JF, Pavlin EG, Heimbach DM. Patients with burns are resistant to atracurium. Anesthesiology 1986; 65: 517–520
123 Mills AK, Martyn JA. Evaluation of atracurium neuromuscular blockade in paediatric patients with burn injury. Br J Anaesth 1988; 60: 450–455
124 Mills AK, Martyn JA. Neuromuscular blockade with vecuronium in paediatric patients with burn injury. Br J Clin Pharmacol 1989; 28: 155–159
125 Tatman AJ, Wrigley SR, Jones RM. Resistance to atracurium in a patient with an increase in plasma alpha globulins. Br J Anaesth 1991; 67: 623–625
126 Martinez S, Achauer B, Dobkin-de-Rios M. Ketamine use in a burn center: hallucinogen or debridement facilitator? J Psychoactive Drugs 1985; 17: 45–9
127 Galizia JP, Cantineau D, Selosse A, Crepy A, Scherpereel P. Essai comparatif du propofol et de la ketamine au cours de l'anesthésie pour bain des grands brules. Ann For Anesth Réanim 1987; 6: 320–323
128 Cote CJ, Petkau AJ. Thiopental requirements may be increased in children reanesthetized at least one year after recovery from extensive thermal injury. Anesth Analg 1985; 64: 1156–1160
129 Gronert GA, Schaner PJ, Gunther RC. Multiple halothane anesthesia in burn patients. JAMA 1968; 205: 878–880
130 Marvin JA, Heimbach DM. Pain control during the intensive care phase of burn care. Crit Care Clin 1985; 1: 147–157
131 Meyer RA, Campbell JN. Myelinated nociceptive afferents account for the hyperalgesia that follows a burn to the hand. Science 1981; 213: 1527–1529
132 Klein RM, Charlton JE. Behavioral observation and analysis of pain behavior in critically burned patients. Pain 1980; 9: 28–40
133 Denson DD, Concilus RR, Warden G, Raj PP. Pharmacokinetics of continuous intravenous infusion of methadone in the early post-burn period. J Clin Pharmacol 1990; 30: 70–75
134 Concilus R, Denson DD, Knarr D, Warden G, Raj PP. Continuous intravenous infusion of methadone for control of burn pain. J Burn Care Rehabil 1989; 10: 406–409
135 Desai MH, Herndon DN, Abston S. *Candida* infection in massively burned patients. J Trauma 1987; 27: 1186–1188
136 Lamb JD. Anaesthetic considerations for major thermal injury. Can Anaesth Soc J 1985; 32: 84–92
137 Larson SM, Parks DH. Managing the difficult airway in patients with burns of the head and neck. J Burn Care Rehabil 1988; 9: 55–56
138 Cote CJ, Drop LJ, Hoaglin DC, Daniels AL, Young-ET. Ionized hypocalcemia after fresh frozen plasma administration to thermally injured children: effects of infusion rate, duration, and treatment with calcium chloride. Anesth Analg 1988; 67: 152–160

20. Anaesthesia for major organ transplantation

R. A. Wiklund   J. A. Fabian   R. L. Keenan

Starzl and colleagues[1-3] noted that the entire approach to disease in patients with end-stage organ failure has changed with the advent of major organ transplantation. Previously, physicians aimed at restoring or enhancing the remaining function of diseased tissues or organs but when function of the organ deteriorated beyond the minimum required to maintain homeostasis for the individual, death was inevitable. Major organ transplantation offers an alternative approach which can restore homeostasis for some patients. However, transplantation programmes impose severe demands on patients, their families, physicians and health care systems with resources that are already limited.

The first successful major organ transplantation, a living related renal homograft, was performed at the Peter Bent Brigham Hospital in Boston, Massachusetts in 1954, and 9 cases were reported[4] in 1956. Prolonged survival of the recipient occurred when renal homograft transplantation was performed between identical twins. In 1963, Starzl et al[5] performed the first orthotopic liver transplantation (OLT) and in 1967, Barnard[6] undertook the first heart transplantation. The availability of histocompatible organs limited the success of major organ homografts until the phenomenon of organ rejection could be controlled with the introduction of cyclosporin A[7,8] in 1976, for immunological suppression of the recipient.

Several advances led to the development of transplantation programmes at centres worldwide. Control of acute rejection was improved with cyclosporin A. Improved extracorporeal preservation of the transplanted organ was possible with preservatives such as that developed at the University of Wisconsin (UW solution).[9,10] Technical advances improved the surgical and anaesthetic management of the brain-dead donor and transplanted organ,[11] as well as the recipient.[12,13] However, despite an increased public awareness of the possibility of organ donation following death, organ availability continued to be the limiting resource for most transplantation programmes.

Although the anaesthesia team is not directly involved in many aspects of a transplantation programme, its members need to understand and be familiar with preoperative and postoperative problems involved in transplantation because of the impact of the events in the operating room on homograft and recipient survival. Some of the problems are exemplified by transplantation at the simplest level, a blood transfusion or blood 'transplantation'. Histocompatibility, harvesting, tissue preservation, storage, support of the recipient and prevention of rejection are principles applicable to blood transfusion as well as major organ transplantation. The complexity of these issues increases as the list of organs suitable for organ transplantation grows. Organs suitable for homograft today include heart, lung, heart and lung, liver, kidney, pancreas, small bowel, bone marrow, cornea, skin, blood and blood products.

Organs may be transplanted to the site occupied by the native organ — orthotopic (heart, liver) — or may be placed in adjacent or even remote areas of the recipient — heterotopic (kidney, islet cells, potentially heart). Most organs are derived from the same species (homografts) or even the same individual (allografts) but the future of transplantation may include organs from other species (xenografts), particularly if the problem of donor organ salvage cannot be solved. Xenografts may offer the only future for the large number of newborn patients who need organ transplantation for immediate survival.

Transplantation, as addressed in this chapter, is performed at the organ level, but there is potential for transplantation at the tissue, cellular and molecular level for diseases such as Parkinson's disease, type 1 diabetes mellitus and muscular dystrophy. Molecular engineering may permit transplantation without the need for immunosuppression.

We will review several topics common to all major organ homografts, including brain death, organ availability, organ procurement, recipient selection and economic impact of major organs. For an in-depth review of the anaesthetic management for specific homografts, reviews,[14-16] chapters[17-19] and monographs[20] are available. This chapter will review the three stages of transplantation common to all organs: end-stage disease, absence of the native organ and the neotransplantation period. These stages will be reviewed for the three commonly performed major organ transplantation (liver, kidney and heart), with the strongest emphasis on OLT.

GENERAL CONSIDERATIONS

Organ procurement

All transplantation programmes suffer from a lack of suitable organs for transplantation despite the availability of suitable donors. Public awareness has been increased by initiatives such as universal donor declarations appended to drivers' licences, legislative efforts to presume consent for organ donation and publicity campaigns suggesting 'Don't take your heart to heaven, heaven knows we need it here!'

Pilot programmes for organ procurement in the USA were organized in 1968 in Boston and Los Angeles as part of the federally controlled end-stage renal disease programme. Since then, organ availability and utilization have been maximized by a programme established under the National Organ Transplant Act of 1968 and controlled by the Secretary of Health and Human Services. The Secretary awarded a contract to the United Network for Organ Sharing (UNOS, 1100 Boulders Parkway, Suite 500, PO Box 13770, Richmond, Va 23225) for a registry of patients awaiting organ transplantation and required all medical centres performing major organ transplantation to participate and co-operate with UNOS in allocation of donor organs and recipient selection. UNOS now works with 71 organ procurement organizations in matching compatible donors and recipients. UNOS maintains a database of the recipient histocompatibility profile, physical status, location and availability. In addition, urgency of transplantation for patients awaiting transplantation (Table 20.1) is co-ordinated with organ availability.

The first organ procurement organization in Europe was set up in the Netherlands. Eurotransplant serves the Netherlands, Belgium, Luxemburg, Germany and Austria. UK Transplant Services serves the UK and Ireland. The Scandinavian countries allocate organs through Scandia Transplant. Similar services exist in France and Italy. Co-ordination of transplantation in most other countries is not organized and donor organs are procured locally.

Table 20.1 United Network for Organ Sharing classification of liver transplant recipient status

Status	Clinical features
I	At home, working full-time, disease well-compensated
II	At home, unable to work because of the clinical features of liver disease
III	In the hospital, liver disease inadequately compensated
IV	In an intensive care unit, may be in respiratory or renal failure, may be coagulopathic or encephalopathic

Once a donor has been identified, organ harvesting is performed by a surgical team, usually from the centre where the transplantation will be performed. With a minimum of warm ischaemia time, immediate perfusion with hypothermic UW solution and simplified topical hypothermia, organs can be transported by the harvesting team over long distances without loss of organ viability. Recipients may be required to travel an equally long distance for emergency admission to their medical centre for transplantation.

Suitable potential donors for major organs are plentiful; it has been estimated that there are between 20 000 and 25 000 per year in the USA.[21] In 1990, over 22 000 patients remained on the waiting list for major organs because there were only 4357 cadaver donors (Table 20.2). The Uniform Anatomical Act has provided an opportunity for individuals to express their permission for organ donation in the event of death without the need for additional authorization by surviving family members. However, physicians continue to be reluctant to harvest organs without family consent because of fear of legal liability in addition to

Table 20.2 Number of patients on United Network for Organ Sharing waiting list versus donors

Homograft	1987	1988	1989	1990
Heart	699	1032	1324	796
Heart–lung	155	205	240	226
Kidney	12 099	13 944	16 363	17 955
Liver	454	617	830	1248
Lung	16	70	94	309
Pancreas	63	164	322	474
Total	13 396	16 032	19 173	22 008
Cadaver donors			3923	4357
Living donors			1874	1788
Total			5797	6145

concerns of adverse publicity, strain on the surviving family and misunderstanding about brain death.

Criteria for allocation of organs by UNOS may include histocompatibility, physical match, urgency of transplantation for the recipient, chances of recovery following transplantation, time on the waiting list, logistics of procurement and transplantation and survival of the preserved organ. In kidney transplantation, highest priority is given to a perfect histocompatibility match because an organ can be transported over long distances without compromise of graft survival, allowing optimum recipient selection.[22] Medical urgency of the recipient and graft survival are the highest priorities in heart transplantation, although ABO blood group compatibility is necessary to avoid hyperacute rejection. Since heart homografts do not tolerate cold ischaemia time, hearts are allocated first to local patients, then to regional medical centres within a few hours of transport time. Hearts are seldom transported over long distances. Physical match is a concern in liver transplantation because the liver of a large male donor will not fit the space available following native hepatectomy in a small female or a child; however, transplantation of a segment of adult liver into a child has been performed. Histocompatibility is less important in liver transplantation, but ABO matching is sought. Liver homografts can be transported over long distances if cold ischaemia time can be kept to less than 24 h.[8]

Brain death

Head trauma, subarachnoid haemorrhage and coma from severe hypoxia are the leading causes of brain death in suitable organ donors. The criteria for determining brain death are complex and vary among institutions, states, countries and cultures.[23] The lack of cortical brain function is insufficient to declare a potential donor as brain-dead. Most institutions require evidence of absent brainstem function for a patient to be declared brain-dead. If the electroencephalogram (EEG) is used as a criterion, it should meet the guidelines of the American EEG Society. However, the EEG cannot establish absence of brainstem function and is not reliable in patients who are hypothermic, have a history of drug intoxication, or are being treated aggressively with central nervous system (CNS) depressants. CNS depressants and muscle relaxants used to control intracranial pressure (ICP) limit the usefulness of tests of reflex activity.

Intracranial blood flow can be assessed using angiography but this is invasive and technically difficult. Radio-active isotopes can estimate cerebral blood flow but must distinguish between intracranial blood flow and scalp perfusion. Computed tomography with contrast injection and ultrasonography of the intracranial blood vessels can establish absence of intracranial blood flow.

The apnoea test is used in many centres to assess the absence of brainstem function.[24] Adequate oxgen supply to the brain is achieved with apnoeic oxygenation (at least 10 min of controlled ventilation with an $FIO_2 = 1.0$). Ventilation is discontinued and $PaCO_2$ is monitored while a T-piece with 100% oxygen is attached to the tracheal tube. Brainstem function is deemed to be absent when no spontaneous respiratory effort occurs with a $PaCO_2$ of 8 kPa (60 mmHg). It is essential that all reversible causes of coma and treatment protocols for elevated ICP, capable of suppressing ventilatory drive, be excluded before apnoea testing is used for determination of brain death.

The determination of brain death is most difficult in patients with drug overdose or with hypothermic, hypoxic brain injury such as cold-water drowning. Paediatric patients[25] represent an extremely limited and near ideal potential source of organs for children. An increased demand for donor organs for these infants and children has occurred as technical problems of transplantation in small children continue to be resolved.[26]

Potential donors with coma of undetermined cause present another difficult problem. Reversible causes of coma must be ruled out and screening for infectious and toxic causes of coma that may destroy homograft function must be undertaken. Alcoholics, cocaine addicts and intravenous drug abusers have a high incidence of associated hepatitis B, hepatitis C and human immunodeficiency viral (HIV) infections and are not suitable organ donors. Similarly, other viral infections (encephalitis, meningitis) can be causes of coma and brain death in which organs cannot be used for transplantation into patients who will be immunosuppressed.

Head-injury patients are the most frequent source of donor organs at most transplant centres. In general, they are young and free of systemic disease. Haemodynamic stability can be established in the head-injury patient for a number of days while the determination of brain death is made. At our institution, we have developed a simplified system for evaluating head-injury patients that accurately predicts their survival and rehabilitation[27] (Table 20.3). Grade IV head-injury patients show no sign of brain function and have no cerebral blood flow secondary to markedly increased ICP. If these patients do not have injuries to the organs that are potential homografts, and are free

Table 20.3 Medical College of Virginia (MCV) grading of head injury

MCV grade	Clinical features of head injury	Glasgow coma scale
Grade I	Alert, oriented, no history of loss of consciousness	12–14
Grade II	Able to follow simple commands or alert with focal neurological deficit, history of loss of consciousness	9–11
Grade III	Unable to follow simple commands because of impaired consciousness	6–8
Grade IV	No evidence of brain function, potential organ donor	3–5

From Narayan,[27] with permission.

from contamination from bowel injury, every effort should be made to stabilize blood pressure and urine output while permission for harvesting of organs is obtained. Grade III patients have a high mortality rate and may progress to brain death if ICP and cerebral perfusion pressure (CPP) cannot be controlled.[28]

Treatment of comatose patients with increased ICP (>20 mmHg) and decreased CPP (<40 mmHg) is counterproductive to the pre-operative optimization of the potential donor for organ harvesting. At our institution, CPP is estimated in patients with head injury or intracranial haemorrhage by means of a jugular bulb catheter, arterial line and intraventricular catheter or cranial bolt. Brain compliance curves are established by tracking the effects of small increments in intracranial volume. ICP is controlled with diuretics, mannitol, steroids, dehydration, CNS depressants, muscle relaxants and hyperventilation. Barbiturate coma (alternatively etomidate in the haemodynamically unstable patient) has not proved to be of major benefit for brain injury.[29] The intraventricular catheter has an advantage over subarachnoid bolts because of the ease with which small volumes of intraventricular cerebrospinal fluid can be drained to decrease ICP. However, intracranial bolts are associated with a lower risk of intracranial haemorrhage in the patient with a coagulopathy and are preferred in paediatric patients with brain injury.

Our institution is involved in clinical trials of superoxide dismutase, a scavenger for cytotoxic free radicals, for patients with grade III head trauma. Ischaemia injury results in the breakdown of adenosine triphosphate (ATP) to xanthine and hypoxanthine and subsequent generation of cytotoxic superoxides on reperfusion of the brain. Similar biochemical mechanisms are important in the reperfusion injury (see below) of donor organs following transplantation.

Management of the organ donor

Once brain death has been determined and certified according to institutional and community standards, counselling of the donor's family and permission for organ harvesting are urgent. Organs, not donors, should be transported to the recipient. Demise of major organs becomes imminent with progressive hypothermia, haemodynamic instability, sepsis, renal shut-down and multi-organ failure associated with adult respiratory distress syndrome (ARDS).[30,31] Once brain death has been established, brain resuscitation measures which compromise heart, lung, liver and kidney function must be discontinued. Intravascular volume should be replaced, cardiac output supported and urine output maintained.[32] Diabetes insipidus can be treated with vasopressin and fluid replacement. Renal perfusion may require administration of dopamine or dobutamine. Vasoconstrictors, particularly α-adrenergic agonists, which reduce both renal and hepatic blood flow, should be avoided.[33]

Ventilation is maintained to assure normal blood gases and the patient is transferred to the operating room for organ harvesting through an extensive, bilateral subcostal incision and median sternotomy. Multiple teams from different (and differing) institutions or services may be involved in the harvesting of organs. Anaesthetic support is usually provided by local anaesthetists who find themselves working with surgeons they have never met before in a difficult thoracoabdominal procedure in an unstable patient! The abdominal and thoracic great vessels and the branches to the liver and kidneys are isolated. Mannitol, frusemide (furosemide), heparin and chlorpromazine may be requested immediately before the organs are perfused with cardioplegic and hypothermic preservatives. Manipulation of the heart and great vessels and the associated blood loss make control of systemic pressures and heart rate difficult. Communication between the anaesthetists and the various surgeons on this issue should be clear before harvesting is begun.

Hypothermic perfusion of the harvested liver and kidneys with UW solution eliminates the need for complicated haemoperfusion devices. Organs may be perfused *in vivo* by means of aortic cannulation or *ex vivo* by cannulation of the arterial or venous vessels. The anaesthetist may be asked to record the warm ischaemia time — the time from cross-clamping of the homograft's blood supply, or the time from cardioplegia to the time of cold perfusion.

Acceptable ischaemia time for hearts is only 4 h; it begins with cross-clamping of the donor's aorta and ends with unclamping of the recipient's aorta. UW solution allows livers to be used up to 24 h, and kidneys up to 2 days, after harvesting. UW solution is hyperkalaemic (30 mmol.l^{-1}) and contains buffers (pH 7.4), antibiotic (co-trimoxazole), insulin, raffinose, magnesium sulphate, adenosine, glutathione and allopurinol (Table 20.4).

Living related organ transplantation is common for kidney transplantation but is performed at only a few centres for liver transplantation in children. With a living related donor, histocompatibility can be maximized for kidney transplantation.[34] Arteriography is used to define renal vessels. Nephrectomy is performed in a room immediately adjacent to the transplant recipient and warm ischaemia time is minimized. Living related kidney transplantation leads to better allograft survival than cadaver kidney transplantation.[35] Living related liver segmental grafts (see below) are taken from a parent for a child with end-stage liver disease.[36] Transplanted lobes grow and conform to the size of the child while regeneration occurs in the donor.

Reperfusion injury

Major organs for transplantation are stored for periods of a few hours to 2 days in a cold, ischaemic and hypoxic environment. All organ homografts suffer reperfusion injury once the vascular anastomoses to the organ are completed and warm, oxygenated recipient blood flow from the recipient is begun. Reperfusion injury has been defined by Pretto[37,38] in general terms applicable to all organs, as tissue and cellular injury resulting from the re-establishment of blood flow and oxygen to a previously ischaemic or anoxic organ. It is characterized by two features: the 'no-reflow' phenomenon and the production of excess oxygen-derived free radicals (ODFR). The no-reflow phenomenon has been documented mainly in transplanted hearts and is a microvascular phenomenon in which areas of the myocardium are transiently devoid of blood flow despite adequate perfusion pressure with normothermic, oxygenated blood. ODFRs are produced with reperfusion in all organs studied. Re-oxygenation leads to the production of superoxide free radicals to a level which normal scavenging mechanisms cannot control. Superoxide, hydrogen peroxide and free hydroxyl radicals are ODFRs. They contain an unmatched electron in their outer electron orbit and produce homograft organ injury by oxidation of lipids, proteins and nucleic acids. They are produced from high-energy substrates by xanthine oxidase and NADPH oxidase as well as by auto-oxidation of semiquinone. Xanthine oxidase is normally present as xanthine dehydrogenase in a variety of tissues, including vascular endothelium. In the ischaemic state, xanthine dehydrogenase is converted to xanthine oxidase which liberates free radicals during the conversion of xanthine to urate. The conversion of xanthine dehydrogenase to xanthine oxidase is calcium- and protease-dependent and can be prevented by calcium antagonists and protease inhibitors. Xanthine oxidase production of superoxides can be limited by allopurinol, an inhibitor of xanthine oxidase. Adkinson and colleagues[39] and Nordstrom et al[40,41] have shown that superoxide dismutase, catalase and allopurinol are all effective in preventing reperfusion injury of the liver. Xanthine is freely available in the ischaemic, hypoxic organ from the hydrolysis of ATP, adenosine diphosphate and monophosphate. Superoxide dismutase is a free radical scavenger and has been used to protect ischaemic organs. Other effective scavengers include catalase, glutathione peroxidase, mannitol and dimethylsulphoxide.

Clinically, reperfusion of the ischaemic and anoxic transplanted liver is associated with acute myocardial dysfunction.[42] It is unclear whether this is caused by the presence of superoxides in the venous effluent from the liver, hyperkalaemia associated with washout of preservative from the liver, or the effect of hypothermic, acidotic venous return. Calcium chloride and sodium bicarbonate are usually effective in restoring normal myocardial function. In kidney transplantation,

Table 20.4 University of Wisconsin solution ViaSpan (Belzer UW); the solution is precooled to 2–6°C

Pentafraction	50.0 g.l^{-1}
Lactobionic acid	35.83 g.l^{-1}
Potassium phosphate	3.4 g.l^{-1}
Magnesium sulphate	1.23 g.l^{-1}
Raffinose	17.83 g.l^{-1}
Adenosine	1.34 g.l^{-1}
Allopurinol	0.136 g.l^{-1}
pH	7.40
Penicillin G	200 000 units
Regular insulin	40 units
Dexamethasone	16 mg
Adult ex vivo infusion	
Kidney	300–500 ml
Liver	1200 ml
Child ex vivo infusion	
Kidney	50 ml.kg^{-1}
Liver	150–250 ml

the anaesthetist must be prepared to maximize the immediate function of the homograft. Renal perfusion can be increased with dopamine and mannitol, and renal tubular metabolic requirements decreased with frusemide. Reperfusion of the heart may be associated with the microcirculatory changes noted above. Reperfusion is characterized by a combination of left and right ventricular dysfunction that is not influenced by normal autonomic control.

Histocompatibility

Histocompatibility is most important in candidates for renal transplantation. Patients are screened for six human leukocyte antigens (HLAs) for class 1 at the A and B loci of chromosome 6 and two class 2 antigens at the HLA-DR locus.[43] In addition, recipients are screened at intervals for reactivity to antigens in the population at large. Patients who are highly sensitized to a panel of antigens in the population (per cent panel reactive antibody) are less likely to have a successful kidney transplantation. Histocompatibility of these antigens greatly improves renal allograft survival. Histocompatibility is not as important with heart or liver transplantation, although patients are matched for ABO blood group compatibility with the donor.

Social issues

Brain death has been accepted by religions and societies, medical staff and hospital personnel as the essential feature of the death of the individual. Individuals, however, continue to be reluctant to designate themselves as organ donors in the event of brain death and families continue to be distressed about authorizing organ donation with brain death of a loved one. Physicians, particularly those practising at medical centres without an active transplant programme, continue to be concerned about legal liability when declaring an individual brain-dead. UNOS continues to address these issues in the USA with public awareness programmes and legislative efforts.

Transplantation as treatment for end-stage organ failure is extremely expensive. Average hospital charges for cardiac tansplantation in the USA during 1988 were $148 000, liver transplantation $235 000 and kidney transplantation $51 000. These charges did not include physicians' fees, charges related to organ procurement or the cost of supportive therapy such as long-term haemodialysis. In addition to these charges, patients on health care systems must face the cost of long-term medical care related to transplantation, especially the cost of medications for immunosuppression.

SELECTION AND PREPARATION FOR TRANSPLANTATION

Transplantation is appropriate in the presence of end-stage organ failure. The clinical picture of end-stage organ failure is different for patients with liver disease, heart disease and kidney disease.

Liver

Indications

Liver transplantation is indicated for a variety of end-stage diseases.[44] The most common diagnoses are postnecrotic cirrhosis (46%), followed by biliary cirrhosis (18%), sclerosing cholangitis (11%) fulminant hepatic necrosis (8%), primary liver malignancy (7%), metabolic diseases (6%) and miscellaneous other liver diseases (4%). Ascher[45] noted that the risk to the recipient in OLT was related to primary non-function of the donor liver, technical difficulties in harvesting the donor liver with injury to the vascular pedicles, preservation injuries (prolonged warm ischaemia and excessive cold preservation times), donor–recipient size mismatches, ABO incompatibility and residual disease transmitted from the recipient to the donor liver, especially hepatitis.

Selection of recipients

Selection of patients for OLT is controversial. Shaw & Wood[46] noted that application of the Child's classification, even as modified by Pugh, was not helpful in correlating success of OLT with severity of liver disease. They used the criteria developed in Pittsburgh for patients in Nebraska and reported survival rates better than those reported in Pittsburgh (Table 20.5).

Van Thiel et al[47,48] feel that alcoholic liver disease is an acceptable indication for OLT. It is the most common cause of chronic liver failure, with an estimated prevalence of 9 000 000 cases in the USA and 450 000

Table 20.5 Survival following orthotopic liver transplantation

Pittsburgh classification	Pittsburgh experience	Nebraska experience
Well-controlled	74%	90.4%
Moderately severe liver failure	73%	85.2%
Advanced liver failure	22%	44.5%

From Shaw & Wood,[46] with permission.

deaths annually. The average age of these patients is 48.2 years. Therefore, there is reasonable expectation of a productive life-span following succesful transplantation. In their series of patients transplanted after introduction of cyclosporin, 74% of patients with alcohol-related liver failure found gainful employment following OLT and 89.5% remained abstinent. They recommend completion of an alcohol withdrawal programme followed by abstinence from alcohol for 3–6 months prior to OLT. Recidivism following OLT in patients with a history of alcohol abuse who have undergone a programme of abstinence and rehabilitation is low.

Patients in our programme who have a history of alcohol abuse or dependence must demonstrate abstinence from alcohol for at least 6 months prior to being listed for liver transplantation. Abstinence must be corroborated by family members or by the patient's participation in an alcohol treatment programme. Random blood testing must remain negative. If transplantation for the alcohol-dependent patient is urgent (status III or IV), evaluation must suggest that the patient will acknowledge the role of alcohol as a cause of disease and that the patient has coping skills, a record of stability in personal relationships and support from family members before being listed for OLT. Similar criteria are applied to patients with a history of drug abuse.

Liver transplantation for hepatic failure following viral-related infection is controversial because of the high incidence (near 100%) of re-infection with hepatitis B and co-incident infection with hepatitis C.[49,50] Further, patients with long-standing chronic active hepatitis have a 200-fold increased risk of hepatocellular cancer. This susceptibility to development of malignancy is enhanced by immunosuppression. Luketic and colleagues[51] reported one patient who developed recurrent hepatitis B infection after OLT which led to hepatocellular carcinoma 4 years later.

Features of hepatic failure

Fulminant hepatic failure is caused by exposure to hepatotoxins (halothane, isoniazid, methyldopa, paracetamol/acetaminophen) or may be secondary to viral infection.[52] Encephalopathy occurs within 8 weeks of the onset of the disease. With the onset of encephalopathy, transplantation should be considered as urgent. These patients may be transferred with deteriorating mental status from other hospitals. Since the transition from grade II to grade III and IV hepatic coma is insidious, the transferring team should consider control of the airway and begin therapy aimed at reducing ICP.[53] Charcoal haemofiltration produces only limited improvement in patients with advanced hepatic coma.[54] The mortality rate of grade III–IV hepatic coma is over 80%[55] without liver transplantation's whereas Peleman et al[56] reported 53% survival with OLT in fulminant hepatic failure. Schafer & Shaw[57] reported long-term survival of 58% in 24 patients with fulminant hepatic failure with ages ranging from 2 weeks to 57 years. They recommend the use of intracranial epidural pressure monitoring for all patients with grade III or IV coma. Epidural pressure monitoring was used in 14 of their patients. Only one of these developed an intracranial haemorrhage thought to be related to the technique. If cerebral oedema secondary to fulminant hepatic failure results in a flat EEG or a CPP of >40 mmHg, liver transplantation is contraindicated.

Clinically evident hepatobiliary cancer is associated with an extremely poor prognosis; usually survival is less than 3–6 months.[58,59] OLT has been shown to provide a 30% survival after 3 years.[60] However, incidental hepatocellular carcinoma is not uncommon in patients undergoing OLT for postnecrotic or biliary cirrhosis and survival for these patients may be as high as 70–90% at 5 years. Koneru et al[61] reported results with OLT in children with hepatoblastoma. Half of the children were alive 24–70 months following surgery.

Patients with postnecrotic or biliary cirrhosis may present with well-compensated liver failure. These patients have the highest survival rate following OLT,[62] approaching 90% after 5 years.

Assessment and preparation

At our institution, all candidates for OLT are reviewed by a multidisciplinary panel of transplant surgeons, hepatologists, pathologists, anaesthesiologists, social workers, nurse co-ordinators, psychologists and financial advisers. In addition to evaluation of the nature of their liver disease, they are evaluated for anatomical suitability for transplantation (height, weight, chest and abdominal measurements, angiography and ultrasound with duplex scanning). Patients are evaluated for evidence of other systemic diseases, especially heart disease. If electrocardiogram and echocardiogram are abnormal, persantine or stress thallium testing and coronary angiography, may be performed. Portal hypertension[63] and hepatic anatomy[64] can be defined accurately by magnetic resonance imaging; this is of particular value in children, in whom invasive studies should be avoided. Pulmonary function tests and arterial blood gases are obtained. Patients and their families are advised of the difficulties related to organ transplantation. They develop a strong relationship with all members of the transplant team. All patients awaiting transplantation and those in the immediate post-transplant period are reviewed by the team at weekly meetings. Typically, we have 20–30 patients awaiting transplantation, in addition to 10 or more in the medical centre awaiting discharge. At major centres with approved liver transplantation programmes, transplant surgery has evolved as a surgical subspecialty distinct from vascular surgery.

Prior to transplantation, ascites should be controlled with diuretics but not to the point of limiting renal function. Because oesophageal varices or other sources of gastro-intestinal bleeding lead to anaemia, ammonia intoxication and hyperbilirubinaemia, non-invasive imaging should be used to evaluate the presence or absence of varices and portal hypertension. Coagulation profiles are abnormal, with reduced fibrinogen concentration, and prolonged prothrombin and activated thromboplastin times. If splenomegaly secondary to portal hypertension is present, patients may have marked thrombocytopenia. These defects in coagulation can be overcome partially by pre-operative administration of fresh frozen plasma and pooled platelets. Anaemia should raise suspicion of gastro-intestinal bleeding secondary to portal hypertension. Nitrogen balance can be controlled by limiting intake and altering metabolism with nitrogen-consuming bacteria. These steps limit ammonia production and help to control impending hepatic coma, which increases the risk of operative and postoperative death from cerebral oedema.

Renal failure (hepatorenal syndrome) occurs in patients with advanced liver disease because of the reduction in effective renal blood flow related to ascites and excessive concentrations of aldosterone and antidiuretic hormone. Hepatorenal syndrome, although poorly understood, is reversible. Maddrey et al[12] emphasized the importance of renal failure in patients awaiting liver transplantation. In their series, a pre-operative plasma creatinine concentration greater than 120 $\mu mol.l^{-1}$ (1.73 $mg.dl^{-1}$) predicted death accurately in 79% of patients who did not survive OLT. Kidneys from donors with hepatorenal syndrome function normally when transplanted to patients with normal liver function. Similarly, hepatorenal syndrome responds rapidly to successful OLT. It is difficult to decide whether to transplant a kidney from the same donor to a patient with combined hepatic and renal failure undergoing OLT. Some believe that the transplanted liver offers immunological protection to the kidney. However, the window of opportunity to use the kidneys from the donor of the liver is short. Renal function is supported aggressively during OLT by the administration of appropriate intravenous fluids and electrolytes, fresh frozen plasma, albumin, mannitol, frusemide and dopamine.

Patients with end-stage liver disease have a typical hyperdynamic cardiovascular profile, with tachycardia, high cardiac output, increased stroke volume, low systemic vascular resistance and increased mixed venous oxygen saturation.[65] Fluid shifts are common. Patients with ascites and pleural effusions may have borderline respiratory function with an increased alveolar–arterial oxygen gradient that improves as soon as the abdomen is decompressed. Cardiovascular disease is not as common a problem with end-stage liver disease as it is with end-stage renal disease. However, patients with alcoholic cardiomyopathy are an exception. These patients have biventricular failure, do not respond readily to cardiovascular resuscitation, and are at particular risk during reperfusion of the new liver.

Heart

Indications

A patient is a candidate for heart transplantation if he or she has end-stage cardiac disease with severely limited prognosis.[66] Although the majority of patients are New York Heart Association class IV status, class III patients are considered for transplantation when the potential exists for an abrupt change to a class IV status.[67]

More than 90% of heart transplants are performed for patients with dilated cardiomyopathy.[33] Both ischaemic and idiopathic cardiomyopathy are sub-populations of this broader category,[68,69] and the 30-day mortality rates after transplantation are the same for both.

Clinical features

The hallmark of dilated cardiomyopathy is a profound reduction in left ventricular ejection fraction (LVEF). A complex set of compensatory mechanisms ensues which may be initially supportive in maintaining performance, but ultimately exacerbates decompensation.[70]

Significant impairment of left ventricular diastolic function results in left ventricular dilation (Frank–Starling mechanism) to maintain stroke volume. Although the right ventricle may dilate, this does not necessarily occur. Left ventricular end-diastolic pressure (LVEDP) increases. However, the pressure–volume relationship is variable, and the LVEDP, although increased, may be lower than normal for a given diastolic volume.[71] As a result, left atrial pressure (LAP) may or may not increase, and cardiac output may be normal or low. Although the cardiac output may be normal, the dilated cardiomyopathic heart cannot increase cardiac output in response to exercise.

Activation of the renin–angiotensin system causes sodium and water retention and, therefore, increased blood volume. This may improve pump function initially through the Frank–Starling mechanism. However, pump function ultimately becomes exhausted and no further increase in stroke volume occurs with increased end-diastolic volume. Excessive fluid retention may lead to pulmonary congestion. The pulmonary capillary wedge pressure (PCWP) at which pulmonary oedema develops is higher in patients with long-standing elevations.[72]

Sympathetic activity increases in response to pump failure to maintain cardiac output. Chronic activation leads to catecholamine depletion and decreased adrenergic receptors (down-regulation).[73]

Pre-operative management

Medical management of the patient with congestive heart failure falls into three categories:

1. alleviating sodium and water retention
2. improving cardiac contractility
3. reducing the workload of the heart.

Loop diuretics are used to reduce preload of the failing heart. The goal of diuretic therapy is an optimal filling pressure which permits maximum cardiac output without pulmonary congestion. This may be quite high in patients with chronic congestive failure. Contractility is improved by the use of positive inotropic agents. Digitalis, unless contra-indicated, is usually part of the initial medical regimen for patients with severe congestive failure. When more support is required, dopamine, dobutamine and amrinone are used widely.

Arteriolar vasodilators increase cardiac output and decrease the workload of the heart by reducing systemic vascular resistance. Angiotensin-converting enzyme inhibitors such as captopril and enalapril improve survival of patients with congestive cardiomyopathy.[74] They also partially reverse β-adrenergic receptor down-regulation.[75] Sodium nitroprusside and intravenous nitroglycerine are used singly or in combination in the acutely ill patient with congestive cardiomyopathy.

Mechanical circulatory support (intra-aortic balloon counterpulsation, left and/or right ventricular assist devices, total artificial hearts) may be used to sustain life in the moribund patient awaiting a donor heart. Of the 219 patients receiving circulatory support for staged cardiac transplantation in 1988, 73% were transplanted. Although rates of transplantation were not dependent upon types of support employed, 76% of patients receiving univentricular support, 67% receiving biventricular support and 48% receiving total artificial heart support were discharged from the hospital.[76]

Less than 10% of adult heart transplants are performed for conditions other than the dilated cardiomyopathies. These include graft rejection, end-stage valve disease and congenital disease. Survival rates are not as good in patients with these diagnoses when compared to patients with ischaemic or idiopathic cardiomyopathy.

Kidney

End-stage renal disease

End-stage renal disease is most commonly the result of glomerulonephritis, hypertension or diabetes mellitus.[77] It is more frequent in the American black population than the Caucasian population. This is a reflection of the threefold greater incidence of hypertension in the American black population as well as the higher incidence of nephrosclerosis complicating hypertension in blacks.[78]

Kidney disease may progress from decreased renal reserve to renal insufficiency and, finally, to renal failure or end-stage renal disease. Patients with diminished renal reserve show a decreased creatinine clearance but are usually asymptomatic. As their disease progresses to renal insufficiency, elevations of serum creatinine and blood urea nitrogen occur. At this stage, they are unable to cope with large loads of either salt or water. Conversely, haemorrhage or dehydration may result in acute renal failure. With end-stage renal disease, extracellular fluid volume is directly related to intake, and metabolic waste products lead to uraemia.[79]

End-stage renal disease produces systemic effects related to regulation of body water, serum electrolyte concentrations (including sodium, chloride, potassium, calcium and phosphorus), acid–base balance and systemic blood pressure. Although many of these can be corrected by long-term haemodialysis, patients scheduled for kidney transplantation have anaesthetic management problems related to each.

Haemodialysis

Long-term haemodialysis has lessened the urgency for transplantation in patients with renal failure. Unfortunately, similar technology is not available for patients with cardiac or liver failure. Long-term haemodialysis is dependent on vascular access through arteriovenous shunts placed in a variety of locations in the body. A long surgical history of arteriovenous fistula placement, revision, declotting and removal because of infection is typical. Functioning fistulae limit the use of extremities.

Arteriovenous access procedures can be performed with ease using supraclavicular nerve blocks. We use a perivascular or an interscalene approach to the brachial plexus with insulated needles (22-gauge Teflon-coated, Professional Instruments, Houston, TX) and a peripheral nerve stimulator (Digi Stim II, Neurotechnology, Houston, TX) capable of delivering defined currents less than 1 mA. Sedated patients tolerate the procedure well. Consistent sensory anaesthesia is achieved when stimulation evokes a median nerve finger flexor response. Our choice of local anaesthetic is either mepivicaine (5–7 mg.kg^{-1}) or bupivacaine (2 mg.kg^{-1}) with adrenaline (5 µg.ml^{-1}, 1 : 200 000). Alkalinization with sodium bicarbonate (0.1 mmol.ml^{-1} of local anaesthetic solution) leads to rapid onset of a profound block with no apparent decrease in vasoconstrictor effect of adrenaline. Since patients with end-stage renal disease are hypoproteinaemic and anaemic, the total dose of local anaesthetic should be limited to avoid CNS and cardiovascular toxicity.

Ideally, haemodialysis should be performed less than 24 h before kidney transplantation and serum electrolyte and haemoglobin concentrations should be measured following dialysis. Although hyperkalaemia may be controlled by haemodialysis pre-operatively, dextrose and insulin or calcium chloride and sodium bicarbonate may be necessary during transplantation. If hyperkalaemia cannot be controlled pre-operatively, haemodialysis should be anticipated during transplantation.

Secondary features

Anaemia is so common with end-stage renal disease that the experience with these patients has altered the approach of most anaesthetists to transfusion therapy. While the electrolyte abnormalities and fluid balance of patients with end-stage renal disease can be controlled with haemodialysis, anaemia is not corrected. Transfusion is controversial. Sutherland et al[80] have shown that routine pretransplant random blood transfusion increases graft and patient survival in both children and in diabetic adults. The benefit of pre-transplantation blood transfusion is thought to be greatest when a cadaver homograft is anticipated.[81] Transfusion risks include transmission of viral illness[82] and sensitization to donor antigens. Multiparous females, patients with systemic lupus erythematosus and patients who have previously rejected a renal transplant are at high risk of developing widely reactive antibodies. Transfusion is not recommended for those patients.

Hyperparathyroidism with hypercalcaemia is common in the patient with end-stage renal disease and total parathyroidectomy may be necessary. When this is performed, one of the parathyroid glands can be transplanted, usually into the forearm, for easy access should further reduction in the amount of parathyroid tissue be necessary.

Hypertension is a common feature of, as well as a cause of, end-stage renal disease and may result in left ventricular failure. Philipson et al[83] reviewed their experience with cardiovascular complications in diabetic patients with end-stage renal disease. Sixty patients with type 1 diabetes mellitus were evaluated prior to renal transplantation. Thallium stress testing and cardiac catheterization were used to separate patients into five categories ranging from no evidence of cardiac disease to evidence of severe cardiac disease. The overall mortality rate for patients without cardiac disease was 5.4%. With moderate cardiac disease, the mortality rate was 20% and with severe cardiac disease, 62%. Their recommendation was that diabetic patients with severe cardiac disease determined by cardiac catheterization should not be considered as candidates for renal transplantation.

Nephrectomy

Bilateral nephrectomy is indicated in patients with end-stage renal disease who have recurrent infections secondary to pyelonephritis or structural abnormalities, renin-induced hypertension, some cases of glomerulonephritis, Goodpasture's syndrome or symptomatic polycystic kidney disease. Excessive morbidity and mortality from bilateral nephrectomy are avoided by a posterior surgical approach and by adequate blood volume and fluid replacement aimed at maintaining a central venous pressure between 5 and 10 cmH$_2$O.

ANAESTHETIC MANAGEMENT FOR MAJOR ORGAN TRANSPLANTATION

Liver

Our protocol for the management of adults undergoing OLT is similar to that of Kang at the University of Pittsburgh.[15]

Intravenous access

Patients are brought to the operating room with existing intravenous access, and general anaesthesia is induced prior to the placement of other venous or arterial cannulae. A large-bore cannula, 14-gauge Teflon catheter or 7.5 FG introducer sheath, is placed in the left brachial or cephalic vein for connection to one infusion limb of the Sorensen Rapid Infusion Device (RID).[84] Two introducer sheaths (Double IJ) are placed in the right internal jugular vein and the side-arm of one is used for the second infusion limb of the RID. Potassium and citrate concentrations are reduced, and cellular debris removed, from packed red cells by washing prior to mixing with fresh frozen plasma in the RID (see below). Introducer sheaths are available in 9 FG coupled with stopcocks designed to avoid turbulent flow (Walrus High Flow, Medical Parametrics, Woburn, MA). We use an anterior approach at the apex of the triangle formed by the heads of the sternocleidomastoid muscle to minimize risk of inadvertent carotid puncture in a coagulopathic patient. This system allows us to administer as much as 3 l.min^{-1} of reconstituted blood. An oximetric thermodilution pulmonary artery catheter is passed through one of the introducer sheaths and a triple-lumen catheter is passed through the other. The presence of these catheters in sheaths, particularly the 9 FG sheaths, does not significantly limit our ability to provide high-flow rates via the RID. The triple-lumen catheter, the side-arm of the second introducer sheath and the proximal port of the pulmonary artery catheter are used for continuous infusions of platelets, fresh frozen plasma, opioid/muscle relaxant solution, dopamine and other vasoactive infusions.

Monitoring

An arterial cannula (20-gauge) is placed in each radial artery. One, which is unheparinized, is used for all blood samples. Blood samples for thrombelastography (TEG; see below) and coagulation profiles (prothrombin time (PT), partial thromboplastin time (PPT), factors V, VII and VIII and platelet count) are drawn from the unheparinized arterial line (Table 20.6). Both arterial lines are used for continuous blood pressure monitoring. Haemodynamic profiles are determined from thermodilution cardiac output, central venous pressure, PCWP and systemic and pulmonary arterial pressures. Thermodilution cardiac output determination can be difficult during OLT if moderate hypothermia occurs during the anhepatic phase of the operation. We use room-temperature injectate for determination of cardiac output to avoid exacerbation of hypothermia. Patients with end-stage liver disease have pulmonary and systemic shunts with haemodynamic profiles that include a high cardiac index, high mixed venous oxygen saturation, and low systemic vascular resistance. Mixed venous oxygen saturation parallels thermodilution cardiac output measurements during OLT.

New modalities of assessing ventricular function have been described but are not used routinely in liver transplantation. Some centres utilize a rapid-response thermocouple right ventricular catheter (Swan–Ganz thermodilution ejection fraction/volumetric catheter)

Table 20.6 Coagulation factors of concern monitored during orthotopic liver transplantation

Factor	Name	Half-life (h)	Normal or minimal haemostatic level	Replacement blood product
I	Fibrinogen*	36–90	1.7–4.0 g.l^{-1}	Cryoprecipitate
II	Prothrombin*	60–70	PT = 11–13 s	Vitamin K
V	Labile factor*	12–36	5–10%	Fresh frozen plasma
VII	Stable factor*	4–7	5–10%	Fresh frozen plasma
VIII	Anhaemophilic factor†*	10–12	30%	Fresh frozen plasma Cryoprecipitate Factor VIII concentrate
IX	Christmas factor	24	30%	Fresh frozen plasma
X	Stuart–Power factor	48	8–10%	Fresh frozen plasma
XI	Plasma thromboplastin antecedent	60	20–30%	Fresh frozen plasma
XIII	Fibrin-stabilizing factor	336	1%	Fresh frozen plasma Cryoprecipitate

* Monitored during orthotopic liver transplantation.
† Production not limited to the liver.
PT = Prothrombin time.
Table produced with Dr Lyman Fisher, Hemostasis Laboratory, Medical College of Virginia.

that allows calculation of cardiac output and right ventricular stroke volume.[85] Lichtor et al[86] describe transoesophageal echocardiography (TEE) during OTL for assessment of right and left ventricular function. They have shown that TEE may identify changes in ventricular function not predicted by PCWP. Furthermore, TEE is a sensitive monitor of venous air embolism which may occur during isolation and manipulation of the inferior vena cava. Abrams et al[87,88] used transtracheal Doppler signals in animals and in humans to measure cardiac output continuously. When they had free access to the head in patients under general anaesthesia, they were able to obtain a strong correlation ($r = 0.835$) between transtracheal Doppler cardiac output and standard thermodilution determination. Also, transtracheal Doppler signals measured the diameter of the ascending aorta accurately when compared to data obtained from pre-operative B-mode echocardiography ($r = 0.817$). We have tried to use this device in a number of patients during elective surgery. Positioning of the head to obtain an adequate signal was critical and adequate signal was lost with head movement. When a strong and stable signal was obtained, correlation with thermodilution cardiac output was good. If the positioning difficulties could be resolved, this technique could provide continuous assessment of cardiac output.

Venovenous bypass

Other than the arterial cannula, no other lines are inserted in the patient's right arm. Venous cannulae are inserted in the portal vein via the inferior mesenteric vein and the right femoral vein via the saphenous branch and are connected to the inflow limb of venovenous bypass. Use of the inferior mesenteric vein permits continued portal decompression during anastomosis of the portal vein. Venous blood is returned to the patient by means of a cannula in the right axillary vein.

Venovenous bypass is begun immediately before occlusion of the inferior vena cava. With heparin-bonded cannulae and flow rates in excess of 1.5 l/min, systemic heparinization is not necessary. Haemodynamic stability is consistent if venovenous bypass flow is greater than 2 l/min in adults. Venous thromboembolism is not a problem if a minimum flow of 1 l/min is maintained. During venovenous bypass, we reduce the volume of fresh frozen plasma and platelets administered to prevent thrombus formation and do not give cryoprecipitate until the large venous cannulae have been removed. Recently, we have found that a heat exchanger (Omnitherm Model A-19-38, Scimed, Minneapolis, MN) in the venovenous bypass system enables us to warm patients during the anhepatic phase of OLT.

ICP monitoring during OLT for patients with clinical signs of hepatic encephalopathy is controversial because of the risk of intracranial haemorrhage following placement of intraventricular catheters when the patient is coagulopathic. However, brain herniation from marked increases in ICP secondary to hepatic encephalopathy is fatal. ICP monitoring is recommended for patients with grade 3 or 4 hepatic encephalopathy.[57]

Hypothermia is a major problem during OLT.[89] Standard and innovative means of warming the patient are not effective in maintaining normal body temperature during the anhepatic and reperfusion phases of OLT. A warming blanket is used throughout the procedure. Heat-conserving devices are placed in the breathing system and plastic bags are used to insulate the scalp and feet. Warming coils are used for intravenous lines and heat exchangers are used with the RID and venovenous bypass. Cardiac output is determined using injectate at room temperature. Despite these measures, body temperature may fall to 33–34°C during the anhepatic and reperfusion phases of OLT. As mentioned, with the use of a warming coil during venovenous bypass, we have been able to restore body temperature to 36–37°C during the anhepatic stage.

Metabolic acidosis, hyperkalaemia and hypoglycaemia occur during the native hepatectomy and anhepatic phases of OLT because of limited or absent liver function, hypothermia and the administration of large amounts of blood and blood products.[90] Arterial blood gases, sodium, potassium, ionized calcium and sugar concentrations are measured hourly or more often during OLT. Sodium bicarbonate is given to maintain pH and base excess near normal but sodium bicarbonate therapy may contribute to the hypernatraemia that occurs commonly during the neohepatic phase.

Hyperkalaemia may warrant administration of additional sodium bicarbonate, calcium chloride, glucose and insulin. We routinely wash all packed cells prior to administration through the RID. Belani & Estrin[91] have shown that this reduces the serum concentration of potassium from 16.6 to 3.4 mmol.l^{-1}. In addition, washing reduces the free plasma haemoglobin and citrate concentrations.

Excess citrate from stored blood can cause marked decreases in serum ionized calcium concentration. Administration of calcium chloride has theoretical advantages over calcium gluconate in that it does not require hepatic metabolism to release calcium. Calcium should be given to maintain an ionized calcium concentration of between 1.0 and 1.5 mmol.l^{-1}.

Blood loss can be a major problem during the isolation of the native liver if the patient has varices.[92] Blood loss is increased in patients with prior surgery, extensive adhesions and portal hypertension. However, the RID allows the anaesthetists to maintain blood volume with relative ease, even when replacement approaches as much as 30–50 l.

Coagulopathy associated with end-stage liver disease and the pre-anhepatic, anhepatic and neohepatic phases of OLT is a major problem. Clinical laboratory studies of fibrinogen, PT, PTT, factors VI, VII and VIII and platelet count are needed to guide administration of fresh frozen plasma, cryoprecipitate and pooled platelets.

TEG is a useful tool to evaluate coagulation and clot lysis during OLT. A sample of blood from the unheparinized arterial line (0.36 ml) is placed in a cuvette, covered with a drop of mineral oil, and a shear pin is lowered into the cuvette (Fig. 20.1). A strip recorder displays the magnitude of shear forces generated by rotation of the pin in the sample with clot formation and lysis.[93] Alternatively, an analogue-to-digital converter can be used to display and quantify shear forces at a video terminal. Calculation of the reaction time (R-value), coagulation time (RK) and the angle between

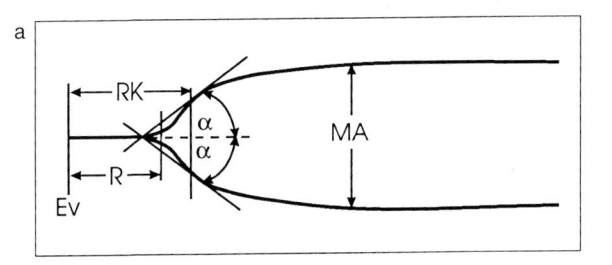

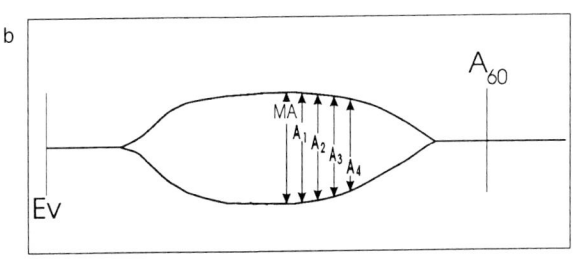

Fig. 20.2 (a) Native thrombelastograph profile. The sample is placed in the cup at Ev. R = Re-active time; RK = clot time; MA = maximum amplitude; α = angle; Ev = event marker. (b) Fibrinolytic profile. Amplitudes at 5-min intervals after maximum amplitude (MA) are compared to MA. With fibrinolysis, there is progressive decrease in amplitude, usually within 30–60 min. A_{60} = Amplitude at 60 min; A_1–A_4 = amplitude at 5-min (10-mm) intervals after MA.

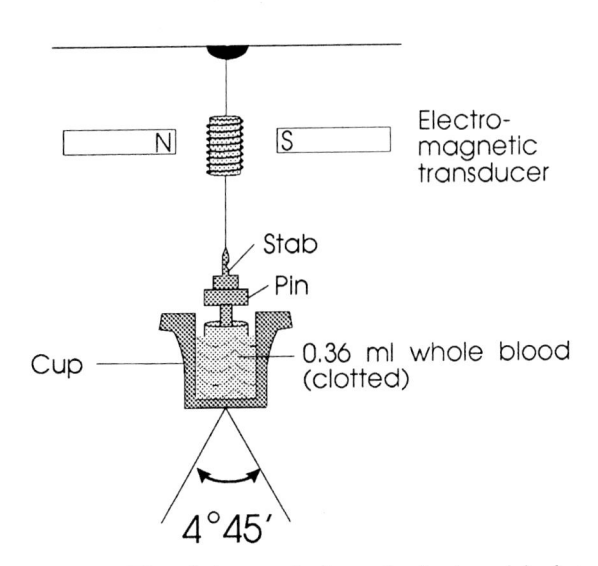

Fig. 20.1 Thrombelastograph. A sample of unheparinized blood is placed in the cup and covered with a layer of mineral oil. A pin, suspended from a torsion wire, is lowered into the cup. The cup rotates through an arc, generating tension on the wire as clot is formed. The torque on the wire produced by the rotating cup is converted to a graphic display, the thrombelastograph.

the R-value and an amplitude of 20 mm gives indices of dynamic clot formation (Fig. 20.2). The R-value correlates with partial thromboplastin time. The coagulation time and the angle, α, correlate with normal clot formation. The maximum amplitude of the TEG correlates with platelet function. The appearances of TEGs associated with normal and abnormal clotting are characteristic (Fig. 20.3). Abnormal fibrinolytic activity is identified by comparing the amplitude at 60 min with the maximum amplitude.

Kang et al[94] and Spiess et al[95] have shown that the TEG can identify abnormal fibrinolytic activity and in vitro reversibility with ϵ-aminocaproic acid (EACA). In 20 patients with abnormal fibrinolytic activity that was reversible in vitro, EACA produced a return of the TEG to normal with no evidence of continued haemorrhage or thrombotic complications. However, Ratnoff[96] has warned of the adverse effects of EACA. Mallett et al[97] have used aprotinin in a similar manner and have reported diminished blood loss in 6 consecutive patients undergoing OLT. However, the control group for that study comprised 6 consecutive prior patients who had not received aprotinin. Aprotinin has been used more extensively to reduce blood loss in patients undergoing cardiopulmonary bypass.[98]

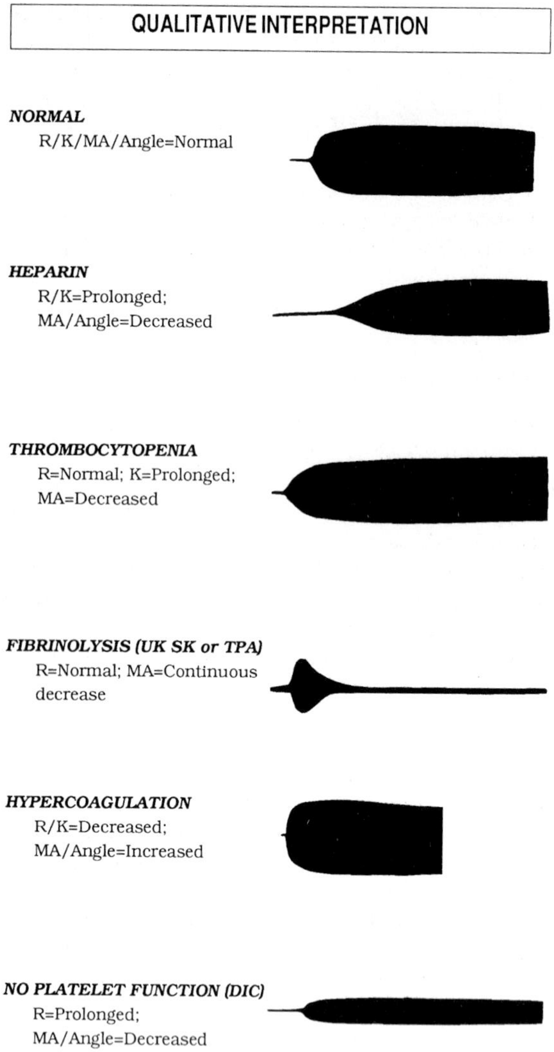

QUALITATIVE INTERPRETATION

NORMAL
R/K/MA/Angle=Normal

HEPARIN
R/K=Prolonged;
MA/Angle=Decreased

THROMBOCYTOPENIA
R=Normal; K=Prolonged;
MA=Decreased

FIBRINOLYSIS (UK SK or TPA)
R=Normal; MA=Continuous decrease

HYPERCOAGULATION
R/K=Decreased;
MA/Angle=Increased

NO PLATELET FUNCTION (DIC)
R=Prolonged;
MA/Angle=Decreased

Fig. 20.3 Thrombelastograph patterns seen in normal and abnormal clinical conditions. R = Re-active time; = R/K = coagulation time; MA = maximum amplitude; UK = urokinase; SK = streptokinase; TPA = tissue plasminogen activator; DIC = disseminated intravascular coagulation.

Anaesthetic technique

Airway management. Kang[15] has emphasized the need to consider OLT as an emergency procedure for patients who have a full stomach. Additionally, intragastric pressure may be elevated by the presence of ascites. We prefer a modified rapid-sequence induction and intubation technique using vecuronium 0.5 mg.kg^{-1} with head-up position, pre-oxygenation and cricoid pressure. Although our patients require postoperative mechanical ventilation, we do not use nasotracheal tubes because of the risk of epistaxis. A nasogastric tube is carefully inserted after the airway is secured, but if oesophageal varices are present, this can be delayed until after the portal system has been decompressed.

Induction agents. Thiopentone, etomidate or ketamine can be used in patients with end-stage liver disease. If haemodynamic stability is of concern, we use etomidate. We premedicate adult patients with lorazepam (2–4 mg) immediately before entering the operating room to ensure amnesia during the procedure. Massive volume replacement can alter the kinetics of amnesic agents during OLT to the point of awareness. Midazolam has a shorter duration of action and offers no advantage. Scopolamine produces amnesia with minimal cardiopulmonary effects.

Maintenance agents. Isoflurane has not been associated with hepatic toxicity and does not produce significant haemodynamic depression at low end-tidal concentrations (0.4–0.6%). We use isoflurane in combination with opioids and muscle relaxants during OLT. The place of desflurane, an agent with only a fraction of the metabolism of isoflurane, remains to be evaluated.

Nitrous oxide should not be used because of the risk of fatal air embolism during manipulation of the inferior vena cava and during venovenous bypass. In patients with right-to-left shunts, venous air embolism may result in systemic embolism.

Muscle relaxants. Suxamethonium has been used without adverse effect. Theoretically, patients with end-stage liver disease may have low concentrations of plasma cholinesterase and may have an abnormal response to suxamethonium. However, all of these patients receive fresh frozen plasma which contains serum cholinesterase. Furthermore, the time frame required for OLT and the blood volume replacement given precludes any significant residual effect of suxamethonium. We do avoid suxamethonium, however, in patients with end-stage organ failure (liver and kidney) associated with hyperkalaemia.

Atracurium has a theoretical advantage compared with other non-depolarizing muscle relaxants in that it undergoes Hofmann degradation as an alternative method of elimination. It is indicated for use in patients with end-stage renal disease. There is concern about the accumulation of laudanosine with long-term administration of atracurium. However, this does not appear to be clinically significant and should not preclude its use in patients with end-stage renal disease. Vecuronium is our choice of muscle relaxant for OLT because of its lack of cardiovascular effects.

The intubating dose (0.5 mg.kg^{-1}) for rapid-sequence intubation is followed by an infusion of 10 µg.kg^{-1} per h.

Opioids. The choice of opioid is a matter of preference. We induce anaesthesia with a bolus dose of sufentanil (1–2 µg.kg^{-1}) followed by an infusion (1 µg.kg^{-1}.h^{-1}). Haemodynamic stability is consistent and there is little need to alter infusion rates. We combine sufentanil with vecuronium (100 mg vecuronium plus 1000 µg sufentanil in 1000 ml of diluent) and administer it as a single infusion. The technique is simple, requires little attention, and the addition of vecuronium solves any problem of substance abuse with left-over infusions at the end of the procedure.

Medications

Methylprednisolone and azathioprine are administered before surgery. OKT-3, a murine monoclonal antibody directed against the T3 locus on human lymphocytes,[99] is given during the anhepatic phase of OLT. This immunosuppressant may produce pulmonary hypertension, bronchospasm and acute respiratory failure. Ranitidine is given pre-operatively and continued postoperatively because of the risk of peptic ulcer disease, gastritis and hiatus hernia in patients with advanced disease. Ranitidine H$_2$ also serves to block H$_2$-mediated effects of OKT-3. An H$_1$-blocker (diphenhydramine 50 mg) and methylprednisolone (300 mg) are given 15 min before OKT-3. Hydrocortisone is given 5 min after OKT-3. Azathioprine (200 mg) is given during the anhepatic phase. Cyclosporin therapy is begun several days after surgery.

A dopamine infusion (2–4 µg.kg^{-1}.min^{-1}) is begun after induction of general anaesthesia to support renal blood flow. Rarely, the dopamine infusion may be increased to rates that provide β-adrenergic support of cardiac function. Dobutamine is added if myocardial function is inadequate. Mannitol (1 g.kg^{-1} up to 50 g) and frusemide (1 mg.kg^{-1}) are given approximately 1 h prior to the beginning of venovenous bypass in an effort to increase renal blood flow, decrease renal tubular oxygen consumption and preserve renal function. The diuresis that occurs must be balanced by adequate intravenous fluid administration.

We use a continuous infusion of magnesium sulphate (0.2 g.h^{-1}) throughout the period of native hepatectomy, the anhepatic phase and reperfusion for haemodynamic stability and inhibition of sympathetic nervous system-mediated ventricular arrhythmia, particularly during reperfusion of the liver. Vasopressin (5–10 units.h^{-1}) can be used to decrease splanchnic blood flow and to decrease portal hypertension prior to portal decompression with venovenous bypass. It is important to discontinue the vasopressin infusion well before reperfusion of the liver. We begin an infusion of prostaglandin E$_1$, starting at 10 µg.h^{-1} and increasing to 40 µg.h^{-1}, after haemodynamic stability has been achieved following reperfusion. Prostaglandin E$_1$ serves to increase liver blood flow.

Dextran may be administered to patients who have evidence of hypercoagulability by TEG or during OLT when there is concern over the adequacy of hepatic artery blood flow, particularly in infants and children with near normal coagulation factors.

Reperfusion of the liver

Blood flow to the transplanted liver can be re-established following completion of the anastomoses of the suprahepatic vena cava, infrahepatic vena cava and the portal vein. Immediately before reperfusion, iced balanced salt solution is infused through the hepatic artery to remove the UW solution and any air bubbles that might have entered venous sinusoids during harvesting. In addition, the liver may be flushed with the recipient's blood by unclamping the caval anastomoses prior to completion of the portal vein anastomosis. The aim is to reduce the efflux of potassium from the new liver and the adverse effects of hyperkalaemia on cardiac rhythm. The hepatic artery anastomosis can be performed either before or after reperfusion of the liver. Delaying hepatic artery anastomosis reduces the warm ischaemia time of the new liver.

Reperfusion of the liver allows cold, acidotic, hyperkalaemic blood to enter the inferior vena cava and can result in severe myocardial depression and ventricular arrhythmias.[100,101] The reperfusion phenomenon can be limited by control of metabolic acidosis during the anhepatic phase, and administration of large amounts of calcium chloride. Myocardial depression associated with reperfusion of the liver is transient and responds well to calcium and sodium bicarbonate.[102,103] Ionized serum calcium and serum electrolyte concentrations are measured hourly during the native hepatectomy and every 30 min during the anhepatic phase and during reperfusion. Ionized calcium concentrations during native hepatectomy require supplementation if large volumes of citrated blood products have been administered. We administer calcium chloride in an effort to maintain ionized calcium concentration greater than 1.0 mmol.l^{-1}. During the first few minutes of reperfusion, calcium chloride is administered in doses of 1–4 g depending on the haemodynamic response to reperfusion. Sodium bicarbonate is given as well, in doses of 50–200 mmol. Hypernatraemia (150–158 mmol.l^{-1})

may occur during the first few hours following reperfusion but this can be limited if hypotonic intravenous fluids are used after haemodynamic stability has returned.

Fluids and blood products should not be given in an attempt to increase preload and improve blood pressure because excessive volume increases central venous pressure and causes engorgement of the new liver. Should this occur, nitroglycerine should immediately be available to reduce central venous pressure and decompress the new liver. If myocardial depression persists, dobutamine (5–10 µg.kg^{-1}.min^{-1}) or adrenaline (10–100 µg) can be used to increase contractility.

Neohepatic phase

With good management, haemodynamic stability returns within 30 min of reperfusion of the new liver. Once it has been determined that there is adequate perfusion of the new liver and that the vena caval, portal and hepatic anastomoses are secure, the cannulae used for venovenous bypass should be removed promptly to prevent venous thrombosis. Aggressive correction of coagulation factor deficits should be withheld until these cannulae have been removed. Every effort should be made to optimize the warming of the new liver to normal body temperature. Warm and cold ischaemia times should be documented. Warm ischaemia time includes the time during harvesting in which the vessels to the transplanted liver were unperfused by warm, native blood (i.e. when the vessels were cross-clamped) to the time of perfusion with cold UW solution, plus the time from the new liver being placed in the recipient's abdomen until the time of reperfusion. Warm ischaemia time should be as short as possible, but averages 1–2 h. Cold ischaemia time should be less than 24 h.

Neohepatic function can be estimated by the appearance of the liver, metabolic changes, serum potassium concentrations, normalization of coagulation factors, appearance of bile production, and measurement of monoethylglycine xylidide (MEGX) formation following the administration of intravenous lignocaine (1 mg.kg^{-1}). The new liver should be the colour of a normal liver. It should not be distended, the margins should be sharp and the substance soft. As the new liver returns to normal body temperature, restored metabolic function is demonstrated by the development of metabolic alkalosis. However, this is not apparent if there is continued loss of large volumes of blood following reperfusion.

Although severe hyperkalaemia can be a major feature of reperfusion, hypokalaemia occurs during the several hours required for completion of the OLT following reperfusion if the new liver functions as expected. We give supplemental potassium if the serum concentration is less than 3.0 mmol.l^{-1}.

Splenomegaly with thrombocytopenia is a frequent finding in patients with portal hypertension.[104] If the platelet count continues to decrease during the neohepatic phase, splenectomy may be required. If possible, splenectomy should be avoided because of the risk of increased bleeding during the remaining part of the procedure and because of the impact of asplenism in the immunocompromised patient.[105]

Coagulation factors can be used to assess adequacy of coagulation and efficacy of the new liver's production of clotting factors. We monitor factors V, VII, VIII and fibrinogen, platelet count, PT and PTT. Coagulation parameters are measured during the native hepatectomy, the anhepatic phase and the neohepatic phase of OLT. Factor VII has a half-life of 4–7 h, and a rapid increase in factor VII concentration in the neohepatic phase is a good index of neohepatic function.[106,107]

OLT for infants and children is significantly different from that in adults. Biliary atresia is the leading indication for OLT in children. Inborn errors of metabolism, of which α_1-antitrypsin deficiency is the most frequent, are the second commonest indication for OLT in children.[108]

Availability of appropriately sized livers for OLT is a major problem, especially in infants. It is estimated that 20% of children with end-stage liver disease will die while awaiting a suitable whole organ for transplantation.[109] Reduced-sized livers, split liver transplants and living related donation offer hope of increased organ availability for infants and children. Initially, reduced liver transplants resulted in a higher mortality than whole-organ transplantation. However the overall reduction in mortality for end-stage liver disease in children was improved because fewer children died while waiting for a whole organ. With increased experience, Broelsch et al[110] showed no significant difference in survival with reduced livers (79%) compared with whole livers (82%). Split liver transplants are associated with different problems. By definition, the medical centre performing the transplantation may be performing two liver transplantations simultaneously if the donor liver can be dissected into two (or more) suitable homografts. Unfortunately, technical considerations of the utilization of the donor blood vessels and biliary tree result in two homografts unequal in quality and potential for graft survival.

Patient survival with split liver transplantation is 67%, and graft survival 50%. Biliary complications, particularly bile leak with subdiaphragmatic collection, are frequent (27%). Hepatic artery thrombosis is a major problem in children weighing less than 10 kg because of the small size (3 mm) of the whole-organ hepatic artery. With reduced-size liver segments, the donor hepatic artery (or branch) is larger and the risk of thrombosis less. Retransplantation is required for graft failure in 24% of children receiving the whole organ, 17% who receive a reduced transplant and 35% of those in whom split liver transplantation is performed.

Infants receiving whole, reduced or split liver grafts present the same problems of coagulopathy, blood loss and reperfusion as adults. In addition, OLT in infants may require cross-clamping of the aorta during anastomosis of the hepatic artery. Coagulation needs must be balanced not only to prevent blood loss but also to prevent thrombosis of the hepatic artery and clot embolus of venovenous bypass.

Carlier et al[109] have shown that OLT can be performed and haemodynamic stability maintained in children without the use of venovenous bypass. It is technically difficult in children less than 10 kg in weight. However, portal engorgement may contribute to the adverse haemodynamic events seen on reperfusion.

Closure of the abdomen in infants with a large transplanted organ results in a restrictive respiratory defect that may require high peak airway pressures, with the risk of barotrauma and the need for prolonged respiratory support.

Living related liver transplants for children are associated with significant risks for the donor (1–2% mortality and 5% serious complication rate). Split livers and reduced-size livers are associated with much greater blood loss during reperfusion than whole-organ transplantation. In these children, it is important to monitor and control clotting factors closely. These issues were addressed by Broelsch's group in Chicago.[111] Partial hepatectomy for other purposes has a reported mortality of up to 11%. Centres with considerable experience in performing partial hepatectomy have not experienced donor deaths.

Broelsch and colleagues conclude that living related liver transplantation should be performed when children with advanced liver disease are relatively stable and the donor has ample opportunity to review the risks and benefits of organ donation. Parents, mature siblings and grandparents are considered suitable donors. This procedure offers the advantages of a new ideal organ for transplantation and possible immunological advantage from genetic relationship. In 5 children undergoing living related OLT by Broelsch et al, survival rate of the grafts and the patients was 100%.

Neurosurgical complications were reported by Mawk et al[112] to occur in 18.6% of 43 children in their series. Of these 8 children (aged 4–42 months), 5 recovered, 2 died and 1 was vegetative. Complications included haemorrhage/infarction, hydrocephalus, cerebral oedema and fungal brain abscess.

Cyclosporin renal toxicity is a greater problem in children than in adults.[113] Additionally, it may interfere with the immune response of children to immunizations or common viral and bacterial infections. Moulin et al[114] reported that 47 of 50 patients (mean age 4.25 years) developed cyclosporin-related hypertension. Two of these patients developed hypertensive encephalopathy. Steroids used for immunosuppression may interfere with the growth and development of children following OLT.

Ryckman et al[115] described an immunosuppressive protocol for children (mean age 5.3 years) that involves OKT-3, azathioprine and methylprednisolone and gives good survival, avoids rejection and preserves renal function. In other protocols, aminoglycosides have been used in combination with cyclosporin A without renal toxicity.[116,117]

Other problems faced by children after OLT include bleeding, infection, ascites, fistula formation, need for secondary abdominal procedures (e.g. drainage of bile collections or haematomas), right hemidiaphragm paralysis, atelectasis and pleural effusions.[118] Hypertension and bradycardia secondary to cyclosporin therapy is a major postoperative problem.[119]

The outlook for children following OLT is positive. They return to near-normal lifestyle, re-enter school, compete academically with their peers and establish normal growth and development. While the cost of paediatric OLT is high (in excess of $250 000), it is less than medical care without transplantation.

Heart transplantation

Patients presenting for heart transplantation range from those who are compensated and waiting at home for a suitable heart, to those who are decompensated and on inotropic and, possibly, ventilatory and/or mechanical circulatory support. Pre-operative sedation is omitted or decreased in those who are at the sicker end of the spectrum. Antacid therapy is commonly administered because of the possibility of delayed gastric emptying, recent food ingestion prior to notification of surgery or oral administration of cyclosporin A.

A 20-gauge Teflon catheter is placed in the radial artery for direct measurement of systemic blood pressure and determination of blood gases. We perform double left internal jugular cannulation with a 7 FG triple-lumen central venous catheter and an 8 FG sheath through which is inserted an oximetric pulmonary artery catheter. It is preferable to preserve the right internal jugular vein for repeated access for heart biopsies after transplantation.

Some have argued against the use of a pulmonary catheter for heart transplantation because of the theoretical increased risk of infection and the lack of any requirement for pulmonary artery measurement in the absence of pulmonary hypertension.[120,121]

Recently, some investigators have suggested the use of a modified right ventricular ejection fraction catheter. They have shown that right ventricular monitoring is useful in demonstrating the continuing need for postoperative pharmacological support of the right ventricle in patients who had normal pulmonary artery pressures prior to transplantation.[122,123]

The anaesthetic agent employed is less important than the ability to control haemodynamic stability in patients with little or no cardiac reserve. We use a modified rapid-sequence induction technique with vecuronium (0.5 mg.kg^{-1}) and sufentanil (2–7 µg.kg^{-1}) or fentanyl (25–50 µg.kg^{-1}) with or without midazolam (15–70 µg.kg^{-1}). Additional muscle relaxant is administered as required. Others have employed thiopentone,[124,125] ketamine, etomidate or high-dose opioid[126] with success. Inotropic support may need to be increased or added to avoid further cardiac decompensation in the pre-bypass period. If the patient has had a previous median sternotomy, blood and/or other volume support may be required.

For cardiopulmonary bypass, the inferior and superior venae cavae are cannulated separately. If a pulmonary artery catheter has been inserted, it should be withdrawn into the sterile sleeve before the snares around the caval cannulae are tightened. Many, if not most, heart transplant patients require diuretic therapy prior to surgery, and it may be necessary to administer additional diuretic during cardiopulmonary bypass to maintain urine output. Management of cardiopulmonary bypass is not different from that of other operations, except that a longer rewarming period is required because of the more profound cooling of the donor heart and more prolonged ischaemia time than for the usual cardiac operation.

Because the transplanted heart is denervated, it typically develops a sinus bradycardia or atrioventricular block and requires chronotropic support.[127] We routinely initiate an isoprenaline infusion at 10–50 µg.kg^{-1}.min^{-1} prior to separation from cardiopulmonary bypass in order to maintain the heart rate at 100–120 beats.min^{-1}. Performance of the transplanted heart is also compromised to some degree because it is post-ischaemic, and isoprenaline augments its performance.

Amrinone, adrenaline or noradrenaline infusions may be used to augment a poorly contracting right ventricle. In situations where the newly transplanted right ventricle fails due to transient pulmonary vasospasm, prostaglandin E_1 infusion has been shown to unload the right heart.[128]

Kidney transplantation

There is greater opportunity for pre-operative preparation of the patient with end-stage renal disease for kidney transplantation than for either heart or liver transplantation because of long-term haemodialysis and the longer viability of a renal homograft.

Dialysis

Haemodialysis should be performed in anticipation of renal transplantation. Dialysis should be undertaken with a hypokalaemic dialysate in anticipation of hyperkalaemia associated with reperfusion of the kidney. Post-dialysis serum electrolyte concentrations and blood counts should be available prior to transplantation. The anticoagulation which may be caused by heparin administration during dialysis can be measured by activated clotting time.

Intravenous access

Intravenous access is one of the major difficulties with patients scheduled for renal transplantation. Most patients have had repeated procedures on their upper extremities for haemodialysis access. We insert a triple-lumen catheter into either the right subclavian or internal jugular vein. This allows us to monitor central venous pressure, administer necessary blood products and to use one port for intravenous fluids and medications.

Monitoring

Non-invasive haemodynamic monitoring is adequate for many patients undergoing renal transplantation. While the procedure may take several hours, the surgery is not traumatic and there is minimal blood loss. Radial artery cannulation should be avoided unless the patient has a history of uncontrolled hypertension, diabetes mellitus, coronary artery disease or uncontrolled uraemia with metabolic acidosis and hyperkalaemia. Radial artery cannulation in the immunosuppressed patient can lead to infection of arteriovenous fistulae that may be necessary for haemodialysis if the homograft does not function promptly. Central venous pressure can be used as an adequate indicator for intravenous fluid administration and blood volume replacement when there is no evidence that the patient has left ventricular dysfunction. Central venous pressure should be approximately 10 cmH$_2$O and systolic blood pressure should be greater than 130 mmHg when renal blood flow is restored to the homograft.[129] These parameters can be achieved by control of anaesthetic depth, augmentation of extracellular fluid volume or administration of dopamine.

Patients with end-stage renal disease who have type 1 diabetes mellitus may have hypertension and coronary artery disease with a history of stroke or congestive heart failure. These patients need invasive haemodynamic monitoring with an arterial line and pulmonary artery catheter.

Anaesthetic agents

If the renal transplantation patient does not have evidence of heart disease or liver dysfunction, there is little to recommend one anaesthetic technique over another. Patients with end-stage renal disease have altered pharmacokinetics related to renal clearance, altered volume of distribution for many drugs and decreased protein binding because of hypoproteinaemia. Therefore, opioids, hypnotics and anxiolytic medications should be administered carefully and respiratory depression anticipated. Pethidine is metabolized to a toxic metabolite and should not be used in patients with end-stage renal disease.

Pre-operative hyperkalaemia is a relative contraindication to the use of suxamethonium for induction because increases in serum potassium concentration of 0.5–0.7 mmol.l^{-1} may be associated with its administration.[130] Even minimal increases in serum potassium concentration can lead to fatal arrhythmias during induction of anaesthesia in the patient with end-stage renal disease. Atracurium has the theoretical advantage of not relying on renal excretion as its undergoes Hofmann degradation. However, the other commonly used muscle relaxants can be used safely when there is normal hepatic function. Fahey et al[131] showed that patients with end-stage renal disease have higher levels of laudanosine following the administration of 0.5 mg.kg^{-1} atracurium when compared with patients without renal failure. Although laudanosine causes CNS excitation in animals,[132] none of the patients in Fahey's study exhibited evidence of CNS toxicity. If the patient has been dialysed recently and has evidence of a reduced extracellular fluid volume, etomidate may be indicated as an induction agent because of its better haemodynamic stability compared with thiopentone.

Regional anaesthesia can offer some advantages to the patient with end-stage renal disease, such as profound abdominal muscle relaxation, decreased bowel distension, maintenance of spontaneous ventilation and an unintubated airway. Continuous epidural anaesthesia or analgesia can be combined with minimal general anaesthesia, and provides postoperative pain relief as well. However, uraemia is associated with platelet dysfunction and the insertion of an epidural catheter may be associated with a risk of epidural bleeding. Although Smith[133] has reported the use of spinal anaesthesia in over 300 patients undergoing renal transplantation, he has abandoned the use of the technique because of a high failure rate.

Medications

Mannitol (1 g.kg^{-1}) and frusemide (1000 mg) are administered prior to reperfusion of the transplanted kidney in order to maximize renal blood flow and renal function.

A variety of protocols have been described for immunosuppression following kidney transplantation. Most include the administration of methylprednisolone prior to unclamping the renal artery.

Living related renal transplantation

Living related renal transplantation is associated with the lowest mortality and morbidity and highest rate of graft survival for the recipient.[134] However, nephrectomy remains a major abdominal procedure for the donor. Pre-operatively, renal arteriography is performed to define the vascular anatomy of the donor and determine if the kidney is an anatomical match for the recipient. Anaesthesia for the donor may be delayed until it is known that the recipient has tolerated induction and intubation. Regional anaesthesia can be used for the donor nephrectomy either alone or in conjunction with general anaesthesia and for postoperative pain relief.

POSTOPERATIVE MANAGEMENT

Liver transplant

Since patients require postoperative ventilatory support for several days, no attempt is made to reverse muscle relaxants or to discontinue opioids. Patients are watched closely for evidence of primary non-function of the transplanted liver, which is reported by Ascher[135] to occur in 7–10% of transplants. Primary non-function is characterized by rising transaminase concentrations, minimal bile production, severe coagulopathy, hypoglycaemia, hepatic encephalopathy and acute renal failure. The mortality rate with primary non-function is 80%, not only because of the severe metabolic consequences of acute liver failure, but because treatment requires emergency retransplantation; it is often difficult to obtain a second suitable liver in a timely period. When primary non-function is clearly evident from the appearance of the transplanted liver, continued coagulopathy and metabolic acidosis after reperfusion, hepatectomy and retransplantation should be performed immediately if a second liver is available. Prostaglandin therapy can reverse primary non-function of the transplanted liver. Greig et al[136] reported improvement in coagulopathy and decreased serum transaminases in 8 of 10 patients with primary non-function between 4 and 34 h after treatment with prostaglandin E_1. Improvement in neohepatic function with prostaglandin treatment is presumed to be related to improved liver blood flow. Prostaglandin E_1 can be started in the neohepatic phase at $10\,\mu g.h^{-1}$ and increased to $40\,\mu g.h^{-1}$ as long as there is no adverse effect on systemic haemodynamics. Acute hepatic failure secondary to primary non-function can be improved temporarily by hepatectomy while awaiting retransplantation.

Neohepatic function is assessed by coagulation profile, control of acid–base balance and bile formation. MEGX can be measured in the donor prior to harvesting of organs as well as in the recipient to gauge the recovery of the new liver from cold and warm ischaemic injury. A MEGX level greater than $100\,ng.ml^{-1}$ during the neohepatic or postoperative periods indicates adequate neohepatic function. Low MEGX levels in the donor should raise doubts about suitability of the liver for transplantation. Neohepatic liver injury is monitored by serum concentrations of transaminases, coagulation factors, electrolytes (especially potassium and calcium) and acid–base status.

Plevak and colleagues[137] reported that liver transplantation patients at the Mayo Clinic had a mean intensive care unit length of stay of 5.9 days and an additional length of stay of 6.2 days if re-admission was required for postoperative complications. They recognized hypothermia and hyperglycaemia as consistent problems in the intensive care unit for all of their liver transplantation patients. Other common problems included renal insufficiency and a variety of bacterial, viral and fungal infections. Intensive care unit stays could be limited by selective bowel decontamination to reduce Gram-negative and fungal infections and control of hypertension and coagulopathy to reduce the incidence of intracranial haemorrhage.

Renal failure (hepatorenal syndrome) and hepatic encephalopathy often improve immediately after OLT. However, coagulopathy may require continued replacement of platelets, fresh frozen plasma or cryoprecipitate as indicated by coagulation profiles, TEG or factor analysis.

Infection and rejection are the major postoperative problems faced by liver homograft recipients. Immunotherapy, which is continued throughout the postoperative course in an effort to prevent rejection of the homograft, is associated with a high incidence of opportunistic infections, including fungi (*Candida* and *Aspergillus*), cytomegalovirus, Epstein–Barr virus, as well as a variety of unusual bacterial infections. Pneumonitis and septicaemia with *Candida* or *Aspergillus* is a fatal complication. Apparently innocuous sources of fungal infection include leafy vegetables in the diet. Castaldo et al[138] reported 91 episodes of fungal infection in 72 patients (23.8%) after OLT. *Candida* was the fungal organism in 83.5% of cases, with infection becoming evident about 16 days after surgery. Fungal infection was associated with a decrease in patient survival from 83.5 to 50%. Bacterial and fungal infections are the leading postoperative complications of OLT.

Espstein–Barr viral infection may be associated with hepatic fibrosis as well as the lymphoproliferative syndrome. Cytomegalovirus is another leading cause of morbidity following OLT. It may cause pneumonitis, hepatitis and retinitis in the immunosuppressed patient. Viral infections may be treated with immunoglobulins but recurrence of clinical infection occurs when immunotherapy is stopped. Acyclovir and other antimetabolites may be useful in controlling viral infections.[139] Prolonged immunotherapy with cyclosporin may put patients at risk of developing malignant diseases, including lymphoma.

A second dose of OKT-3 may be requested prior to the completion of OLT and may be continued in the postoperative period to control acute rejection using the percentage of T3 cells as a guide for repeated administration. OKT-3 has been shown to be more effective than cyclosporin in controlling acute rejection and results in less renal dysfunction and improved patient survival.[91]

Survival following OLT is related to the primary cause of end-stage liver disease. Best results follow OLT for sclerosing cholangitis[140] and biliary cirrhosis,[141] while the poorest are associated with malignant diseases of the liver.[58] However, sclerosing cholangitis is associated with a 30% incidence of cholangiocarcinoma that may not be diagnosed until a frozen section is performed on the common bile duct after native hepatectomy.[142] Survival with cholangiocarcinoma extending beyond the common duct is so low that an alternative recipient should be available when transplantation is considered for these patients.

Overall 1-year survival following OLT in approximately 2000 patients in 1988 was 76%. Five-year survival for non-malignant disease is approximately 70%. One-year survival following OLT for primary malignant disease of the liver is only 30%, but exceeds the survival associated with other forms of treatment. Busuttil et al[143] reported on the results of OLT at the University of California at Los Angeles. In the last year of their series, patient survival was 88% at 1 year following OLT. Severe acute rejection and the need for renal dialysis were the leading indicators of non-survival. Shaw et al summarized the factors that influenced survival at 6 months in the Pittsburgh series.[144] First, no patient with grade IV hepatic coma survived OLT. With the advent of venovenous bypass, prior abdominal surgery did not influence survival following OLT. They noted that there was no margin for technical errors in the performance of the vascular anastomoses. The historical date of surgery was significant for improved patient survival. They felt that this related to two historical events in their programme. First was the routine use of venovenous bypass to reduce bleeding and improve haemodynamics. The second was the development of dedicated anaesthesia teams for transplantation.

Postoperative ventilatory support is routine following OLT. Weaning from ventilatory support is begun only after coagulopathy has been controlled, neohepatic function is returning towards normal, body temperature is normal, renal function is normal and there is no evidence of sepsis or pulmonary congestion.

Heart transplant

Postoperative management of the heart transplant patient is directed at three goals: cardiovascular support, prevention of rejection and prevention of infection.

Haemodynamic stability of the newly transplanted heart is influenced strongly by two factors; the heart is post-ischaemic and it is denervated. In the immediate postoperative period, cardiac index and diastolic compliance are reduced.[125] Right- and left-sided filling pressures are elevated, but gradually recede.[145] It is essential to recognize the need to maintain an adequate preload since the denervated heart is isolated from the baroreceptor control loop and is unable to increase heart rate or cardiac output in response to hypovolaemia. In one series,[146] nearly two-thirds of patients had tricuspid regurgitation and right ventricular enlargement immediately after transplant. This may have been due to ventricular ischaemia and the response to pulmonary hypertension.

The transplanted heart is controlled by the donor sino-atrial node, which is devoid of all normal autonomic innervation. Resting heart rate is 90–100 beats.min^{-1}, similar to the rate which can be achieved in the innervated heart with vagal and β-adrenergic blockade. Drugs such as atropine, suxamethonium, edrophonium, neostigmine, pancuronium and digoxin, which affect vagal tone, have no effect on the denervated heart rate. However, chronic exercise training does result in a slight decrease in resting heart rate.[147] The acute response of the denervated heart to exercise is a delayed increase in heart rate, which also requires a longer time to decrease after completion of exercise. Attenuation of this response by β-blockade indicates circulating catecholamines as the probable cause.[148]

The myocardium of the transplanted heart is depleted of noradrenaline and adrenaline because of interruption of postganglionic cardiac nerves.[149] An increase in β-receptor up-regulation leads to a postsynaptic form of β-adrenergic hypersensitivity.[150]

Infection remains one of the major complications following heart transplantation. However, the incidences of both infection and death attributable to infection in the first year after transplantation have declined since the advent of cyclosporin A therapy.[151]

Most infections are bacterial, and the most common site of infection is the lungs.[152] Cytomegalovirus infections occur in most transplant patients and produces no definite symptoms. Patients who are seronegative for cytomegalovirus before transplantation may acquire their infection from seropositive organ donors or blood products.[153] Other infections may be fungal (candidiasis) or protozoal (*Pneumocystis carinii*). The most common minor infections are due to the herpes simplex and herpes zoster viruses.

Rejection of the donor organ in cardiac transplantation may be defined as hyperacute, acute or chronic. Hyperacute rejection occurs because of preformed HLA antibodies in the recipient serum that are specific for donor HLAs. These antibodies are formed as a result of previous exposure to human antigens through prior blood transfusion, pregnancy or previous transplantation. True hyperacute rejection is rare, and the response to any combination of therapy is poor.[154]

Acute rejection is mediated by a T-lymphocyte response to the donor heart and occurs sporadically over days or weeks. Clinically, the patient may be asymptomatic. Symptoms of ventricular failure in the postoperative period may be due to other factors, but should be considered to be due to acute rejection until proven otherwise. Until the technique of endomyocardial biopsy was introduced by Stanford University for the early diagnosis of acute rejection,[155] reduction of the QRS voltage on the surface electrocardiogram was the primary method of detection.[156] This correlation with electrocardiographic voltage has not proven valid in patients on cyclosporin therapy.[157] Sampling errors may occur with endomyocardial biopsy due to presence of scar tissue from previous biopsies, the non-homogeneous nature of the cellular infiltrate in the right ventricle and myopic reactions which do not meet conventional pathological standards. Some other tests which may be adjuncts to, but do not substitute for, endomyocardial biopsy are Doppler echocardiography, magnetic resonance imaging and cytoimmunological monitoring.

Maintenance immunosuppression of heart transplant patients consists usually of cyclosporin, azathioprine and either antithymocyte globulin or prednisone.[158] Rejection episodes are generally treated with oral or intravenous corticosteroids. OKT-3 has been used successfully for the treatment of refractory rejection.[159,160]

Chronic rejection is a fibro-intimal proliferation which is manifested clinically as coronary arteriosclerosis. It is characterized by diffuse vessel involvement, concentric intimal thickening, absence of calcification and involvement of small, intramyocardial arteries.[161] The incidence appears to be 40–50% at 5 years following transplantation.[162] Presenting symptoms usually include malaise and decreasing exercise tolerance, although silent myocardial infarction, symptoms of congestive failure and sudden death may occur. Anginal pain is not present due to sympathetic denervation of the transplanted heart. The only treatments available are percutaneous transluminal coronary angioplasty of discrete lesions and retransplantation. Because of the nature of the arteriosclerosis, angioplasty is infrequently an option.

Renal transplantation

Patient and homograft survival in renal transplantation is greatest with living related donors and recipients with negative B-cell and T-cell cross-matches and HLA tissue compatibility.[35] With donor-specific blood transfusions and triple immunosuppression (cyclosporin, azathioprine and prednisone), 1-year graft survival is between 85 and 90%.[35,80] Influential factors include histocompatibility, pre-operative transfusions, aetiology of renal failure, medical conditions of the patient prior to transplantation, history of no prior transplantation or graft survival greater than 1 year with prior transplantation, and the experience of the medical centre in the management of renal transplant patients.

Postoperatively, patients are followed closely for signs of homograft rejection.[163,164] Hyperacute rejection occurs immediately after reperfusion of the new kidney and is analogous to the Arthus phenomenon with the intravascular coagulation limited to the kidney. Although hyperacute rejection occurs in less than 1% of cases, it usually causes graft failure. Acute rejection occurs 1 week to 1 year following transplantation. This predominantly cellular rejection is characterized by interstitial inflammation and responds rapidly to prednisone. Humoral rejection is associated with intravascular changes similar to hyperacute rejection and does not respond to drug therapy. Chronic rejection occurs several months to years after transplantation and is characterized by interstitial fibrosis, glomerular thickening and arteriolar narrowing. When transplantation has been performed for end-stage glomerulonephritis, recurrent glomerulonephritis may occur in up to 25% of patients.[165] Other systemic diseases may recur as well. However, rejection is the leading factor in the requirement for a second and possibly a third transplant in patients with ESRD.

Renal transplant nephrectomy is not a benign procedure. Intra-operative bleeding was the major problem encountered in one series.[166] It was necessary to remove the transplanted kidney in 32% of patients. In 72% of these patients, the kidney was removed within 3 months of transplantation for uncontrolled acute rejection, in 25% for chronic rejection, and in 3% for other reasons.

The immunosuppressed renal transplant patient is at risk of numerous other postoperative complications that have anaesthetic implications. Gastro-intestinal ulceration and bleeding have been reported in approximately 7% of renal transplant patients.[167,168] This complication had a mortality rate of 83% related mostly to sepsis and rejection. These patients had a high incidence of cytomegalovirus infection, possibly related to aggressive treatment of rejection. A similar relationship to cytomegalovirus infection and gastro-duodenal ulceration or erosive gastritis in renal transplant patients was reported by Cohen et al.[168]

Opportunistic respiratory infections are another cause of postoperative morbidity. Hariharan et al[169] reported 46 episodes of symptomatic tuberculosis in 550 renal transplant recipients. Hesse et al[170] reported a slightly lower incidence of, and mortality from, pulmonary infections in patients receiving cyclosporin immunosuppression compared to those receiving azathioprine. The organisms reported included *Candida*, *Aspergillus*, cytomegalovirus and mixed bacteria.

Pneumococcal vaccination is effective in immunosuppressed renal transplant patients. However, the duration of an effective antibody level is much shorter in both haemodialysis and renal transplant patients.[171] As mentioned above, Seale et al[139] showed that acyclovir prophylaxis was effective in controlling the development of active herpetic lesions in renal transplant patients with serum antibody to the herpes simplex virus.

Risk of HIV transmission and development of acquired immunodeficiency syndrome (AIDS) appears to be low in transplant recipients.[172] However, cadaver donors need to be screened carefully if the brain-dead donor comes from a high-risk group.

FUTURE TRENDS IN TRANSPLANTATION

The future for transplantation depends on the development of more effective immunosuppressants associated with lower incidences of side-effects, opportunistic infections and predisposition to lymphoproliferative disorders. FK 506, developed in Japan, has undergone clinical trials in kidney, liver and heart transplantation patients as well as in patients receiving islet cell and bone marrow transplants.

UNOS and similar organizations continue to explore the problem of donor organ availability. Universal donor programmes and presumed consent laws have not resolved the shortage. Xenografts may represent the only potential source of organs for infants and children. However, this concept has not been accepted by the public. Future growth in transplant surgery is also dependent on the development of plans to control cost of transplantation and the willingness of federal and private insurance programmes to defray hospital and physician charges for transplantation services.

The list of organs suitable for transplantation, and the degree of success, are limited only by the imagination and technical skill of transplant surgeons (Table 20.4). Pancreas grafts and islet cells grafts are being performed in clinical trials. Multiple organ grafts (heart, liver, kidney, pancreas) are complex procedures but are of real potential benefit for the patient with systemic disease and multi-organ failure.

UW solution has greatly extended the viability of liver and kidney homografts but prolonged preservation of heart and lung grafts has not been achieved. Studies of new preservatives aim not only to extend the useful cold ischaemia time of organs for transplantation, but also to control the problems of reperfusion injury.

Table 20.4 One-year survival rate recorded by United Network for Organ Sharing in 1988

Homograft	Patient survival	Homograft survival
Heart	83%	82%
Heart–lung	57%	57%
Kidney (cadaver)	92%	81%
Kidney (living)	97%	91%
Liver	76%	69%
Lung	48%	48%
Pancreas	89%	71%

REFERENCES

1. Starzl TE, Demetris AJ, Van Thiel DH. Medical progress: liver transplantation (part I). N Engl J Med 1989; 321: 1021–1022
2. Starzl TE, Demetris AJ, Van Thiel DH. Medical progress: liver transplantation (part II). N Engl J Med 1989; 321: 1092–1099
3. Starzl TE, Iwatsuki S, Van Thiel DH et al. Evolution of liver transplantation. Hepatology 1982; 2: 614–636
4. Merrill JP, Murray JE, Harrison JH, Guild WR. Successful homo-transplantation of human kidney between identical twins. JAMA 1956; 160: 227–282
5. Starzl TE, Marchioro TL, von Kaulla KN, Herman G, Brittain KS, Waddell WR. Homotransplantation in humans. Surg Gynecol Obstet 1963; 117: 659–676
6. Barnard CN. A human cardiac transplant: an interim report of a successful operation performed at Groote Schuur Hospital. S Afr Med J 1967; 41: 1271–1274
7. Borel JF, Feurer C, Gubler HO, Stahelin H. Biological effects of cyclosporine A: a new antilymphocytic agent. Agents Actions 1976; 6: 468–475
8. Heimbecker RO. Transplantation: the cyclosporine revolution. Can J Cardiol 1985; 1: 354–357
9. Todo S, Nery J, Yanaga K et al. Extended preservation of human liver grafts with U.W. solution. JAMA 1989; 216: 711–714
10. Jamieson NV, Sundberg R, Lindell S et al. Preservation of the canine liver for 24–48 hours using a simple cold storage with UW solution. Transplantation 1988; 46: 517–522
11. Salter DR, Dyke CM. Cardiopulmonary dysfunction following brain death. In: Fabian J, ed. Issues in organ transplantation. Philadelphia, PA: JB Lippincott. 1991
12. Maddrey WC, Friedman LS, Munoz SJ, Hahn EG. Selection of the patient and timing of surgery. In: Maddrey WC, ed. Transplantation of the liver. New York: 1988: pp 40–45
13. First MR. Pre-transplant evaluation and preparation of donors and recipients. In: Jacobson HR, Striker GE,

Klahr S, eds. The principles and practice of nephrology. Philadelphia, PA: BC Decker. 1991
14 Cook DR. Anesthetic considerations for organ transplantation. In: Annual refresher course lectures. Park Ridge: American Society of Anesthesiology. 1989
15 Kang Y. Anesthesia for liver transplantation. Anesthesiol Clin North Am 1989; 7: 551–580
16 Borland LM. Anesthesia considerations for pediatric orthotopic liver transplantation. Refresher Course in Anesthesiol 1986; 14: 29–41
17 Keown PA, Stiller CR. Kidney transplantation. Surg Clin North Am 1986; 66: 517–539
18 Kang YG, Gelman S. Liver transplantation. In: Gelman S, ed. Anesthesia and organ transplantation. Philadelphia, PA: Saunders. 1987
19 Gelman S, Kang YG, Pearson JD. Anesthetic considerations in liver transplantation. In: Fabian JA, ed. Issues in organ transplantation. Philadelphia, PA: JB Lippincott. 1991
20 Gelman S, ed. Anesthesia and organ transplantation. Philadelphia, PA: WB Saunders. 1987
21 Cate FH, Laudicina SS. Transplantation white paper. The Annenberg Washington Program and UNOS. 1991
22 Colombe BW, Garovoy MR. Clinical histocompatibility testing. In: Milford EL, Brenner BM, Stein JH, eds. Renal transplantation. New York: Churchill Livingstone, 1989; pp 21–43
23 Pallis C. Brainstem death: the evolution of a concept. In: Morris PJ, ed. Renal transplantation: principles and practice, 3rd edn. Philadelphia, PA: WB Saunders, 1988: pp 123–150
24 Milhaud A, Riboulot M, Gayet H. Disconnecting tests and oxygen uptake in the diagnosis of total brain death. Ann NY Acad Sci 1978; 315: 241–251
25 Sommerauer JF. Brain death determination in children and the anencephalic donor. Clin Transplant 1991; 137–145
26 First MR, Schroeder TJ. Solid-organ transplantation in the pediatric population. Clin Transplant 1991; 5: 132–136
27 Narayan RK. Emergency room management of the head-injured patient. In: Becker DB, Gudeman SK, eds. Textbook of head injury. Philadelphia, PA: WB Saunders. 1989
28 Alberico AM, Ward JD, Choi SC, Marmarou A, Young HF. Outcome after severe head injury. Relationship to mass lesions, diffuse injury, and ICP course in pediatric and adult patients. J Neurosurg 1987; 67: 648–656
29 Ward JD, Becker DP, Miller JD et al. Failure of prophylactic barbiturate coma in the treatment of severe head injury. J Neurosurg 1985; 62: 383–388
30 Novitzky D, Cooper DKC, Wicomb WN, Reichart B. Brain death-induced hemodynamic changes resulting in cardiac and pulmonary injury in the baboon. Transplant Proc 1986; 18: 1190–1192
31 Darby JM, Stein KS, Grenvik A, Stuart SA. Approach to management of the heartbeating 'brain dead' organ donor. JAMA 1989; 261: 2222–2228
32 Novitzky D, Cooper DKC, Reichart B. Hemodynamic and metabolic responses to hormonal therapy in brain-dead potential organ donors. Transplantation 1987; 43: 852–854
33 Whelchel JD, Diethelm AG, Philips MG, Rhyder WR, Schein LG. The effect of high-dose dopamine in cadaver donor management on delayed graft function and graft survival following renal transplantation. Transplant Proc 1986; 18: 523–527
34 Terasaki PI, Vredevoe DL, Mickey MR et al. Serotyping for homotransplantation — VI, selection of kidney donors for 32 recipients. Ann NY Acad Sci 1966; 129: 500–520
35 Najarian JS, So SKS, Simmons RL et al. The outcome of 304 primary renal transplants in children (1968–1985). Ann Surg 1986; 204: 246–258
36 Broelsch CE, Emond JC, Thistlethwaite JR, Rouch DA, Whitington PF, Lichtor JL. Liver transplantation with reduced-size donor organs. Transplantation 1988; 519–524
37 Pretto EA. The effect of hepatic ischemia–anoxia and reperfusion injury on myocardial function in the rat. A new experimental model. Crit Care Med 1990; 18: S180
38 Pretto EA. Cardiac function after hepatic ischemia–anoxia and reperfusion injury: a new experimental model. Crit Care Med 1991; 19: 1184–1194
39 Adkinson D, Hollwarth ME, Benoit JN, Parks DA, McCord JM, Granger DN. Role of free radicals in ischemia–reperfusion injury to the liver. Acta Physiol Scand 1986; (suppl 548): 101–107
40 Nordstrom G, Seeman T, Hasselgren PO. Beneficial effect of allopurinol in liver ischemia. Surgery 1985; 97: 679–684
41 Nordstrom G, Saljo A, Hasselgren PO. Studies on the possible role of oxygen-derived free radicals for impairment of protein and energy metabolism in liver ischemia. Circ Shock 1988; 26: 115–126
42 Kang YG, Freeman JA, Aggarwal S, DeWolf AM. Hemodynamic instability during liver transplantation. Transplant Proc 1989; 21: 3489–3492
43 Krensky AM, Weiss A, Crabtree G, Davis MM, Parham P. T-Lymphocyte-antigen interactions in transplant rejection. N Engl J Med 1990; 322: 510–517
44 Carithers RL, Yee YS, Mills AS, Posner MP, Mendez-Picon G. Liver transplantation. In: Gitnik G, ed. Current hepatology, vol 10. Chicago, IL: Yearbook Medical Publishers, 1990: pp 226–249
45 Ascher NL. Selection criteria for liver transplantation donors. Transplant Proc 1989; 21: 3483–3483
46 Shaw BW, Wood RP. The operative procedures. In: Waddrey WC, ed. Current topics in gastroenterology, transplantation of the liver. New York: Elsevier, 1988: pp 87–110
47 Van Thiel DH, Gavaler JS, Tarter RE et al. Liver transplantation for alcoholic liver disease: a consideration of reasons for and against. Alcohol: Clin Exp Res 1989; 13: 181–184
48 Kumar S, Stauber R, Basista M et al. Orthotopic liver transplantation for alcoholic liver disease. Hepatology 1990; 11: 159–164
49 Demetris AJ, Jaffe R, Sheahan DG et al. Recurrent hepatitis B in liver allograft recipients: differentiation between viral hepatitis B and rejection. Am J Pathol 1986; 125: 161–172
50 Fagan EA, Yousef G, Brahm J et al. Persistence of hepatitis A virus in fulminant hepatitis and after liver transplantation. J Med Virol 1990; 30: 131–136

51 Luketic VA, Shiffman ML, McCall JB, Posner MP, Mills AS, Carithers RL. Primary hepatocellular carcinoma after orthotopic liver transplantation for chronic hepatitis B infection. Ann Intern Med 1991; 114: 212–213

52 Vickers C, Neuberger J, Buckels J, McMaster P, Elias E. Transplantation of the liver in adults and children with fulminant hepatic failure. J Hepatol 1988; 7: 143–150

53 Ware AJ, D'Agostino AN, Combes B. Cerebral edema: a major complication of massive hepatic necrosis. Gastroenterology 1971; 61: 877–884

54 O'Grady JG, Gimson AE, O'Brien CJ et al. Controlled trials of charcoal hemoperfusion and prognostic factors in fulminant hepatic failure. Gastroenterology 1988; 94: 1186–1192

55 Tygstrup N, Ranek L. Fulminant hepatic failure. Clin Gastroenterol 1981; 10: 191–208

56 Peleman RR, Gavaler JS, Van Thiel DH et al. Orthotopic liver transplantation for acute and subacute hepatic failure in adults. Hepatology 1987; 7: 484-489

57 Schafer DF, Shaw BW. Fulminant hepatic failure and orthotopic liver transplantation. Semin Liver Dis 1989; 9: 189–194

58 O'Grady JG, Polson RJ, Rolles K, Calne RY, Williams R. Liver transplantation for malignant disease. Results in 93 consecutive patients. Ann Surg 1988; 207: 373–379

59 Pilchmayer R. Is there a place for liver grafting for malignancy? Transplant Proc 1988; 20 (suppl 1): 478–482

60 O'Grady JG, Polson RJ, Rolles K, Calne RY, Williams R. Liver transplantation for malignant disease. Results in 93 consecutive patients. Ann Surg 1988; 207: 373–379

61 Koneru B, Flye MW, Busuttil RW et al. Liver transplantation for hepatoblastoma: the American experience. Ann Surg 1991; 213: 118–121

62 Markus BH, Dickson ER, Grambsch PM et al. Efficacy of liver transplantation in patients with primary biliary cirrhosis. N Engl J Med 1989; 320: 1709–1713

63 Williams DM, Cho KJ, Aisen AM, Eckhauser FE. Portal hypertension evaluated by MR imaging. Radiology 1985; 157: 703–706

64 Bisset GS, Strife JL, Balistreri WF. Evaluation of children for liver transplantation: value of MR imaging and sonography. Am J Radiol 1990; 155: 351–356

65 Moreau R, Lee SS, Soupison T, Roche-Sicot J, Sicot C. Abnormal tissue oxygenation in patients with cirrhosis and liver failure. J Hepatol 1988; 7: 98–105

66 Copeland JG, Emery RW, Levinson MM et al. Selection of patients for cardiac transplantation. Circulation 1987; 75: 2–9

67 Hastillo A, Hess ML. Selection of patients for cardiac transplantation. Cardiovasc Clin 1990; 20: 107–120

68 Johnson RA, Palacios I. Dilated cardiomyopathies of the adult (part I). N Engl J Med 1982; 307: 1051–1058

69 Johnson RA, Palacios I. Dilated cardiomyopathies of the adult (part II). N Engl J Med 1982; 307: 1119–1126

70 Parmley WW. Pathophysiology of congestive heart failure. Am J Cardiol 1985; 56: 7A–11A

71 Dodge HT, Baxley WA. Hemodynamic aspects of heart failure. Am J Cardiol 1968; 22: 24–34

72 Pierpont GL, Francis GS. Medical management of terminal cardiomyopathy. Heart Transplant 1982; 2: 18–27

73 Bristow MR, Ginsburg R, Mionbe W et al. Decreased catecholamine sensitivity and beta-adrenergic receptor density in failing human hearts. N Engl J Med 1982; 307: 205–211

74 Kramer BL, Massie BM, Topic N. Controlled trial of captopril in chronic heart failure: a rest and exercise hemodynamic study. Circulation 1983; 67: 807–816

75 Bristow MR, Port JD, Hershberger RE, Gilbert EM, Feldman AM. The beta adrenergic receptor–adenylate cyclase complex as a target for therapeutic intervention in heart failure. Eur Heart J 1989; 10 (suppl B): 45–54

76 Pae WE, Parascandola SA, Miller CA, Pierce WS. Results of mechanical circulatory support as a 'bridge' to cardiac transplantation — combined registry report. In: Cooper DKC, Novitsky D, eds. The transplantation and replacement of thoracic organs. Boston: Kluwer Academic Publishers, 1990: pp 445–449

77 Keown PA, Stiller CR. Kidney transplantation. Surg Clin North Am 1986; 66: 517–539

78 Rostand SG, Kirk KA, Rutsky EA, Pate BA. Racial differences in the incidence of end stage renal disease. N Engl J Med 1982; 306: 1276–1279

79 Graybar GB, Tarpey M. Kidney transplantation. In: Gelman S, ed. Anesthesia and organ transplantation. Philadelphia, PA: Saunders, 1987: pp 61–110

80 Sutherland DER, Fryd DS, Payne WD, Ascher N, Simmons RL, Najarian JS. Kidney transplantation in diabetic patients. Transplant Proc 1987; 19: 90–94

81 Salvatierra O, Melzer J, Potter D et al. A 7-year experience with donor specific blood transfusions: results and considerations for maximum efficacy. Transplantation 1985; 40: 654–659

82 Chou S, Kim DY, Normal DJ. Transmission of cytomegalic virus by pretransplant leukocyte transfusions in renal transplant candidates. J Infect Dis 1987; 155: 565–567

83 Philipson JD, Carpenter BJ, Itzkoff J et al. Evaluation of cardiovascular risk for renal transplantation in diabetic patients. Am J Med 1986; 81: 630–634

84 Sassno JJ. The rapid infusion system. In: Winter PM, Kang YG, eds. Hepatic transplantation: anesthetic and perioperative management. New York: Praeger, 1986: pp 120–134

85 Dhainaut JF et al. Bedside evaluation of right ventricular performance using a rapid computerized thermodilution method. Crit Care Med 1987; 15: 148–152

86 Lichtor JL, Ellis JE, Uitvlugt A et al. Transesophageal echocardiography during liver transplantation. Anesth Analg 1987; 66: abstract S104

87 Abrams JH, Weber RE, Holmen KD. Transtracheal Doppler: a new method of continuous cardiac output measurement. Anesthesiology 1989; 70: 134–138

88 Abrams JH, Weber RE, Holmen KD. Continuous cardiac output determination using transtracheal Doppler: initial results in humans. Anesthesiology 1989; 71: 11–15

89 Aldrete JA, Clapp HW, Starzl TE. Body temperature changes during organ transplantation. Anesth Analg 1970; 49: 384–388

90 Carmichael FJ, Lindop MJ, Farman JV. Anesthesia for hepatic transplantation: cardiovascular and metabolic alterations and their management. Anesth Analg 1985; 64: 108–116
91 Belani KG, Estrin JA. Biochemical, metabolic and hematologic effects of intraoperative processing of CPDA-1 and AS-1 packed red cells. Anesthesiology 1987; 67: A156
92 Bontempo FA, Lewis JH, Van Thiel DH et al. The relation of preoperative coagulation findings to diagnosis, blood usage, and survival in adult liver transplantation. Transplantation 1985; 39: 532–536
93 Thrombelastograph Coagulation Analyzer, Haemoscope Corp, Morton Grove IL.
94 Kang YG, Martin DJ, Marquez J et al. Intraoperative changes in blood coagulation and thrombelastographic monitoring in liver transplantation. Anesth Analg 1985; 64: 888–896
95 Spiess BD, Logas WG, Tuman KJ et al. Thromboelastography used for detection of perioperative fibrinolysis: a report of four cases. J Cardiothorac Anesth 1988; 2: 666–672
96 Ratnoff OD. Epsilon aminocaproic acid — a dangerous weapon. N Engl J Med 1969; 280: 1124–1125
97 Mallett S, Rolles K, Cox D, Burroughs A, Hunt B. Intra-operative use of aprotinin (Trasylol) in orthotopic liver transplantation. In: First symposium of the International Society for Perioperative Care in Liver Transplantation. Pittsburgh, PA: 1990
98 Royston D, Bidstrup BP, Taylor KM, Sapsford RN. Effect of aprotinin on need for blood transfusion after repeat open-heart surgery. Lancet 1988; ii: 1289–1291
99 First MR, Schroeder TJ, Melvin DB et al. OKT3 therapy in kidney, liver, heart, and pancreas transplantation. Clin Transplant 1988; 2: 185-189
100 Kang YG, Freeman JA, Aggarwal S, DeWolf AM. Hemodynamic instability during liver transplantation. Transplant Proc 1989; 21: 3489–3492
101 Aggarwal S, Kang YG, Freeman JA, Fortunato FL, Pinsky MR. Post reperfusion syndrome: cardiovascular collapse following hepatic reperfusion during liver transplantation. Transplant Proc 1987; 19 (suppl 3): 54–55
102 Estrin JA, Belani KG, Ascher NL et al. Hemodynamic changes in liver transplant recipients during reperfusion of the homograft. Anesthesiology 1988; 69: A172
103 Gelman S. Hemodynamic support in patients with liver disease. In: First symposium of Perioperative Care in Liver Tranplantation. Pittsburgh, PA: 1991
104 Toghill PJ, Green S, Ferguson R. Platelet dynamics in chronic liver disease with special reference to the role of spleen. J Clin Pathol 1977; 30: 367–371
105 Alexander JW, First MR, Majeski JA et al. The late adverse effect of splenectomy on patient survival following cadaveric renal transplantation. Transplantation 1984; 37: 467–470
106 Groth CG. Changes in coagulation. In: Starzl TE, ed. Experience in hepatic transplantation. Philadelphia, PA: WB Saunders, 1969: pp 159–175
107 Stremple JF, Hussey CV, Ellison EH. Study of clotting factors in liver homotransplantation. Am J Surg 1966; 111: 862–869
108 A-Kader HH, Ryckman FC, Balistreri WF. Liver transplantation in the pediatric population: indications and monitoring. Clin Transplant 1991; 161–167
109 Carlier M, van Obbergh L, Veyckemans F et al. Intraoperative haemodynamic modifications during paediatric orthotopic liver transplantation. Intensive Care Med 1989; 15 (suppl 1): S73–S75
110 Broelsch CE, Emond JC, Thistlethwaite JR, Rouch DA, Whitington PF, Lichtor JL. Liver transplantation with reduced-size donor organs. Transplantation 1988; 45: 519–524
111 Singer PA, Siegler M, Whitington PF et al. Occasional notes: ethics of liver transplantation with living donors. N Engl J Med 1989; 321: 620–622
112 Mawk JR, Shaw BW, Wood RP, Williams L. Neurosurgical complications of pediatric orthotopic liver transplantation. Childs Nerv Syst 1988; 4: 26–29
113 Iwatsuki S, Esquivel CO, Klintmalm GBG, Gordon RD, Shaw BW, Starzl TE. Nephrotoxicity of cyclosporin in liver transplantation. Transplant Proc 1985; 117 (suppl 1): S191–S195
114 Moulin D, de Clety SC, Reynaert M et al. Intensive care for children after orthotopic liver transplantation. Intensive Care Med 1989; 15(suppl 1): S71–S72
115 Ryckman FC, Schroeder TJ, Pedersen SH et al. OKT3 induction therapy in pediatric liver transplant recipients. Hepatology 1990; 12: 863
116 Leach CT, Kuhls TL, Brill JE, Busuttil RW, Cherry JD. Use of aminoglycosides during cyclosporine A immunosuppression after liver transplantation in children. Pediatr Infect Dis J 1989; 8: 354–357
117 Zitelli BJ, Gartner JC, Malatack JJ et al. Pediatric liver transplantation: patient evaluation and selection, infectious complications, and life-style after transplantation. Transplant Proc 1987; 19: 3309–3316
118 Moulin D, de Clety SC, Reynaert M et al. Intensive care for children after orthotopic liver transplantation. Intensive Care Med 1989; 15: S71–S72
119 Lawless S, Ellis D, Thompson A, Cook DR, Esquivel C, Starzl TE. Mechanisms of hypertension during and after orthotopic liver transplantation in children. J Pediatr 1989; 115: 372–379
120 Demas K, Wyner J, Mihm FG et al. Anaesthesia for heart transplantation — a retrospective study and review. Br J Anaesth 1986; 58: 1357–1364
121 Garman JK. Anesthesia for cardiac transplantation. Cleve Clin Q 1981; 48: 142–146
122 Gasior T, Armitage J, Stein K, Jacquet L, Miyamoto Y. Right ventricular performance in the transplanted heart. Anesthesiology 1989; 71: A86
123 Nakatsuka M, Colquhoun AD, Barhnart G. Right ventricular function of the denervated heart immediately after heart transplantation. Soc Cardiovasc Anesth 1989; A291
124 Ozinsky J. Cardiac transplantation — the anaesthetist's view: a case report. S Afr Med J 1967; 41: 1268–1270
125 Keats AS, Strong MJ, Girgis KZ, Goldstein A. Observations during anesthesia for cardiac homotransplantation in 10 patients. Anesthesiology 1969; 30: 192–198
126 Hensley FA, Martin DE, Larach DR, Romanoff ME. Anesthetic management for cardiac transplantation in North America — 1986 survey. J Cardiothorac Anesth 1987; 1: 429–437

127 Stinson EB, Caves PK, Griepp RB, Oyer PE, Rider AK, Shumway NE. Hemodynamic observations in the early period after human heart transplantation. J Thorac Cardiovasc Surg 1975; 69: 264–270
128 Armitage JM, Hardesty RL, Griffith BP. Prostaglandin E$_1$: an effective treatment of right heart failure after orthotopic heart transplantation. J Heart Transplant 1987; 6: 348–351
129 Carlier M, Squifflet J, Pirson Y, Gribomont B, Alexandre GPJ. Maximal hydration during anesthesia increases pulmonary arterial pressures and improves early function of human renal transplants. Transplantation 1982; 34: 201–204
130 Koide M, Waud BE. Serum potassium concentrations after succinylcholine in patients with renal failure. Anesthesiology 1972; 36: 142–145
131 Fahey MR, Rupp SM, Canfell C et al. Effect of renal failure on laudanosine excretion in man. Br J Anaesth 1985; 57: 1049–1051
132 Duncan PW. A problem with atracurium. Anaesthesia 1983; 38: 597
133 Smith BE. Renal failure, renal transplantation and anesthesia. In: Annual Refresher Course Lectures. Park Ridge, IL: American Society of Anesthesiologists. 1990
134 Keown PA, Stiller CR. Kidney transplantation. Surg Clin North Am 1986; 66: 517–539
135 Ascher NL. Selection criteria for liver transplantation donors. Transplant Proc 1989; 21: 3482–3483
136 Greig PD, Woolf GM, Abecassis M et al. Treatment of primary liver graft non-function with prostaglandin E$_1$: results in increased graft and patient survival. Transplantation 1989; 21: 2385–2388
137 Plevak DJ, Southorn PA, Narr BJ, Peters SG. Intensive-care unit experience in the Mayo liver transplantation program: the first 100 cases. Mayo Clin Proc 1989; 64: 433–445
138 Castaldo P, Stratta RJ, Wood RP et al. Clinical spectrum of fungal infections after orthotopic liver transplantation. Arch Surg 1991; 126: 149–156
139 Seale L, Jones CJ, Kathpalia S et al. Prevention of herpesvirus infections in renal allograft recipients by low-dose oral acyclovir. JAMA 1985; 254: 3435–3438
140 Marsh JW, Iwatsuki S, Makowka L et al. Orthotopic liver transplantation for primary sclerosing cholangitis. Ann Surg 1988; 207: 21–25
141 Markus BH, Dickson ER, Grambsch PM et al. Efficacy of liver transplantation in patients with primary biliary cirrhosis. N Engl J Med 1989; 320: 1709–1713
142 Foster JH, Berman MM. Solid liver tumors, 1st edn. Philadelphia, PA: WB Saunders. 1977
143 Busuttil RW, Colonna JO, Hiatt JR et al. The first 100 liver transplants at UCLA. Ann Surg 1987; 206: 387–402
144 Shaw BW, Wood RP, Gordon RD, Iwatsuki S, Gillquist WP, Starzl TE. Influence of selected patient variables and operative blood loss 6-month survival following liver transplantation. Semin Liver Dis 1985; 5: 385–393
145 Young JB, Leon CA, Hort HD et al. Evolution of hemodynamics after orthotopic heart and heart–lung transplantation: early restrictive patterns persisting in occult fashion. J Heart Transplant 1987; 6: 34–43
146 Bhatia SJS, Kirschenbaum JM, Shemin RJ et al. Time course of resolution of pulmonary hypertension and right ventricular remodeling after orthotopic cardiac transplantation. Circulation 1987, 76: 819–826
147 Kavanagh T, Yacoub M, Mertens D et al. Cardiorespiratory responses to exercise training after orthotopic cardiac transplantation. Circulation 1988; 77: 162–171
148 Donald DE, Ferguson DA, Milburn SE. Effect of beta-adrenergic blockade on racing performance of greyhounds with normal and with denervated hearts. Circ Res 1968; 22: 127–134
149 Mohanty PK, Sowers JR, Thames MD, Beck FWJ, Kawaguchi A, Lower RR. Myocardial norepinephrine, epinephrine and dopamine concentrations after cardiac autotransplantation in dogs. J Am Coll Cardiol 1986; 7: 419–424
150 Lurie KG, Bristow MR, Reitz BA. Increased beta-adrenergic receptor density in an experimental model of cardiac transplantation. J Thorac Cardiovasc Surg 1983; 86: 195–201
151 Hofflin JM, Potasman I, Baldwin JC, Oyer PE, Stinson EB, Remington JS. Infectious complications in heart transplant recipients receiving cyclosporine and corticosteroids. Ann Intern Med 1987; 106: 209–216
152 Dummer JS, Hardy A, Poorsattar A, Ho M. Early infections in kidney, heart and liver transplant recipients. Transplantation 1983; 36: 259–267
153 Chou S. Cytomegalovirus infection and reinfection transmitted by heart transplantation. J Infect Dis 1987; 155: 1054–1056
154 Cooper DKC. Diagnosis and management of acute rejection. In: Cooper DKC, Novitsky D, eds. The transplantation and replacement of thoracic organs. Boston; MA: Kluwer Academic Publishers, 1990: pp 127–142
155 Vaves PK, Stinson EB, Graham AF, Billingham ME, Grehl TM, Sumway NE. Percutaneous transvenous endomyocardial biopsy. JAMA 1973; 225: 288–291
156 Stinson EB, Dong E, Bieber CP, Schroeder JS, Shumway NE. Cardiac transplantation in man. I. Early rejection. JAMA 1969; 207: 2233–2247
157 Schroeder JS, Hunt S. Cardiac transplantation: update 1987. JAMA 1987; 258: 3142–3145
158 Bolman RM, Elick B, Olivari MT, Ring WS. Improved immunosuppression for heart transplantation. Heart Transplant 1985; 4: 315–318
159 Gilbert EM, DeWitt CW, Eiswirth CC et al. Treatment of refractory cardiac allograft rejection with OKT3 monoclonal antibody. Am J Med 1987; 82: 202–206
160 Sweeney MS, Sinnott JT, Cullison JP et al. The use of OKT3 for stubborn heart allograft rejection: an advance in clinical immunology? J Heart Transplant 1987; 6: 324–328
161 Billingham ME. Cardiac transplant atherosclerosis. Transplant Proc 1987; 19: 19–25
162 Barnhart GR, Pascoe EA, Mills AS et al. Accelerated coronary atherosclerosis in cardiac transplant recipients. Transplant Rev 1988; 1: 31–46
163 Sibley RK, Rynasiewicz J, Ferguson RM et al. Morphology of cyclosporine nephrotoxicity and acute rejection in patients immunosuppressed with cyclosporine and prednisone. Surgery 1983; 94: 225–234
164 Dunnill MS. Histopathology of rejection in renal transplantation. In: Morris PJ, ed. Kidney

transplantation: principles and practice. London: Academic Press, 1979; p 225
165 Hamburger J, Crosnier J, Noel LH. Recurrent glomerulonephritis after renal transplantation. Annu Rev Med 1978; 29: 67–72
166 Chiverton SG, Murie JA, Allen RD, Morris PJ. Renal transplant nephrectomy. Surg Gynecol Obstet 1987; 164: 324–328
167 Sutherland DER, Chan FY, Foucar E, Simmons RL, Howard RJ, Najarian JS. The bleeding caecal ulcer in transplant patients. Surgery 1979; 86: 386–398
168 Cohen EB, Komorowski RA, Kauffman HM, Adams M. Unexpectedly high incidence of cytomegalovirus infection in apparent peptic ulcers in renal transplant recipients. Surgery 1985; 97: 606–612
169 Hariharan S, Date A, Gopalakrishnan G, et al. Tuberculosis after renal transplantation. Dialysis & Transplantation 1987; 16: 311–312
170 Hesse UJ, Fryd DS, Chatterjee SN, Simmons RL, Sutherland DE, Najarian JS. Pulmonary infections. Arch Surg 1986; 121: 1056–1060
171 Linnemann CC, First MR, Schiffman G. Revaccination of renal transplant and hemodialysis recipients with pneumococcal vaccine. Arch Intern Med 1986; 146: 1554–1556
172 Feduska NJ, Perkins HA, Melzer J et al. Acquired immune deficiency (HTLV/LAV) and Epstein–Barr virus. Observations relating to the incidence of the acquired immune deficiency syndrome and other possibly associated conditions in a large population of renal transplant recipients. Transplant Proc 1987; 19: 2161–2166

21. Anaesthesia for the neurosurgical patient

J. M. Borthwick   W. Fitch

The anaesthetist in a neurosurgical unit can expect to administer anaesthesia to a wide range of patients for a variety of procedures. These may be invasive or non-invasive neuroradiological investigations, diagnostic or definitive surgical procedures or manipulations aimed at alleviating pain. In addition, the anaesthetist has an important role to play in the management of patients in the neurosurgical intensive care unit, especially those with severe head injury.

Neurosurgeons operate on patients with a variety of pathological conditions of the brain and spinal cord, and of their surrounding and supporting tissues. In order to administer safe anaesthesia to these patients, and simultaneously provide the surgeon with good operating conditions, the anaesthetist must be fully conversant with the pathophysiology of the patient's disease. It is essential to understand the interrelationships between cerebral metabolic rate for oxygen ($CMRO_2$), cerebral blood flow (CBF) and intracranial pressure (ICP), and their application to neuro-anaesthetic practice.

The $CMRO_2$ in normal, awake human brain remains very stable and is 3.0–3.8 ml.min^{-1} per 100 g. CBF is normally coupled to $CMRO_2$ and is also fairly stable (45–65 ml.min^{-1} per 100 g). CBF remains constant over a range of mean arterial pressures of approximately 50–150 mmHg. This process of autoregulation is generally assumed to be due to myogenic and chemical mechanisms. In patients with intracranial pathology, autoregulation is impaired or lost altogether. Flow then becomes pressure-dependent; an increase in arterial pressure causes increases in CBF, cerebral blood volume (CBV) and ICP. Decreased flow, if substantial, leads to cerebral ischaemia and hypoxic brain injury.

Another major determinant of CBF is the arterial partial pressure of carbon dioxide (Pa_{CO_2}). A twofold increase in Pa_{CO_2} causes approximately a twofold increase in CBF before reaching a plateau. Similarly, if the Pa_{CO_2} is halved, CBF is approximately halved before reaching a plateau. In the pathological brain, this cerebrovascular reactivity to carbon dioxide may be impaired or lost. As a consequence, hypercapnia may cause a 'steal' of CBF from the region of pathology by dilating normal blood vessels. Conversely, hypocapnia may cause 'inverse steal'; the vessels in the region of the pathology are unresponsive, and the pathological region receives excess perfusion.

Hyperoxia has little effect on CBF. When the arterial partial pressure of oxygen (Pa_{O_2}) decreases to less than 6.5 kPa, CBF increases acutely. This is probably due to the accumulation of acid metabolites caused by the hypoxia.

Hypothermia produces a decrease in $CMRO_2$ of 5–7%/°C. At 27°C, $CMRO_2$ is about 50% of normal. At this temperature, both autoregulation and carbon dioxide reactivity remain intact and CBF and $CMRO_2$ remain coupled in the 'normal' brain if Pa_{CO_2} is maintained at 5.3 kPa, using a non-temperature – corrected measurement technique. A reduction in temperature to 17°C produces an iso-electric electroencephalograph (EEG) in unanaesthetized brain. The hypothermic brain should withstand total ischaemia for longer than the normothermic brain.

THE EFFECTS OF ANAESTHETIC DRUGS

Inhaled agents

Nitrous oxide (N_2O)

Under conditions of normocapnia, N_2O causes an increase in CBF in humans by a mechanism of vasodilatation. This has the potential for raising ICP.[1] The increase in CBF can be attenuated if vessel calibre is maintained by reducing Pa_{CO_2}. When N_2O is added to anaesthesia with volatile agents, a marked increase in CBF may occur, even when total minimum alveolar concentration (MAC) is maintained.[2] This increase may be a direct effect of N_2O on cerebral vasculature, and not mediated by a change in $CMRO_2$.[3] This may indicate that the use of N_2O should be contra-indicated in patients with raised ICP. However, infusions of propofol at clinical concentrations may obtund the metabolic activation and subsequent increases in CBF and ICP which may be associated with N_2O.[4] In clinical practice hyperventilation also overcomes this increase in CBF, as confirmed by its successful use in many thousands of patients over the years.

Halothane

Halothane causes cerebral vasodilatation and increases CBF at normocapnia and with a normal perfusion pressure.[5] In patients with intracranial pathology and reduced brain compliance, the use of halothane induces an increase in ICP. These effects are overcome by hyperventilation to a Pa_{CO_2} of 3.3 kPa before introduction of halothane.[6] Clinical concentrations of halothane cause dose-related reductions in $CMRO_2$ with progressive EEG suppression. Halothane can produce an iso-electric EEG, but not until a halothane concentration in blood equivalent to 4.5% is achieved.[7] Above 2.3% halothane, there is evidence of a toxic effect on oxidative phosphorylation.[7] A decrease in metabolic rate also occurs with enflurane and isoflurane but to different degrees.[8] Halothane may enhance cerebrovascular reactivity to carbon dioxide[9] but may also impair autoregulation, and at concentrations of 1.5 MAC or greater may abolish it.[10] Halothane decreases the rate of re-absorption of cerebrospinal fluid (CSF).[11]

Enflurane

This anaesthetic ether causes less cerebrovascular dilatation and more metabolic suppression than does halothane.[12,13] Its use in concentrations of 1.5 MAC or greater in hyperventilated subjects may induce seizure activity.[12] Under clinical conditions, this effect is not significant and does not preclude its use in patients with seizure susceptibility. Enflurane increases the rate of CSF production and decreases the rate of re-absorption.[11]

Isoflurane

Although a structural isomer of enflurane, isoflurane has less effect on CBF than does either halothane or enflurane.[14–16] It also reduces $CMRO_2$ to a greater degree than do the other two agents.[15,16] At approximately 2 MAC it has the capacity to produce an iso-electric EEG[17] with a reduction in $CMRO_2$ of approximately 40%. There is evidence from studies in baboons that coupling between flow and metabolism is maintained when low concentrations of isoflurane are used.[18,19] At twice the concentration required to produce an iso-electric EEG (4 MAC), $CMRO_2$ did not decline further and normal brain metabolites were preserved. While the ICP effects of halothane are overcome by prior hyperventilation of the lungs, simultaneous hyperventilation is adequate to prevent an increase in ICP using isoflurane.[20] Isoflurane does not alter either the rate of production or re-absorption of CSF.[11] These characteristics may mean that the use of isoflurane imparts some degree of neuroprotection and makes it the volatile agent of choice for neuro-anaesthesia.

Intravenous agents

Barbiturates

The commonly available intravenous barbiturates, thiopentone and methohexitone, cause a dose-related decrease in $CMRO_2$ and parallel decreases in CBF.[21] This effect has caused them to be known as cerebral vasoconstrictors, in contrast to the effect of the volatile anaesthetic agents. Autoregulation is maintained even when $CMRO_2$ is reduced by 50%.[22] Cerebrovascular reactivity to carbon dioxide is attenuated but not abolished.[23] Barbiturates can produce an iso-electric EEG.[8,23]

Thiopentone is still a popular choice of induction agent in neuroanaesthesia. Methohexitone may be associated with epileptiform EEG activity, but this has not precluded its successful use. Barbiturates have been used by infusion but recovery times are prolonged, even with the shorter half-life of methohexitone. Their effects on EEG, $CMRO_2$, CBF, CBV and ICP make the barbiturates the most potent drugs available to the neuroanaesthetist.

Etomidate

This agent has similar effects to thiopentone on the intracranial volume–pressure relationship.[24] As with barbiturates, additional drug administered after the production of iso-electricity does not reduce the $CMRO_2$ any further. It has been shown to be effective in reducing ICP without reducing cerebral perfusion pressure in head-injured patients.[25] Its relatively short half-life indicates that it should be useful for infusion but its interference with adrenocortical function causing reduced steroid production may contra-indicate this use.[26]

Propofol

The pharmacology and clinical uses of this relatively new agent have been reviewed.[27] Propofol reduces $CMRO_2$, CBF and ICP[28,29] and is used extensively in neuroanaesthesia. It has been used for induction of anaesthesia, maintenance of anaesthesia, sedation for neuroradiological investigations and for sedation of severely head-injured patients in the intensive care unit without compromising cerebral perfusion.[30] Autoregulation is preserved during infusions in baboons.[31] Propofol has been implicated in central nervous system (CNS) excitability. There are reports of grand mal seizures, rigidity and opisthotonus associated with its use.[32] However, there is also evidence of its anticonvulsant activity in mice[33] and it has been shown to reduce the duration of seizures in electroconvulsive therapy.[34,35]

Ketamine

The administration of ketamine causes increases in $CMRO_2$, CBF and ICP.[36,37] However, these effects may be controlled by the simultaneous use of lignocaine, either as a bolus or as an infusion.[38] Ketamine is postulated to exert its anaesthetic effect by an interaction with the N-methyl-D-aspartate (NMDA) receptor complex.[39] Antagonism at this receptor site may block the release of those excitatory amino acids which facilitate cellular membrane damage and calcium entry to neurones. Other agents aimed specifically at producing cerebral protection by this action are at present undergoing evaluation.

Benzodiazepines

Midazolam is the member of this group of γ-hydroxybutyric acid type A ($GABA_A$) receptor antagonist drugs which is most commonly used in neuroanaesthetic practice. $CMRO_2$ and CBF are reduced in parallel by the use of midazolam. An iso-electric EEG is not produced but the EEG is stabilized, with a mixture of high amplitude θ and δ waves. The presence of normal brain metabolites indicates a lack of toxic effects.[40] The use of midazolam in patients with a brain tumour has no effect on ICP.[41] In a recent study in patients with supratentorial tumours, the use of flumazenil to reverse the effects of midazolam did not affect $CMRO_2$ or CBF.[42] These properties make midazolam a useful agent, especially as an infusion for sedation in the intensive care unit.

Opioids

There are many reports of studies involving the measurement of cerebral blood flow in association with the use of opioids. There appear to be conflicting results but these can be accounted for by the variations in the background anaesthesia. In a recent study using fentanyl,[43] it was clear that large doses of this opioid had little effect on $CMRO_2$ or CBF. Opioids do not alter carbon dioxide reactivity.[44] Canine studies have shown that fentanyl does not cause an increase in ICP[45] or in CSF production if Pa_{CO_2} is controlled.[46] Alfentanil has been used successfully in neuroanaesthesia and maintains a stable cardiovascular system. No changes in $CMRO_2$, CBF, carbon dioxide responsiveness, autoregulation or the CBF response to hypoxia were observed when alfentanil was administered to anaesthetized dogs.[47] A comparison of fentanyl, sufentanil and alfentanil in humans with brain tumours indicated that alfentanil may increase CSF pressure compared with a slight reduction caused by fentanyl. Sufentanil appeared to cause an even greater increase in ICP.[48]

Neuromuscular blocking agents

The use of neuromuscular-blocking agents is common in neuroanaesthetic practice. Their use prevents coughing and bucking and any other movement which could be detrimental to delicate surgical techniques. The drugs do not cross the blood–brain barrier and thus have no direct cerebral effects. Pancuronium has the potential to increase arterial pressure and cause tachycardia. This may be detrimental to patients with reduced intracranial compliance and loss of autoregulation. However, in dogs, pancuronium has no significant effect on $CMRO_2$, CBF, ICP or EEG.[49] Vecuronium given to patients with an intracranial tumour produces modest reductions in ICP and mean arterial pressure, with no significant change in cerebral perfusion pressure (CPP).[50] Atracurium given to similar patients has no effect on ICP or mean arterial pressure.[51] Atracurium releases histamine, and this may be a disadvantage. One of atracurium's metabolites, laudanosine, may be epileptogenic but this has not proved to be a problem in clinical practice.

Suxamethonium causes an increase in ICP. This is short-lived and may be attenuated by pretreatment with a competitive neuromuscular blocking agent.[52] This action is thought to be due to muscle spindle activity which increases cerebral afferent input. Suxamethonium is usually administered after a 'sleep dose' of induction agent which should attenuate this effect. Suxamethonium releases large amounts of potassium from denervated muscle, such as may occur in spinal cord transection. Although it is usually safe to use suxamethonium during the first 2 days after injury, the period of risk may extend for 6 or 12 months after the injury. The use of suxamethonium in these patients may cause cardiac arrest.

Local anaesthetic agents

All local anaesthetic agents rapidly cross the blood–brain barrier to cause dose-related sedation, excitation and then severe CNS depression. Lignocaine in a dose of 1.5 mg.kg^{-1} causes reductions in $CMRO_2$ and CBF. This effect is often used in patients with low intracranial compliance at the time of anaesthetic induction, and permits a reduction in the dose of induction agent required to produce loss of consciousness.

MONITORING

Most neurosurgical procedures are complex and interfere directly or indirectly with normal physiology. Continuous electrocardiography (ECG) and pulse oximetry are required for all patients undergoing anaesthesia or sedation. Although automatic non-invasive measurement of arterial pressure may be adequate for some procedures, the use of an arterial cannula and the constant display of systolic, mean (MAP) and diastolic pressures is essential in many cases. Central venous pressure can be transduced and is of use in situations associated with major blood loss or fluid shifts. The presence of a catheter in the right atrium may permit the aspiration of air in the event of air embolism (see below). Peroperative measurement of pulmonary artery pressure may be useful but is not used routinely in British neuroanaesthetic practice.

Hyperventilation is an inherent part of neuroanaesthesia; thus continuous measurement of end-tidal carbon dioxide tension (PE'_{CO_2}) permits adjustment of CBF and intracranial volume. Capnography and pulse oximetry reduce the frequency with which blood gas analysis is required. Inspired oxygen concentration monitoring allows accurate adjustment of air/oxygen or oxygen/N_2O mixtures. Knowledge of inspired and end-tidal concentrations of anaesthetic agents is useful, but not essential.

Many neurosurgical procedures are prolonged, and a method of measuring core temperature is essential, especially if hypothermia is to be used in the anaesthetic technique. A nasopharyngeal probe is effective.

Intracranial pressure monitoring

ICP may be increased as a result of a space-occupying lesion, hydrocephalus, cerebral oedema or an increase in CBV. The importance of its measurement is in the maintenance of an adequate CPP (CPP = MAP – ICP). The 'gold standard' to which all methods of measurement are compared is the fluid-filled intraventricular catheter. The pressure can be displayed on a continuous paper print-out which allows observation of the pressure waveforms. Withdrawal of CSF is possible using this technique, but there is a risk of ventriculitis (up to 10%).[53] Other techniques, such as subdural bolts, subdural catheters and extradural transducers, have been used with varying degrees of success.

More recently, a fibre-optic catheter with a transducer at its tip (Camino) has become available.[54] This is inserted using a twist drill and the tip can be placed in the extra- or subdural space, or more commonly in the brain parenchyma. The pressures measured by this technique correlate well with those measured using an intraventricular catheter, and the use of this technique is becoming routine in many centres.

Neurophysiological monitoring

Electroencephalography

The EEG reflects the spontaneous electrical activity of the cerebral cortex. A montage of 20 electrodes (the international 10–20 system) is placed over the scalp and the standard recordings are made on a 16-channel recorder. Clinical interpretation of the EEG involves assessment of frequency, amplitude, form and distribution of the electrical activity. These continuous displays are recorded on paper and produce records which require considerable expertise in interpretation. Consequently, there is little application of standard EEG recording in clinical surgical and anaesthetic practice. In order to overcome some of these practical drawbacks, attempts have been made to process the EEG signals into a more easily comprehensible format.

The cerebral function monitor compresses all frequency and amplitude information into a single value. A continuous paper record displays power against time; increasing distance above the baseline indicates increased activity and decreases towards zero indicate decreasing activity.

The cerebral function analysing monitor produces a more detailed analysis of the frequencies and the amplitude distribution of the EEG waveform but may be difficult to interpret.[55]

All EEG signals are compilations of sine waves of differing frequencies. Computers using fast Fourier transformation can break down a complex wave into its component frequencies (power spectrum analysis). In a predetermined period of time, for example a 2-3s epoch, the computer can calculate the distribution of energy (power) at each interval of frequency. The frequency spectrum derived by this analysis can then be displayed in a variety of ways. Compressed spectral array provides a pseudo-three-dimensional display of frequency against power distribution over time. Sequentially derived spectra are displayed in a stack with the appearance of a range of mountains. If the majority of the power is in low-frequency bands then the peaks are to the left of the display and if the majority of the power is in the higher frequencies then the peaks appear further to the right.

Further simplifications can be made to aid interpretation. The spectral edge frequency is the frequency below which 95% of the power is distributed. The peak power frequency is the frequency at which the highest power is found. The median power frequency can be calculated easily.

Density spectral array[56] is similar to compressed spectral array, but instead of peaks of power, the amount of power is represented by the density of the display; the greater the power present at a particular frequency, the greater the density of the displayed signal. A similar device (Lifescan, Braun Melsungen, Germany) produces an array of rods, the heights of which relate to the power of the signal received.

Various physiological conditions may affect the EEG. These include hypoxaemia, hypocapnia and hypothermia. Alterations in depth of anaesthesia may also affect the EEG. Attempts to use the processed EEG to determine absolute depth of anaesthesia have not as yet been successful, although changes in depth may be observed.

Cerebral ischaemia may be recognized by the use of EEG monitoring during carotid artery surgery.[57,58] Prolonged ischaemia results in an iso-electric EEG but early recognition and correction reinstate electrical activity. Changes in anaesthetic depth and physiological variables must be taken into account in interpreting the data. Processed EEG techniques have been used in cerebral aneurysm surgery to detect local ischaemia[59] and in cardiopulmonary bypass surgery to detect cerebral ischaemia (either globally, or focal ischaemia caused by emboli).

The EEG may be used in the intensive care unit to monitor patients with seizure activity. If pharmacological muscle paralysis is being used, seizure activity can still be detected.[60] The efficacy of anticonvulsant therapy can also be monitored.

Evoked potentials

Sensory evoked potentials (SEPs) are electrophysiological responses to a stimulus. They are usually recorded at the scalp but electrodes may be placed on the cortex (although this may interfere with the surgical procedure). They can be classified as somatosensory evoked potentials (SSEP), auditory evoked potentials (AEP) and visual evoked potentials (VEP). Many factors affect SEPs, including anaesthetic drugs. Halothane, enflurane and isoflurane all cause dose-related decreases in amplitude and increases in latency. Diazepam, fentanyl, thiopentone and etomidate all affect the SEP, but acceptable recordings can still be obtained. It is advisable to avoid altering the patient's pharmacological condition during, or just prior to, any surgical manipulation when SEPs are being monitored. Hypothermia, hyperthermia, alterations in Pa_{CO_2} and alterations in cerebral or spinal cord blood flow can all affect SEPs.

SSEPs may be used to assess the patency of sensory pathways during surgery. This may include scoliosis surgery, surgery for cervical spondylosis and surgery for tumours or vascular lesions of the spinal cord.

AEP recording may be carried out when the eighth cranial nerve or the brainstem is at risk, for example during resection of an acoustic neuroma or other cerebellopontine angle tumour. AEPs have been used as indicators of anaesthetic depth. In patients breathing spontaneously a mixture of nitrous oxide and oxygen, surgical anaesthesia can be achieved by a computer-driven system which infuses propofol to maintain the AEP amplitude response at approximately 40% of pre-anaesthetic values.[61]

VEPs may be used during surgery on lesions compressing the visual pathways. There is a relatively high frequency of false-positive and false-negative results. This may be due to difficulty in providing an adequate stimulus in the anaesthetized patient.

Motor evoked potentials (MEP) may provide information on the integrity of areas of the spinal cord which cannot be assessed using SSEPs. Either direct stimulation or transcranial stimulation of the motor cortex may be used. Both electrical and magnetic sources of stimulation have been employed.

Other monitors

Transcranial Doppler ultrasonography allows non-invasive determination of blood flow velocity profiles in the vessels in and adjacent to the circle of Willis. This technique has been used to identify the onset of vasospasm in patients with a cerebral aneurysm.[62]

Jugular venous oxygen saturation (Sj_{VO_2}) measurement is used in the management of patients with severe head injury. It permits the detection of impending global cerebral ischaemia, the monitoring of the effects of increasing ICP on CBF and $CMRO_2$, and monitoring of the effect of therapeutic intervention. The continuous measurement of Sjv_{O_2} can be carried out using the Oximetrix 3 monitor and fibre-optic catheter.[63] This technique also permits intermittent blood sampling for the measurement of cerebral metabolites.

SUPRATENTORIAL SURGERY

Cerebral artery aneurysms

Cerebral artery aneurysms occur at, or near to, junctions of vessels. The weakness in the vessel wall may be due to a congenital defect, often with a family history (e.g. polycystic disease or co-arctation of the aorta), or may be acquired due to arteriosclerotic disease.

Diagnosis is usually made after the rupture of an aneurysm causes a subarachnoid haemorrhage which presents as an acute, severe headache with or without signs of meningism, focal deficit or reduction in conscious level. The diagnosis is usually confirmed by the presence of uniformly blood-stained CSF at lumbar puncture. Computer tomography (CT) can verify the presence of subarachnoid blood, the presence or absence of an intracerebral haematoma, or hydrocephalus. Cerebral angiography can confirm the site of the ruptured aneurysm and the presence or absence of any other unruptured aneurysms, and is essential prior to surgical intervention.

The Hunt & Hess grading[64] put forward in 1968 is still used as the basis for classifying the patient's condition following subarachnoid haemorrhage (Table 21.1). As a general rule, those in higher grades (I and II) have a better prognosis than those in lower grades (III–V).

Table 21.1 The grading of patients with subarachnoid haemorrhage

Grade	Description
Grade I	Asymptomatic, or minimal headache and slight neck stiffness
Grade II	Moderate to severe headache, neck stiffness, no neurological deficit other than cranial nerve palsy
Grade III	Drowsiness, confusion or mild focal deficit
Grade IV	Stupor, moderate to severe hemiparesis, possible early decerebrate rigidity and vegetative disturbances
Grade V	Deep coma, decerebrate rigidity, moribund appearance

From Hunt & Hess,[64] with permission.

Following subarachnoid haemorrhage, 30–70% of patients develop vasospasm of a large cerebral artery. Up to 50% of these patients develop neurological deficits, which may or may not be permanent. The vasospasm is thought to be due to the presence of blood in the CSF and the presence of vaso-active substances. The presence of a large intraventricular blood load is associated with a higher incidence of vasospasm. Alterations in calcium homeostasis may play a major part in the production of vasospasm. The use of nimodipine, a calcium antagonist with a preferential action on cerebral vessels, is beneficial in subarachnoid haemorrhage.[65] Onset of neurological deficit due to vasospasm is not instantaneous; the period of greatest risk is between 4 and 14 days after the haemorrhage, with the peak at 7 days.[66]

Another major complication following subarachnoid haemorrhage is rebleeding, which results in neurological deterioration or death in the majority of patients in whom it occurs. The period of risk from rebleeding is greatest in the first few days after the original haemorrhage. During the first week, the risk is 10–17%; this reduces to 10–12% in the second week.

The poor outcome of patients who suffer a rebleed has stimulated interest in attempting to clip aneurysms soon after the initial haemorrhage. Some centres progress to surgery directly after angiography. However, there is usually brain swelling and raised ICP in the period immediately after subarachnoid haemorrhage; this makes surgery more difficult and may increase the risk of intra-operative aneurysm rupture. The timing of surgery is a balance between operating early to reduce the risk of rebleeding and later to avoid the peak period of vasospasm.

Anaesthetic management

Pre-operative assessment. The pre-operative assessment of patients undergoing cerebral artery aneurysm surgery must include an evaluation of their general medical condition as well as their neurological status. Common problems such as ischaemic heart disease and pulmonary disease must be assessed, and the patient's condition optimized promptly. The grade of the patient's condition, the time since subarachnoid haemorrhage, the presence of an intracerebral haematoma or hydrocephalus, and the amount of subarachnoid blood should be assessed. Some patients may have received large amounts of intravenous fluids pre-operatively and some may have been treated with diuretics for neurogenic pulmonary oedema or raised ICP. Patients who have suffered subarachnoid haemorrhage may develop hyponatraemia or hypovolaemia without diuretic therapy; it is therefore essential to measure electrolyte concentrations.

When subarachnoid haemorrhage has been diagnosed, nimodipine should be prescribed in a dose of 60 mg by mouth every 4 h and this should be continued until the patient is transferred to the anaesthetic room.

ECG abnormalities are noted frequently in association with subarachnoid haemorrhage, commonly without a history of myocardial ischaemia. The usual changes are in the T wave and the ST segment, but other changes have been reported. Investigation of patients with ECG changes after subarachnoid haemorrhage using echocardiography has shown that poor myocardial function is related to the severity of the neurological condition, and not to the ECG abnormalities.[67]

Alert patients may be anxious about surgery and should be premedicated with a small dose of a sedative agent such as a benzodiazepine. Those with any reduction in the level of consciousness seldom require any premedicant drugs. All concurrent medication should be continued until the patient is transferred to the anaesthetic room.

Anaesthesia. Induction of anaesthesia is one of the most critical periods of the procedure. A smooth transition from the conscious, anxious state to the anaesthetized, intubated and ventilated state is required. ECG and oxygen saturation are monitored before any intervention. Adequate venous access should be achieved before induction; an additional large-bore cannula can be inserted after the patient has been anaesthetized. The insertion of an arterial cannula is essential for management and may be performed under local anaesthesia before induction. Modern automated arterial pressure monitors can produce rapid measurements at short intervals, and may be adequate if arterial access is difficult.

The best induction agent is the one with which the anaesthetist is most familiar. Thiopentone, methohexitone, etomidate and propofol have all been used. The authors' preference is to administer propofol several minutes after giving intravenous lignocaine and a small dose of fentanyl. Neuromuscular blockade is achieved using the non-depolarizing agent of choice. The cardiovascular characteristics of vecuronium make it a suitable agent, and it can be continued as an intravenous infusion, its effects being monitored using a peripheral nerve stimulator.

Immediately after induction, ventilation is controlled, and a mixture of oxygen, oxygen and air or oxygen and nitrous oxide is delivered, with isoflurane. It is vitally important to maintain manual ventilation until full neuromuscular blockade is achieved. During this period of manual ventilation, Pa_{CO_2} should be kept only slightly lower than normal. Excessive hyperventilation before the dura is opened reduces ICP and may increase the transmural pressure of the aneurysm and the risk of rupture.

The combination of lignocaine, fentanyl and propofol is usually adequate to attenuate the pressor response to laryngoscopy and intubation. An orotracheal tube is inserted and fixed firmly to the patient's face with adhesive tape to avoid possible venous obstruction from tape around the neck. The eyes should be protected using ointment and padding. Any further invasive monitoring should now be inserted.

If the surgeon has requested the insertion of a spinal CSF drain, the patient may be turned to the lateral position at this stage. An extradural catheter can be inserted into the CSF via the lumbar route using a Tuohy needle, and the catheter secured to the skin. The drain should remain closed until the dura is opened.

Anaesthesia may be maintained using an intravenous infusion technique, a nitrous oxide/opioid technique or one based on isoflurane with or without nitrous oxide. A comparison of an air/oxygen/propofol infusion technique with a nitrous oxide/oxygen/isoflurane technique demonstrated no difference in surgical conditions or outcome.[68] Pa_{CO_2} should be maintained slightly below normal and is easily monitored using measurements of end-tidal carbon dioxide concentration. Periods of increased stimulation such as the insertion of the three-pin head-rest and scalp infiltration with local anaesthetic may be managed by giving bolus doses of an opioid such as fentanyl. When the dura is open, hyperventilation and opening the spinal drain reduce brain bulk and facilitate surgery. Mannitol, with or without frusemide, may be requested by the surgeon as another method of reducing brain bulk.

In the past, induced arterial hypotension was routinely used to aid aneurysm clipping. The reduction in pressure reduced the wall tension, and so the risk of rupture. The use of the operating microscope and the placement of temporary clips on the vessel for short periods have virtually removed the requirement for hypotension. Some surgeons ask for a cerebral protective agent such as a barbiturate to be given immediately before temporary clipping. Prevention of hypotension caused by such a manoeuvre must be achieved.

The use of intentional hypothermia is no longer routine practice; however, it has been used in combination with cardiopulmonary bypass in operations on giant aneurysms of the posterior cerebral circulation.

If the aneurysm ruptures intra-operatively, and control of haemorrhage cannot be achieved using a temporary clip on the feeding vessel, the anaesthetist may be asked to lower the arterial pressure rapidly to reduce the amount of bleeding, thereby assisting the surgeon to regain control. The technique and drugs with which the anaesthetist is most familiar should be employed.

The circulating blood volume should be maintained throughout the operation and a combination of crystalloid and colloid usually proves suitable. Overtransfusion with blood is inadvisable; indeed, hypervolaemic haemodilution may be effective in overcoming the neurological sequelae of vasospasm.

At the end of the operation, neuromuscular blockade is antagonized and anaesthesia discontinued. A smooth transition to spontaneous ventilation and extubation is required. This should be followed by a smooth, rapid return to consciousness in order to assess the patient's neurological condition.

Postoperative management. Postoperatively, the patient should be monitored in a high-dependency nursing unit. Arterial oxygenation should be maintained with supplemental oxygen by mask. Circulating volume should be maintained by infusing 125.ml.h^{-1} of a balanced crystalloid solution and analgesia provided by appropriate doses of an opioid such as dihydrocodeine. Hourly (or more often, if indicated) neurological nursing observations should be carried out and any signs of deterioration treated appropriately and aggressively. Oral nimodipine therapy must be continued in the postoperative period.

Vasospasm may present as a deficit such as dysphasia or hemiparesis. When a transcranial Doppler technique is used to measure the flow velocities in the cerebral vessels, a markedly increased velocity is seen in the vessel with vasospasm. Treatment consists of ensuring good oxygenation, normal pulmonary ventilation, an adequate arterial pressure and a full circulating volume using a mixture of crystalloid, colloid and blood.[69,70] There is some evidence that monitoring these patients using a pulmonary artery catheter is beneficial.[71] Maintenance of an adequate left atrial filling pressure and a normal or increased cardiac output (with the use of inotropic agents if necessary) may improve outcome. Nimodipine may be administered intravenously if there is any doubt about absorption from the gastro-intestinal tract.

Arteriovenous malformations

Arteriovenous malformations (AVMs) are congenital lesions. They consist of groups of dilated arteries and veins with high blood flows. Most are usually situated in the cerebral hemispheres and may present as a subarachnoid or intracerebral haemorrhage, or as epilepsy.

Operative excision can be carried out on the smaller and more accessible AVMs. Peroperative angiography is helpful. In larger lesions, pre-operative embolization under local anaesthesia reduces the vascularity and improves surgical conditions. Morbidity and mortality associated with deep AVMs are sufficiently high to consider conservative management.

Anaesthesia

The anaesthetic management of patients undergoing surgical resection of an AVM is similar to that for cerebral aneurysms. Blood loss may be high. It may be appropriate to monitor venous central or pulmonary artery pressure in patients with a large AVM.

When surgical excision is in progress, hyperventilation may be used to reduce brain bulk; diuretics and CSF drainage may also be employed. Hypotension may be induced to reduce operative blood loss.

Percutaneous embolization using isobutyl, 2-cyanoacrylate (a fast-setting glue) under heavy sedation has proved to be successful.[72] After induction of anaesthesia with propofol and the insertion of a laryngeal mask airway, the patient is sedated with intravenous midazolam, fentanyl and droperidol and breathes oxygen-enriched air spontaneously. Arterial pressure is controlled meticulously to prevent hypertensive episodes during embolization. Light sedation and manipulation of the arterial pressure are continued for 24 h in the postoperative period when the patient is still at risk from surges in arterial pressure. The mean arterial pressure is maintained below 100 mmHg, but the systolic arterial pressure is kept above 80 mmHg.

Supratentorial tumours

Tumours that occur within the cranium may be benign, malignant or metastatic. Tumours within the skull are space-occupying lesions. They are sometimes diagnosed by their local effects, for example deafness due to an acoustic neuroma. A tumour may cause a first seizure and the patient presents as a potential epileptic. Investigation of female infertility may uncover the presence of a microprolactinoma without there being any space-occupying effects.

More commonly, the effect of space occupancy is to cause an increase in ICP and a generalized decrease in the level of consciousness. This may be due to the tumour itself, or to obstructive hydrocephalus produced by the tumour preventing CSF from leaving the ventricular system. An impaired level of consciousness indicates that the patient's position on the ICP/volume compliance curve is far to the right. A very small additional increase in intracranial volume may cause the patient to 'cone'.

Surgery in these patients may involve different approaches. It may be directed at attempting to obtain a tissue diagnosis via a burr-hole biopsy. In the case of hydrocephalus, drainage may be carried out by inserting a ventriculoperitoneal shunt. Definitive surgery may be required to decompress the tumour with or without a previous tissue diagnosis, or to produce a cure by excising a benign tumour. This is achieved through a craniotomy.

Anaesthesia

In all cases, the principles of anaesthetic management are the same. These are to induce and maintain anaesthesia in a patient with raised ICP in whom the perfusion pressure of the brain is critical and in whom autoregulation of CBF is almost certainly absent.

Pre-operatively, the patient with intracranial hypertension due to tumour should have been treated with dexamethasone to decrease the oedema which surrounds the tumour. The conscious level may have improved with this therapy by pushing the position on the compliance curve a variable distance to the left. Anticonvulsant therapy may have been instituted. Patients with a large meningioma frequently bleed profusely at operation; however, pre-operative embolization should reduce blood loss.

In the anaesthetic room, the patient is monitored using ECG, pulse oximetry and direct measurement of arterial pressure (preferably prior to induction of anaesthesia). A wide-bore intravenous cannula should be inserted under local anaesthesia so that a rapid infusion of fluid can be given if arterial pressure decreases after induction of anaesthesia. The drugs used for induction should be selected with the aim of maintaining arterial pressure, reducing ICP (or at least not increasing it) and attenuating the pressor response to laryngoscopy and tracheal intubation. The authors' choice is the same as that employed in intracranial vascular surgery, namely lignocaine, fentanyl, propofol and vecuronium for neuromuscular blockade, in appropriate doses for the patient. If hypotension develops, prompt treatment with intravenous fluids and vasopressors is required.

When the patient is anaesthetized and stable, additional intravenous cannulae may be inserted, as indicated. The expected blood loss from a large meningioma may warrant the measurement of central venous pressure. A urinary catheter should be inserted for all but the briefest of procedures. A nasopharyngeal temperature probe can be inserted, and protection for the eyes must be provided. Peri-operative antibiotics and additional steroids should be administered, as indicated.

Anaesthesia may be maintained using either an inhalational or an intravenous technique. However, in patients with critically increased ICP and marginal CPP, it is theoretically beneficial to avoid any potential causes of further increases in CBF. Hyperventilation with an air/oxygen mixture and the maintenance of anaesthesia with an intravenous infusion of propofol may avoid the potential hazards of N_2O and volatile anaesthetic agents. In clinical practice there is little evidence of any benefit from such a technique, but attention to detail is all-important and any alteration to cardiovascular indices must be detected and managed with the utmost of care.

The lungs should be hyperventilated to produce a Pa_{CO_2} of about 3.3 kPa. Further hyperventilation may be required if the brain is found to be very swollen. Mannitol may be required to reduce brain bulk and should be given after dural opening in a dose of about 0.25 g.kg^{-1}. Blood loss should be replaced, and maintenance fluids administered throughout the operation. Emergence from anaesthesia should be smooth and prompt; the trachea should be extubated before the patient bucks or coughs.

Postoperatively, the patient should be nursed in a high-dependency area with careful assessment of the neurological state. If the tumour has been decompressed, ICP should not be problematic and CPP should be maintained easily. There is a risk that the patient may develop a postoperative intracranial haematoma and any sign of clinical deterioration should be investigated by CT scanning.

Pituitary surgery

Pituitary tumours may present with headache, cranial nerve palsies, visual disturbances due to pressure on the optic chiasma or as endocrine dysfunction. The commonest endocrine problems involve prolactin, growth hormone and adrenocorticotrophic hormone. Endocrine effects due to compression and hyposecretion produce panhypopituitarism, requiring hormone replacement before surgery. Pressure effects on the posterior pituitary may cause diabetes insipidus (due to failure to secrete antidiuretic hormone).

Endocrine assessment must be carried out pre-operatively. Patients with Cushing's disease are susceptible to hypertension, hyperglycaemia, hypokalaemia and overhydration. Acromegalics may suffer from hypertension, hyperglycaemia, organomegaly and altered airway anatomy, resulting in intubation difficulties.

Anaesthesia

Surgery involves resection of the tumour by the transsphenoidal route under general anaesthesia. The patient is monitored using ECG, pulse oximetry and, usually, non-invasive measurement of arterial pressure. If the tumour extends into the suprasellar region, anaesthesia should be managed as for other intracranial tumours. Following induction, the trachea is intubated orally with an armoured tracheal tube. The patient's head and neck are maximally extended during the operation and kinking of the tube may occur. This position allows the surgeon to stand at the patient's head and therefore have clear access to the operating microscope and image intensifier (which allows verification of the direction of the surgical approach). A throat pack is inserted to absorb blood in the pharynx.

Anaesthesia may be maintained by an inhalational or intravenous technique and ventilation is controlled. The surgeon usually prepares the nose with cocaine, and local anaesthetic and adrenaline solutions, and this influences the choice of anaesthetic agent. Deliberate hypotension is seldom required but control of arterial pressure during particularly stimulating stages reduces the amount of blood in the operating field. Occasionally, procedures are deferred because of venous bleeding, which is not amenable to arterial pressure control.

At the end of the operation, it may be necessary to insert a spinal drain if a CSF leak has been produced by the surgery. Any residual neuromuscular blockade is antagonized, the throat pack removed and the pharynx examined for blood and secretions. When the patient can maintain adequate ventilation, the trachea may be extubated but the patient must be placed in the recovery position until full pharyngeal reflexes return.

Postoperative alterations in endocrine function may occur and should be assessed. All patients are prescribed a reducing regimen of dexamethasone and maintained on a small dose until biochemical investigation confirms re-instatement of the pituitary–adrenal axis. Urine output should be monitored for the occurrence of diabetes insipidus, and fluid losses replaced. The use of exogenous vasopressin may be required.

INFRATENTORIAL SURGERY

Infratentorial surgery is carried out for tumours which may be benign, malignant or metastatic. Developmental abnormalities such as the Arnold–Chiari malformation may require decompression. Trigeminal neuralgia due to vascular compression of the fifth cranial nerve root may be alleviated by surgical decompression.

Surgery may be performed with the patient in a horizontal position (prone or park-bench) or in a sitting position. There are advantages and disadvantages to each (Table 21.2). The choice of position depends on the experience of the surgeon and the anaesthetist. There are two particular problems for the anaesthetist if the patient is in the sitting position — postural hypotension and venous air embolism.

Table 21.2 The advantages and disadvantages of the sitting position compared with the horizontal position for posterior fossa surgery

Advantages
Better physical access to the operative site

More neck flexion allows easier access

Improved gravitational drainage of blood, cerebrospinal fluid and debris from the operative site

Less venous distension and brainstem pulsation

Reduced transfusion requirement

Better access to the face for monitoring evoked twitch responses

Better access to the anterior chest for monitoring purposes

Disadvantages
Increased potential for postural hypotension

Increased risk of venous air embolism

Postural hypotension

Postural hypotension may occur when the anaesthetized patient is transferred from the horizontal position to the upright position. This must be prevented in order to maintain CPP. Preloading the circulation, binding the legs, the use of a G-suit and altering the patient's position slowly reduce the risk of postural hypotension. If it does occur, it must be treated promptly by returning the patient to the horizontal position and administering a vasopressor. When stability returns, a further attempt at positioning the patient may be made.

Venous air embolism

Venous air embolism may occur when a vein in which the pressure is subatmospheric is opened to the atmosphere. In the sitting position, all the veins in the scalp and the neck muscles are well above the heart, as are the diploic veins and the venous sinuses. Consequently, the pressure of blood in these veins is subatmospheric.

Both the total volume of air and the rate of entry into the circulation are important. A high rate of entry may overcome the ability of the lungs to dissipate the air. Air in the right atrium and ventricle causes turbulence which is heard as the classical 'millwheel murmur'. Pulmonary oedema and reflex brochoconstriction may occur due to air in the pulmonary vasculature. Pulmonary artery pressure increases, central venous pressure increases, cardiac output is reduced, hypotension develops and arrhythmias occur. Gas exchange is impaired and carbon dioxide excretion is reduced. Death is due to acute right heart failure and anoxia. If air enters the systemic circulation by way of an intracardiac right-to-left shunt, such as a patent foramen ovale, paradoxical air embolism occurs. Air may then enter the coronary and cerebral arteries.

Various forms of monitoring are available for the detection of venous air embolism. An oesophageal or precordial stethoscope may allow auscultation of the mill-wheel murmur but this is a late occurrence and the technique is insensitive. Arterial hypotension occurs soon after significant venous air embolism but is variable and may be detected too late. The use of pulmonary artery or central venous pressure monitoring may help detection but, although better than auscultation, both are relatively insensitive and occur late in the process of events. Continuous monitoring of Pe'_{CO_2} permits detection of a reduction in carbon dioxide excretion within a few breaths of a significant venous air embolism and before cardiovascular changes occur.

A precordial Doppler ultrasound probe can be positioned over the fourth intercostal space to the right of the sternum. It permits continuous monitoring of the heart sounds and can detect the presence of small amounts of air entering the right atrium. However, the Doppler instruments are very sensitive to surgical diathermy and it is difficult to detect changes in signal when diathermy is in use. The period of greatest risk of venous air embolism is during opening and closing of the wound and these are the times when surgical diathermy is most likely to interfere with the signal.

Transoesophageal echocardiography is becoming more widely available for clinical use. This is very sensitive and allows visualization of the cardiac chambers. Air can be detected in the the right atrium by this method and it also allows detection of paradoxical air emboli. This may be the method of choice in the future.

It is better to prevent venous air embolism than to have to treat it. Careful haemostasis by the surgeon, using diathermy and bone wax, should minimize air entry. If there is the suspicion of an open vessel then the field should be flooded with saline until the vessel is closed. The venous pressure may be increased by intermittent manual compression of the jugular veins in the neck at the request of the surgeon, and this may permit identification of the open vein.

The use of positive end-expiratory pressure (PEEP) is controversial. The values of PEEP used clinically may be ineffective in increasing the venous pressure significantly. In addition, the risk of paradoxical air embolus[73] is greater if right atrial pressure is increased towards or above left atrial pressure. The effects of PEEP on haemodynamic variables in a patient at risk of postural hypotension must be taken into account in considering its role.

Aspiration of the central venous pressure catheter may produce a quantity of air and may be life-saving. This is probably only effective in cases of massive venous air embolism. Aspiration of a pulmonary artery pressure catheter is unlikely to be effective because of the small calibre of its lumen. If N_2O is being used as part of the anaesthetic technique, its use should be discontinued on diagnosing venous air embolism. N_2O causes an increase in the volume of the embolized air and worsens the clinical situation. Infusion of intravenous fluids and the administration of vasopressors may be required to maintain cardiac output. It may be necessary to return the patient to the horizontal position in order to carry out effective resuscitation but by the time this is achieved, the prognosis may be hopeless.

In a retrospective study,[74] the incidence of intraoperative hypotension was no different between patients in the horizontal position and those in the sitting position. The incidence of venous air embolism as detected by Doppler was greater in those who were sitting than in those in the horizontal position but the need for blood transfusion was significantly less in the sitting patients. There were no differences in postoperative cardiac or respiratory complications.

Anaesthesia

Monitoring consists of ECG, pulse oximetry and invasive arterial pressure with the transducer at the level of the occiput. In order to detect the occurrence of venous air embolism, continuous capnography allows observation of Pe'_{CO_2} precordial Doppler ultrasonography permits continuous access to the heart sounds and a central venous pressure catheter allows access to the right atrium for aspiration of air. Posterior fossa operations are long, and the insertion of a urinary catheter and a temperature probe is beneficial. A nasogastric tube should be passed if bulbar problems are anticipated.

If the patient is prone or in the park-bench position,

the anaesthetic considerations are similar to those for supratentorial surgery. The patient's neck may be flexed or rotated to achieve the best access for surgery, and the use of an armoured tracheal tube is advantageous.

The choice of an inhalational or intravenous technique is available to the anaesthetist. Smooth control of anaesthetic depth and rapid awakening postoperatively are easily achieved using isoflurane as the major anaesthetic component. The requirement for intra-operative nerve stimulation may preclude the use of continuous neuromuscular blockade. It is reasonable to administer a fairly large dose of a competitive neuromuscular blocking agent for tracheal intubation and to allow it to wear off during positioning of the patient and the formation of the craniectomy. A technique using controlled ventilation with N_2O/oxygen and isoflurane has proved to be acceptable.

In patients who are to undergo surgery in the sitting position, the principles of anaesthetic management are the same. After careful induction to maintain CPP, the trachea is intubated with an armoured tube. The use of N_2O in patients in the sitting position is controversial. The author's choice is to use an air/oxygen/isoflurane mixture. If nerve stimulation is not required, then muscular relaxation is maintained with an infusion of a medium-acting neuromuscular blocking agent, such as vecuronium or atracurium.

Spontaneous ventilation has been used as a monitor of motor tract continuity and preservation of the respiratory centre. If venous air embolism occurs in a spontaneously breathing patient, entrainment of air is greater because of the lower intrathoracic and venous pressures. It is preferable to control ventilation and to rely on cardiovascular changes to warn of brainstem damage. Electrophysiological monitoring may prove useful in this situation.

Measures to prevent postural hypotension as described above should be used. Infusion of crystalloid or colloid to maintain a full circulating intravascular volume reduces the incidence of hypotension. Movement from the supine to the sitting position must be carried out slowly and smoothly. If hypotension occurs, the patient must be returned to the supine position and intravenous fluids and/or vasopressors administered. When stability returns, a further attempt may be made to reposition the patient.

Once the patient's body is positioned, the knees and hips must be flexed to prevent sciatic nerve strain, the arms placed on the patient's lap, and pressure areas protected. The patient's head is positioned for the best surgical access, while permitting access by the anaesthetist to the anterior neck. Patency of the tracheal tube is checked and the head is fixed in position using a three-pin fixator.

Intra-operative problems of venous air embolism, hypotension and surgically induced arrhythmias must be continuously monitored and treated appropriately. Severe bradycardia or asystole may occur as a result of brainstem retraction or surgical stimulation. Atropine must be immediately available. Prophylactic treatment may be effective but its use may remove an important sign of impending damage.

At the end of the procedure, any residual neuromuscular blockade is antagonized and anaesthesia discontinued. The patient is returned to the supine or lateral position and the airway cleared in anticipation of emergence and tracheal extubation. If a bulbar problem exists, the tracheal tube should be left in situ until recovery occurs and the patient can protect his or her own airway. If the deficit is permanent, tracheostomy should be performed at an appropriate time.

STEREOTACTIC NEUROSURGERY

Stereotactic neurosurgery involves surgery on a very localized area of the brain. The commonest procedures are biopsies of deep-seated lesions in which conventional open biopsy may produce a significant degree of damage to surrounding normal brain.

Functional stereotactic surgery describes the formation of a lesion in a pathway in order to interrupt that pathway. Parkinsonian tremor which does not respond to medical treatment may respond to surgery. The surgeon produces a temporary radiofrequency lesion by the application of an electrode to the designated site. The patient is then examined for changes in the tremor and, if the side of treatment is dominant, for speech changes. If the generated lesion produces the desired reduction in the tremor within acceptable levels of side-effects, the surgeon makes a permanent lesion. It is clear that the patient must be awake and co-operative to comply with this form of treatment.

To isolate the lesion or the target site, imaging techniques are employed to define the site in relation to reproducible reference points. CT imaging or magnetic resonance imaging may be appropriate and some centres use angiography, depending on the lesion and its site. The reproducible reference points are on a frame which the surgeon fixes to the patient's head. The three-dimensional co-ordinates of the target site are then calculated from the result of the imaging.

Armed with the target co-ordinates, the surgeon decides on the approach. A large protractor which holds the biopsy needle or radiofrequency electrode is then attached to the frame on the patient's head. Its position is adjusted so that the target co-ordinates can be accommodated, and an appropriately placed burr-hole is drilled. The operating instument is then advanced to the correct depth and the surgery performed.

Anaesthesia

In some units, imaging is not undertaken on the same day as surgery. In these units, the frame is usually fixed to the patient's skull under local anaesthesia with or without sedation. The patient is transferred to the scanner, where the image is produced. The frame is then removed, note having been taken of the micrometer readings on the fixation pins so that they may be replaced in exactly the same position when surgery is to be performed.

If functional surgery is planned immediately after imaging, the patient is transferred back to the operating theatre. The procedure is then performed under local anaesthesia with the minimum of sedation to allow for compliance.

Stereotactic biopsies which follow imaging may be performed under general anaesthesia. The anaesthetic technique depends on the effect of the lesion on the patient's neurological state. If ICP is elevated, measures should be taken to maintain CPP, as described above. It is useful to use an intravenous technique for maintenance of anaesthesia in these patients. Anaesthesia is induced in the anaesthetic room; the patient is then transferred to the scanning room (at a variable distance from the operating theatre) and then returned to the operating suite for surgery. A continuous infusion of propofol from a battery-operated pump is a suitable technique. The intermittent or continuous use of neuromuscular blocking agents prevents coughing when the patient is being moved on and off trolleys. Controlled ventilation using an air/oxygen mixture from a transport ventilator avoids the necessity to transport N_2O cylinders around the hospital.

Some patients may present to the anaesthetist awake with a frame in place. The frame may have been attached to the patient's head with the neck in such a position that tracheal intubation would be difficult or impossible by conventional methods. An awake/sedated fibre-optic intubation with an armoured tracheal tube is the technique of choice in this situation.

SPINAL SURGERY

Neurosurgeons are usually involved in spinal surgery in order to decompress neural tissue which is being encroached upon by a pathological process. This may occur at any level from the first cervical vertebra to the sacrum. Surgery may involve either a posterior or an anterior approach. An anterior approach is relatively straightforward in the cervical region but more difficult in the thoracic and lumbar regions.

Odontoid surgery is usually undertaken for myelopathy in patients with rheumatoid disease. Atlanto-occipital subluxation causes compression of the cord or, if vertical, of the lower brainstem. The surgical approach is either transoral or transmaxillary. Both routes may involve difficulties in tracheal intubation. There may be cervical instability, and access may be limited due to temporomandibular joint disease. Posterior fixation as part of the same procedure stabilizes the cervical spine.

The authors' choice of management is fibre-optic intubation under local anaesthesia, by the nasal route, in a sedated patient. Anaesthesia is maintained using a volatile agent and an intravenous opioid with the patient breathing spontaneously. This allows monitoring of the descending pathways of the spinal cord. Evoked potential monitoring may be of use for this procedure. Intra-arterial pressure monitoring allows early detection of brainstem trauma.

Posterior approaches to the cervical, thoracic and lumbar spine require the patient to be in the prone position. (Some centres prefer to carry out cervical laminectomy in the sitting position: see the section on anaesthesia for posterior fossa surgery.) Care must be taken to prevent abdominal compression to avoid restriction of venous return and consequent reduction in cardiac output. Extradural venous congestion caused by abdominal compression can also cause considerable bleeding in thoracic and lumbar operations.

An anaesthetic technique involving mechanical ventilation using a volatile agent and an opioid analgesic is the method of choice. Non-steroidal anti-inflammatory drugs reduce postoperative opioid analgesic requirements.

Anterior cervical decompression and fixation (Cloward's procedure) is usually required for degenerative disease with osteophyte compression of the cord or for removal of a prolapsed intervertebral disc. Some patients suffer from instability of the cervical spine but the majority have a relatively rigid neck which may cause some difficulty in intubation. The authors use a similar anaesthetic technique for this procedure to that for posterior decompression.

The anterior approach to the thoracic spine is required for decompression and replacement of vertebral bodies. This may require the passage of a double-lumen tube and the use of one-lung anaesthesia. Blood loss may be considerable and elective postoperative ventilation may be beneficial. (For details of one-lung anaesthetic techniques, see Chapter 10.)

A retroperitoneal approach to the anterior aspect of

HEAD INJURIES

The treatment of severe head injury should start as soon as possible after the event. Traumatic brain injury is a primary event and the severity of damage is related to the speed of impact. A relatively minor primary injury may be converted into a severe injury by secondary events which may be avoidable. These secondary events include hypoxaemia, hypercapnia, hypotension and untreated seizure activity.

Resuscitative measures include maintenance of a clear airway by the removal of any debris, the insertion of an oral airway or tracheal intubation. Tracheal intubation with an appropriately sized cuffed tube may help to protect the airway from further soiling. Many head-injured patients hyperventilate spontaneously but may still be hypoxaemic. Oxygen should be administered to achieve adequate haemoglobin saturation. The injured brain may lose its ability to autoregulate so that CBF depends on mean arterial pressure. An adequate perfusion pressure is required and intravenous fluid resuscitation should be achieved. Persistent hypotension does not occur in a patient with an isolated head injury. The source of hidden haemorrhage must be found and treated. Peritoneal lavage may be indicated. Fractured long bones must be splinted. A urinary catheter may be inserted into the bladder and all indicated investigations completed, including cervical spine imaging.

Specific therapy aimed at reducing ICP includes hyperventilation of the lungs, the administration of sedative agents (without reducing arterial pressure) and the use of osmotic diuretics. Mannitol is the most commonly used agent, and reduces ICP in doses of 0.25–0.5 g.kg^{-1} intravenously. The concomitant use of a loop diuretic may have a synergistic effect.

It is important to document the patient's neurological condition before administration of any sedative or neuromuscular blocking agent; the arterial pressure and state of oxygenation should also be recorded. The Glasgow coma scale[75] is a simple scale of responses to auditory and painful stimuli and allows a clear and reproducible picture of the patient's condition to be communicated to other clinicians (Table 21.3). Patients with a very low Glasgow coma scale score may improve neurologically when adequate resuscitation is complete. At this stage, the further management of the patient may be discussed with the neurosurgical unit, and transfer planned.

Table 21.3 Glasgow coma scale

Action	Score
Eye opening	
Spontaneously	4
To verbal command	3
To painful stimulus	2
None	1
Best verbal response	
Oriented	5
Confused	4
Inappropriate words	3
Incomprehensible sounds	2
None	1
Best motor response	
To verbal command	
Obeys commands	6
To painful stimulus	
Localizes	5
Flexion — withdrawal	4
Flexion — abnormal	3
Extension	2
None	1
Maximum total	15

From Teasdale & Jennett,[75] with permission.

During transfer to a neurosurgical unit, it is imperative to avoid the causes of secondary brain injury. It is the responsibility of the referring centre to care adequately for the patient until the patient is accepted by the receiving neurosurgical unit. The experience of the transferring member of the medical staff must be adequate to deal with any changes in the patient's condition during transfer.

If it is considered that the trachea should be intubated before transfer, all precautions to prevent further increases in ICP must be taken (see below). Sedation should be continued during transfer because of the beneficial effects on $CMRO_2$ and ICP.

On arrival at the neurosurgical unit, the patient is examined and transferred to the radiology department for CT scanning. Further management depends on the diagnosis.

Depressed skull fracture

Patients with depressed skull fractures are often conscious unless additional brain injuries are present. Both closed and compound depressed fractures require elevation under general anaesthesia. Anti-staphylococcal therapy, and tetanus toxoid if indicated, should be administered. In patients with evidence of raised ICP, the anaesthetic technique should be chosen appropriately.

Intracranial haematoma

Extradural, acute subdural and intracerebral haematomas that occur as a result of trauma are neurosurgical emergencies. Small haematomas will produce minimal compression in patients who are otherwise well; these may not require immediate evacuation but may be observed closely for a variable period. The morbidity and mortality associated with the removal of an intracerebral haematoma are high and it may be preferable to avoid surgery in the first instance.

The anaesthetic management of this condition is very similar to the management of any other intracranial space-occupying lesion with raised ICP. The patient in whom tracheal intubation and mechanical ventilation have been instituted for transfer to the neurosurgical unit undergoes CT scanning on arrival, and may then be transferred to theatre where a craniotomy and immediate haematoma removal can be carried out under general anaesthesia.

The urgency of the removal of the haematoma dictates the level of monitoring instigated before surgery. The insertion of intra-arterial pressure monitoring should not delay the start of surgery in a rapidly deteriorating patient. Modern non-invasive arterial pressure monitors are adequate in the first instance. A urinary catheter can be inserted when the operation has started, if it has not been inserted before transfer.

Patients who are not already anaesthetized require careful induction of anaesthesia and intubation of the trachea using agents to reduce ICP and maintain CPP. Many patients with head injury are intoxicated with alcohol at the time of injury, and those who are not may still be at risk of regurgitation and aspiration. The use of a rapid-sequence induction of anaesthesia and tracheal intubation with the aid of cricoid pressure is advised. The transient increase in ICP produced by suxamethonium causes a lesser secondary brain injury than does hypoxaemia associated with the aspiration of gastric contents.

It may be advisable to avoid all agents which are liable to increase CBF and ICP, at least until the dura is open. An intravenous infusion of propofol in a patient who is pharmacologically paralysed and whose lungs are moderately hyperventilated with a mixture of air and oxygen is a suitable technique. This may be continued for the duration of the procedure or can be converted to a technique which includes N_2O and a volatile agent after the dura is open.

If the brain is slack and obviously decompressed at the end of the procedure, the patient may be allowed to emerge from anaesthesia. If there is concern about the condition of the brain, it is advisable to insert an ICP monitor, and to sedate the patient and ventilate the lungs in the postoperative period. Blood loss may be heavy, and good venous access is required; blood must be replaced if appropriate.

Chronic subdural haematomas usually occur in the elderly as a result of minimal trauma and may not be diagnosed until many hours or days after the incident. These haematomas are liquid and are removed by washing them out through burr-holes. This can be performed under local anaesthesia with or without sedation, or under general anaesthesia.

Diffuse brain injury

Patients in coma caused by diffuse brain injury may have raised ICP and are best managed in an intensive care unit. The benefits of such a unit are that the patients can be monitored closely and various manipulations carried out in order to optimize the delivery of oxygen to the brain. Patients with severe injuries cannot be monitored using the Glasgow coma scale alone, and more invasive techniques are required.

Monitoring

Patients with severe diffuse head injury require many variables to be monitored and a complex computerized system can be very helpful.[76] The indices monitored are shown in Table 21.4.

The trachea is intubated, the lungs ventilated mechanically, and the patient is sedated and paralysed. The aim is to maintain Pa_{O_2} greater than 15 kPa and Pa_{CO_2} in the range of 4.5–5.0 kPa with a minimum CPP of 60 mmHg. Some patients, especially children, have a high CBF in response to the injury. The high flow rate allows little time for oxygen extraction from the blood, resulting in a high Sjv_{O_2} (normal range 55–75%). These patients can then be subjected to

Table 21.4 Indices monitored in the management of severe diffuse (and other) head injuries

Electrocardiogram
Intra-arterial pressure (including mean)
Intracranial pressure
Derived cerebral perfusion pressure
Arterial oxygen saturation
Continuous jugular venous oxygen saturation
Arterial blood gas tensions
Central venous pressure and pulmonary artery pressures (if indicated)
Urine output
Electroencephalogram

hyperventilation to reduce CBF and to allow better oxygen extraction (with a reduction in Sjv_{O_2}).

Patients with low Sjv_{O_2} are extracting as much oxygen as they can, so that a reduction in CBF only reduces the delivery of oxygen to the cells. Increasing the level of sedation to reduce $CMRO_2$ as monitored using the EEG reduces the oxygen demand, and jugular venous saturation increases. Increasing the sedation may depress arterial pressure and CPP, and may require inotropic support of the cardiovascular system. The drugs used in our unit at present are infusions of propofol, morphine and midazolam for sedation, atracurium for neuromuscular blockade, dobutamine for inotropic support and noradrenaline as a vasoconstrictor. Recent work may indicate a place for etomidate.

There is evidence from animal studies to indicate that competitive NMDA antagonists reduce ischaemic damage in head injury and so provide some degree of cerebral protection.[77] This unit has completed a study with the use of one of these experimental agents in severely head-injured patients. If these drugs prove to be effective they could have many uses in neurosurgery, cardiac surgery, cerebrovascular surgery and possibly many more areas.

The patient is maintained in this condition for as long as is necessary to control ICP and CBF. When stability or improvement has been achieved, neuromuscular blocking agents are withdrawn, Pa_{CO_2} values adjusted to normal and the sedative agent discontinued. Mechanical ventilation is stopped when spontaneous ventilation is adequate, and the patient's trachea is extubated when the tracheal tube is no longer tolerated.

Patients suffering from other causes of raised ICP have also benefited from this form of management. These have included those with meningitis and encephalitis.

It must always be remembered, however, that some injuries are so severe that the brain cannot recover, irrespective of the degree of physiological and pharmacological intervention. Consequently, it is not unusual to have a higher mortality rate in neurosurgical intensive care units than in a general unit.

Brainstem death

Death has traditionally been diagnosed by the irreversible cessation of ventilation and heartbeat, which lead inevitably to anoxia and cessation of function of all other organs. Modern technology has made it possible to support ventilation and cardiac output, despite permanent loss of brainstem function. Brainstem death leads to vital function failure within 2 weeks and usually within a few days.[78,79] Criteria for the diagnosis of brainstem death have been laid down by the Conference of Medical Royal Colleges and Faculties of the UK,[80] but additional criteria are required in some other countries before the diagnosis can be made.

Certain preconditions must be met before the diagnosis can be considered. The patient must be deeply comatose. Coma must not be due to depressant drugs or primary hypothermia. Metabolic and endocrine disturbances which can cause coma must be excluded.

The patient is maintained on a ventilator because of previous inadequacy or cessation of spontaneous ventilation. Sedative or neuromuscular blocking drugs must be excluded as a cause of the requirement for support of ventilation.

There should be no doubt that the patient's condition is due to irremedial structural brain damage and that a diagnosis which can lead to brain death has been established. Common examples of such diagnoses are severe head injury or massive subarachnoid haemorrhage.

If these criteria are fulfilled, then diagnostic tests are carried out to confirm brainstem death. These involve attempts to elicit brainstem reflexes. In the presence of brainstem death, the following signs are present:

1. The pupils are fixed and dilated.
2. There is no corneal reflex.
3. The vestibulo-ocular reflexes (caloric testing) are absent.
4. There is no motor response within the cranial nerve distribution to adequate stimulation of any somatic area.
5. There is no gag reflex or reflex response to bronchial stimulation by a suction catheter passed into the trachea.
6. When the patient is disconnected from the ventilator and the Pa_{CO_2} is 6.65 kPa or greater under conditions of apnoeic oxygenation, there is no spontaneous respiratory effort.

If there are any positive findings, brainstem death cannot be diagnosed.

In the UK, these tests should be carried out by two experienced clinicians, at least one of whom should be a consultant. It is usual to allow a period of 6 h to elapse between the time of onset of coma and the time when brainstem death testing is carried out. It is customary to repeat the tests but there is no fixed time interval between the two sets of tests. Spinal reflexes may persist, or return after being absent, in the presence of brainstem death. In the UK, it is not regarded as necessary to use other confirmatory tests such as

EEG or carotid angiography to diagnose brainstem death. Concise reviews of brain death are available.[81]

When the diagnosis of brainstem death has been made, it is recognized that death has occurred and the time of death is the time of confirmation of the diagnosis. If the relatives of the deceased agree to cadaveric organ donation, support of physiological function is maintained until the organs are retrieved.[82] If donation is declined, the ventilator may be switched off and anoxia will follow, leading to cessation of heart beat.

REFERENCES

1. Barker J. Nitrous oxide in neurosurgical anaesthesia. Br J Anaesth 1987; 59: 146–147
2. Hansen TD, Warner DS, Todd MM, Vust LJ. Effects of nitrous oxide and volatile anaesthetics on cerebral blood flow. Br J Anaesth 1989; 63: 290–295
3. Reasoner DK, Warner DS, Todd MM, McAllister A. Effect of nitrous oxide on cerebral metabolic rate in rats anaesthetized with isoflurane. Br J Anaesth 1990; 65: 210–215
4. Fitch W, Van Hemelrijck J, Mattheusson M, Lawers T, Van Aken H. Effect of nitrous oxide on cerebral blood flow, cerebral metabolism and intracranial pressure during the infusion of propofol. Eur J Anaesthesiol 1990; 7: 339
5. McDowall DG. The effects of clinical concentrations of halothane on the blood flow and oxygen uptake of the cerebral cortex. Br J Anaesth 1967; 39: 186–196
6. Adams RW, Gronert GA, Sundt TM, Michenfelder JD. Halothane, hypocapnia and cerebrospinal fluid pressure in neurosurgery. Anesthesiology 1972; 37: 510–517
7. Michenfelder JD, Theye RA. In vivo toxic effects of halothane on canine cerebral metabolic pathways. Am J Physiol 1975; 229: 1050–1055
8. Stullken EH, Milde JH, Michenfelder JD, Tinker JH. The non-linear responses of cerebral metabolism to low concentrations of halothane, enflurane, isoflurane and thiopental. Anesthesiology 1977; 46: 28–34
9. Drummond JC, Todd MM. The response of feline cerebral circulation to Pa_{CO_2} during anesthesia with isoflurane and halothane and during sedation with nitrous oxide. Anesthesiology 1985; 62: 268–273
10. Miletich DJ, Ivankovich AD, Albrecht RF et al. Absence of autoregulation of cerebral blood flow during halothane and enflurane anesthesia. Anesth Analg 1976; 55: 100–109
11. Artru AA. Effects of enflurane and isoflurane on resistance to reabsorption of cerebrospinal fluid in dogs. Anesthesiology 1984; 61: 529–533
12. Michenfelder JD, Cucchiara RF. Canine cerebral oxygen consumption during enflurane anesthesia and its modification during induced seizures. Anesthesiology 1974; 40: 575–580
13. Moss E, Dearden NM, McDowall DG. Effects of 2% enflurane on intracranial pressure and cerebral perfusion pressure. Br J Anaesth 1983; 55: 1083–1088
14. Eintrei C, Leszniewski W, Carlsson C. Local application of ^{133}xenon for measurement of regional cerebral blood flow during halothane, enflurane and isoflurane anaesthesia in humans. Anesthesiology 1985; 63: 391–394
15. Newman B, Gelb AW, Lam AM. The effect of isoflurane induced hypotension on cerebral blood flow and cerebral metabolic rate for oxygen in humans. Anesthesiology 1986; 64: 307–310
16. Murkin JM, Farrar JK, Tweed WA, Guiraudon G. Cerebral blood flow, oxygen consumption and the electroencephalogram during isoflurane anesthesia. Anesth Analg 1986; 65: S107
17. Newberg LA, Milde JH, Michenfelder JD. The cerebral metabolic effects of isoflurane at and above concentrations that suppress cortical electrical activity. Anesthesiology 1983; 59: 23–28
18. Van Aken H, Fitch W, Brussel T, Graham DI. Responsiveness of the cerebral circulation to alterations in the mean arterial pressure during isoflurane-induced hypotension in baboons. Anesthesiol Rev 1985; 12: 42–43
19. Van Aken H, Fitch W, Graham DI, Brussel T, Themann H. Cardiovascular and cerebrovascular effects of isoflurane-induced hypotension in the baboon. Anesth Analg 1986; 65: 565–574
20. Campkin TV. Isoflurane and cranial extradural pressure. A study of neurosurgical patients. Br J Anaesth 1984; 56: 1083–1087
21. Pierce EC, Lambertsen CJ, Deutsch S et al. Cerebral circulation and metabolism during thiopental anesthesia and hyperventilation in man. J Clin Invest 1962; 41: 1664–1671
22. Donegan JH, Traystman RJ, Koehler RC et al. Cerebral vascular hypoxic and autoregulatory responses during reduced brain metabolism. Am J Physiol 1985; 249: 421–429
23. Kassell NF, Hitchon PW, Gerk MK et al. Influence of changes in arterial P_{CO_2} on cerebral blood flow and metabolism during high dose barbiturate therapy in dogs. J Neurosurg 1981; 54: 615–619
24. Artru AA. Intracranial volume–pressure relationships following thiopental or etomidate. Anesthesiology 1989; 71: 763–768
25. Dearden NM, McDowall DG. Comparison of etomidate and althesin in the reduction of increased intracranial pressure after head injury. Br J Anaesth 1985; 57: 361–368
26. Ledingham IMcA, Watt I. Influence of sedation on mortality in critically ill multiple trauma patients. Lancet 1983; i: 1270
27. Sebel PS, Lowdon JD. Propofol: a new intravenous anesthetic. Anesthesiology 1989; 71: 260–277
28. Ravussin P, Guinard JP, Ralley T, Thorin D. The effect of propofol on cerebrospinal fluid pressure and cerebral perfusion pressure in patients undergoing craniotomy. Anaesthesia 1988; 43 (suppl): 37–41
29. Vandesteene A, Trempont V, Engelman E et al. Effect of propofol on cerebral blood flow and metabolism in man. Anaesthesia 1988; 43 (suppl): 42–43
30. Farling PA, Johnston JR, Coppel DL. Propofol infusion for sedation of patients with head injury in intensive care. A preliminary report. Anaesthesia 1989; 44: 222–226
31. Fitch W, Van Hemelrijck J, Mattheussen M, Van Aken

H. Responsiveness of the cerebral circulation to acute alterations in mean arterial pressure during administration of propofol. J Neurosurg Anesthesiol 1989; 1: 375–376
32. Shearer ES. Convulsions and propofol. Anaesthesia 1990; 45: 255–256
33. Lowson S, Gent JP, Goodchild CS. Anticonvulsant properties of propofol and thiopentone: comparison using two tests in laboratory mice. Br J Anaesth 1990; 64: 59–63
34. Dwyer R, McCaughey W, Lavery J, McCarthy G, Dundee JW. Comparison of propofol and methohexitone as anaesthetic agents for electroconvulsant therapy. Anaesthesia 1988; 43: 459–462
35. Rouse EC. Propofol for electroconvulsant therapy. A comparison with methohexitone. Anaesthesia 1988; 43 (suppl 3): 61–64
36. Dawson B, Michenfelder JD, Theye RA. Effects of ketamine on canine cerebral blood flow and metabolism. Modification by prior administration of thiopental. Anesth Analg 1971; 50: 443–447
37. Gardner AE, Dannemillar FJ, Dean D. Intracranial cerebrospinal fluid pressure in man during ketamine anesthesia. Anesth Analg 1972; 51: 741–745
38. Barker J, Nimmo WS. Althesin, ketamine and lignocaine infusions for neurosurgery. Br J Anaesth 1984; 56: 1309P–1319P
39. Yamamura T, Harada K, Okamura A, Kemmotsu O. Is the site of ketamine anesthesia the N-methyl-D-aspartate receptor? Anesthesiology 1990; 72: 704–710
40. Fleischer JE, Milde JH, Moyer TP, Michenfelder JD. Cerebral effects of high dose midazolam and subsequent reversal with Ro15-1788 in dogs. Anesthesiology 1988; 68: 234–242
41. Giffin JP, Cottrell JE, Shwiry B et al. Intracranial pressure, mean arterial pressure and heart rate following midazolam or thiopental in humans with brain tumors. Anesthesiology 1984; 60: 491–494
42. Knudsen L, Cold GE, Holdgard HO, Johansen UT, Jensen S. Effects of flumazenil on cerebral blood flow and oxygen consumption after midazolam anaesthesia for craniotomy. Br J Anaesth 1991; 67: 277–280
43. Shah N, Long C, Marx W et al. Cerebrovascular response to CO_2 in oedematous brain during either fentanyl or isoflurane anesthesia. J Neurosurg Anesthesiol 1990; 2: 11–15
44. McPherson RW, Traystman RJ. Fentanyl and cerebral vascular responsivity in dogs. Anesthesiology 1984; 60: 180–186
45. Artru AA. Relationship between cerebral blood volume and cerebrospinal fluid pressure during anesthesia with isoflurane or fentanyl in dogs. Anesthesiology 1984; 60: 575–579
46. Artru AA. Effect of halothane and fentanyl on the rate of CSF production in dogs. Anesth Analg 1983; 62: 581–585
47. McPherson RW, Krempasanka E, Eimerl D et al. Effects of alfentanil on cerebral vascular reactivity in dogs. Br J Anaesth 1985; 57: 1232–1238
48. Marx W, Shah N, Long C et al. Sufentanil, alfentanil and fentanyl: impact on cerebrospinal fluid pressure in patients with brain tumors. J Neurosurg Anesthesiol 1989; 1: 3–7
49. Lanier WL, Milde JH, Michenfelder JD. The cerebral effects of pancuronium and atracurium in halothane-anesthetized dogs. Anesthesiology 1985; 63: 589–597
50. Stirt JA, Maggio W, Haworth C et al. Vecuronium: effect on intracranial pressure and hemodynamics in neurosurgical patients. Anesthesiology 1987; 67: 570–572
51. Rosa G, Orfie P, Sanfilippo M et al. The effects of atracurium besylate on intracranial pressure and cerebral perfusion pressure. Anesth Analg 1986; 65: 381–384
52. Minton MD, Grosslight K, Stirt JA, Bedford RF. Increases in intracranial pressure from succinylcholine. Prevention by prior non-depolarizing blockade. Anesthesiology 1986; 65: 165–169
53. Clark WC, Muhlbauer MS, Lowrey R, Hartman M, Ray MW, Watridge CB. Complications of intracranial pressure monitoring in trauma patients. Neurosurgery 1989; 25: 20–24
54. Chambers IR, Mendelow AD, Sinar EJ, Modha P. A clinical evaluation of the Camino subdural screw and ventricular monitoring kits. Neurosurgery 1990; 26: 421–423
55. Maynard DE, Jenkinson JL. The cerebral function analysing monitor. Anaesthesia 1984; 39: 678–690
56. Fleming RA, Smith NT. An inexpensive device for analysing and monitoring the electroencephalogram. Anesthesiology 1979; 50: 456–461
57. Michenfelder JD, Sundt TM, Fode N, Sharbrough FW. Isoflurane when compared to enflurane and halothane decreases the frequency of cerebral ischemia during carotid endarterectomy. Anesthesiology 1987; 67: 336–340
58. Rampil IJ, Holzer JA, Quest DO, Rosenbaum SH, Correll JW. Prognostic value of computerized EEG analysis during carotid endarterectomy. Anesth Analg 1983; 62: 186–192
59. Tempelhoff R, Modica PA, Rich KM, Grub RL. Use of computerized electroencephalographic monitoring during aneurysm surgery. J Neurosurg 1989; 71: 24–31
60. Shearer ES, O'Sullivan EP, Hunter JM. An assessment of the Cerebrotrac 2500 for continuous monitoring of cerebral function in the intensive care unit. Anaesthesia 1991; 46: 750–755
61. McFadzean WA, Mantzaribis H, Kenny GNC. Assessment of anaesthetic depth. Adv Hosp Technol 1992; 2: 22–25
62. Harders AG, Gilsbach JM. Time course of blood velocity changes related to vasospasm in the circle of Willis measured by transcranial doppler ultrasound. J Neurosurg 1987; 66: 718–728
63. Andrews PJD, Dearden MN, Miller JD. Jugular bulb cannulation: description of a cannulation technique and validation of a new continuous monitor. Br J Anaesth 1991; 7: 553–558
64. Hunt WE, Hess RM. Surgical risk related to time of intervention in the repair of intracranial aneurysms. J Neurosurg 1968; 28: 14–20
65. Pickard JD, Murray GD, Illingworth R et al. Effect of oral nimodipine on cerebral infarction and outcome after subarachnoid haemorrhage. British aneurysm nimodipine trial. Br Med J 1989; 298: 636–642
66. Kassel NF, Sasaki T, Colohan ART, Nazar G. Cerebral vasospasm following aneurysmal subarachnoid haemorrhage. Stroke 1985; 16: 562–572
67. Davies KR, Gelb AW, Manninen PH, Boughner DR,

Bisnaire D. Cardiac function in aneurysmal subarachnoid haemorrhage: a study of electrocardiographic and echocardiographic abnormalities. Br J Anaesth 1991; 67: 58–63

68 Farling PA, Unni VKN, Aitken HA et al. Total intravenous anaesthesia for intracranial aneurysm surgery. In: Prys-Roberts C, ed. Focus on infusion: intravenous anaesthesia. London: Current Medical Literature, 1991: pp 164–167

69 Kassel NF, Peerless SJ, Durward QJ, Beck DW, Drake CG, Adams HP. Treatment of ischaemic deficits from vasospasm with intravascular volume expansion and induced arterial hypertension. Neurosurgery 1982; 11: 337–343

70 Soloman RA, Fink ME, Lennihan L. Early aneurysm surgery and prophylactic hypervolaemic hypertensive therapy for the treatment of aneurysmal subarachnoid haemorrhage. Neurosurgery 1988; 23: 699–704

71 Finn SS, Stephensen SA, Miller CA, Drobnich L, Hunt WE. Observations on the perioperative management of aneurysmal subarachnoid hemorrhage. J Neurosurg 1986; 65: 48–62

72 Burke AM, Dervin J. Personal communication, 1992

73 Black S, Cucchiara RF, Nishimura RA, Michenfelder JD. Parameters affecting the occurrence of paradoxical air embolism. Anesthesiology 1989; 71: 235–241

74 Black S, Ockert DB, Oliver WC, Cucchiara RF. Outcome following posterior fossa craniectomy in patients in the sitting and horizontal positions. Anesthesiology 1988; 69: 49–56

75 Teasdale GM, Jennett B. Assessment of coma and impaired consciousness; practical scale. Lancet 1974; ii: 81–84

76 Rafferty C, Hanson S, Bullock R, Teasdale GM, Fitch W, Jamal GA. Intensive care monitoring of severe head injury. Clin Intensive Care 1992; 3 (suppl 2): 107

77 Chen M, Bullock R, Graham DI, Miller JD, McCulloch J. Ischaemic neuronal damage after acute subdural haematoma in the rat: effects of pretreatment with a glutamate antagonist. J Neurosurg 1991; 74: 944–950

78 Jennett B, Gleave J, Wilson P. Brain death in three neurosurgical units. Br Med J 1981; 282: 533–539

79 Pallis C. Prognostic significance of a dead brainstem. Br Med J 1983; 286: 123–124

80 The Conference of Royal Colleges and Faculties of the United Kingdom. Diagnosis of brain death. Br Med J 1976; ii: 1187–1188. Lancet 1976, ii: 1069–1070

81 Fitch W. Brain death. In: Fitch W, Barkewr J, eds. Head injury and the anaesthetist. New York: Elsevier Science. 1985

82 Odom NJ. Organ donation. Br Med J 1990; 300: 1571–1575

22. Anaesthesia for paediatric surgery

S. G. E. Lindahl

The development of successful but complicated surgical treatment in neonates, infants and children would not have been possible without excellent co-operation between paediatric surgeons and paediatric anaesthetists. Because of the development of improved skills in paediatric anaesthesia, surgeons have felt more comfortable to expand into areas in which patients with more complicated diseases and malformations can enjoy a good quality of life or even be surgically cured.

There are also areas in which improved communication has been a key issue in paediatric anaesthesia. The 1980s saw the evolution of improved parental communication which undoubtedly has led to improvements in nursing and medical care. For example, pain symptoms in neonates, infants and children are interpreted better, and therefore possibilities have developed for more appropriate pain treatment.

PHYSIOLOGY

There are three neonatal conditions that are not related to any specific major organ system and which do not correlate with similar physiological conditions in the adult. They are prematurity, transitional circulation and non-shivering thermogenesis. All three share the potential of being life-threatening.

Prematurity

It is not only gestational age that is of importance, but also the weight and size of the baby (Fig. 22.1). The premature child may be classified as preterm with a body size that is small, appropriate or large for gestational age.[1] Generally, survival is better in the near-term, small-for-date baby, than in the severely premature of appropriate weight.

A neonate is considered to be premature if born before the 37th gestational week. Those that are born after the 30th week are classified as moderately premature, whereas those born earlier than the 31st week

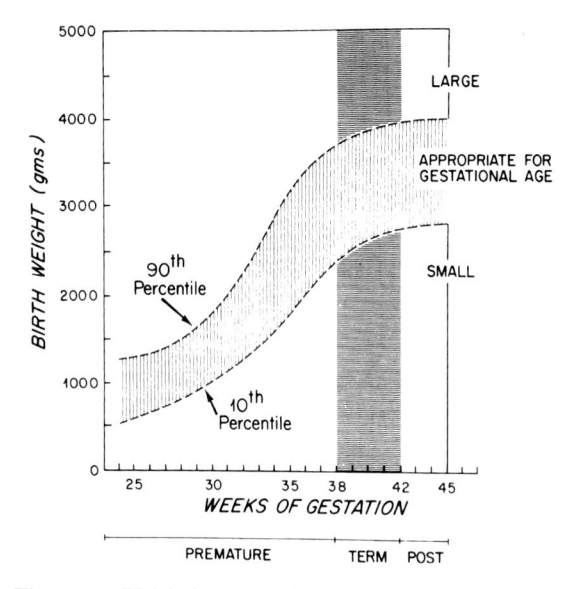

Fig. 22.1 Weight in grams related to gestational age in weeks. Birth weights outside the 90th and 10th percentiles indicate large and small, respectively, for gestational age. From Battaglia,[1] with permission.

are severely premature. This classification is based on outcome and is therefore related to mortality, which is close to 5% between the 30th and the 32nd week and is similar to the overall perinatal mortality at a gestational age of 36 or 37 weeks.[2,3] It is in the group of severely premature babies (<31st week), which constitute about 1% of all live-born infants, that the majority (70%) of all neonatal deaths occur.[3,4] This is due to incomplete organ development, particularly of the respiratory and nervous systems.

Immaturity of the regulation of breathing causes an increased incidence of apnoea after general anaesthesia at term.[5-7] Therefore, premature babies, as well as full-term newborns that are younger than 46 gestational weeks, should be observed in hospital for 24 h after any operation. These patients cannot be operated upon on a day-stay basis, even for minor surgical procedures such as hernia repair or circumcision. In fact, the postoperative risks after general anaesthesia are so high in preterm babies that an increasing number in need of hernia repair, including 'graduates' from neonatal intensive care, have their operations performed under regional anaesthesia alone, in order to avoid the need for postoperative mechanical ventilatory support.

Another problem that is very much related to prematurity and immature organ development is retinopathy of prematurity. In premature babies weighing less than 1000 g it occurs in at least every fifth baby and it results in blindness in as many as 10% of these.[8-11] In premature infants weighing more than 1500 g the incidence is less than 0.5%. Since it is thought that retinopathy of prematurity is caused by the vulnerability of growing retinal arteries, it is important to bear in mind that those arteries are not completely developed until at least a month after birth, even in term neonates. The pathogenic mechanism for retinopathy of prematurity has not been determined yet, although hyperoxia has been related to the incidence. However, hypoxia may also be a trigger, which indicates clearly that more basic knowledge is needed to explain retinopathy of prematurity. Clinically, it is wise to avoid both hyperoxia and hypoxia, particularly in the very premature small-for-date baby.

Transitional circulation

After the termination of placental circulation, the systemic vascular resistance increases. Simultaneously, expansion of the lungs and an increased alveolar oxygen tension contribute to the reduction of pulmonary vascular resistance. During the first 24 h of life, it is not unusual for pulmonary arterial pressure to decrease from 60 to 30 mmHg.[12,13] With concomitant increases in left atrial, left ventricular and aortic pressures, significant right-to-left shunting of blood via the foramen ovale and ductus arteriosus is terminated, although the ductus arteriosus remains anatomically open in a large number of babies up to 8–12 weeks after birth.[12,13] Thus, during these months, there remains the possibility for a relapse into fetal circulation if pulmonary artery pressure increases, aortic pressure decreases, or if both conditions occur simultaneously. Reactivity in the pulmonary vasculature to increased sympathetic activity and to hypercapnia or acidosis is brisk at this age, and may cause resumption of the fetal circulation, initiating a vicious cycle of hypoxia and acidosis.

Non-shivering thermogenesis

Heat loss is exaggerated in newborns, compared with older infants and young children. Many factors contribute, including a relatively large body surface area in relation to weight, and a thin insulating subcutaneous layer of fat. It is also known that the muscle mass is less and heat compensation via shivering thermogenesis is almost negligible. Instead, non-shivering mechanisms are of great importance; in the newborn these occur mainly as thermogenesis from brown adipose tissue (BAT). This tissue is of mesenchymal origin, being formed around the 20th gestational week[14] and is located in special areas[15,16] surrounding major vessels in order to deliver heat efficiently (Fig. 22.2). It has its normal peak effect at about 4 weeks of life but remains a significant factor for thermogenesis for at least 5–6 months.[17] BAT comprises only about 3% of body weight but its metabolic rate can, on a weight basis, exceed the whole body resting metabolic rate by at least 30–40 times. Heat production from BAT therefore contributes significantly to temperature balance in the newborn and young infant.

Normally, neonates increase heat production in a linear fashion at skin temperatures less than 35°C.[18] This makes them dependent on environmental temperature. During general anaesthesia,[19] the normal awake linear response of oxygen consumption (i.e. heat production) at skin temperatures less than 35°C is eliminated (Fig. 22.3). This is most likely explained by the effect of anaesthetics on BAT thermogenesis since

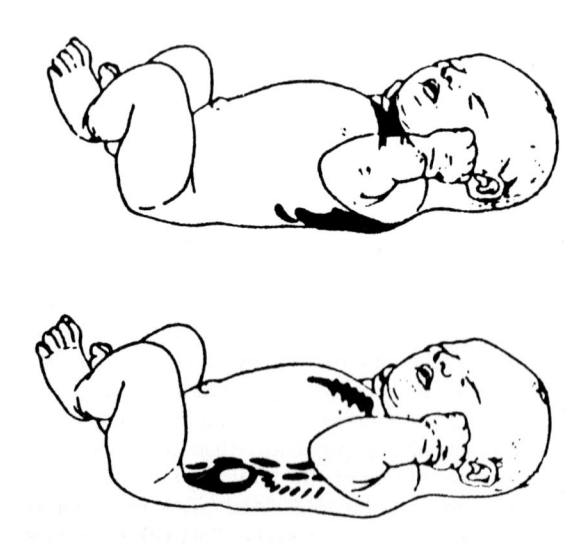

Fig. 22.2 Distribution of brown adipose tissue in the newborn. From Dawkins & Hull,[15] with permission.

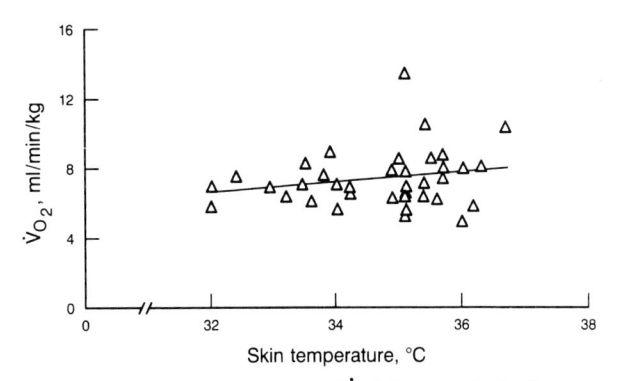

Fig. 22.3 Oxygen consumption ($\dot{V}_{O_2}$) in anaesthetized infants and children related to skin temperature. Note that there is no increase in $\dot{V}_{O_2}$ at skin temperatures lower than 35°C, which is the case when awake.

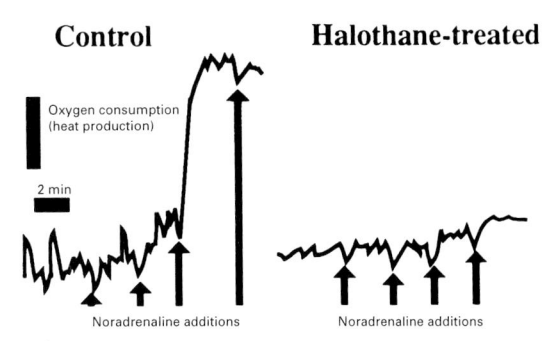

Fig. 22.4 Oxygen consumption (heat production) in brown fat cells. Arrows indicate the addition of increasing concentrations of noradrenaline and maximal consumption is reached in control cells, whereas 3% halothane eliminates this response.

brown fat cells, exposed to volatile anaesthetic agents, demonstrate[20] a dose-dependent inhibition of noradrenaline-stimulated oxygen consumption (Fig. 22.4). It is therefore concluded that the normal delicate temperature balance at lower environmental temperatures is depressed during anaesthesia, due to the effect of volatile anaesthetic agents in depressing the compensatory heat production from BAT. Hence, to avoid hypothermia, environmental temperature must be at the optimal level for each neonate, who should never be left naked on the operating table. Heating lamps should be used prior to surgery, and fluids must be warmed before infusion. In addition, heated gases from an efficient heat and moisture exchangers should be employed to eliminate heat loss from the lungs.

ORGAN FUNCTION AND PAEDIATRIC ANAESTHESIA

Paediatric anaesthetists can seldom influence pre-existing primary diseases in the various organ systems. However, the anaesthetist can have a positive influence on outcome by predicting, preventing or treating secondary malfunctions. Thus, it is of the utmost importance that the anaesthetist has a firm knowledge of applied physiology in order to interpret and treat various conditions that appear during and immediately after surgery.

Central nervous system

Increased intracranial pressure (ICP) is a common secondary malfunction after neurosurgery. The most reliable physiological variable in respect of significant brain ischaemia is cerebral perfusion pressure (CPP), which is the difference between mean arterial pressure (MAP) and ICP. This should be maintained above approximately 50 mmHg. When MAP and ICP are the same, brain death occurs. In neonates and young infants, ICP increases if volume expansions occur in brain tissue, cerebrospinal fluid or cerebral blood. Even in infants with open fontanelles and suture lines, the cranium is relatively rigid and does not allow a rapid expansion without increasing the ICP.

The most important factor which influences ICP is cerebral blood flow (CBF), although blood contributes only about 10% of the total intracranial volume.[21,22] It is necessary to measure CBF in order to assess the influence of various treatment regimens for the control of ICP. Traditionally, the Kety–Schmidt technique has been used.[23] Normal values for CBF, arterial to jugular vein oxygen differences and cerebral metabolic oxygen consumption ($CMRO_2$) have been measured in children aged 3–11 years.[24] The average CBF in that study was approximately 100 ml.min^{-1} per 100 g and the mean $CMRO_2$ was 5.2 ml.min^{-1} per 100 g. Corresponding values in the adult are 50–60 ml.min^{-1} per 100 g for CBF and 3.5–4.5 ml.min^{-1} per 100 g for $CMRO_2$. The recent development of transcranial Doppler techniques will make measurements of relative changes in CBF more readily available for clinical use. Provided that careful evaluation of these new techniques confirms their accuracy, it is likely that they will be recommended for routine use whenever ICP disturbances might occur in order to prepare treatment plans and to initiate early treatment.

Hyperventilation is a rapid and predictable method of reducing CBF in the short term. It is well-documented in the adult that CBF is reduced by 2 ml.min^{-1} per 100 g for each 1 mmHg (0.13 kPa) reduction in $Paco_2$.[25] The effects in neonates and young infants are at least as potent as that in the adult. In the adult, it is also suggested that volatile anaesthetic agents inhibit autoregulation and result in vasodilatation and increased cerebral blood volume. Although this has not been studied as extensively in the paediatric patient, many paediatric anaesthetists avoid the use of volatile anaesthetic agents in patients with reduced intracranial compliance.

CBF can also be diminished by a reduction in cerebral metabolic rate using barbiturate infusions or hypothermia. The rationale of these techniques is that reductions in cerebral metabolic rate should protect the ischaemic brain enclosed in the skull at an increased pressure. To date, clinical benefit has not been clearly demonstrated in controlled studies.[26-28]

Clinical considerations

Before anaesthesia and surgery in patients with intracranial pathology, it is important to evaluate the ICP. Will the intracranial compliance be low, with an increased risk of tentorial or foramen magnum herniation? If so (often suspected because of a variable state of consciousness and the presence of papilloedema), preparations should be made for active treatment of sudden increases in ICP. The therapeutic choices include corticosteroids and an infusion of mannitol which, together with barbiturates and hyperventilation, will contribute to control of sudden increases in ICP in the pre-operative period. If premedication is to be used, potent respiratory depressants such as the opioids should be avoided and the doses of sedatives and anxiolytics should be reduced in relation to those used in patients with no risk of intracranial hypertension. The technique for induction of anaesthesia in neurosurgical patients at risk of increased ICP should avoid carbon dioxide retention and ensure stress-free laryngoscopy and tracheal intubation.

An oxygen–nitrous oxide technique with opioids and muscle relaxation is usually employed for maintenance of anaesthesia because these drugs are not associated with significant changes in CBF or ICP. Ketamine increases CBF and $CMRO_2$ and should be avoided. As indicated above, many paediatric anaesthetists also believe that volatile anaesthetic agents are contraindicated because they are claimed to increase cerebral blood volume.[29] If the use of a volatile agent is required, current documentation favours the use of isoflurane.[30,31]

In addition to standard monitoring with an oesophageal stethoscope, electrocardiography pulse oximetry and capnography, the use of invasive arterial pressure and central venous pressure monitoring is frequently indicated. Insertion of a central venous catheter is indicated particularly if craniotomy is to be performed in the sitting position, when there is a high risk of air embolism. Considering the high rate with which air embolism occurs, it is dubious whether the sitting position should be used at all for paediatric neurosurgery.

Respiratory system

Lung growth and maturation

There is now increasing evidence that growth and maturation of the lungs are two separate phenomena.[32] Thus, lungs can be mature but hypoplastic and vice versa. It has been demonstrated that surfactant activity and alveolar stability increase with glucocorticoid treatment in late gestation.[33] At the same time, however, the number of cells and the lung weight may decrease, making the lung more mature but hypoplastic.[34] A series of complex structural changes occur during late fetal and early postnatal life. There is a rapid decline in the thickness of the interstitium between gestational weeks 20 and 32, whereas the respiratory surface area during the same period shows only small changes. From the 32nd gestational week until term, there is a rapid increase in the respiratory surface area (Fig. 22.5). These structural changes normally accompany each other so that cell multiplication and maturation result in increased lung weight. The lung also has the unique ability to increase in size without increasing in weight. This occurs during the first years of life; the lungs at birth contain about 3 ml of air per gram of lung tissue, but by the age of 6 years, the adult value of 8 ml.g^{-1} has been achieved.[35]

Growth and maturation of the lungs continue as active processes well into the postnatal period. Thus, the lungs of neonates with some of the most complicated congenital malformations, such as congenital diaphragmatic hernia with pulmonary hypoplasia, may continue to develop postnatally, and attain a sufficient number of alveoli to achieve normal gas exchange.

Regulation of breathing

The function of the entire motor system of respiration is altered by the state of consciousness. During rapid eye movement (REM) sleep, tonic postural muscle activity ceases[36] and lung volumes decrease.[37] There is a marked irregularity in the rate of breathing during REM sleep. In contrast, non-REM sleep is characterized by a more regular breathing pattern, with greater tidal volumes and a lower respiratory rate.[38] These matters

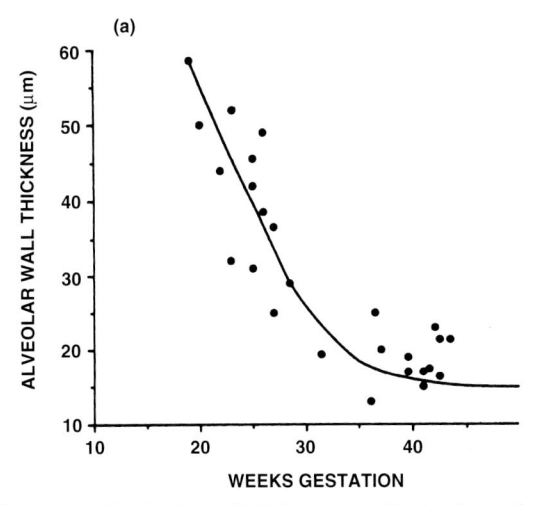

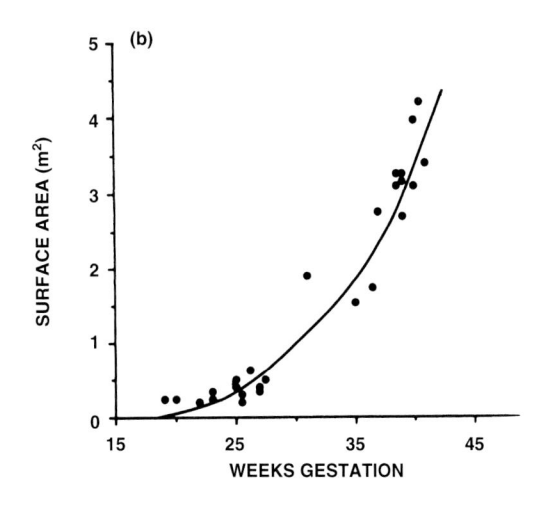

Fig. 22.5 (a) Alveolar wall thickness and (b) alveolar surface area related to gestational age. Data from Brody & Thurlbeck.[32]

deserve special attention in premature infants. More than 50% of neonates born before the 32nd gestational week have significant apnoea, with pauses lasting longer than 20 s, and frequently associated with bradycardia.[39] Peripheral chemoreceptors demonstrate altered sensitivity during the first few days of life, and Hertzberg recently emphasized that stimulation of laryngeal reflexes during hypoxia elicited bradycardia.[40,41] He stressed that simultaneous stimulation of different reflex systems in the newborn results in an exaggerated response that may be life-threatening.

Mechanics of breathing

Ventilation is influenced by mechanical properties of airways, lungs and chest wall. Airway resistance is greater in infants than in adults due to the smaller size of the airways; resistance, by application of Poiseuille's law, is inversely proportional to the fourth power of the radius of the airways. In addition, the Bernouille phenomenon of decreasing lateral forces at increased flow rates means that if a higher airflow occurs, the effective airway diameter becomes narrower, resulting in even higher airway resistance and increased work of breathing.[42] Clinically, it is sometimes valuable to analyse flow–volume curves in patients suffering from diseases which may cause airway obstruction[43] in order to identify whether the obstruction is intra- or extrathoracic (Fig. 22.6).

Compliance of the total pulmonary system is related to the compliance of the chest wall as well as to that of the lungs. The compliance of the chest wall, which to a large extent is determined by the properties of the ribcage, is very high in the newborn and young infant, indicating that the lung compliance is closer to the total compliance than later in life.[44] This predisposes to paradoxical breathing, which also occurs in a dose-dependent manner during halothane anaesthesia and which is uninfluenced by carbon dioxide stimulation.[45] At a light level of halothane anaesthesia, paradoxical breathing disappears and a ventilatory ribcage response occurs (Fig. 22.7). Lung mechanics in neonates and young infants support the routine use of moderate positive end-expiratory pressure during anaesthesia.

Ventilation volumes and respiratory pattern during anaesthesia

During anaesthesia, the respiratory pattern of the neonate, infant and child is regular, and tidal volume is

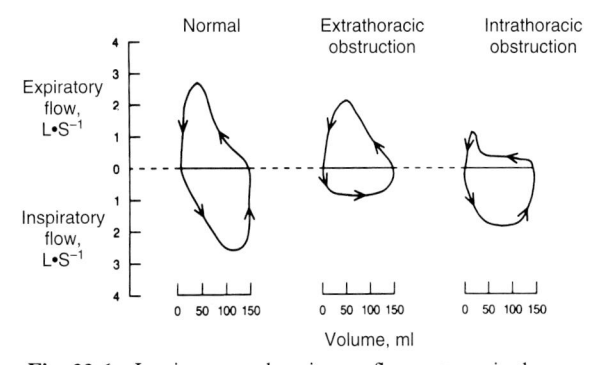

Fig. 22.6 Inspiratory and expiratory flow patterns in the normal subject as well as in patients with extrathoracic or intrathoracic airway obstruction. Note that extrathoracic obstruction restricts inspiratory flow while expiratory flow is depressed with an intrathoracic obstruction.

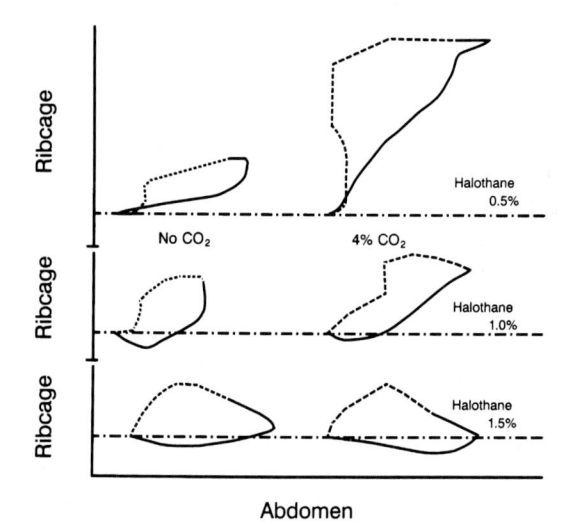

Fig. 22.7 The vertical axis represents movements of the ribcage and the horizontal axis movements of the abdomen. The broken lines depict the resting ventilatory level. The loops to the left show movements during unstimulated breathing and those to the right during 4% carbon dioxide provocations. In the loops, continuous lines illustrate inspiration and broken lines expiration. At end-tidal halothane concentrations of 1.5 and 1.0%, paradoxical breathing is shown. Note the impressive stimulation of ribcage movements during carbon dioxide stimulation at 0.5% halothane.

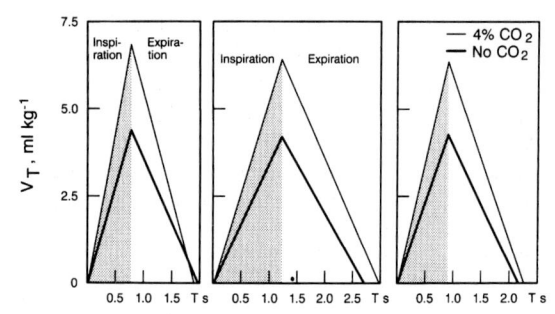

Fig. 22.9 The vertical axis represents tidal volume (V_T) in millilitres per kilogram body weight and the horizontal axis time in seconds. The shaded area illustrates the duration of inspiration. Thin lines show the mean ventilatory response to 4% carbon dioxide stimulation of breathing in infants and children during inhalation of halothane (left panel), enflurane (middle panel) or isoflurane (right panel) at equi-anaesthetic concentrations (1 minimum alveolar concentration, or MAC). There was no shortening of the duration of expiration during carbon dioxide breathing, which is normally seen in the awake state.

related almost linearly to body weight (Fig. 22.8) provided that the depth of anaesthesia is stable.[46] The ventilatory motor response to carbon dioxide stimulation is maintained, although depressed in a dose-dependent manner, irrespective of age and volatile anaesthetic agent used.[36,47,48] However, the normal awake respiratory rate response to carbon dioxide, with shortening of the duration of expiration, is eliminated (Fig. 22.9) during anaesthesia with halothane, enflurane or isoflurane.[47,48]

Because of the low functional residual capacity (FRC) and high oxygen consumption in infants,[49,50] the oxygen reserve is consumed more rapidly than in children. Thus, hypoxaemia occurs more rapidly during apnoea in the youngest patients.

Circulation

The right ventricle is the systemic ventricle in fetal life. Immediately after birth, the left ventricle is required to take over the systemic circulation, although it is relatively weak. However, its strength improves markedly during the first month of life.

Although adjustments of neonatal cardiac output are accomplished predominantly by changes in heart rate, the basal rate is already high and close to that at which inefficiency occurs.[51] One of the reasons for the more rate-dependent cardiac output in the neonate is the presence of a higher proportion of connective tissue, and less contractile elements.[52] The neonate's heart is not as compliant as later in life. Consequently, the maximal increase in stroke volume is achieved at an end-diastolic pressure of 5–10 mmHg in the newborn, whereas filling pressures up to 20 mmHg generally continue to increase stroke volume in children and adults.[53,54]

In response to hypoxaemia, the neonate is capable of redistributing cardiac output to organs that are important to survival.[55] It has been suggested that the

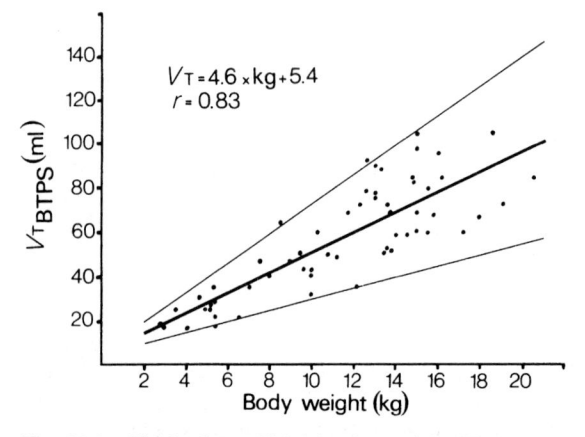

Fig. 22.8 Tidal volume (V_T) related to weight. The regression line (bold line) is given as well as the regression equation. The two thin lines illustrate ± 2 s.d.

neonate is able to redistribute central circulation at low cardiac output, irrespective of its cause. However, newborn babies have an immature baroreflex response, which is depressed still further by volatile anaesthetic agents.[56,57] This means that compensatory mechanisms for hypotension are less efficient in infants than in children and adults, particularly during anaesthesia. Thus, vasopressors should be administered to minimize the negative effects of low cardiac output. Fetal haemoglobin contains lower concentrations of 2,3-diphosphoglycerate (DPG), resulting in an increased affinity for oxygen and a shift of the dissociation curve to the left. This compromises oxygen supply to the tissues and contributes to the narrow margins of safety for oxygen delivery in the neonate.

Congenital cardiac malformations

Neonates with congenital cardiac malformations create special problems that sometimes have to be dealt with on an emergency basis. Neonates with preductal co-arctation of the aorta, pulmonary atresia with an intact ventricular septum and those who have an extremely tight pulmonary stenosis are frequently in a reasonable clinical condition until the ductus arteriosus starts to close. Previously, these patients died at this stage or were brought to the operating theatre in an extremely poor condition. However, anaesthesia and surgery can now be conducted with the neonate in a much better condition because an infusion of prostaglandin (prostaglandin E_1 or E_2, initial dose 0.05–0.1 $\mu g.kg^{-1}.min^{-1}$) is capable of keeping the ductus arteriosus open.

Usually, infants and children with congenital cardiac malformations can be categorized into two groups, cyanotic and acyanotic, based on arterial oxygenation. During a balanced anaesthetic with controlled ventilation, there is no difference in oxygen consumption between cyanotic and acyanotic infants.[58] The same is also true for carbon dioxide elimination[58] and energy expenditure (Fig. 22.10). However, when breathing spontaneously during halothane anaesthesia, tidal volume and respiratory effort, reflected by airway occlusion pressures, are greater in cyanotic than in acyanotic infants.[58] This is caused by a greater dead-space ventilation in cyanotic patients, also reflected by a greater arterial to end-tidal carbon dioxide difference.[59–61]

When infants and children with a congenital heart malformation present for elective non-cardiac surgery, it is always wise to establish whether the non-cardiac surgical procedure could be postponed until cardiac failure is controlled. Particular caution should be exercised in patients with tight aortic stenosis or tight pulmonary stenosis. The anaesthetic risk in patients with clinically insignificant patent ductus arteriosus, or atrial or ventricular septal defects, is not increased during minor or intermediate non-cardiac surgical procedures. However, injection of intravenous air bubbles must be avoided, and antibiotic prophylaxis is essential.

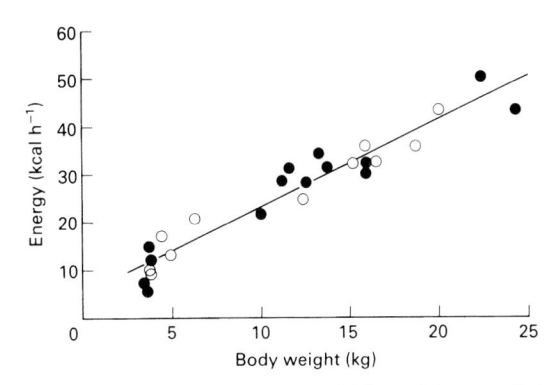

Fig. 22.10 Energy expenditure in children with congenital heart malformations during balanced anaesthesia, related to weight. Open circles represent children with acyanotic and closed circles with cyanotic congenital heart malformations.

FLUID BALANCE AND ENERGY EXPENDITURE

Physiology

Because of physiological differences in the neonate and young infant, fluid management must be undertaken with precision.

Body fluid volumes

In relation to weight, the body content of fluids is greater in younger than in older children. In the premature baby, 80% of body weight is water. Approximately two-thirds of the total volume of water is extracellular fluid (ECF). By 6 months of age, the volume of ECF has diminished in relative terms, and represents only one-third of total body water.[62] Already at this age, the volume of ECF is lower than that of intracellular fluid (ICF), and the distribution of fluid is more similar to that of the adult (Fig. 22.11).

Consequences

The relatively large volume of ECF in infants younger than 6 months of age means that fluid losses and hypovolaemia may develop rapidly, resulting in low blood pressure and inadequate peripheral circulation. Consequently, neonates and young infants must not be

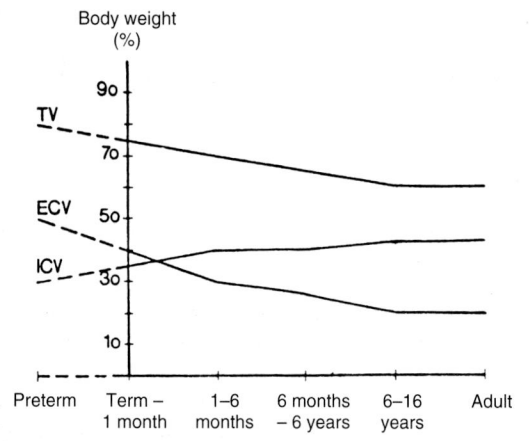

Fig. 22.11 Total body fluid volume (TV), and extracellular (ECV) and intracellular volume (ICV) at different ages and given as a percentage of body weight. Modified from Friis-Hansen,[62] with permission.

anaesthetized until sufficiently rehydrated. During major surgery, fluid loss must be replaced early. Severe hypotension during the first 2 months of life is of particular interest because a patent ductus arteriosus may exist; the combination predisposes to the recurrence of fetal circulation, resulting in reduced lung perfusion, hypoxaemia and acidosis.

The large ECF volume also means that drugs that are mainly distributed in the ECF should be administered in higher doses per kilogram body weight than later during childhood. For example, for complete correction of metabolic acidosis with bicarbonate, the dose (mmol) in an adult is based on the formula: $0.3 \times$ body weight (kg) $\times$ base deficit (mmol.l^{-1}). The coefficient (0.3) should be replaced by the value of 0.5 in the premature baby and 0.4 at term and during the first 6 months of life.

Renal function

All healthy neonates should produce urine during the first 36–48 h of life. A volume of 25–30 ml of urine per 24 h is not unusual during the first few days, but should be 100–200 ml at 1 week of life. In the intensive care unit, infants older than 1 week of age should have an average urinary output of approximately 1 ml.kg^{-1}.h^{-1}.

Renal vascular resistance is high immediately after birth, but decreases rapidly, and is low after 2 weeks of life. The glomerular filtration rate is low in the neonate and increases steadily during childhood[63] (Table 22.1). The loop of Henle is short, and this interferes with the ability of the kidneys to retain sodium via the ascending loop of Henle.[64] Even at a low glomerular filtration rate, a net loss of sodium may occur easily.

Table 22.1 Glomerular filtration rates and age

Age	ml.min^{-1} per 1.73 m^2 body surface area
1–2 days	20–25
1 week	35–40
3 months	55–60
Adult	120

The enzyme carbonic anhydrase is present at birth in the proximal tubules, but is sparse in the distal tubules. Together with lower concentrations of buffering ions, this reduces the capacity of the kidneys to eliminate acids.[65]

Consequences

Because of the reduced length of the loop of Henle, the capacity for sodium preservation is less than in the adult. Sodium-free solutions should not routinely be used in neonates and infants. The diminished activity of carbonic anhydrase in the distal tubules predisposes to acidosis because of a reduced capacity to re-absorb bicarbonate ions.

Energy expenditure, fluid and electrolyte needs

In neonates and infants, perspiration via the skin is an important source of fluid and energy losses because the ratio of body surface area to weight is up to three times greater than in the adult. In a healthy neonate in a temperate climate, fluid loss via perspiration is 1 ml.kg^{-1}.h^{-1} and in a premature baby values of 2–3 ml.kg^{-1}.h^{-1} are not uncommon.

Because of the high energy expenditure and fluid turnover in neonates and infants, periods of fasting and fluid restriction before anaesthesia should be kept as short as possible. Acceptable pre-operative fasting periods are shown in Table 22.2.

Energy needs determine fluid requirements; 1.6 ml fluid is evaporated and vaporized per kilocalorie.[66,67] During anaesthesia, energy balance is similar to that in a basal metabolic state[67,68] and is calculated according to the formula:[67]

Table 22.2 Periods for fasting and fluid restrictions

Age	Milk and solid food hours	Clear fluids hours
Neonates	4	2
1–6 months	4	2
6 months and older	6	4

Energy expenditure (kcal.h^{-1}) = 1.5 × body weight (kg) + 5.0

Basal fluid requirements during anaesthesia may be calculated from the formula:

Fluid volume (ml.h^{-1}) = 2.5 × body weight (kg) + 10.0

During surgery, it is necessary to administer additional volumes of fluid to take account of extra losses by evaporation and for accumulation of 'third-space' fluid. A volume of 2 ml.kg^{-1}.h^{-1} should be added in children undergoing a minor surgical procedure, 4 ml.kg^{-1}.h^{-1} for laparotomy or thoracotomy and 6 ml.kg.$^{-1}$.h^{-1} for major surgical procedures such as abdominoperineal or thoraco-abdominal operations.

Choice of fluids

Care must be exercised in the choice of fluids in all premature babies, and in infants and children scheduled for cardiac procedures during deep hypothermia and cardiac arrest. In these cases, it is mandatory to measure blood glucose frequently and it is recommended that solutions containing glucose should be avoided, because the incidence of intraventricular haemorrhage is higher in premature babies in the presence of hyperglycaemia, and because neurological sequelae are believed to occur at a higher rate after cardiac arrest during deep hypothermia if pre-bypass hyperglycaemia existed.[2,69]

In all other patients, the use of solutions containing 2.5–5% glucose is recommended as there is no scientific evidence that moderately high blood glucose concentrations for short periods have any negative metabolic effects, whereas it is beyond any doubt that profound hypoglycaemia results in severe neurological damage. As a response to major surgical procedures, trauma and shock, hyperglycaemia is, in the acute phase, most probably a purposeful physiological response. Hyperglycaemia is a rapid means of increasing plasma osmolality in order to mobilize fluids so that the circulatory volume is maintained at an adequate level.

Electrolyte needs

Based on energy expenditure and evidence that 3 mmol of sodium and 2 mmol of potassium are required per 100 kcal,[70,71] the hourly electrolyte requirements during anaesthesia and surgery can be estimated from the following formulae:

sodium (mmol.h^{-1}) = (4.5 × body weight (kg) + 10) × 10^{-2}

potassium (mmol.h^{-1}) = (3.0 × body weight (kg) + 10) × 10^{-2}

Rehydration

The degree of dehydration is sometimes difficult to estimate. However, it is important to evaluate dehydration carefully so that the volume of fluid required for adequate rehydration can be calculated. A simple schematic scale for estimation of dehydration is given in Table 22.3.

Rehydration with intravenous fluids should be employed if the degree of dehydration is estimated to amount to more than 5% of calculated total body water. Rehydration volumes (RV) are calculated according to the formula:

RV (ml) = 10 × weight (kg) × % dehydration

Basal fluid requirements during the period of infusion must be added to the calculated rehydration volume. It is common practice to administer half of the rehydration volume during the first hour and the second half during the next 3 h, although longer infusion periods are required if dehydration is severe.

Burn injuries

The surface area that is burned has to be estimated correctly in order to calculate replacement volumes of fluids. Adult standards for relative surface areas from head and lower extremities are not valid in children. Figure 22.12 presents a simple, easily memorized modification of adult standards for use in infants and children.

The extra fluid volume required in paediatric burn injuries may be calculated according to the guidelines shown in Table 22.4. This schedule for fluid replacement may be practical to use, but it is necessary to exercise care in administration of blood or fluids which

Table 22.3 Estimates of dehydration in children

Degree of dehydration (% of body weight)	Symptoms
5	Dry skin and mouth
10	Sunken fontanelle, tachycardia, oliguria
15	Sunken eyeballs, hypotension, decreased peripheral circulation

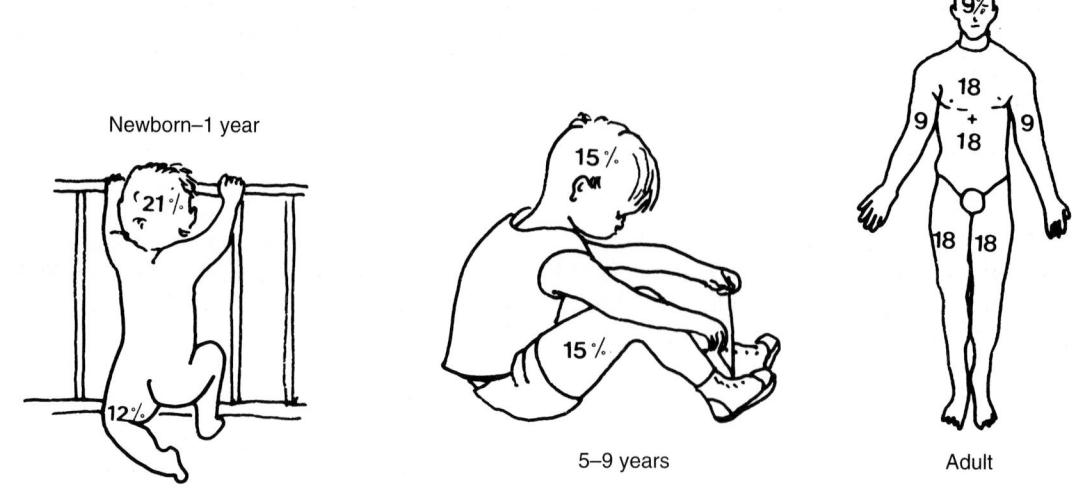

Fig. 22.12 Changes in head and lower-limb contribution to body surface with regard to age.

contain potassium during the first days after a burn injury. The use of solutions which contain glucose may result in hyperglycaemia which, if moderate, and in the absence of ketosis and metabolic acidosis, is acceptable.

BLOOD REPLACEMENT

The blood volume (BV) ranges from 90 ml.kg^{-1} in a premature baby to 65 ml.kg^{-1} in a teenager. Frequently, a value of 80 ml.kg^{-1} is used to estimate blood volume in preschool children (see Table 22.5). The acceptable blood loss during surgery is based on the haematocrit (Hct). Hct reductions of 15% are usually acceptable. If a Hct of 33% is regarded as acceptable in a patient, the following calculations can be employed.

The initial volume of red blood cells (RBC) is:

$$RBC = \frac{BV \times \text{initial Hct}}{100}$$

At a Hct of 33, the volume of red blood cells is:

$$RBC_{33} = \frac{BV \times 33}{100}$$

The acceptable loss of red blood cells (ALRBC) is:

$$ALRBC = RBC - RBC_{33}$$

and the acceptable blood loss volume (ABLV) is

$$ABLV \text{ (ml)} = ALRBC \times 3$$

The factor 3 varies with the acceptable level of Hct. For example, if the acceptable Hct is 50% (as it might be in a neonate), the factor is 2 (100 divided by 50); the factor would be 2.5 if the acceptable Hct was 40%.

A simple schedule for blood replacement regimens is shown in Table 22.6.

Table 22.4 Additional fluid requirements for infants and children with burn injuries related to percentage burned body surface area

	< 5 years	> 5 years	Fluids
First 24 h	4 ml.kg^{-1} per % burn	2–3 ml.kg^{-1} per % burn	Glucose 25 mg.ml^{-1} with sodium
Second 24 h	2–3 ml.kg^{-1} per % burn	1–2 ml.kg^{-1} per % burn	Glucose 25 mg.ml^{-1} with sodium, plasma or albumin
48 h	2 ml.kg^{-1} per % burn	1 ml.kg^{-1} per % burn	Glucose 50 or 100 mg.ml^{-1} with sodium, plasma or albumin and blood if needed

Table 22.5 Some normal values in infancy and childhood

Age	0–1 week	3 months	6–12 months	Preschool
Haemoglobin (g.dl^{-1})	17.0–22.0	10.5–12.0	11.0–12.0	11.5–12.5
Haematocrit (%)	55–70	35–40	34–41	37–41
Blood volume (ml.kg^{-1})	80 (preterm 90)	80	75	70

PRE-OPERATIVE ASSESSMENT

Normal children

In the normal child, minor surgical procedures such as circumcision, repair of inguinal hernia and adenoidectomy can all be performed on a day-stay basis and without laboratory tests and urine analysis, provided that the physical examination and previous medical and family histories are normal.

The child with a runny nose could be suffering from an allergic disease; if no exacerbation of the allergy is present, it is appropriate to undertake routine surgical procedures after instituting symptomatic treatment. If the runny nose is caused by an infection, anaesthesia and surgery should be postponed because airway problems during induction of anaesthesia occur more frequently and tracheal intubation may infect the lower respiratory tract. A period of 1 month should elapse after the last symptoms of an upper respiratory tract infection, croup or one of the acute exanthematous diseases have subsided.

In intermediate and major paediatric surgical cases, laboratory tests (haemoglobin concentration, serum urea and electrolyte concentrations and urinalysis) are frequently indicated. In addition, it is necessary to consider the need for cross-matching blood for transfusion.

A scheme for pre-operative evaluation and preparation of normal children subjected to elective minor, intermediate and major surgical procedures is shown in Table 22.7. Age-dependent variation of normal values of haemoglobin, Hct and BV must be taken into account (Table 22.5).

Table 22.6 Example of blood replacement routines

Blood loss as a % of blood volume	Replacement fluid
<5%	Crystalloid, 3–4 ml/ml blood loss
5–10%	Crystalloid, 3–4 ml/ml blood loss or colloids 1 ml/ml blood loss
>10–15%	Red blood cells + colloids 1 ml/ml blood loss

Complicated children

In the complicated child, potential anaesthetic problems are frequently prevented by proficient pre-operative examination and preparation.

Anaemia and sickle-cell disease

A haemoglobin (Hb) concentration below 10 g.dl^{-1} is abnormal and may require investigation. Surgery should not be delayed if Hb is marginally below this value, but this may be an indication for earlier intra-operative blood transfusion.

A sickle-cell screening test should be performed on all patients of African origin after the age of 3 months. If this is positive, quantitative electrophoresis should follow to determine precisely the haemoglobinopathy present. Patients with sickle-cell disease (HbSS) for planned surgery may be given two transfusions with fresh blood, the first 3 weeks and the second 3 days pre-operatively, to raise the Hb to not more than 12 g.dl^{-1}. Repeat electrophoresis should show a pattern more like that of the heterozygous form (HbSA), which carries a very low risk with general anaesthesia.

Craniofacial malformations and upper airway obstruction

These malformations are often associated with congenital malformations in other organ systems. The most common deformities are uni- or bilateral cleft lip and palate, but conditions such as the Pierre Robin syndrome (with micrognathia, macroglossia and a cleft palate), and the Treacher Collins syndrome (with micrognathia, microstomia, aplastic zygomatic arches, choanal atresia, as well as congenital lymph- and haemangiomata in the neck and face) are also relatively common. In such patients, pre-operative information concerning the breathing pattern and the child's ability to maintain a clear airway is vitally important. In the neonatal period, awake intubation of the trachea may be appropriate in the most difficult cases. Otherwise, intubation is generally performed under inhalation anaesthesia, with spontaneous breathing being maintained. If difficult intubation is anticipated in older children, preparations should be made for fibre-optic intubation.

Table 22.7 Pre-operative preparation routines in children scheduled for elective surgical procedures

	Physical examination, family & medical histories	Haemoglobin	BG CM	Electrolytes	Urea	Liver function	Coagulation system	Blood gases
Minor procedures	+	–	–	–	–	–	–	–
Intermediate or major procedures	+	+	+	(+)	(+)	(–)	(–)	(–)

BG = Blood grouping; CM = cross-matching.
(+) = Cases where disturbances might be anticipated or where postoperative total parenteral nutrition will be needed.
(–) = Only in special cases.

Acquired conditions such as haematoma in the mouth or throat, bleeding tonsillar bed, peritonsillar abscess, acute epiglottitis and foreign body are all emergency cases, and the time for pre-anaesthetic evaluation is often limited. In these situations, as well as for some craniofacial malformations, it is wise to co-operate with an experienced ear, nose and throat specialist during induction of anaesthesia and intubation of the trachea, and to have easy access to equipment for a possible emergency tracheostomy.

Pulmonary disorders

Pulmonary complications are more frequent in patients with asthma or cystic fibrosis. It is important that such patients are anaesthetized and operated upon under optimal conditions. The treatment of the asthmatic patient or the child with cystic fibrosis should be intensified for at least 2 weeks before anaesthesia. For the asthmatic child, repeated lung function tests should be used to assess the effect of inhalation therapy, selective β_2-agonists and perhaps also corticosteroids. For the child with cystic fibrosis, postural drainage treatment and physiotherapy need to be intensified.

Cerebral palsy

For the paediatric anaesthetist, the most common problems related to cerebral palsy are associated with patients who suffer from the most complicated cerebral palsy syndromes. One of the principal features of these children is increased salivation. They may also suffer from cerebral convulsions requiring treatment with one or more anticonvulsant drugs. The anticonvulsant treatment should not be terminated before anaesthesia; the normal doses should be administered on the morning of the operation with a sip of water.

Rheumatoid arthritis

The child with rheumatoid disease may have suffered from the illness for many years, although still young. Joints are progressively destroyed and may require surgery, which is usually performed under general anaesthesia in childhood. In some cases, laryngeal involvement and restricted movements of the mandible create difficulties with tracheal intubation. All rheumatoid children should be investigated with an X-ray of the cervical spine to show possible pathological movements of the atlanto-occipital and atlanto-axial joints. There may also be myocardial involvement, and an electrocardiogram should also be available pre-operatively.

Endocrine disease

The most common endocrine disorder is diabetes mellitus, which is nearly always insulin-dependent in childhood. The well-controlled diabetic patient does not need to be admitted to the hospital until the day before surgery. Measurement of acid–base balance, blood glucose concentration and urinalysis (for ketone bodies and glucose) should be performed.

Patients undergoing minor surgery may be managed by omitting the morning dose of insulin, together with breakfast on the day of surgery. For more complex surgery, an infusion of insulin is more satisfactory; soluble insulin 0.1 unit.kg^{-1}.h^{-1} is infused with hourly fluid requirements given as glucose 5% (+ 10 mmol K$^+$ in 500 ml). Frequent blood sugar and potassium estimations are mandatory. Neuropathy may be present even in young diabetics, and cardiomyopathy may also exist.

Reduced adrenocortical function may be caused by adrenal haemorrhage, hypoplasia, adrenocorticotrophic hormone (ACTH) insufficiency, congenital unresponsiveness to ACTH, fulminating infection, Addison's disease or iatrogenic adrenal insufficiency. One of the most common forms of adrenocortical hypofunction is 21-hydroxylase deficiency, which gives rise to the adrenogenital syndrome. These patients are treated with subcutaneous implantation of desoxycortisone acetate (DOCA) pellets. When DOCA pellets are not used, or when the child is unable to take medication orally, DOCA should be administered intramuscularly. It is of the utmost importance that plasma electrolyte concentrations are measured pre-operatively in patients with adrenocortical hypofunction. Hydrocortisone 25 mg should be given on the evening before operation, 25 mg on the morning of surgery and 25 mg before induction of anaesthesia.

Approximately 90% of children suffering from phaeochromocytoma are hypertensive. Multiple tumours occur more frequently (30%) than in adults (5%).[72] These children often have a decreased circulating BV. Pre-operative treatment with an adrenergic blocking agent should be undertaken for 2 weeks. The most frequently used drug is phenoxybenzamine; the usual starting dose is 5–10 mg, and the dose is then gradually increased over 2–3 days until orthostatic hypotension occurs. If tachycardia occurs in response to this treatment, it may be necessary to add a β-blocker such as propranolol or atenolol.

Liver disease and coagulopathies

Liver disease may, in advanced cases, decrease glycogen storage and predispose to hypoglycaemia. Furthermore, plasma concentrations of albumin and coagulation factors may be low. Liver enzymes, bilirubin (conjugated and unconjugated) and serum protein concentrations should be measured, and clotting studies performed pre-operatively.

A coagulopathy frequently occurs in the neonatal period. This is due in part to vitamin K deficiency in the neonatal liver, and consequently is treated by injections of vitamin K_1. Coagulation disorders may also be inherited, with specific deficiencies in the production of coagulation factors. Pre-operatively, a complete laboratory coagulation profile should be undertaken, and evidence of fibrinolysis, as well as thrombocytopenia, sought. Pre-operatively, specific clotting factors (e.g. factor VIII), fresh frozen plasma (which contains coagulation factors) or fresh blood should be available. If there is evidence of fibrinolysis, inhibitors such as ∈-aminocaproic acid should be given. Platelets should be available for thrombocytopenic patients, and may be given pre-operatively or kept in reserve for intra-operative bleeding.

PRE-OPERATIVE PSYCHOLOGICAL PREPARATION AND PREMEDICATION

There are now many sophisticated methods of informing children and parents about anaesthesia, surgery and postoperative recovery. It is my personal experience that photograph albums containing realistic pictures from the operating theatre are superior to videos; they are easier to update so that they always give a true reflection of the personnel and atmosphere in the operating department. The nursing personnel must spend time with children and parents to explain what the pictures illustrate, and this guarantees an allotted time for questions from children and parents. The information must be adapted for the child's age, and this is easily achieved with an album of photographs.

Children scheduled to undergo surgery on an inpatient basis should always be visited by an anaesthetist on the day before surgery. Detailed information related to anaesthesia is provided, and personal contact is achieved.

The need for pre-operative anxiolytic treatment varies from individual to individual. With an efficient and complete pre-operative information and preparation programme, only a light anxiolytic is needed. In many cases, premedication may be regarded as unnecessary. In many countries, midazolam is regarded as the best choice for premedication and can be administered nasally, orally or rectally.[73-75] A rectal dose of 0.3 mg.kg^{-1} (maximum 7.5 mg) given 15 min before induction of anaesthesia (frequently combined with atropine 0.02 mg.kg^{-1} to a maximum dose of 0.5 mg) is practical and satisfactory premedication.

Intramuscular injections for premedication hurt, and should be avoided in infants and children.

Heavy premedication (sometimes used as a routine technique for induction of anaesthesia) can be achieved using rectal methohexitone (25 mg.kg^{-1}, maximum dose 600 mg) or thiopentone (30 mg.kg^{-1}, maximum dose 700 mg). The rectal absorption of these drugs is unpredictable and the dose is sometimes not enough for the induction of sleep; however, a proportion of patients have a prolonged postoperative sleep. In spite of these disadvantages, this technique has a long tradition at some major centres for paediatric anaesthesia, and in these centres appears to work satisfactorily.

In recent years, the introduction of EMLA (eutectic mixture of local anaesthetics) cream for topical anaesthesia has changed the attitude among paediatric anaesthetists with respect to intravenous induction of anaesthesia. Application of EMLA cream over the two best veins at least 60 min before planned venepuncture has been adopted as a routine part of pre-operative preparation and medication in many centres. Pain-free venous access can be achieved in nearly all children.[76] This has permitted the advantages of intravenous induction of anaesthesia, with its safe and predictable effects, to be made available routinely to paediatric patients. This in turn means that salivation, breath-holding, coughing and the stage of excitement associated with the second stage of anaesthesia are eliminated, and heavy premedication with sedative and anticholinergic drugs is no longer necessary. Despite the benefits of sevoflurane for inhalation induction, it is likely that induction of anaesthesia by face mask will continue to become less frequent, and that pre-anaesthesia preparation will be focused more on anxiolysis. However, if inhalation induction is planned, the anaesthetist should remember that careful and adequate pre-anaesthetic medication reduces airway problems and the incidence of cardiac arrhythmias.[77,78]

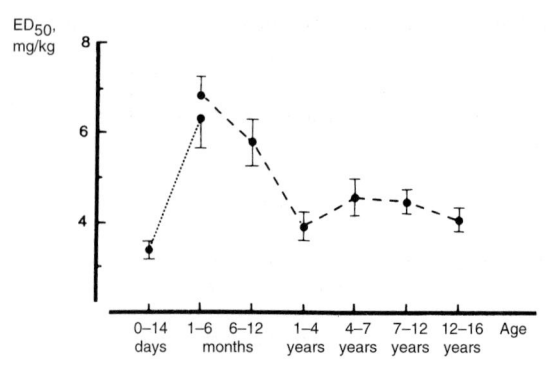

Fig. 22.13 Median effective dose (ED$_{50}$) of thiopentone for induction of anaesthesia in infants and children. Note that requirements reach a peak between 1 and 6 months of age and that they are lowest in the neonate. Dotted line: from Jonmarker et al;[79] broken line: from Westrin et al;[80] with permission.

AGE-RELATED PHARMACOLOGICAL ASPECTS

Newborn babies have a reduced glomerular filtration rate (Table 22.1) and the capacity of the liver to metabolize drugs is diminished in comparison with later in life. In addition, plasma proteins such as albumin and α_1-acid glycoprotein bind less drug in neonates, leaving a higher proportion of drug in the unbound active form. When these specific conditions are taken together, it is obvious that the half-life of drugs is prolonged in neonates. Since more of the drug is in its active and unbound state, toxicity concentrations extrapolated from pharmacokinetic data in the adult are invalid. However, the larger proportion of body water in neonates (Fig. 22.11) dilutes the drugs, resulting in a lower plasma concentration. But renal function and liver enzyme capacity are higher after the age of 6 months, when body fluid volumes also are approaching adult values (Fig. 22.11).

Clinically, the effects of anaesthetic agents are age-related. Intravenous (Fig. 22.13) and inhalation anaesthetic agents (Fig. 22.14) have, in the premature and term neonate, equipotent effects at lower dosages than in the infant who is 6 months old.[79–86] Interestingly, at 6–12 months of age, drug requirements are higher than later in life.

SPONTANEOUS BREATHING DURING PAEDIATRIC ANAESTHESIA

To estimate minute ventilation ($\dot{V}_E$) in spontaneously breathing children during halothane anaesthesia, the following formula can be used[46] (Fig. 22.8):

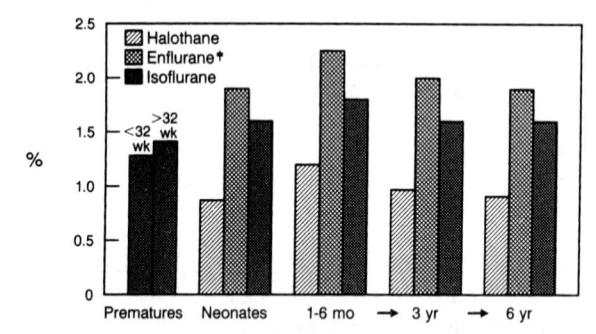

Fig. 22.14 Age-related minimum alveolar concentration values (vertical axis) for halothane, enflurane or isoflurane. ‡ Values for enflurane are estimated from measurements made in the adult by Gion & Saidman.[82] Values for isoflurane are from Cameron et al[85] and Le Dez & Lerman.[86] Values for halothane are from Gregory et al[81] and Lerman et al.[84]

$$\dot{V}_E \text{ (ml.min}^{-1}\text{)} = 5 \times \text{body weight (kg)} \times \text{respiratory rate}$$

There are many different aspects of spontaneous breathing which warrant discussion. Spontaneous breathing is the most physiological way to achieve gas exchange, although other considerations, such as age, difficulties in maintaining a clear airway and the nature of surgery, influence the decision concerning the most appropriate mode of ventilation in paediatric anaesthesia.

Most young infants (<6 months of age) benefit from tracheal intubation in order to maintain the airway, even if only a minor surgical procedure is to be undertaken. Infants are capable of spontaneous breathing via a tracheal tube for short periods, but ventilation

Table 22.8 Criteria of rebreathing — one or more must be fulfilled

---

A rise in minute or tidal volume by 10% or more, not accompanied by a corresponding fall in end-tidal carbon dioxide tension

An increase in end-tidal carbon dioxide tension of 5 mmHg or more, which could not be accounted for by a decrease in ventilation

An increase in ventilation of 5% or more, accompanied by an increase in end-tidal carbon dioxide tension of 2 mmHg or more

---

should always be assisted in infants if controlled mechanical ventilation is not used.

Usually, a partial rebreathing system, such as the Mapleson D, E or F, is used in paediatric anaesthesia.[87–89] Ever since the introduction of the T-piece by Phillip Ayre in 1934,[90] rebreathing has been a subject for clinical research and debate. If the criteria for clinically significant rebreathing set by Kain & Nunn[91] in 1968 (Table 22.8) are used, fresh gas flows of 1.5–2 times the estimated minute ventilation are adequate.[91] At these fresh gas flow rates, inspired carbon dioxide concentrations of up to 1.5% occur late during inspiration.[92] However, for rebreathing to be of any clinical significance, it is necessary for the inspired carbon dioxide to reach the alveoli. Because rebreathing at fresh gas flows of 1.5–2.0 times minute ventilation occurs late during inspiration, carbon dioxide does not reach the alveoli. Consequently, these fresh gas flow rates are acceptable.

However, when the dead space of the anaesthesia system is increased, rebreathing of carbon dioxide occurs early during inspiration, resulting in a rapid increase in the alveolar carbon dioxide tension.[93] It is therefore of the utmost importance during spontaneous breathing to keep the apparatus dead space as small as possible.

It is also of great value to know whether the ventilatory response to partial airway obstruction is maintained or not during anaesthesia. It has been demonstrated that the immediate reflex response is not present.[94] However, over a 5-min period, a gradual adaptation to resistive breathing occurs, which indicates compensation caused by chemical stimulation and/or by complex reflexes from joint receptors and muscle spindles involved in ventilation.[94]

In anaesthetized, spontaneously breathing children with a congenital heart malformation, those with a right-to-left shunt and underperfusion of the lungs have a high minute ventilation volume and use increased ventilatory efforts to achieve alveolar ventilation that is comparable with that in children without a congenital heart malformation. This is because of greater dead space ventilation, reflected by a larger gradient between arterial and end-tidal carbon dioxide tensions, than in those with a left-to-right shunt and those with normal lung perfusion.[59,61]

Traditionally, partial rebreathing systems are used for paediatric anaesthesia. This is due to a postulated increase in resistance to breathing in a circle system with a carbon dioxide absorber. However, a recent comparison between a paediatric circle system and a partial rebreathing system demonstrated that use of the circle system was associated with less work of breathing because of lower expiratory elastance.[95] Therefore, for surgical procedures in which spontaneous breathing is deemed to be appropriate, the paediatric circle system appears to be a reliable alternative. The practice of low-flow anaesthesia using a circle system with carbon dioxide absorption is appropriate in children, provided that oxygen saturation, end-tidal carbon dioxide tension and inspired oxygen and anaesthetic gas concentrations are monitored accurately.

CONTROLLED VENTILATION

There are in reality four different techniques for controlling ventilation during anaesthesia and surgery. One is the use of manually controlled ventilation, which was regarded for many years as the most appropriate and safest technique in small children. However, in a recent publication, the manual control of ventilation was found to be inferior to mechanical ventilation.[96] Mechanically controlled ventilation may be delivered by three different techniques which are related to the anaesthesia system selected.

1. If a non-rebreathing system is selected, the minute volume required to achieve normocapnia may be calculated from the formula:

$$\dot{V}_E \text{ (ml.min}^{-1}) = 10 \times \text{body weight (kg)} \times \text{respiratory rate}$$

which, at rates between 20 and 25 breaths.min^{-1}, results in normoventilation.[97,98] However, it is important to note that the compressible volume of gas in the tubing must be added. Using paediatric tubing, this volume is usually 1 ml.cmH$_2$O^{-1}, resulting in the addition of 300 ml.min^{-1} if the respiratory rate is 20 breaths.min^{-1} at an end-inspiratory tracheal pressure of 15 cmH$_2$O.

2. If a paediatric circle system with carbon dioxide absorption is employed, low flow rates of anaesthetic gases can be selected, and the total minute volume is delivered according to the formula given above.

3. If mechanical ventilation is delivered via a partial rebreathing system, the arterial carbon dioxide tension is dependent on the fresh gas flow rate. If fresh gas flows are set at 1.8–2.0 times the minute ventilation,[99] end-tidal carbon dioxide tension remains stable (Fig. 22.15).

Controlled mechanical ventilation in children with congenital heart malformation does not impair gas exchange compared with that during spontaneous breathing in children who have a right-to-left shunt and oligaemic lungs. Furthermore, in these patients, short (25% of respiratory cycle) and long (50%) inspirations do not influence gas exchange.[100] In children with a left-to-right shunt and hyperperfused lungs, the most efficient gas exchange occurs if inspiratory time occupies 50% of the respiratory cycle.[100]

It is important to keep in mind that there is a discrepancy between arterial and end-tidal carbon dioxide tensions in cyanotic children with oligaemic lungs.[60] Recently, attention has been drawn to the fact that each 10% decrease in oxygen saturation is equivalent to a difference of 3–4 mmHg between arterial and end-tidal carbon dioxide tensions; this information is useful in estimating the appropriate settings on the ventilator when capnography is used to estimate the adequacy of ventilation. However, it is good practice to measure arterial carbon dioxide tension directly by intermittent blood gas analysis in complex or prolonged procedures.[101]

NEONATAL SURGICAL EMERGENCIES

The enormous development of neonatal intensive care during the last decade has improved not only the possibility of survival for the very small preterm neonate, but also for the term newborn with an anatomical malformation that needs urgent surgical treatment. The outcome after major neonatal surgery is related to factors such as prematurity, hypothermia, associated congenital malformation(s) and pulmonary complications. The three most common conditions usually considered as neonatal surgical emergencies are:

1. oesophageal atresia with or without tracheo-oesophageal fistula
2. gastroschisis
3. congenital diaphragmatic hernia.

Oesophageal atresia

The incidence is 1 in 3000 births and the most common type is oesophageal atresia with a distal fistula entering the trachea close to the carina (Fig. 22.16).

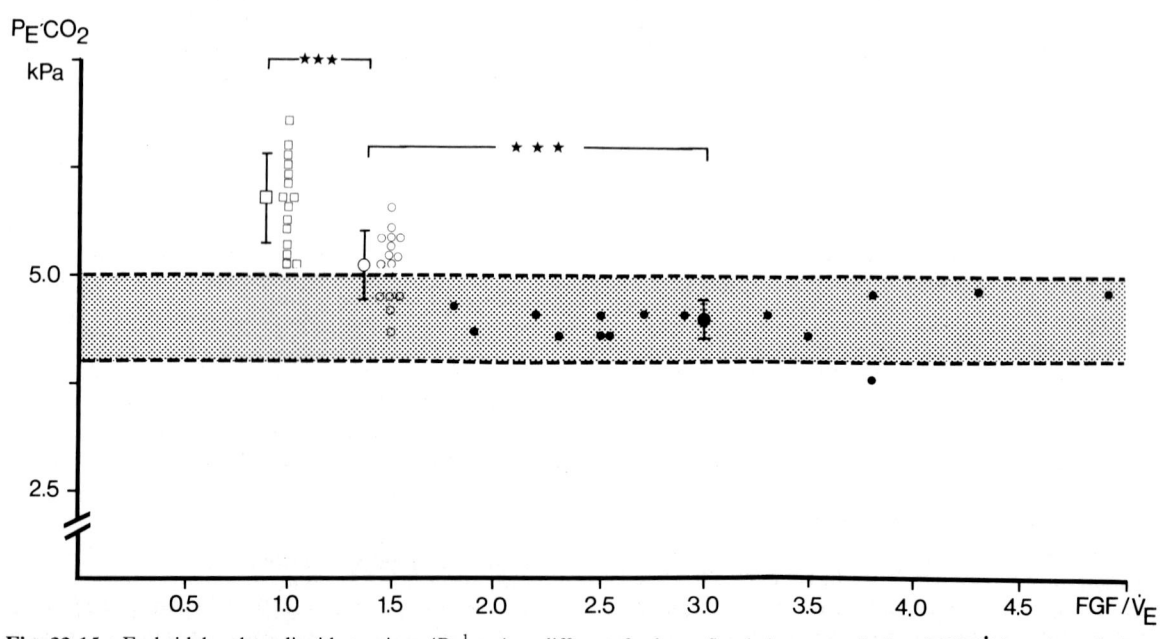

Fig. 22.15 End-tidal carbon dioxide tensions ($P_E'{CO_2}$) at different fresh gas flow/minute ventilation (FGF/$\dot{V}_E$) settings during controlled mechanical ventilation using a partial rebreathing system. Filled circles represent data from high fresh gas flow settings with minimal rebreathing: open circles show $P_E'{CO_2}$ values at 1.5 × FGF/$\dot{V}_E$ and open squares at 1.0 × FGF/$\dot{V}_E$. Large filled and open circles and open squares indicate mean values (± 1 s.d.). Shaded area shows a $P_E'{CO_2}$ range between 4.0 and 5.0 kPa. ***$P < 0.001$ for the differences indicated.

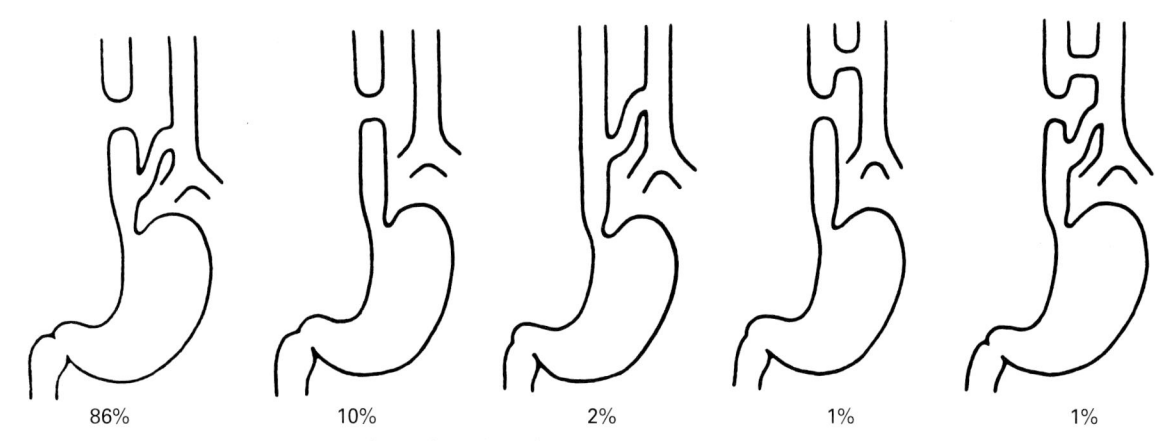

Fig. 22.16 The most frequent types of oesophageal atresia. (86%, 10%, 2%, 1%, 1%)

Cardiovascular anomalies co-exist in about 35% of patients, musculoskeletal in 30% and gastro-intestinal in 20%.

Pre-operatively, the major goal is to avoid pulmonary complications by constant suctioning of the atretic end of the oesophagus and by nursing the baby in a semi-upright position to minimize regurgitation.

Anaesthetic management focuses on prevention of hypothermia and of gaseous distension of the stomach. After administration of atropine 0.02 mg.kg^{-1}, anaesthesia is induced using thiopentone or ketamine and the trachea is intubated, preferably after administration of suxamethonium. Although Salem et al in 1973[102] advocated bronchial intubation initially, followed by repositioning of the tracheal tube just proximal to the carina, the author's preference is to position the tip of the tube in the mid-tracheal position, which causes less complications during surgical manipulations of the fistula.

Successful outcome for the term neonate with the common type of oesophageal atresia, and without associated abnormalities and pulmonary complications, is almost 100%. For the preterm neonate with severe pneumonia or serious associated abnormalities, the survival rate is less than 50%.

Gastroschisis

The incidence is 1 in 10 000 births, and it is caused by a failure in the development of the abdominal wall lateral to the umbilicus. It is almost always associated with a malrotation of the intestines, and in about 20% of the cases there is also an associated cardiac abnormality.

Pre-operatively, the principal aims are the avoidance of hypothermia, hypovolaemia and septicaemia; the intestines are not protected because of the defect in the peritoneal cavity, and have a brown and leathery appearance secondary to fetal peritonitis. If the neonate is not in optimal condition, surgery should be delayed.

Anaesthetic management in the warmed operating room (after gastric decompression, application of monitors and pre-oxygenation) comprises initially the administration of atropine and induction of anaesthesia with ketamine; intubation of the trachea should be facilitated by administration of suxamethonium. Prolonged postoperative mechanical ventilation should be anticipated because the hypoplastic abdomen is usually not large enough to accommodate the intestines, and postoperative spontaneous ventilation is frequently impaired. Nitrous oxide must not be used because it dilates the gastro-intestinal tract. A neuromuscular blocking agent is administered before the start of surgery, and the compliance of the total respiratory system is noted; this is a valuable guide in evaluating the possibility of closing the abdomen at the end of surgery. Irrespective of whether abdominal closure is possible or not, a prolonged stay in the neonatal intensive care unit is usually needed. Intestinal function often remains abnormal for many days, and total parenteral nutrition is usually required.

Outcome in the absence of serious associated abnormalities is good, although intestinal malfunction can exist for a long time.

Congenital diaphragmatic hernia

The incidence is 1 in 5000 births. A posterolateral defect on the left side of the diaphragm (foramen of Bochdalek) is the most common and occurs in about 80%. These defects also produce the most significant degree of respiratory problems. Associated abnormalities in the central nervous system occur in about 30% of patients, in the gastro-intestinal tract in about 20% and in the cardiovascular system in 15%.

Pre-operative considerations focus primarily on management of the co-existing pulmonary hypoplasia. On the side of herniation, fetal development of the lung is disrupted. The number of generations of airways is reduced, and fewer alveoli exist. The newborn with grave cyanosis immediately after birth usually has severe pulmonary hypoplasia and presents with a combination of metabolic and respiratory acidosis due to hypercapnia and hypoxaemia. Intubation of the trachea and mechanical ventilation are required early; ventilation by mask should be avoided. Mechanical ventilation should be at a high rate (40–80 breaths.min^{-1}) in order to keep tracheal pressures low so that the risk of pneumothorax is minimized. It is important that sufficient pre-operative time is allowed to optimize the baby's condition and to evaluate the degree of pulmonary hypoplasia.

Anaesthetic management requires extensive monitoring and constant evaluation of ventilation, demanding the use of a sophisticated mechanical ventilator which allows analysis of pulmonary function and gas exchange. If the trachea is not intubated before arrival in the operating room, it is likely that the degree of herniation is mild, and normal intravenous induction of anaesthesia may be employed; the trachea should be intubated after administration of suxamethonium. After the repair, it may be difficult to close the abdomen. If the abdomen is closed under tension, prolonged postoperative mechanical ventilation is often required. Extubation of the trachea should not normally be attempted in the operating room, but should be delayed until the baby's condition has stabilized in the intensive care unit.

Postoperatively, the main goal is to evaluate the degree of pulmonary hypoplasia by the alveolar–arterial oxygen tension gradient. It is also vital to keep pulmonary artery pressures low, i.e. not to allow acidosis and deep hypoxaemic periods. Alveolar–arterial gradients of 400 mmHg or less are predictive of survival, while those above are predictive of non-survival. Some babies with this condition may require treatment with extracorporeal membrane oxygenation when other means of treatment have failed.

The mortality rate is heavily influenced by associated abnormalities, and has been reported to be as high as 60% in babies with severe pulmonary hypoplasia. The long-term prognosis among survivors is encouraging. Normal lung volumes are usually achieved, although perfusion of the affected side remains impaired. This is an indication that lung hypoplasia most probably remains throughout life, but it does not seem to affect the quality of life.

PAEDIATRIC REGIONAL ANAESTHESIA

Although Bainbridge used spinal anaesthesia in children at the beginning of the 20th century,[103] and anaesthetists in Montreal gave more than 1000 spinal anaesthetics to children between 1940 and 1947,[104] it is only in the last 15 years that the use of regional anaesthesia in paediatric practice has become widespread. Interest was fuelled by reports of the effective use of caudal anaesthesia for the relief of postoperative pain after genito-urinary procedures. Simultaneously, new long-acting local anaesthetics were discovered, outpatient surgery became more frequent and respiratory complications were described after general anaesthesia in the high-risk neonate discharged from the neonatal intensive care unit.

There are several important considerations relating to paediatric regional anaesthesia that differ from the common practice of regional anaesthesia in the adult. These include anatomical age variations, myelinization of the nervous system, metabolism of local anaesthetics and the plasma drug-binding capacity to albumin and to α_1-acid glycoprotein. In addition, regional block in the paediatric patient is most frequently established during general anaesthesia; this demands dexterity, caution and alertness to the possibility of complications.

Developmental factors

At the end of the fifth gestational month, the lower end of the spinal cord lies at the first sacral segment (S1); at term, it usually lies at the lower border of the third lumbar vertebra (L3). By the end of the first year of life, the spinal cord ends at L1–2, nearly in the adult position. At term, the dural sac is at the level of S3 (Fig. 22.17).

Ligaments and fasciae are thinner and therefore easier to pierce. Frequently, a distinct loss of resistance is felt. The epidural space is much more superficial in children, and special epidural needles are required. Epidural fat tissue is sparse, and local anaesthetic agents spread more evenly.

The less myelinated central and peripheral nerve tracts in infants permit faster diffusion of local anaesthetics, but the propagation of the nerve impulse is slower. Structurally, local anaesthetic agents are either esters or amides. The esters are metabolized by plasma cholinesterase, which is present in low concentrations for the first 6 months of life; consequently, elimination of these drugs may be prolonged. Amides are metabolized in the liver, which has a reduced enzyme capacity in the neonate and young infant, resulting in a longer half-life. Furthermore, plasma concentrations of

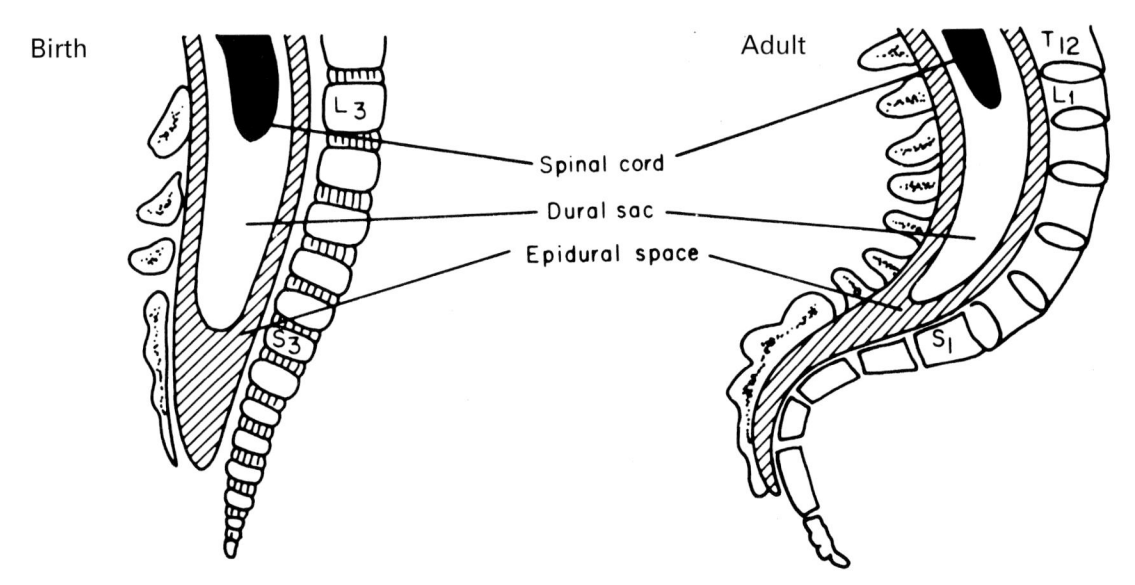

Fig. 22.17 Positions of spinal cord and dural sac related to lumbar and sacral bones at birth and in the adult. From Yaster & Maxwell,[106] with permission.

α_1-acid glycoprotein are lower in the neonate and young infant, resulting in a larger fraction of unbound drug in plasma. Theoretically, this could increase toxicity. However, the pharmacological effect of the larger fraction of unbound drug is offset by the larger volume of distribution in young children, which reduces total plasma concentration of drug.

Potencies and dosages

The potency of local anaesthetics is determined by their fat solubility. Procaine and chloroprocaine both have a low fat solubility, are of a low potency and have a short duration of action. Fat-soluble drugs such as amethocaine (tetracaine), bupivacaine and etidocaine are all more potent, and have a longer duration of action. Lignocaine (lidocaine), prilocaine and mepivacaine are intermediate. The classification of the local anaesthetic drugs, and maximum doses for epidural, spinal and peripheral blocks, are summarized in Tables 22.9 and 22.10. In infants and children older than 6 months, the half-life of bupivacaine is of the order of 250 min,[105] but it is longer in the neonate and young infant.[106] The consequences of this are that the second dose of local anaesthetic at this young age should be given either after a longer interval or in reduced quantity. If a continuous infusion is employed, one-third to one-half of the recommended hourly dose in adult patients (adjusted for body weight) should be given to infants younger than 6 months of age.

Bupivacaine is by far the most frequently used local anaesthetic drug in paediatric practice. It has a reasonably short onset of action in children, has an acceptable duration and gives an effective sensory block.

Table 22.9 Maximal dosages of some commonly used local anaesthetics for epidural and peripheral blocks

Potency	Drugs	Dose without adrenaline (mg.kg^{-1})	Dose with adrenaline (mg.kg^{-1})
Low	Procaine	10	15
	Chloroprocaine	15	15
Intermediate	Lignocaine	5	10
	Mepivacaine	5	7
	Prilocaine*	5	7
High	Amethocaine	2	2
	Bupivacaine	3	3
	Etidocaine	3	3

*Prilocaine should not be used at the dosages given in the table for infants younger than 6 months of age due to the risk of methaemoglobinaemia.

Table 22.10 Maximal dosages of local anaesthetics for spinal anaesthesia in paediatric patients

Drug	Dose without adrenaline (mg.kg^{-1})	Dose with adrenaline (mg.kg^{-1})
Lignocaine	1	2
Amethocaine	0.25	0.5
Bupivacaine	0.3	0.4

The side-effects of different epidural doses of morphine have been evaluated. Epidural morphine in a dose of 100 µg.kg^{-1} resulted in apnoea in 1 patient, and a high incidence of pruritus was noted.[107] The recommended dose of preservative-free morphine injected into the epidural space is 30–50 µg.kg^{-1}. Patients who receive epidural morphine must be observed closely for apnoea for at least 12 h after the last dose.

Regional blocks used in children

Caudal epidural anaesthesia

This is the most frequently used block in paediatric anaesthesia. Its indications are for pain relief following circumcision, hypospadias repair, anal surgery and surgery for clubbed feet. It can also be used for operations such as orchidopexy, hernia repair and implantation of ureters in the bladder.

After induction of general anaesthesia, and at a stable depth of anaesthesia, the child is placed in the lateral position with the hips flexed at 90°. The sacral ligament is pierced with a 22- or 23-gauge cannula. A dorsal approach to the epidural space is preferred in order to avoid the anterior veins. Before the drug is injected, it is important to ensure that the tip of the cannula is not positioned intravascularly or intrathecally.

A dose of 0.5 ml.kg^{-1} of bupivacaine 0.25% with adrenaline (epinephrine) is always enough for circumcision, hypospadias repair, anal procedures and operations for clubbed feet. This dose does not result in high incidences of postoperative paralysis of the lower extremities, or urinary retention. If the operation lasts more than 2–3 h, the caudal injection can be repeated after surgery with two-thirds of the initial dose, provided that the patient is older than 6 months of age. For orchidopexy or hernia repair, a dose of 0.75–1 ml.kg^{-1} is usually required; this results in more frequent problems with lower-limb paralysis and urinary retention.

Lumbar epidural anaesthesia

This block is indicated for major abdominal and/or thoracic procedures as well as for hip and knee surgery. It can be used in infants weighing as little as 5 kg due to the development of high-quality 18-gauge epidural needles through which a 20-gauge epidural catheter passes easily. It is important to appreciate that the epidural space is usually no more than 1–1.5 cm deep to the skin. A midline approach is recommended. Since the epidural block is almost always established in a patient who is already under general anaesthesia, it is important to be especially cautious in order to avoid complications. Bupivacaine 0.25% with adrenaline is frequently used for the initial dose. A total dose of 0.5 ml.kg^{-1} is enough to achieve a sufficient level of block for abdominal surgery; one-quarter of this dose should be given as a test dose.

The epidural catheter is usually retained to provide postoperative analgesia, and it is important to secure the catheter in a safe and comfortable position.

Spinal anaesthesia

Spinal block is used by some paediatric anaesthetists for many surgical procedures in the lower half of the body. It has gained popularity in some countries in the awake high-risk neonate who has recently been discharged from the neonatal intensive care unit. Since these babies have borderline respiratory function, it is wise not to flex the head and thorax while performing the block. Short 25-gauge spinal needles are used; recommended doses of local anaesthetic are shown in Table 22.10.

High-risk neonates and caudal epidural block

It is not uncommon for premature neonates to develop an inguinal hernia while in the neonatal intensive care unit. Premature babies have reduced lung function, with paradoxical breathing. Some also develop bronchopulmonary dysplasia with cor pulmonale. These neonates will not survive an incarcerated hernia with intestinal gangrene, which may occur if the hernia is not repaired. Consequently, elective surgery is necessary before discharge from hospital. Even then, the risks are high.

One major threat is that, after a general anaesthetic with tracheal intubation, it may be necessary to readmit the baby to the neonatal intensive care unit. Consequently, many paediatric anaesthetists prefer surgery to be performed under caudal anaesthesia, with the baby awake. Commonly, bupivacaine 0.25% is used in a volume of 1 ml.kg^{-1}. It is essential that these babies are anaesthetized by a specialist paediatric anaesthetist who is familiar with the technique and who is capable of dealing with any problems which may occur.

Haemodynamic effects of epidural and spinal blocks in children

For reasons which are not completely understood, bradycardia and hypotension occur rarely in association with caudal, epidural or spinal anaesthesia in children younger than 6–8 years.[108] In our practice, we have seen a few cases of hypotension associated with caudal anaesthesia in the premature respiratory acidotic child with fully developed bronchopulmonary dysplasia. Extreme caution is advised in these patients, and steps should be taken to ensure that volume resuscitation with up to 10 ml.kg^{-1} of 5% albumin can be provided if necessary.

Ilio-inguinal block

This is an excellent nerve block for hernia repair and surgery for undescended testicles. First, the anterior superior iliac spine is identified. A 22- or 23-gauge needle is inserted approximately 1 cm medial and 0.5 cm caudal to the anterior superior iliac spine, and directed dorsally. The needle must pass two fasciae, one for the external and the other for the internal oblique muscle. After aspiration, local anaesthetic is injected ventral to the transverse muscle in order to block the ilio-inguinal nerve. The needle is then retracted while injecting local anaesthetic. When it has returned to a subcutaneous position, the tip of the needle is redirected at a 45° angle to the skin, and the tip of the needle is directed medially. Two losses of resistance must be felt and a new injection started. Before finishing, a subcutaneous fan-shaped injection is given, starting at the anterior superior iliac spine. In total, not more than 0.5 ml.kg^{-1} of 0.25% bupivacaine should be given.

Penile block

This block is useful for circumcision. With a 22- or 23-gauge needle, the pubic bone is identified in the midline. The needle is then advanced caudally and laterally, piercing Buch's fascia, first on one and then on the other side. Bupivacaine 0.25% is injected in a volume of 1–2 ml. Finally, a subcutaneous injection around the penis is given. Under no circumstances should local anaesthetic solutions which contain adrenaline be used for a penile block.

Axillary plexus block

The arm to be blocked is positioned as in the adult patient. The axillary artery is identified and the sheath around nerve and vessels is pierced with a blunt needle. Usually, only one injection is needed. The most frequent reason for an insufficient axillary block in a child is that the injection is made too deep; the nerve is very superficial in children. Up to 0.5 ml.kg^{-1} of 0.25% bupivacaine is injected.

EMERGENCE AND RECOVERY FROM ANAESTHESIA

The quality of emergence is related primarily to the standard of the anaesthetic given. It is a direct reflection of the stability of the depth of anaesthesia, the ventilatory level, the temperature and replacement of fluid losses. It is a major goal to have the patient as alert as possible at the end of the procedure, and this requires a considerable degree of skill and experience on the part of the anaesthetist. It is most important that, although alert in the immediate postoperative period, patients are not in pain. If it is impossible to give a regional block, an alternative strategy for pain relief should be employed, for example treatment with a non-steroidal anti-inflammatory agent or, after major surgery, an intravenous morphine infusion. Following major procedures, a bolus dose of morphine 0.1 mg.kg^{-1} is appropriate in most children older than 6 months, followed by a continuous infusion of 0.02 mg.kg^{-1}.h^{-1}. If large doses of analgesia were given during surgery, the bolus dose should be reduced, and if the infant is less than 6 months old, the bolus dose and infusion rate should be halved.

It is important that the recovery unit is well-equipped with pulse oximeters and apnoea alarms. It must also be staffed with personnel who are trained in the management of paediatric patients. Parents should be allowed into the postoperative recovery unit soon after surgery.

REFERENCES

1. Battaglia FC. Intrauterine growth retardation. Am J Obstet Gynecol 1970; 106: 1103
2. Usher RH. Clinical implications of perinatal mortality statistics. Clin Obstet Gynecol 1971; 14: 885
3. Gregory GA. Anesthesia for premature infants. In: Gregory GA, ed. Pediatric anesthesia. New York, NY: Churchill Livingstone. 1989
4. Usher RH. The special problems of the premature infant. In: Avery GB, ed. Neonatology. Philadelphia, PA: J B Lippincott. 1981

5. Gregory GA, Steward DJ. Life-threatening perioperative apnea in the 'ex-premie'. Anesthesiology 1983; 59: 495
6. Liu LM, Cote CJ. Goudsouzian NG et al. Life-threatening apnea in infants. Anesthesiology 1983; 59: 506
7. Kurth CD, Spitzer AR, Broennle AM, Downes JJ. Postoperative apnea in premature infants. Anesthesiology 1987; 66: 483
8. Patz A. The effect of oxygen on immature retinal vessels. Invest Ophthalmol 1965; 4: 988
9. Ashton N. Oxygen and the growth and development of retinal vessels. Am J Ophthalmol 1966; 62: 412
10. Baum JD. Retrolental fibroplasia. Dev Med Child Neurol 1979; 21: 385
11. Lucey JF, Dongman B. A re-examination of the role of oxygen in retrolental fibroplasia. Pediatrics 1984; 73: 82
12. Rudolph AM. The changes in the circulation after birth. Their importance in congenital heart disease. Circulation 1970; 41: 343
13. Friedman WF, Hirschklau MJ, Previtz MP et al. Pharmacologic closure of patent ductus arteriosus in the premature infant. N Engl J Med 1976; 295: 526
14. Barnard T, Skála J. The development of brown adipose tissue. In: Lindberg O, ed. Brown adipose tissue. New York, NY: Elsevier. 1986
15. Dawkins MJR, Hull D. The production of heat by fat. Sci Am 1965; 213: 62
16. Lean MEJ, James WPT. Brown adipose tissue in man. In: Lindberg O, ed. Brown adipose tissue. New York, NY: Elsevier. 1986
17. Cannon B, Johansson BW. Non-shivering thermogenesis in the newborn. In: Baum H, Gergely J, eds. Molecular aspects of medicine. Oxford: Pergamon Press. 1980
18. Hey EN. The relation between environmental temperature and oxygen consumption in the newborn baby. J. of Physiol (London) 1969; 200: 589–603
19. Lindahl SGE, Grigsby EJ, Meyer DM, Beynen FMK. Thermogenic response to mild hypothermia in anaesthetized infants and children. Paediatr Anaesth 1992; 2: 23
20. Ohlsson K, Lindahl SGE, Mohell N et al. Thermogenesis in Brown Adipocytes is Inhibited by Volatile Anaesthetic Agents. A Factor contributing to Hypothermia in Infants? Anesthesiology 1994; 81: 176
21. Kuhl DE, Revich M, Alavi A et al. Local cerebral blood volume determined by three dimensional reconstructions of radionuclide data. Circ Res 1975; 36: 610
22. Swedlow DB. Anesthesia for neurosurgical procedures. In: Gregory GA, ed. Pediatric anaesthesia. New York, NY: Churchill Livingstone. 1989
23. Kety SS, Schmidt CF. The determination of cerebral blood flow in man by the use of nitrous oxide in low concentrations. Am J Physiol 1945; 143: 53
24. Kennedy C, Sokoloff L. An adaptation of the nitrous oxide method to the study of the cerebral circulation in children: normal values for cerebral blood flow and cerebral metabolic rate in childhood. J Clin Invest 1957; 36: 1130
25. Grubb RL, Raichle MES, Eichling JO et al. The effects of changes in Pa_{CO_2} on cerebral blood volume, blood flow and vascular mean transit time. Stroke 1974; 5: 630

26. Schwartz ML, Tator CH, Rowed DW et al. The University of Toronto head injury treatment study: a prospective, randomized comparison of pentobarbital and mannitol. Can J Neurol Sci 1984; 11: 434
27. Ward JD, Becker DP, Miller JD et al. Failure of prophylactic barbiturate coma in the treatment of severe head injury. J Neurosurg 1985; 62: 383
28. Trauner DA. Barbiturate therapy in acute brain injury. J Pediatr 1986; 109: 742
29. Drummond JC, Todd MM, Toutant SM et al. Brain surface protrusion during enflurane, halothane and isoflurane anesthesia in cats. Anesthesiology 1983; 59: 288
30. Grosslight K, Foster R, Colohan AR et al. Isoflurane for neuroanesthesia: risk factors for increases in intracranial pressure. Anesthesiology 1985; 63: 533
31. Artru AA. Partial preservation of cerebral vascular responsiveness to hypocapnia during isoflurane-induced hypotension in dogs. Anesth Analg 1986; 65: 660
32. Brody JS, Thurlbeck WM. Development, growth and aging of the lung. In: Fishman AP, ed. Handbook of physiology. The respiratory system, section 3, Mechanics of breathing part I. Baltimore, MD: Williams & Wilkins. 1986
33. Kotas RV, Avery ME. Accelerated appearance of pulmonary surfactant in the fetal rabbit. J Appl Physiol 1971; 30: 358
34. Kotas RV, Mims L, Hart L. Reversible inhibition of lung cell numbers after glucocorticoid injection. Pediatrics 1974; 53: 358
35. Stigol LC, Vawter GF, Mead J. Studies on elastic recoil of the lung in a pediatric population. Am Rev Respir Dis 1972; 105: 552
36. Jouvet M. Neurophysiology of the states of sleep. Physiol Rev 1967; 47: 117
37. Stark AR, Cohlan BA, Waggener TB et al. Regulation of end-expiratory lung volume during sleep in premature infants. J Appl Physiol 1987; 62: 1117
38. Eichenwald EC, Stark AR. Respiratory motor output. Effect of state and maturation in early life. In: Haddad GG, Farber JP, eds. Developmental neurobiology of breathing. New York, NY: Marcel Dekker. 1991
39. Henderson-Smart DJ. The effect of gestational age on the incidence and duration of recurrent apnoea in newborn babies. Aust Paediatr J 1981; 17: 273
40. Wennergren G, Hertzberg T, Milerad J et al. Hypoxia reinforces laryngeal reflex bradycardia in infants. Acta Paediatr Scand 1989; 78: 11
41. Hertzberg T. Postnatal adaptation of peripheral arterial chemoreceptors. Reflex responses and biochemical characteristics with special reference to the carotid body. Thesis. Karolinska Institute. 1990
42. Comroe JH Jr. Physiology of respiration, 2nd edn. Chicago, IL: Yearbook Medical Publishers. 1974
43. Miller RD, Hyatt RE. Obstructing lesions of the larynx and trachea: clinical and physiological characteristics. Mayo Clin Proc 1969; 44: 145
44. Auld PAM. Concepts in pulmonary physiology. In: Scarpelli EM, ed. Pulmonary physiology of the fetus newborn and child. Philadelphia, PA: Lea & Febiger. 1975
45. Lindahl SGE, Yates AP, Hatch DJ. Respiratory depression in children at different end tidal halothane concentrations. Anaesthesia 1987; 42: 1267

46 Lindahl SGE, Hulse MG, Hatch DJ. Ventilation and gas exchange during anaesthesia and surgery in spontaneously breathing infants and children. Br J Anaesth 1984; 56: 121

47 Lindahl SGE, Olsson AK. Respiratory drive and timing before and during CO_2 inhalation in infants anaesthetized with halothane. Eur J Anaesthesiol 1986; 3: 427

48 Lindahl SGE, Johannesson GP. Ventilatory CO_2 response, respiratory drive and timing in children anaesthetized with halothane, enflurane or isoflurane. Eur J Anaesthesiol 1987; 4: 313

49 Lindahl SGE. Oxygen consumption and carbon dioxide elimination in infants and children during anaesthesia and surgery. Br J Anaesth 1989; 62: 70

50 Thorsteinsson A, Jonmarker C, Larsson A et al. Functional residual capacity in anesthetized children: normal values and values in children with cardiac anomalies. Anesthesiology 1990; 73: 876

51 Brett CM. Cardiovascular physiology in pediatrics. In: Gregory GA, ed. Pediatric anesthesia. New York, NY: Churchill Livingstone. 1989

52 Friedman WF. The intrinsic properties of the developing heart. In: Friedman WF, Lesch M, Sonnenblick EH, eds. Neonatal heart disease. Orlando, FL: Grune & Stratton. 1973

53 Romero TE, Friedman WF. Limited left ventricular response to volume overload in the neonatal period: a comparative study in the adult animal. Pediatr Res 1979; 13: 910

54 Strobeck JE, Sonnenblick EH. Myocardial and ventricular function. Herz 1981; 6: 275

55 Hommes FA, Drost YM, Geraets WXM, Reijenga MAA. The energy requirement for growth: an application of Atkinsons's metabolic price system. Pediatr Res 1975; 9: 51

56 Gregory GA. The baroresponses of preterm infants during halothane anaesthesia. Can Anaesth Soc J 1982; 29: 105

57 Wear R, Robinson S, Gregory GA. The effect of halothane on the baroresponse of adult and baby rabbits. Anesthesiology 1982; 56: 188

58 Grigsby EJ, Beynen FMK, Lindahl SGE. Gas exchange, metabolic rate and fluid requirements during anaesthesia of acyanotic and cyanotic infants and children with congenital heart malformations. Paediatr Anaesth 1991; 1: 25

59 Lindahl SGE, Olsson AK. Congenital heart malformations and ventilatory efficiency in children. Effects of lung perfusion during halothane anaesthesia and spontaneous breathing. Br J Anaesth 1987; 59: 410

60 Lindahl SGE, Yates AP, Hatch DJ. Relationship between invasive and noninvasive measurements of gas exchange in anesthetized infants and children. Anesthesiology 1987; 66: 168

61 Fletcher R. Carbon dioxide production and ventilatory efficiency during controlled ventilation in children with cyanotic heart disease. Br J Anaesth 1988; 61: 743

62 Friis-Hansen B. Body composition during growth. In vivo measurements and biochemical data correlated to differential anatomic growth. Paediatrics 1971; 47: 264

63 Kenney RA. Renal function. Paediatr Clin North Am 1976; 23: 651

64 Roy RN, Chance GW, Radde IC et al. Late hyponatremia in very low birth weight infants. Paediatr Res 1976; 10: 526

65 Edelman CM Jr, Soriano JR, Boichis II et al. Renal bicarbonate reabsorption and hydrogen ion excretion in normal infants. J Clin Invest 1967; 46: 1309

66 Lowe HJ. Monitoring metabolism during closed circuit anesthesia. In: Lowe H, ed. The quantitative practice of anesthesia. Baltimore, MD: Williams & Wilkins. 1981

67 Lindahl SGE. Energy expenditure and fluid and electrolyte requirements in anesthetized infants and children. Anesthesiology 1988; 69: 377

68 Talbot FB. Standards of basal metabolism in normal infants and children. Am J Dis Child 1921; 21: 519

69 Newberg-Milde L. Cerebral protection. In: Cucchiara RF, Michenfelder JD, eds. Clinical neuroanesthesia. New York, NY: Churchill Livingstone. 1990

70 Darrow DC, Pratt EL. Fluid therapy; relation to tissue composition and expenditure of water and electrolyte. Council on Food and Nutrition. JAMA 1950; 143: 365

71 Holliday MA, Segar WE. The maintenance need for water in parenteral fluid therapy. Pediatrics 1957; 19: 823

72 Heikkinen ES, Akerblom HK. Diagnostic and operative problems in multiple pheochromocytomas. J Pediatr Surg 1977; 12: 157

73 Greenblatt DJ, Abernethy DR, Locniskar A et al. Effect of age, gender and obesity on midazolam kinetics. Anesthesiology 1984; 61: 27

74 Saint-Maurice C, Meistelman C, Rey E et al. The pharmacokinetics of rectal midazolam for premedication in children. Anesthesiology 1986; 65: 536

75 Saint-Maurice C, Landais A, Delleur MM et al. The use of midazolam in diagnostic and short surgical procedures in children. Acta Anaesthesiol Scand 1990; 34: (suppl 92): 39

76 Hallén B, Uppfeldt A. Does lidocaine-prilocaine cream permit painfree insertion of i.v. catheters in children? Anesthesiology 1982; 57: 340

77 Sigurdsson GH, Lindahl SGE, Nordén NE. Influence of premedication on sympathetic and endocrine responses and cardiac arrhythmias during halothane anaesthesia in children undergoing adenoidectomy. Br J Anaesth 1983; 55: 961

78 Johannesson GP, Lindahl SGE, Sigurdsson GH, Nordén NE. Halothane, enflurance and isoflurane anaesthesia for adenoidectomy in children using two different premedications. Acta Anaesthesiol Scand 1987; 31: 233

79 Jonmarker C, Westrin P, Larsson S, Werner O. Thiopental requirements for induction of anesthesia in children. Anesthesiology 1987; 67: 104

80 Westrin P, Jonmarker C, Werner O. Thiopental requirements for induction of anesthesia in neonates and in infants 1 to 6 months of age. Anesthesiology 1989; 71: 344

81 Gregory GA, Eger EI II, Munson ES. The relationship between age and halothane requirement in man. Anesthesiology 1969; 30: 488

82 Gion H, Saidman LJ. The minimum alveolar concentration of enflurane in man. Anesthesiology 1971; 35: 361

83 Quasha AL, Eger EI II, Tinker JH. Determination and applications of MAC. Anesthesiology 1980; 53: 315

84 Lerman J, Robinson S, Willis MM, Gregory GA. Anesthetic requirements for halothane in young children 0–1 month and 1–6 months of age. Anesthesiology 1983; 59: 421
85 Cameron CB, Robinson S, Gregory GA. The minimum anesthetic concentration of isoflurane in children. Anesth Analg 1984; 63: 418
86 Le Dez MB, Lerman J. The minimum alveolar concentration (MAC) of isoflurane in preterm neonates. Anesthesiology 1987; 67: 301
87 Mapleson WW. Theoretical considerations of the effect of rebreathing in two semiclosed systems. Br Med Bull 1958; 14: 64
88 Willis BA, Pender JW, Mapleson WW. Rebreathing in a T-piece: volunteer and theoretical studies of the Jackson–Rees modification of Ayre's T-piece during spontaneous respiration. Br J Anaesth 1975; 47: 1239
89 Conway CM, Seeley HF, Barnes PK. Spontaneous ventilation with the Bain anaesthetic system. Br J Anaesth 1977; 49: 1247
90 Ayre P. Anaesthesia for harelip and cleft palate in babies. Br J Surg 1937; 25: 131
91 Kain ML, Nunn JF. Fresh gas economies of the Magill circuit. Anesthesiology 1968; 29: 964
92 Lindahl SGE, Charlton AJ, Hatch DJ. Ventilatory responses to rebreathing and carbon dioxide inhalation during anaesthesia in children. Br J Anaesth 1985; 57: 1188
93 Charlton AJ, Lindahl SGE, Hatch DJ. Ventilatory responses of children to changes in deadspace volume. Studies using the T-piece (Mapleson F) system. Br J Anaesth 1985; 57: 562
94 Lindahl SGE, Charlton AJ, Hatch DJ, Phythyon J. Ventilatory responses to inspiratory mechanical loads in spontaneously breathing children during halothane anaesthesia. Acta Anaesthesiol Scand 1986; 30: 122
95 Conterato JP, Lindahl SGE, Meyer D, Bires JA. Assessment of spontaneous ventilation in anesthetized children with use of a pediatric circle or a Jackson–Rees system. Anesth Analg 1989; 69: 484
96 Spears RS Jr, Yen A, Fisher DM, Zwass MS. The 'educated hand'. Can anesthesiologists assess changes in neonatal pulmonary compliance manually? Anesthesiology 1991; 75: 693
97 Lindahl SGE, Okmian L, Thomson DA. Artificial ventilation in children during anaesthesia using a tidal volume ventilator. Acta Anaesthesiol Scand 1979; 23: 587
98 Hulse MG, Lindahl SGE, Hatch DJ. Comparison of ventilation and gas exchange in anaesthetized infants and children during spontaneous and artificial ventilation. Br J Anaesth 1984; 56: 131
99 Hatch DJ, Yates AP, Lindahl SGE. Flow requirements and rebreathing during mechanically controlled ventilation in a T-piece (Mapleson E) system. Br J Anaesth 1987; 59: 1533
100 Olsson AK, Lindahl SGE. Spontaneous versus controlled ventilation in anaesthetized children with congenital cardiac malformations. Acta Anaesthesiol Scand 1987; 31: 87
101 Fletcher R. The relationship between the arterial to endtidal P_{CO_2} difference and hemoglobin saturation in patients with congenital heart disease. Anesthesiology 1991; 75: 210
102 Salem MR, Wong AY, Lin YH et al. Prevention of gastric distension during anesthesia for newborns with tracheo-esophageal fistulas. Anesthesiology 1973; 38: 82
103 Bainbridge WB. Analgesia in children by spinal injection with a report of a new method of sterilization of the injected fluid. Med Record 1900; 58: 937
104 Leigh MD. Spinal anaesthesia in infants and children. Int Anaesthesiol Clin 1963; 1: 825
105 Ecoffey C, Desparment J, Maury M et al. Bupivacaine in children: pharmacokinetics following caudal anesthesia. Anesthesiology 1985; 63: 447
106 Yaster M, Maxwell LG. Pediatric regional anesthesia. Anesthesiology 1989; 70: 324
107 Krane EJ. Delayed respiratory depression in a child after caudal epidural morphine. Anesth Analg 1988; 67: 79
108 Murat I, Delleur MM, Esteve C et al. Continuous epidural anaesthesia in children: clinical and haemodynamic implications. Br J Anaesth 1987; 59: 1441

23. Local anaesthetic techniques

T. M. Murphy   D. Fitzgibbon

Controversy exists as to the advantages of regional as opposed to general anaesthesia.[1] When anaesthetists today counsel patients regarding the most desirable anaesthetic, the decision is based most often on techniques learned in training, institutional tradition, medicolegal fears and perceived time constraints, rather than factual data supporting the method. The acceptance by patients of a proposed anaesthetic technique is based on many factors, including the anaesthetist's and surgeon's recommendations, nursing staff input, previous experience with anaesthetics, and community expectations and standards. Originally, the arguments in favour of regional anaesthesia were the experienced comments proffered by seasoned practitioners in the field who, having persevered with it over the years, were impressed by the excellent peri-operative conditions of a regional anaesthetic.[2-4] In reality, there are few studies clearly documenting that either regional or general anaesthesia is safer for an individual surgical patient. Few randomized studies have been designed to compare regional and general anaesthesia directly. The studies which have been undertaken involve principally evaluation of deep venous thrombosis, mental status changes or surgical blood loss.

Evidence of direct benefits from regional anaesthesia exist in the following situations:

1. Fewer haemodynamic changes in hypertensive patients[5]
2. Decreased surgical blood loss[6]
3. Reduced incidence of thrombo-embolism[7]
4. Reversal of ischaemic events in patients with ischaemic heart disease[8]
5. Use in patients with malignant hyperpyrexia.[9]

The ability to compare anaesthetic techniques, regional or general, is limited primarily by the remarkable safety of both methods. In the healthy, elective, surgical patient undergoing non-body cavity operation, the risk of dying from a primary anaesthetic cause is probably no more frequent than 1 in 100 000. The difficulty in determining relative risk is highlighted in a report by Tiret and colleagues,[10] who analysed nearly 200 000 patients who received anaesthesia in France between 1978 and 1982; although the analysis included all anaesthetics, no comment could be made regarding differences between regional and general techniques. Pre-existing disease, magnitude of operation and postoperative care have more influence over morbidity and mortality, and it is virtually impossible to show that one anaesthetic technique is significantly different from another in terms of outcome, provided that each technique is founded on sound physiological principles. There are few circumstances in which general anaesthesia offers clear advantages over regional anaesthesia when the surgical procedure is appropriate to either technique.

Judicious use of regional anaesthesia is associated with significant postoperative analgesia. Peripheral nerve blockade has long been known to provide excellent postoperative relief and has been used with enthusiasm by individual practitioners since its discovery. Organ function appears to be better preserved, and there is a decreased morbidity in critically ill patients in whom prolonged epidural analgesia is used in the intensive care unit.[11] McQuay and colleagues[12] demonstrated in a wide group of patients undergoing orthopaedic surgery that postoperative analgesia could be produced for a period of approximately 8 h by judicious use of analgesia of the operative area with regional nerve blocks coupled with an appropriate opioid premedication. The duration of pain relief was four times that of comparable control groups who received neither of these forms of treatment (Fig. 23.1).

Tverskoy et al[13] found that, in patients undergoing inguinal herniorrhaphy, significant pain relief could be obtained by peripheral (ilioinguinal–inguinal nerve block) or central (subarachnoid) block. Both of these were superior to general anaesthesia in the immediate postoperative period. Of interest is that the patients who received the peripheral nerve block prior to the

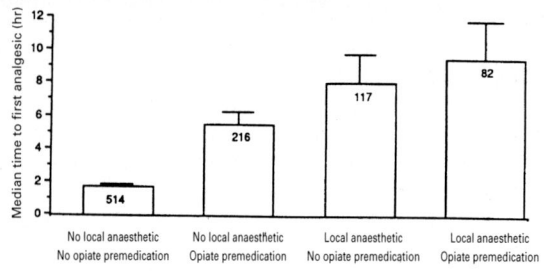

Fig. 23.1 Duration of postoperative analgesia in a variety of surgical operations with different combinations of opioid premedication and local anaesthetic blockade. Note that maximal postoperative analgesia is achieved with a combination of both, but local anaesthesia alone still affords significant analgesic duration. From McQuay et al,[12] with permission.

surgical trespass had significantly less pain on wound pressure 2 weeks after the operation compared with the other groups. It would appear that, by denying access of the nociceptive stimulus to the central nervous system, analgesic benefits may accrue for a significant period of time. Bach et al[14] used a preoperative regional anaesthetic in patients scheduled for amputation of a painful limb, and showed that the incidence of phantom limb pain was absent in the experimental group a year after the event, but occurred in a percentage of the control patients. There may be some clinical benefit in diminishing the duration of post-nociceptive pain by denying access of these stimuli to the dorsal horn and preventing subsequent escalation and preservation of pain via mechanisms central to this site.[15]

CENTRAL BLOCKADE

History

Subarachnoid injection of cocaine in humans was first performed in 1899 by Bier,[16] and epidural analgesia by Siccard[17] and Cathelin[18] in 1901. Central blockade soon became widely accepted as a safe, convenient and effective anaesthetic method. By the mid 1940s, subarachnoid anaesthesia had peaked in popularity. However, the fear of neurological complications resulting from a series of widely publicized, but scientifically unsound, articles on the high incidences of neurological sequelae following subarachnoid block,[19] and the increase in popularity of intravenous anaesthetics and neuromuscular relaxants, led to a decline and almost a demise in the widespread use of central blockade, especially in the UK. Factors which resulted in renewed popularity of central blockade included studies by Dripps & Vandam,[20] the introduction of new amide-type local anaesthetics, and the gradual acceptance that there were also hazards associated with general anaesthesia. Although continuous lumbar epidural anaesthesia was first used for surgical procedures and postoperative pain,[21] the sustained use of the technique occurred as a result of its application in obstetrics. Dawkins[22] used regional and peripheral blockade for surgery and postoperative pain relief in the UK, and Bonica[2] and Moore[3] in the USA. Central and peripheral blockade is now commonly used for surgical anaesthesia, for obstetric patients and for patients with acute and chronic pain.

Fundamental considerations

Subarachnoid and epidural techniques can produce profound anaesthesia over large areas of the body. The mechanism by which local anaesthetics produce reversible blockade of nerve pathways to and from, and even within, the neuraxis is incompletely understood. During subarachnoid anaesthesia, local anaesthetics are deposited in close proximity to the neural target and are found both in nerve roots and within the substance of the spinal cord.[23] The major cause of loss of sensation and muscle relaxation during subarachnoid anaesthesia is the presence of local anaesthetics in spinal nerve roots and in dorsal root ganglia, not within the spinal cord. The duration of blockade is determined by the rate at which local anaesthetics are removed from the subarachnoid space by vascular absorption.[24] Other factors influencing the duration and intensity of neural blockade include the total dose of drug, baricity, vasoconstrictors, cord blood flow and lipid solubility. In contrast, epidural injection deposits local anaesthetic some distance from the neural target, so that diffusion across tissue barriers is very important.

Epidural local anaesthetic comes in contact with a number of different structures:

1. Spinal nerves in paravertebral spaces
2. Dorsal root ganglia
3. Anterior and posterior spinal nerve roots with dural cuffs
4. Spinal roots as they exit from the cord (cerebrospinal fluid (CSF) transfer)
5. Peripheral regions of the spinal cord (CSF transfer).

Bengtsson and colleagues[25] demonstrated the effect of zones of differential sensory blockade in which different types of sensory afferent fibres have different sensitivities to local anaesthetics. At the same sensory level, the physiological responses to epidural and subarachnoid anaesthesia are often quite different. The onset of sympathetic blockade is usually slower with epidural anaesthesia, thus permitting adequate compensatory vasoconstriction in the unblocked segments of the body. This difference tends to be more evident in the older, less vasoreactive age groups. In addition, drugs injected epidurally can produce a systemic effect after vascular uptake from the injection site, in contrast to the much smaller doses used for subarachnoid blockade, which have little or no systemic effect. Overall, these differences between subarachnoid and epidural anaesthesia help to explain the clinical variations observed between the two techniques in terms of volume of drug required, time of onset of anaesthesia, intensity of blockade and side-effects encountered. A disadvantage of epidural anaesthesia is the requirement for larger volumes and doses of local anaesthetic agents, which may result in pharmacologically active plasma concentrations with resultant additive circulatory depressant effects and potential adverse effects on the fetus in obstetric anaesthesia. One major advantage of continuous epidural analgesia is the ability to maintain prolonged anaesthesia during unexpectedly protracted surgical procedures. This is of particular importance in the light of recent evidence of potential neurological sequelae associated with the use of continuous spinal catheter techniques.[26,27]

It is possible to produce segmental anaesthesia with epidural techniques; selected dermatomes and myotomes may be anaesthetized for intra-operative anaesthesia or postoperative analgesia. In specific types of upper abdominal procedure, such as gastric bypass, in which the surgical field is limited to a few dermatomes, small doses of local anaesthetic administered via a thoracic epidural catheter can give very satisfactory post-operative segmental analgesia.[28] In addition, the efficacy of continuous infusions of mixtures of epidural opioids and low-concentration epidural local anaesthetics is being used increasingly in the management of patients with postoperative pain[29] and of those with chronic cancer pain.[30] Animal and human studies have shown that these drugs have a synergistic effect. Local anaesthetic requirements are reduced when such combinations are used, with the additional advantage of reduced cardiovascular instability.

Applied anatomy

The spinal canal extends from the foramen magnum to the sacral hiatus. It is bounded anteriorly by the vertebral bodies, laterally by the pedicles and posteriorly by the laminae. Intervertebral discs and the ligamentous connections between the laminae and spines provide additional boundaries. The only openings in the canal are the intervertebral foramina, through which segmental nerves and blood vessels pass. The spinal cord lies within the canal surrounded by three membranes — the pia mater, arachnoid mater and the dura mater. The dura, or theca, is a direct continuation of the fibrous layer of dura in the cranium, and extends from the foramen magnum to S2. The arachnoid mater lies within the dura and is separated from it by only a thin layer of lymph. The pia mater surrounds, and is adherent to, the spinal cord.

Traditionally, the dura is considered to be the significant barrier to the transfer of drugs (opioids and local anaesthetics) from the epidural space to the CSF. Recent evidence[31] suggests that the arachnoid may be the regulating barrier, and that the dura is a relatively inert structure which provides little impedance to drug transfer. The spinal cord extends the length of the canal in the fetus (at birth it is found at the level of L3), and reaches its final position at L1/2 by the second decade of life. The conus medullaris is the tapered final limit of the cord. The dura maintains its embryological attachments at the S2 level. Below the conus medullaris is a relatively large subarachnoid compartment stretching from L1 to S2, which contains the cauda equina consisting of spinal nerve roots destined for body levels below L1. Subarachnoid and epidural punctures are classically performed between the upper border of L2 (conus medullaris) and the upper border of the sacrum at L5/S1. However, puncture may be performed at other levels of the spinal canal, but with a risk of spinal cord trauma; that risk is probably related to the skill and experience of the anaesthetist performing the puncture.

The epidural space is the compartment between the dura and the bony and ligamentous walls of the spinal canal, and its anatomy has been reviewed recently.[32] The space is filled with extradural fat and the internal vertebral plexus of veins, arranged in two paramedian chains throughout the length of the extradural space. Segmental nerves, as they leave the dura, cross the space before exiting from the canal through the intervertebral foramina. Epidural anaesthesia is usually performed in the lumbar region, but can be used in other regions of the canal if indicated clinically[28] (Fig. 23.2).

The following vertebrae are used as classical landmarks for identification of spinal levels:

1. C7 vertebra (the only vertebra identified with certainty)
2. L4 vertebra or the L4–5 interspace (located by joining the iliac crests with a transverse line)
3. T7 (with the arms by the side, a horizontal line

Dermatomes and myotomes

The proper conduct of central blockade and the correct interpretation of its effects and complications require a thorough knowledge of the sensory, motor and autonomic distribution of the different spinal nerves. This requires knowledge of the dermatomes and myotomes of the body. A dermatome is the area of skin supplied by a single spinal nerve. The dermatome distribution is shown in Figure 23.3.

Like skin, muscles are also supplied by segmental nerves. Last[33] pointed out that there appear to be spinal centres for joint movements and that these spinal centres tend to occupy four continuous segments in the cord. The two higher segments innervate one

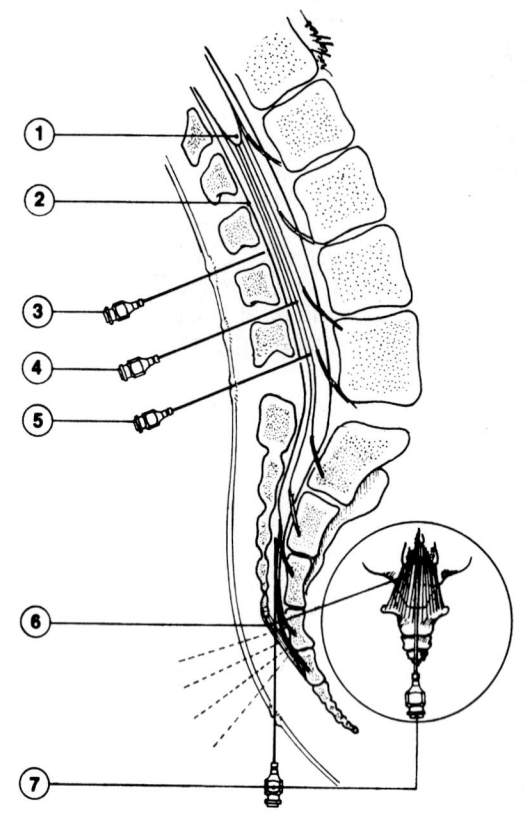

Fig. 23.2 Subarachnoid and epidural approaches to the neuraxis. Longitudinal section through the lumbar and sacral areas, showing the options for subarachnoid and epidural needle placement. (1) Conus medullaris of the distal cord at the level of L2 (below this point the spinal canal contains the cauda equina); (2) the dura mater; (3) a lumbar epidural needle positioned at the L3/L4 interspace, with the needle point situated in the epidural space; (4) subarachnoid needle at L4/L5 interspace; (5) subarachnoid puncture at L5/S1 interspace (Taylor approach); (6) sacrococcygeal ligament showing site of puncture for caudal epidural needle placement. The dashed lines represent the initial placement of the needle with a vertical approach to detect sacrococcygeal ligament puncture and the bony end-point of the dorsal aspect of the ventral plate of the sacrum prior to assuming a steeper angle for advancement into the terminal (caudal) epidural canal; (7) care is exercised to prevent the needle being advanced cephalad to the S2 level (where the dura mater terminates) to prevent inadvertent subarachnoid puncture.

joining the lower end of both scapulae usually passes through T7).

Other vertebrae are located clinically by counting from these levels. This may be inaccurate anatomically, but it is clinically practical in all but the most sophisticated diagnostic and therapeutic nerve blocks.

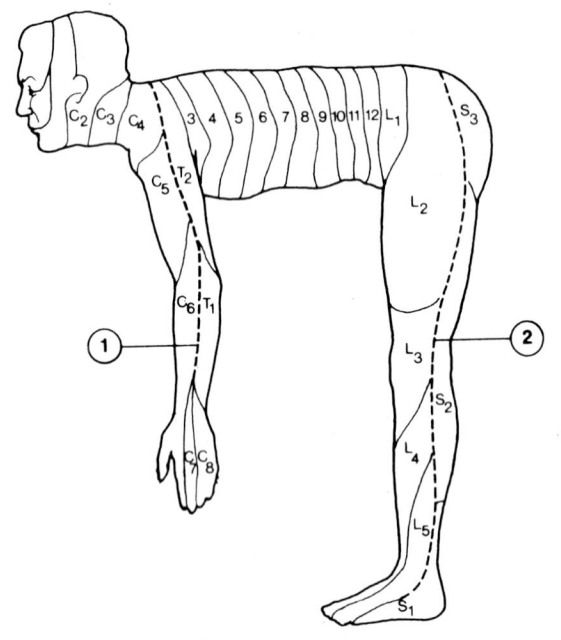

Fig. 23.3 Dermatomes of the body. Note the orderly crandiad to caudad sequence of dermatomes by positioning the body as shown. Note that C1 has no dermal distribution. Note on the extremities that the dermatomes are distributed symmetrically about an axial line (1 and 2 for the upper and lower limbs respectively). Note that the upper-extremity dermatomes are distributed symmetrically pre- and post-axially with symmetrical borrowing of trunk skin from C4 and T2 dermatomes. Note that the central dermatome C7 is most distally distributed to the middle finger.

The dermatomal distribution of the lower extremity is complicated by an asymmetrical pre-axial 'borrowing' of large amounts of skin from the body wall L2, 3, bringing its lumbar plexus nerve supply with it. The central dermatome of the true lower extremity (S1) is also distributed most peripherally (on the lateral plantar surface of the foot), with the pre-axial L4 and 5 dermatomes and postaxial S2 and S3 dermatomes distributed accordingly. From Foerster,[34] with permission.

LOCAL ANAESTHETIC TECHNIQUES 561

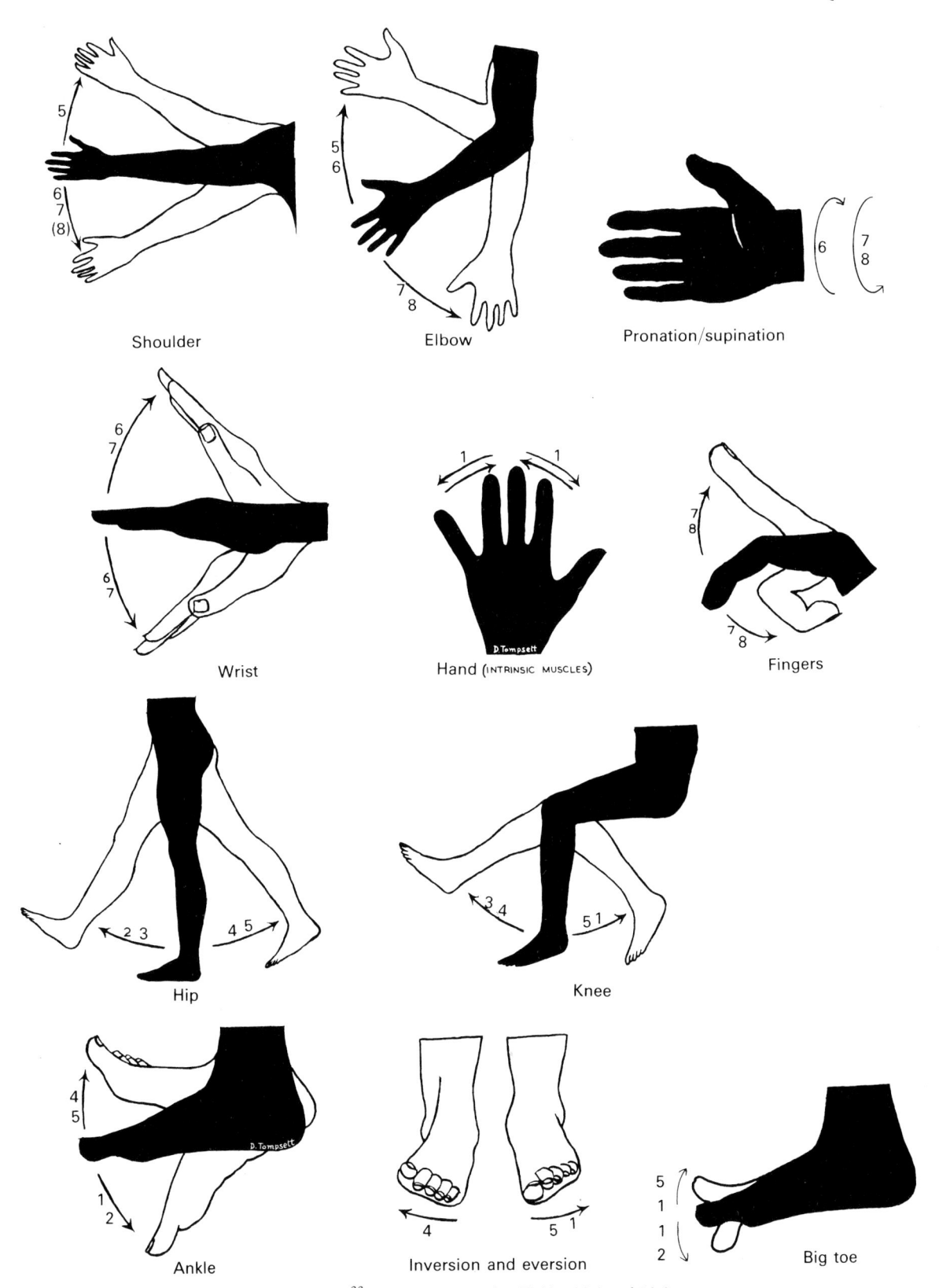

Fig. 23.4 Myotomes of the Body. From Last,[33] with permission. See Tables 23.1 and 23.2.

movement of the joint and the two lower segments innervate the opposite movement. For example, the centre for the hip joint is L2, L3, L4 and L5. Hip flexion is supplied by L2 and L3, while extension is supplied by L4 and L5 (Fig. 23.4, Tables 23.1 and 23.2).

The anatomic nervous system

Efferent fibres for the sympathetic nervous system exit in the anterior roots of spinal nerves T1–L2. Sympathetic fibres leave the nerve roots in the white ramus communicans to enter the sympathetic trunk. The trunk consists of three cervical ganglia, 11 thoracic, four lumbar and four sacral. Only ganglia from T1 to L2 receive white rami. The sympathetic trunk has both somatic and visceral branches. Somatic branches leave the ganglia as grey rami communicantes and enter the segmental somatic nerves, conveying vasoconstrictor, sudomotor and pilomotor fibres to the area of distribution of the nerve. Visceral branches leave the trunk and form plexuses, for example coeliac, for various visceral destinations. The cardiac, oesophageal, pulmonary and coeliac plexuses receive a parasympathetic supply from the vagus, whereas the inferior hypogastric and pelvic plexuses receive parasympathetic efferents from the pelvic parasympathetic outflow of S2–4.

The sympathetic nervous system also contains many visceral afferent sensory fibres. These travel to the neuraxis via the sympathetic pathway and plexuses described above. Somatic afferent fibres usually travel along blood vessels and somatic spinal nerves. There appear to be spinal levels for these different sympathetic innervations which serve as useful guides when determining appropriate levels of anaesthesia required for surgery on viscera. The duration of sympathetic blockade is often shorter than either sensory or motor blockade.[25]

Clinical aspects

Pre-operative evaluation and assessment of the patient in whom a regional technique is planned should be as detailed as that undertaken in any patient scheduled to undergo general anaesthesia. The need for premedication and monitoring should not be influenced by the planned anaesthetic technique, but should be determined by the physical status of the patient and the nature of the surgical procedure planned. Perioperative anxiety and apprehension may be reduced by explaining the degree of sensory and motor loss to be expected, the absence of nociception and potential benefits in terms of diminished postoperative pain and morbidity. Premedication, if needed, is usually with a short-acting benzodiazepine such as temazepam. The use of intra-operative sedation, titrated to a level which is not associated with impairment of the patient's upper airway reflexes or ventilation, has become easier with the introduction of continuous infusions of propofol. An infusion of propofol in the range of 1–3 mg.kg^{-1}.h^{-1} usually results in adequate sedation without excessive cardiovascular or respiratory depression. The pharmacokinetics and pharmacodynamics of this agent appear to be superior to those of others used for intra-operative sedation. Wilson et al[35] compared propofol with midazolam in 40 patients undergoing orthopaedic surgery under subarachnoid block, and concluded that immediate postoperative recovery and restoration of higher mental function were significantly more rapid in the propofol group. However, amnesia for the immediate postoperative period was significantly greater in patients who received midazolam ($P < 0.001$).

Caplan et al[36] recently evaluated 14 cases of cardiac arrest in young, healthy patients during spinal anaesthesia, which resulted in death or severe neurological injury. In half of these cases, unappreciated respiratory insufficiency seemed to have contributed to the cardiac arrest. In the other half, respiratory insufficiency was not evident and cardiac arrest seemed to have evolved against a background of apparently stable haemodynamics. An inadequate appreciation of the interaction between high sympathetic blockade and the role of α-adrenergic tone during resuscitation may have con-

Table 23.1 Myotomes of the lower extremity

Hip		Knee		Ankle	
Flex	L2/3	Extend	L3/4	Dorsiflex	L4/5
Extend	L4/5	Flex	L5/S1	Plantarflex	S1/2

Modified from Last.[33]

Table 23.2 Myotomes of the upper extremity

Shoulder		Elbow		Wrist		Digits	
Flex	C5	Flex	C5/6	Flex/extend	C6/7	Flex/extend	C7/8
Extend	C6/7/8	Extend	C7/8			Adduct/abduct	T1

LOCAL ANAESTHETIC TECHNIQUES 563

tributed to a poor outcome in these cases. In any event, the patient's cardiovascular and respiratory systems need to be monitored closely for the duration of all perioperative sedation.

Positioning and approaches for central blockade

Three positions may be adopted for lumbar puncture — sitting, lateral decubitus or lumbosacral (Taylor approach).

Sitting

The patient is positioned sitting on the operating table, with the knees bent and the feet resting comfortably on a stool. The patient is instructed to fold the arms and to rest them on a suitable stand, or to lean on an assistant. These manoeuvres position the patient's spine optimally for performing either a midline or paramedian lumbar puncture. This position is particularly effective when hyperbaric spinal techniques are used for procedures confined to the perineal area. The central position of the vertebrae in the seated patient facilitates dural puncture in the presence of obesity or other conditions in which palpation of spinous processes and identification of bony landmarks, or even the midline, is difficult. Depending on the level of anaesthesia required, the patient either remains seated for a limited period, or assumes the supine position following completion of the puncture.

Lateral decubitus

This is probably the most common position for subarachnoid and epidural anaesthesia in surgical and obstetric practice. Ideally, the patient's back is parallel to the edge of the table, and the shoulders and iliac crests vertical. The thighs, head and neck are flexed. This produces maximal curvature of the spine and maximizes the interspinal distance. If a hyperbaric technique is planned, the region to be operated on should be dependent. In situations where a midline approach results in repeated difficulty, the paramedian approach should be used. In the paramedian approach, the needle is introduced 1–2 cm (a finger's breadth) from the midline. The needle is advanced parallel to the spine until the bony end-point of lamina is encountered. This provides an indication of the depth of the ligamentum flavum. 'Walking' the needle in a cephalad and medial fashion along the lamina results in the needle entering the ligamentum flavum. Further advancement results in penetration of the epidural space, and ultimately the subarachnoid space.

Lumbosacral (Taylor approach)

Described by Taylor in 1940,[37] the approach is at the L5–S1 interspace, and is a variation of the conventional paramedian approach. The L5–S1 interspace is the largest interspace in the vertebral column. The needle is introduced 1 cm medial and 1 cm cephalad to the posterior superior iliac spine. The needle is directed cephalad and medially. If the bony surface of the sacrum is encountered, the needle is walked cephalad until it slips off the surface and pierces the ligamentum flavum and then the dura (Fig. 23.5).

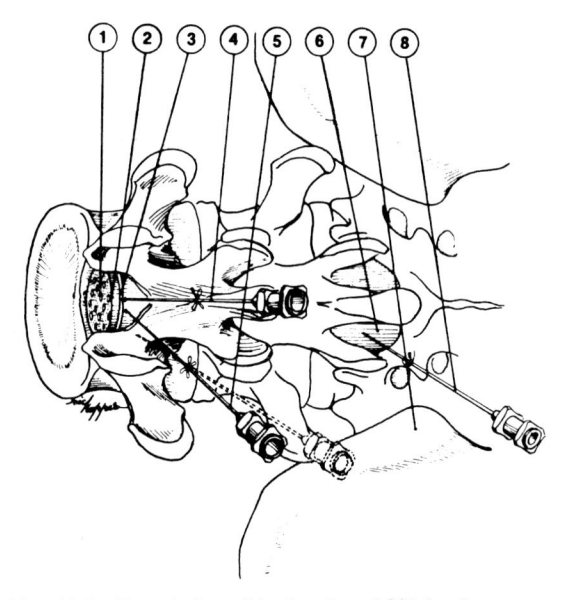

Fig. 23.5 Dorsal view of the fourth and fifth lumbar vertebrae and their relationship to the sacral and iliac bones. This shows the most frequently used approaches for needle puncture in both subarachnoid and lumbar epidural techniques. (1) Cauda equina; (2) dura mater; (3) ligamentum flavum at L3/4 interspace; (4) a needle in the midline position for both subarachnoid and epidural techniques where the needle is introduced between the spines of L3 and L4 vertebrae traversing the supra- and interspinous ligaments to pierce the ligamentum flavum; (5) paramedian approach at the same level where the dermal needle puncture site is 1–2 cm lateral to the midline approach — if the initial approach results in contacting the lamina of the vertebra, as shown in the silhouettes with the dashed lines, then the needle is repositioned more cephalad and medially until it slips off the lamina, contacting ligamentum flavum as shown; (6) the large interspace between S5 and L1 is approached by needle puncture at a site 2 cm medial and cephalad from the posterior/superior iliac spine; (7) the needle (8) is introduced via the L5/S1 interspace in the Taylor approach for either subarachnoid or epidural puncture.

Subarachnoid block

Different terms, such as spinal anaesthesia/analgesia and subarachnoid anaesthesia/analgesia, have been used to describe the injection of local anaesthetic into the subarachnoid space. In this chapter, we use the term *subarachnoid block* to describe the production of anaesthesia by injection into the spinal subarachnoid space. Few anaesthetic techniques offer such excellent operating conditions, proven patient safety or economy of anaesthetic effort and resources, especially for operations involving the lower abdomen, the perineum and the lower extremities (Table 23.3).

Needles and bevels

A variety of sizes of needle are available for subarachnoid puncture. The usual gauges are 18-, 22-, 25- and 26-gauge. In addition, 29- and 32-gauge needles are available. These very thin needles are associated with an unacceptably high failure rate on attempted puncture, precluding their use in other than exceptional circumstances.[38] Recent reports indicate that the incidence of spinal headache may not be significantly diminished in comparison to that associated with the use of 26- and 25-gauge needles, especially in the obstetric population. The 25-gauge needle is probably the most popular gauge in current use.

Needles are also classified according to the shape of the bevel. The most popular are the Quincke–Babock, Greene and Whitacre. Quincke–Babock needles (the standard needle) have a sharp point with a medium-length cutting bevel. The Greene needle has a rounded point and a rounded non-cutting bevel of medium length. The Whitacre, or pencil-point needle, has a rounded non-cutting bevel with a solid tip, the opening being 2 mm proximal to the tip. To facilitate the introduction of the small-bore needles, a variety of introducers are available.

Drugs used for subarachnoid block

Modern local anaesthetics used for subarachnoid block are safe and not neurotoxic.[39] The two drugs used most commonly are lignocaine and bupivacaine, and the choice is determined primarily with regard to their duration of action. The duration of action may be enhanced by the addition of adrenaline (epinephrine). However, Chambers et al[40,41] suggested that the addition of adrenaline over a spectrum of doses produced little or no prolongation of subarachnoid block with either lignocaine or bupivacaine, although the duration of action of amethocaine (tetracaine) appears to be prolonged.[42] Initial fears that vasoconstrictors might produce cord ischaemia sufficient to cause postoperative neurological complications have proved groundless.[20] Adrenaline and phenylephrine are the vasoconstrictors used most widely to prolong the duration of subarachnoid block. Doses of adrenaline vary from 0.2 to 0.5 mg (0.2–0.5 ml of 1 : 1000 adrenaline), and of phenylephrine from 0.5–5 mg (0.05–0.5 ml of 1% solution). Unless amethocaine is the agent of choice, there is probably little need for the addition of vasoconstrictors for subarachnoid block.

Local anaesthetic solutions used for subarachnoid administration may be classified according to baricity into hypobaric (specific gravity < CSF), isobaric (specific gravity = CSF) and hyperbaric (specific gravity > CSF). Standard solutions of lignocaine and bupivacaine are made hyperbaric by the addition of glucose 5 or 8%. The most usual concentrations of lignocaine and bupivacaine used for subarachnoid block are 5 and 0.5% respectively. A solution of 1% amethocaine is made hyperbaric by mixing with an equal volume of glucose 10% to produce a 0.5% solution. The concept of combining low doses of opioids with local anaesthetics to prolong and improve analgesia while reducing the risks of adverse effects of each is not new. In a blinded study, Abouleish et al[43] evaluated the effects of adding morphine 0.2 mg to intrathecal bupivacaine for Caesarean section, and demonstrated a significant improvement in both intraoperative and postoperative analgesia. In view of potentially serious respiratory depression associated with the use of intrathecal opioids, this technique should be reserved for units capable of adequate levels of postoperative monitoring.

Table 23.3 Level of subarachnoid block required for common surgical procedures

Level	Surgical procedure
T4–5	Upper abdominal
T6–8	Intestinal (including appendicectomy)
	Gynaecological pelvic
	Ureter and renal pelvic
T10	Transurethral resection of the prostate
	Vaginal delivery of fetus
	Hip
	Lower-extremity procedures with tourniquet
L1	Transurethral resection of the prostate (no bladder distension)
	Lower-limb amputations, etc. (without tourniquet)
L2–3	Foot
S2–5	Perineal
	Haemorrhoidectomy
	Anal dilation, etc.

Greene reviewed the factors influencing the distribution of local anaesthetics within the CSF.[44] Many factors have been implicated. The determinants of subarachnoid distribution of local anaesthetic solutions may be classified in the following manner.

Major determinants

1. Baricity of the local anaesthetic solution
2. Position of the patient during injection when using non-isobaric solutions
3. Dose of local anaesthetic
4. Site of injection.

Minor determinants (except in extreme situations)

1. Patient age
2. Patient height
3. Anatomical configuration of the spinal column
4. Direction of the spinal needle during injection
5. Volume of CSF

Controversial determinants

1. Volume of local anaesthetic solution
2. Changes in posture after completion of subarachnoid administration of non-isobaric solutions.

These factors are interdependent. The total dose of the agent used may have a more profound effect on the duration of the anaesthetic than on dermatomal spread.[45] A study by Shesky et al attempted to resolve these difficulties.[46] In a double-blind study, age, height, position and other factors influencing distribution were controlled. Seventy-two patients given glucose-free bupivacaine were divided into six equal groups. The concentrations, volumes and doses (mg) of bupivacaine injected are shown in Table 23.4. Levels of anaesthesia were significantly higher (T2–4) in patients who received 15 or 20 mg of bupivacaine (groups II, III, V, VI) than in patients given 10 mg (T5–8; groups I and IV). Levels of anaesthesia were similar in patients given the same dose of bupivacaine (groups I and IV), even though the concentration of bupivacaine and the volume injected differed. Patients given the same volume of injectate (2 ml) had levels of anaesthesia significantly higher when a concentration of 0.75% was injected (group V) than when 0.5% solution was used (group I). The dose of bupivacaine seems to be more important than the volume or concentration of injectate in affecting distribution. Volume, although a factor, is probably of secondary importance to dosage. This view has been confirmed by other studies.[47,48] In a study comparing the subarachnoid administration of bupivacaine 12.5 mg in a volume of either 2.5 or 10 ml, the maximum levels of sensory block were similar, demonstrating that subarachnoid distribution is determined by dose even when large variations in volume are employed.[49,50] Of course, dose, volume and concentration of anaesthetic solution have an inseparable relationship with each other, since dose is the product of volume and concentration.

Baricity of the anaesthetic solution is determined by the density of the solution relative to the density of CSF. Since the distributions of hypo- and hyperbaric solutions injected into CSF are subject to the effects of gravity, the baricity of the anaesthetic solution affects the distribution within the subarachnoid space. The use of posture to control the subarachnoid distribution of a hyperbaric solution has recently been questioned. Using non-isobaric solutions, the position of the patient at the time of injection affects the direction of subarachnoid spread, at least initially. Whether changes in posture after subarachnoid injection has been completed can be used to extend or limit subarachnoid distribution of the local anaesthetic is still controversial. In a study using hyperbaric bupivacaine 0.5%, the effect of a 15° head-down tilt for 10 min after injection was compared with the level after injection of the same volume with the patient maintained in the horizontal position; the average maximum levels of sensory block, although higher in the head-down group, did not differ significantly.[51] It appears that non-isobaric local anaesthetic solutions initially spread under the effect of gravity, but the extent to which posture can be used to direct subarachnoid distribution of a hyperbaric solution after injection has been completed remains controversial.

An isobaric solution is truly isobaric only when it is isobaric at 37°C and injected at 37°C. Plain solutions of bupivacaine injected at 37°C behave as hypobaric solutions, the resulting maximum levels of sensory block being both high and predictable[52] (Table 23.5).

Table 23.4 Concentration and dose of glucose-free bupivacaine and volume of solution used in six groups of 12 patients

Group	Concentration (%)	Volume (ml)	Dose (mg)
I	0.5	2.0	10
II	0.5	3.0	15
III	0.5	4.0	20
IV	0.75	1.3	10
V	0.75	2.0	15
VI	0.75	2.7	20

From Logan et al,[47] with permission.

Table 23.5 Doses of drugs (in mg) commonly used in hyperbaric blocks. These doses apply to solutions mixed in 2 ml of glucose 10%

Drug	Low block to L1	Mid-block to T10	High block to T6
Lignocaine	25	50	75
Bupivacaine	7	10	12
Amethocaine	5	10	12

Effects of subarachnoid block

The injection of local anaesthetic solutions into the subarachnoid space produces important and often widespread physiological responses. The key to successful management of central somatic blockade is an understanding of the aetiology and significance of these physiological responses.

Cardiovascular. The response of the cardiovascular system to central blockade is a result of the combined effects of autonomic denervation and, with higher levels of neural blockade, the unopposed added effects of vagal nerve activity. Sympathetic denervation is complete at the T1 level. Plasma concentrations of local anaesthetics during subarachnoid block are much lower than those required to produce direct effects on either the myocardium or peripheral vascular smooth muscle. Sympathetic denervation produces arterial and arteriolar denervation, but following acute pharmacological sympathetic denervation, the arterial side of the circulation retains a significant degree of autonomous tone. Consequently, the total decrease in systemic vascular resistance is of the order of 15–18% in normal, normovolaemic subjects even in the presence of total sympathetic denervation, provided that cardiac output is kept normal.[53] The venous circulation retains no significant tone following acute pharmacological denervation and venous return depends on the position of the patient, especially during high spinal anaesthesia. Thus, severe hypotension is due to decreases in preload associated with peripheral pooling of blood in vasodilated capacitance vessels, or to hypovolaemia, or both.

Respiratory. The height of the spinal anaesthetic determines the degree of effect on respiratory function. Low subarachnoid block has no effect on function. As the height of blockade ascends, there is a progressive increase in intercostal muscle paralysis. However, this has very little effect on respiratory efficiency in the supine resting surgical patient.[54] Even with profound blockade up to high thoracic or low cervical areas, arterial blood gases are usually normal (except in the grossly obese) because of adequate diaphragmatic excursion. However, these patients are compromised in their ability to expectorate effectively as a result of abdominal and thoracic wall muscle paralysis. Failure of ventilation is usually due to significant hypotension, with resultant inadequate perfusion of the respiratory centre. Although the clinical situation should not be allowed to deteriorate to this degree, if necessary, treatment of such failure should focus on ventilatory assistance, airway protection and reversal of hypotension.

Other. The degree of reduction in hepatic blood flow during subarachnoid blockade is reflected by the degree of reduction of arterial pressure.[55] There is insufficient evidence to demonstrate beneficial or adverse effects of subarachnoid block in patients with pre-existing liver disease. Renal blood flow is protected by autoregulatory mechanisms, and in the absence of severe hypotension (mean arterial pressure <50 mmHg), renal blood flow is unaffected. The effect of subarachnoid block on suppression of the stress response is related to the duration of block, and when sensation returns, metabolic and hormonal responses to surgical stimulation become indistinguishable from those in patients who have received general anaesthesia. To date, no study has demonstrated conclusively that regional anaesthesia has a significant modifying effect on metabolic and endocrine responses to surgery relative to any other anaesthetic technique.[56] Preganglionic fibres from T5 to L1 are inhibitory to the gut. Mid thoracic anaesthesia results in excellent operating conditions for intra-abdominal procedures due to the combination of a contracted gut (unopposed vagal activity) and complete relaxation of the abdominal wall musculature.

Complications of subarachnoid block

Hypotension. The indications for treatment of arterial hypotension during subarachnoid block should be considered with respect to the effects on the organs most susceptible to diminution in oxygenation — the heart and the central nervous system. A decrease in mean arterial pressure of the order of 15–20% is acceptable in both normotensive and hypertensive subjects during subarachnoid blockade. Recognition of the fact that myocardial work and oxygen requirements diminish to essentially the same extent as does myocardial oxygen supply during moderate levels of arterial hypotension has altered previous concepts of when and how hypotension should be treated during subarachnoid anaesthesia. Physiological treatment of hypotension during subarachnoid anaesthesia consists of restoration of preload by increasing venous return to the heart.

This is accomplished simply by placing the patient in a Trendelenburg position of 20°. Extreme Trendelenburg positions should be avoided as extensive distension of the jugular venous system may be counterproductive. Failure to restore arterial pressure to acceptable levels by physiological means requires rapid infusion of intravenous fluids such as compound sodium lactate (1.5–2 l) or a synthetic colloid such as Haemaccel (0.5–1 l). In addition, a vasopressor may be required. The ideal vasopressor would be one acting selectively to produce venoconstriction, without effects on afterload, heart rate and myocardial contractility. Unfortunately, such an agent is not currently available. If heart rate is rapid, incremental doses of an agent such as methoxamine or metaraminol, titrated to effect, are appropriate. If heart rate is slow, or if the patient is taking a β-blocker, an agent such as ephedrine is suitable. Attention to voiding of urine peri-operatively is required if the patient receives large volumes of fluid intravenously during subarachnoid block.

Nausea and vomiting. Nausea and vomiting during anaesthesia have many causes. However, if they occur during the early stages of establishing a block, hypotension is usually the cause, and the best treatment is reversal of hypotension. Atropine often helps if bradycardia is present. The occurrence of nausea and/or vomiting during established block is usually due either to an inadequate level of anaesthesia, or to unrecognized hypotension.

Post-dural puncture headache. Post-dural puncture headache (PDPH) occurs when leakage of CSF through a dural hole lessens the cushioning effect on the brain, allowing it to sag within the intracranial vault and causing traction on pain-sensitive cerebral structures. The incidence of headache varies from 0.2 to 24% and appears to be dependent on a number of factors.

1. *Needle diameter.* Tourtellotte et al[57] demonstrated a threefold decrease in the incidence of headache with a 26-gauge compared with a 22-gauge needle of the same tip design.
2. *Needle tip design.* Standard sharp-point spinal needles, such as the Quincke tip, cut dural tissue and allow dural tears to persist. Blunt or rounded-point needles (Greene, Whitacre, Sprotte) are believed to spread dural fibres and allow rebound closure after withdrawal of the needle. One study alleges an incidence of headache as low as 0.02% using 24-gauge Sprotte needles for 7175 diagnostic and surgical lumbar punctures.[58] This remarkably low incidence has been confirmed as less than 1% in a smaller study of patients undergoing Caesarean section.[59] A recent study[60] comparing the incidence of PDPH with 29-gauge Quincke and 22-gauge Whitacre needles indicated that the incidences of headache were 2 and 3.5% respectively. These studies indicate that improved needle-tip designs reduce but do not eliminate the incidence of PDPH.
3. *Needle bevel direction.* Needle punctures that part dural fibres longitudinally seem to produce less headache than those that cut fibres transversely (Fig. 23.6).
4. *Age.* The younger the patient, the higher the incidence of headache. Elderly patients are less prone to develop PDPH, and needle size and design may be less important as a factor.

PDPH is characteristically postural in nature, exacerbated by sitting upright, coughing or straining, and usually relieved by remaining supine. The onset of the headache is classically in the first or second day after puncture, but may occur within several hours of the puncture. The headache is described as typically bifrontal and occipital, and frequently involves the neck and upper shoulders. Associated symptoms may include nausea and loss of appetite, photophobia, tinnitus and depression. In more severe cases, diplopia and cranial nerve palsies are attributed to traction on cranial nerves, and indicate urgent treatment. The nerves most commonly affected are the abducent, the oculomotor and the trochlear. A variety of treatments have been used for PDPH including analgesics, non-steroidal anti-inflammatory drugs, steroids, abdominal binders, forced hydration and lying prone, none of which has been demonstrated consistently to be of benefit. Bed rest, analgesics and hydration constitute

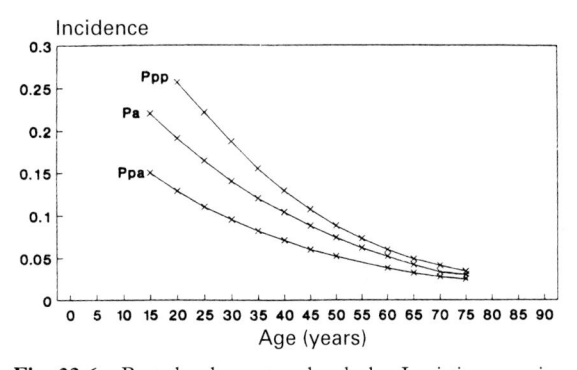

Fig. 23.6 Post-dural puncture headache. Logistic regression of incidence of post-dural puncture headache (Pa) in relation to age of patient. Note the different incidences when the needle is inserted parallel (Ppa) or perpendicular (Ppp) in relation to the longitudinal fibres of the dura mater. From Lybecker et al,[61] with permission.

accepted conservative treatment. There are three additional forms of treatment which are favoured.

1. *Epidural saline.* This usually involves a 24-h continuous infusion of saline 0.9% into the epidural space. Proponents claim a success rate of up to 90%, but a high relapse rate limits the technique.

2. *Caffeine therapy.* Caffeine probably relieves headache by reversing reflex vasodilatation of cerebral vessels. Oral and intravenous forms of caffeine have been used. Intravenous caffeine sodium benzoate 500 mg is 96% effective in treating PDPH, but over half of these patients experience recurrence of symptoms.[62]

3. *Epidural blood patch (EBP).* This remains the 'gold standard' for the treatment of refractory PDPH. The average success rate is 90–99%. Within 36 h of EBP, there is an 8% recurrence of PDPH, necessitating a second EBP.[63] Volumes of up to 20 ml of autologous blood are injected under sterile conditions into the epidural space, although Szeinfeld and colleagues[64] suggest injecting 12–15 ml, stopping when the patient complains of either back or leg pain. Some of the theoretical complications resulting from EBP are infection (meningitis or epidural abscess), adhesive arachnoiditis and radiculitis. Provided that a proper aseptic technique is used, EBP is considered a safe procedure, as complications are both infrequent and transient. The contra-indications to EBP are usually the same as those applicable to epidural block, the more important being evidence of back inflammation or infection, and septicaemia.

Urinary retention. Urinary retention occurs frequently in the postoperative period and is often due to persistent block of the nerve supply to the bladder. If large amounts of intravenous fluids have been administered, bladder distension may occur; this should be treated by urethral catheterization.

Backache. The incidence of backache following lumbar puncture varies from 2 to 25%.[65] The likely reason underlying this problem is probably the flattening of the normal lumbar curve secondary to relaxation of the muscles and ligaments of the back. The complaint of backache following atraumatic lumbar puncture is probably no more common than in patients who have received general anaesthesia.[66] Backache is ubiquitous in society with or without spinal puncture[67] and symptomatic treatment is generally all that is required.

Infection. Infection is an exceedingly rare complication of subarachnoid anaesthesia. The occurrence of infection, either localized or generalized (meningitis), usually implies a breakdown in the sterile technique.[68] A review by Kilpatrick & Girgis[69] of the incidence of meningitis following spinal anaesthesia detected the organism *Pseudomonas aeruginosa* in 17 out of 14 029 patients. Treatment necessitates meticulous bacteriological examination and administration of appropriate antibiotics.

Neurological sequelae. Reports of neurological damage[70,71] following subarachnoid anaesthesia are exceedingly rare, although concern has been expressed recently regarding the use of intrathecal catheters for continuous anaesthesia and the development of neurological sequelae.[26,72] Lund[65] reviewed over 500 000 cases of subarachnoid anaesthesia between the years 1948 and 1958, and found no cases of permanent motor paralysis associated with the technique. Nevertheless, awareness for the potential of this complication must exist, and all cases of claimed neurological impairment following subarachnoid anaesthesia must be evaluated critically. The important first step in any neurological complication is accurate diagnosis and treatment, and to this end early consultation with a neurologist is important. Anatomically, injuries following anaesthesia and surgery may be categorized into peripheral or central. Central injuries may be subdivided into cauda equina, spinal cord and intracranial. A complication in a unilateral peripheral nerve distribution is more likely to be secondary to trauma (direct or operative) or to positioning than to subarachnoid block. In contrast, bilateral involvement, whether cauda equina or higher up the spinal cord, is more indicative of a subarachnoid injury.

Preventive measures are obviously very important to avoid spinal or peripheral nerve injury. Strict attention to aseptic technique, injection of correct doses and concentrations of drugs and vasopressors, and careful positioning of the patient are of the utmost importance. However, unexplained neural deficits continue to occur after both regional and general anaesthesia.

Visual and auditory dysfunction. Vandam & Dripps[73] originally described a syndrome of decreased intracranial pressure following 9277 spinal anaesthetics. Leakage of CSF through a dural opening left by a spinal needle may result in a headache and associated symptoms of visual and auditory disturbance, probably as a result of decreased intracranial pressure. Ocular difficulties reported were double vision, blurring, difficulty in focusing, spots before the eyes, photophobia and difficulty in reading. Auditory complaints included decreased hearing, popping, tinnitus, buzzing and roaring. Additional reports followed of cranial nerve palsies after dural puncture, usually with involvement of the abducent nerve.[74] Ocular nerve palsy may appear 1 week after puncture and persist for weeks to months, usually with eventual return of functional vision. Minor hearing deficits after spinal anaesthesia have been observed on the second postoperative day in 42% of patients who underwent transurethral resection of the prostate.[75] Based on complaints of deafness (major hearing deficit), the incidence of vestibulocochlear dysfunction after spinal anaesthesia varies between 0.2 and 8%.[76,77] In addition to hearing deficits, hyperacusis following spinal anaesthesia has also been described.[78] The aetiology of auditory dysfunction after dural puncture is unclear. It may result from a decrease in CSF pressure that follows a leak in the lumbar dura which is transmitted through the cochlear aqueduct to the inner ear, resulting in endolymphatic hydrops. Hearing loss after subarachnoid anaesthesia is related to the size of the spinal needle; the larger the needle, the higher the incidence of hearing loss.[79] Hearing deficits are transient, although deficits may take several months to resolve[73] (Fig. 23.7).

Contra-indications to subarachnoid block

There are few absolute contra-indications to subarachnoid block, and the majority of contraindications are probably relative.

Usual contraindications include the following:

1. refusal by the patient, or patients who are psychologically or psychiatrically unsuitable
2. significant hypovolaemia or shock
3. infection at the site of injection
4. septicaemia or bacteraemia
5. raised intracranial pressure
6. abnormality of clotting.

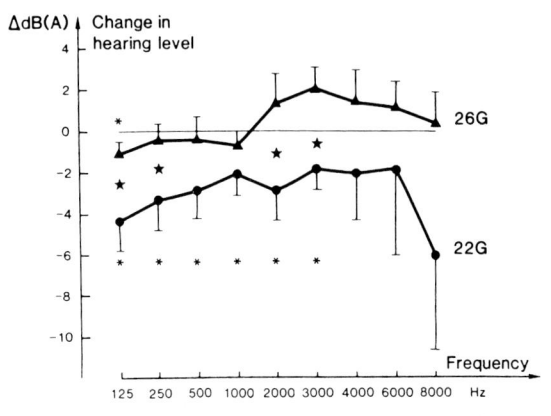

Fig. 23.7 Hearing loss after subarachnoid anaesthesia. Mean changes in hearing level ± standard error of the mean on the 'worse side' shown at each frequency. Negative values indicate decreased hearing. * Statistically significant changes in hearing level compared with pre-operative values.
★ Statistically significant intergroup differences. From Fog et al,[79] with permission.

At the present time, subarachnoid anaesthesia is *relatively* contra-indicated in patients receiving antiplatelet medications, aspirin, prophylactic low-dose heparin (Minihep), and other medications for deep venous thrombosis prophylaxis, even if there is no detectable abnormality of haemostasis on conventional testing, as the safety of performing regional anaesthesia remains unresolved. All forms of spinal nerve block are *absolutely* contra-indicated in any patient with demonstrable gross abnormalities in clotting, irrespective of treatment modality (see the section on *haemorrhagic complications and neuraxial block*, below).

Indications for subarachnoid block

Subarachnoid block has the advantage of being relatively easy to perform, rapidly induced and, even in untrained hands, predictable in spread. A disadvantage of the single-shot subarachnoid block is the relatively short duration of effect, which has potentially serious implications for the unexpectedly long surgical procedure. Some surgical procedures, such as transurethral resection of the prostate and repair of fractured neck of femur, are particularly suited to the use of a regional technique (usually subarachnoid block) to reduce intra-operative blood loss and to provide excellent early postoperative analgesia. Potential advantages of subarachnoid block in the area of operative delivery in obstetrics exist, not only from rapidity in onset of excellent anaesthesia, but also from an absence of placental drug transfer to the fetus. Anaesthetists trained in both epidural and subarachnoid anaesthesia recognize the advantages and disadvantages of both techniques, and very often the selection of one technique over another is a matter of individual preference and time.

Epidural block

The study of epidural block sustained interest in central neural blockade techniques in 1950 at a time when they seemed doomed to obscurity. For many years, caudal rather than lumbar epidural blockade was the preferred method of pain relief. The adaptation of Tuohy's spinal needle and the gradual recognition of the greater efficacy and safety of lumbar techniques led to a resurgence in popularity of epidural anaesthesia. By the early 1970s, there was increased understanding of the advantages of segmental block, with minimal local anaesthetic dosage, and thus reduced toxicity. Prolonged analgesia associated with minimal motor blockade with bupivacaine by a continuous epidural catheter technique became popular in both surgery and obstetrics. The advent of prolonged analgesia by the administration of opioids via the neuraxial route in the late 1970s extended the applications of epidural techniques into the area of chronic pain. The implantation of epidural catheters on a more permanent basis is currently increasing in popularity. There are important salient differences between epidural and subarachnoid techniques. The disparity between motor and sensory levels is usually more marked with epidural anaesthesia than with subarachnoid anaesthesia. The site of action of the local anaesthetic agents in producing sensory block during epidural anaesthesia is a matter of controversy. It is a segmental effect peripheral to the central conduits of the cord, probably at the level of the spinal ganglia[80] or on the nerves as they traverse the epidural space.

As with high subarachnoid block, the ability to cough is compromised by intercostal and abdominal wall muscle paralysis. Opinion is divided as to the potential beneficial effects postoperatively of epidural anaesthesia or opioid use.[81,82] In patients with severe pain, epidural block probably improves vital capacity and functional residual capacity as well as Pa_{CO_2}, at least in the early postoperative period. This may result in improved respiratory exchange and more effective coughing[83] (Table 23.6).

Epidural injection is commonly performed at lumbar sites. The caudal approach was, and still is, popular and useful. Cervical and thoracic approaches are used much less frequently, but do have indications for circumstances that require segmental block. The most popular site for injection is the mid lumbar area, as this is generally the easiest and safest point of entry to the epidural space. Because of the extreme angulation of the spinous processes in the mid thoracic area, midline puncture is difficult, and the paramedian approach is preferable. Because of the potential for traumatizing the underlying spinal cord, and a narrower epidural space than in the lumbar region, high thoracic and cervical epidurals should not be performed by the novice. Although trauma to the spinal cord is a possibility, neurological deficits after this procedure are rare if performed by an experienced operator. Anatomically, there is an additional safety feature if blocks are restricted to the mid thoracic area because the spinal cord is at its thinnest in the area between the two enlargements of the brachial plexus and lumbosacral plexuses. Thus there is a greater distance from ligamentum flavum to the dorsum of the cord in the mid thoracic than in the lower or upper thoracic areas.

The epidural space is identified by one of two methods:

1. *The loss of resistance technique.* This is perhaps the most frequently employed. A Tuohy or Crawford needle with stilette in situ is introduced into the ligamentum flavum via a midline or paramedian approach. The stilette is then removed and the resistance to injection is checked either intermittently or continuously as the needle is advanced slowly through the ligamentum flavum. As the needle enters the epidural space, there is sudden loss of resistance to injection of either air or fluid. A negative aspiration test for blood or CSF suggests that the tip of the needle is in the epidural space. Indicators such as spring-loaded pistons, small air-filled balloons, etc. have been described occasionally, and used to assist in demonstrating loss of resistance. However, none of these indicators is an improvement on appropriate manual dexterity.

2. *The hanging drop technique.* This consists of placing a fluid drop on the hub of the needle when the point is in the ligamentum flavum. The needle is advanced slowly through the ligament, and on entry into the epidural space, the drop is suddenly sucked into the needle, due to the negative pressure which is usually present in the epidural space. This method is not consistently reliable due to generation of a positive pressure in the space during manoeuvres such as breath-holding.

With the midline approach in the lumbar area, the ligamentum flavum is commonly encountered at a depth of 3–7 cm.[84] Once the needle has been inserted by 3 cm, continuous testing of resistance to injection is necessary. With paramedian approaches, the needle is inserted lateral to the spinous processes below the space selected for puncture. The needle is inserted parallel to the line of the vertebral spine, and the lamina of the vertebra is usually located at a depth of 4–7 cm. By 'walking' the needle in a cephalad and medial direction off the bony lamina, the ligamentum flavum is usually detected as a more pliant sensation.

Upon location of the epidural space, the distance

Table 23.6 Boundaries of the epidural space

Level	
Superior	Foramen magnum (fusion of periosteum of spinal canal and dura)
Inferior	Sacral hiatus + sacrococcygeal membrane
Anterior	Posterior longitudinal ligament
Posterior	Periosteum of anterior surfaces of laminae, articular processes, roots of vertebral spines, interlaminar spaces, ligamentum flavum

from the skin to the space is noted, and a nylon or Teflon catheter is advanced into the space. After withdrawal of the needle, the catheter is withdrawn until approximately 2–3 cm remains within the space. If more extensive threading of the catheter is planned, it should be performed under X-ray control with a radiopaque catheter to ensure accuracy. Without this, it is impossible to have any control over the direction of an epidural catheter (Table 23.7).

Epidural blockade often entails the use of the maximum safe dose of local anaesthetic, with resultant blood concentrations approaching toxic levels.[85] Consequently, a prerequisite to safe epidural anaesthesia is knowledge of both the pharmacokinetics and the toxicity of local anaesthetics. In contrast to subarachnoid block, local anaesthetics are deposited some distance from the neural target. Diffusion across tissue barriers is of great importance. Agents with a pKa close to physiological pH (e.g. lignocaine, pKa = 7.87) are most effective in terms of both lipid and water solubility. Epidural fat provides a potential reservoir for deposition of fat-soluble local anaesthetics such as bupivacaine. Less fat-soluble agents such as lignocaine tend not to accumulate. Repeated injections of lignocaine may result in a gradually increasing plasma concentration.[86] The epidural venous system provides a means for rapid absorption of local anaesthetic. The inclusion of adrenaline in the shorter-acting local anaesthetic solutions (usually 1 : 200 000 concentration) may greatly reduce vascular absorption, enhancing blockade and reducing the possibility of systemic toxicity. However, with the longer-acting agents, such as bupivacaine, the adrenaline effect dissipates before that of the local anaesthetic and there is little, if any increase, in duration of effect. Ideally, adrenaline should be added to the local anaesthetic solution immediately before use; the lower pH of commercially available adrenaline-containing solutions may result in reduced release of local anaesthetic base and reduced penetration of neural tissue because acidic solutions, containing anti-oxidants to stabilize adrenaline, release anaesthetic base poorly.

In order to facilitate onset and quality of blockade, carbonation of local anaesthetic agents readily releases base and has superior penetrating ability.[87] Evaluation of carbonated lignocaine in the epidural space[88] has shown that the addition of carbon dioxide to produce lignocaine hydrocarbonate improves the quality of sensory analgesia, particularly in the L5, S1 segments, which are often inadequately blocked using conventional lignocaine solutions in lumbar epidural anaesthesia.[89] Carbonation of lignocaine is associated with higher plasma levels of circulating lignocaine. DiFazio et al[90] demonstrated the desirable characteristics of epidural local anaesthetic solutions when the pH was adjusted towards the physiological range by the addition of 1 mmol of sodium bicarbonate per 10 ml of local anaesthetic solution. They demonstrated a more rapid onset of both analgesia and surgical anaesthesia, and a more rapid spread of the local anaesthetic solution in the epidural space, permitting very early identification of adequate levels of anaesthesia. Although the final levels achieved with local anaesthetics at 30 min are independent of pH adjustment, the rapidity of onset of adequate surgical anaesthesia with pH adjustment suggests that this method of administering local anaesthesia offers distinct advantages. However, this topic has been discussed for at least a decade and the use of pH adjustment has yet to find universal acceptance.

The agents used most commonly for epidural blockade are lignocaine and bupivacaine with or without adrenaline.

Lignocaine

Lignocaine is an excellent drug for epidural anaesthesia. Use of a 1% solution produces analgesia but a 2% solution is needed for operative procedures. It has a relatively rapid onset of action, and is of medium duration. Doses vary from 1.6 ml per segment of a 2% solution for young adults to half that for elderly patients.[91] Motor blockade with 2% is often limited to the myotomes adjacent to the site of injection; the further the myotome from the injection site, the less satisfactory the motor block.

Consequently, for lumbar epidural anaesthesia, there

Table 23.7 Dose, latency and duration of local anaesthetic-induced epidural anaesthesia. Data are for agents without adrenaline, which increases the duration of action of lignocaine by 50%

Drug	Concentration (%)	Dose (mg) per segment	Latency (min)	Duration (min)
Lignocaine	2	31	16	46
Bupivacaine	0.5	7	18	120

is often profound motor block of the hip flexors, but the patient can still actively produce plantar flexion of the feet. Tachyphylaxis (increasing dose requirements for maintenance of the same segmental spread of blockade) is common with shorter-acting agents such as lignocaine. Beneficial effects in terms of lowering local anaesthetic plasma concentrations and duration of block are seen when adrenaline is added to lignocaine,[92] although additional benefits do not occur if adrenaline concentrations in excess of 1 : 200 000 are used.

Bupivacaine

Bupivacaine is characterized by a slower onset of action than lignocaine. Anaesthesia at the upper and lower limits of the block recedes earlier, but persists for a considerably longer period at the level of the block. Ideally, for postoperative analgesia, positioning of the catheter centrally in the dermatomal area of maximal discomfort results in maximal analgesia, with minimal spread of local anaesthetic to areas not requiring blockade. This facilitates early postoperative ambulation. With lumbar anaesthesia, bupivacaine often does not penetrate into the central core of the large S1 and L5 nerves,[89] which frequently results in a sparing of sensation in the distal distribution of the nerves over the foot.

Anaesthetic sparing of lower lumbar and sacral segments

The use of long-acting agents such as bupivacaine in lumbar epidural anaesthesia may result in inadequate anaesthesia in the lower leg and foot. This is almost certainly due to lack of penetration of the drug into the larger L5 and S1 nerve roots. This lack of penetration is less evident with lignocaine.[93] However, if adrenaline is not included in the lignocaine solution, satisfactory caudal analgesia frequently does not result.[92] If a block is required in the L5 and S1 dermatomes, a low lumbar approach should be used and the catheter directed caudally. Alternatively, a caudal approach to the epidural space may be used (Fig. 23.2).

Epidural anaesthesia occasionally results in prolonged postoperative motor block, contributing to immobilization and anxiety, and extended stay in the recovery room. In such cases, it is desirable to reverse or antagonize motor block. Until recently, it was believed that regional block was not amenable to reversal techniques. However, in vitro studies[94] demonstrate that local anaesthetic-induced neural blockade can be rapidly reversed by washing isolated nerve preparations with crystalloid solutions. Johnson et al[95] recently demonstrated clinically that the duration of motor (but not sensory block) can be reduced by 50% by washing out the epidural space with aliquots of 15 ml injections of crystalloid solutions on three occasions in the immediate recovery period.

Choice of local anaesthetic

Great flexibility of sensory and motor block can be obtained by careful choice of both type and concentration of drug. The requirements for profound sensory block with excellent muscle relaxation (e.g. operative obstetrics) are best met with lignocaine 2% with adrenaline. Bupivacaine 0.5% (with or without adrenaline) is probably the drug of choice for long surgical procedures necessitating repeated top-ups. Satisfactory postoperative analgesia is accomplished with minimal motor block by intermittent or continuous administration of bupivacaine. For intermittent injections, concentrations of bupivacaine varying from 0.125 to 0.25% are adequate, and for continuous infusions, concentrations from 0.08 to 0.25% (with or without fentanyl 4 $\mu g.ml^{-1}$) have been used. The capability of local anaesthetics to block sensory and motor fibres differentially has been described.[96] Different concentrations of anaesthetic may be used to obtain selective block of sympathetic, sensory and motor fibres. Lignocaine 0.5–2% is useful for diagnostic and therapeutic blockade; 0.5% results in sympathetic block, 1% in sensory block and 2% in motor block. For diagnostic blockade requiring a prolonged duration of sensory block with no motor block, bupivacaine 0.25% is useful. Local anaesthetic mixtures (amide–amide, amide–ester) enjoyed a period of popularity because of perceived improvement in rapidity of onset combined with increased duration of analgesia. However, there is less need for use of mixtures, particularly if an epidural catheter is used.[97] Nevertheless, the amide–ester (lignocaine–amethocaine) mixture does have a long history of successful use for a fast onset and long-acting effect.

Assessment of epidural block

Evaluation of an adequate level of anaesthesia is essential before surgical incision. Clinical modalities commonly used to assess the level of anaesthesia include determination of extent of sensory, sympathetic and motor block and the presence or absence of reflex responses.

Sensory block. Two methods commonly used to assess sensory loss are loss of pinprick sensation and loss of temperature sensation. Either modality requires testing in each dermatomal area on each side of the body in a sequential fashion. The use of an alcohol swab or ethyl chloride spray to assess loss of temperature is the most sensitive indicator of initial onset of sensory block.

Sympathetic block. Onset of sympathetic block may be indicated clinically by the patient reporting an increase in warmth in both lower limbs, or by observation of cutaneous vasodilatation and palpation of increased skin temperature in the blocked areas. Quantification of sympathetic block may be achieved simply by measurement of temperature rise in the blocked areas. Skin conductance changes can be measured by psychogalvanic responses. More precise methods (but of research application only) are the use of cobalt blue and starch iodine, or the response of skin plethysmography to ice during venous occlusion plethysmography.

Motor block. This is usually assessed by the Bromage scale[98] for motor block in the lower limbs (Table 23.8).

Reflex response. Crude assessment of sensation can be made by use of the reflex response to pinch by a forceps at appropriate segmental levels. Reflexes such as cremaster, anal and abdominal may be useful as a rough guide to the adequacy of block.

Complications of epidural block

The complications of epidural block have been reviewed recently[99] and may be classified in the following manner.

General complications

Local anaesthetic toxicity. This is one of the most common complications reported with all regional techniques. Toxicity may result from allergy, idiosyncracy, local effects or systemic effects. Allergic reactions are very rare and are associated with the preservative in local anaesthetics esters. Local effects of local anaesthetics refer to effects of the drugs or additives on local tissue (nerve or muscle). Cases of adhesive arachnoiditis following subarachnoid injection of 2-chloroprocaine have been associated with the injection of the additive sodium bisulphite.[100] Systemic effects of local anaesthetics account for the majority of side-effects of local anaesthetics. Systemic effects most frequently occur following accidental intravascular injection or gross overdose. Symptoms and signs of local anaesthetic toxicity include peri-oral numbness, tingling, visual and auditory disturbances, twitching, grand mal seizures, coma and death. With proper care and attention, serious toxic effects of local anaesthetic drugs can be minimized during epidural block (see the section on the test dose below). Attempts to reverse an epidural anaesthetic by crystalloid infusion[101] resulted primarily in reduction of motor rather than sensory block (Fig. 23.8).

Neurological. This subject has been discussed above, under complications of subarachnoid block. Permanent neurological injury after epidural block is rare, and transient neurological injury uncommon.

Failure. Failure rates may be reduced by proper selection of patients, timing and the skill of the anaesthetist. Failure of the technique may occur if diminution of neural blockade occurs after repeated epidural injection. A single repeat dose (20% of the total dose) will consolidate the established level of block, but will not extend the level of anaesthesia. A second dose of approximately 50% of initial dosage will maintain the initial segmental level of anaesthesia if given when the upper level of segmental anaesthesia has receded one or two dermatomes. If a segment is missed or a block is inadequate on one side, it is worthwhile turning the patient on that side and injecting 2% lignocaine with 1 : 200 000 adrenaline. Inadequate motor block within

Table 23.8 Bromage scale (percentage motor block)

Degree of block	Action possible
No block (0%)	Full flexion of knees and feet
Partial (33%)	Just able to flex knees, full flexion of feet
Almost complete (66%)	Unable to flex knees, still flexion of feet
Complete (100%)	Unable to move legs or feet

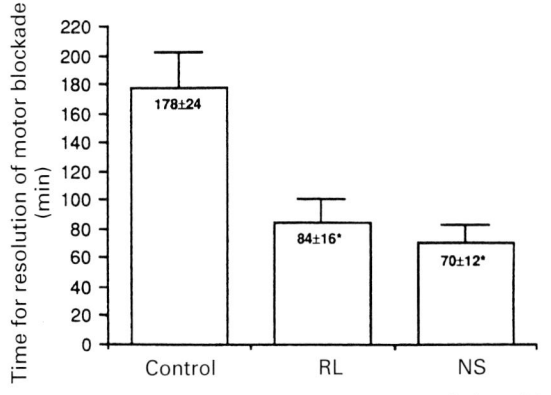

Fig. 23.8 Reversal of motor block by epidural infusion with crystalloid infusion. Duration between end of operation and resolution of motor block in control subjects and the effects of infusion with epidural crystalloids.
RL = Ringers lactate; NS = normal saline. ★P = 0.05. From Johnson et al,[95] with permission.

the segmental area blocked requires further injection, 30 min after the initial injection, of approximately half this dose, preferably as 2% lignocaine with adrenaline.

Total spinal anaesthesia. Total spinal anaesthesia occurs most frequently when a large quantity of local anaesthetic drug intended for the epidural space reaches the subarachnoid space. Total spinal anaesthesia is characterized by a rapid onset of flaccidity, apnoea, unconsciousness and circulatory collapse. Treatment includes ventilation and circulatory support.

Medication errors. These errors usually involve overdose, injection of the wrong solution or injection into the wrong site. Potassium chloride has been injected into the epidural space causing permanent damage.[102] The risk of medication errors may increase because catheter techniques are being used more frequently in the postoperative period.

Catheter techniques. The following problems may occur — threading difficulties, kinking, occlusion, migration (intravascular, intradural), knotting, infection and breakage. These complications may be reduced by observation of the rule that once the catheter is through the needle, it must never be withdrawn with the needle in place; in addition, only a short length of catheter (2–3 cm) should be left within the epidural space.

The issues of backache and headache have been discussed under complications of subarachnoid block, above.

Haemodynamic effects. Hypotension is one of the most consistent complications reported during subarachnoid and epidural anaesthesia. The onset of sympathetic block is usually slower with epidural anaesthesia than with subarachnoid block and this often permits adequate compensatory vasoconstriction in unblocked segments.[103] However, much higher plasma concentrations of local anaesthetic follow induction of epidural block, producing systemic effects. Nevertheless, although mean arterial pressure changes are often similar in both groups, the net effect on tissue perfusion may be increased in the epidural group if adrenaline is added to the local anaesthetic. Due to low circulating concentrations of adrenaline which result from absorption from the epidural space, a marked β-adrenergic stimulating effect stimulates an increase in cardiac output. Doses of adrenaline in the range of 80–130 μg, as used in epidural block, produce a moderate increase in cardiac output and heart rate, and decrease mean arterial pressure.[104] Bonica et al[105] found that normovolaemic human volunteers were well able to compensate for vasodilatation with blocks as high as the fifth thoracic dermatome. However, anaesthesia above this level also blocks cardio-accelerator fibres, with appreciable changes in blood pressure, heart rate and cardiac output. In general, a 30% decrease in systolic blood pressure should be treated by the methods outlined above.

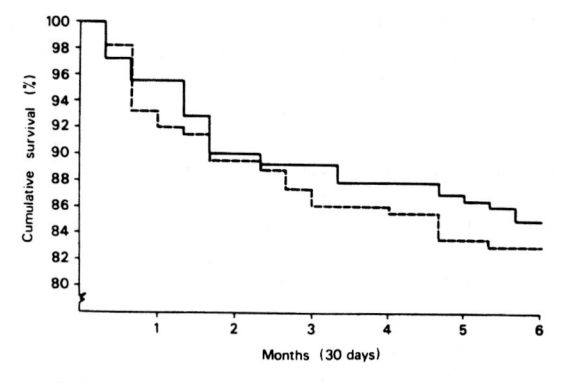

Fig. 23.9 Mortality after surgery for repair of fractured hip. Survival compared between patients who had general anaesthesia (solid line) and patients who had regional anaesthesia (dashed line). There was no difference in this nationwide (New Zealand) multicentre study. From Davis et al,[106] with permission.

Mortality

Although posing significant theoretical advantages at times, no significant improvement in mortality has been demonstrated in studies to date[106] (Fig. 23.9).

The test dose in epidural anaesthesia

A test dose is defined as the injection of a dose of drug sufficient to reveal an effect or the absence of an effect of the drug in question. The dose should be so small that the risk of side-effects or toxic reactions is at a minimum. In epidural anaesthesia, the test dose is classically used to detect intravascular injection or inadvertent subarachnoid injection. The epidural space contains blood vessels situated laterally as well as in the midline; these drain into the inferior vena cava and the azygous system. The catheter tip may lie within an epidural blood vessel in up to 9–11% of cases.[107] Migration of the catheter during the course of a continuous block may also occur.[108] The frequency of inadvertent perforation of the dura varies with the experience of the anaesthetist and may occur in up to 2.5% of cases. As a result, the catheter may be placed in either a subdural or a subarachnoid position. The consequences of intravascular and subarachnoid injection are described above. Subdural injection may be more common than previously believed. A very extensive block, usually of slow onset and associated with respiratory impairment, usually results.[109] Ideally, the test dose should be large enough to produce a distinct subarachnoid block if deposited intrathecally, yet small enough for the block to be limited. Doses of lignocaine of 60–100 mg or bupivacaine 10–15 mg should be sufficient for this purpose. In epidural anaesthesia, a period of at least 3 min is required to manifest an inadvertent subarachnoid block. If injected intravascularly, mild subjective symptoms should be produced without endangering the condition of the patient.

The addition of 15 μg of adrenaline is regarded[110] as sufficient to cause an increase in heart rate of >20 beats.min^{-1}. The effects of intravascular injection usually appear within 2 min. The reliability of the test dose has been questioned, especially in the area of obstetrics.[111,112] The suggested test dose with adrenaline does not appear to be an ideal procedure. It does not guarantee identification of the two most serious complications of epidural anaesthesia — intravascular and subarachnoid injection. However, there is no single measure that detects these complications absolutely. Alternative test doses have been suggested, including the use of air.[113] Advocates of this technique suggest that the injection of 1 ml of air into an epidural vein produces clearly audible changes in heart sounds monitored with a precordial stethoscope.

In general, the test dose can be of help in certain circumstances, but the performer of the block must be aware of its limitations. The use of a test dose does not exclude other precautions. Any injection should be preceded by an aspiration test. The administration of local anaesthetic by slow injection and the use of fractional doses with close observations of the patient's reactions are very important safety features.

Haemorrhagic complications and neuraxial block

Serious neurological sequelae following epidural analgesia are rare; the incidence of paraplegia is probably less than 1 in 10 000 procedures.[114] One of the more important factors contributing to paraplegia is extradural bleeding with the formation of haematoma.[115] Patients receiving anticoagulation and/or thrombolytic therapy pre-operatively are not considered suitable for a regional technique because of the risk of potential haemorrhagic complications.

The risk of developing spinal haematoma requires clarification in patients who:

- receive low-dose standard or low-molecular-weight heparin (LMWH) for thromboprophylaxis
- are anticoagulated intra-operatively
- receive thrombolytic therapy pre-operatively
- receive oral anticoagulants and antiplatelet medications preoperatively.

The use of regional anaesthesia in patients on low-dose standard heparin (heparin, 5000 IU subcutaneously every 8–12 h) has been questioned.[116] Following subcutaneous administration, the anticoagulation effect is observed in 40–50 min and usually returns to baseline in 4–6 h. A wide variation in the response of activated partial thromboplastin time (APTT) to subcutaneous heparin makes it difficult to formulate a generalized recommendation for regional anaesthesia.[117] A number of studies[118,119] report the safe use of epidural and subarachnoid anaesthesia in patients receiving pre- and postoperative low-dose heparin. However, there are at least two reported cases[116,120] of epidural haematoma occurring in patients who had received low-dose heparin. The conflicting results of these studies and the rarity of complications make it difficult to assess the relative risk of the use of low-dose heparin in regional anaesthesia. Several studies[121,122] have reported on the use of heparinization intra-operatively approximately 1 h after epidural and/or subarachnoid injection, without neurological sequelae. However, Ruff & Dougherty[123] studied 342 patients who received a diagnostic lumbar puncture for evaluation of acute cerebral ischaemia and were subsequently anticoagulated. Seven patients developed a documented spinal haematoma (5 with paraperesis, 2 with severe back pain). Eighteen patients complained of radicular pain lasting more than 48 h. Traumatic needle placement, initiation of anticoagulation within 1 h of puncture or aspirin treatment at the time of puncture were identified as potential risk factors.

LMWHs have theoretical advantages over standard heparin as peri-operative thromboprophylactic agents with low bleeding potential. Distinguishing pharmacodynamic properties of LMWHs over standard heparin include a longer biological half-life, less variable anticoagulant response to weight-adjusted doses, and close to 100% bio-availability after subcutaneous administration. LMWHs have a more selective mode of action on the coagulation cascade, resulting in a selective inhibition of factor Xa without accelerated inhibition of thrombin. Consequently, the effects of LMWHs cannot be monitored by routine tests such as prothrombin time, APTT and thrombin clotting times, but may require determination of antifactor Xa level.[124] Recent reports[125] document potential clinical advantages of LMWHs, particularly in patients undergoing orthopaedic procedures, which may result in increased use of these agents in the peri-operative period. The overall safety of LMWHs, and in particular assessment of the risk of spontaneous haemorrhagic complications, has not yet been determined. However, a recent case report[126] of a spontaneous spinal subdural haematoma in a patient receiving LMWH suggests the need for caution. Further research is required in this area.

Thrombolytic agents commonly used clinically include streptokinase and recombinant tissue plasminogen activator (rTPA). These agents act primarily by decreasing plasminogen levels and by antiplatelet effects. After thrombolytic therapy, fibrinogen and plasminogen levels are maximally depressed at 5 h and remain depressed for at least 24 h. Generally, invasive procedures should be avoided in patients receiving thrombolytic therapy.

Occasionally, patients present for surgery while taking oral anticoagulants (warfarin, dicoumarol). The anticoagulant effect of these drugs is not immediate, but is dependent on the reduction of the level of vitamin K-dependent clotting factors. Even with high loading doses of warfarin, anticoagulation is not therapeutic for 48–72 h. The anticoagulant effect persists for 4–6 days after therapy is terminated. Patients who have received one or two doses of an oral anticoagulant will not have an increased prothrombin time and may safely undergo regional anaesthesia.

Antiplatelet therapy includes medications such as aspirin, Naprosyn and dipyridamole. Horlocker and colleagues[127] reviewed the records of 805 patients who had received pre-operative antiplatelet therapy, and in whom a total of 1013 spinal or epidural anaesthetics had been performed. No patient developed signs of spinal haematoma or postoperative neurological deficit. Prolongation of the bleeding time may theoretically increase the risk of haematoma formation with these agents. Benzon et al[128] noted that in patients taking aspirin in a variety of doses, those with a bleeding time of up to 10 min did not develop a haematoma after epidural or spinal anaesthesia. However, bleeding time is not always a reliable indicator of platelet function.[129] Although bleeding time may normalize within 3 days after aspirin ingestion, platelet function may take up to a week to return to normal. Ferraris & Swanson[130] demonstrated a lack of correlation between aspirin-induced prolongation of the bleeding time and surgical blood loss. The risk of neuraxial blockade in patients receiving antiplatelet therapy remains controversial and largely unstudied. Of the available studies,[127,131] the results are conflicting. The risk of developing haemorrhagic complications appears to be increased in difficult or traumatic needle placement, and if an epidural technique rather than subarachnoid block is used in elderly patients. Analysis of thrombo-elastography yields qualitative information about platelet function, thromboplastin generation and their interaction with the intrinsic cascade to form a stable clot. Additional information is obtained from fibrinogen and factor XIII levels as well as the fibrinolytic system. It is conceivable that thrombo-elastography may play an important role in detection of bleeding diatheses in patients undergoing regional techniques in the future. In the interim, patients should be evaluated on an individual basis in terms of the risks and/or[132] benefits of receiving prophylactic deep venous thrombosis therapy and the risks and/or benefits of a regional technique as opposed to a general anaesthetic technique.

Recommendations for patients receiving or about to receive anticoagulant therapy

1. Spinal/epidural anaesthesia is contra-indicated within 24 h of:
   (a) receiving thrombolytic therapy
   (b) identification of a coagulopathy
   (c) significant thrombocytopenia.

2. Central block should be avoided in fully anticoagulated patients. Patients who have received one to two doses of an oral anticoagulant may undergo a regional procedure, but preferably, these patients should have a prothrombin time measured initially.

3. Patients fully anticoagulated with continuous intravenous heparin should have the infusion discontinued at least 4–6 h prior to needle or catheter placement, and the APTT should be measured. Subcutaneous heparin should not be administered 4–6 h before a regional technique is performed.

4. Epidural/spinal anaesthesia followed by systemic heparinization is probably safe provided that the following precautions are taken:
   (a) Heparin is not administered for at least 1 h after catheter placement or needle puncture.
   (b) The necessity to proceed with the surgical procedure should be reconsidered in patients receiving antiplatelet therapy and in those who will require subsequent heparinization after a difficult or traumatic catheter placement or needle puncture.
   (c) The catheter should not be removed for 4–6 h after the last heparin dose and further anticoagulation should not be initiated for at least 1 h.

5. Regional anaesthesia can be performed safely in patients receiving antiplatelet therapy. However, if a history of easy bleeding or bruising is obtained pre-operatively, the bleeding time should be determined.

6. A medium-duration local anaesthetic should be considered to facilitate postoperative neurological evaluation. Epidural block should be allowed to regress sufficiently before initiating continuous local anaesthetic infusion for postoperative analgesia. In these

Table 23.9 Pharmacological parameters of anticoagulants and antiplatelet agents

Agent	Bleeding time	Prothrombin time	Activated thromboplastin time	Time to peak effect	Time to normal haemostasis post-therapy
Intravenous heparin	↑	↑	↑↑↑	Minutes	4–6 h
Subcutaneous heparin	↑	↑	↑↑	40–50 min	4–6 h
Warfarin	—	↑↑↑	↑	4–6 days (3 days after loading dose)	4–6 days
Aspirin	↑↑↑	—	—	Hours	7 days
NSAID	↑↑↑	—	—	Hours	3–5 days
Thrombolytic agent	↑↑↑	↑	↑	Minutes	1–2 days

NSAID = non-steroidal anti-inflammatory drug.
Modified from Horlocker & Wedel,[133] with permission.

patients, use of neuraxial opioids is probably more appropriate.

7. The risk of developing spinal haematoma during central block in patients receiving thromboprophylactic LMWH is undetermined (Table 23.9).

If subarachnoid or epidural regional anaesthesia is used, it is prudent to wait for at least 1 h before intravenous heparin is administered following insertion of the needle. The effects of subcutaneous heparin on haemostasis may be monitored by measurement of activated clotting time and APTT. Elderly patients receiving aspirin or other non-steroidal anti-inflammatory drugs may be at increased risk of minor epidural haemorrhage following epidural anaesthesia.

Continuous subarachnoid anaesthesia

The first continuous subarachnoid anaesthetic was performed by Dean[134] in 1907, by leaving the spinal needle in place during the operation. The popularity of the continuous subarachnoid technique has not surpassed that of epidural methods, largely because of the high incidence of spinal headache from the large needles required to insert the catheter.

Advantages

1. Anaesthesia may be prolonged indefinitely.
2. Administration and careful titration of the anaesthetic can be achieved after the patient is positioned, minimizing cardiovascular instability.
3. The facility to use short-acting local anaesthetics shortens the recovery period.
4. Neuraxial narcotics may be administered for long-lasting postoperative analgesia.

Disadvantages

1. There is a high incidence of headache when large-bore needles are used to insert a large-diameter catheter.
2. Additional time is required for catheter (especially microcatheter) placement, which occasionally may be difficult or impossible.
3. There is an increased potential for infection, nerve injury and haemorrhage.

Advantages of continuous subarachnoid over continuous epidural block are that visualization of CSF flow increases the incidence of successful block, and the risk of systemic toxic reactions is eliminated by a significant reduction in the total dose of local anaesthetic required.

Indications and contra-indications for continuous subarachnoid anaesthesia are similar to those for single injection subarachnoid anaesthesia, but further indications are for critically ill patients, in whom slow incremental dosing minimizes haemodynamic changes, and whenever the duration of the operation might exceed the duration of the single injection technique (Table 23.10).

Polyamide catheters have an embedded stainless steel stilette that remains in place after insertion. This design is necessary to prevent kinking after insertion. Catheters of 27, 28 and 32 gauge require a special threading aid to be placed in the hub of the needle to guide and stiffen the catheter as it passes through the hub. Resistance may be felt as the catheter passes through the tip of the needle. Markings on the catheter aid in estimating the distance that the tip of the catheter has passed beyond the tip of the needle. Inserting the catheter by 2–3 cm is sufficient. Any of

Table 23.10 Types of continuous subarachnoid catheter

Type	Material	Gauge	Needle
Epidural	Nylon, Teflon	19, 20	17, 18
Spinal	Polyurethane	27	22
Spinal	Nylon	28	22
Spinal	Polyamide	28	22
Spinal	Polyamide	32	26, 27

the local anaesthetics used for single-injection anaesthesia may be used for continuous subarachnoid anaesthesia. Lignocaine 20–25 mg lasts approximately 30 min. For long procedures, bupivacaine 5 mg lasts for 30–60 min, and may be used to decrease the redosing interval.

Instances of inadequate anaesthesia may occur when small-gauge catheters are used.[132] This could be due to trapping of the catheter between the cauda equina nerves, so that the distribution of the local anaesthetic is not uniform. Another possibility is that, instead of being positioned cephalad and at the peak of the lumbar lordosis, the catheter tip is located too low in the intrathecal sac. Pooling of hyperbaric local anaesthetic is likely, and inadequate anaesthesia possible.

Recently, a number of reports have commented on the incidence of neurological deficits associated with continuous subarachnoid anaesthesia with microspinal catheters, characterized by perineal sensory loss and changes in sphincter function.[26] Cauda equina syndrome is a prolonged and possibly permanent neurological deficit characterized by one or more of the following: loss of bladder and/or bowel control; loss of perineal sensation; decreased sensation or mobility of the lower extremities. The Food and Drug Administration (FDA) in the USA recently issued a safety alert on the use of microspinal catheters based on 11 reports of cauda equina syndrome in which small-bore catheters (27-gauge or smaller) were used to deliver 5% lignocaine with 7.5% glucose to the intrathecal space. This compared with only 1 reported case of cauda equina syndrome associated with the use of large-bore catheters since 1984.

Review of these reports indicated the following similarities:

1. the use of 5% lignocaine (50 mg/ml) in 7.5% glucose
2. less than the expected anaesthetic effect for a given dose
3. an initial lignocaine dose of 100 mg or more to establish anaesthesia
4. a total lignocaine dose exceeding 100 mg.

A possible mechanism for these neurological deficits is maldistribution of 5% lignocaine in 7.5% glucose. Hurley[135] and Lambert[26] suggest that non-uniform distribution of the local anaesthetic results from low flow as the local anaesthetic leaves the catheter tip owing to the high resistance of the microcatheter.

To reduce the risk of neurological deficit, the following advice may be appropriate.

1. Do not thread the catheter more than 2 cm beyond the tip of the needle.
2. Limit the use of lignocaine 5% in 7.5% glucose to less than 100 mg in establishing the initial block.
3. If inadequate anaesthesia results, use a solution of different density and alter the patient's position to direct the local anaesthetic to the poorly blocked nerves.
4. Use less concentrated local anaesthetic.
5. Limit the total dose of drug administered in a manner consistent with the duration of the operation.

All anaesthetic methods have potential for complications. Although continuous subarachnoid anaesthesia is no exception, the advantages of this technique have much to offer in terms of improved patient comfort and safety.

PERIPHERAL NERVE BLOCKS

Upper extremity nerve blocks

As in other areas of the body, a critical understanding of the applied anatomy of the upper extremity is necessary, not only to accomplish the initial block procedure successfully, but also to identify what deficits, if any, remain following initial attempts at brachial plexus block, and to correct them.

Applied anatomy of upper extremity

The segmental nerve supply of the upper extremity is C5–8 and T1 and there is both craniad and caudad borrowing of the innervation of the skin supply from C4 (supraclavicular) on the craniad side and T2 in the armpit caudally (intercostobrachial nerve; Fig. 23.3).

After leaving the intervertebral foramina, the anterior primary rami of these nerves lie in the groove between the anterior scalene and the middle scalene muscles. They emerge in the posterior triangle of the neck posterior to the sternocleidomastoid muscle, pass through this area and exit the posterior triangle under the midpoint of the clavicle, to reach the axilla. Here, the nerves arrange themselves circumferentially around the subclavian artery, which acts as an identifying landmark when using the axillary approach to perform nerve block.

As the plexus emerges between the scalene muscles, it pushes forward a 'funnel' of prevertebral fascia. This well-defined layer of the cervical fascia surrounds the plexus circumferentially,[136] although there appear to be many septa dividing the interfascial compartment into several discrete, but probably communicating, entities.[137,138]

The main branches of the distal brachial plexus start to leave this fascial funnel quite high in the axilla.

The *musculocutaneous nerve* is the first to exit and, having left the fascial compartment, it plunges into the body of the coracobrachialis muscle, one of the smaller adductor muscles which attaches the coracoid process of the scapula to the upper humerus. Exiting this muscle, it emerges from its anterior surface beneath the biceps brachialis muscle, and continues down in the flexor compartment of the arm between the biceps muscle in front and the brachialis muscle behind. The nerve emerges from the lateral border of the biceps tendon at or near the flexion crease of the elbow and supplies sensation to the lateral border of the fore-arm from elbow to the snuff box.

The radial nerve leaves the brachial plexus in the axilla, curves around the posterior aspect of the humerus and, in slim individuals, can be palpated (and blocked) as it crosses the lateral aspect of the humerus at the junction of its upper two-thirds and lower third. It gives off most of its muscular branches in the arm prior to making a brief appearance in the lateral aspect of the antecubital fossa before proceeding down the forearm to emerge at the wrist where it can be blocked lateral to the pulsations of the radial artery. At the level of the flexion creases of the wrist, some terminal branches have already left the main trunk, and are proceeding dorsally and distally over the lateral aspect of the dorsum of the wrist and hand to supply the dorsal aspects of the lateral $3\frac{1}{2}$ digits (with the exception of the nail beds).

The *median nerve* leaves the brachial plexus and continues peripherally down the flexor compartment of the arm to emerge in the medial aspect of the antecubital fossa, immediately medial to the pulsations of the brachial artery. The nerve can be readily located and easily blocked at this site. It pursues a deeply situated course in the fore-arm and, proximal to the flexor retinaculum of the wrist, gives the superficial cutaneous branch which passes superficial to the retinaculum supplying an area over the proximal thenar eminence. However, the main branch of the median nerve passes deep to the dense flexor retinaculum along with the long flexor tendons of the digits, eventually supplying the ventral surface of the lateral $3\frac{1}{2}$ digits and also the nail beds (these being ventral structures that have migrated dorsally and carried their nerve supply with them).

The *ulner nerve* forms in the axilla and pursues a deep course in the arm, to emerge at the site familiar to most, at the medial aspect of the dorsal surface of the elbow sited between the olecranon and the medial epicondyle of the humerus (the 'funny bone' or 'crazy bone'). The ulnar nerve is readily blocked at this site; it is suggested the injection is made somewhat proximal to its actual site in the ulnar groove, to prevent any pressure effects from the expanding injection. The nerve then follows a deep course in the medial aspect of the forearm and is located peripheral to the ulnar artery (i.e. medial) at the level of the flexion creases of the wrist. Further peripherally (at the hook of the hamate), it divides into a deep muscular (motor) branch (supplying predominantly the deep muscles of the medial aspect of the palm) and its anaesthetically important cutaneous branches which supply sensation to the medial $1\frac{1}{2}$ digits on both ventral and dorsal aspects.

Nerve blocks for upper extremity procedures

The dense and compact nature of the brachial plexus and the relatively superficial and easily identified peripheral branches lend themselves well to regional anaesthesia procedures, which have been conducted extensively by practitioners since the discovery of local anaesthetics at the turn of the century. Some of these initial injections were performed after open dissection, but when percutaneous techniques were developed, a variety of approaches were described, and have been perfected and promulgated by many enthusiasts.

The initial attempts were to anaesthetize the brachial plexus at its most dense and compact site as it crosses the first rib, but because of the proximity of this site to the dome of the pleura, it results in a risk of pneumothorax; this risk should be about 1% in good hands but may be very much higher in less experienced hands. The supraclavicular approach is still a most effective form of anaesthetizing the upper extremity[139] and has been perfected over the years by a variety of protagonists. The technique most commonly used involves placing a needle over the mid-point of the clavicle, at a site 1–2 cm dorsal and craniad, inserting the needle in a vertically caudad direction, and attempting to find the first rib as an end-point.[140] There have been several variations added to this approach, each with its own enthusiasts, but the 1% or so incidence of pneumothorax remains. This has tended to encourage anaesthetists to seek and perfect alternative approaches and these have mainly pursued a more craniad approach (interscalene) or a more caudad approach (axillary) to avoid trespass on the pleura.

Interscalene block

The scalene muscles are δ-shaped muscles in the neck, with their base attached to the anterior or posterior tubercles of the middle cervical vertebrae. The apex of the anterior scalene muscle is attached to the first rib at the scalene tubercle, and the middle scalene muscle attached to more posterior aspects of the first rib. Their attachments are separated by the subclavian groove, which is occupied by the artery of the same name. The five segmental nerves (C5–8 and T1) which form the roots of the brachial plexus pass in this groove with the artery between the two scalene muscles, cross the first rib and enter the axilla.

The dense prevertebral fascia (which covers those muscles attached to the vertebrae in the neck, and separates them from the mobile viscera of trachea and oesophagus) covers the scalene muscles, and as the brachial plexus emerges through the gap between these muscles it pushes a funnel of fascia ahead of it, forming the brachial plexus sheath.

The branches of the plexus are stacked vertically as they emerge between the scalene mucles. A needle can be inserted between these scalene muscles, cephalad to the traditional supraclavicular approach; local anaesthetic can be deposited around these more craniad elements of the brachial plexus and, hopefully, it diffuses sufficiently caudad to give a satisfactory block. Alas, the caudad spread can often be deficient, so that surgical procedures involving the C8 and T1 components of the brachial plexus may be left with defective analgesia. However, craniad spread is more efficient than in the supraclavicular approach and the anaesthetic that is introduced into the interscalene groove (depending on the position of the patient) can spread cephalad to anaesthetize C4, C3 and even C2, providing analgesia of all of the ipsilateral neck and posterior scalp up to the areas innervated by the trigeminal nerve. Because of this spread, interscalene brachial plexus block lends itself well to surgery in and around the shoulder area (e.g. shoulder joint replacement) or along the pre-axial (thumb side) border of the upper extremity (e.g. Colles fracture repair).

Technique. The interscalene groove is identified at the level of the cricoid cartilage (C6) at the posterior border of the sternocleidomastoid muscle. This muscle can usually be identified easily in slim, long-necked individuals; in more corpulent, short-necked patients, it can be palpated by asking the patient to attempt forcefully to approximate the mastoid process to the supraclavicular fossa. Posterior to the sternomastoid muscle at the C6 (cricoid) level, the anaesthetist palpates for the interscalene groove. The scalene muscles are accessory muscles of respiration; with the spine fixed, they elevate the first rib. In normal respiratory patterns, they are not easily palpated, but if the patient takes forced inspirations (e.g. by asking the patient to gasp or sniff), then the scalene muscles are brought into action and can be palpated easily in all but the most corpulent (bull-necked) individuals. It is also possible to identify the interscalene groove in slim individuals by palpating the subclavian artery at the mid-point of the clavicle and following the groove craniad and medially.

With the interscalene groove identified, a short-bevel, short needle (i.e. a 22-gauge short-bevel $1\frac{1}{2}$ in (4 cm) needle) is inserted at the site where the posterior border of the sternomastoid muscle intersects with the horizontal line drawn from the cricoid cartilage. The needle is inserted in the skin at right angles to the slope of the neck, making a determined effort to have a distinctly caudad angle to its insertion, so that if its intended nerve contact does not occur, the needle will contact the vertebral bodies, rather than enter the intervertebral foramina. These pass downwards and outwards; thus, if the needle is inserted inwards then downwards, it is less likely to enter the intervertebral foramen, epidural and/or subarachnoid space or the spinal cord. If the procedure is undertaken for analgesia in the distal forearm or hand, then it is performed optimally with the patient in a semirecumbent position so that gravity assists the caudad spread of local anaesthetic solution. Paraesthesia to the C5 or C6 dermatomes (i.e. lateral aspect of fore-arm or thumb) confirms correct placement. If a nerve stimulator is used, contractions of the biceps muscle suggests appropriate placement.

The drug of choice is determined by the requirements of the operation. If the operation is of relatively short duration, lignocaine 1% with adrenaline 1:200 000 is appropriate; this produces a block that will last 2–4 h. If longer analgesia is required, bupivacaine 0.375% with adrenaline 1:200 000 would be appropriate, but the onset latency period is longer than that of lignocaine. For rapid onset and long duration, the author prefers lignocaine 1% plus amethocaine 0.1% (with adrenaline 1:200 000), and use 40–50 ml of this solution for a 70 kg individual.

The spread of anaesthesia is probably proportional to the volume of local anaesthetic injected. Because the drug is deposited near the smaller roots of the plexus, rather than the much larger trunks and cords, a weaker solution is frequently effective. Lignocaine 0.75% and/or bupivacaine 0.25% often provide excellent analgesia and permit the use of larger volumes which help to promote the more caudad spread for those surgical procedures that involve the postaxial border of the forearm.

If surgery involves the elbow joint or medial forearm and arm, it is essential to check specifically that the block has been effective in anaesthetizing this area. If it has not, then it is best to supplement analgesia by blocking the medial cutaneous nerves of arm and forearm; these are most easily blocked by the traditional axillary approach on the medial side of the axillary artery, high in the axilla (as for ulnar nerve analgesia in axillary block; see below).

Complications. Because the needle is inserted very close to the vertebral foramen, it is possible for drugs (even catheters) to enter the epidural space,[141] and if large volumes of local anaesthetic solution are used, it is not uncommon to produce a segmental epidural block. If unilateral segmental epidural block could be produced predictably, this would be an excellent form of anaesthesia. However, bilateral segmental epidural block can occur,[142] and if trespass of the dura mater occurs, either via a dural sleeve that extends peripheral to the foramen, or by inserting the needle too far centrally into the foramen, high (even total) subarachnoid (spinal) anaesthesia can occur. The other critical structure in this area is the vertebral artery as it passes through the foramina transversaria of the cervical vertebrae. It is possible, with a high placement in the interscalene groove and a less caudad angle to the needle, to enter the lumen of the vertebral artery[143,144] and even a very small volume of local anaesthetic (0.25 ml)[145] injected into this vessel can produce quite profound convulsions because it is a direct conduit to the brain. Fortunately, because the vertebral artery enters the foramina transversaria at C6, the needle contact is caudad to this entry site, and penetration of the vertebral vein (which enters the foramen at C7) is more likely, with less dire consequences.

Any of the other structures in this part of the neck may be involved in the spread of local anaesthetic. Recent studies have shown that the phrenic nerve is blocked whenever the interscalene approach is used.[146] However, because the patient is lying still on an operating table and not subject to any respiratory demands, this usually passes unnoticed. The diaphragm is dually innervated, its central fibres emanating from the phrenic nerve and its peripheral fibres from intercostal nerves. Consequently, unilateral phrenic block in a person at rest usually creates little or no respiratory difficulty.

If significant amounts of the drug are deposited anterior to the prevertebral fascia, then sympathetic block in the form of Horner's syndrome develops. If this occurs rapidly, then the anaesthetist should consider whether significant amounts of the drug have been placed superficial to the prevertebral fascia, and therefore that the quantity of drug around the plexus may be insufficient to produce an effective block. With a successful interscalene block, the later onset of Horner's syndrome is not unexpected, because the drug deposited in the interscalene groove tracks caudally in the paravertebral groove, eventually reaching the sympathetic nerves at T1 and T2.

If significant quantities of the drug are deposited superficial to the prevertebral fascia, the drug can pass on to other neural elements such as the recurrent laryngeal nerve, producing a hoarse voice; this happens infrequently, but when it occurs, the patient should be reassured of its temporary nature.

Axillary block

This block is used very commonly for surgical procedures distal to the elbow. It obviates the risk of pneumothorax and also the potential for central nervous system (neuraxial) spread of drug with its subsequent compromise of cardiovascular and respiratory stability. Because the drug is deposited more distally in the plexus, the more proximally supplied parts of the upper extremity are often spared in this block, and it is frequently unsatisfactory in surgery involving the proximal arm and elbow, and for the added nociceptive input of an inflated proximal tourniquet.

Initially, this block was performed by separate infiltration of the different neural elements of the brachial plexus as they clustered around the axillary artery. The medial cord (ulnar) lies on the medial side of the vessel, the lateral cord (median) on the lateral side of the artery and the posterior cord (radial) lies deep to the vessel in the axilla. The remaining fourth important branch to the upper extremity is the musculocutaneous nerve, which leaves the main brachial plexus group at a higher level in the axilla.

As indicated above, the brachial plexus carries with it a fascial sheath as it pierces the scalene muscles, and this sheath forms an envelope around the plexus and its derivatives. It does not appear to be the single-lumen tube described originally, but is probably divided by many septa.[126] Although a single injection into this sheath has been recommended to produce block,[136] it often fails to produce a complete block of all of the elements of the plexus.[139] For this reason, many anaesthetists (including the author) like to obtain subjective and/or objective evidence of placement of the drug alongside at least two, and preferably three, of the main neural components supplying the upper extremity.

Technique. This block is performed optimally with the arm at right angles to the body, with the patient's hand tucked behind the head if possible. It is feasible to perform axillary block in patients who cannot abduct their upper extremity to the desired 90°, but this requires innovation in technique and is usually performed optimally by individuals who already have a degree of expertise with the conventional approach.

The pulsations of the axillary artery are critical to obtaining a satisfactory location for needle placement. Although this artery is eminently palpable in the vast majority of subjects, there are some individuals in whom palpation is very difficult, especially the obese patient with large axillary folds of subcutaneous fat. Sometimes the artery cannot be palpated, and it is necessary to perform the block either by wide infiltration (less satisfactory and frequently inadequate) or by using a nerve stimulator.

Having pinned the vessel between the middle and index fingers of the non-dominant hand, a skin weal is made over the vessel. A needle is inserted through the weal, and manipulated to the medial and lateral aspects of the vessel while paraesthesiae are sought in the ulnar (little finger) or median (thumb) nerve distributions; 10 ml of local anaesthetic solution is injected at each site, with a further 10 ml injected posterior to the vessel. Ideally, paraesthesiae are obtained on the dorsum of the hand, indicating proximity to the radial nerve. However, having injected at least 20 ml into the sheath, it is probably less appropriate to seek further paraesthesia because of the risk of damaging a nerve whose peripheral fibres may already be anaesthetized.

In attempting to locate initial paraesthesiae and to detect the 'pop' through the axillary sheath, the axillary artery itself is penetrated occasionally; the flow of blood into the syringe is easily detected. If this occurs, it is best to insert the needle further, until it emerges from the posterior aspect of the artery, and then to inject a bolus of 15 ml of drug with a degree of confidence that it will be within the sheath. It is best then to seek ulnar and/or medial nerve paraesthesia, having withdrawn the needle back out through the anterior aspect of the artery. Some authors deliberately puncture the artery, depositing boluses of drug superficial and deep, and claim success.[147] The above manoeuvres usually produce satisfactory anaesthesia of the arm for the intended surgery.

The musculocutaneous nerve leaves the plexus proximal to the needle sites described. It can be blocked at one of two sites. The first site is in the axilla, where the nerve, having left the plexus proximal to the needle site, plunges into the substance of the coracobrachialis muscle, which is a relatively poorly defined muscle lying under the lateral aspects of the insertion of the pectoralis major muscle; although it can readily be palpated in some patients, it can be difficult to identify in others. A nerve stimulator used in exploring this muscle mass under the insertion of pectoralis major can help to locate the musculocutaneous nerve and a bolus of 10 ml of local anaesthetic will produce analgesia of the muscles of the anterior flexor compartments of the arm, and analgesia of the skin of the lateral aspect of the fore-arm from elbow to base of thumb. The second site is at the elbow. Since the musculocutaneous nerve is only sensory to the fore-arm, deficiencies of its block can be resolved by blocking just this sensory component. The nerve descends down the arm between brachialis and biceps muscles, emerging at the lateral aspect of the biceps tendon usually at or about the flexion crease at the elbow. The biceps tendon is easily palpated (if the nerve is not blocked) by active flexion of the arm. If the patient cannot flex the arm, then the nerve is presumably well on its way to being blocked. The nerve may be 1–2 cm above or below this line, and therefore can be blocked at the lateral aspect of the biceps tendon over an area 2 or 3 cm above and below the flexion crease. Because it pierces the deep fascia at a variable point in this course, it is optimally blocked by infiltrating a cuff of subcutaneous anaesthesia along the biceps tendon at that site (either superficial or deep to the deep fascia). This block can be performed quite successfully for anaesthetizing the radial border of the fore-arm in connection with teaching intravenous puncture and catheter placements in the cephalic vein.

As with all regional anaesthesia, it is critical to ascertain if the block is producing the desired effects before surgery starts, and therefore it is necessary to test the efficacy of the block as it develops so that deficiencies can be supplemented earlier rather than later. Different anaesthetists use different techniques to achieve this. Usually, motor weakness precedes sensory block. Lanz et al[139] claim that 90% of successful blocks show signs of motor weakness within 5 min. Clearly, testing flexion and extension at the elbow will determine the relative success of the musculocutaneous and radial nerve blocks, and testing the patient's grip will define motor weakness of median and ulnar nerves. We validate sensory block (which is obviously the most essential) with a relatively blunt pin. A safety pin is the optimal convenient instrument. Knowing the anatomy of the area, it is important to test along the ulnar side of the arm and fore-arm for block of the medial cutaneous nerve of arm and fore-arm respectively (which usually occurs quite early as the block spreads proximal to distal) to check the distribution of the ulnar nerve in the palm on the little finger and hypothenar aspect, and to test the median nerve on the thenar eminence and the volar aspects of the lateral $3\frac{1}{2}$ digits. Successful radial nerve block can be determined by checking sensation in the dorsal aspect of the interval between the thumb and the first metacarpal bone.

As mentioned above, the bête noir of axillary blocks is a deficiency of anaesthesia in the distribution of the musculocutaneous nerve. Consequently, flexion of the arm due to intact biceps and brachialis muscle power often persists, and should warn that the sensory component of the musculocutaneous nerve may be inadequately blocked; this can be confirmed by pinprick testing over the lateral (i.e. pre-axial) border of the fore-arm.

Rescuing inadequate blocks

Blocks at the elbow

Deficiencies of block of the main nerves of the arm can be easily identified using the techniques described above. Inadequate blocks may be salvageable by performing supplementary peripheral blocks. The *median nerve* can be located at the level of the flexion crease of the elbow, as the most medial content of the antecubital fossa, immediately medial to the pulsations of the brachial artery. At this point, with an appropriate skin weal and an infiltration of 5 ml of the anaesthetic of your choice, a median nerve block can be accomplished fairly predictably (it often occurs in infiltration for intra-arterial trespass at this point). The *ulnar nerve* is readily identifiable at the elbow. The nerve can be rolled and identified in the ulnar groove. Supplemental block is usually undertaken proximal to that groove, taking due care not to trespass on the nerve or to inject intraneurally. The *radial nerve* has very little sensory distribution in the upper extremity, and inadequate block can usually be supplemented adequately at the wrist. However, the nerve can be located in the arm above the elbow. Block at this site is performed approximately four fingers' breadth above the lateral epicondyle, where the nerve courses round the posterior aspect of the humerus in the radial groove, and can be rolled against the humerus in thin subjects. If the nerve cannot be identified by palpation, a needle is inserted at a site four fingers above the lateral epicondyle until the humerus is located, and 'walked' proximally and distally until radial paraesthesiae are obtained or appropriate twitching of the dorsal extensors of the wrist is seen when a nerve stimulator is used. Block of the *musculocutaneous nerve* has been described above.

Nerve blocks at the wrist

From the description of the anatomy above, it is relatively simple to produce blocks at the wrist. The radial nerve lies radial to the radial artery and the ulnar nerve is ulnar to the ulnar artery at the levels of the flexion creases at the wrist; a bolus of approximately 3 ml of local anaesthetic in appropriate relation to the artery can anaesthetize these two nerves effectively. However, the radial nerve has already given off dorsal cutaneous branches proximal to this site; these supply the posterior aspect of the lateral third of the hand and can be anaesthetized by extending the radial block at the radial aspect of the radial artery with dorsal infiltration over the lateral aspect of the wrist. The median nerve gives off a superficial palmar cutaneous branch which crosses superior to the flexor retinaculum and is usually adequately anaesthetized by the superficial infiltration with a skin weal performed in preparation for the main median nerve block. The median nerve lies more deeply between the long flexor tendons of the thumb and fingers. In the 75% of individuals who have a palmaris longus tendon, the needle should be inserted just on the medial side of this tendon. It punctures the flexor retinaculum with a very definite give, somewhat akin to a ligamentum flavum puncture. The needle is now sitting in the flexor tunnel along with all the flexor tendons, and a bolus of 3 ml of the local anaesthetic of your choice should anaesthetize the median nerve at this site.

Metacarpal and digital blocks

Individual fingers can be blocked by producing a wall of anaesthesia from dorsal to palmar skin on either side of the appropriate metacarpal bone, usually just proximal to its distal end (the knuckles). This can be a useful manoeuvre if a digit remains unblocked (and surgical trespass is imminent) while waiting for distal spread of the anaesthesia from a more proximally placed axillary or interscalene block.

Lower-extremity nerve blocks

In contrast to the upper limb, the nerve supply of the lower limb is much less compact, receiving contributions from much more widely spaced vertebral levels. The reason for this is that, as human beings have assumed the upright gait, large amounts of tissue have been 'borrowed' from the trunk into the substance of the thigh and have brought their nerve supply with them.

The skin and muscle of the anterior thigh are supplied by the lumbar plexus, whereas the posterior thigh and virtually all of the true leg (i.e. the lower extremity below the knee) are supplied from the sacral plexus via the sciatic nerve and is branches. Thus, the origins of the nerve supply of the lower extremity extend from L2 to S3. Because of this wide origin, the peripheral nerve supply of the lower extremity does not lend itself to single-needle techniques peripheral to the neuraxis. Therefore, in those patients in whom the elegant simplicity of single-needle subarachnoid or epidural anaesthesia is not appropriate, peripheral block usually needs to be accomplished with at least two, and usually more, separate needle insertions.[148] For this reason, these blocks are performed less commonly than upper-extremity blocks and are usually reserved for patients who have some pathological or personal contra-indication to more central needle insertion (e.g. spinal cord tumour, previous vertebral surgery, unstable spine, patient's preference, anticoagulation, etc.).

Basic anatomy

Lumbar plexus

This plexus is formed from the second, third and fourth lumbar nerves between the psoas major muscle and the quadratus lumborum muscles.

The major branch of this plexus is the *femoral nerve*, forming at the lateral border of psoas major muscle and passing behind the inguinal ligament lateral to the femoral artery. This supplies the main muscle mass of the thigh and the skin over the anterior aspects, plus a terminal twig (the *saphenous nerve*) which supplies skin on the medial aspect of the leg below the knee down to the ankle and beyond. The lateral part of the thigh has a separate nerve supply from the purely sensory *lateral femoral cutaneous nerve*, also emerging on the lateral border of psoas, passing around the pelvic brim and emerging into the lower extremity, a couple of centimetres medial and caudad to the anterior superior iliac spine, either behind or piercing the inguinal ligament at this point, and supplying an area of skin on the lateral thigh from hip to knee.

The most deeply situated branch of the lumbar plexus is the *obturator nerve* which enters the pelvis medial to the psoas major muscle and exits through the obturator foramen into the medial thigh where it lies within and supplies the adductor muscle mass, a variable area of skin over the medial aspect of the thigh, and a terminal articular twig to the knee joint by its deep muscular branch.

The sciatic nerve

This nerve originates in the branches of L4, L5 and S1–3 on the anterior concave surface of the sacrum and leaves the pelvis through the greater sciatic notch. It usually passes below the piriformis muscle, although in some instances the sciatic nerve divides into the medial and lateral popliteal nerves within the pelvis, in which case the lateral popliteal branch may sometimes pierce the piriformis muscle. The sciatic nerve then passes from its central gluteal position down the midline of the thigh to the popliteal fossa. At this point, it divides into a medial popliteal branch which continues as the *posterior tibial nerve* supplying, and deeply situated within, the calf muscles, as far as the foot, which it enters behind the medial malleolus to supply the medial part of the sole of the foot via its terminal plantar branches. The lateral popliteal nerve or *peroneal nerve* exits the popliteal fossa laterally, curving around the head of the fibula where it may be palpated (and easily blocked) subcutaneously. This nerve primarily provides motor distribution to the dorsiflexors of the distal extremity and provides sensation to the skin over the dorsum of the foot.

The lateral aspect of the foot is supplied by the *sural nerve* (a branch of the posterior tibial nerve) which exits the muscle mass of the calf to pass behind the lateral malleolus, supplying the lateral border of the foot.

These nerves can be blocked at various points, from their immediate origins in the paravertebral gutter through to the distal digital branches.

Traditional lower-extremity nerve blocks

These are usually accomplished by individual blocks of the branches of the femoral plexus as they emerge at the level of the inguinal ligament, with separate needle insertions for the obturator nerve, femoral nerve and lateral cutaneous nerve of thigh, together with a separate needle insertion in the buttock to anaesthetize the sciatic nerve.

The inguinal ligament extends from the anterior superior iliac spine to the pubic tubercle. To perform these blocks, the ligament is identified, and the pulsations of the femoral artery noted at the mid-point. The femoral nerve enters the thigh immediately lateral to the artery at this site, and has often divided into its terminal branch system about this point. A shallow bevel short 3–4 cm needle is usually satisfactory in normal-sized individuals. The nerve lies below the superficial skin structures and immediately deep to fascia lata. Paraesthesia in the anterior medial thigh may be elicited; if a nerve stimulator is used, contraction of the anterior thigh muscles can be produced. Femoral nerve block usually requires a volume of approximately 15 ml of local anaesthetic, although by forcing larger volumes into this site, proximal spread of the drug and more extensive femoral plexus block can be accomplished (see below).[149]

Lateral femoral cutaneous nerve

This entirely sensory nerve supplies the lateral aspect of the thigh, and emerges below the inguinal ligament 2 cm medial and caudad to the anterior superior iliac spine. Blockade can be accomplished by infiltration at this site (two finger breadths in and down from the anterior superior iliac spine) after seeking paraesthesiae in the lateral thigh, or by means of a fan-like infiltration of approximately 5 ml of local anaesthetic superficially at this site. If the injection here is delivered above the inguinal ligament by accident or intent, then the injected drug can spread along the fascial planes, and if sufficient volume is administered, can track proximally to produce variable degrees of block of the femoral and even obturator nerves.[150]

Obturator nerve

This is the most deeply situated branch of the femoral plexus. The nerve pursues an intrapelvic course, exiting into the medial thigh through the medial and superior aspects of the obturator foramen. It is blocked by inserting a needle approximately two finger breadths lateral and caudad to the pubic tubercle at the medial attachment of the inguinal ligament. This nerve is deeply situated, and usually requires a needle insertion of 3–4 cm, and sometimes more in large subjects, before neural contact is achieved. After entering the thigh, the obturator nerve divides into a superficial and a deep branch. It is the superficial branch that usually carries most of the sensory supply to the skin of the thigh. This sensory supply is variable but usually includes an area about the size of the palm of a hand over the middle third of the medial side of the thigh. The obturator is primarily a motor nerve supplying the adductors of the thigh, and location can be helped by using a nerve stimulator in this socially threatening anatomical area. Because it gives an articular twig to the knee joint, it is usually deemed appropriate to ensure block of the deep branch of the obturator nerve if surgery on the joint is to be performed under a peripheral nerve block. A dose of approximately 10 ml of local anaesthetic should be sufficient to anaesthetize both superficial and deep divisions of this nerve.

Alternative techniques. In an attempt to reduce the extent and degree of needle trespass, alternative methods have been sought to produce satisfactory anaesthesia of the lumbar plexus contribution to the lower extremity. Lumbar paravertebral block of the L2–4 nerves can be performed in the paravertebral gutter. Because of the communications among the paravertebral spaces, injection into one of these paravertebral locations usually creates spread to adjacent nerves. Paravertebral block is produced by inserting a 3–4 cm needle approximately 2 cm lateral to the craniad end of the lumbar spine of L3 and inserting the needle until it contacts the transverse process, when the needle is 'walked off' the caudad aspect, seeking paraesthesia of the anterior thigh (or myotomal contractions of the quadriceps and/or adductor thigh muscles with a nerve stimulator).

Other attempts to anaesthetize the lumbar plexus have been performed at more peripheral sites (between the paravertebral origins and the terminal branch sites described above) where the plexus is forming posterior to the psoas major muscle and anterior to the quadratus lumborum muscle. Attempts to enter this anatomical area, where the plexus is most compact, have been made from below (by endeavouring to force local anaesthetic proximal to the femoral nerve injection site, as described above) to the formation of the lumbar plexus at the pelvic rim between the psoas and quadratus lumborum muscles, with spread to the lateral femoral cutaneous and the obturator nerves.[149] A posterior approach to the same location has been described by Chayne and colleagues,[157] who introduced the needle paravertebral to the L5 spine superior to the L5 transverse process, and medial to the posterior superior iliac spine, attempting to detect a loss of resistance between the quadratus lumborum and psoas major muscles. There is a subtle loss of resistance that can be detected by the educated hand. A more predictable way of locating the plexus at this site is to use a nerve stimulator, seeking responses in the quadriceps or obturator muscle mass. Because of its intramuscular location, the end-point for performing this psoas compartment block is not predictable and this procedure has not been widely adopted. However, it can be useful in patients in whom a peripheral lower-extremity block is indicated, but access to the anterior thigh is compromised; the psoas compartment block permits satisfactory regional anaesthesia of the lower extremity with dorsal injections for both femoral plexus and sciatic nerves. It has special applicability in traumatized patients in whom the necessity to move the patient from supine to prone positions to accomplish peripheral block would be difficult.

Sciatic nerve

The sacral origins of the sciatic nerve are joined by the lumbosacral trunks of L4 and L5 to produce the sacral plexus. The sciatic nerve is the largest nerve in the body (about as wide as a thumb). It is situated deeply in the buttock, having left the pelvis through the greater sciatic notch; depending upon how well-padded the buttock is, it can sometimes be palpated in thin individuals. It is necessary to relax the gluteal muscle mass by turning the patient's toes in and heels out, which is an appropriate instruction prior to attempting to block the sciatic nerve. Usually, it is necessary to rely on superficial landmarks for finding the sciatic nerve. The mid-point of a line joining the posterior superior iliac spine and the tip of the greater trochanter is identified. The point of entry of the needle lies at a point 3–4 cm in a caudad direction, where a line bisecting the first line at right angles intersects with a third line joining the sacral hiatus to the great trochanter.

Depending on the degree of steatopygia, a longer or shorter needle may be needed, but usually a 6–8 cm needle is adequate to reach the sciatic nerve. If the nerve is not located at the first attempt, then paraesthesiae can be sought by directing the needle along a path at right angles to the sciatic nerve projection; if a nerve stimulator is used, muscle twitches in the hamstrings or calf muscles are identified. Because of the size of the nerve, approximately 20 ml of local anaesthetic solution is needed and it often takes 20–30 min to penetrate the nerve to produce satisfactory anaesthesia of the distal limb, because the nerve fibres to this area are situated in the central core of the nerve.

An alternative landmark for blocking the sciatic nerve is approximately halfway between the greater trochanter and the ischial tuberosity. This tuberosity (like the pubic tubercle) is, of course, a socially threatening area and many practitioners and patients prefer the more traditional landmarks.

Alternative approaches to the sciatic nerve. Just as the lumbar plexus can be anaesthetized from the rear, so the sciatic nerve can be anaesthetized by anterior approaches. This site is found by drawing a line along the inguinal ligament from pubic tubercle to the anterior superior iliac spine, and a second line parallel to this passing through the greater trochanter. A perpendicular line is dropped from the junction of the medial third and lateral two-thirds of the inguinal ligament line and the point at which this crosses the more caudad line passing through the greater trochanter is the site for needle entry. The needle is inserted and contact with the anterior surface of the femur is anticipated. The needle is 'walked' off the medial aspect of the femur, seeking contact paraesthesia (and/or dorsiflexion or plantar flexion of the foot if a nerve stimulator is used) as confirmation of nerve contact.[152] A long needle (at least 8 cm) is needed. Because of the dorsal position of the posterior cutaneous nerve of the thigh relative to the sciatic nerve, analgesia in the posterior thigh is often defective when the anterior approach to the sciatic nerve is used.

A lateral approach to the sciatic nerve has also been described.[153] This is rarely used but is possible by passing a needle posterior to the femur from a lateral site and seeking paraesthesia and/or motor stimulation.

Distal blocks of the lower extremity

These are not often used in anaesthetic practice, although in peripheral surgery of the foot, orthopaedic practitioners frequently use ankle block. This provides excellent anaesthesia for surgery in this region, assuming that a tourniquet is not needed. It is possible to accomplish peripheral block at both the knee and the ankle as elective techniques, or these blocks may be used to supplement a deficient proximal block.

Blocks at knee

The medial and lateral popliteal branches of the sciatic nerve are located centrally in the popliteal fossa, and usually are still travelling together at the apex of that fossa. A needle inserted at this site, where the medial and lateral posterior muscle masses of the thigh are starting to separate, can bring about contact with, and anaesthesia of, the sciatic nerve components distal to the knee.[154] The point of needle insertion is determined by locating the mid-point of the skin crease in the popliteal fossa and drawing a 10 cm line proximally in the midline. Satisfactory anaesthesia here provides numbness over all of the area below the knee with the exception of the strip of skin on the medial side of the leg from knee to medial malleolus (and sometimes beyond) supplied by the saphenous branch of the femoral nerve. This runs with the long saphenous vein, which can serve as a landmark for blocking the nerve, usually just below the medial aspect of the knee joint. If the vein cannot be seen readily, a horizontal subcutaneous arc of local anaesthetic infiltration across the medial aspect of the tibial condyle should anaesthetize the saphenous nerve.

Ankle blocks

There has been renewed interest in these blocks because of the trend to outpatient surgery; these blocks can be very useful for accomplishing anaesthesia for surgical procedures in the foot, and for permitting both postoperative comfort and early discharge.[155] The nerves supplying the foot are five in number and enter the foot circumferentially. The saphenous (as mentioned above) is a terminal branch of the femoral, and the remainder are branches of the sciatic nerve. An ankle block is almost a ring block of the lower extremity at, or usually just proximal to, the malleoli. However, an effort should be made to distribute the analgesic drug more anatomically and correctly.

The *plantar* aspects of the foot are supplied by branches of the posterior tibial and sural nerves. The posterior tibial nerve can be located 1–2 cm behind, i.e. dorsal to the medial malleolus. It runs with, and can be located by, feeling the pulsations of the posterior tibial artery site, which is usually approximately one-third of the distance from the malleolus to the tip of the calcaneum. Injection of 3–5 ml of local anaesthetic will anaesthetize the medial and lateral plantar nerves, producing analgesia over most of the sole of the foot.

The *lateral* aspect of the foot and part of the lateral sole are supplied by the sural nerve, which enters the foot approximately halfway between the lateral malleolus and calcaneum. This nerve is quite superficial, and infiltration of local anaesthetic superficially at this site should anaesthetize these areas.

The *dorsum* of the foot is mostly supplied by the superficial peroneal (anterior tibial) nerve, most of which enters the foot superficial to the extensor retinaculum and can be blocked by infiltrating a cuff of anaesthesia from medial to lateral malleoli. The medial aspect of this cuff should anaesthetize any terminal branches of the saphenous nerve that proceed beyond the medial malleolus. The only remaining unblocked area is the first interdigital web space, supplied by the deep peroneal nerve, which is more deeply situated between the tendons of tibialis anterior and extensor hallucis longus muscles. This nerve can be blocked by placing a needle between these two easily identified tendons and 'popping' through the extensor retinaculum.

These peripheral nerve blocks are used infrequently, although anaesthetists accomplished in their use will find increasing opportunities, especially in day-case surgery and in patients for whom epidural or subarachnoid anaesthesia techniques may be contra-indicated. They are enjoying a renewed popularity[148] and have even been used in paediatric practice.[156] It is possible to insert catheters into some of the nerve block sites described above,[157] and better guidelines are needed in this regard, particularly to enable more stability of the catheter when patients are mobilized after surgery. For the anaesthetist who has the skills and inclination to perform these blocks, there will be many opportunities to do so.

PERIPHERAL NERVE STIMULATION

Continued popularity of regional anaesthesia depends upon a high success rate. The use of peripheral nerve stimulation is a valuable aid to nerve localization. Although a useful adjunct, peripheral nerve stimulation is not a substitute for sound anatomical knowledge.

Principles of nerve stimulation

A threshold stimulus must be applied to a nerve fibre to result in nerve impulse propagation. Below this threshold, no impulse is propagated; above this threshold, no increase is produced in the impulse. If a square pulse of current is used to stimulate a nerve, the total charge applied to the nerve is the product of the current (strength) and the length of the pulse (duration). The current needed to stimulate a nerve depends on the pulse width or duration of the stimulus. A pulse width of 50–100 µs is ideal. The optimal frequency of stimulation is 0.5–2.0 Hz. It is possible to stimulate large Aα motor fibres without stimulating the smaller Aδ or C pain fibres.[158] This implies that a mixed peripheral nerve can be located by a muscle twitch without causing pain.

Less current is needed to generate a muscle twitch if the cathode (negative) rather than the anode (positive) is adjacent to the nerve. If the stimulating needle is negative, the current flow which alters the resting membrane potential adjacent to the needle to produce an area of depolarization easily triggers an action potential. If the stimulating needle is the anode, the current causes an area of hyperpolarization, resulting in a more limited area of depolarization.

Stimulus current (at a fixed stimulus duration) varies with the distance from the nerve. As the stimulating tip moves away from the nerve, the relationship between the stimulus intensity and the distance from the nerve is governed by Coulomb's law — $E = K \cdot Q/r^2$, where E = current required, K = constant, Q = minimal current, r = distance. If the tip is some distance from the nerve, a very high stimulus is required. The current delivered should be displayed on a clearly legible digital meter. With the stimulating needle on the nerve, only a very small current (in the region of 0.5 mA) is needed to stimulate the nerve (Fig. 23.10).

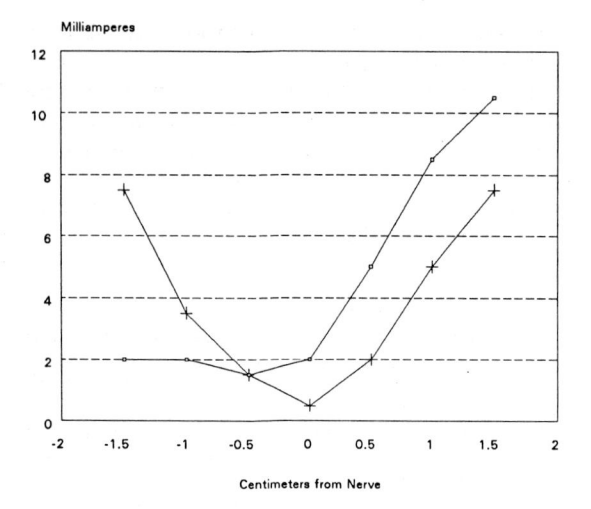

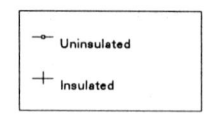

Fig. 23.10 Comparison of current required to stimulate the nerve against distance from nerve for insulated and uninsulated needles. The insulated needle requires less current throughout. Modified from Pither et al,[159] with permission.

Technique

Using appropriate local infiltration, the needle is inserted through the skin and advanced a short distance. An assistant connects the nerve stimulator with the negative electrode attached to the needle. The stimulator is turned on, with a current of 5–10 mA shown on the meter. This often produces a localized muscle twitch. The needle is advanced towards the nerve and movement is sought in the appropriate muscle groups. When movement is elicited in the appropriate muscles, the needle tip is likely to be 1–2 cm from the nerve. As the needle is advanced towards the nerve, the twitch increases in intensity. The assistant reduces the current strength. If the twitch decreases with advancement, the needle is probably to one side of the nerve and should be redirected. The needle is manipulated until a twitch occurs at minimal current (0.5–1.0 mA). When the point of optimal muscle twitch at minimal current has been obtained, a test dose of 2 ml of local anaesthetic is injected. The twitch should considerably diminish or disappear within 10 s after the test injection (probably due to mechanical displacement of the stimulating tip from the nerve). If it does not, the needle should be withdrawn and redirected until the muscle twitch is maximal at 0.5–1.0 mA and the 2 ml test dose abolishes the twitch. Only then should the full calculated dose of local anaesthetic be given. The onset of the block occurs initially in the region supplied by the nerve to the muscles that were twitching. Proximal muscle groups appear to be paralysed earlier than the occurrence of sensory loss or sympathetic block. Stimulation of pure sensory nerves results in a radiating paraesthesia, with every pulsation in the distribution of the nerve.

TOURNIQUET PAIN

Tourniquets are generally used to provide bloodless operating conditions and prevent unnecessary blood loss during surgery of the extremities. After the extremity has been exsanguinated, the tourniquet is inflated to average pressures of 300 mmHg. Prolonged inflation times (>60 min) during either general or regional anaesthesia may cause an increase in blood pressure or complaints of vague, dull pain in the limb; the pain is resistant to analgesics, and usually resolves on deflation of the tourniquet. The average time of pain tolerance after inflation of the tourniquet in conscious patients is 30 min, and 45 min in those who are sedated.[160,161] Tourniquet-induced pain is frequently reported when surgery is performed during subarachnoid or epidural anaesthesia, usually during an otherwise adequate block.[162] Smaller cuffs tend to be endured longer than larger cuffs.

Pain occurs less frequently when bupivacaine is employed for subarachnoid anaesthesia compared to amethocaine (incidence of pain is 25 versus 60%). This difference between the two drugs is unrelated to baricity, dose or level of sensory anaesthesia.[163] The mechanism of tourniquet pain is controversial. The pain is thought to be mediated by slow conducting C fibres which are usually inhibited by the earlier arriving fast pain impulses conducted by Aδ fibres. After approximately 30 min, the larger Aδ fibres may be blocked by cuff compression, leaving the C fibres, which are still functioning, uninhibited. Previous theories suggesting that tourniquet pain is caused by sympathetic transmission appear ill-founded, as regional sympathetic blocks do not relieve the pain.[164,165] To minimize the incidence of tourniquet pain, subarachnoid anaesthesia is the technique of choice. When using subarachnoid anaesthesia, the occurrence of tourniquet pain indicates that subarachnoid anaesthesia is not complete, i.e. the presence of a satisfactory high level of sensory block notwithstanding, nociceptive stimuli originating in blocked dermatomes well below the maximum level of sensory block as determined by pinprick are still transmitted to the central nervous system. To achieve complete subarachnoid anaesthesia and prevent tourniquet pain, plain bupivacaine should be used rather than hyperbaric bupivacaine or amethocaine.[166] To minimize the pain further, adrenaline 15 µg or clonidine 150 µg may be added to the bupivacaine solution.[167,168] The subarachnoid administration of morphine 0.3 mg added to hyperbaric bupivacaine has been shown to prevent tourniquet pain, although its use is associated with side-effects.[169] For upper-extremity pain, a study applying a eutectic mixture of prilocaine and lignocaine (Emla) to the skin underlying the tourniquet demonstrated a better tolerance of the tourniquet.[170] However, in spite of these studies, tourniquet pain remains a difficult and perplexing problem in the presence of otherwise adequate regional anaesthesia.

REFERENCES

1. Murphy TM. When is regional anesthesia the anesthetic of choice? Adv Anesth 1990; 7: 1–14
2. Bonica JJ. Regional anesthesia in private practice. Anesthesiology 1960; 21: 554
3. Moore DC. Regional block, 1st edn. Springfield, IL: CC Thomas. 1953
4. Atkinson RS, Rushman GB, Lee JA. A synopsis of anaesthesia. Bristol: Wright, 1987: pp 593–735
5. Selwyn AP, Braunwald E. Ischemic heart disease. In: Braunwald E, Isselbacher KJ, Petersdorf RG, et al. Harrison's principles of internal medicine, 11th edn. New York: McGraw-Hill, 1987: p 978
6. Keith I. Anaesthesia and blood loss in total hip replacement. Anaesthesia 1987; 32: 444
7. Modig J, Borg T, Karlstrom G et al. Thromboembolism after total hip replacement: role of epidural and general anaesthesia. Anesth Analg 1983; 62: 174
8. Urmey WF, Lambert DH. Spinal anesthesia associated with reversal of myocardial ischaemia. Anesth Analg 1986; 65: 908
9. Adragna MG. Professional Advisory Council adopts new policy statement on local anesthetics. MHAUS (Malignant Hyperthermia Association of the United States) Communicator 3, Spring 1985 [Published by MHAUS, Box 3231, Daren, CT 06820 USA]
10. Tiret L, Desmonts JM, Hatton F et al. Complications associated with anaesthesia. A prospective survey in France. Can Anaesth Soc J 1986; 33: 336
11. Yeager MP, Glass DD, Neff RK, Brinck-Johnsen T. Epidural anaesthesia and analgesia in high risk surgical patients. Anesthesiology 1987; 66: 729–736
12. McQuay HJ, Carrol D, Moore RA. Postoperative orthopedic pain: the effect of opiate premedication and local anaesthetic blocks. Pain 1988; 33: 291–296
13. Tverskoy M, Cozacov C, Ayache M et al. Postoperative pain after inguinal herniorrhaphy with different types of anaesthesia. Anaesth Analg 1990; 70: 29
14. Bach S, Noreng MF, Tjellden NU. Phantom limb pain in amputees during the first 12 months following limb amputation after pre operative lumbar epidural blockade. Pain 1988; 33: 297
15. Dubner R, Hargreaves KM. The neurobiology of pain and its modulation. Clin J Pain 1989; 5 (suppl): S1
16. Bier A. Versuche über cocainisirung des rückenmarkes. Dtsch Z Chir T 1899; 51: 361, as translated in Surv Anesth 1962; 6: 352
17. Siccard A. Les injections medicamenteuses extradurales par voie sacro-coccygienne. CR Soc Biol (Paris) 1901; 53: 396
18. Cathelin MF. Une novelle voie d'injection rachidienne. Methode des injections epidurales par le procede du canal sacre applications l'homme. CR Soc Biol (Paris) 1901; 53: 452
19. Kennedy F, Effron AS, Perry G. The grave spinal cord paralyses caused by spinal anaesthesia. Surg Gynecol Obstet 1950; 91: 385
20. Dripps RD, Vandam LD. Long term follow-up of patients who received 10 098 spinal anesthetics. I. Failure to discover major neurologic sequelae. JAMA 1954; 156: 1486
21. Cleland JGP. Continuous peridural and caudal analgesia in surgery and early ambulation. Northwest Med J 1949; 48: 26
22. Dawkins CJM. Discussion on extradural spinal block. Proc R Soc Med 1945; 38: 299
23. Cohen EN. Distribution of local anesthetic agents in the neuraxis of the dog. Anesthesiology 1968; 29: 1002
24. Burm AG, van Kleef JW, Gladines MP et al. Plasma concentrations of lidocaine and bupivacaine after subarachnoid administration. Anesthesiology 1983; 59: 191
25. Bengtsson M, Lofstrom JB, Malmquist LA. Skin conductance responses during spinal analgesia. Acta Anesthesiol Scand 1985; 29: 67–71
26. Lambert DH, Hurley RL. Cauda equina syndrome and continuous spinal anaesthesia. Anesth Analg 1991; 72: 817–819
27. Rigler ML, Drasner K, Krejcie TC et al. Cauda equina syndrome after continuous spinal anesthesia Anesth Analg 1991; 72: 275–281
28. Buckley FP, Robinson NB, Simonowitz DA et al. Anesthesia in the morbidly obese. Anaesthesia 1983; 38: 840
29. Schnider SM. Epidural and subarachnoid opiates in obstetrics. ASA refresher course, New Orleans vol 235. American Society of Anesthesiology 1989
30. DuPen SL, Ramsey D. Compounding local anesthetics and narcotics for epidural analgesia in cancer outpatients. Anesthesiology 1988; 69: 1405
31. Bernard CM, Hill HF. The spinal nerve root sleeve is not a preferred route for redistribution of drugs from the epidural space to the spinal cord. Anesthesiology 1991; 75: 827–832
32. Hogan Q. Lumbar epidural anatomy: a new look by cryomicrotome section. Anesthesiology 1991; 75: 767
33. Last RJ. Anatomy, regional and applied, 6th ed. Edinburgh: Churchill Livingstone, 1978; pp 37–47
34. Foerster I, Brain 1933; 56:
35. Wilson E, David A, MacKenzie N, Grant IS. Sedation during spinal anaesthesia: comparision of propofol and midazolam. Br J Anaesth 1990; 64: 48–52

36. Caplan RA, Posner K, Ward RJ, Cheney FW. Adverse respiratory events in anesthesia: a closed claims analysis. Anesthesiology 1990; 72: 828
37. Taylor JA. Lumbosacral approach subarachnoid tap. J Urol 1940; 43: 561
38. Dahl JB, Schultz P, Anker-Moller E, Christensen EF, Staunstrup HG, Carlsson P. Spinal anaesthesia in young patients using a 29-gauge needle: technical considerations and an evaluation of postoperative complaints compared with general anaesthesia. Br J Anaesth 1990; 64: 178
39. Greene NM. Present concepts of spinal anesthesia. Refresher Courses Anesthesiol 1979; 7: 131
40. Chambers WA, Littlewood DG, Logan MR et al. Effect of added epinephrine on spinal anesthesia with lidocaine. Anesth Analg 1981; 60: 417
41. Chambers WA, Littlewood DG, Scott DD. Spinal anesthesia with hyperbaric bupivacaine: effect of added vasoconstrictors. Anesth Analg 1982; 61: 49
42. Park WY, Balingot PE, McNamara TE. The effects of patient age, pH of cerebrospinal fluid and vasopressor on onset and duration of spinal anesthesia. Anesth Analg 1975; 54: 455
43. Abouleish E, Rawal N, Fallon K, Hernandez D. Combined intrathecal morphine and bupivacaine for Cesarean section. Anesth Analg 1988; 67: 370–374
44. Greene NM Distribution of local anesthetic solutions within the subarachnoid space. Anesth Analg 1985; 64: 715–730
45. Wildsmith JAW, McClure JH, Brown DT et al. Effects of posture on the spread of isobaric and hyperbaric amethocaine. Br J Anaesth 1981; 53: 273
46. Shesky MC, Rocco AG, Bizzarri-Schmidt M et al. A dose–response study of bupivacaine for spinal anesthesia. Anesth Analg 1983; 62: 931
47. Logan MR, McClure JH, Wildsmith JAW. Plain bupivacaine: an unpredictable spinal anaesthetic agent. Br J Anaesth 1986; 58: 292
48. Mukkada TA, Bridenbaugh PO, Singh P, Edstrom HH. Effects of dose, volume, and concentration of glucose-free bupivacaine in spinal anesthesia. Reg Anesth 1986; 11: 98
49. Vanzudert AA, DeWolf AM. Extent of anesthesia and hemodynamic effects after subarachnoid administration of bupivacaine with epinephrine. Anesth Analg 1988; 67: 784
50. Nielsen TH, Kristoffersen E, Olsen KH et al. Plain bupivacaine: 0.5% or 0.25% for spinal analgesia? Br J Anaesth 1989; 62: 164
51. Sinclair CJ, Scott DB, Edstrom HH. Effect of the trendelenberg position in spinal anaesthesia with hyperbaric bupivacaine. Br J Anaesth 1982; 54: 497
52. Stienstra R, Van Poorten JF. The temperature of bupivacaine 0.5% affects the sensory level of spinal anesthesia. Anesth Analg 1988; 67: 272
53. Greene NM. Physiology of spinal anesthesia, 3rd edn. Baltimore, MD: Williams & Wilkins. 1981
54. Freund FG, Bonica JJ, Ward RJ et al. Ventilatory reserve and level of motor block during high spinal and epidural block. Anesthesiology 1967; 8: 834
55. Kennedy WF Jr, Everett GB, Cobb LA, Allen GD. Simultaneous systemic and hepatic hemodynamic measurements during spinal anesthesia in normal man. Anesth Analg 1970; 49: 1016
56. Kehlet H. The modifying effect of anesthetic technique on the metabolic and endocrine responses to anesthesia and surgery. Acta Anaesthesiol Belg 1988; 3: 143
57. Tourtellotte WW, Henderson WG, Tucker RP et al. A randomized, double-blind clinical trial comparing the 22 versus 26 gauge needle in the production of the post-lumbar puncture syndrome in normal individuals. Headache 1972; 12: 73
58. Sprotte G, Schedel R, Pajunk H et al. Eine atraumatische Universalkanule fur einzeitige Regionalanaethesien. Regional-Anaethesie 1987; 10: 104
59. Cesarini M, Torrielli R, Lahaye F et al. Sprotte needle for intrathecal anaesthesia for Caesarian section. Incidence of post-lumbar-puncture headache. Anaesthesia 1990; 45: 656
60. Lynch J, Arhelger S, Krings-Ernst I. 1992 Post-dural puncture headache in young orthopaedic in-patients: comparision of a 0.33 mm (29-gauge) Quincke-type with a 0.77 mm (22-gauge) Whitacre spinal needle in 22 patients. Acta Anaesthesiol Scand 1992; 36: 58
61. Lybecker H, Møller JT, May O, Neilsen HK. Incidence and prediction of postdural puncture headache: a prospective study of 1021 spinal anesthetics. Anesth Analg 1990; 70: 389–394
62. Abboud TK, Zhu J, Reyes A et al. Efficacy of intravenous caffeine for post dural puncture headache. Anesthesiology 1990; 73: A936
63. Abouleish E. Epidural blood patch for the treatment of chronic post-lumbar-puncture cephagia. Anesthesiology 1978; 49: 291
64. Szeinfeld M, Ihmeidan IH, Moser MM et al. Epidural blood patch: evaluation of the volume and spread of blood injected into the epidural space. Anesthesiology 1986; 64: 820
65. Lund PC. Principles and practice of spinal anesthesia. Springfield, IL: Charles C Thomas. 1971
66. Brown EM, Elman DS. Postoperative backache. Anesth Analg 1961; 40: 683
67. Loeser JD, Bigos SJ, Fordyce WE, Volinn E. Low back pain. In: Bonica JJ, ed. The management of pain. Philadelphia, PA: Lea & Febiger, 1990: pp 1448–1483
68. Burman RS, Eisele JH. Bacteremia, spinal anesthesia and the development of meningitis. Anesthesiology 1978; 48: 378
69. Kilpatrick ME, Girgis NI. Meningitis — a complication of spinal anesthesia. Anesth Analg 1983; 62: 513
70. Mantia AM. Clinical report of the occurrence of an intracerebral hemorrhage following post lumbar puncture headache. Anesthesiology 1981; 55: 684
71. Wedel DJ, Mulroy ME. Hemiparesis following dural puncture. Anesthesiology 1983; 59: 475
72. Rigler ML, Drasner K, Krejchi TC, et al. Cauda equina syndrome after continuous spinal anaesthesia. Anesth Analg 1991; 72: 275–281
73. Vandam LD, Dripps RD. Long term follow-up of patients who received 10098 spinal anesthetics. Syndrome of decreased intracranial pressure (headache and ocular and auditory difficulties). JAMA 1956; 161: 586
74. Bryce-Smith RM, Macintosh RR. Sixth-nerve palsy after lumbar puncture and spinal analgesia. Br Med J 1971; 1: 275
75. Wang LP, Fog J, Bove M. Transient hearing loss

76. Panning B, Mehler D, Lehnhardt E. Transient low-frequency hypoacousia after spinal anesthesia. Lancet 1983; ii: 582
77. Collins JV. Principles of anesthesiology. Philadelphia, PA: Lea & Febiger, 1976: pp 690–697
78. Gordon AG. Hyperacusis after spinal anesthesia. Anesth Analg 1991; 73: 502
79. Fog J, Wang LP, Sundberg A, Mucchiano C. Hearing loss after spinal anaesthesia is related to needle size. Anesth Analg 1990; 70: 517–522
80. Frumin MJ, Schwartz H, Burns JJ et al. Sites of sensory blockade during segmental spinal and segmental peridural anesthesia in man. Anesthesiology 1953; 14: 576
81. Bromage PR. Epidural anesthesia. Philadelphia, PA: WB Saunders. 1978
82. Haljanae H, Stefansson T, Wickstrom I. Influence of anesthetic technique on postoperative pulmonary complications in geriatric patients. Reg Anesth 1982; 7 (suppl): S122
83. Wahba WM, Don HF, Craig DB. Postoperative epidural analgesia: effects on lung volumes. Can Anaesth Soc J 1975; 22: 519
84. Currie JM Measurement of the depth to the extradural space using ultrasound. Br J Anaesth 1984; 56: 345
85. Tucker GT, Mather LE. Pharmacokinetics of local anaesthetic agents. Br J Anaesth 1975; 47: 213
86. Morikawa KI, Bonica JJ, Tucker GT, Murphy TM. Effect of acute hypovolaemia on lignocaine absorption and cardiovascular response following epidural block in dogs. Br J Anaesth 1974; 46: 631–635
87. Catchlove RFH. The influence of CO_2 and pH on local anesthetic action. J Pharmacol Exp Ther 1972; 181: 298
88. Martin R, LaMarche Y, Tetreault L. Comparison of the clinical effectiveness of lidocaine hydrocarbonate and lidocaine hydrochloride with and without epinephrine in epidural anesthesia Can Anaesth Soc J 1981; 28: 217
89. Gallindo A, Hernandez J, Benevides O et al. Quality of spinal and extradural anaesthesia: the influence of spinal nerve root diameter. Br J Anaesth 1975; 47: 41
90. DiFazio CA, Carron H, Grosslight KR, Moscicki JC, Bolding WR, Johns RA. Comparision of pH-adjusted lidocaine solutions for epidural anesthesia. Anesth Analg 1986; 65: 760
91. Bromage PR. Ageing and epidural dose requirements. Segmental spread and predictability of epidural analgesia in youth and extreme age. Br J Anaesth 1969; 41: 1016
92. Murphy TM, Mather LE, Stanton-Hicks MA, Bonica JJ, Tucker GT. Effects of adding adrenaline to etidocaine and lignocaine in extradural anaesthesia. 1. Block characteristics and cardiovascular effects. Br J Anaesth 1976; 48: 893–898
93. Gissen AJ, Covino BG, Gregus J. Differential sensitivities of mammalian nerve fibres to local anaesthetics agents. Anesthesiology 1980; 53: 467
94. Benzon HT, Gissen AJ, Strichartz GR, Avram MJ, Covino BG. The effect of polyethylene glycol on mammalian nerve impulses. Anesth Analg 1987; 66: 553
95. Johnson MD, Burger GA, Mushlin PS, Arthur GR, Datta S. Reversal of bupivacaine epidural anesthesia by intermittent epidural injections of crystalloid solutions. Anesth Analg 1990; 70: 395
96. Wildsmith JAW, Gissen AJ, Gregus J, Covino BG. Differential nerve blocking activity of amino-ester local anesthetics. Br J Anaesth 1985; 57: 612
97. Seow LT, Lips FJ, Cousins MJ, Mather LE. Lidocaine and bupivacaine mixtures for epidural blockade. Anesthesiology 1982; 56: 177
98. Bromage PR. A comparison of the hydrochloride and carbon dioxide salts of lidocaine and prilocaine in epidural analgesia. Acta Anaesth Scand 1965; 16 (suppl): 55
99. Murphy TM, O'Keeffe D. Complications of spinal, epidural and caudal anesthesia. In: Benumof JL, Saidman LJ, eds. Anesthesia and perioperative complications. St Louis MO: Mosby Yearbook, 1992: pp 38–51
100. Ravindran RS, Bond VK, Tasch MD et al. Prolonged neural blockade following regional anesthesia with 2-chloroprocaine. Anesth Analg 1980; 59: 447
101. Johnson MD, Burger GA, Mushlin PS et al. Reversal of bupivicaine epidural anesthesia by intermittent epidural injections of crystalloid solutions. Anesth Analg 1990; 70: 395–399
102. Shanker KB, Palker NV, Nishkala R. Paraplegia following epidural potassium chloride. Anaesthesia 1985; 40: 45
103. Shimosato S, Etsten BE. The role of the venous system in cardiocirculatory dynamics during spinal and epidural anesthesia in man. Anesthesiology 1969; 30: 619
104. Bonica JJ, Akamatsu TJ, Berges PU, Morikawa K, Kennedy WF. Circulatory effects of peridural block. II. Effects of epinephrine. Anesthesiology 1971; 34: 514
105. Bonica JJ, Berges PU, Morikawa K. Circulatory effects of peridural block. I. Influence of level of analgesia and dose of lidocaine. Anesthesiology 1970; 33: 619
106. Davis FM, Woolner DF, Frampton C et al. Prospective multicenter trial of mortality following general or spinal anaesthesia for hip fracture surgery in the elderly. Br J Anaesth 1987; 59: 1080–1088
107. Verniquet AJW. Vessel puncture with epidural catheters. Experience with obstetric patients. Anaesthesia 1980; 35: 660
108. Philips DC, MacDonald R. Epidural catheter migration during labour. Anaesthesia 1987; 42: 661
109. Lubenow T, Keh-Wong E, Dristof K, Ivankovich O, Ivankovich AD. Inadvertent subdural injection: a complication of an epidural block. Anesth Analg 1988; 67: 175–179
110. Moore DC, Batra M. The components of an effective test dose prior to an epidural block. Anesthesiology 1981; 55: 693
111. Leighton BL, Norris MC, Sosis M, Epstein R, Chayen B, Larijani GE. Limitations of epinephrine as a marker of intravascular injection in laboring women. Anesthesiology 1987; 66: 688
112. Tom WC. The epidural test dose and the identification of rare events. Can J Anaesth 1988; 35: 327
113. Leighton BL, Norris MC, DeSimone CA et al. The air test as a clinically useful indicator of intravenously placed epidural catheters. Anesthesiology 1990; 73: 610
114. Gustafson H, Rutberg H, Bengtsson M. Spinal haematoma following epidural analgesia. Anaesthesia 1988; 43: 220

115 Kane RE. Neurologic deficits following epidural or spinal anesthesia. Anesth Analg 1981; 60: 150
116 Parnass SM, Rothenberg DM, Fischer RL et al. Spinal anesthesia and minidose heparin. JAMA 1990; 263: 1496
117 Poller L, Taberner DA, Sandilands DG et al. An evaluation of APTT monitoring of low-dose heparin dosage in hip surgery. Thromb Haemostas 1982; 47: 50
118 Allemann BH, Gerber H, Gruber UF. Peri-spinal anesthesia and subcutaneous administration of low-dose heparin-dihydergot for prevention of thromboembolism. Anaesthesist 1983; 32: 80
119 Lowson SM, Goodchild CS. Low-dose heparin therapy and spinal anaesthesia. Anaesthesia 1989; 44: 67
120 Dean WM, Woodside JR. Spinal hematoma compressing cauda equina. Urology 1979; 13: 575
121 Rao TLK, El-Etr AA. Anticoagulation following placement of epidural and subarachnoid catheters: an evaluation of neurologic sequelae. Anesthesiology 1981; 55: 618
122 Matthews ET, Abrams LO. Intrathecal morphine in open heart surgery. Lancet 1980; ii: 543
123 Ruff RL, Dougherty JH. Complications of lumbar puncture followed by anticoagulation. Stroke 1981; 12: 879
124 Levine MN, Plane A, Hirsh J et al. The relationship between anti-factor Xa level and clinical outcome in patients receiving enoxaparine low molecular weight heparin to prevent deep venous thrombosis after hip replacement. Thromb Haemost 1989; 62: 940
125 Nurmohamed MT, Rosendaal FR, Buller HR et al. Low-molecular-weight heparin versus standard heparin in general and orthopaedic surgery: a meta-analysis. Lancet 1992; 340: 152
126 Metzger G, Singbartl G. Spinal epidural hematoma following epidural anesthesia versus spontaneous spinal subdural hematoma. Two case reports. Acta Anaesthesiol Scand 1991; 35: 105
127 Horlocker TT, Wedel DJ, Offord KP. Does perioperative antiplatelet therapy increase the risk of hemorrhagic complications associated with regional anesthesia? Anesth Analg 1990; 70: 631
128 Benzon HT, Brunner EA, Vaisrub N. Bleeding time in nerve blocks after aspirin. Reg Anesth 1984; 9: 86
129 Hindman BJ. Usefulness of the post-aspirin bleeding time. Anesthesiology 1986; 64: 368
130 Ferraris VA, Swanson E. Aspirin usage and peri-operative blood loss in patients undergoing unexpected operations. Surg Gynecol Obstet 1983; 156: 439
131 Owens EL, Kasten GW, Hessel EA. Spinal hematoma after lumbar puncture and heparinization. Anesth Analg 1986; 65: 1201
132 Mallett SV, Platt M. Role of thrombelastography in bleeding diatheses and regional anaesthesia. Lancet 1991; 338: 765–766
133 Horlocker TT, Wedel DJ. Anesthesiol Clin North Am 1992; 10: 1–9
134 Dean HP. Discussion on the relative value of inhalation and injection methods of inducing anesthesia. Br Med J 1907; 5: 869
135 Hurley RJ, Lambert DH. Continuous spinal anesthesia with a microcatheter technique: preliminary experience. Anesth Analg 1990; 70: 97
136 Winnie AP. Interscalene brachial plexus block. Anesth Analg 1974; 49: 455
137 Thompson GE, Rorie DK. Functional anatomy of the brachial plexus sheath. Anesthesiology 1983; 59: 117–122
138 Partridge BL, Katz J, Benirschke K. Functional anatomy of the brachial sheath: implications for anaesthesia. Anesthesiology 1987; 66: 743–747
139 Lanz E, Theiss D, Jankovic D. The extent of blockade following various techniques of brachial plexus block. Anesth Analg 1983; 62: 55–58
140 Moore DC. Regional anaesthesia, 4th edn. Springfield, IL: Charles C Thomas. 1978
141 Cook LB. Unsuspected extradural catheterization in an interscalene block. Br J Anaesth 1991; 67: 473–475
142 Lombard TP, Couper JL. Bilateral spread of analgesia following interscalene brachial plexus block. Anesthesiology 1983; 58: 472
143 Tuominen MK, Pere P, Rosenberg PH. Unintentional arterial catheterization and bupivacaine toxicity associated with continuous interscalene brachial plexus block. Anesthesiology 1991; 75: 356–358
144 Durrani Z, Winnie AP. Brainstem toxicity with reversible locked-in syndrome after intrascalene brachial plexus block. Anesth Analg 1991; 72: 249–252
145 Kozody R, Ready LB, Barsa JE, Murphy TM. Dose requirement of local anaesthetic produce grand mal seizure during stellate ganglion block? Can Anaesth Soc J 1982; 29: 489
146 Urmey WF, Talts KH, Sharrock NE. One hundred percent incidence of hemidaphragmatic paresis associated with interscalene brachial plexus anesthesia by ultrasonography. Anesth Analg 1991; 72: 498–503
147 Cockings E, Moore P, Lewis RC. Transarterial brachial plexus blockade using high doses of 1.5% mepivacaine. Reg Anesth 1987; 12: 159
148 Murphy TM. Lower extremity nerve blocks. In: Rogers MC, ed. Current practice in anesthesiology, 2nd edn. St Louis, MO: Mosby Year Book, 1990: pp 195–199
149 Winnie AP, Ramamurthy S, Durrani Z. The inguinal paravascular technique of lumbar plexus anaesthesia: 'The 3-in-1 block'. Anesth Analg 1973; 52: 989
150 Sharrock NE. Inadvertent three in one block following injection of the lateral cutaneous nerve of the thigh. Anesth Analg 1989; 59: 887–888
151 Chayne D, Nathan H, Chayne N. The psoas compartment block. Anesthesiology 1976; 45: 95–99
152 Beck GP. Anterior approach to sciatic nerve block. Anesthesiology 1963; 24: 222
153 Ichiyanigi K. Sciatic nerve block: lateral approach with patients supine. Anesthesiology 1959; 20: 601–604
154 Rorie DK, Byer DE, Nelson DO, Sittipong R, Johnson KA. Assessment of block of the sciatic nerve in the popliteal fossa. Anesth Analg 1980; 59: 371–376
155 Schurman DJ. Ankle block anesthesia for foot surgery. Anesthesiology 1976; 44: 348–352
156 Dalens W, Tangey A, Vanneville G. Sciatic nerve blocking in children: comparison of the posterior, anterior and lateral approaches in 180 pediatric patients. Anesth Analg 1990; 70: 131–137
157 Ben-David B, Lee E, Croitoru M. Psoas block for surgical repair of hip fracture: case report and description of the catheter technique. Anesth Analg 1990; 71: 298–301

158 Ranck JB. Which elements are excited in electrical stimulation of mammalian central nervous system? A review. Brain Res 1975; 98: 417
159 Pither CE, Ford DJ, Raj PP. Peripheral nerve stimulation with insulated and uninsulated needles: efficacy of characteristics. Reg Anesth 1984; 9: 42–43
160 Hagenouw RRPM, Bridenbaugh PO, Van Egmond J, Stuebing R. Tourniquet pain: a volunteer study. Anesth Analg 1986; 65: 1175
161 Fuselier CO, Binnig T, Dobbs BM et al. A study of the use of a double tourniquet technique to obtain hemostasis in combination with local standby sedation during podiatric surgery. J Foot Surg 1988; 27: 515
162 Valli H, Rosenberg PH. Effects of three anaesthesia methods on haemodynamic responses connected with the use of thigh tourniquet in orthopaedic patients. Acta Anaesthesiol Scand 1985; 29: 142
163 Bridenbaugh PO, Hagenouw RR, Gielen MJ, Estrom HH. Addition of glucose to bupivacaine in spinal anesthesia increases incidence of tourniquet pain. Anesth Analg 1986; 65: 11-81–1185
164 Valli H. Lumbar sympathetic blockade does not prevent tourniquet-induced hypertension during general anesthesia. Reg Anesth 1988; 13: 152
165 Farah RS, Thomas PS. Sympathetic blockade and tourniquet pain in surgery of the upper extremity. Anesth Analg 1987; 66: 1033
166 Bridenbaugh PO, Hagenouw RRPM, Gielen MJM, Edstrom HH. Addition of glucose to bupivacaine in spinal anesthesia increases the incidence of tourniquet pain. Anesth Analg 1986; 65: 1181
167 Gielen MJM, Meulman H, Van Beem H, Bridenbaugh PO. Does the addition of epinephrine to hyperbaric bupivacaine 0.5% in spinal analgesia decrease the incidence of tourniquet pain? Proceedings of the meeting of the European Society of Regional Anaesthesia, Malmo, F3 1986
168 Bonnet F, Diallo A, Saada M et al. Prevention of tourniquet pain by spinal isobaric bupivacaine with clonidine. Br J Anaesth 1989; 63: 93
169 Horlocker TT, Wedel DJ, Anticoagulants, antiplatelet therapy and neuraxis blockade. Anesth Clin North Am 1992; 10: 1–11 (Table 23.9)
170 Foerster O. The dermatomes of man. Brain 1933; 56: 1–39 (Fig. 23.3)

24. Intra-operative complications

A. J. Cunningham

CARDIOVASCULAR SYSTEM

Acute homeostatic control of vital organ blood flow during general anaesthesia requires alterations in heart rate, myocardial contractility, venous tone and arterial resistance. These responses are mediated by the sympathetic and parasympathetic nervous systems. Since autonomic reflexes are under the control of the central nervous system, it can be expected that general anaesthetic agents will alter baroreflex control of heart rate, contraction of cardiac muscle and vascular smooth-muscle reactivity.[1]

Acute changes in heart rate

Traditionally, heart rate responses have been attributed to a balance effect involving parasympathetic stimulation and β-adrenergic activity.[2] Cardiac conduction begins with depolarization of the sino-atrial (SA) node which initiates the electrical impulse that is conducted to the atrioventricular (AV) node. In addition to neurogenic stimuli, SA node depolarization is influenced by humoral and metabolic factors, e.g. endogenous catecholamines and temperature/thyroid hormone influences.

Haemorrhage-induced reduction of arterial blood pressure results in baroreceptor-mediated reflex increases in heart rate and myocardial contractility. Baroreceptor sensitivity is defined by the slope of the relationship between arterial blood pressure and R–R interval.[3]

Acute changes in heart rate are observed commonly during general anaesthesia.

Bradycardia during anaesthesia

A differential diagnosis of intra-operative bradycardia is outline in Table 24.1.

Sinus bradycardia. This may be pre-existing, vagally mediated, drug-induced, hypothermia-related or as a result of β-adrenergic blockade. The degree of bradycardia which will be tolerated by an individual patient is not always predictable. For heart rates in the range

Table 24.1 Bradycardia — intra-operative differential diagnosis

Physiological
Athletes

Surgery-related
Intra-abdominal
Laparoscopic
Gynaecological
Ophthalmic
Electroconvulsive therapy

Anaesthetic drug-induced
Non-depolarizing agents — vecuronium/atracurium
Inhaled agents — halothane
Opioids — fentanyl

Pre-operative drug-related
β-Adrenoceptor blockers
Parasympathomimetic agents

Temperature and metabolism
Hypothermia
Hypothyroidism

40–60 beats.min^{-1}, no treatment is usually indicated unless hypotension, low cardiac output or escape rhythms (junctional or ventricular) appear. Sinus bradycardia associated with hypotension or evidence on the electrocardiogram (ECG) of myocardial ischaemia warrants immediate treatment with atropine 0.3–0.6 mg intravenously. In general, a heart rate of less than 40 beats.min^{-1}, even without obvious adverse effects, warrants treatment because progression to sinus arrest may ensue.[4]

Junctional bradycardia. This is usually an escape rhythm caused by suppression of SA node depolarization by anaesthetic agents, e.g. halothane, vecuronium and fentanyl. A reduction in the administered concentration of volatile anaesthetic agent, an alteration in anaesthetic depth or anticholinergic treatment usually causes resumption of normal sinus rhythm.

Atrioventricular block. This may be associated with drug-induced delay in AV node conduction, a slow ventricular response to atrial fibrillation or flutter or more advanced second- or third-degree heart block.

Effects of anaesthetic drugs. The newer non-depolarizing neuromuscular blocking agents vecuronium and atracurium have their site of action mainly at the nicotinic receptors, with little muscarinic activity. These agents have achieved widespread popularity for, among other reasons, their cardiovascular stability. However, these agents, lacking vagolytic effects, may facilitate the development of drug- or reflex-induced bradycardia during surgery.[5] Numerous case reports have described the development of bradycardia, sinus arrest and asystole with vecuronium[6,7] and atracurium.[8] The administration of the anticholinergic agent atropine usually restores sinus rhythm. In contrast, older neuromuscular blocking agents such as pancuronium have intrinsic vagolytic effects which help to mask vagally mediated cardiovascular effects.[9] Because vecuronium has no vagolytic property, an anticholinergic agent such as atropine or glycopyrronium should be considered when vecuronium is used in high-risk situations, e.g. ophthalmic or intraperitoneal surgery.[10]

Inhaled anaesthetic agents influence heart rate by altering the rate of sinus node depolarization, by changing myocardial conduction times or by influencing autonomic nervous system activity. At concentrations of 0.5–1.5 minimum alveolar concentration (MAC), halothane decreases the contractile rate of isolated heart atria.[11] Thus, the bradycardia sometimes seen with halothane may result from a direct depression of atrial rate.

Intravenous injection of fentanyl produces bradycardia in animals and humans. In this respect, fentanyl is similar to other opioids, with the exception of pethidine (meperidine), which often causes tachycardia.[12] The mechanism of fentanyl-induced bradycardia is not completely understood, although there is experimental evidence to suggest stimulation of the central vagal nucleus.[13] Fentanyl-induced bradycardia is more marked during anaesthesia than in the conscious subject, and when breathing 100% oxygen than when nitrous oxide is used with oxygen.[14] Second and subsequent doses of fentanyl cause less bradycardia than initial doses. Infusion experiments in dogs have indicated that most of the decrease in heart rate occurs with the first 5 $\mu g.kg^{-1}$ of fentanyl. The degree of bradycardia may be related to the speed of injection.[15] Slow administration of fentanyl, anticholinergic premedication and prior administration of pancuronium 0.5–2.0 mg intravenously before induction of anaesthesia with high-dose fentanyl may attenuate bradycardia and reduce the extent of muscle rigidity.[16]

Reflex bradycardia, hypotension and surgical procedures. Acute reductions in heart rate and arterial blood pressure, attributable to vagal reflexes, have been observed during a wide range of procedures including ophthalmic, abdominal, gynaecological and laparoscopic surgery, and electroconvulsive therapy. Bradycardia and hypotension have been observed with surgical manipulation of intra-abdominal contents: traction of the peritoneum, displacement of the liver, insertion of surgical packs, bowel evisceration and bowel retraction.[17]

The oculocardiac reflex, associated with traction of the orbit and recti muscles, is well-recognized.[18] Bradycardia and asystole, attributable to parasympathetic stimulation from both peritoneal stretching and cervical dilatation, have been reported in association with dilatation and curettage of the cervix, and during laparoscopy.[19] There have been numerous reports of bradycardia during electroconvulsive therapy.[20] Although atropine has been used routinely before this procedure, its administration may not prevent bradycardia and, by relaxing the cardiac sphincter, may increase the risk of regurgitation.[21]

Anaesthesia and baroreceptor control of heart rate. Inhaled anaesthetic agents attenuate the baroreceptor control of heart rate in humans, this depressant effect is more marked with halothane and enflurane than with isoflurane.[22-24] Halogenated agents probably have multiple sites of action leading to depression of baroreflex function. Benzodiazepines and most intravenous anaesthetic agents, with the exception of ketamine and etomidate, depress or modify the baroreflex response.[25,26] Impairment of baroreceptor-mediated changes in heart rate during anaesthesia in response to hypovolaemia markedly decrease the tolerance to haemorrhage. Alterations of baroreflex responses during general anaesthesia appear to be related mainly to a non-specific anaesthetic effect rather than a specific receptor-mediated modification.[1]

Sinus tachycardia

This is generally considered to apply to a heart rate greater than 100 beats.min^{-1} with normal complexes on the ECG. Sinus tachycardia may be considered physiological when associated with exercise or emotional stress, and pathological when associated with fever, hypovolaemia, anaemia, heart failure, cardiogenic and septic shock, thyrotoxicosis and following drug administration, e.g. adrenaline (epinephrine).

During anaesthesia, increases in heart rate have a deleterious effect on both myocardial oxygen supply (decreased diastolic filling time) and myocardial oxygen demand (increased myocardial work). Studies in anaesthetized patients undergoing cardiac[27] and non-cardiac surgery[28] have consistently demonstrated a relationship between intra-operative tachycardia and myocardial ischaemia. Conditions predisposing to intra-operative tachycardia are outlined in Table 24.2.

Intra-operative acute increases in heart rate should prompt the anaesthetist to determine the cause. Pain, light anaesthesia, hypovolaemia, hypoxaemia and hypercapnia are all associated with sympathetic nervous system stimulation and endogenous catecholamine release. Thyrotoxicosis, fever and malignant hyperpyrexia are all associated with increased metabolism. If the heart rate exceeds 160 beats.min^{-1}, differentiation from atrial tachycardia may be difficult. Treatment of intra-operative tachycardia includes treatment of the underlying cause, e.g. administering opioids or deepening the level of anaesthesia, and correction of any associated hypovolaemia, hypoventilation or hypoxaemia. In the case of unexplained tachycardia associated with ECG evidence of myocardial ischaemia, immediate pharmacological treatment with an intravenous β-adrenergic blocker such as esmolol may be necessary.

Acute changes in blood pressure

Acute regulation of arterial blood pressure during anaesthesia is mediated by arterial baroreceptors, resulting in changes in heart rate, cardiac contractility and peripheral sympathetic outflow. Volatile anaesthetic agents diminish the baroreceptor reflex and, together with the influence of altered $Pa\text{CO}_2$ and intrathoracic pressure, combine to decrease venous return, cardiac contractility and peripheral vascular resistance.[29] Aetiological factors involved in intra-operative hypotension are shown in Table 24.3.

The effect of inhaled anaesthetics on the circulation

The overall influence on inhaled anaesthetic agents is

Table 24.2 Conditions predisposing to intra-operative tachycardia

Surgical stimulation
Pain
Light depth of anaesthesia

Sympathetic nervous system stimulation
Hypovolaemia
Hypoxaemia
Hypercapnia

Anaesthetic drug-related
Non-depolarizing relaxants — pancuronium
Opioids — pethidine
Anticholinergics — atropine, glycopyrronium
Inhaled agents — isoflurane, desflurane

Peri-operative drug-related
Sympathomimetics

Temperature and metabolism
Fever
Thyrotoxicosis
Malignant hyperpyrexia

Table 24.3 Intra-operative hypotension

Decreased cardiac preload
Hypovolaemia — blood loss, plasma or extracellular fluid deficit
Surgical positioning
Positive intrathoracic pressure — IPPV/pneumothorax
Vasodilatation — drug-induced
Pericardial effusion

Decreased heart rate

Decreased cardiac contractile function
Myocardial-depressant drugs
    Volatile anaesthetic agents
    Intravenous induction agents
    β-Adrenoceptor blockers
    Calcium antagonists
Myocardial ischaemia/infarction
Hypoxaemia
Hypocalcaemia
Acidosis
Major regional anaesthesia (high epidural/spinal)

Decreased cardiac afterload
Vasodilating agents
    Volatile anaesthetics
    α-Adrenoceptor blockers
    Calcium antagonists
Anaphylaxis
Major regional anaesthesia (epidural/spinal anaesthesia)

IPPV = Intermittent positive-pressure ventilation.

to decrease mean arterial pressure (MAP).[30] Halothane,[31] enflurane[32] and isoflurane[33] decrease MAP in direct proportion to the inspired concentration. At 2 MAC, MAP is approximately 50% of the control (awake) value. Halothane and enflurane reduce cardiac output to a degree which parallels their effect on arterial pressure. In contrast, the increased heart rate associated with isoflurane tends to maintain cardiac output, despite a decrease in MAP. Overall, systemic vascular resistance is unchanged by halothane, decreased by enflurane and markedly diminished by isoflurane. The effects of sevoflurane are similar to those of isoflurane. Desflurane produces slightly less myocardial and peripheral vascular depression, but a greater increase in heart rate.[30] With all agents, the hypercapnia which is associated with spontaneous ventilation during anaesthesia may enhance heart rate and cardiac output.[34] Nitrous oxide has direct myocardial depressant effects; however, indirect sympathetic stimulation may attenuate its direct depressant effects.[35] Thus, the overall effect of the potent inhaled agents is a decrease in cardiac output (enflurane ≈ halothane ≫ isoflurane ≈ sevoflurane > desflurane) and a decrease in systemic vascular resistance (isoflurane ≈ sevoflurane > desflurane > enflurane ≫ halothane), leading to a reduction in MAP.

Inhaled agents may depress myocardial contractility by decreasing inward movement of calcium through the sarcolemma, by increasing calcium release from the sarcoplasmic reticulum, by decreasing intracellular calcium availability, or by decreasing the calcium sensitivity of the contractile actin and myosin proteins.[29]

Hypotension induced by inhaled anaesthetics is due, in part, to a decrease in peripheral vascular resistance. The anaesthetic influences on regional vascular resistance depend on the specific vascular bed involved. For example, halothane and isoflurane have very different effects on the cerebral and coronary vascular beds.[36]

Intra-operative implications

Logical treatment of intra-operative hypotension involves prompt determination of the cause.

Hypovolaemia. This may occur following loss of blood, plasma or extracellular fluid.

Decreased cardiac preload. This may be related to surgical positioning, major regional anaesthesia, positive intrathoracic pressure (due to intermittent positive-pressure ventilation or pneumothorax), pericardial effusion, etc.

Decreased heart rate.

Decreased cardiac contractile function. In addition to the effects of potent anaesthetic agents, this may occur in association with myocardial ischaemia/infarction, hypoxaemia, hypocalcaemia, acidosis, cephalad spread of local anaesthetic agents with major regional anaesthesia, β-adrenoceptor blockers and direct myocardial depressant agents.

Decreased cardiac afterload. In addition to the effects of potent inhaled agents, this may occur with major regional anaesthesia (epidural and subarachnoid), anaphylactic or anaphylactoid reactions, drugs with α-receptor or calcium channel-blocking properties and direct vasodilating agents.

Hypertension

Intra-operative hypertension may result from a multiplicity of causes (Table 24.4). Patients with untreated, poorly treated or labile pre-operative hypertension may be at greater risk of peri-operative blood pressure lability, arrhythmias and myocardial ischaemia.[37] Withdrawal of pre-operative antihypertensive medication, such as β-blockers, calcium antagonists or clonidine, may be associated with greater blood pressure lability.[38]

Intra-operative hypertension may be associated with:

- inadequate depth of anaesthesia
- intense surgical stimulation
- sympathetic nervous system activation and

Table 24.4 Intra-operative hypertension

Pre-operative factors
Inadequate hypertension control
Withdrawal of antihypertensive therapy
  α_2-Agonists, e.g. clonidine
  β-Adrenoceptor blockers
  Calcium antagonists

Surgery-related
Reflex sympathetic responses — mesentery, peritoneum, bile ducts
Vascular surgery
  Thoracic/abdominal aortic cross-clamp
  Carotid endarterectomy

Surgical stimulation
Pain
Light depth of anaesthesia

Sympathetic nervous system stimulation
Hypoxaemia
Hypercapnia

Endogenous catecholamine release
Phaeochromocytoma

Drug-related
α- and β-adrenoceptor agonists

Intravenous and blood replacement
Hypervolaemia

endogenous catecholamine release associated with hypoxaemia, hypercapnia, acidosis and hypermetabolic states or
- the administration of drugs with α- or β-adrenoreceptor agonist activity.

Intra-operative hypertension may also be associated with overzealous hydration during anaesthesia and exaggerated replacement of blood loss.

A number of surgical interventions may produce significant acute elevations in arterial blood pressure. Small-bowel evisceration, traction on visceral or parietal peritoneum, manipulation of the bladder or common bile duct, or traction on the mesentery may all cause reflex sympathetic responses characterized by tachycardia, hypertension, sweating and cutaneous pallor.[39] These reflex cardiovascular responses of noxious surgical stimuli may be attenuated or prevented by deep levels of anaesthesia associated with administration of volatile anaesthetic agents, high-dose opioids administered before the onset of surgery, or in specific cases, by the appropriate use of regional anaesthesia.

Cross-clamping of the thoracic or abdominal aorta to facilitate thoracic or abdominal aortic aneurysm resection or during corrective procedures for aortoiliac occlusive disease may be associated with significant haemodynamic consequences[40] (see Chapter 9). Conflicting findings have been reported by different groups in respect of plasma renin activity during experimental and human aortic vascular surgery. Depending on the extent of intra-operative hydration, plasma renin activity may be increased or remain unchanged following aortic cross-clamping.[41] Peri-operative blood pressure lability quickly follows carotid endarterectomy and may be related to pre-operative hypertension, altered baroreceptor activity and abnormal plasma volume.[42]

Myocardial ischaemia

The extent of the problem

The relationship between intra-operative myocardial ischaemia and peri-operative cardiac morbidity has been evaluated by Mangano in a review.[43] Myocardial ischaemia has been reported in 18–74% of patients with coronary artery disease who undergo non-cardiac surgery. The wide variability in incidence has been attributed to differences in study populations, study protocols and methods. Classically, intra-operative ischaemia is thought to be precipitated either by increases in myocardial oxygen demand caused by tachycardia, hypertension, sympathetic nervous system stimulation, sympathomimetic drugs and the discontinuation of β-adrenoceptor blocking agents, or by decreases in myocardial oxygen supply caused by hypotension, tachycardia, anaemia, hypoxaemia and increased ventricular filling pressures. Recent data suggest that up to 50% of episodes of intra-operative myocardial ischaemia may be 'non-demand'-related, i.e. not associated with increases in heart rate or blood pressure.[44] The aetiology of this reduced-supply ischaemia has been attributed to atherosclerotic plaque rupture with accelerated thrombosis and vessel spasm (Fig. 24.1).

Techniques to detect myocardial ischaemia

Haemodynamic indices. Several techniques have been advocated to detect and quantify myocardial ischaemia including haemodynamic indices, multiple-lead ECG, transoesophageal echocardiography and myocardial lactate production (Table 24.5). It has been suggested that the rate–pressure product (RPP = systolic blood pressure × heart rate) may be a valid index for myocardial oxygen consumption. RPP appears to correlate well with myocardial oxygen consumption in exercising patients,[45] but these variables agree poorly during general anaesthesia.[46] The worst clinical scenario for myocardial ischaemia, i.e. hypotension and tachycardia, results in a normal RPP.[47]

External
- Hypotension
- Tachycardia
- Hypoxaemia
- Anaemia

Internal
- Atherosclerotic plaque rupture
- Thrombosis
- Vessel spasm

- Tachycardia
- Hypertension
- Sympathetic nervous system stimulation
- Sympathomimetic drugs
- Discontinuation β-blockers

Supply / Demand

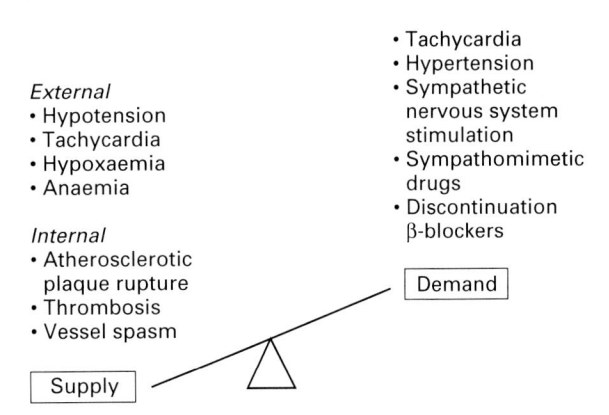

Fig. 24.1 Intra-operative myocardial ischaemia: myocardial supply/demand imbalance

Buffington et al,[48] in experimental studies, proposed an alternative haemodynamic risk index, the pressure/rate ratio (P/R = MAP/HR, where HR = heart rate). Myocardial ischaemia was associated with a P/R ratio <1 (decreased MAP, increased heart rate or both).

The value of the pulmonary artery catheter for the diagnosis of myocardial ischaemia may be limited. Kaplan & Wells[49] suggested that an elevation of pulmonary capillary wedge pressure (PCWP) associated with abnormal waves (*a*, *c* or *v*) was a more sensitive index of myocardial ischaemia than V5 ECG ST segment changes. Vascular surgery patients whose PCWP increased by 8 mmHg or more, associated with an abnormal wave form, had a 92% likelihood of developing ischaemia.[50] However, only 13% of all PCWP measurements and 21% of all ischaemic events were associated with an abnormal wave form. The absence of a change in PCWP does not ensure the absence of ischaemia.

Table 24.5 Intra-operative detection of myocardial ischaemia

Haemodynamic indices
Rate–pressure product (systolic blood pressure × heart rate)
Pressure/rate ratio (mean arterial pressure ÷ heart rate)

Pulmonary capillary wedge pressure
Elevation
Abnormal waves

ECG ST segment abnormalities

Transoesophageal echocardiography
Decreased myocardial wall thickening
Wall motion abnormalities

Biochemical markers
Lactate production

ECG = Electrocardiogram.

ECG ST segment abnormalities. ECG ST segment changes of myocardial ischaemia depend on electrode placement, the band width and calibration of the ECG signal, the selection and number of leads monitored, the ECG signal display and the extent of pre-existing ST segment abnormalities. Pre-existing ST segment changes may be associated with ventricular hypertrophy, myocardial infarction, digitalis and diuretic therapy, hypokalaemia, etc. Most changes involve ST depression; ST elevation appears to be uncommon. Reversible ST changes are most likely to be ischaemic in origin.[44] The V5 lead has been reported to detect about 85% of ST segment abnormalities recorded by the 12-lead ECG.[51] A combination of leads II, V4 and V5 detects 96% of new ST segment abnormalities observed on the 12-lead ECG.[44] Definitive outcome studies relating to intra-operative ischaemia during non-cardiac surgery are pending. Is there any correlation between ischaemic time, magnitude of ischaemia as detected by the extent of ST depression and adverse outcome? Are other ECG changes, e.g. new T-wave inversion, uni- or multifocal premature ventricular contractions or new nodal rhythms predictive of adverse outcome?

Transoesophageal echocardiography. Transoesophageal echocardiographic changes are earlier and more sensitive indices of myocardial ischaemia than ECG ST segment changes. The earliest changes noted are decreased myocardial wall thickening during systole (M-mode assessment of the anterior left ventricular wall) followed by two-dimensional wall motion abnormalities progressing from hypokinesia to akinesia to dyskinesia.[52] Preliminary data suggest that transoesophageal wall motion and wall thickening as changes indicative of ischaemia, even without ECG changes, are associated with increased peri-operative cardiac morbidity.[53] The specificity of wall motion changes is not clearly established. Such changes may be influenced by heart rate, left ventricular loading conditions and afterload.

Biochemical markers. Various biochemical markers of intra-operative myocardial ischaemia have been advanced. Production of lactate in the territory of the myocardium deprived of oxygen has been advocated as the 'gold standard' for identifying myocardial ischaemia. Myocardial release of inosine or hypoxanthine has also been used.[54] However, because of the complex relationship between myocardial lactate uptake and production, and the regional nature of myocardial ischaemia, serum lactate is an insensitive marker for myocardial ischaemia.[55]

Major arrhythmias

The ECG is monitored routinely in contemporary anaesthetic practice to identify myocardial ischaemia as well as to recognize intra-operative arrhythmias. Standard limb lead II is usually used because the P wave is best observed and because the lead's electrical axis parallels the electrical axis of the heart.[56]

Incidence

Studies evaluating intra-operative arrhythmias have been limited by intermittent rather than continuous recordings, and the failure to compare intra- and post-operative arrhythymias with the pre-operative baseline rhythm pattern. The reported incidence of intra-operative arrhythmias has ranged from 13 to 84%, with ventricular arrhythmias ranging from 6 to 60%.[57-59] Bradycardias and tachycardias must be diagnosed with respect to their site of origin, possible aetiologies and clinical importance. The ability to separate supraventricular from ventricular arrhythmias, and to assess the haemodynamic consequences of the rhythm disturbance, is crucial in management. Wandering atrial pacemaker, AV dissociation with halogenated anaesthetic agents and drug-induced bradyarrhythmias are observed commonly and may not produce significant haemodynamic changes. The incidence of serious arrhythmias (persistent multifocal premature ventricular contractions, ventricular tachycardia, ventricular fibrillation) has been reported to range between 0.9%[57] and 6%.[59]

Predisposing factors

Conditions predisposing to the development of intra-operative haemodynamically significant arrhythmias are outlined in Table 24.6. The association between bradyarrhythmias and volatile anaesthetic agents, neuromuscular blocking agents and opioids has been discussed previously. Intra-operative arrhythmias may be associated with hypoxaemia, hypercapnia and respiratory acidosis, acute hypokalaemia, myocardial ischaemia or infarction, hypermetabolic states (fever, malignant hyperpyrexia, hyperthyroidism, phaeochromocytoma) and exogenous catecholamine administration. Arrhythmias are more common at the times of tracheal intubation and extubation. Intra-operative ventricular arrhythmias have been reported to be more common in patients with known heart disease (60 versus 37%).[58] Other factors associated with intra-operative arrhythmias include surgery, which may produce sinus bradycardia and permit ventricular escape rhythms to evolve (e.g. the oculocardiac reflex may produce severe rhythm disturbances during ophthalmic surgery) and the insertion of vascular catheters into the right atrium or into the pulmonary artery.[56]

Table 24.6 Intra-operative arrhythmias — predisposing causes

Pre-existing coronary artery disease
Tracheal intubation
Right and left cardiac monitoring catheters
Myocardial ischaemia/infarction
Gas exchange abnormalities
    Hypoxaemia
    Hypercapnia
Biochemical and metabolic disturbances
    Acute acidosis/alkalosis
    Hypokalaemia
Surgical factors — autonomic reflexes
Anaesthetic factors — depth of anaesthesia
Drug-related — exogenous catecholamine administration
Hypermetabolic states
    Fever
    Malignant hyperpyrexia
    Phaeochromocytoma
    Thyrotoxicosis

Management

In assessing an intra-operative rhythm disturbance the anaesthetist should seek the answers to the following questions:

- what is the associated heart rate?
- is the rhythm regular (constant R–R interval)?
- is there sinus rhythm, i.e. a P wave before each QRS complex?
- is the QRS complex normal?
- is there haemodynamic instability?
- is there any obvious cause, e.g. hypoxaemia, hypercapnia, myocardial ischaemia, pyrexia, surgical stimulation, hypokalaemia or drug effect?

The treatment required for an individual intra-operative arrhythmia depends on its aetiology, the patient's underlying cardiac status and any associated haemodynamic disturbance.

Premature atrial contractions, usually with a different P wave, irregular rhythm and normal QRS complex, have little clinical significance and treatment is usually unnecessary. In contrast, a run of rapidly repeating supraventricular beats from a site other than the SA node characterizes paroxysmal atrial tachycardia (PAT). The inclusion of tachycardias originating in the AV node (junctional rhythms) permits the useful classification of paroxysmal supraventricular tachycardia (SVT). These rhythms may be abrupt in both their onset and termination. PAT (with heart rates varying from 120 to 250 beats/min, a P wave hidden in the QRS complex, a normal QRS, or ST segment changes) may be associated with pre-existing Wolff–Parkinson–White syndrome and other aberrant conduction pathway syndromes. PAT may also be associated with ischaemic heart disease, chronic obstructive lung disease, thyrotoxicosis, digitalis toxicity and pulmonary embolism. Changes in autonomic nervous system function, drug effects and intravascular volume shifts may precipitate PAT and significant haemodynamic changes. This arrhythmia requires active intervention. Appropriate forms of treatment include:

- vagal manoeuvres such as carotid sinus massage
- administration of a calcium antagonist, e.g. verapamil 2.5–5.0 mg intravenously (not in patients with known Wolff–Parkinson–White syndrome)
- administration of a β-adrenoceptor blocker, e.g. esmolol 1 mg.kg^{-1} followed by an infusion at a rate of 50–100 μg.kg.min^{-1}
- intravenous digitalization, e.g. digoxin 0.5–1 mg intravenously or
- cardioversion with appropriate synchronization.

Calcium antagonists and β-adrenoceptor blockers should be used with extreme caution during halothane anaesthesia because of the risk of precipitating complete heart block due to the additive effects of the changes on AV nodal conduction.

Atrial flutter or fibrillation usually indicates the presence of significant coronary artery disease, chronic obstructive pulmonary disease, hyperthyroidism, mitral valve disease, pulmonary embolism, myocardial contusion or myocarditis. In addition, atrial fibrillation may predispose to atrial thrombi formation with the possibility of pulmonary and systemic embolization. Treatment may include pharmacological reduction of ventricular rate with digitalis, verapamil 2.5–5 mg intravenously, esmolol 0.5–1 mg.kg^{-1} or synchronized direct current cardioversion with low voltage (10–50 J).

Premature ventricular contractions (PVCs), to be differentiated from PACs with aberrant ventricular conduction, may be ominous arrhythmias during anaesthesia. The onset of new PVCs may progress to ventricular tachycardia or fibrillation, especially in the context of myocardial ischaemia or infarction, hypoxaemia, hypercapnia, hypermetabolic states, digitalis toxicity with hypokalaemia, and halothane anaesthesia. Progression of PVCs to ventricular fibrillation is more likely with frequent, multifocal bigeminal rhythm or with complexes firing near the vulnerable period of the preceding ventricular depolarization (the R-on-T phenomenon). Treatment priorities include correction of any underlying cause (e.g. hypoventilation, hypoxaemia, hypokalaemia) and prompt anti-arrhythmic treatment with lignocaine 1.5 mg.kg^{-1} intravenously followed by an infusion of 1–4 mg.min^{-1}, if required.

Cardiovascular drug interactions during anaesthesia

A number of drugs given in the pre-operative period may have significant adverse effects on heart rhythm and haemodynamic function during anaesthesia. These drugs include antihypertensive, antidepressant and anti-anginal medications.

Antihypertensive agents

Antihypertensive agents such as β-adrenoceptor blockers, calcium antagonists and other vasodilators should be continued up to the day of surgery. Pharmacologically controlled hypertensive patients have less intra-operative blood pressure lability compared with untreated or poorly controlled hypertensives.[37] The administration of anaesthetic or other vasodilating drugs to treated hypertensive patients may produce hypotension which may necessitate judicious intravenous volume infusion or administration of an α-adrenergic agonist. Pre-operative clonidine (an $α_2$-adrenoceptor agonist) withdrawal before surgery may precipitate peri-operative rebound hypertension.[38]

Antidepressant drugs

Antidepressant agents with significant cardiovascular implications include tricyclics and monoamine oxidase inhibitors (MAOIs). Tricyclic antidepressants have peripheral and central anticholinergic effects and inhibit the amine pump responsible for noradrenaline re-uptake at the adrenergic nerve terminal. The anticholinergic and adrenergic effects are responsible for the potentially undesirable tachycardia, decreased atrioventricular conduction and hypertension during anaesthesia. MAOIs, e.g. tranylcypromine, alter the synthesis, release, re-uptake and metabolism of noradrenaline at adrenergic nerve terminals. Interactions between MAOIs and anaesthetic agents, e.g. pethidine, include unpredictable hypertension, hyperrigidity and adrenergic effects.[60]

Anti-anginal medication

Anti-anginal medication, including β-adrenoceptor blockers and calcium antagonists, may have interactive cardiovascular effects, especially with volatile anaesthetic agents. β-adrenergic blockers, e.g. propranolol, metoprolol, may possibly potentiate myocardial depression while calcium entry blockers such as nifedipine and verapamil may be associated with hypotension (nifedipine), and varying degrees of heart block (verapamil).[61]

RESPIRATORY SYSTEM

Aspiration

Vomiting and regurgitation of gastric contents, with subsequent aspiration into the tracheobronchial tree, is still an important cause of morbidity and mortality in patients undergoing general anaesthesia. Reports attribute acid aspiration syndrome as the cause of 25% of maternal deaths associated with anaesthesia and 19% of total deaths associated with general anaesthesia.[62]

Incidence

Silent regurgitation of gastric contents into the oropharynx has been reported in 4–14.5% of adult general anaesthetic administrations, depending on the anaesthetic agents and technique used, the site of surgery and the position of the patient.[62–64] Subsequent pulmonary aspiration of regurgitated gastric contents occurs in a variable proportion of these patients. Published mortality rates associated with massive aspiration have varied from 30 to 50%, depending on the extent of the lung injury.[65,66] Mortality may occur at any age, but is most likely in elderly or debilitated patients.[67] Bacterial contamination of the aspirate, as may occur in a patient with bowel obstruction, is associated with a very high mortality rate. Aspiration of particulate matter, such as partially digested food, causes severe physiological derangements.[68] Aspiration pneumonia has been cited as the anaesthetic-related cause of death in 0.008–0.2 deaths per 1000 anaesthetic administrations.[62,69]

Associated features

Clinically significant aspiration is most likely in patients at the extremes of age undergoing emergency surgery. Patients with excess gastric acid and delayed gastric emptying (e.g. hypovolaemia, opioid administration, pregnancy, obesity) and gastro-intestinal pathology (e.g. hiatus hernia, bowel obstruction) are predisposed to regurgitation and aspiration (Table 24.7).

The acidity of the aspirate, often pH <2.5, is probably the most important factor contributing to the severity of pneumonitis. In numerous experimental studies, increasing acidity, whether alone or in combination with food particles, results in increasing tracheal mucosal and lung parenchymal damage.[70,71] Recovery and healing of lung injury are faster if the acidity of the aspirate is reduced. The critical volume of aspirate (usually considered to be >0.4 mg.kg^{-1}) needed to cause severe lung damage is also dependent on the pH of the

Table 24.7 Patient population at risk of gastric aspiration

Delayed gastric emptying and excess gastric acid
Pregnancy, labour, delivery and postpartum
Morbid obesity
Unpremedicated outpatients
Emergency surgery: trauma, hypovolaemic shock, pain
Opioid administration

Gastro-intestinal disorders
Gastro-oesophageal reflux
Upper gastro-intestinal bleeding
Gastric outlet obstruction
Small or large intestinal obstruction

Table 24.9 Treatment of acid aspiration

Immediate endotracheal suctioning or bronchoscopy
Supplemental oxygen therapy ± CPAP
Ventilatory support: IMV and PEEP
Frequent arterial blood gas analysis
Restoration of intravascular volume
Haemodynamic monitoring
    Pulmonary artery catheter
        PCWP
        Cardiac output
        Pulmonary and systemic vascular resistance
Intra-arterial pressure monitoring

CPAP = Continuous positive airways pressure; IMV = intermittent mandatory ventilation; PEEP = positive end-expiratory pressure: PCWP = pulmonary capillary wedge pressure.

aspirate. Even small volumes are associated with a high mortality rate if the pH is low.[72] Aspiration of particular matter, e.g. partially digested food particles, results in the immediate onset of severe pulmonary physiological derangements. In the long term, a granulomatous response develops around these particles.[63] Experimental studies have confirmed that pulmonary dysfunction increases as the osmolarity of the aspirate increases.[73]

Prophylaxis and treatment

Guidelines for the prophylaxis and prevention of acid aspiration are shown in Table 24.8. Suggested treatment strategies for peri-operative aspiration are outlined in Table 24.9.

Gas exchange

Hypoxia

Tissue hypoxia occurs when there is cessation of oxidative phosphorylation and mitochondrial Po_2 falls below a critical level. The utilization of anaerobic pathways produces poorly excreted metabolites, e.g. hydrogen and lactate ions. The brain is most sensitive to hypoxia in the awake state and the heart is most sensitive in the anaesthetized patient.

Assuming a normal arterial oxygenation (Pa_{O_2} 12 kPa; 97% oxygen saturation), mild arterial hypoxaemia may be considered as an arterial saturation between 80 and 90%, moderate hypoxaemia an arterial oxygen saturation 60–80% and severe hypoxaemia an arterial oxygen saturation less than 60%.[74]

Conditions associated with intra-operative hypoxaemia. A classification of the conditions associated with intra-operative hypoxaemia is outlined in Table 24.10. Hypoxaemia may be associated with a reduction in alveolar oxygen tension (PA_{O_2}) or an increased alveolar–arterial oxygen tension difference.

A reduction in PA_{O_2} may be associated with reduced or absent inspired oxygen or alveolar hypoventilation. Hypoxaemia due to mechanical failure of the oxygen supply system or the anaesthetic machine is a recognized, but increasingly uncommon, hazard of general anaesthesia. Disconnection of the patient from the oxygen supply system (usually at the tracheal tube connection) and inadvertent excess administration of nitrous oxide are the most common causes of mechanical failure to deliver oxygen to the patient. Empty or depleted oxygen cylinders, incorrectly filled oxygen cylinders, failure of gas pressure in the pipeline oxygen system and crossing of pipelines during construction have all been associated with reported cases of intra-operative hypoxaemia. Technological advances in anaesthetic machine construction and safety features, including the advent of inspired oxygen analysers and continuous monitoring of the arterial oxygen saturation, have reduced the incidence of intra-operative

Table 24.8 Acid aspiration prophylaxis and prevention

Identify patient population at risk

Prophylaxis
High-risk: consider awake tracheal intubation
Pharmacological prophylaxis
    Anticholinergics
    Gastric acid neutralization: 0.3 molar sodium citrate
    H_2-Receptor antagonists
    Promote gastric emptying: metoclopramide
Consider regional anaesthesia

All at-risk patients require tracheal intubation

Rapid-sequence induction of anaesthesia
Cricoid pressure to occlude oesophagus
Lateral head-down position

Awake extubation

Table 24.10 Intra-operative hypoxia

$P_{A_{O_2}} \downarrow$
$F_{I_{O_2}} \downarrow$
Mechanical failure of anaesthetic apparatus to deliver sufficient oxygen

Hypoventilation
Mechanical ventilation — inadequate $\dot{V}_E$: tidal volume/respiratory rate

Spontaneous ventilation
　Altered chemical control of breathing
　Increased airways resistance
　Decreased lung compliance

Alveolar–arterial oxygen tension difference $\uparrow$

Shunt $\uparrow$
Endobronchial intubation

Functional residual capacity and atelectasis $\downarrow$
General anaesthesia — change in thoracic cage muscle tone changes in thoracic blood volume

Supine position

Paralysis

$P\bar{v}_{O_2} \downarrow$

Anaemia

Cardiac output $\downarrow$
　Hypovolaemia
　Myocardial depression

Oxygen consumption $\uparrow$
　Sympathetic nervous system stimulation
　Pyrexia
　Shivering

$P_{A_{O_2}}$ = Partial pressure of alveolar oxygen; $F_{I_{O_2}}$ = fraction of inspired oxygen; $\dot{V}_E$ = minute ventilation; $P\bar{v}_{O_2}$ = Mixed venous oxygen saturation

---

hypoxaemia due to mechanical failure of anaesthetic apparatus. However, hypoxic gas delivery is still possible if flowmeters fracture or stick, if rotameter tubes are transposed or if liquid oxygen reservoirs are filled incorrectly. Intra-operative hypoxaemia may be observed, despite the presence of a normally adequate inspired oxygen concentration, if significant hypoventilation occurs in spontaneously breathing patients, or if the preset minute ventilation is inadequate for the metabolic requirements of the patient. All inhaled anaesthetics depress minute ventilation and the ventilatory response to carbon dioxide. The degree of ventilatory depression varies with the anaesthetic agent (greatest with enflurane)[75] and the expired anaesthetic concentration. Kinking of the tracheal tube, blockage with secretions, and a herniated or ruptured cuff may all cause significant hypoventilation and hypoxaemia.

An increased alveolar–arterial oxygen tension difference may be associated with intra-operative hypoxaemia. This is associated most commonly with increased intrapulmonary shunting and decreased mixed venous oxygen tension. Inadvertent endobronchial intubation, often associated with the Trendelenburg position and head flexion, results in intra-operative hypoxaemia. A reduction in functional residual capacity (FRC) relative to closing volume (due to the cephalad shift of the diaphragm associated with the supine position,[76] the loss of inspiratory muscle tone, the appearance of end-expiratory tone in the abdominal expiratory muscles, changes in intrathoracic blood volume associated with induction of anaesthesia,[77] and the influence of muscle relaxants on diaphragmatic excursion[78]) all favour the development of intra-operative atelectasis and intrapulmonary shunting. A decreased cardiac output (associated with hypovolaemia and myocardial depression) in the presence of constant oxygen consumption or increased oxygen consumption (due to pyrexia, sympathetic nervous system stimulation, shivering, etc.) in the presence of a constant cardiac output reduces mixed venous oxygen tension. The larger the intrapulmonary shunt, the greater the reduction in Pa_{O_2} because more venous blood with lower oxygen tension mixes with oxygenated end-capillary blood in the lungs.

Hypercapnia

Hypercapnia comprises an increased arterial carbon dioxide tension (Pa_{CO_2}) with an associated respiratory acidosis. A classification of the intra-operative conditions associated with hypercapnia is shown in Table 24.11. These conditions include increased carbon dioxide production, increased alveolar dead space, hypoventilation and mechanical failure of anaesthetic apparatus.[74]

If minute alveolar ventilation remains constant, an increase in Pa_{CO_2} results from increased carbon dioxide production (caused by shivering, pyrexia, sympathetic nervous system stimulation, hypermetabolic states, etc.) Specific intra-operative events may be associated with increased alveolar dead space; these include reduced pulmonary artery pressure associated with position or hypovolaemia, positive intrathoracic pressure associated with intermittent positive-pressure ventilation, with or without positive end-expiratory pressure (PEEP), and mechanical interference with pulmonary artery blood flow associated with venous air embolism (VAE), fat or pulmonary embolism.

Hypoventilation results in an increase in Pa_{CO_2} if carbon dioxide production remains constant. Hypoventilation during anaesthesia may result from reduced ventilatory drive, increased resistance to air flow in

Table 24.11 Intra-operative hypercapnia

Anaesthetic apparatus
Inadequate fresh gas flow
Carbon dioxide rebreathing
Increased anatomical dead space

Hypoventilation ↓ $\dot{V}_E$:
Medullary ventilatory drive ↓
    Volatile agents
    Opioids
    Sedatives/hypnotics
Air flow resistance ↑
    Upper airway obstruction
    Anaesthetic circuit
    Tracheal tube diameter
    Tracheal tube kinking, blockage or cuff herniation
Airway resistance ↑
    Laryngospasm
    Bronchospasm

Alveolar deadspace ↑
Pulmonary blood flow ↓
    Patient position
    Hypovolaemia
    Cardiac output ↓
    Mechanical distribution of blood flow
    Pulmonary embolism
    Venous air embolism
    Fat embolism

Carbon dioxide production ↑
Hypermetabolic states
Pyrexia
Shivering

$\dot{V}_E$ = minute ventilation.

external anaesthesia equipment, the tracheal tube and the tracheobronchial tree, or decreased pulmonary compliance. Volatile anaesthetic agents, opioids, sedatives and hypnotics may exert potent depressant effects on the medullary centres involved in the control of ventilation. Hypoventilation may be caused by increased resistance to air flow through the tracheal tube (kinking, obstruction with secretions and herniated or ruptured cuff) and through external breathing apparatus and circuits. Hypoventilation secondary to upper airway obstruction must be considered in the unintubated patient. Airway resistance is increased and pulmonary compliance is decreased during anaesthesia because of the reduction in the airway calibre and tendency towards airway collapse associated with general anaesthesia. Finally, the anaesthetic apparatus may be associated with hypercapnia because of rebreathing of carbon dioxide. The breathing system may increase the anatomical dead space, the carbon dioxide absorber may be depleted or inadvertently switched off, and the fresh gas flow may be inadequate to prevent rebreathing with the breathing system in use. The order of increasing rebreathing and fresh flow requirements for spontaneously breathing patients with non-rebreathing Mapleson circuits is A (Magill) >D>C>B.

Intra-operative bronchospasm

The large central airways — the trachea, main stem and segmental bronchi — account for approximately 80% of the measurable resistance to air flow.[79] Bronchoconstriction in these airways results in significant air flow obstruction. Bronchial smooth-muscle tone reflects a balance of constrictor tone, maintained by efferent vagal innervation, and dilator tone, maintained by the sympathetic nervous system. A direct sympathetic inhibitory pathway to human airway smooth muscle is speculative but a non-adrenergic inhibitory pathway does exist and recent evidence points to the neuropeptide vasoactive intestinal polypeptide as the neurotransmitter at this site.[80] Within the epithelial walls of the airway are three types of sensory receptors whose activity alters bronchial muscle tone, principally via parasympathetic pathways.[81] These include pulmonary stretch receptors, juxtapulmonary j receptors and rapidly adapting irritant receptors. The last of these respond to mechanical irritation, thermal stimuli and irritants such as inhaled particles and gases.

Precipitating causes

The potential aetiologies of intra-operative bronchospasm are shown in Table 24.12.

The bronchial hyperreactivity associated with asthmatic patients and patients with chronic obstructive lung disease has been attributed to reduced resting airway calibre, hypertrophy of airway smooth muscles and increased accessibility of stimuli to the target cell. Increased tracheobronchial mucus and airway oedema compound the problem. Removal of the epithelial barrier by viral respiratory tract infections allows greater access of irritant stimuli (e.g. from tracheal tube or cold inspired gases) to the subepithelial receptors.[82] Airway hyperreactivity persists for 3–4 weeks following upper respiratory tract infection. The presence of rapidly adapting receptors in the mucosa of cartilaginous airways may explain the bronchoconstrictor response to mechanical irritation during anaesthesia (e.g. pulmonary aspiration of gastric contents, tracheal tube placement during inadequate depth of anaesthesia or the administration of cold and dry anaesthetic gases).[83] Bronchospasm during anaesthesia may be associated with an immunological response related to mediator release from mast cells or circulating basophils.[84] The specific mediators involved in anaphylactoid reactions

Table 24.12 Intra-operative bronchospasm — predisposing causes

Bronchial hyperreactivity
Associated viral infections
Chronic obstructive pulmonary disease
Asthma

Irritant receptor response
Mechanical — tracheal tube
Thermal

Pulmonary aspiration

Mediator release — allergy/anaphylaxis
Histamine
Leukotrienes
Eicosanoids (TXA$_2$; PGI$_2$; PGF$_{2\alpha}$)

Pharmacological responses
β-Adrenoceptor blockers

Differential diagnosis during anaesthesia
Endobronchial intubation
Pneumothorax
Pulmonary embolism
Pulmonary oedema

TXA$_2$ = Thromboxane A$_2$; PGI$_2$ = prostacyclin; PGF$_{2\alpha}$ = prostaglandin F$_{2\alpha}$.

will be discussed later, but histamine released from airway mast cells, leukotrienes derived from arachidonic acid by the action of lipo-oxygenase, thromboxane A$_2$, prostaglandin F$_{2\alpha}$ (PGF$_{2\alpha}$) and prostacyclin (PGI$_2$) produced from arachidonic acid by the action of cyclo-oxygenase, and bradykinin formed by the action of kallikrein on a plasma precursor are all potent bronchoconstrictors which may be associated with the development of intra-operative bronchospasm.[85] These mediators may be involved in occasional bronchospasm associated with the administration of induction agents (e.g. thiopentone[86] and propofol), neuromuscular blocking agents (e.g. *d*-tubocurarine[87] and suxamethonium) and opioids (e.g. morphine[88]).

A number of pharmacological agents which alter bronchomotor tone or influence mediator release may be implicated in the development of intra-operative bronchospasm if these agents are taken in the pre-operative period, e.g. β-adrenoceptor blocking agents and prostaglandin inhibitors (aspirin, indomethacin). Important components of the differential diagnosis in the event of intra-operative bronchospasm include endobronchial intubation, pneumothorax, pulmonary embolism and pulmonary oedema secondary to left ventricular failure.

Prevention and management

An outline of the therapeutic options available to treat intra-operative bronchospasm is presented in Figure 24.2. Because most bronchoconstrictor reflexes are vagally mediated, administration of an anticholinergic agent (e.g. atropine 0.6 mg or glycopyrronium 0.2 mg) intravenously prior to induction of anaesthesia may be

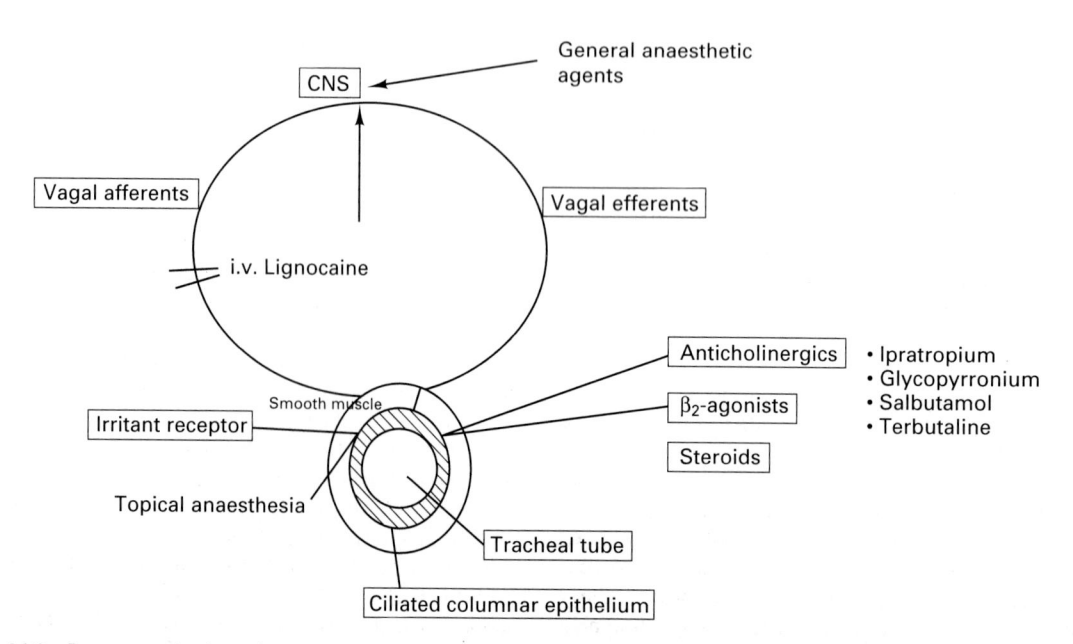

Fig. 24.2 Intra-operative bronchospasm: mechanisms and prevention. CNS = Central nervous system.

appropriate.[89] Intravenous lignocaine 1 mg.kg⁻¹ to produce a clinically useful plasma concentration (1–2 μg.ml⁻¹) may prevent reflex bronchoconstriction at the time of induction.[90]

Ketamine may be the intravenous induction agent of choice for patients with reactive airways disease.[91] Thiopentone may be associated with bronchospasm if premature instrumentation of the airway occurs or if depth of anaesthesia is inadequate. The volatile anaesthetic agents directly relax airway smooth muscle.[92] Both enflurane and isoflurane are equally effective in preventing and reversing bronchospasm when an adequate concentration (>1.5 MAC) is used.[93] Halothane potentiates the arrhythmogenic potential of hypercapnia, endogenous catecholamines or drugs such as β_2-agonists which may be administered to treat established bronchospasm.

Management of intra-operative bronchospasm involves establishing the diagnosis, ensuring adequate depth of anaesthesia, altering inspiratory oxygen concentration, flow rates and inspiration/expiration (I/E) ratio and pharmacological intervention. Low inspiratory flows and high I/E ratios have been advocated to minimize peak airway pressure and cardiovascular effects, and to improve the distribution of ventilation during intra-operative bronchospasm.[94] However, most published data favour a high inspiratory flow and low I/E ratio to maximize expiratory time, reduce pulmonary hyperinflation and improve gas exchange.[95] A cornerstone in the management of intra-operative bronchospasm is the administration of nebulized β_2-sympathomimetics (e.g. terbutaline or salbutamol 0.5 mg in 2 ml normal saline). The use of the phosphodiesterase inhibitor aminophylline 5 mg.kg⁻¹ intravenously to treat intra-operative bronchospasm may be ineffective and may be associated with potentially hazardous cardiac arrhythmias, especially in the presence of hypercapnia and halothane administration.[96] Hydrocortisone 1–2 mg.kg⁻¹ may be administered, although its mechanism of action has not been established and its onset time may be delayed.

Pneumothorax

The clinical conditions associated with intra-operative pneumothorax are outlined in Table 24.13. Pneumothoraces may be divided into spontaneous, which occur without prior trauma or other obvious causes, and traumatic, which occur as a result of direct or indirect chest trauma. Spontaneous pneumothoraces may be further divided into primary and secondary. Primary spontaneous pneumothorax occurs in otherwise healthy individuals (usually following rupture of

Table 24.13 Intra-operative pneumothorax — associated conditions

SPONTANEOUS
Primary
Otherwise healthy patients

Secondary
Complicating lung disease
  COPD
  Asthma
  Bullous emphysema
  Congenital cystic lung disease
  Cystic fibrosis
  Pneumatocele
Neoplastic
  Bronchogenic carcinoma
  Sarcoma
Interstitial lung disease
  Interstitial fibrosis
  Sarcoidosis
  Eosinophilic granuloma
Infectious disease
  Anaerobic pneumonia
  Tuberculosis
  Atypical pneumonia

TRAUMATIC
Indirect
IPPV/PEEP

Direct
Intravascular catheters — TPN
Surgery — mediastinoscopy, monitoring
Penetrating/non-penetrating trauma — fractured ribs, flail chest, pulmonary contusion
Intercostal nerve blocks

COPD = Chronic obstructive pulmonary disease; IPPV = intermittent positive-pressure ventilation; PEEP = positive end-expiratory pressure; TPN = total parenteral nutrition.

subpleural emphysematous blebs); secondary spontaneous pneumothorax occurs as a complication of clinically manifest lung disease.[97]

Two quite different mechanisms may lead to intra-operative spontaneous pneumothorax. The first is a visceral pleural tear (i.e. bronchopleural fistula) that results from rupture of a subpleural bleb, parenchymal pulmonary trauma or a process which erodes the visceral pleura (e.g. necrotizing pneumonia, intravascular catheters, etc.). The second mechanism is a partial bronchial obstruction which may behave as a check valve leading to progressive hyperinflation of distal air spaces. Eventually, air dissects along the bronchovascular spaces into the lung hilum and directly into the mediastinum (pneumomediastinum). If the process continues, air ruptures in one of two directions — either through fascial planes in the neck resulting in subcutaneous emphysema, or through the visceral pleura into one or both pleural spaces, resulting in pneumothorax. A tension pneumothorax implies air in the pleural space under sufficient positive pressure to inhibit venous return, displace mediastinal structures and restrict the inflation of the contralateral lung.

A number of special considerations regarding intra-operative pneumothorax should be emphasized. Pulmonary barotrauma is defined as extra-alveolar air arising from lung damage secondary to changes in intrathoracic pressure.[98] Clinical manifestations of barotrauma associated with intermittent positive-pressure ventilation and PEEP include pneumothorax, bronchopleural fistula, pneumomediastinum and subcutaneous emphysema. Peak inspiratory pressures greater than 60–80 cmH$_2$O are associated with an increased incidence of barotrauma.[99] The high peak inspiratory pressures associated with barotrauma may reflect the severity of the underlying lung disease. There is no conclusive evidence that maintaining constant minute ventilation by manipulating peak inspiratory pressures (reversed I/E ratio, decreased flow rate, decreased tidal volume with increased respiratory rate, etc.) has any effect on the incidence of barotrauma.

A pneumothorax is a potential complication of central venous cannulation performed for total parenteral nutrition or haemodynamic monitoring. Pneumothorax is a relatively frequent complication of mediastinoscopy, but is not usually apparent until the postoperative period and seldom requires decompression by insertion of an intrapleural drain. As in the case of central venous cannulation, a chest radiograph following the procedure is mandatory. Pneumothoraces normally contain nitrogen (from air), a gas with low solubility (blood:gas partition coefficient 0.015), which limits its removal by blood. Nitrous oxide, a more soluble gas (blood:gas partition coefficient 0.47), is transported in blood in substantial quantities, and has the potential to double the volume of a pneumothorax in 10 min and to triple it in 30 min[100] (assuming a nitrous oxide concentration of 75%).

A pneumothorax that occurs intra-operatively, as evidenced by increased peak inspiratory pressure, tracheal shift, distant breath sounds, unilateral bronchospasm, hypotension and cyanosis, requires immediate treatment with needle aspiration or chest tube insertion, usually in the second intercostal space in the mid clavicular line.

Embolization

Potential embolic complications during anaesthesia include VAE, fat and pulmonary embolism.

Venous air embolism

Venous air entrainment is a gravity-related phenomenon, and is associated with risks of pulmonary and/or systemic air embolism. It is a potential hazard confronting a patient placed in the sitting position for cervical spine or posterior fossa surgery, or patients placed in a significant head-up tilt for thyroid or head and neck surgery. Additional cardiovascular monitoring to detect and treat VAE is indicated in neurosurgical patients placed in the sitting or head-up position. Continuous measurement of arterial blood pressure is required in this position and the transducer must be zeroed at skull level; the central venous pressure should be recorded at heart level, and the cerebral perfusion pressure should be calculated.[101]

Decreasing sensitivity	Physiological function	
• Transoesophageal echocardiography • Doppler ultrasound	Normal
• ↓ End tidal CO$_2$ • ↑ Pulmonary artery pressures	↑ Dead space
• ↑ Central venous pressure • 'Mill-wheel' murmer – oesophageal stethoscope • Hypotension • ECG changes	• Clinical changes • Cardiovascular collapse

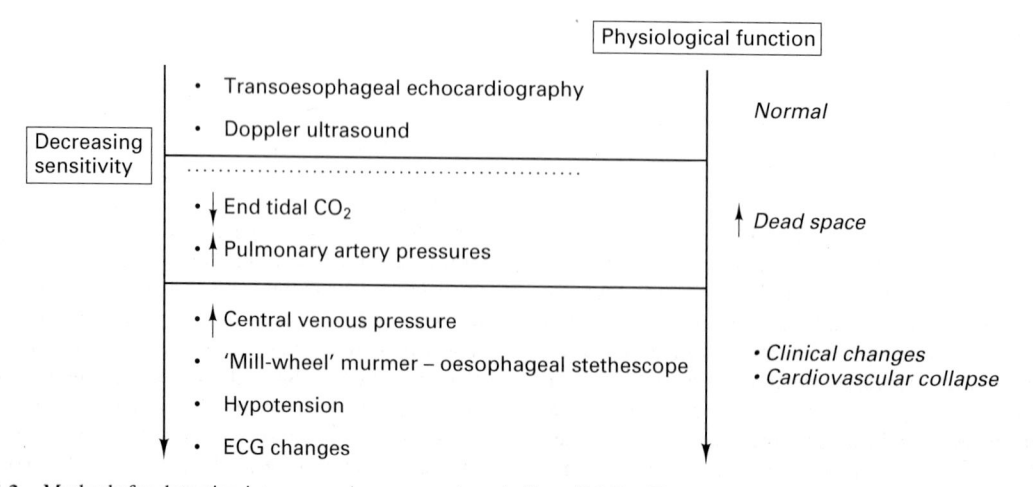

Fig. 24.3 Methods for detecting intra-operative venous air embolism. ECG = Electrocardiogram.

The sensitivities of the various clinical and technological devices to detect intracardiac air are listed in Figure 24.3. Transoesophageal echocardiography is the most sensitive technique for detection of air in the right atrium and paradoxical embolization to the left atrium through a patent foramen ovale.[102] However, the technique is not specific for VAE; fat emboli and blood micro-emboli are also detected. The most sensitive generally available monitoring technique to detect intracardiac air is Doppler ultrasound.[103] Air is an excellent acoustic reflector, and its passage through the heart is heralded by a change from a regular swishing signal to an erratic roaring noise. Air in the pulmonary microcirculation leads to a reduction in lung perfusion relative to ventilation and an increased physiological dead space. A sudden decrease in end-tidal carbon dioxide tension accompanied by increased pulmonary artery pressure may provide a semiquantitative estimate of the volume of VAE.[104] Auscultation of a 'mill-wheel' murmur with an oesophageal stethoscope implies the presence of large volumes of intracardiac air. Finally, hypotension, elevations in central venous pressure and ECG changes indicate the existence of severe VAE.

A central venous pressure catheter tip located near the superior vena cava/right atrial junction is the most efficacious site for air removal. Accurate central venous pressure catheter tip placement may involve chest X-ray or the confirmation of a right ventricular pressure pattern followed by withdrawal of the catheter into the right atrium.

Fat embolism

Intra-operative fat embolism may complicate the use of autotransfusion systems, and may occur in association with long bone or pelvic fractures and during orthopaedic surgery procedures, e.g. total hip replacement and open reduction, interval fixation of hip fractures, etc. Following insertion of the freshly prepared bone cement (methyl methacrylate polymer) into the acetabular cup, or more commonly the femoral canal, an increased heart rate, hypotension or increased airway pressure may be observed. These responses may be due to absorption of the still liquid or vaporized monomer via the raw bony surfaces.[105] Bone cement monomer is a known peripheral vasodilator and direct myocardial depressant. The hypotensive response may result from an exothermic reaction or air/fat embolization with cement impregnation.[106] Concurrent hypovolaemia, deep anaesthesia and the relative size of the exposed raw bony surface to which the cement is applied may also contribute.

CENTRAL NERVOUS SYSTEM

Awareness

The problem of awareness during general anaesthesia became prominent with the introduction in the 1940s of muscle relaxants which permitted lighter levels of general anaesthesia. The problem intensified in the 1970s when opioids began to be used as the primary or sole anaesthetic agents and subsequently in the 1980s with the advent of total intravenous anaesthesia.

The scope of the problem

Only a small amount of information which evokes a neural response is stored in long-term memory. Information held in long-term memory is wholly unconscious — this information induces awareness only when small portions of it are transferred into conscious memory.[107] As the depth of anaesthesia is increased, the patient's state changes from conscious awareness with grossly impaired recall of peri-operative events to unconscious awareness, where some stimuli perceived by the brain may be stored in the long-term memory, but do not subsequently enter consciousness. Finally, the perception of stimuli by the brain is severely attenuated, and registration in both short-term and long-term memory is abolished.

What exactly constitutes anaesthesia has been the subject of correspondence and editorial comment. Pinsker[108] claimed that paralysis, unconsciousness and attenuation of the stress response were the necessary and sufficient components of the anaesthetized state, and that control of these three components constituted general anaesthesia. Paralysis and attenuation of stress responses are easily determined. However, unconsciousness remains ill-defined and includes amnesia and hypnosis. Unfortunately, there is no current end-point that serves as a basis for the rational administration of drugs to achieve unconsciousness. Presently, the absence of recall is the only objective criterion of unconsciousness/hypnosis/amnesia used routinely. Anaesthetists cannot guarantee lack of recall and similarly cannot guarantee that intra-operative events and conversations will not have adverse long-term psychological effects.

Prys-Roberts[109] has sought to redefine anaesthesia in terms of the response of the patient to the trauma of surgery, and the suppression of those responses by a wide variety of drugs. The essential premiss of his argument is that pain is the conscious perception of a noxious stimulus; it follows that anaesthesia is defined, in his view, as a state in which, as a result of drug-induced unconsciousness, the patient neither perceives nor recalls noxious stimuli. The response to noxious stimuli (mechanical, chemical, thermal or irradiation, causing actual or potential cell damage) involves somatic (sensory and motor) and autonomic (haemodynamic, sudomotor and hormonal) responses.

Monitoring depth of anaesthesia

At present, the anaesthetist's principal monitor of depth of anaesthesia is the patient's somatic and autonomic responses to surgical stimuli. Many of these clinical signs depend on muscle activity (e.g. respiratory changes, movement in response to stimulation and muscle tone) and autonomic responses (changes in blood pressure and pulse rate, sweating and lacrimation). These responses are modified by neuromuscular-blocking agents and by drugs which act on the cardio-vascular system. The presence or absence of these responses does not, however, correlate with conscious awareness. They are inadequate indicators of a satisfactory depth of anaesthesia.[110]

A wide variety of techniques have been advocated to assess depth of anaesthesia during surgery (Table 24.14). Whereas the concentration of volatile agents in end-tidal gas, and hence blood level, bears a predictable relationship, after equilibration, to the administered concentration, the relationship between dose rate and plasma concentration of intravenous agents varies widely between individuals. The motor response to somatic noxious stimulation is characterized by reflex withdrawal of the affected part.[109] Suppression of the reflex is the basis of the two quantitative indices of anaesthetic potency — the MAC for volatile agents and the minimum infusion rate for intravenous agents.[111] These indices involve movement of 50% of patients in response to surgical incision. Such movements are not subsequently recalled. Therefore the blood concentration of volatile or intravenous agent required to suppress movement is higher than that required to induce unconsciousness and amnesia.

A number of mechanical techniques may be used to monitor depth of anaesthesia. Tunstall[112] demonstrated responses to commands in patients undergoing Caesarean section by isolating the forearm from access by neuromuscular blocking agents. A positive response might indicate awareness. However, the majority of responders had no subsequent recall. A progressive decrease in spontaneous and evoked contractions of the lower oesophagus is seen with increasing depth of anaesthesia. Wide interindividual variation and drug effects have limited the application of this technology.[113]

A number of electrical techniques have been advocated as indicators of depth of anaesthesia. Electromyogram contraction of the frontalis muscle may reflect the transition from wakefulness to anaesthesia.[114] The frontalis muscle is more resistant to neuromuscular blocking agents than the adductor pollicis. An increased amplitude with decreasing frequency has been observed in electroencephalogram (EEG) signals with increasing depth of anaesthesia. These changes, however, differ quantitatively and qualitatively for different agents[115] and are non-specific (i.e. similar changes may be observed with hypocapnia, ischaemia, hypoglycaemia or hypothermia). Computer assessment of the EEG in a given time epoch and display as power versus various frequency bands allows measurement of the spectral edge (the frequency below which 95% of the EEG power lies). Similar monitoring of depth of anaesthesia with frequency edge on aperiodic analysis has been advocated.

The auditory evoked response is the EEG response to a sound stimulus. It is extracted from the raw EEG by computer averaging and consists of a series of waves representing the passage of electrical activity through the acoustic nerve, superior olivary complex, lateral lemniscus, medial geniculate body, auditory radiation and auditory cortex.[116] The volatile anaesthetic agents produce minimal or no change in brainstem responses and large graded changes in amplitude and latency of the early cortical waves. The changes in early cortical waves are similar whether produced by intravenous or inhaled agents, and these observations may prove to be sensitive indicators of depth of anaesthesia.

Table 24.14 Monitoring depth of anaesthesia

Motor response to noxious stimuli
Minimum alveolar concentration (MAC)
Minimum infusion rate (MIR)

End-tidal volatile agent concentration

Autonomic changes
Heart rate
Blood pressure
Lacrimation
Sweating

Mechanical
Isolated limb
Oesophageal contraction

Electrical
Frontalis EMG
EEG
   Unprocessed
   Processed — Compressed and density-modulated
     spectral array
   Aperiodic analysis
Evoked potentials — auditory

EMG = Electromyogram; EEG = electroencephalogram.

Cerebral ischaemia

The brain has a high rate of energy utilization and very limited energy storage capacity. It is therefore extremely vulnerable in the event of interruption of substrate (oxygen, glucose) supply. No currently available cerebral function monitor demonstrates cerebral ischaemia as clearly as ECG ST segment changes indicate myocardial ischaemia. Advances in monitoring of cerebral ischaemia, particularly electrophysiological monitoring, together with new understanding of the pathophysiology of cerebral ischaemia, may make intra-operative recognition and treatment of potential neurological damage feasible in the near future.[117]

Mechanisms and classification of ischaemic injury

Blood is supplied to the brain via the two internal carotid and vertebral arteries. There is an extensive collateral circulation both intracranially through the circle of Willis and extracranially from the external carotid artery, mainly through the ophthalmic artery.

Cerebral blood flow is closely related to the metabolic rate of brain tissue under normal circumstances. The normal brain autoregulates cerebral blood flow with variations in MAP varying from 60 to 140 mmHg to provide cerebral blood flow of 40–60 ml.min^{-1} per 100 g and cerebral oxygen consumption of 3–5 ml.min^{-1} per 100 g. In hypertensive patients, this autoregulation curve is shifted to the right, and signs of cerebral ischaemia may occur at a higher MAP. Cerebral perfusion pressure, the effective pressure perfusing the brain, is the difference between MAP and intracranial pressure.

Two patterns of cell death may occur after a cerebral ischaemic insult: immediate infarction or delayed neuronal necrosis. Delayed neuronal damage may be related to reperfusion injury following ischaemia. During reperfusion, neuronal damage may be mediated by free radicals (oxidants).

Cerebral ischaemia may be global or focal, complete or incomplete (Table 24.15). Complete global ischaemia (no cerebral blood flow) occurs during cardiac arrest, whereas incomplete global ischaemia (reduced cerebral blood flow) occurs at a cerebral perfusion pressure <40 mmHg because of decreased MAP or increased intracranial pressure, e.g. during carotid endarterectomy with ipsilateral internal carotid clamping and reduced collateral pressure from the contralateral internal carotid across the circle of Willis. Complete focal ischaemia occurs when the blood supply to a localized area of brain is completely arrested, e.g. in cerebrovascular occlusion during intracerebral aneurysm clipping. Incomplete focal ischaemia occurs when cerebrovascular stenosis and decreased cerebral perfusion pressure co-exist.

Table 24.15 Classification of cerebral ischaemia

Global	
Complete global ischaemia	Cardiac arrest
Incomplete global ischaemia	Hypotension
Focal	
Complete focal ischaemia	Cerebrovascular occlusion
Incomplete focal ischaemia	Cerebrovascular stenosis + hypotension

Threshold values of cerebral blood flow

There is a substantial reserve below normal cerebral blood flow (50 ml.min^{-1} per 100 g) before signs of ischaemia become manifest. Loss of spontaneous electrical activity occurs at a cerebral blood flow of 15–20 ml.min^{-1} per 100 g, and at 15 ml.min^{-1} per 100 g the cortical EEG becomes iso-electric. Evoked potentials persist until the cerebral blood flow is reduced to 15 ml/min per 100 g, but with reduced amplitudes and increased latencies. A cerebral blood flow of 15 ml.min^{-1} per 100 g is referred to as the flow threshold of electrical failure. Cerebral blood flow in the range of 6–10 ml.min^{-1} per 100 g is associated with irreversible membrane failure and cell death.

Cerebral ischaemic injury involves a process by which energy supply falls short of energy demands and in which the intracellular environment changes significantly. Calcium may be central to the cerebral ischaemic insult. Cerebral ischaemia may cause excess excitatory neurotransmitters, e.g. glutamate, to activate the various calcium influx mechanisms,[118] e.g. *N*-methyl-D-aspartate gated and voltage-dependent channels. There is a failure of adenosine triphosphate production which is necessary to allow re-uptake of intracellular calcium, and free intracellular calcium concentration increases. The sustained effects of calcium's intracellular actions (liberation of fatty acids from cell membranes, chemically reactive free radicals and lactic acid from anaerobic glycolysis) contribute to the neuronal injury. In addition, while adenosine triphosphate depletion may occur homogeneously throughout the ischaemic brain, neuronal damage may be focal, with some anatomical areas such as the hippocampus and cerebellum being more sensitive to ischaemia than others.[119]

TEMPERATURE AND HORMONAL RESPONSES

Hypothermia

Hypothalamic thermoregulation control systems normally maintain core body temperature within 0.4°C of the normal 37°C temperature in humans. Hypothermia is a common intra-operative observation, and is caused by inhibition of hypothalamic thermoregulation induced by anaesthesia, and exposure to the cold operating theatre environment and to cold inhaled gases.[120]

Moderate hypothermia (34–35°C) is common during anaesthesia and surgery. Following induction of anaesthesia, core temperature decreases by 0.5–1°C due to vasodilatation-induced mixing of cool peripheral blood with warm central blood. Core temperature may decline further with time to a steady state around 34.5–35°C as heat is lost to the environment. Inhaled anaesthetic agents depress the thermoregulatory threshold (the temperature at which thermoregulatory mechanisms become active) from approximately 37°C in the normal state to 34.5°C.[121] The only thermoregulatory responses available to an anaesthetized, paralysed, hypothermic patient are vasoconstriction and non-shivering thermogenesis. Hypothermic anaesthetized patients demonstrate profound peripheral cutaneous vasoconstriction, which is not associated with haemodynamic changes.

Control of the operating theatre environmental temperature is the most crucial factor in limiting intra-operative heat loss because most metabolic heat is lost by radiation and convection from the skin and surgical incisions. The most effective way of maintaining body temperature is to ensure an ambient temperature ≥21°C and to cover exposed parts. Skin heat loss may be minimized by using reflective covers (space blankets). Heat loss due to tracheobronchial rewarming may be minimized by using low fresh gas flows with a circle rebreathing system or by adding an active heater-humidifier to the airway. Alternatively, a heat- and moisture-exchanging filter may be incorporated instead of active systems to maintain airway humidity. Heat loss due to cold intravenous fluids and blood transfusion may be minimized by the use of fluid/blood warmers.

Intra-operative hypothermia may be associated with postoperative shivering. The associated increases in metabolic rate and oxygen consumption may produce hypoxaemia. In addition, hypothermia reduces hepatic drug biotransformation and renal excretion. Hypothermia is most commonly a clinical problem during long surgical procedures, with extensive incisions and infusion of large volumes of blood and other intravenous fluids. In these cases, the warming techniques referred to above should always be employed.

Hormonal responses

The surgical stress response includes an increase in plasma concentrations of catecholamines, cortisol, antidiuretic hormone and human growth hormone, with concomitant increases in plasma concentrations of glucose, lactate and pyruvate.[12] Increases in plasma concentrations of these stress hormones occur during general anaesthesia with most inhaled and intravenous agents[122] and are further increased by surgical stimulation. Increases in plasma glucose and cortisol concentrations induced by surgery are related to the severity of the operative trauma[123] and are greater during intra-abdominal surgery than body surface procedures.[124] They are considered undesirable because they promote haemodynamic instability and intra-operative and postoperative metabolic catabolism. Postoperative analgesia provided by epidural local anaesthetics and/or opioids combined with light general anaesthesia has been reported to reduce the stress hormone response and to diminish operative mortality and postoperative morbidity due to myocardial infarction and congestive cardiac failure.[125]

INTRA-OPERATIVE DRUG EFFECTS

Anaesthesia and allergic drug reactions

The pathophysiology and clinical manifestations of allergic drug reactions during anaesthesia have been highlighted in a review.[126] Allergic drug reactions during anaesthesia are potentially life-threatening. Untoward physiological responses (with manifestations varying from mild urticaria and pruritus to severe angioneurotic oedema, bronchospasm and hypotension) can be produced by an immunologically mediated anaphylactic reaction as well as by a non-immune direct drug response (anaphylactoid reaction). The use of an ever-increasing number of drugs in the peri-operative period (antibiotics, chymopapain, intravascular contrast media, plasma volume expanders, protamine, blood and its products, etc.) has resulted in an increased incidence of allergic drug reactions during anaesthesia.[127] In addition, a large spectrum of anaesthetic drugs may initiate an allergic response. Anaphylactic reactions to latex released from the surgeon's gloves may occur during operations. The clinical manifestations and treatment are essentially identical, irrespective of whether the reaction is anaphylactic or anaphylactoid.

Anaesthetic drugs

Both anaphylactic and anaphylactoid drug reactions have been reported following the administration of thiopentone and methohexitone.[128,129] A much higher incidence of allergic reactions was associated with Althesin and propanidid than with thiopentone.[130]

These agents, which are no longer available, were dissolved in Cremophor EL, and the high incidence of allergic reactions was attributed to this solvent. Similarly, a higher incidence of drug reactions was noted following diazepam administration, when Cremophor was substituted for propylene glycol.[131] Reactions to etomidate differ from those with other intravenous induction agents in that the symptoms are mostly cutaneous and gastro-intestinal rather than the more serious cardiovascular and respiratory manifestations.[132]

Opioids may induce adverse reactions because of direct histamine release from basophils and mast cells. Anaphylactic reactions have been reported with pethidine (meperidine). The synthetic opioids fentanyl and alfentanil may produce histamine-induced bronchospasm and vasodilatation, but true anaphylactic or anaphylactoid reactions have not been reported.[126] Both anaphylactic and anaphylactoid reactions have been reported in association with the use of depolarizing and non-depolarizing muscle relaxants. Factors associated with allergic reactions to muscle relaxants include a female predominance, with significantly higher incidences in patients with atopy, asthma, penicillin sensitivity and cosmetic allergy.[133] Sensitivity may have been higher with the older non-depolarizing agents, tubocurarine and gallamine, while the preservative methylparaben has been implicated in allergic reactions to suxamethonium.[134] The incidence of allergic responses to local anaesthetic agents has been confined mainly to ester agents which produce metabolites related to the highly antigenic para-aminobenzoic acid. Some local anaesthetic solutions also contain methylparaben, a preservative with bacteriostatic and fungistatic properties.

Management

Histamine is the principal mediator involved in allergic reactions during anaesthesia. Other mediators include neutrophil and eosinophil chemotactic factors, slow-reacting substance of anaphylaxis, platelet-activating factor and prostaglandins. Prevention of allergic reactions during anaesthesia involves identification of the patient at risk, pre-operative preparation of susceptible patients with corticosteroids and H_1- and H_2-receptor antagonists and avoidance of drugs which, either alone or in association with a solvent or additive, have a high potential for allergic reactions. Immediate treatment of an established anaphylactic or anaphylactoid reaction involves:

- discontinuation of the offending allergenic drug
- administration of 100% oxygen
- intravascular volume expansion with crystalloids or, preferably, colloid solution
- intravenous administration of adrenaline 1–5 µg.kg^{-1} titrated to the desired clinical effect.

Secondary management includes treatment with an antihistamine, e.g. diphenhydramine 50 mg intravenously or orally, and corticosteroids, e.g. hydrocortisone 1 g intravenously, if complement activation is suspected.

After recovery, the reaction should be investigated fully in an attempt to identify the drug responsible.[135] The patient should be warned to inform the anaesthetist about the results of these investigations if anaesthesia is required subsequently.

Drug interactions

Cardiovascular interactions associated with antihypertensive, antidepressant and anti-anginal drug medications during anaesthesia have been discussed above. A miscellaneous group of drugs may impair acetylcholine transmission or non-competitively alter cholinergic receptor function, thereby potentiating the action of non-depolarizing muscle relaxants. These drugs are involved in two clinically important situations, receptor desensitization and channel blockade. The volatile anaesthetic agents, anti-arrhythmic agents, some antibiotics (e.g. aminoglycosides and polymyxin), local anaesthetic agents, phenothiazines and calcium antagonists (e.g. verapamil[136]) are amongst the drugs implicated in reducing prejunctional acetylcholine release, desensitization of nicotinic cholinergic receptors or blocking ionic flow through transmembrane channels.

REFERENCES

1. Marty J, Reves JG. Cardiovascular control mechanisms during anesthesia. Anesth Analg 1989; 69: 273–275
2. Leon DF, Shaver JA, Leonard JJ. Reflex heart rate control in man. Am Heart J 1970; 80: 729–739
3. Seagard JZ, Hopp FA, Donegan JH, Kalbfleisch JH, Kampine JP. Halothane and the carotid sinus reflex: evidence for multiple sites of action. Anesthesiology 1982; 57: 191–202
4. Doyle DJ, Mark PWS. Reflex bradycardia during surgery. Can J Anaesth 1990; 37: 219–222
5. Higgins M, Thorp JM. Non-vagolytic anaesthetic sequence — sinus arrest. Anaesthesia 1986; 41: 89
6. Pollok AJP. Cardiac arrest immediately after vecuronium. Br J Anaesth 1986; 58: 936–937
7. May JR. Vecuronium and bradycardia. Anaesthesia 1985; 40: 710
8. Hardy PAJ. Atracurium and bradycardia. Anaesthesia 1985; 40: 504–505

9. Cozanitis DA, Powttu J, Rosenberg PH. Bradycardia associated with the use of vecuronium. A comparative study with pancuronium with and without glycopyrronium. Anaesthesia 1987; 42: 192–194
10. Coventry DM, McMenemin I, Lawrie S. Bradycardia during intra-abdominal surgery. Modification by preoperative anticholinergic agents. Anaesthesia 1987; 42: 835–839
11. Price ML, Price HL. Effects of general anesthesia on contractile responses of rabbit aortic strips. Anesthesiology 1962; 23: 16–21
12. Bovill JG, Sebel PS, Stanley TH. Opioid analgesics in anesthesia: with special reference to their use in cardiovascular anesthesia. Anesthesiology 1984; 61: 731–755
13. Reitan JA, Stangert KB, Wymore ML, Martucci RW. Central vagal control of fentanyl induced bradycardia during halothane anesthesia. Anesth Analg 1978; 57: 31–36
14. Liu WS, Bidwai AV, Stanley TH, Loeser EA. Cardiovascular dynamics after large doses of fentanyl and fentanyl plus N_2O in the dog. Anesth Analg 1976; 55: 168–172
15. Stanley TH, Webster LR. Anesthetic requirements and cardiovascular effects of fentanyl-oxygen and fentanyl-diazepam-oxygen anesthesia in man. Anesth Analg 1978; 57: 411–416
16. Sebel PS, Bovill JG, Boekhorst RAA, Rog P. Cardiovascular effects of high dose fentanyl anaesthesia. Acta Anaesthesiol Scand 1982; 26: 308–315
17. Seltzer JL, Ritter DE, Starsnic MA, Marr AT. The hemodynamic response to traction on the abdominal mesentery. Anesthesiology 1985; 63: 96–99
18. Moonie GT, Rees DL, Elton D. The oculocardiac reflex during strabismus surgery. Can Anaesth Soc J 1964; 11: 621–632
19. Doyle DJ, Mark PWS. Laparoscopy and vagal arrest. Anaesthesia 1989; 44: 448
20. Marks RJ. Electroconvulsive therapy: physiological and anaesthetic considerations. Can Anaesth Soc J 1984; 31: 541–548
21. Wyant GM. Electroconvulsive therapy. Can Anaesth Soc J 1981; 5: 491
22. Duke PC, Fownes D, Wade JG. Halothane depresses baroreflex control of heart rate in man. Anesthesiology 1977; 46: 184–187
23. Morton M, Duke PC, Ong B. Baroreflex control of heart rate in man awake and during enflurane and enflurane-nitrous oxide anesthesia. Anesthesiology 1980; 52: 221–223
24. Kotrly KJ, Ebert TJ, Vucins EF, Igler FO, Barney JA, Kampine JP. Baroreceptor reflex control of heart rate during isoflurane anesthesia in humans. Anesthesiology 1984; 60: 173–179
25. Marty J, Gauzit R, Lefevre P et al. Effects of diazepam and midazolam on baroreflex control of heart rate and on sympathetic activity in humans. Anesth Analg 1986; 65: 113–119
26. Bernards C, Marrone B, Priano L. Effect of anesthetic induction agents on baroreceptor function. Anesthesiology 1985; 63: A31
27. Slogoff S, Keats AS. Does perioperative myocardial ischemia lead to postoperative myocardial infarction? Anesthesiology 1985; 62: 107–114
28. Rao TK, Jacobs KH, El-Etr AA. Reinfarction following anesthesia in patients with myocardial infarction. Anesthesiology 1983; 59: 499–505
29. Pavlin EG, Su JY. Cardiopulmonary pharmacology. In: Miller RD, ed. Anesthesia, 3rd edn. Churchill Livingstone 1990: pp 105–134
30. Hickey RF, Eger EI. Circulatory pharmacology of inhaled anesthetics. In: Miller RD, ed. Anesthesia, 2nd edn. Churchill Livingstone 1986: pp 649–666
31. Eger EI, Smith NT, Stoelting RK, Cullen DJ, Whitcher CE. Cardiovascular effects of halothane in man. Anesthesiology 1970; 32: 396–408
32. Calverley RK, Ty Smith N, Prys-Roberts C, Eger EI, Jones CW. Cardiovascular effects of enflurane anesthesia during controlled ventilation in man. Anesth Analg 1978; 57: 619–628
33. Stevens WC, Cromwell TH, Halsey MJ, Eger EI, Shakespeare TF, Bahlman SH. The cardiovascular effects of a new inhalation anesthetic, Forane, in human volunteers at constant arterial carbon dioxide tension. Anesthesiology 1971; 35: 8–16
34. Calverley RK, Ty Smyth N, Jones CW, Prys-Roberts C, Eger EI. Ventilatory and cardiovascular effects of enflurane anesthesia during spontaneous ventilation in man. Anesth Analg 1978; 57: 610–618
35. Ty Smyth N, Eger EI, Stoelting RK, Whayne TF, Cullen D, Kadis LB. The cardiovascular and sympathomimetic responses to the addition of nitrous oxide to halothane in man. Anesthesiology 1970; 32: 410–421
36. Reiz S, Balfors F, Sorensen MB, Ariola S, Friedman A, Truedsson H. Isoflurane — a powerful coronary vasodilator in patients with coronary artery disease. Anesthesiology 1983; 59: 91–97
37. Prys-Roberts C, Meloche R, Foex P. Studies of anaesthesia in relation to hypertension: 1 Cardiovascular responses to treated and untreated patients. Br J Anaesth 1971; 43: 122–137
38. Bruce DL, Croley TF, Lee JS. Preoperative clonidine withdrawal syndrome. Anesthesiology 1979; 51: 90–92
39. Cunningham AJ, Synnott A. Blood pressure measurement and monitoring in anesthesia. In: O'Brien E, O'Malley K, eds. Handbook of hypertension, vol 14. Amsterdam: Elsevier Science Publishers. 1991
40. Cunningham AJ. Anaesthesia for abdominal aortic surgery — a review (part 1). Can J Anaesth 1989; 36: 426–444
41. Gal TJ, Cooperman LH, Berkowitz HD. Plasma renin activity in patients undergoing surgery of the abdominal aorta. Ann Surg 1974; 179: 65–69
42. Asiddao CB, Donegan JH, Whitesell RC, Kalbfleisch JH. Factors associated with perioperative complications during carotid endarterectomy. Anesth Analg 1982; 61: 631–637
43. Mangano DT. Perioperative cardiac morbidity. Anesthesiology 1990; 72: 153–184
44. London MJ, Hollenberg M, Wong MG et al. Intraoperative myocardial ischemia: localization by continuous 12 lead electrocardiography. Anesthesiology 1988; 69: 232–241
45. Weiner DA. Accuracy of cardiokymography during exercise testing: results of a multicenter study. J Am Coll Cardiol 1985; 6: 502–509
46. Kotrly KJ, Kotter GS, Mortara D, Kampine JP.

Intraoperative detection of myocardial ischemia with an ST segment trend monitoring system. Anesth Analg 1984; 63: 393–397
47 Gobel FL, Nordstrom LA, Nelson RR. The rate pressure product as an index of myocardial oxygen consumption during exercise in patients with angina pectoris. Circulation 1978; 57: 549–556
48 Buffington CW, Bashein G, Sivarajan M. Blood pressure and heart rate predict ischemia in collateral-dependent myocardium. Anesthesiology 1987; 67: A5
49 Kaplan JA, Wells PH. Early diagnosis of myocardial ischemia using the pulmonary artery catheter. Anesth Analg 1981; 60: 789–793
50 Haggmark S, Hohner P, Ostman M et al. Comparison of hemodynamic, electrocardiographic, mechanical and metabolic indicators of intraoperative myocardial ischemia in vascular surgical patients with coronary artery disease. Anesthesiology 1989; 70: 19–25
51 Blackburn H, Katigbak R. What electrocardiographic leads to take after exercise. Am Heart J 1964; 67: 184–188
52 Hauser AM, Gangadharan V, Ramos RG, Gordon S, Timmis GC, Didlets P. Sequence of mechanical, electrocardiographic and clinical effects of repeated coronary artery occlusion in human beings: electrocardiographic observations during coronary angioplasty. J Am Coll Cardiol 1985; 5: 193–197
53 Smith JS, Cahalan MK, Benefiel DJ et al. Intraoperative detection of myocardial ischemia in high risk patients: electrocardiography versus two dimensional transoesophageal echocardiography. Circulation 1985; 72: 1015–1021
54 Kugler G. Myocardial release of lactate, inosine and hypoxanthine during atrial pacing and exercise-induced angina. Circulation 1979; 59: 43–49
55 Gertz EW, Wisneski JA, Neese R, Bristow JD, Searle GL, Hanlon JT. Myocardial lactate metabolism: evidence of lactate release during net chemical extraction in man. Circulation 1981; 63: 1273–1279
56 Kaplan JA, Thys DM. Electrocardiography. In: Miller RD, ed. Anesthesia, 3rd Edn. Churchill Livingstone 1990; pp 1101–1127
57 Kuner J, Enescu V, Utsu F, Boszormenyi E, Bernstein H, Corday E. Cardiac arrhythmias during anesthesia. Dis Chest 1967; 52: 580–587
58 Bertrand CA, Steiner NV, Jameson AG, Lopez M. Disturbances of cardiac rhythm during anesthesia and surgery. JAMA 1971; 216: 1615–1617
59 Vanik PF, Davis HS. Cardiac arrhythmias during halothane anesthesia. Anesth Analg 1968; 47: 299–307
60 Cullen BF, Miller MG. Drug interactions and anesthesia: a review. Anesth Analg 1979; 58: 413–423
61 Reves JG, Kissin I, Lell WA, Tosone S. Calcium entry blockers: uses and implications for anesthesiologists. Anesthesiology 1984; 57: 504–518
62 Cunningham AJ. Acid aspiration: Mendelson's syndrome. Annals RCPSC 1987; 20: 335–339
63 Turndorf H, Rodis ID, Clark TS. 'Silent' regurgitation during general anesthesia. Anesth Analg 1974; 53: 700–703
64 Blitt CD, Gutman HL, Cohen DD. 'Silent' regurgitation and aspiration during anesthesia. Anesth Analg 1970; 49: 707–712
65 Berson W, Adriani J. 'Silent' regurgitation and aspiration during anesthesia. Anesthesiology 1954; 15: 644–649
66 Le Frock JL, Clarke TS, Davies B, Klaniner AS. Aspiration pneumonia: a 10 year review. Am J Surg 1979; 45: 305–313
67 Stewardson RH, Nyhus M. Pulmonary aspiration. Arch Surg 1977; 112: 1192–1197
68 Wynne JW, De Marco FJ, Hood CL. Physiological effect of corticosteroids in foodstuff aspiration. Arch Surg 1981; 116: 46–49
69 Gibbs CP, Modell JH. Aspiration pneumonitis. In: Miller RD, ed. Anesthesia, 2nd edn, vol 3. Churchill Livingstone 1986: pp 1013–1050
70 Awe WC, Fletcher WS, Jacob SW. The pathophysiology of aspiration pneumonitis. Surgery 1966; 60: 232–239
71 Wynne JW, Ramphal R, Hood CL. Tracheal mucosal damage after aspiration. Am Rev Respir Dis 1981; 124: 728–731
72 James CF, Modell JH, Gibbs CP, Kuck EJ, Ruiz BC. Pulmonary aspiration — effects of volume and pH in the rat. Anesth Analg 1984; 63: 665–668
73 Rogers MA, Toung JK, Gurtner G, Rogers MC, Traystman RJ, Cameron JL. The effects of osmolarity on pulmonary damage in aspiration. Anesthesiology 1984; 61: A490
74 Benumof JL. Respiratory physiology and respiratory function during anesthesia. In: Miller RD, ed. Anesthesia, 3rd edn. Churchill Livingstone 1990: pp 505–549
75 Pavlin EG. Respiratory pharmacology of inhaled anesthetics. In: Miller RD, ed. Anesthesia, 2nd edn. Churchill Livingstone 1986: pp 667–699
76 Slocum HC, Hoeflich EA, Allen CR. Circulatory and respiratory distress from extreme positions on the operating table. Surg Gynecol Obstet 1947; 84: 1065–1068
77 Craig DB. Postoperative recovery of pulmonary function. Anesth Analg 1981; 60: 46–51
78 Froese AB, Bryan CA. Effects of anesthesia and paralysis on diaphragmatic mechanics in man. Anesthesiology 1974; 41: 242–248
79 Macklem PT, Mead J. Resistance of the central and peripheral airways measured by a retrograde catheter. J Appl Physiol 1967; 22: 395–401
80 Nadel JA. Autonomic control of airway smooth muscle and airway secretions. Am Rev Respir Dis 1977; 115 (suppl 2): 117
81 Hammouda M, Wilson WH. Reflex slowing of respiration accompanying the changes in intrapulmonary pressure. J Physiol 1937; 88: 284–289
82 Empey DW, Laitinen LA, Jocobs L, Gold WM, Nadel JA. Mechanism of bronchial hyperreactivity in normal subjects after upper respiratory tract infection. Am Rev Respir Dis 1976; 113: 131–139
83 Dohi S, Gold MK. Pulmonary mechanics during general anaesthesia — the influence of mechanical irritation of the airway. Br J Anaesth 1979; 51: 205–214
84 Laitinen LA, Empey DW, Poppius H. Effects of intravenous histamine on static lung compliance and airway resistance in normal man. Am Rev Respir Dis 1976; 114: 291–295
85 Kingston HGG, Hirshman CA. Perioperative

85 management of the patient with asthma. Anesth Analg 1984; 63: 844–855
86 Schnider SM, Papper EM. Anesthesia for the asthmatic patient. Anesthesiology 1961; 22: 886–892
87 Crago RR, Bryan AC, Laws AK, Winestock AE. Respiratory flow resistance after curare and pancuronium measured by forced oscillations. Can Anaesth Soc J 1972; 19: 607–614
88 Rosow SE, Moss J, Philbin DM, Savarese JJ. Histamine release during morphine and fentanyl anesthesia. Anesthesiology 1982; 56: 93–96
89 Gal TJ, Surratt PM. Atropine and glycopyrrolate effects on lung mechanics in normal man. Anesth Analg 1980; 60: 85–90
90 Downes H, Gerber N, Hirshman CA. IV lignocaine in reflex and allergic bronchoconstriction. Br J Anaesth 1980; 52: 873–878
91 Hirshman CA, Downes H, Farbood A, Bergman NA. Ketamine block of bronchospasm in experimental canine asthma. Br J Anaesth 1979; 51: 713–718
92 Hirshman CA, Edelstein G, Peetz S, Wayne R, Downes H. Mechanism of action of inhalational anesthesia on airways. Anesthesiology 1982; 56: 107–111
93 Hirshman CA, Bergman NA. Halothane and enflurane protect against bronchospasm in an asthma dog model. Anesth Analg 1978; 57: 629–633
94 Darioli R, Perret C. Mechanical controlled hypoventilation in status asthmaticus. Am Rev Respir Dis 1984; 129: 385–387
95 Tuxen DV, Lane S. The effects of ventilatory pattern on hyperinflation, airway pressures, and circulation in mechanical ventilation of patients with severe airflow obstruction. Am Rev Respir Dis 1987; 136: 872–879
96 Roizen MF, Stevens WC. Multiform ventricular tachycardia due to the interaction of aminophylline and halothane. Anesth Analg 1978; 57: 738–741
97 O'Neill S. Spontaneous pneumothorax: aetiology, management and complications. Ir Med J 1987; 80: 306–311
98 Shapiro BA, Cane RD. Respiratory care. In: Miller RD, ed. Anesthesia. Churchill Livingstone 1990; pp 2169–2209
99 Peterson GW, Baier H. Incidence of pulmonary barotrauma in medical ICU. Crit Care Med 1983; 11: 67–70
100 Hunter AR. Problems of anaesthesia in artificial pneumothorax. Proc R Soc Med 1955; 4: 765
101 Shapiro HM, Drummond JC. Neurosurgical anesthesia and intracranial hypertension. In: Miller RD, ed. Anesthesia. Churchill Livingstone 1990: pp 1737–1789
102 Cucchiara RF, Seward JB, Nishimira RA, Nugent M, Faust RJ. Identification of patent foramen ovale during sitting position craniotomy by transesophageal echocardiography with positive airway pressure. Anesthesiology 1985; 63: 107–109
103 Michenfelder JD, Miller RH, Gronert GA. Evaluation of an ultrasonic device (Doppler) for the diagnosis of venous air embolism. Anesthesiology 1972; 36: 164–167
104 Breckner VL, Bethune RUM. Recent advances in monitoring pulmonary air embolism. Anesth Analg 1971; 50: 255–259
105 Newens AF, Volz RG. Severe hypotension during prosthetic hip surgery with acrylic bone cement. Anesthesiology 1972; 36: 298–300
106 Schuh FT, Schuh SM, Vignera MG, Terry RN. Circulatory changes following implantation of methyl methacrylate bone cement. Anesthesiology 1973; 39: 455–458
107 Johnes JG, Konieczko K. Hearing and memory in anaesthetised patients. Br Med J 1986; 292: 1291–1292
108 Pinsker MC. Anesthesia: a pragmatic construct. Anesth Analg 1986; 65: 819–820
109 Prys-Roberts C. Anaesthesia: a practical or impractical construct? Br J Anaesth 1987; 59: 1341–1345
110 Blacher RS. Awareness during surgery. Anesthesiology 1984; 61: 1–2
111 Prys-Roberts C, Sear JW. Non-barbiturate intravenous anaesthetics and continuous infusion anaesthesia. In: Pharmacokinetics of anaesthesia. Oxford: Blackwell Scientific 1984: p 128
112 Tunstall ME. Detecting wakefulness during general anaesthesia for caesarian section. Br Med J 1977; 1: 1321
113 Evans JM, Bithell JF, Vlachonikolis IG. Relationship between lower oesophageal contractility, clinical signs and halothane concentration. Br J Anaesth 1987; 59: 1346–1355
114 Edmonds HL, Paloheimo M. Computerized monitoring of the EMG and EEG during anaesthesia: an evaluation of the anaesthesia and brain function monitor. Int J Clin Monit Comput 1985; 1: 201–210
115 Clark DL, Rosner BS. Neurophysiologic effects of general anesthesia. Anesthesiology 1973; 38: 564–582
116 Thornton C, Newton DEF. The auditory evoked response: a measure of depth of anaesthesia. Baillières Clin Anaesthesiol 1989; 3: 559–585
117 O'Sullivan K, Cunningham AJ. Intra-operative cerebral ischaemia. Br J Hosp Med 1989; 42: 286–296
118 Greenmyre A. The role of glutamate in neurotransmission and in neurologic disease. Arch Neurol 1986; 43: 1058–1063
119 Kirino T. Delayed neuronal death in the gerbil hippocampus following ischemia. Brain Res 1982; 239: 57
120 Sessler DI. Temperature monitoring. In: Miller RD, ed. Anesthesia, 3rd edn. Churchill Livingstone 1990: pp 1227–1242
121 Sessler DI, Olofsson CI, Rubinstein EH, Beebe JJ. The thermoregulatory threshold in humans during halothane anesthesia. Anesthesiology 1988; 68: 836–842
122 Stanley TH, Berman L, Green O, Robertson D. Plasma catecholamine and cortisol responses to fentanyl oxygen. Anesthesia for coronary artery operations. Anesthesiology 1980; 53: 250–253
123 Clarke RSJ. The hyperglycaemic response to different types of surgery and anaesthesia. Br J Anaesth 1970; 42: 45–53
124 Clarke RSJ, Hohnston H, Sheridan B. The influence of anaesthesia and surgery on plasma cortisol, insulin and free fatty acids. Br J Anaesth 1979; 42: 295–299
125 Yeager MP, Glass DD, Neff RK, Brinck-Johnsen T. Epidural anesthesia and analgesia in high risk surgical patients. Anesthesiology 1987; 66: 729–736
126 Moudgil GC. Anaesthesia and allergic drug reactions. Can Anaesth Soc J 1986; 33: 400–414

127 Parker CW. Drug allergy. N Engl J Med 1975; 242: 732–736
128 Westacott P, Ramachandran PR, Jancelewicz Z. Anaphylactic reaction to thiopentone: a case report. Can Anaesth Soc J 1984; 31: 434–438
129 Hirshman CA, Peters J, Cartwright-Lee I. Leukocyte histamine release to thiopental. Anesthesiology 1982; 56: 64–67
130 Evans JM, Keogh JAM. Adverse reactions to intravenous anaesthetic induction agents. Br Med J 1977; 2: 735–736
131 Huttel MS, Schou Olesen A, Stoffersen E. Complement-mediated reaction to diazepam with cremophor as solvent (Stesolid MR). Br J Anaesth 1980; 52: 77–79
132 Beamish D, Brown DT. Adverse responses to iv anaesthetics. Br J Anaesth 1981; 53: 55–57
133 Fisher MMcD, Munroe I. Life threatening anaphylactoid reactions to muscle relaxants. Anesth Analg 1983; 59: 559–564
134 Morrow JG. Allergy to succinylcholine. Anesth Analg 1981; 60: 456
135 Suspected anaphylactic reactions associated with anaesthesia. Report of a working party of the Association of Anaesthetists of Great Britain and Ireland and the British Society of Allergy and Clinical Immunology. London: Association of Anaesthetists of Great Britain and Ireland, 1995.
136 Jones RM, Cashman JN, Casson WR, Broadbent MP. Verapamil potentiation of neuromuscular blocakde: failure of reversal with neostigmine but prompt reversal with edrophonium. Anesth Analg 1985; 64: 1021–1025

25. Postanaesthesia care

E. A. M. Frost

In 1863, Florence Nightingale wrote about the use of special areas designated in county hospitals for the recovery of patients from the immediate effects of surgery.[1] Dandy and Firor opened a three-bed unit at the Johns Hopkins hospital in 1923, specifically for the care of postoperative neurosurgical patients.[2] By 1943, the annual report from the Mayo Clinic noted the establishment of a post-anaesthesia observation room that cared for 2000 patients annually.[3] Today, hospitals frequently have not one but several postanaesthesia care units (PACU) offering expertise for specific situations such as obstetrics, cardiac surgery and neurosurgery, among others.

The currently recognized importance of the PACU was summarized in a North American supreme court decision in 1969.[4]

The function of this room is to provide highly specialised care, frequent and careful observation of patients who are under the influence of anesthesia. They remain in this room until they have regained consciousness and their bodies return to their normal functions. The nurses in this room are there for the purpose of promptly recognising any respiratory problem, cardiovascular problem, or hemorrhaging. The patient is more prone to crises after the operation than while in the operating room where the respiration is being controlled. This is the most important room in a hospital and one in which the patient requires the greatest attention because it is fraught with the greatest potential dangers to the patient. As the dangers or risks are ever-present there should be no relaxing of vigilance.

Nevertheless, PACUs have not been established universally to date, for several reasons. In rare instances, specialized and adequate nursing care or personal care by relatives may provide reasonably safe postoperative care in general wards. Surgeons and administrators have argued that few data are available to prove that disasters are prevented by PACU observation; rather, this area represents increased expense and hampers operating room utilization if blockages occur. Of course, the argument that successful outcome from surgery has been generally realized without PACUs for years, and therefore that establishment of such areas is unnecessary, has been raised repeatedly.

However, standards established by the American Society of Anesthesiologists' (ASA) House of Delegates in 1988 are strongly worded.

The first standard is as follows:

All patients who have received general anesthesia, regional anesthesia or monitored anesthesia care shall receive appropriate postanesthesia management.

A Postanesthesia Care Unit (PACU) or an area which provides equivalent postanesthesia care shall be available to receive patients after surgery and anesthesia. All patients who receive anesthesia shall be admitted to the PACU except by specific order of the anesthesiologist responsible for the patient's care.

The medical aspects of care in the PACU shall be governed by the policies and procedures which have been reviewed and approved by the Department of Anesthesiology.

The design, equipment and staffing of the PACU shall meet requirements of the facility's accrediting and licensing bodies.

The nursing standards of practice shall be consistent with those approved in 1986 by the American Society of Postanesthesia Nurses (ASPAN).

In general, patients are transferred directly from the operating room to the ward only under the following circumstances.

1. Local anaesthesia only was used, and the patient's condition is stable.
2. The patient is an infection risk, and no isolation area is available.
3. There is an intensive care unit specially designed for specific care (for example, after cardiac surgery or for premature babies).
4. By agreement with the surgeon and anaesthetist, the patient makes arrangements for special care on a regular nursing unit.

If the patient is returned directly to the surgical ward postoperatively, the standards of nursing care during this period must equal those of the PACU. Otherwise, all patients who receive a general or regional anaes-

ADMISSION ASSESSMENT

A further standard of postanaesthetic care of the ASA states that:

Upon arrival in the PACU the patient shall be re-evaluated and a verbal report provided to the responsible PACU nurse by the member of the Anesthesia Care Team who accompanies the patient.

The patient's status on arrival in the PACU shall be documented.

Information concerning the pre-operative condition and the surgical/anaesthetic course shall be transmitted to the PACU nurse.

The member of the Anesthesia Care Team shall remain in the PACU until the PACU nurse accepts responsibility for the nursing care of the patient.

When the patient is accepted to the PACU, a short form can be inserted in the medical record (Fig. 25.1). PACU orders are either included on a routine form or may be written by the surgeon or anaesthetist (Fig. 25.2). Assessment of recovery from anaesthesia may be made by applying the Aldrete score, which is based on the Apgar score (Table 25.1).[5] The range is 10 for complete recovery to zero in comatose patients. The score should be recorded on admission and at intervals of 15–30 min to document improvement or deterioration. Limitations of the score are apparent when the patient receives a score of 10 but is oliguric, severely nauseated, vomiting or develops arrhythmias.

The Carignan post-anaesthesia score (Table 25.2) is rarely applicable in the PACU setting, as assessments are made on the second, fifth and 15th day of surgery.[6]

The patient's status should be judged by the nurse and anaesthetist immediately on arrival in the PACU and at a minimum of 15-min intervals until discharge. Documentation is essential.

Table 25.1 The Aldrete score. Trending of the Aldrete score is generally accepted as an indication of recovery or deterioration after anaesthesia

Activity	
Voluntary movement of all limbs to command	2
Voluntary movement of two extremities to command	1
Unable to move	0
Respiration	
Breathing deeply and coughing	2
Dyspnoeic, hypoventilating	1
Apnoeic	0
Circulation	
Blood pressure ± 20% of pre-anaesthetic level	2
Blood pressure ± 20–50% of pre-anaesthetic level	1
Blood pressure ± 50% of pre-anaesthetic level	0
Consciousness	
Fully awake	2
Arousable	1
Unresponsive	0
Colour	
Pink	2
Pale, blotchy	1
Cyanotic	0

From Aldrete & Kronlik,[5] with permission.

MONITORING

Monitoring in the PACU is essential to adequate evaluation and good outcome. Respiratory, cardiovascular, neuromuscular, thermoregulatory and renal systems, in addition to state of consciousness and fluid and electrolyte balance, are routinely evaluated.

Cardiorespiratory assessment

Common measurements of respiratory function are listed in Table 25.3. Good, careful auscultation is irreplaceable in the initial assessment of adequate respiration. Rate should be recorded on admission and

---

```
                          PACU Admission

Vital signs:  temperature _____ BP _____ PR _____ RR _____
Anaesthesia:  regional _____ general _____ other _____
   Regional:  level of analgesia _____
    General:  unresponsive _____ drowsy _____ awake _____
              airway oral _____ nasal _____ none _____
              endotracheal tube _____ tracheostomy _____
```

Fig. 25.1 A form or rubber stamp inserted in the chart that the postanaesthesia care unit (PACU) nurse may complete to record patient data at the time of admission. BP = Blood pressure; PR = pulse rate; RR = respiratory rate. Adapted from Bristow & Giesecke,[7] with permission.

```
                    Routine PACU Orders

1. O₂ administration: Give O₂ @ _____ l/min _____ mask _____ cannula
2. Vital signs q 15 min
3. Endotracheal tube care
    a. Suction prn
    b. Administer O₂ mist/T tube @ _____ %
    c. May be extubated when PACU written scoring criteria are met
    d. Obtain ABGs _____ minutes after admission to unit
4. Continue operating room IV _____ unless otherwise ordered by surgeon
5. Cardiac monitor
6. Pulse oximetry
7. Medications
    a. Atropine 0.5-1 mg IV bolus if cardiac rate is less than _____
    b. Ligncaine 50 mg IV bolus stat for development of PVCs 6 per minute Ventricular
       tachycardia or bigeminy: call anaesthetist.
    c. _____ IV for pain
8. Notify anaesthetist if:
    Blood pressure _____ or _____
    Respiration _____ or _____
    Heart rate _____ or _____
```

Fig. 25.2 Postoperative orders to be completed by the anaesthetist in consultation with the postanaesthesia care unit (PACU) nurse. ABGs = Arterial blood gases; IV = intravenous; PVCs = premature ventricular contractions.

at 15-min intervals. Respiratory pattern, which normally has a regular inspiratory to expiratory ratio of 1:3, should be noted. Pulse oximetry is a simple and accurate means of assessing oxygen saturation and volume status. Routine use of oximetry is recommended strongly in the early recovery period, especially after head and neck injuries, in patients cared for in the prone position, in those who have not recovered from the effects of anaesthetic drugs, in patients with chronic lung disease and in children with sleep apnoea syndromes. In many PACUs, one or two stations are equipped to monitor inspired and expired gases (mass spectroscopy or infrared gas analyses). Continuous measurement of expired carbon dioxide levels (capnography), especially in the patient whose trachea is still intubated, provides early warning of respiratory or

Table 25.2 Carignan's postanaesthetic scoring system.

	0	1	2	3	4
Circulation	BP stable, pulse always <100 beats.min⁻¹	BP change <30%, pulse 100–200 beats.min⁻¹	Vasopressors or digitalis	BP <100 mmHg in spite of treatment	Decompensated
Respiration	Rate < 15 breaths. min⁻¹, breath-holding more than 25 s	Rate 15–20 breaths. min⁻¹, productive cough	Rate >20 breaths. min⁻¹, rales or temperature up to 37.8°C	Temperature >37.8°C, partial atelectasis	Major
CNS	Amnesic, satisfied	Confused or recalls induction	Dissatisfied with anaesthesia for any reason	Extrapyramidal signs	Major neurological complications
Gastro-intestinal tract	Nothing	No more than 3 episodes of nausea	Nausea, vomited once only	Vomiting	Ileus
Renal	Voids >800 ml	Over 800 ml per catheter	Voids 500–800 ml	500–800 ml per catheter	Under 500 ml

BP = Blood pressure; CNS = central nervous system.
From Carignan et al,[6] with permission.

Table 25.3 Common indicators used to assess respiratory function in the recovery room. Deviations from normal in one of these variables indicates respiratory distress and corrective action should be taken

Indicator	Normal range
Auscultation	Bilaterally equal
Rate	10–35 breaths.min^{-1}
Pattern	Regular
Pulse oximetry	>94% oxygen saturation
Capnography	<5.2% (5.3 kPa; 40 mmHg)
Tidal volume	4–5 ml.kg^{-1}
Vital capacity	20–40 ml.kg^{-1}
Inspiratory force	−40 cmH$_2$O
Arterial blood gases (breathing 30% oxygen)	Pa_{O_2} ≥ 13.3 kPa (100 mmHg) Pa_{CO_2} 4.7–6.0 kPa (35–45 mmHg)

cardiac depression if previously stable levels deteriorate.

Inadequate ventilation and hypoxaemia are common postoperatively. Frequent causes include the residual effects of anaesthetic agents, especially muscle relaxants and opioids, fluid overload, pain at the operation site, shivering, pre-existing disease (especially related to smoking) and, less commonly, aspiration or intra-operative complications.

Abnormalities of respiratory pattern, such as phasic variations (Cheyne–Stokes respiration), use of accessory muscles, diaphragmatic breathing and sternal retraction, indicate residual effects of anaesthetic drugs, neurological complications, or respiratory obstruction. Prompt re-establishment of an adequate airway is required. This may be achieved simply by support of the chin, or by insertion of an oral or nasal airway; however, in some cases, it is necessary to re-intubate the trachea and to apply assisted ventilation. Probably the best measurement of the adequacy of ventilation is obtained from blood gas analysis. Accurate interpretation must take the inspired oxygen concentration into consideration. If an arterial cannula is not in place and monitoring of gases requires repeated arterial puncture, continuous monitoring of oxygen saturation by pulse oximetry is an acceptable alternative.

In assessing the adequacy of circulation, blood pressure, pulse and heart sounds are monitored (Table 25.4). Blood pressure variations of more than 25% of pre-operative values usually require therapy, either to reduce arterial hypertension (e.g. labetalol infusion) or to treat hypotension (fluids, blood, vasopressors, depending on cause).[8]

Arterial hypotension may be due to inadequate volume replacement, drug overdose, intra-operative catastrophe or acute cardiopulmonary disease. Cardiac arrhythmias may be precipitated by myocardial ischaemia, hypoxaemia or drugs. Diagnosis requires a careful review of the chart and examination of the patient. Therapy is determined by the underlying cause.

Continuous electrocardiographic monitoring coupled with the availability of a printer to obtain a permanent record should be routine. Not only does this monitor afford a visual and auditory indication of rate and rhythm, but it may indicate hypoxia of cardiac muscle if the ST segment is deflected by more than 1 mm from baseline. Electrolyte abnormalities (especially potassium) may be apparent from wave changes. Serum estimations of such changes are more accurate.

Temperature

Temperature is decreased during operation by administration of cold fluids and gases, exposure of both the interior and the exterior of the body to a cool environment, vasodilatation and depression of the thermoregulatory centre by anaesthetic agents.[9] Although moderate hypothermia can be protective by decreasing oxygen consumption, shivering during the recovery period can increase oxygen demand by up to 400%, which may be catastrophic for critically ill patients with coronary or cerebrovascular disease.[10] The depressant effects of all anaesthetic agents are exaggerated by hypothermia. Radiant heat may be useful in controlling shivering rapidly.[11]

Warming must be performed gradually to prevent skin burns in areas of low perfusion. The electrocardiogram must be monitored for ventricular arrhythmias. Care must be taken to avoid sudden elevations of the limbs, which might push large quantities of relatively cold peripheral blood into the heart. Respiratory status must be monitored closely, particularly if the patient has received a muscle relaxant, because recurarization may occur as the body is warmed.

Postoperative hyperthermia may be due to pre-existing disease, an infective process, seizures, drug reaction or malignant hyperthermia. This last syndrome may be triggered by pain or stress, but is related more commonly to the administration of volatile anaesthetic agents or suxamethonium. It is associated with persistent coma, high fever, supraventricular tachycardia, hyperventilation, unstable blood pressure, acute pulmonary and cerebral oedema and acute renal failure. Therapy requires cardioventilatory support, sodium bicarbonate, external and internal cooling, dantrolene sodium, procaine hydrochloride, steroids, diuretics and insulin in glucose.

Fluid and electrolyte balance

Close monitoring of fluid and electrolyte balance is important in the PACU. There may be residual abnormalities from the intra-operative period, and continuing changes in distribution of water and electrolytes as a result of the trauma of surgery and the changing catecholamine concentrations which follow the reduction in stimulation after skin closure and extubation of the trachea. Routine postoperative intravenous fluid orders may not be adequate to maintain the normal status, and close co-operation of PACU physicians and nurses is essential. Most electrolyte measurements are performed in the appropriate laboratories in a separate area in the hospital, although we have found the immediate availability of Na^+, K^+, Ca^{2+} and haematocrit determinations useful in both the operating theatre and the PACU. Urine output is a guide to the adequacy of renal perfusion, and as such reflects the general haemodynamic status. However, the lack of urine output may reflect primary kidney malfunction and not perfusion deficits.

Disturbances of fluid and electrolyte balance occur most often in elderly or debilitated patients, in treated hypertensives, in severe diabetics or after major intracranial surgery or head injury. Peri-operative use of diuretics predisposes to hypokalaemia, hyponatraemia and hypochloraemia. During bowel manipulation particularly, large volumes of fluid may be lost from the circulation and may not have been replaced adequately during operation. Non-ketotic hyperosmolar hyperglycaemic coma may complicate anaesthetic recovery in patients with overt diabetes mellitus, normal patients under stressful conditions or elderly, debilitated patients who have been unable to drink or who have received insufficient intravenous fluid replacement. This condition differs from diabetic keto-acidosis in that there is no ketosis, but shares the characteristics of hyperglycaemia, hyperosmolality and electrolyte and fluid disequilibrium. There is usually marked cerebral dysfunction, which may present as stupor or with localizing signs. The lack of ketosis results from the level of circulating insulin, which is sufficient to suppress fat metabolism but unable to control the blood glucose concentration. The associated osmotic diuresis results in hypovolaemia, with haemoconcentration, hypotension and, potentially, poor peripheral perfusion. The syndrome has been seen in patients receiving parenteral hyperalimentation, presumably because hypertonic infusions have been given during a stressful event.

DISCHARGE CRITERIA

In all instances, a physician should assess the patient before discharge from the PACU. The policy in many hospitals requires that an anaesthetist examines the patient or writes the discharge note. Although such a circumstance pertains in many situations, it is not a workable solution in all institutions. There is considerable variability in the characteristics of patients and procedures, availability of physician staff and level of nursing expertise. Each PACU is responsible for establishment of appropriate written criteria for discharge.

A number of parameters have been generally accepted.

1. The patient can maintain the airway, clear secretions, breathe deeply and cough on command. He or she can turn to the side if vomiting occurs, and can call for help.
2. The haemodynamic status is stable and close to pre-operative values.
3. The fluid balance is equilibrating. Urinary output is adequate (about 25–50 ml.h^{-1}) and electrolyte concentrations are close to normal.
4. The post-surgical status is controlled with no evidence of active bleeding. Drains and intravenous cannulae are patent and functioning.
5. All physician orders in the PACU have been initiated, the patient has been observed for a reasonable period of time and no untoward effects have been observed.
6. The temperature is stable and within defined limits.

Table 25.4 Approximate normal ranges for cardiac measurements obtained in the recovery room

Variable	Normal range
Heart rate	55–120 beats.min^{-1}
Blood pressure	$\frac{90}{50} - \frac{160}{100}$ mmHg
Central venous pressure	3–8 mmHg
Right atrial pressure	1–6 mmHg
Right ventricular pressure	$\frac{20}{0} - \frac{30}{5}$ mmHg
Pulmonary artery pressure	$\frac{20}{8} - \frac{30}{12}$ mmHg
Pulmonary capillary wedge pressure	4–12 mmHg
Cardiac output	4–8 L.min^{-1}
Cardiac index (cardiac output/ body surface area)	2.5–3.5 L.min^{-1}.m^{-2}

7. Following regional anaesthesia, the patient must recover enough motor strength to change position in bed and sufficient sensory function to prevent possible injury.

Several minimum waiting periods have been recommended on the basis that, if complications develop, it is most probable that they will do so within these periods. The recommendations include a 60-min period after intramuscular administration of an opioid, anti-emetic or antibiotics, a 60-min period after extubation of the trachea, and a 30-min period after discontinuation of oxygen therapy. Special, additional discharge criteria must be applied to day-case patients who are discharged home.[12] These additional recommendations are addressed in Chapter 16.

POSTANAESTHETIC COMPLICATIONS

Although administration of anaesthesia is considered safe and serious complications are rare, minor morbidity is relatively common, and problems related to anaesthesia and surgery are seen frequently in the PACU (Table 25.5).

Postoperative nausea and vomiting (PONV)

These are common causes of postoperative morbidity, and occur in 20–70% of all surgical patients. Causative factors include opioids, pain, obesity, hypotension, history of motion sickness, previous postoperative nausea, long duration of anaesthesia/surgery, sudden position change and possibly the use of nitrous oxide. PONV occurs more frequently in females and after specific surgical procedures (e.g. strabismus repair, laparoscopy).[13]

In at-risk patients the prophylactic administration of an anti-emetic as part of the anaesthetic technique is indicated. Droperidol (1.5–3.0 mg) or a 5-HT$_3$ antagonist, such as ondansetron (4 mg), is usually effective and associated with minimal side-effects. If prophylaxis is ineffective, which is uncommon, treatment of PONV is most appropriate by using a drug with a different receptor activity than that used for prophylaxis. Although the use of nitrous oxide often appears to increase the incidence of PONV — perhaps by increasing pressure in distensible cavities such as the middle ear and stomach — administration may not necessarily increase the incidence of vomiting postoperatively.[14]

Persistent nausea and vomiting of clear or bile-stained material may be treated in the PACU by the intravenous administration of any of the following agents:[13]

1. metoclopramide 5 mg intravenously
2. prochlorperazine 12.5 mg intramuscularly
3. ondansetron 4 mg intravenously.

Myalgias

Postoperative muscle pain has been reported in 10–72% of ambulatory surgical patients.[15,16] Suxamethonium (succinylcholine) has been implicated as the causative agent but this generally held belief has been disputed.[17,18] Whatever the cause, the muscle aches are generally short-lasting (1–2 days) and may be treated readily by simple analgesics.

Pain

The treatment of postoperative pain is discussed in detail in Chapter 26. The recent acceptance of patient-controlled analgesic techniques, epidural and subarachnoid instillation of opioids and intra-operative nerve blocks has greatly decreased the suffering of the post-surgical patient. Also, an increased awareness and understanding of the need for analgesia in the paediatric population has improved patient care in this situation.

Sore throat

Approximately 50% of patients complain of sore throat postoperatively, related predominantly to tracheal intubation and the use of artificial airways.[15] The complication is usually short-lived and may be treated successfully by anaesthetic lozenges, gargling with local anaesthetic solutions, analgesics and reassurance.

Delayed return of consciousness

Most patients regian consciousness promptly after general anaesthesia. However, a few remain comatose for longer periods. The commonest cause of prolonged

Table 25.5 Postanaesthetic complications

Nausea and vomiting
Myalgias
Pain
Delayed return of consciousness
Sore throat
Hepatorenal problems

Several problems may arise in the postanaesthetic care unit and contribute to complications in the recovery phases after anaesthesia.

somnolence in the PACU is a prolonged effect of anaesthetic drugs. Other causes include drug interaction, respiratory depression, cardiovascular abnormalities, hypothermia, fluid and electrolyte imbalance, intra-operative catastrophe and pre-operative state.

Clearly the differential diagnosis must be considered and appropriate therapy applied to correct the situation.

Prolonged anaesthetic effect

Diagnosis and treatment of prolonged anaesthetic effect in the PACU are summarized in Table 25.6. A premedicant drug such as diazepam has a half-life of 12 h (even longer in the elderly) and effects often extend into the postoperative period. Midazolam also has marked individual variation in response (especially in the geriatric population) and may occasionally exert long-lasting effects. If a combination of drugs has been administered pre-operatively, a synergistic effect or interaction may result in prolonged hypnosis.[19] A particularly marked synergistic effect has been described between midazolam and fentanyl, drugs which are often used together during monitored anaesthetic care.[20] Therapy is both supportive and specific.

The volatile anaesthetic agents in common use are usually associated with rapid awakening when they are discontinued (i.e. within 10 min). Recovery is not usually delayed even in markedly obese patients if anaesthetic time is less than 3 h. However, the anaesthetic effect may persist after longer administration or because of interactions with other drugs. Delayed awakening is most marked with the more soluble agents and least marked with relatively insoluble agents such as desflurane and sevoflurane.

Intravenous techniques involve the administration of several drugs (barbiturates, opioids, tranquillizers, muscle relaxants). Several factors can combine to prolong the action of these agents. Thiopentone has a very short duration of action when it is used only as a single bolus for induction. However, it is extremely fat-soluble and, when used as a continuous infusion over several hours, as a bolus for cerebral protection or during emergence to control blood pressure, coma may persist. Moreover, thiopentone is re-absorbed by the renal tubules and recirculated. In extreme cases, peritoneal dialysis may be required to remove the drug.

Other factors that contribute to increased hypnotic effects of barbiturates include decreased cardiac output and blood volume, poor renal function, competitive binding of protein sites (e.g. by X-ray contrast material), acute alcoholism (decreased microsomal enzyme activity) and synergism with opioids.[21] The paralysed patient may not be anaesthetized but differentiation between neuromuscular paralysis and postoperative coma may be difficult. Causes of prolonged effects of neuromuscular blocking agents include presence of atypical cholinesterase (about 1 : 3000 cases), puerperium, acid–base imbalance (acidosis), hypothermia (recurarization may occur during rewarming), frank overdose and combinations of different types of drug.[22] In patients with clinical evidence of residual paralysis, monitoring of muscle power may be assessed more comfortably in the awake patient by using the train-of-four response (a series of four supramaximal single shocks delivered to the ulnar nerve at 2 Hz for 2 s) than by using tetanic stimulation. Using train-of-four, decreased response from the first to the fourth twitch (ratio of 4 to 1 twitch of up to 50%) indicates marked residual non-depolarizing block. Edrophonium chloride 20 mg and atropine 0.5 mg may be used as a clinical test and as an indicator of the effectiveness of

Table 25.6 Common drug causes of prolonged unresponsiveness

Anaesthetic drugs	Diagnosis	Treatment
Premedication	Order sheet in chart	Supportive
Inhaled agents	Anaesthetic record	Assist ventilation
Barbiturates		Maintain cardiovascular stability Maintain normothermia
Benzodiazepines		Flumazenil
Opioids	Anaesthetic record	Naloxone or nalmafene
Muscle relaxants	Peripheral nerve stimulator	Neostigmine and atropine or glycopyrrolate Correct acid–base imbalance Maintain normothermia

Prolonged anaesthetic effect, often due to absolute or relative overdose, is the commonest cause of delayed return to consciousness in the postanaesthetic care unit.

neostigmine (a longer-acting drug). A train-of-four value of 75–80% indicates return of adequate neuromuscular function.

Drug interactions

Surgical patients recieve an average of 13–20 drugs, many of which are multicomponent preparations. The relationship between the number of drugs administered and the incidence of reactions is not linear. If fewer than six drugs are used, the reaction rate approximates to 4%. However, if more than 11 drugs are given, the complication rate increases out of proportion to the number of drugs consumed (e.g. 20 drugs have a 45% reaction rate). Some of the commonly used drugs that interact with anaesthetic agents to cause increased sedation are listed in Table 25.7.

The list of possible drug interactions increases almost daily. A computer program available through the *Physician's Desk Reference* (publisher Medical Economics Data, Oradell, NJ) may be used to identify problem areas and interactions of up to 20 drugs at one time or screen out the source of a side-effect.

Intra-operative complications

Several untoward events may occur intra-operatively that are reflected as continued postoperative coma. In diagnosis and therapy, the most important factors are early and continued communication between the anaesthetist, surgeon and PACU nurse.

Shock may develop intra-operatively following sudden or massive haemorrhage. Massive blood transfusion is often associated with pulmonary and renal problems

Table 25.7 Drugs that interact to increase sedation after anaesthesia with anaesthetics

Maintenance medications
Cardiovascular; antihypertensive drugs, anti-arrhythmic agents, digitalis glycosides

Antibiotics

Psychotropic drugs; lithium, monoamine oxide inhibitors, phenothiazine derivatives, street drugs

Cimetidine

Intravenous agents
Opioids, barbiturates, benzodiazepines, ketamine, trimetaphan

Inhalation agents
Nitrous oxide, halothane, enflurane, isoflurane, desflurane, seroflurane

Muscle relaxants

after a few hours, and these systems must be monitored carefully. Septic shock may develop rapidly, particularly in seriously ill and elderly patients or after manipulation of a large abscess, infarcted bowel or a gangrenous area. The condition is recognized by severe hypotension, tachycardia, often hypothermia, but without overt signs of bleeding. Ventilation and circulation must be supported.

Myocardial infarction (MI) is a possible complication of a hypotensive episode. It also occurs more commonly in patients who have had a previous MI, or who are hypertensive, diabetic or have peripheral vascular disease.

Peri-operative MI is now the leading cause of postoperative death in the elderly undergoing non-cardiac surgery.[23] Some studies[24] indicate a 38% incidence of ischaemia, MI or cardiac death in patients older than 70 years, compared with 7% in those aged 40–49 years; other authors[25] report that age is a significant predictor only when other factors are present.

Another study has indicated that re-infarction occurred in only 1.9% of 733 patients who had had a previous MI.[26] Peri-operative re-infarction occurred in 5.7% of patients who had an MI less than 3 months previously and in 2.3% of those whose MI was 4–6 months earlier. Most outcome studies have been unable to differentiate between inhalational and opioid anaesthesia in patients undergoing coronary bypass surgery in the patient with cardiac disease.

Nitrous oxide tends to decrease cardiac output and increase systemic vascular resistance when given alone or in combination with opioid analgesics. It has been shown that nitrous oxide can induce ischaemia in an area supplied by a critically stenotic coronary artery, thereby inducing regional myocardial dysfunction. Opioid/nitrous oxide relaxant anaesthesia was associated with a significantly higher incidence of myocardial re-infarction (7.0 versus 0.5% for other general anaesthetics).[27]

In patients with cardiac disease, the postoperative period can be stressful because of the onset of pain during emergence from anaesthesia, fluid shifts, temperature changes and alteration of respiratory function. Marked changes occur in plasma catecholamine concentrations, haemodynamics, ventricular function and coagulation following non-cardiac surgery, particularly in patients with pre-existing cardiac disease.

Recent studies in both cardiac and non-cardiac[28] surgery have shown that heart rate commonly increases postoperatively by 25–50% compared with intra-operative values and that tachycardia (heart rate > 100 beats.min^{-1}) occurs in 10–25% of patients. Preliminary studies suggest that ischaemia occurs most commonly during the postoperative period and persists for 48 h or longer.[28] Postoperative ischaemia and most infarcts appear to be silent, and therefore difficult to detect. If postoperative ischaemia is proved to be an important predictor of morbidity, extended postoperative monitoring and aggressive treatment of ischaemia would be indicated.

Intracranial complications may be recognized first in the PACU. Rupture of an intracranial aneurysm intra-operatively prior to clipping has a poor prognosis. If it has been necessary to clip major vessels to control bleeding or if there has been extensive and deep tumour dissection, considerable cerebral oedema may develop.

Another problem that may become obvious in the PACU is that of intracranial air. Intra-operatively, the brain size is decreased by hyperventilation, diuresis and cerebrospinal fluid withdrawal. As the brain re-expands, air trapped intracranially may be put under pressure, resulting in a tension pneumocephalus and coma.

In any patient with altered intracranial dynamics, small increases in $Pa{CO_2}$ may cause marked deterioration in the level of consciousness. Should intracranial hypertension or respiratory or cardiac abnormalities associated with decrease in conscious level occur in any neurosurgical patient, management must include prompt neurosurgical consultation and immediate attempts to control intracranial pressure at less than 20 mmHg (hyperventilation, diuretics, head-up position).

Delayed postanaesthetic complications

Although prompt and complete reversal of anaesthetic effects frequently indicates good recovery without adverse effects, in some instances disease processes may arise days or weeks after surgery. Some organ systems deserve special attention.

Pulmonary complications

The incidence of postoperative pulmonary complications has been reported to be as low as 3% in patients with general surgical procedures, and up to 76% after upper abdominal surgery.[29]

Atelectasis is the most common complication seen after surgery. The pathophysiology is due to an abnormal pattern of breathing. Normally, the respiratory pattern consists of a 400–500 ml tidal volume interrupted every 5–10 min by a maximal deep breath to near total lung capacity.[30] During a breath, a few alveoli collapse at the end of expiration and fail to expand with the ensuing inspiration. These alveoli are eventually expanded by a maximum inflation (a sigh or yawn). The aetiology of atelectasis in the postoperative state, especially after upper abdominal or thoracic surgery, is related to smaller tidal volumes and the inability to take the normal sigh due to postoperative pain, sedative drugs such as opioids and postoperative diaphragmatic dysfunction. If the atelectasis is not resolved at an early stage, complications such as hypoxaemia and pneumonia can occur.

Pulmonary function tests after upper abdominal surgery show a restrictive pulmonary deficit that lasts for more than 1 week.[31] There is a 60% decrease in vital capacity and forced expiratory volume in 1 s/forced vital capacity (FEV_1/FVC) ratio on postoperative day 1, which improves to a 30% decrease from normal by 7 days. Post-thoracotomy operations which do not include pulmonary resection result in a 40% decrease in vital capacity on day 1, with recovery by day 7.[32] Surgery of the lower abdominal cavity causes a 35% decrease in vital capacity on day 1. Conversely, no decrease is seen after extra-abdominal surgery.

In view of the absence of changes in pulmonary function in the non-abdominal and non-thoracic patients, the anaesthetic used probably does not alter postoperative mechanical pulmonary function properties. In descending order, the types of surgery most likely to result in postoperative pulmonary complications are upper abdominal surgery; thoracic surgery with lung resection; thoracic surgery without lung resection; lower abdominal surgery; and extrathoracic and extra-abdominal surgery.

The second most important risk factor in predicting pulmonary complications is the presence of chronic obstructive pulmonary disease. Studies indicate that approximately 26% of patients with pre-existing chronic respiratory disease develop pulmonary complications, compared with 8% of patients without respiratory disease.[33] In patients with normal pulmonary function test results, the incidence of clinically evident postoperative atelectasis is 3%. If tests are abnormal, this figure increases to 70%.[34]

When cigarette smoking is evaluated, patients who smoke 10 cigarettes or more daily have a postoperative pulmonary morbidity rate up to six times that of non-smokers.[35] This correlation with smoking occurs even when pre-operative pulmonary function tests in smokers are not impaired.[36] Obesity increases the pulmonary complication rate from 12 to 35%.[37] However, advanced age alone probably is not a factor.[33,38] Prolonged anaesthesia (more than 3–4 h) may increase the incidence of respiratory difficulties postoperatively.[29]

The best method to treat postoperative atelectasis is

prevention. Pre-operative pulmonary function tests are widely used to identify patients at risk. However, prevention by pre-operative respiratory exercises, bronchodilator therapy, antibiotics and cessation of smoking is only partly successful.

Routine postoperative measures should include:

1. breathing exercises that emphasize a large inspiratory effort of at least 3 s duration, such as incentive spirometry
2. supervision of breathing exercises at least once per hour while awake
3. encouragement, when possible, to be in an upright position in bed
4. sitting upright in a chair as soon as possible
5. adequate pain relief
6. a trial of continuous positive airways pressure (CPAP) by mask, or nasal CPAP, for refractory atelectasis.

Pleural effusion is a rare postoperative complication and occurs in fewer than 2% of patients.[33] The incidence increases after upper abdominal surgery when free peritoneal fluid is present, and in patients with atelectasis.[39] Most effusions resolve without specific therapy. Rarely is thoracocentesis necessary.

Pulmonary embolus is not uncommon postoperatively. In 90% of cases, the origin of the embolus is the deep veins of the legs. The incidence of fatal postoperative pulmonary embolism, in the absence of prophylaxis, depends on the site of surgery.[40] It varies from less than 1% in patients undergoing elective general surgery to 3% in patients undergoing elective hip surgery.[41] Most cases are diagnosed postmortem and two-thirds of patients who die from the disease do so within 30 min after the acute event, before therapy can be started.[42]

Risk factors for pulmonary embolus include obesity, oral contraceptive use, varicose veins, malignancy, prolonged immobility, congestive heart failure, ageing and the type of surgical procedure.[43,44]

Low-dose heparin is usually given as 5000 units 2 h pre-operatively and either every 8 or 12 h postoperatively. Heparin acts by binding to antithrombin III and making it a more effective enzyme in removing activated factors II, X, IX, XI and XII. Since it acts high in the coagulation cascade, much lower doses are needed to inhibit the initiation of a clot than to treat an established thrombosis, because each step in the coagulation cascade amplifies the next step. There appears to be no increased risk of bleeding in general surgical patients.[45] Due to its theoretical potential for bleeding, it should not be used in patients undergoing cerebral, eye or spinal surgery.[46] Low-dose heparin is not effective in the prophylaxis of venous thromboembolism for hip surgery or prostatic surgery. Adjusted-dose heparin therapy given as a dose of 3500 units initially and adjusted to maintain the activated partial thromboplastin time between 31.5 and 36 s markedly reduces the incidence of venous thrombosis in patients undergoing elective hip surgery compared to a lower-dose heparin regimen.[41]

Postoperative wheezing often develops in patients with a prior history of asthma or chronic obstructive pulmonary disease with bronchospasm. The patient is usually on a pre-operative regimen of bronchodilating drugs, with or without steroids. The only danger and therapeutic dilemma occur when there is the possibility that the bronchospasm is related to cardiac disease. Placement of a flow-directed pulmonary artery catheter may be necessary to make the diagnosis.

Treatment of postoperative wheezing can be initiated with a nebulized selective β_2-agonist, which results in the formation of cyclic adenosine monophosphate and bronchial smooth muscle relaxation. The movement of airway mucus is improved. These agents are preferable to adrenaline (epinephrine) and isoprenaline (isoproterenol) due to their lack of cardiac effects at low doses and the minimal systemic effects on inhalation. The major side-effect is tremor, and it is seen more with non-inhalational use. The primary differences between β_2-agents are related to their durations of action. Due to its long duration of action and recent preparations used for inhalation therapy, albuterol is becoming one of the more popular agents in the USA. If subcutaneous therapy is desired, terbutaline 0.25 mg is as effective as adrenaline, and has a much longer duration of action.

Intravenous theophylline, a medium-potency bronchodilator, can be used if bronchospasm is not relieved with β_2-agonists. Intravenous theophylline is administered as the salt form, theophylline plus ethylenediamine or aminophylline. Aminophylline is more soluble in water. The therapeutic activity is due to its theophylline content. Although it was originally thought to increase cyclic adenosine monophosphate through phosphodiesterase inhibition, recent evidence does not support this concept and its mechanism of action is unknown.[47] It causes bronchial smooth-muscle relaxation, decreased diaphragm fatigue and improves airway mucus. The initial dose is 5–6 mg.kg^{-1} with a maintenance infusion rate of 0.2–1 mg.kg.h^{-1}. The maintenance dose should be decreased in the elderly, patients with liver disease or congestive heart failure, or patients simultaneously medicated with cimetidine, erythromycin, troleandomycin, allopurinol, rifampicin, prednisone, carbamazepine, propranolol or oral contraceptives. Maintenance doses should be higher in the young, heavy smokers, patients on high-protein diets, or patients taking barbiturates or isoprenaline. Desired plasma concentrations are between 10 and 20 $\mu g.ml^{-1}$, although lower or even higher levels are acceptable if the desired therapeutic effect is noted without toxicity. The main side-effects include nausea and vomiting, restlessness and irritability, palpitations, tachycardia and ventricular arrhythmias.

Glucocorticoids are used when bronchospasm is not relieved by traditional agents. Their mechanism of action is unknown but possibilities include a decrease in airway inflammation and enhanced responsiveness of β_2-receptors to endogenous catecholamines and administered sympathomimetic drugs.[48] The loading dose for hydrocortisone is 4 $mg.kg^{-1}$ followed by a 3 $mg.kg^{-1}$ bolus every 6 h to achieve a plasma cortisol concentration above 100 $\mu g.ml^{-1}$. Bronchospastic effects are not instantaneous but occur within 6 h of the start of therapy. Therapy is usually continued for 48–72 h and then tapered, stopped or changed to oral therapy depending on clinical indications.

Renal dysfunction

Methoxyflurane, an inhalation agent now withdrawn from clinical use, was associated with postoperative renal abnormalities due to metabolism to high concentrations of inorganic fluoride — a known renal toxin. Most of the anaesthetic agents currently available have few or no long-term renal effects, although enflurane should not be used in patients with pre-existing renal disease, especially if taking any drug which induces liver microsomal enzyme activity (e.g. phenytoin, isoniazid); again, the concern is metabolism to inorganic fluoride ions.

Adequate kidney function is critical for maintaining water and electrolyte homeostasis. The kidney is also involved in the metabolism and excretion of endogenous wastes and exogenously administered medications. In the presence of long-standing renal failure, multiple complications can occur, which may affect central nervous system function. Accelerated hypertension can occur, with cerebrovascular accidents and cardiovascular dysfunction. Volume overload and congestive failure may develop. Electrolyte abnormalities such as hyperkalaemia, hypermagnesaemia and hypocalcaemia can occur. Platelet dysfunction predisposes to a bleeding diathesis, which can affect the central nervous system. Acid–base disturbances resulting from the inability to excrete fixed acid metabolites and uric acid also have the potential of depressing consciousness.

Hepatic abnormalities

As with the kidneys, few adverse effects on liver function are seen with the most commonly used inhalation agents, isoflurane and enflurane. Nevertheless, hepatic dysfunction is a potential cause of delayed emergence. The liver is responsible for multiple functions that maintain the normal homeostasis of the patient, including glucose and protein metabolism and degradation and clearance of toxic metabolites and drugs. As the major site of protein synthesis, dysfunction can decrease albumin concentrations and thus allow increased circulating free drug levels. The liver is responsible for the clearance of nitrogen from protein as urea, and dysfunction can result in elevated levels of ammonia.

Hepatic dysfunction may occur in patients with a history of prolonged hypotension or hypoxaemia, because the liver is sensitive to decreased oxygen supply due to its high metabolic rate. Decreased hepatic function may occur in patients with cardiac dysfunction and congestive failure. Therapy for the cardiac disease may worsen hepatic function if high-dose sympathomimetics and vasopressors are used that decrease hepatic and splanchnic perfusion. Infectious aetiologies such as viral hepatitides (hepatitis A, B, non-A, non-B, Epstein–Barr virus and cytomegalovirus) can damage the liver. Hepatic dysfunction can be caused by anaesthetic agents either directly (halothane hepatitis rarely) or indirectly by hypoperfusion. Extrahepatic problems such as cholelithiasis or bile duct obstruction due to pancreatic tumour can also produce dysfunction.

MULTIPLE TRAUMA

Patients who have sustained multiple trauma often require several teams of surgeons to repair injuries. Consequences are several: anaesthesia is prolonged; blood loss is often significant, requiring repeated transfusions; hypothermia is common; and illicit drug withdrawal symptoms may develop. These problems, which begin intra-operatively, carry over to the postoperative period.

Blood replacement

Blood loss, requiring transfusion of one or more times the total blood volume, often causes coagulopathies. Unless whole blood is administered, the endogenous platelet pool is reduced by infusion of non-platelet-containing blood products, resulting in dilutional thrombocytopenia (the commonest cause of bleeding diathesis following massive transfusion). Signs of coagulopathy include oozing and generalized bleeding from mucosae, puncture sites and wounds. Patients with coagulopathies and thrombocytopenia should be transfused 0.1 unit.kg^{-1} of platelets, which raises the platelet count by 50×10^9 l^{-1} on average.[49] Storing platelets at 4°C causes platelet dysfunction and shortens platelet life span to less than 48 h. In vivo, platelets are sequestered from the circulation during hypothermia, increasing the problem. Coagulopathy from decreased clotting factors V and VIII is much less common and concentrations of as little as 30% of normal levels allow effective coagulation. The formation of a good blood clot in a glass tube within 10 min indicates a normal clotting time and transfusion of fresh frozen plasma is not necessary. Patients who are transfused platelets also receive the clotting factors present in platelet plasma. Infusion of fresh frozen plasma is therefore indicated infrequently.[50]

During rapid blood transfusion, binding of serum ionized calcium by citrate may result in hypocalcaemia (the symptoms and signs include tetany, arterial hypotension, narrow pulse pressure, elevated capillary wedge and central venous pressures), but only if citrate phosphate dextrose blood infusion exceeds 2 ml.kg^{-1}.min^{-1}. Despite transient reductions in serum ionized calcium, euvolaemic patients usually remain haemodynamically stable because the concentration returns to normal within minutes after the infusion is terminated.[51] Factors promoting citrate toxicity (by interfering with hepatic metabolism) include liver disease, liver transplantation and hypothermia.

Bank blood contains an elevated serum potassium concentration. Hyperkalaemia is possible if the infusion rate is greater than 2 ml.kg^{-1}.min^{-1}. Routine or prophylactic calcium administration is not recommended but is indicated if peaked T waves appear when hyperkalaemia results from rapid blood infusion. Although banked blood is acidic (from increased lactate, pyruvate, glycolysis and elevated PaCO_2), it contains ample citrate, and often causes metabolic alkalosis.[51] Bicarbonate administration must not be given routinely and should be based on arterial (or venous) pH and PCO$_2$ values.

Hypothermia

Heat production to heat loss ratio is significantly decreased in the unstable multiple trauma patient during surgery. Preventing hypothermia is more expedient than treatment. Hypothermic patients frequently become management problems in the PACU. Oxygen consumption is elevated by up to 400% during shivering, haemoglobin–oxygen affinity is increased, potassium leaks from red cells, citrate metabolism is impaired, myocardial dysfunction occurs, arrhythmias can be refractory and increased systemic vascular resistance impairs cardiovascular function. Patients with ischaemic heart disease may require sedation and muscle relaxation to prevent the adverse effects of shivering. Hypothermia prolongs pharmacodynamic drug effects and delays awakening. Warm ambient PACU temperature, blankets and radiant heat lamps are necessary.

Organ failure

Multiple trauma frequently leads to organ failure from either direct injury or from shock. The organs most often involved include the lungs and the kidneys. Pulmonary contusion, interstitial oedema and aspiration pneumonitis increase intrapulmonary shunting and require intensive PACU management. Infusions of blood stored longer than 5 days contain fibrin-white blood cell and platelet microaggregates thought to contribute to the development of adult respiratory distress syndrome (ARDS).[52] Micropore (40 µm) filtration of blood transfusion has not significantly decreased the incidence or severity of ARDS as compared to standard (170 µm) filtration.[53] Sepsis and shock (intensity and duration) are more likely to influence the development of ARDS than are microaggregates. Early use of low-level positive end-expiratory pressure (PEEP) is often helpful in minimizing the onset and severity of ARDS. Periodic blood gas analysis in the PACU is used to guide the level of PEEP and the concentration of inspired oxygen. Fluid administration is guided by urine output, haemodynamics, haematocrit and, if necessary, by pulmonary artery wedge pressures.

Prolonged shock is also linked to renal failure. Oliguria often begins in the operating room but is also seen in the PACU, and can be managed according to a protocol suggested by Bristow & Giesecke (Fig. 25.3).[7] Oliguria is defined as urinary output of <0.5 ml.kg^{-1}.h^{-1}. The lower limit of renal autoregulation is reached when the systolic blood pressure is below 80 mmHg. Hypovolaemia results in hormonal changes prolonging oliguria: catecholamines reduce renal blood flow; renin and angiotensin reduce renal cortical blood flow; and increased atrial natriuretic peptide and antidiuretic hormone reduce urinary output. Renal hypoperfusion is improved by maximizing preload, cardiac output and renal blood flow by titration of fluids (crystalloid improves renal cortical ultrafiltration more than colloid), administration of inotropic agents and infusion of low-dose dopamine (3–5 µg.kg^{-1}.min^{-1}), respectively. Primary renal tubular damage is suspected in a haemodynamically stable patient with urinary

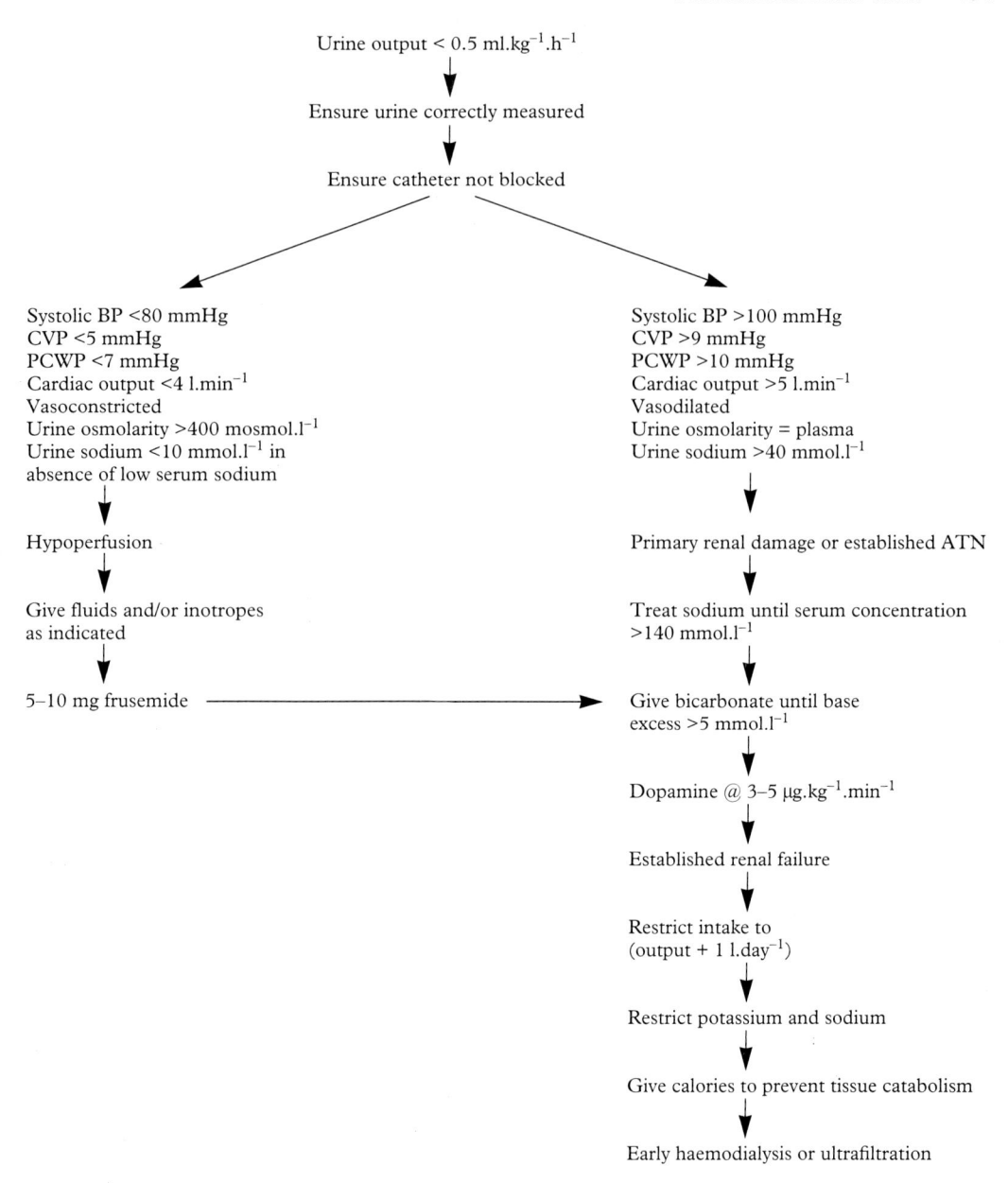

```
                          Urine output < 0.5 ml.kg⁻¹.h⁻¹
                                        ↓
                         Ensure urine correctly measured
                                        ↓
                           Ensure catheter not blocked
                              ↙                    ↘
Systolic BP <80 mmHg                        Systolic BP >100 mmHg
CVP <5 mmHg                                 CVP >9 mmHg
PCWP <7 mmHg                                PCWP >10 mmHg
Cardiac output <4 l.min⁻¹                   Cardiac output >5 l.min⁻¹
Vasoconstricted                             Vasodilated
Urine osmolarity >400 mosmol.l⁻¹            Urine osmolarity = plasma
Urine sodium <10 mmol.l⁻¹ in                Urine sodium >40 mmol.l⁻¹
absence of low serum sodium                           ↓
            ↓                               Primary renal damage or established ATN
      Hypoperfusion                                   ↓
            ↓                               Treat sodium until serum concentration
   Give fluids and/or inotropes             >140 mmol.l⁻¹
      as indicated                                    ↓
            ↓                               Give bicarbonate until base
    5-10 mg frusemide ──────────────────→   excess >5 mmol.l⁻¹
                                                      ↓
                                            Dopamine @ 3-5 μg.kg⁻¹.min⁻¹
                                                      ↓
                                            Established renal failure
                                                      ↓
                                            Restrict intake to
                                            (output + 1 l.day⁻¹)
                                                      ↓
                                            Restrict potassium and sodium
                                                      ↓
                                            Give calories to prevent tissue catabolism
                                                      ↓
                                            Early haemodialysis or ultrafiltration
```

Fig. 25.3 Suggested protocol for the management of oliguria in the trauma patient. BP = Blood pressure; CVP = central venous pressure; PCWP = pulmonary capillary wedge pressure; ATN = acute tubular necrosis. Adapted from Bristow & Giesecke,[7] with permission.

sodium concentration >40 mmol.l⁻¹ prior to administration of frusemide. Early treatment of renal failure includes sodium repletion, alkalinization of the urine (pH over 6.5) and low-dose dopamine. Renal failure in the trauma patient is related most commonly to hypovolaemic shock, although transfusion reactions, disseminated intravascular coagulopathy, nephrotoxic drugs, contrast media, dextrans, sepsis, fat embolism, myoglobin and direct trauma to the kidney are other causes. Severe renal failure requires haemodialysis to maintain intravascular volume, blood urea nitrogen, creatinine and electrolytes in balance.

Non-steroidal anti-inflammatory drugs should be used with caution in the postoperative period, especially if administered intravenously (e.g. ketorolac) as they may precipitate renal failure, particularly in the elderly.

Drug withdrawal

Violent traumatic injury is frequently associated with substance abuse. After a multiple trauma injury requiring prolonged surgery, symptoms of acute drug withdrawal may manifest in the PACU. Victims with an abuse history exhibit bizarre behaviour during withdrawal and demonstrate signs of catecholamine release requiring sedation, opioids, and treatment of hypertension, pulmonary oedema, tachycardia or arrhythmias. Acute intoxication with cocaine ('crack') can result in severe cardiovascular stress culminating in hypertension and intracerebral haemorrhage, myocardial infarction and congestive failure, tachyarrhythmias or sudden death. Chronic alcoholic patients require treatment for impending delirium tremens. Higher concentrations of inhaled agents are often necessary during anaesthesia. Acute alcohol intoxication renders patients more sensitive to anaesthetic agents, predisposing to a delayed recovery period or possible overdosing during anaesthesia.

SEPSIS

Patients with sepsis present difficult problems in the postoperative period. Haemodynamic, metabolic and respiratory complications occur, and mortality is high. The syndrome of sepsis usually consists of hypotension, with normal or elevated cardiac output and low systemic vascular resistance. Septic shock implies organ hypoperfusion, including central nervous system dysfunction, pulmonary failure, renal insufficiency and progressive lactic acidosis.

Sepsis is probably encountered more commonly now for several reasons, including more frequent use of invasive monitoring techniques, aggressive cytotoxic and immunosuppressive therapies, frequent use of corticosteroids, the emergence of multiply resistant strains of micro-organisms and the undertaking of prolonged, intricate surgery on an ageing population often at risk of other diseases such as diabetes and cancer (Table 25.8).

Gram-negative bacteraemia is one of the most common causes of sepsis,[54] accounting for about 150 000 cases annually in the USA. Of these patients, 40–50% develop shock, which is fatal in over half. Sepsis due to Gram-positive organisms, viruses and fungi raises the death toll to 100 000 annually in the USA. Failure to develop a febrile response to bacteraemia and hypo-

Table 25.8 Factors increasing risk of sepsis

Advanced age
Severe debilitating disease
Burns
Instrumentation of body cavities
Invasive monitoring
Mechanical ventilation
Septic abortion
Premature rupture of membranes
Steroids
Cytotoxic drugs
Undrained pus collections
Cirrhosis
Haematological cancer

tension is associated with high mortality.[55] Gram-negative bacteraemia is associated with a mortality of about 10% in the absence of hypotension; if shock is present, mortality increases to 47%.[56] For Gram-positive bacteraemia, corresponding figures approximate to 8 and 33%.[56] In normotensive patients, polymicrobial bacteraemia is associated with a higher mortality than is single-organism bacteraemia. If shock develops, mortality is similar, suggesting that once the fully developed syndrome of sepsis shock is present, the shock state itself is the major determinant of outcome, rather than the source of the bacterial invasion.[56]

Clinical findings postoperatively may be divided into those caused by the infection itself and those related to the sepsis syndrome (i.e. the systemic response to the infection). Patients generally present with fever, and often with tremors if bacteraemia is present. Signs and symptoms related to the infective source may be present (e.g. rales, purulent sputum, urinary infection, abdominal pain). Some or all may be masked by sedation or the residual effects of anaesthetic drugs.

The earliest sign of sepsis is often tachypnoea with respiratory alkalosis. Altered mental state is common, especially in the elderly. Seizures may occur. Oliguria, thrombocytopenia, hypothermia and leukocytosis (or a decreased white blood cell count) may be detected. Hypotension, often a late sign, is associated with acidosis and shock.

Determination of the source of the infection and institution of definitive therapy (i.e. eradication of the infection rather than supportive therapy) are essential.[57] All invasive catheters should be changed. Cultures must be obtained before empirical antibiotic therapy is started. Intra-abdominal sources of infection should be suspected in all surgical or trauma patients who have sustained any violation of intestinal integrity. Ultrasonography and scintigraphy usually correctly diagnose acute acalculous cholecystitis — a not infrequent cause of sepsis in critically ill patients.[58] Abdominal computed tomographic scans demonstrate 80–90% of intra-abdominal abscesses.

The classic description of septic shock defines two phases: warm shock with peripheral vasodilatation, high cardiac output and hypotension, followed by the preterminal phase of cold shock, characterized by cold, clammy skin, low cardiac output and hypotension. However, this picture is rarely seen clinically. Most deaths are from refractory hypotension with normal to high cardiac output maintained until death, or from multiple organ failure. Cardiac output is a poor indicator of global myocardial performance, as the intact organism can alter rate, contractility and loading conditions to maintain output in the face of compromised pump function.

The sepsis syndrome is a major cause of ARDS. Mediators such as endotoxin and protein cascades (complement, kinin, coagulation systems) can all induce damage to the alveolar–capillary membrane.

The initial treatment of septic shock consists of establishing the diagnosis, obtaining cultures, treating the infection, draining abscesses and removing necrotic tissue. If a fluid challenge (1 l of crystalloid) does not restore blood pressure to at least 90 mmHg systolic, haemodynamic monitoring should be initiated by placement of arterial and pulmonary artery catheters. Fluid resuscitation should be maintained until a pulmonary artery wedge pressure of 12–18 mmHg is attained for three reasons: first, these patients are often dehydrated by fever, tachypnoea and decreased intake; second, diffuse capillary leak requires large fluid volumes to establish normal intravascular volume; and third, total body oxygen consumption depends on oxygen delivery over a wide range. Thus, as long as calculated oxygen delivery (equal to the product of cardiac output and arterial oxygen content) to the periphery increases, oxygen uptake increases, presumably reflecting improved metabolic status of the tissues.

If restoration of intravascular volume does not restore blood pressure, vasopressor therapy is indicated. A noradrenaline infusion may be titrated to maintain an adequate systolic blood pressure. Concomitantly, a low-dose dopamine infusion (0.5–2.5 $\mu g.kg^{-1}.min^{-1}$) is initiated to improve renal perfusion. Dobutamine may be titrated to effect on cardiac output.

The work of breathing may be decreased by mechanical ventilation. Standard goals are arterial oxygen saturation of 90% or more at FI_{O_2} of 0.5, with judicious use of PEEP if necessary.

Nutritional support should be started as soon as feasible to minimize the adverse effects of excessive endogenous protein catabolism. Nutritional goals are to provide 35–40 non-protein $kcal.kg^{-1}$ per day and 1.5–2 $g.kg^{-1}$ protein per day. Calories are divided between carbohydrate and fat with two constraints: no more than 60% of total calories is given as lipid and the rate of administration of carbohydrate should not exceed 5–6 $mg.kg^{-1}.min^{-1}$.

At present, no studies have indicated improved survival after steroid administration. Two randomized prospective double-blind placebo-controlled studies failed to demonstrate a beneficial effect.[59,60] More deaths due to secondary infection were noted in the group treated with steroid.[59]

THE ANAESTHETIST IN THE PACU

Clearly the anaesthetist is the physician responsible for admission, care and discharge of patients in the PACU. However, the role of this specialist should extend to include participation in teaching programmes for PACU nurses, and involvement in planning of physical structures, risk management committees and quality assurance programmes.

Currently, several educational programmes have been established for PACU personnel in the USA.[61] Specialization certification is also available for nurses who complete prescribed courses and examinations. Anaesthetists are logical teachers of many aspects of medical assessment and cardiorespiratory evaluation of the postsurgical patient. Courses which should start at a local level can frequently be expanded to include regional and even national meetings.

Many departments and specialists are involved in planning the physical structure of the PACU.[62] All personnel who will be caring for the postanaesthesia patient should have input into decision-making processes. In particular, the area should be in close proximity to the department of anaesthesia to allow immediate access and prompt response in the event of emergencies, and for any consultations. A communication system (telephone, intercom, flashing light) is essential to allow the PACU nurse to contact operating room personnel and anaesthetists.

Risk management and quality assurance committees have become an integral part of hospital life. Although related in concept, in that both are intended to reduce personal injury and financial loss, these programmes are not identical. Risk management focuses more acutely on patients and how they are affected by policies and events with an aim to reduce malpractice situations. Quality assurance examines providers of health care and patterns of practice to ascertain that quality care is delivered. Both processes should improve the standard of care. Risk management mandates legal standard; quality assurance should go even further.

An anaesthetist should serve on both these committees as they pertain to the PACU. In many hospitals, in-house quality assurance meetings are held monthly to review complications and recommend steps that may be taken to avoid their occurrence in the future. Ideally, the anaesthetist, in conjunction with the head nurse in the PACU, should orchestrate these meetings. Documentation of findings is included in monthly reports from many departments of anaesthesia.

SUMMARY

The postanaesthetic period is a critical time. Following surgery, precise monitoring and minute-to-minute supervision by several physicians are halted abruptly and the patient is transferred to a different environment. The anaesthetist's responsibility for the patient does not end with the conclusion of the operation. Thus it is important that this specialist should have a good understanding not only of the residual effects of anaesthetic drugs and how they may affect organ system, but of all other complications that may arise postoperatively.

REFERENCES

1 Nightingale F. Notes on hospitals. London: Longman, Roberts–Green, 1863: p 89
2 Harvey AM. Neurosurgical genius — Walter Edward Dandy. Johns Hopkins Med J 1974; 135–358
3 Dripps RD, Eckenhoff JE, Van Dam LO. The immediate postoperative period: recovery and intensive care. In: Dripps RD, Eckenhoff JE, Van Dam LO (eds) Introduction to anesthesia: the principles of safe practice, 7th edn. Philadelphia, PA: Saunders, 1988; pp 430–440
4 Fischer TL. Responsibility for care in recovery rooms. Can Med Assoc J 1970; 102–934
5 Aldrete JA, Kronlik D. A postanesthetic recovery score. Anesth Analg 1970; 49: 924–934
6 Carignan G, Keeri-Szanto M, Lavelle JP. Postanesthetic scoring system. Anesthesiology 1964; 25: 396–397
7 Bristow A, Giesecke AH. Fluid therapy of trauma. Semin Anesth 1985; 4: 124–133
8 Prys-Roberts C. Cardiovascular action: too much, too little or irregular. In: Frost E, ed. Post anesthesia care unit. St Louis, MO: CV Mosby, 1990: pp 31–43
9 Hammel HT. Anesthetics and body temperature regulation. Anesthesiology 1988; 68: 833–835
10 Bay J, Nunn JF, Prys-Roberts C. Factors influencing arterial Po_2 during recovery from anaesthesia. Br J Anaesth 1968; 398–406
11 Sharkey A, Lipton JM, Murphy MT et al. Inhibition of postanesthetic shivering with radiant heat. Anesthesiology 1987; 66: 249–252
12 Levine RD. The ambulatory surgery patient. In: Frost E, Goldiner P, eds. Postanesthetic care. Connecticut: Appleton Lange, 1990; pp 277–291
13 Prys-Roberts C. Treatment of postoperative pain. In: Frost E, ed. Post anesthetic care unit, 2nd edn. St Louis, MO: CV Mosby, 1990: pp 9–18
14 Hovorka J, Korttila K, Erkola O. Nitrous oxide does not increase nausea and vomiting following gynaecological laparoscopy. Can J Anaesth 1989; 36: 145–148
15 Fahy A, Marshall M. Postanaesthetic morbidity in outpatients. Br J Anaesth 1969; 41: 433–435
16 Melnick B, Chalasani J, Lion Uy NT et al. Decreasing post-succinylcholine myalgia in outpatients. Can Anaesth Soc J 1987; 34: 238–241
17 Sosis M, Goldberg M, Marr AT et al. Succinylcholine does not contribute to postoperative pain after outpatient laparoscopy. Abstract presented at second annual SAMBA meeting, Washington, DC, 1987.
18 Pearce AC, Williams JP, Jones RM. The use of atracurium for short surgical procedure in day-case patients. Anesthesiology 1983; 159: A265
19 Greenblatt DJ, Abernathy DR, Morse DS et al. Clinical importance of the interaction of diazepam and cimetidine. N Engl J Med 1984; 310: 1639–1643
20 Bailey PL, Pace NL, Ashburn MA. Frequent hypoxemia and apnea after sedation with midazolam and fentanyl. Anesthesiology 1990; 73: 826–830
21 Malley RA. Delayed return to consciousness. In: Frost E, Goldiner P, eds. Postanesthetic care. Connecticut: Appleton Lange, 1990: pp 9–21
22 Cullen BF, Miller MG. Drug interactions and anesthesia: a review. Anesth Analg 1979; 58: 413–423
23 Djokovic JL, Hedley-White J. Prediction of outcome of surgery and anesthesia in patients over 80. JAMA 1979; 242: 2301–2306
24 Carliner NH, Fisher ML, Plotnick GD et al. Routine preoperative exercise testing in patients undergoing major noncardiac surgery. Am J Cardiol 1985; 56: 51–57
25 Driscoll AC, Hobika JH, Etsten BE et al. Clinically unrecognized myocardial infarction following surgery. N Engl J Med 1961; 264: 633–639
26 Rao TK, Jacobs KH, El-Etr AA. Reinfarction following anesthesia in patients with myocardial infarction. Anesthesiology 1983; 59: 499–505
27 Philbin DM, Foex P, Drummond G, et al. Post systolic shortening of canine left ventricle supplied by a stenotic coronary artery when nitrous oxide is added in the presence of narcotics. Anesthesiology 1985; 62: 166–174
28 Fegert G, Hollenberg M, Browner W et al. Perioperative myocardial ischemia in the noncardiac surgical patient. Anesthesiology 1988; 69: A49
29 Pesola G, Eissa N, Kvetan V. Pulmonary complications and respiratory therapy. In: Frost E, Goldiner P, eds. Post-anesthetic care. Connecticut: Appleton & Lange, 1990; pp 63–79
30 Bendixen HH, Smith GM, Mead J. Pattern of ventilation in young adults. J Appl Physiol 1964; 19: 195–198
31 Craig DB. Postoperative recovery of pulmonary function. Anesth Analg 1981; 60: 46–52
32 Ali J, Weisel RD, Layug AB et al. Consequences of

33. Wightman JAK. A postoperative atelectasis and pneumonia: diagnosis, etiology and management based upon 1240 cases of upper abdominal surgery. Ann Surg 1946; 124: 94–110
34. Schlenker JD, Hubay CA. The pathogenesis of postoperative atelectasis. A clinical study. Arch Surg 1973; 107: 846–850
35. Pearce AC, Jones RM. Smoking and anesthesia: preoperative abstinence and perioperative morbidity. Anesthesiology 1984; 61: 576–584
36. Chalon J, Tayyab MA, Ramanathan S. Cytology of respiratory epithelium as a predictor of respiratory complications after operation. Chest 1975; 67: 32–35
37. Mircea N, Constantinescu C, Jianu E et al. Risk of pulmonary complications in surgical patients. Resuscitation 1982; 10: 33–41
38. Latimer RG, Dickman M, Day WC et al. Ventilatory patterns and pulmonary complications after upper abdominal surgery determined by preoperative and postoperative computerized spirometry and blood gas analysis. Am J Surg 1971; 122: 622–632
39. Light RW, George RB. Incidence and significance of pleural effusion after abdominal surgery. Chest 1976; 69: 621–625
40. Shepard RM, White HA, Shirkey AL. Anticoagulant prophylaxis of thromboembolism in post-surgical patients. Am J Surg 1966; 112: 698–702
41. Leyvraz PF, Richyard J, Bachmann F et al. Adjusted versus fixed-dose subcutaneous heparin in the prevention of deep-vein thrombosis after total hip replacement. N Engl J Med 1983; 309: 954–958
42. Donaldson GA, Williams C, Scannell G et al. A reappraisal of the application of the Trendelenburg operation to massive fatal embolism. N Eng J Med 1963; 268: 171–174
43. Kelsey JL, Wood PHN, Charnley J. Prediction of thromboembolism following total hip replacement. Clin Orthop 1976; 114: 247–258
44. Salzman EW, Hirsh J. Prevention of venous thromboembolism. In: Coleman RW, Hirsh J, Marder V et al, eds. Hemostasis and thrombosis. Basic principles and clinical practice. Philadelphia, PA: Lippincott, 1982; pp 986–999
45. International Multicentre Trial. Prevention of fatal postoperative pulmonary embolism by low doses of heparin. Lancet 1975; ii: 45–51
46. Hull RD, Raskob GE, Hirsh J. Prophylaxis of venous thromboembolism. An overview. Chest 1986; 89: 374A–383A
47. Miech RF, Stein M. Methylxanthines. Clin Chest Med 1986; 7: 331–340
48. Ziment I. Steroids. Clin Chest Med 1986; 7: 341–354
49. Berman JA. The trauma victim. In: Frost EAM, ed. Preanesthetic assessment 1. Boston, MA: Birkhäuser, 1988; pp 10–20
50. Braunstein AH, Oberman HA. Transfusion of plasma components. Transfusion 1984; 24: 281–286
51. Denlinger JK, Narhwold ML, Gibbs PS et al. Hypocalcaemia during rapid blood transfusion in anaesthetized man. Br J Anaesth 1976; 48: 995–997
52. Miller RD, Brzica SM. Blood, blood components, colloids and autotransfusion therapy. In: Miller RD, ed. Anesthesia, 2nd edn. vol 2. New York: Churchill Livingstone, 1986; pp 1348–1350
53. Durtschi MB, Haisch CE, Reynolds L et al. Effect of micropore filtration on pulmonary function after massive transfusion. Am J Surg 1979; 138: 8–10
54. Greeman RL. Gram-negative bacteremia. In: Gardener LB, ed. Acute internal medicine. New York: Medical Examination, 1986; pp 393–399
55. Kreger BE, Craven DE, McCabe WR. Gram-negative bacteremia IV. Re-evaluation of clinical features and treatment in 612 patients. Am J Med 1980; 68: 344–355
56. Jacoby I. Septic shock. In: Rippe JM, Irwin RS, Alpert JS, Dalen JE, eds. Intensive care medicine. Boston, MA: Little Brown, 1985; pp 666–675
57. Altmeier WA, Todd CA, Wellford WE. Gram-negative septicemia: a growing threat. Ann Surg 1967; 166: 530–542
58. Fox MS, Wilk PJ, Weissmann HS et al. Acute acalculous cholecystitis. Surg Gynecol Obstet 1984; 159: 13–16
59. Bone RC, Fisher CJ, Clemmer TP et al. A controlled clinical trial of high-dose methylprednisolone in the treatment of severe sepsis and septic shock. N Engl J Med 1987; 317: 653–658
60. Hinshaw L, Peduzzi P, Young E et al. Effect of high dose glucocorticoid therapy on mortality in patients with clinical signs of systemic sepsis. N Engl J Med 1987; 317: 659–665
61. Williams DM. Educational programs for PACU personnel. In: Frost E, ed. Post-anesthesia care unit, 2nd edn. St Louis, MO: CV Mosby, 1990; pp 210–214
62. DeFranco M. Planning the physical structure of the PACU. In: Frost E, ed. Post-anesthesia care unit, 2nd edn. St Louis, MO: CV Mosby, 1990; pp 187–198

26. Postoperative pain relief

R. Sharpe   A. Lawson   R. M. Jones

By any reasonable code, freedom from pain should be a basic human right, limited only by our knowledge to achieve it.[1]

Clinical reviews continue to indicate that standard methods of postoperative pain relief fail to relieve pain in up to half of patients.[2,3] This is in spite of the fact that the adverse physiological effects of acute pain following surgery are well-documented (Table 26.1). The adverse effects of acute pain are potentially most harmful at the extremes of age and in frail patients with significant disease processes. Advances in anaesthetic and surgical techniques have led to many more such patients presenting for surgery. With increasing longevity in western societies, the necessity for good pain control in an ageing population can hardly be doubted.

In contrast to the relative neglect of postoperative pain relief, there have been great advances in the provision of pain relief in other areas such as obstetric analgesia. With the current development of patient advocacy and quality assurance review, adequate postoperative analgesia will be an increasingly important issue in humanitarian, ethical and perhaps medicolegal terms.

Recognition of the widespread inadequacy of pain management has resulted in the promulgation of various practice guidelines and statements by a variety of national colleges and government bodies (Joint Report of the Royal College of Surgeons and College of Anaesthetists 1990;[4] National Health and Medical Research Council of Australia 1988; International Association for the Study of Pain 1991; US Department of Health and Human Services 1992). All these bodies have stressed that there is an ethical obligation to minimize the amount of pain suffered in the postoperative period. With the spiralling costs of hospital medicine, it is also of great importance to appreciate that earlier mobilization, decreased morbidity and shortened hospital stay may significantly decrease the cost of a patient's stay in hospital.

The management of postoperative pain has become a high priority for anaesthetists. This has resulted in the formation of acute postoperative pain services in many hospitals. These have a remit to improve the provision of acute pain relief and to raise standards of education of both medical and nursing staff. They also audit the changes that are instituted.

Nevertheless, it should not be forgotten that, in general, the presence of acute pain remains the cornerstone of surgical diagnosis. Due to the paucity of short-acting analgesics in the past, there was a justifiable tendency to avoid ablating pain pre-operatively until a diagnosis had been made or therapy decided upon. Many surgeons also use the development of new pain in the postoperative period as a vital element in the diagnosis of complications. However, the use of shorter-acting opioids and non-opioid analgesics, coupled with improvements in diagnosis, should allow a more humanitarian approach to patients' welfare both pre- and postoperatively.

It is recognized that the response of patients to surgical pain, and the amount of analgesia required, vary considerably.[5] Traditional methods of pain relief, such as intramuscular opioids, cannot respond to this variability. The introduction of individualized pain therapies has allowed the *patient* to control the amount of analgesia received. This has been made possible by the introduction of patient-controlled analgesia (PCA).

The introduction of novel techniques such as epidural opioids, PCA and plexus infusions of local anaesthetics presents a challenge to the anaesthetist. The advantages of these techniques in pain control are acknowledged by many practising clinicians. However, such techniques require close monitoring to provide high-quality pain relief without potentially increasing morbidity and mortality. The establishment of acute pain services is a fundamental part of this process. There are few controlled studies documenting the efficacy of conventional methods of pain relief. However, that does not absolve the anaesthetic community from attempting to quantify the benefits of the individual techniques that we wish

Table 26.1 Adverse physiological effects of acute pain

System	Physiological effect	Clinical consequence
Respiratory system	Decreased ventilation Decreased FVC Decreased FRC	Atelectasis Lobar collapse Pneumonia Hypoxaemia Hypercapnia
Cardiovascular system	Tachycardia Increased SVR Hypertension Increased cardiac work	Myocardial ischaemia Myocardial infarction
Gastrointestinal tract	Gastric stasis Gastric dilation Ileus	Nausea and vomiting Aspiration Third-space losses
Urology	Urinary retention	Pain Hypertension Agitation
Endocrine	Increased ADH Increased aldosterone Increased cortisol	Water retention Sodium retention Hyperglycaemia
Haematology	Platelet aggregation Venous stasis	Deep vein thrombosis Pulmonary embolism
Muscular system	Immobilization	Muscle wasting
Central nervous system	Altered sleep pattern	Anxiety states Psychosis

FVC = Forced vital capacity; FRC = functional residual capacity; SVR = systemic vascular resistance; ADH = antidiuretic hormone.

to see employed. If we can do that, then not only can we influence patient welfare, but also surgical outcome.

THE PHYSIOLOGICAL BASIS OF PAIN MANAGEMENT

The transmission of nociceptive impulses from the periphery to the higher centres can no longer be viewed as a 'hard-wired' system, in which certain patterns of input result in a predictable output. Instead, it is now recognized that nociceptive impulses are *modulated* at various stages of transmission. The result is an ever-changing, dynamic sensory system. The term *plasticity* has been used to describe this process.[6]

Noxious stimuli are defined as chemical, thermal or mechanical. These activate nociceptors, and nociceptive impulses are transmitted to the spinal cord and then on to higher centres. When nociceptive impulses reach the level of conscious awareness, the experience of pain occurs. Pain has been defined by Merskey as 'an unpleasant sensory and emotional experience associated with actual or potential tissue damage'.[7]

Pain has been categorized by Woolf into physiological and pathological pain.[6] Physiological pain results from the application of a noxious stimulus which neither produces tissue damage nor inflammation, e.g. touching a hot plate. The perception of pain produces reflex withdrawal from the potentially hazardous stimulus, and activation of the sympathetic nervous system initiates the 'flight or fight' response, facilitating the organism in removing itself from danger. In this context, pain is a vital defence mechanism. The ill effects of insensitivity to pain, for example diabetic neuropathy, illustrate the protective role of the sensation of pain.

Pathological pain arises as a consequence of either the inflammatory response occurring with extensive tissue injury, or direct damage to the nervous system. It is now evident that this type of pain results in changes in the nervous system that far exceed the duration of the original stimulus. These changes may result in the following:

1. a reduction in the stimulus required to produce nociceptive impulses
2. a widening of the area where pain is felt

3. the sensation of pain even when noxious stimuli are absent.

The nociceptive impulses arising from postoperative surgical trauma produce these modulatory changes. The reduction of the original nociceptive input, which produces these pain-sensitizing and amplification modulations, forms the basis of pre-emptive analgesia.

The physiological sequelae of pain in the postoperative period appear to confer little or no benefit to the patient and are generally adverse in nature (Table 26.1). For example, excessive splanchnic vasoconstriction resulting from sympathetic overactivity may produce tissue hypoxia, with the release of toxic peptides, including interleukins and endotoxin which produce myocardial depression. Thus, in the setting of postoperative pain, our complex physiological responses are in some ways an evolutionary anachronism.

Peripheral nociceptors

Pain is perceived after the stimulation of nociceptors which are the nerve endings of Aδ and C fibre afferents. Aδ fibres are associated with sharp, well-localized pain, and C fibres with dull, burning, poorly localized pain. C fibres also contain sympathetic fibres which increase the sensitivity of peripheral nociceptors. In cutaneous nerves, approximately 50% of fibres originate from nociceptors.

With the ability to perform sophisticated neurophysiological studies on single neurones it has been possible to classify different types of nociceptors.[8]

1. *C-polymodal receptors (C-PMNs)*. These are abundant non-myelinated C fibres which respond to all three noxious stimuli. i.e. thermal, mechanical and chemical.

2. *A-mechano-heat receptors (AMHs)*. These respond to mechanical and heat stimuli, and the afferent stimuli travel in Aδ fibres.

3. *High-threshold mechanoreceptors*. These only respond to intense mechanical stimuli. In humans, these have been recorded from Aδ fibres.

4. *Muscle nociceptors*. These are thought to be the free nerve endings found in the connective tissue between muscle fibres and in tendons and blood vessels.

5. *Silent nociceptors*. These C fibre afferents do not fire in response to any noxious stimulus, however strong, in normal tissue. In the presence of inflammation, they become sensitized, even to the point of being spontaneously active and mechanosensitive. As a consequence, the inflamed tissue becomes very tender and hurts with minimal movement.

Nociceptive neurones exhibit plasticity, i.e. frequency of discharge to a constant stimulus can vary. This increase in sensitivity can be mediated by chemical activators (in particular, the mediators of inflammation) or by sympathetic postganglionic neurones. Sensitization results in a lowering of the threshold to pain in the localized area of tissue damage and is called *primary hyperalgesia*. Secondary hyperalgesia refers to the widening of the receptive field, which occurs at a spinal level (Fig. 26.1). Chemical activators include protons (H^+) and adenosine triphosphate released during the cellular damage which occurs with tissue trauma, and the inflammatory mediators, including serotonin, bradykinin, histamine, cytokines and the prostaglandins PGE_2, PGD_2 and PGI_2. These sensitize the nociceptor by membrane receptor-gated ion channels or by intracellular second messengers.

Capsaicin, found in red hot peppers, acts in a complex manner on mammalian polymodal nociceptors.[9] When applied to primary afferent C fibre neurones, a brief burning pain is experienced, followed by longer-lasting hyperalgesia. Capsaicin opens a membrane ion channel permeable to sodium and calcium ions. Influx of Na^+ depolarizes the neurone towards the threshold for action potential initiation. Evidence exists for a capsaicin membrane receptor and a competitive antagonist, capsazepine, has been isolated. Exposure to high levels of capsaicin blocks C fibre conduction and may produce selective C fibre neurotoxicity. This is thought to be due to osmotic cell lysis as a result of accumulation of Na^+ in the neurone and also as a result of enzyme-mediated damage triggered by the rise in intracellular Ca^{2+}.[9]

Sympathetically mediated nociceptive sensitization has also been demonstrated. This cannot be reproduced by direct application of noradrenaline to intact C fibres and is therefore thought to be an indirect action. It may be due to α-stimulation of local non-neuronal cells, which release PGI_2.

In addition to transmitting nociceptive impulses to the spinal cord, the primary afferents also release neuropeptides, such as substance P, from their free nerve endings. Release of these causes local vasodilatation and increased vascular permeability, resulting in neurogenic inflammation. Substance P also stimulates the release of interleukins and arachidonic acid. These sensitize the primary afferents further, and a positive feedback loop occurs.

Spinal cord transmission

The Aδ and C fibre afferents have their cell bodies in the dorsal root ganglion. From there, they project to

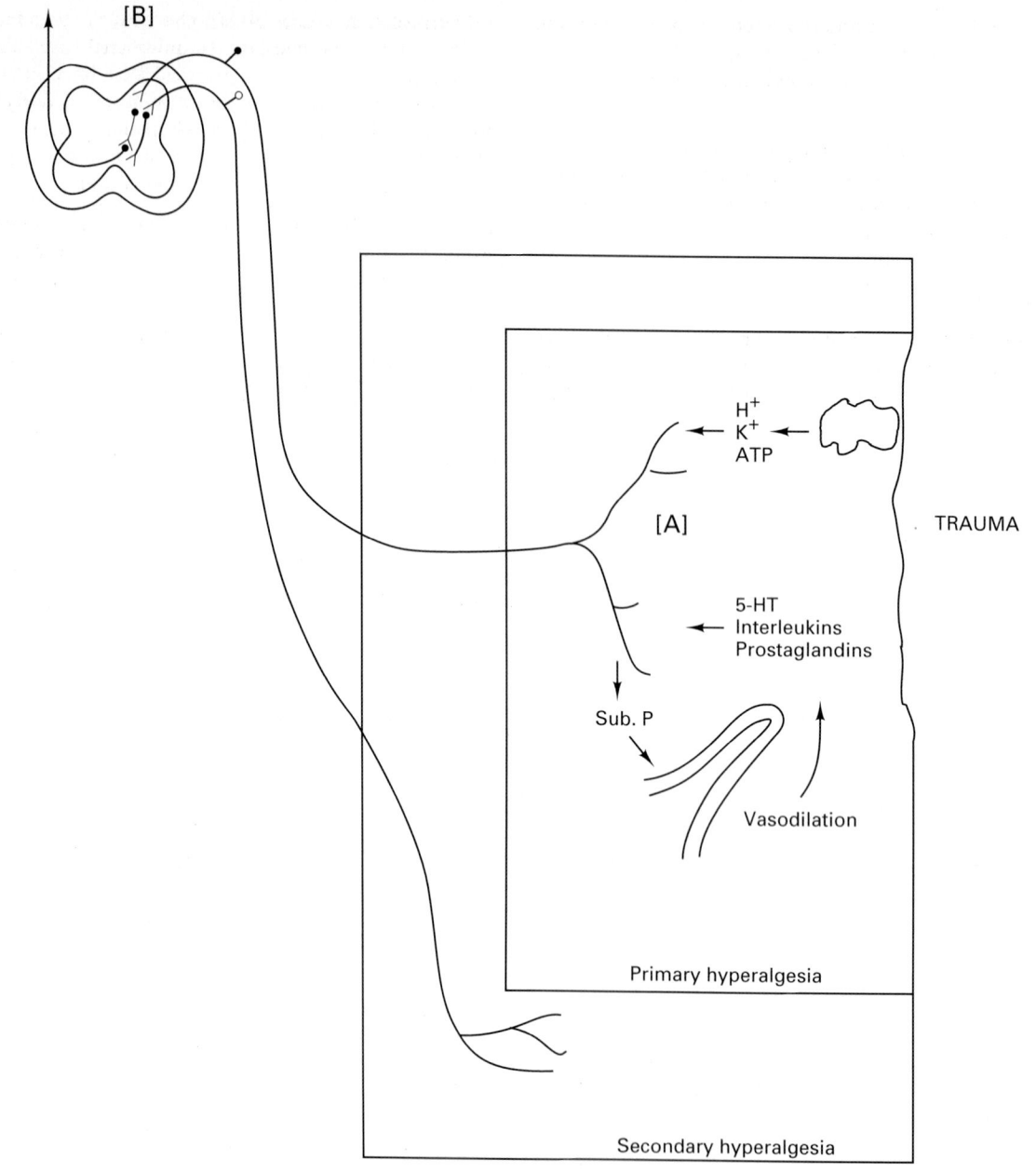

Fig. 26.1 Mechanism of tissue trauma resulting in nociceptor sensitization [A] (primary hyperalgesia) and spinal cord sensitization [B] (secondary hyperalgesia).

the dorsal horn of the spinal cord. The Aδ fibres synapse primarily in Rexed lamina I (lamina marginalis). The C fibres synapse with short fibre interneurones in Rexed laminae II and III (substantia gelatinosa). These interneurones finally synapse with second-order afferents in lamina V.

The incoming Aδ and C fibres synapse with a variety of neurones in the dorsal horn, including:

- various short-fibre relay neurones
- motor neurones forming the monosynaptic withdrawal reflex arc

- ongoing second-order afferents which cross the cord in the anterior commissure and project to the thalamus via the spinothalamic and spinoreticular tracts.

In the dorsal horn, there are multiple excitatory and inhibitory synapses which can modulate ongoing nociceptive transmission. This results in adaptation and plasticity in the system.

Excitatory events

It is evident that repeated C fibre afferent input can produce long-term changes in the excitability of the dorsal horn neurones and alterations in receptive field properties. This *central sensitization* results in an altered perception of peripheral stimuli, called secondary hyperalgesia.

Three mechanisms have been proposed to describe the actions of C fibre afferent action on the dorsal horn (Fig. 26.2).

1. *Fast transmitter release, possibly the amino acid glutamate.* This produces a short postsynaptic excitatory potential lasting 10 ms. This mechanism transfers information of location, onset and duration of the peripheral stimulus.

2. *Neuromodulator release, including aspartate, substance P and calcitonin.* These are co-released from the same terminals as fast transmitters. Their release results in

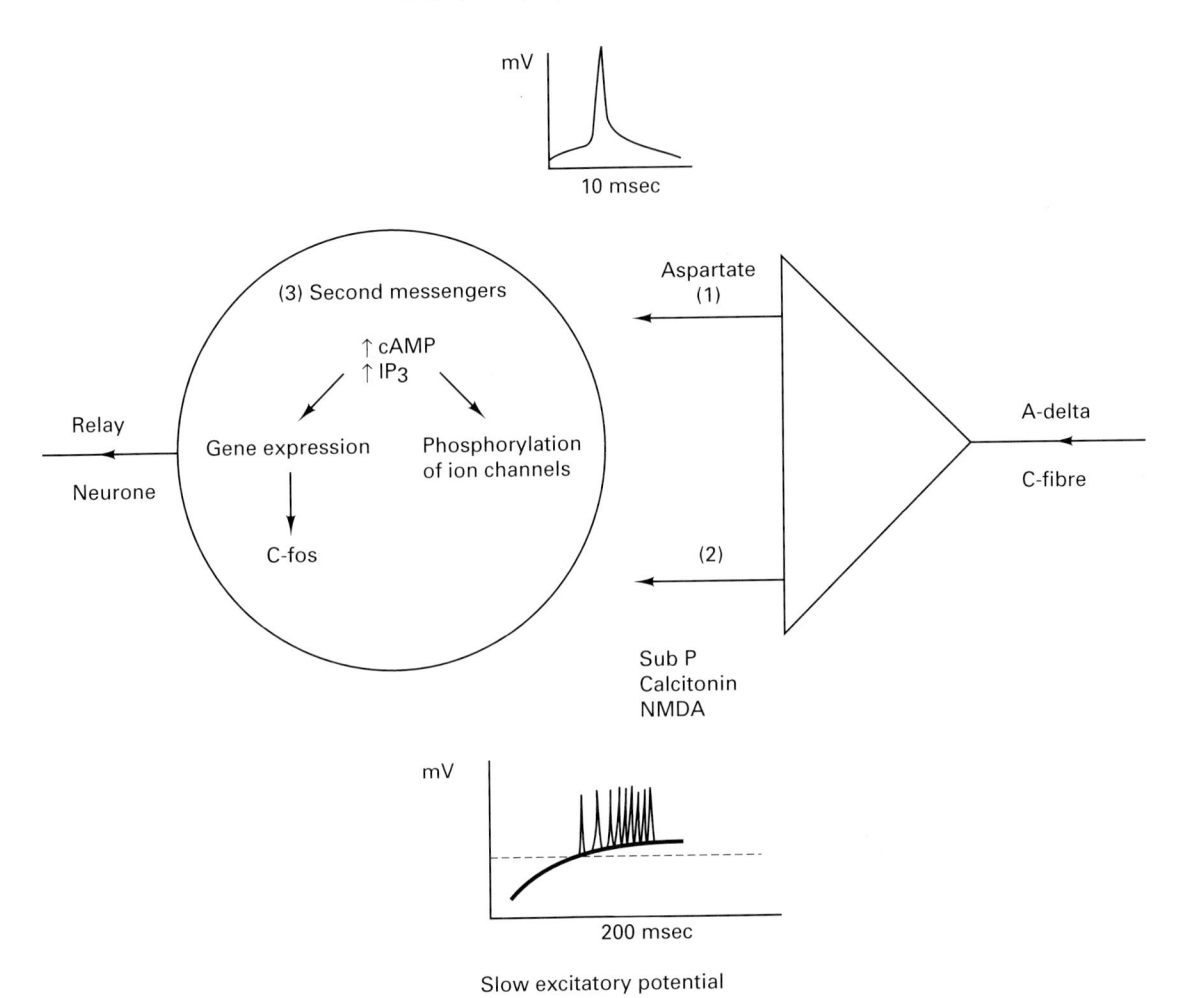

Fig. 26.2 Excitatory events at the nociceptive input to the relay neurons in the dorsal horn. (See text.)

the build-up of slow excitatory potentials due to inward currents of Na^+ and Ca^{2+}, and this produces a sustained depolarization towards the threshold for firing. These potentials may be additive (temporal summation). Repeated stimulation of the same afferent neurone produces a progressive increase in action potential discharge (wind-up) which results in a build-up of pain sensation. Evidence is accumulating that the build-up of slow excitatory potentials is mediated via the *N*-methyl-D-aspartate (NMDA) receptor.[10–12] It has been possible to demonstrate that experimentally induced hyperalgesic states can be blocked by prior administration of NMDA-receptor antagonists such as ketamine.[13]

3. *Second messengers and gene expression.* C fibre afferent stimulation also produces changes in the second messenger systems of the dorsal horn neurones. Increases in intracellular Ca^{2+} concentration produce changes in cyclic adenosine monophosphate, cyclic guanosine monophosphate and inositol triphosphate (IP_3). It is thought that the resultant changes in protein kinases may modify neurone excitability by phosphorylation of ion channels and membrane receptors.

Gene expression in the dorsal horn neurone has been shown to be modified by C fibre afferent stimulation. Hunt et al[14] demonstrated the rapid appearance of c-*fos* protein immunoreactivity in postsynaptic dorsal horn neurones following the application of mustard oil to the hind limb of rats. Immunoreactivity predominated in Rexed laminae I and II. It has been suggested that the proto-oncogene c-*fos* participates in the establishment of prolonged functional changes in the dorsal root neurones.

These adaptive changes can be demonstrated in vivo by the flexion withdrawal reflex to nociceptive input. When the skin is pinched, a flexor withdrawal response occurs. If a cutaneous nerve is stimulated at 1 Hz for 20 s at a current strength high enough to stimulate C fibres, the flexion response becomes more excitable. Eventually, light touch becomes sufficient to trigger the reflex. In addition, the receptive field enlarges, resulting in a larger area of skin in which the reflex can be triggered by light touch.

Inhibitory events

There are also inhibitory influences at the dorsal root level. Inhibitory neurotransmitters include γ-aminobutyric acid (GABA), acetylcholine, $α_2$-agonists, endogenous opioids and serotonin. Many of these are released at the dorsal horn level in response to signals from descending pathways from the higher centres (see below). The influence of the inhibitory neurotransmitters on nociceptive transmission at the dorsal horn is summarized in Figure 26.3.

Opioid receptors

The discovery of opioid receptors was unusual in that the receptors were found first and their endogenous ligands later. Opioid-binding sites were first demonstrated in mammals in 1973 by Pert & Snyder.[15] The theory of multiple opioid receptors was proposed by Martin to explain the differences in the pharmacological actions of morphine and nalorphine.[16]

Five receptors have been isolated. Only three, μ, δ and κ, play a significant role in pain modulation in humans.[17] The later discovery of endogenous opioid peptides and the production of synthetic antagonists have allowed elucidation of the distribution and action of these receptor subtypes.

μ-*Receptors*. These have been subdivided into $μ_1$- and $μ_2$-receptors, based on different affinity states of different radioligands. The significance of such a subdivision (which is not universally accepted[18]) is that it was hoped that a selective $μ_1$-agonist would be able to produce useful analgesic actions without unwanted side-effects, such as respiratory depression. This separation of effects has not been demonstrated, nor a pure $μ_1$-agonist found. Endogenous agonists at μ-receptors are the β-endorphins.

δ-*Receptors*. Highly selective δ-agonists have been demonstrated, including Leu-enkephalin and Met-enkephalin (Try-Gly-Gly-Phe-Met and Try-Gly-Gly-Phe-Leu, respectively).

κ-*Receptors*. The natural κ-agonists are the dynorphins. Exogenous κ agonists, such as pentazocine, produce analgesia at a spinal level, but separation from μ and δ effects is difficult to demonstrate.

All three receptors are found in varying proportions in both the spinal cord (producing spinal analgesia) and brain (producing supraspinal analgesia). Evidence exists for the presence of peripheral opioid receptors in inflammatory states,[19] as it has been demonstrated that opioids have actions on peripheral inflammatory pain.

In order to produce reductions in nociceptive input, and ultimately a reduction in the conscious experience of pain, activation of opioid receptors results in neuronal inhibitory effects. Activation of μ- and δ-receptors results in opening of K^+ channels via G-protein intermediaries in the presynaptic membrane.[20] Opening of these channels allows K^+ efflux, resulting in hyperpolarization. This results in inhibition of nociceptive impulses and a reduction of Ca^{2+} influx at the nerve terminal, which reduces transmitter release. The

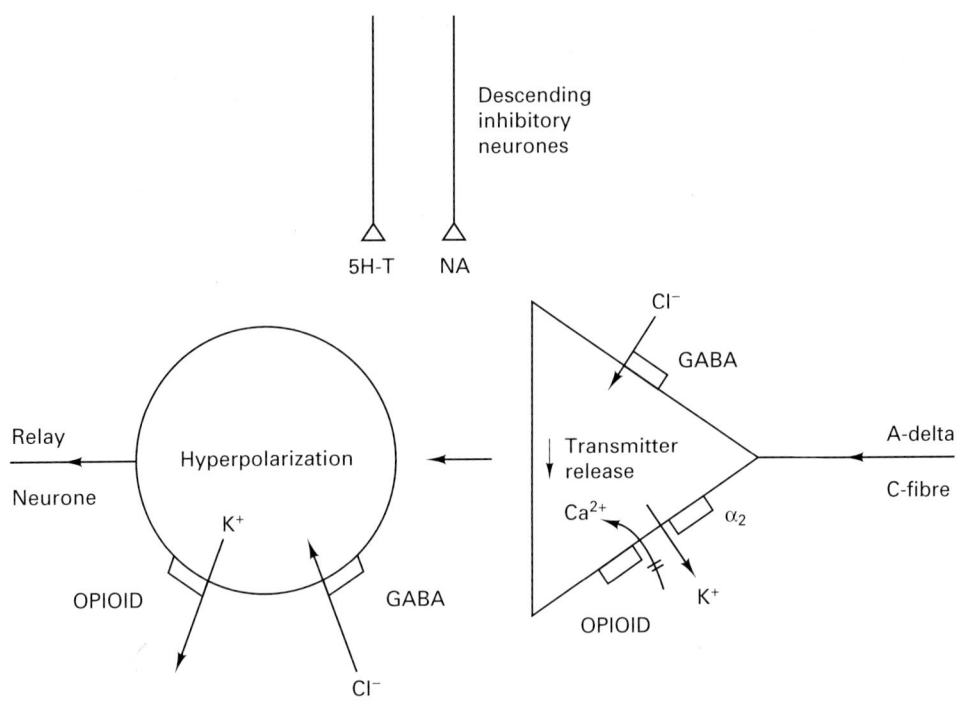

Fig. 26.3 Inhibitory influences on nociceptive transmission in the dorsal horn of the spinal cord. (See text.)

κ receptors seem to have a different action; they close Ca^{2+} channels, resulting in reduced transmitter release from the nerve terminal.

At the spinal level, opioid receptors have been demonstrated at both the pre- and postsynaptic sites in the C fibre input into the substantia gelatinosa.

Opioid-induced hyperpolarization of an *inhibitory neuron* reduces inhibitory input to the next cell in line, which may become excited — an example of disinhibition. Such opioid-induced disinhibitions have been observed in the substantia gelatinosa of the spinal cord[20] and may have a role in the antinociceptive action of opioids.

The excitatory actions of opioids, such as nausea and vomiting, also result from opioid receptor inhibition of inhibitory pathways — a further example of disinhibition.

α-Receptors

$α_2$-Adrenergic receptor activation produces analgesia at both supraspinal and spinal sites.[21] These receptors are linked to transmembrane G-proteins (as are opioid receptors). These coupling proteins may be linked either to a transmembrane ion channel or to an intracellular second messenger system. Efflux of K^+ through an activated channel can hyperpolarize the excitable membrane. This provides an effective means of suppressing neuronal firing. $α_2$-stimulation also decreases Ca^{2+} entry into nerve terminals, resulting in reduced neurotransmitter release.[22] When these mechanisms are considered, together with the demonstration of $α_2$-receptors at spinal and supraspinal sites, it is not surprising that $α_2$-agonists produce analgesia. For example, clonidine produces effective postoperative analgesia when given systemically or directly into the epidural space.[23]

GABA receptors

Both $GABA_A$ and $GABA_B$ receptors have been identified in the dorsal horn at pre- and postsynaptic sites.[24] These are ligand-gated chloride channels. Opening of these channels results in hyperpolarization; as a consequence, there is a reduction in neurotransmitter release and inhibition of postsynaptic neuronal activity. The GABA-receptor agonist THIP (4,5,6,7-tetrahydro, isoxazola -[5,4-c] pyradin-3-ol) has been shown to have potent analgesic effects in animal models.[25]

Descending inhibitory neurones

Descending inhibitory neurones arise from the periaqueductal grey area and the raphe nucleus; they terminate in the dorsal horn, where they exert antinociceptive effects. These descending neurons release serotonin (5-hydroxytryptamine, or 5-HT) and noradrenaline. The antinociceptive effects of these pathways can be blocked by adrenoceptor and serotoninergic antagonists.

Supraspinal nociceptive transmission

As neuronal circuitry becomes more complex, our knowledge becomes more sketchy. We know that the secondary afferents transmit impulses to the thalamus. It is likely that further modulation occurs here. Finally, nociceptive impulses reach the cerebral cortex where the conscious experience of pain is felt. Emotional responses can modify the reactions to pain greatly. For example, it has been described that soldiers in the First World War felt little or no pain following serious wounds to the lower limbs. This has been attributed to the overwhelming sense of relief that the soldier's injury would lead to his removal from the front line.

Endogenous opioids certainly play a role in supraspinal pain modulation. At supraspinal levels, opioid receptor sites have been well-mapped. The highest concentrations of μ- and δ-receptors are found in the midbrain, especially around the raphe nucleus and the peri-aqueductal and periventricular grey matter. The mechanism of action here remains indistinct; it may be due to alterations in the balance of nociceptive to innocuous impulses reaching the higher centres.

$α_2$-Receptor activation also modulates pain transmission at supraspinal sites.

The implications of wind-up and plasticity for postoperative pain relief

The recent expansion in our knowledge of nociceptive transmission and modulation is now being applied to clinical situations.[26] It has been suggested that for adequate management of pain states, treatment should be aimed at treating the neuromodulatory changes in the primary afferents and the dorsal root neurones, rather than merely interrupting the flow of sensory signals.[6] For example, opioids applied to the epidural or subarachnoid spaces can be used in much reduced doses. Excellent analgesia is produced without necessarily producing systemic side-effects. Renewed interest has developed in the use of non-steroidal anti-inflammatory drugs (NSAIDs) which decrease the prostaglandin-mediated sensitization of peripheral nociceptors.[27]

The combination of opioids and NSAIDs has been used in the treatment of cancer pain for many years. Combination therapy is now being considered in acute pain states. It has been demonstrated that pain scores can be reduced almost to zero when a combination of epidural bupivacaine and morphine together with systemic indomethacin is used following cholecystectomy.[28] It is interesting that, many years after the description of the triad of anaesthesia, we are now developing the idea of a triad of analgesia to produce maximal pain reduction.

It is also postulated that the most effective way to treat postoperative pain will be to prevent the development of wind-up in the nervous system. To do this, treatment must be directed at decreasing the *initial* C fibre afferent barrage. The theme of pre-emptive analgesia has evolved from this theory. This will be discussed in detail later.

MEASUREMENT OF PAIN

It is necessary to consider this subject because the clinician must be aware of the methods of pain measurement in order to monitor his or her own practice of pain control, and to interpret clinical trials concerning pain assessment and pain control. Various methods of assessing pain have been designed in an attempt to qualify and quantify the experience of pain.

Objective measurement of physiological indices

These are usually related to measurement of autonomic variables such as pulse rate, skin conductance and skin temperature, or the measurement of biochemical indices such as plasma catecholamine concentrations. Although these variables may be related to pain, they are also strongly influenced by surgical stresses such as haemorrhage, hypovolaemia, hypoxaemia and acute temperature changes. Thus, although these variables can be used in non-surgical volunteers, they are not the ideal way of quantifying pain in postoperative patients. One method that has been used successfully after surgery is the measurement of respiratory function, such as forced expiratory volume in 1 s (FEV_1) and vital capacity, in patients undergoing upper abdominal or thoracic surgery.

Observer assessment of pain

This is performed by trained psychologists who note the frequency of certain behaviours such as grimacing, guarding movements and sighing. The frequency of such behaviour may be used to quantify pain.

Self-assessment of pain

These methods allow the subject to score his or her own experience of pain and permits quantitative and qualitative evaluation.

Pain category rating

The subject is asked to classify the experience of pain according to defined categories, e.g. none, mild, moderate or severe. The problem with this method is that it is difficult to specify the size of each category and whether the categories are of equal spacing.

Visual analogue scales

These usually take the form of a 10 cm line representing a spectrum of pain from no pain to worst pain imaginable. The patient marks the line at a point which represents the intensity of pain which he or she has experienced. The distance along the line can be measured. This ascribes a numerical value to the pain, which can then be used for audit or analysis.

The McGill Pain Questionnaire (MPQ)

This scales pain in three dimensions: sensory, affective and evaluative. The patient selects relevant words to characterize the pain from 20 sets of descriptive terms. Each set contains up to six words in ascending order of the dimension described by the set. The words in each set have been ascribed rank, and therefore scores can be assigned to each dimension of pain. In addition, characteristic patterns of response have been recognized to different pain syndromes such as childbirth and low back pain. The MPQ has been evaluated extensively and is often used in research studies on pain.[29]

Bias and errors may occur when pain is evaluated. For example, observer bias may occur if the observer is familiar with the patient's medical history and diagnosis, or has had prior interaction with the patient before assessment. The patient's assessment of his or her own pain may be influenced by factors such as the presence of relatives, or the cause of the pain, e.g. cancer pain as opposed to benign causes of pain. In addition, the patient may misinterpret, or simply not understand, the method of pain assessment.[30]

In everyday clinical practice, the most commonly used appraisal methods are the visual analogue scores and verbal rating scales. These relatively simple and reasonably effective methods can be applied in clinical audit of pain control methods.

Pre-emptive analgesia

The term pre-emptive analgesia implies that if analgesia is given before a painful stimulus, subsequent pain is reduced, and less analgesia is required.[31] The concept has arisen from increased knowledge of nociceptive transmission from the peripheral nociceptors to the dorsal column in the spinal cord. It is known that repeated firing in the C fibre afferents sensitizes the dorsal horn neurones (wind-up). Wind-up results in a lowering of the threshold for firing nerve action potentials. As a consequence, innocuous inputs may generate pain (allodynia), and increased pain may be felt to suprathreshold stimuli (hyperalgesia). The area in which pain is experienced is widened.

The spinal cord hyperexcitability far outlasts the duration of the initial stimulus. It has been postulated that if the initial afferent barrage could be reduced or prevented, then wind-up could be diminished, thus reducing the quantity of analgesia required subsequently.[32]

Before considering the evidence for and against pre-emptive analgesia, it is important to consider whether wind-up following surgery can be demonstrated in humans. This has been established in only one study to date.[33] Using skin electrodes, the investigation stimulated the sural nerve in surgical patients and volunteers. Pain threshold, nociceptive flexion reflex threshold and response to suprathreshold stimulation were compared pre-operatively and 48 h postoperatively in 15 patients who underwent gynaecological laparotomy. Control measurements were also made at 48-h intervals in non-surgical volunteers. The study showed increased sensitivity to noxious sural nerve stimulation in the postoperative recordings compared with pre-operative measurements. No such differences were seen in the two recordings made in the non-surgical control group.

The first evidence that pre-emptive analgesia may influence postoperative clinical outcome came from a paper from Denmark by Beach et al in 1988.[34] This prospective study of 25 patients compared the occurrence of postoperative phantom limb pain in two different groups of patients. Patients in the first group received epidural lumbar blockade with bupivacaine ± morphine for 72 h pre-operatively to abolish ischaemic pain. Those in the second group were treated with conventional intramuscular analgesia. Both groups received an intra-operative extradural block.

Patients were followed up at 7 days, 6 months and 1 year. At 7 days, 3 patients in the epidural group and 9 in the control group had phantom limb pain ($P < 0.10$). After 6 months, all patients in the epidural group were pain-free, while 5 patients in the control group still had phantom limb pin ($P < 0.05$). After 1 year, the patients treated with epidural block were still pain-free, but 3 control patients had phantom limb pain. The paper concluded that pre-operative lumbar epidural block could reduce the incidence of phantom limb pain for up to 1 year after amputation.

This report stimulated much interest in pre-operative manipulation of postoperative pain states. However, only phantom limb symptoms were studied, and no measurements of pain scores were made. More importantly, there was no evidence that the pre-emptive effect which had been demonstrated could be extrapolated to the majority of surgical patients, who are not in pain pre-operatively.

Further suggestions of prophylactic measures contributing to postoperative analgesia came from a prospective study of 729 orthopaedic patients.[35] Here, the effect of opioid premedication with or without local anaesthetic nerve blocks was studied in respect of the time to first analgesic (TFA) request postoperatively. The median TFA was 2 h in patients who received general anaesthesia alone during surgery, 5 h when opioid premedication was given, 8 h following local anaesthetic nerve block and 9 h if both local anaesthetic nerve block and opioid premedication were used. Again, pain scores were not measured and the study examined only analgesic requirements in the first 24 h.

Since these initial studies, further investigations have provided evidence that pre-operative manipulations may have an effect on postoperative pain and analgesic requirements.[36–38] These trials have included:

- the effects of pre-operative local anaesthetic infiltration
- the effects of pre-operative regional anaesthesia
- the effect of pre-emptive intravenous or intramuscular opioids
- the effect of pre-emptive epidural opioids in addition to general anaesthesia
- the effect of pre-emptive analgesia with NSAIDs.

Studies using pre-operative local anaesthetic wound infiltration have been partly supportive of a pre-emptive effect.[37–39] One study compared pre-operative and postoperative local anaesthetic infiltration for inguinal herniorrhaphy, and showed that the TFA request was prolonged in the pre-emptive group;[39] however, this effect was apparent only in the first 6 h postoperatively. A more prolonged effect has been described,[37] it was demonstrated that infiltration of local anaesthetic before surgical incision for hernia repair performed under general anaesthesia made a significant difference to the pain experienced when a constant measured pressure was applied to the wound for up to 10 days postoperatively. Another study[38] showed that pre-operative infiltration of the tonsillar bed with 0.25% bupivacaine with adrenaline (1 : 200 000) reduced the pain of tonsillectomy for up to 10 days. However, in these two studies, the effects of similar nerve blocks before and after incision were not compared.

In a study by Dierking et al,[40] identical inguinal field blocks were performed either 15 min before or immediately after surgery in patients undergoing herniorrhaphy; no significant differences in visual analogue scale pain scores were noted at rest, during mobilization or during coughing. However, all patient received alfentanil (10 $\mu g.kg^{-1}$) intravenously at induction. It has been shown recently that intravenous opioids at induction can produce a pre-emptive effect,[41] and this may have obscured any potential differences produced by the pre-emptive nerve block.

Studies comparing pre- and postoperative epidural regional block with either bupivacaine alone,[42] or bupivacaine and morphine,[43] have not demonstrated a pre-emptive analgesic effect when visual analogue scores and postoperative morphine requirements were measured. However, in both studies, opioids were given either as premedication or at induction.

A study of 30 thoracotomy patients demonstrated a pre-emptive effect of epidural opioids.[44] Patients were allocated randomly to one of two groups. In group 1 (pre-emptive group), epidural fentanyl 4 $\mu g.kg^{-1}$ in 20 ml saline was given before thoracotomy, and 20 ml saline alone was given 15 min after incision. In group 2 (control group), saline was given before incision and fentanyl 15 min after incision. No other analgesics were given intra-operatively. Postoperative pain was assessed by visual analogue scales and the amount of morphine administered by PCA. Visual analogue scores were significantly lower 6 h after surgery in the pre-emptive group; in addition, PCA morphine consumption was significantly less 12–24 h after surgery. During this time period, visual analogue scores were not significantly different between groups, which may have been due to the increased PCA morphine administration in the control group. Unfortunately, the pain scores beyond 48 h were not reported.

A recent double-blind, randomized trial compared the effects of morphine 10 mg given parenterally at three different stages of surgery in 60 patients who underwent total abdominal hysterectomy.[41] Morphine 10 mg was given either by intramuscular injection 1 h before surgery as premedication, by intravenous injection at induction of anaesthesia or by intravenous injection at closure of the peritoneum. Significantly less morphine was administered by PCA in the first 24 h after operation in patients who received morphine at induction of anaesthesia than in those to whom the drug was given during closure of the peritoneum (38 mg versus 48.4 mg; $P < 0.05$). This is the first study to show that a small dose of morphine has a greater effect if given intravenously at induction compared with the same dose administered at the end of the operation.

Trials studying the pre-emptive use of NSAIDs *alone* have not demonstrated a convincing effect.[45] Perhaps this is because prostaglandins are only one of many agents which sensitize peripheral nociceptors (see above). In addition, central dorsal horn sensitization would not be blocked by NSAIDs.

The value of pre-emptive analgesia continues to be debated. It has been argued that hard reproducible evidence for pre-emptive analgesia is still lacking.[36] There may be several explanations for this.

The timing and duration of the pre-emptive action may be crucial. For example, adequate time for nerve blocks to take full effect may be necessary before the first incision is made. In addition, the duration of action of the pre-emptive analgesic treatment should be sufficient to suppress the afferent barrage associated with surgery. For major surgery, this may last for several hours, and analgesia may need to extend well into the postoperative period to show long-term measurable effects.[46]

The study design should be such that specific interventions (be it opioid, local anaesthetic, NSAID, or combinations of these) should be compared with identical treatments made either before or after incision, and a placebo group must be included (Fig. 26.4). Most trials to date have only shown benefits of treatments given before surgery compared with no treatment at all. This does not prove a pre-emptive action, since it is not known whether the same treatment given after incision would have the same effect. The type of trial design required to demonstrate a pre-emptive effect[31] is outlined in Figure 26.4.

The methods of measuring outcome have varied in different trials, making comparisons difficult. For example, the TFA has been used to establish pre-emptive analgesic actions. However, TFA may be influenced by residual effects of the pre-emptive intervention (e.g. time for a nerve block to wear off) rather than an effect on central hypersensitivity. It has been suggested that the total postoperative analgesic requirement would be a better outcome measure.[31]

The majority of studies examined the analgesic effect only in the first 24–48 h after operation. It would be interesting to establish whether pre-emptive analgesia can produce a prolonged benefit, and whether this could influence surgical outcome (e.g. reduced pain might lead to earlier mobilization, resulting in a reduction in the morbidity associated with immobility).

Since wind-up in the dorsal horn is influenced by several neuromodulatory factors, it may be that combination pre-emptive therapeutic measures may show enhanced actions.

In conclusion, although there is a strong theoretical and physiological basis for using pre-emptive analgesic techniques in our present-day anaesthetic practice, results of adequate well-designed clinical trials are still awaited.

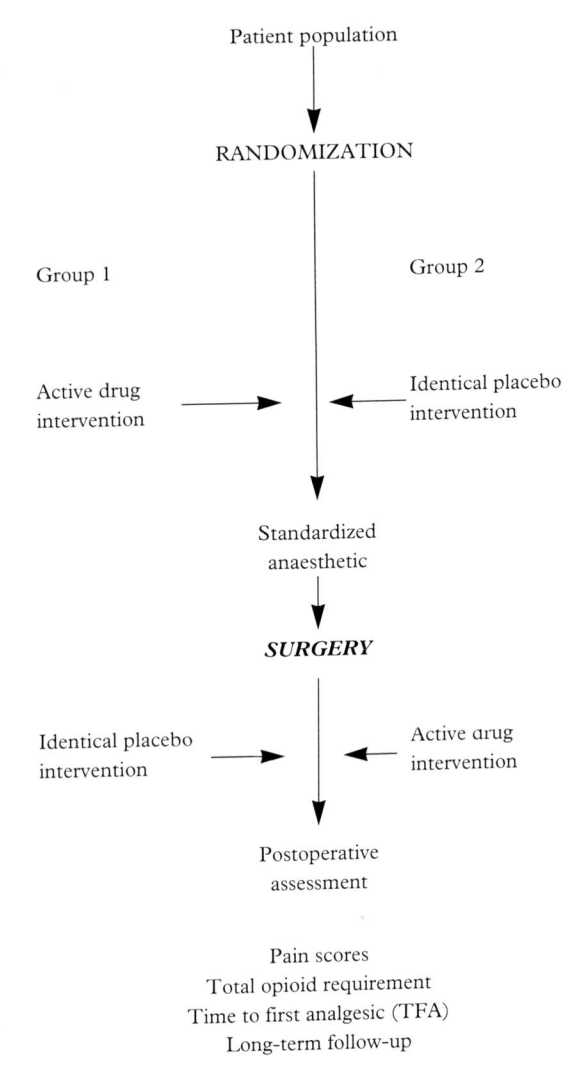

Fig. 26.4 Trial design to demonstrate pre-emptive analgesic effect.

METHODS OF POSTOPERATIVE PAIN RELIEF

The practice of good postoperative pain relief begins pre-operatively. Ideally, it should begin even before the patient's admission, with discussion of the planned procedure and options for postoperative pain relief in the outpatient department. The value of a pre-operative visit by the attending anaesthetist was documented by Egbert and colleagues.[47,48] Compared with patients who were not visited by the anaesthetist, informed subjects were released from hospital 2.7 days earlier than controls, had lower opioid use in the 5 days after operation and were judged by an independent anaesthetist to be in less pain. The anaesthetist's pre-operative visit also reduces anxiety,[49] which in turn is associated with lower pain scores.

Patients should be informed of the procedural details of the planned operation. Discussion of postoperative pain and other aspects of postoperative management should be included in the pre-operative visit. The transitory nature of the pain, together with a realistic estimation of the severity of pain to be expected, should be explained. Treatment options, such as epidural opioids or PCA, can be discussed at this time. A detailed pain history (Table 26.2) helps the anaesthetist to advise the patient on optimum methods of analgesia. The patient may need reassurance about the safety of potent analgesics in respect of addiction, and counselling with regard to the benefits of not being in pain.

Conventional management of acute postoperative pain

For the majority of surgical patients, conventional postoperative opioid therapy has traditionally involved intermittent pro re nata (PRN) intramuscular injections. A few patients managed in the intensive care unit or in a high-dependency area have received intravenous bolus doses or opioid infusions. In 1990, the Royal College of Surgeons of England and the College of Anaesthetists published a report on pain after surgery.[4] It was noted that the incidence of 'insufficient analgesia' and 'moderate to severe pain' in postoperative patients had not changed in the previous 40 years, despite increased knowledge of the physiology of pain and of the pharmacology of opioid drugs. There are a number of reasons why conventional regimens are often ineffective.

Interpatient variability

Age, gender and body weight. These have been assumed to be important variables when prescribing postoperative analgesia. The introduction of PCA has allowed these variables to be studied without observer bias. Elderly patients obtain effective analgesia for longer periods of time, and with smaller doses, when compared with young people. This has been confirmed in a study using self-administration of morphine by PCA.[50] A significant decrease in morphine consumption with increasing age was demonstrated. Studies on the effect of gender have produced conflicting results. Initial studies were limited to small numbers of patients and found no difference.[51,52] In a more recent study of 100 patients undergoing upper abdominal surgery,[50] PCA morphine consumption was significantly higher in males (71.4 versus 48.5 mg). In clinical practice, opioid dose regimens are often calculated on a body weight basis. However, no correlation between body weight and opioid requirement has been demonstrated in adults.[50]

Pharmacokinetics. Drug uptake, distribution, metabolism and excretion vary considerably among patients. Following intramuscular injection, peak plasma concentrations of pethidine or morphine may occur any time between 10 and 90 min. Plasma concentrations achieved vary by up to four times. In many situations, pharmacokinetic variables are altered; this may be as a result of ageing. For example, in the elderly, pethidine and diamorphine have an increased volume of distribution, and a reduced clearance due to a decline in renal function, resulting in a prolonged duration of action. Pharmacokinetic variables are altered in many disease states. For example, in congestive cardiac failure, absorption may be impaired by congestion of the intestine, distribution may be affected by altered tissue perfusion, and hepatic clearance and renal excretion reduced due to poor blood flow.

Pharmacodynamics. The lowest opioid concentration that will produce analgesia with minimal side-effects is known as the *minimum effective analgesic*

Table 26.2 The acute pain history

Previous experience of postoperative pain
Treatment modalities used in the past
Current pain problems
Intercurrent pain problems, e.g. chronic backache
Previous substance abuse
Attitudes to drug use
Previous and present coping responses
Expectations and beliefs concerning postoperative pain

concentration (MEAC). MEAC values can vary widely among postoperative surgical patients. As these individual variations are unpredictable, it is impossible to predict a dosage regimen for an individual patient.

The known side-effects of opioids, such as respiratory depression, suppression of cough reflex, nausea and vomiting, delayed gastric emptying, sedation, dysphoria and arterial and venous vasodilatation may all result in reduced efficacy of analgesia. These side-effects may occur irrespective of the route of administration.

Medical and nursing misconceptions

There has been a paucity of discussion of pain and its relief in medical and nursing education. Misconceptions have developed, resulting in further failures in pain provision.[53] The following are examples of common misconceptions.

1. The doctor and nurse believe that they, rather than the patient, are the authority on the patient's pain.
2. Comparable operations produce comparable pain severity in all patients, and equal doses of analgesics will produce the same degree of analgesia for every patient.
3. Postoperative pain cannot be prevented.
4. Opioid analgesics are addictive, and patients who request analgesia are becoming addicted.

Questionnaires have been used to highlight these misconceptions. In a survey of 302 nurses,[54] 24% thought that they should not give intramuscular injections for postoperative pain occurring 36 h after operation, and 72% would not give intramuscular injections after 48 h. Only 7% of nurses thought that intramuscular analgesia should be given for as long as the patient needed it, and 57% stated that they would not give prescribed analgesics if the patient was not complaining of pain; this results in poor pain relief as the optimum pain control is achieved if the analgesic is repeated before the previous dose has worn off. Amazingly, 52% of nurses thought that the patient would rather suffer the postoperative pain than the pain of the injection; this phenomenon is seen particularly in paediatrics.

Nurses may not be competent at evaluating their patient's pain. Patients may not be asked about their pain, but if they are, the nurse's perception of the pain may be different from the patient's. Frequently, the nurse's evaluation of the patient's pain is lower than the patient's evaluation.

Postoperative pain control is usually managed by the surgical houseman or resident. Apart from pharmacology lectures on opioids, the resident may have had little teaching on practical aspects of pain control. Inappropriate doses may be prescribed because of lack of clinical experience and fear of side-effects. The resident tends to seek advice from the nursing staff, and learns their misconceptions.

Logistics

Responsibility for the management of postoperative pain is delegated by the anaesthetist to the junior surgical staff, who in turn delegate the responsibility to the nursing staff.

The nursing staff may be too busy to deal immediately with analgesic requests; time is needed for checking and administration of controlled drugs. These delays, together with the delay of 15–45 min before the intra-muscular injection becomes effective, may result in the patient being in pain for an hour or more before relief occurs. This may happen every 3–4 h after major operations, resulting in the patient being in pain for a significant proportion of the day.

In order to improve provision of postoperative pain relief, dosage schedules need to be adjusted to take account of interpatient variables. This entails *individualized* treatment regimens. There is a requirement for efficacy and side-effects to be monitored frequently. Pain control should be discussed with the patient before and after surgery, with a greater emphasis on prevention rather than treatment. To a large extent, the establishment of acute pain services (see below) has addressed many of these problems.

Conventional use of opioids

Intramuscular injections

As indicated above, this technique results in widely varying plasma concentrations; peaks and troughs occur which result in fluctuations in pain control. The injection is unpleasant and painful, and the patient may feel unduly dependent on the nursing staff. Despite the disadvantages, there is vast clinical experience with this form of analgesia, resulting in familiarity and safety. It requires no specialized equipment (which may fail) and is inexpensive.

Oral opioids

This route of administration is used widely in terminal care, but is employed rarely for postoperative pain because absorption is particularly unpredictable as a result of delayed gastric emptying, ileus and vomiting in the immediate postoperative period.

Subcutaneous injection

This route is also unpredictable, due to changes in tissue perfusion that may occur with hypovolaemia, dehydration, temperature control and pain itself. Boluses of opioids given into poorly perfused subcutaneous tissue will be ineffective and form a depot which may be absorbed when skin perfusion improves. When this occurs, the patient may be pain-free and the additional opioid can result in excess sedation and respiratory depression.

Intravenous infusion

This technique can provide satisfactory analgesia once steady-state plasma concentrations are achieved. This usually occurs after 3–5 half-lives of the drug. The main advantage of this technique is that the peaks and troughs of intermittent-dose regimens are avoided. Nevertheless, there are significant disadvantages. It may take several hours for steady-state plasma concentrations to be achieved, particularly when opioids with a long half-life, such as morphine, are used. Respiratory depression may develop insidiously and therefore monitoring of ventilation is essential.

Rectal opioids

Formulations are available, but this route of administration is not popular in the UK. Drug absorption is variable and the efficacy of this route has not been established.

Opioid agonist/antagonists

It is well-known that increasing the dose of a pure μ-receptor opioid agonist increases analgesia, but also results in increasing respiratory depression and sedation. For this reason, partial agonist/antagonists have been used. It is assumed that analgesia at δ- and κ-receptors with partial agonist/antagonist effects at μ-receptors will result in opioid analgesia without respiratory depression. Drugs used have included buprenorphine, meptazinol, pentazocine and nalbuphine. In general, the use of these drugs produces disappointing analgesia without many advantages. There are several reasons for this. First, due to the differing relative affinities of agonist/antagonist actions, the dose–response curves are not linear and may even be bell-shaped or U-shaped.[3] Consequently, at low doses, analgesia may occur, but at higher doses, antagonist effects predominate. These actions are unpredictable. Second, the analgesic ceiling of partial agonists is lower than that of morphine, and the pain relief attained is inadequate for major surgery. Third, although respiratory depression may be less likely, other side-effects may be troublesome. These include nausea and vomiting, hallucinations and dysphoria.

Pentazocine is thought to be an agonist at κ-receptors. Doses of 30–50 mg produce analgesia and respiratory depression comparable to the effects of morphine 10 mg. Increasing the dose does not increase the analgesic effect. Pentazocine produces increases in heart rate, pulmonary artery pressure and cardiac work and is therefore best avoided in patients with pulmonary hypertension or ischaemic heart disease. The use of pentazocine is limited by the high incidences of dysphoria and hallucinations.

Nalbuphine acts as a κ-agonist with potent μ-receptor antagonist actions. It has a low analgesic ceiling effect, and produces marked sedation at higher doses. For these reasons, it has not been recommended for treatment of severe postoperative pain.[55]

Buprenorphine is a partial μ-receptor agonist; thus, its ceiling analgesic effect is not as high as that of morphine. Its high lipid solubility makes it suitable for sublingual administration (see below). Significant respiratory depression may occur at doses used clinically. Because of its high affinity for the μ-receptor, this effect may be difficult to antagonize with naloxone. Dysphoria and hallucinations are relatively rare. When used for acute severe postoperative pain, the incidence of nausea and vomiting is not significantly greater than that associated with morphine. The clinical impression that the incidence of nausea and vomiting is a major problem with buprenorphine may be due to the fact that it is used frequently for moderate or mild pain.[3] Of the partial agonist/antagonist opioids, buprenorphine is probably the most useful.

Meptazinol has partial agonist effects at μ-receptors. It also has other obscure analgesic actions, which may be mediated through cholinergic systems. Given parenterally, meptazinol had half the potency of pethidine but the incidence of nausea and vomiting is significantly higher.[56]

Tramadol has a mechanism of action which is not entirely clear. It appears to be either a partial μ-agonist or a pure μ-agonist of low potency.[57] In addition, non-opioid mechanisms of action may contribute to its analgesic activity, since its antinociceptive effects are only partly antagonized by naloxone.[58] It requires further evaluation before its place in anaesthetic practice is defined.

In summary, the partial agonist/antagonist opioids have not gained the widespread popularity of the pure μ-receptor agonist opioids. The latter are used in preference by many anaesthetists because their side-effects are predictable, and because of the accumulated clinical experience with their use.

Novel delivery routes for opioids

In order to increase flexibility in drug use, various novel routes of administering opioids have been introduced in the last few years. This approach has been aided by recent advances in biopharmaceutical technology which have produced sophisticated delivery systems that allow drug input into the body by hitherto unorthodox routes of administration. These methods may be useful in patients in whom parenteral injections are difficult and painful, such as children, and patients with bleeding disorders, inaccessible veins or muscle wasting.

Transdermal fentanyl

The transdermal therapeutic system of fentanyl delivery is a transparent patch containing four layers[59] (Fig. 26.5). The outer layer is an impermeable polyester film. Underneath this is the drug reservoir, containing fentanyl (250 μg.cm^{-2}) and ethyl alcohol, to enhance absorption, in a gel.

The third layer contains a microporous rate-controlling membrane. The fourth layer is a silicone skin adhesive containing a bolus of fentanyl to allow absorption as soon as the patch is applied.

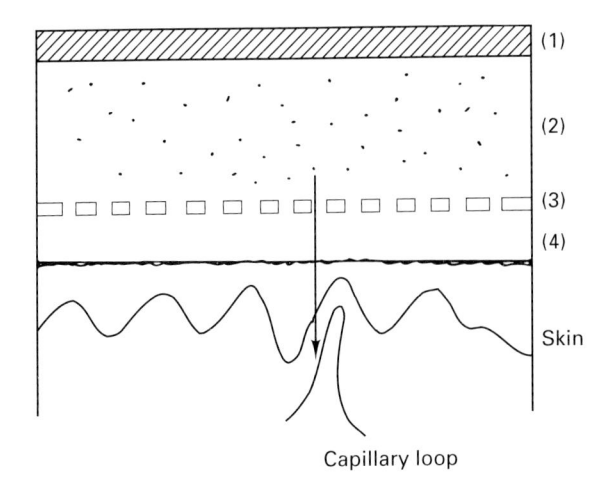

Fig. 26.5 The transdermal fentanyl patch. Layer 1: impermeable polyester film; Layer 2: drug reservoir (fentanyl and alcohol in a gel film); Layer 3: microporous rate-controlling membrane; Layer 4: adhesive, containing a 'bolus' of fentanyl.

Pharmacokinetic studies show that the transdermal fentanyl patch can produce a stable plasma concentration of fentanyl over a 24-h period.[60] However, initial absorption is slow, and steady-state levels occur only after 12–14 h. When the patch is removed, plasma concentrations decline slowly over the next 36 h. This is due to continuing absorption from a depot of fentanyl in the stratum corneum. Transdermal fentanyl patches have been studied in surgical patients after upper abdominal surgery.[61] In this study, it was shown that the application of a transdermal fentanyl patch reduced PCA morphine consumption and improved pain scores.

When used for postoperative pain, supplementary analgesics are often needed in the first 12 h, reflecting the lag phase in achieving therapeutic plasma levels. In the USA, transdermal patches have not been approved for use in acute postoperative pain because plasma concentrations rise and fall too slowly to meet rapidly changing states of postoperative pain.

Iontophoresis

This technique enhances transdermal drug delivery by introducing ions of soluble salts along an electrical current. Its use with morphine has been described in patients undergoing total hip or total knee replacement.[62] The advantage compared with passive transdermal fentanyl is that the dose of drug delivered can be adjusted by altering the current. In addition, drug delivery stops when the current is switched off. At present, it seems unlikely that this method of opioid delivery will become popular as the safety of iontophoresis for periods greater than 6 h is unknown.

Transmucosal drug administration

Nitrates have been given via the sublingual mucosa for the treatment of angina for over a century. Transmucosal administration has a number of advantages in comparison to conventional routes.

1. The high vascularity of mucosa aids rapid absorption into the systemic circulation.
2. This route avoids first-pass hepatic metabolism.
3. It is simple, painless and non-invasive.
4. The oral/nasal mucosa is more permeable than skin and so a greater number of drugs can be given by this route.

Buccal and sublingual morphine. No special formulation exists, but standard formulations have been used. Studies concerning bio-availability have demonstrated highly variable absorption which may be due to disparate chemical properties of different formulations.[63] Due to its low lipid solubility, bitter taste and the lack of an optimized formulation, morphine seems to be a poor choice for transmucosal opioid administration.

Sublingual buprenorphine. Buprenorphine is lipophilic and highly potent, making it suitable for transmucosal administration. It is absorbed rapidly from mucosal membranes and has been used successfully for postoperative pain relief. Any drug which is accidentally swallowed is metabolized by first-pass liver metabolism. The analgesic effect of sublingual buprenorphine lasts for 8–10 h, and produces postoperative analgesia which is as effective as a comparable dose of intra-muscular morphine.[63]

Intranasal buprenorphine. Pharmacokinetic studies show that absorption via this route is fast; maximum plasma concentrations occur after approximately 30 min and bio-availability is comparable to that of sublingual buprenorphine.[64] However, there are no reports of clinical experience in patients with postoperative pain.

Oral transmucosal fentanyl. This new formulation, oral transmucosal fentanyl citrate, consists of a sweetened lozenge on a stick containing fentanyl 100–800 µg. When sucked, the fentanyl dissolves in saliva and is absorbed through the oral mucosa. If sedation becomes excessive, the patient stops sucking the lozenge. A rapid onset of action, which occurs in 20 min,[65] makes this preparation suitable for acute pain relief. It has also been shown to be an effective premedicant in children.[66]

Intranasal fentanyl. Commercially available fentanyl (50 µg.ml^{-1}) has been used in a nasal spray delivering 4.5 µg per puff.[67] Using 6 puffs (27 µg), onset of analgesia occurred within 10 min, and was nearly as effective as the same dose given intravenously. Further clinical evaluation is necessary to study the effect of fentanyl administration on the nasal mucosa.

Intranasal sufentanil. Sufentanil has high potency and lipid solubility, making administration by this route possible. No special formulation exists, but the parenteral solution given as drops has been studied.[68] Rapid absorption suggests a place in acute pain management, but its use in this area is not well-documented at present.

All of these delivery systems may be used in patients when intramuscular opioids are undesirable. At the present time, it remains to be determined whether the use of these systems (with the exception of sublingual buprenorphine) will be accepted in routine practice. However, because of the perceived failure of traditional postoperative analgesic regimens, three techniques have rapidly increased in popularity within recent years: PCA infusion, epidural or subarachnoid opioids and the use of NSAIDs as adjuncts to opioid therapy. In addition, the establishment of acute pain services has increased education and awareness in the provision of postoperative pain, and provides the means for auditing changes in clinical practice.

Patient-controlled analgesia

As noted above, many of the failures of postoperative analgesia result from the lack of individualized treatment regimens. In addition, medical and nursing protocols fail to prescribe and administer the analgesia the patient needs. These problems can largely be overcome by the use of PCA pumps to deliver intravenous, subcutaneous or epidural opioids.

The concept of PCA has existed since the late 1960s. The first description relied on a nurse administering a bolus of 1 mg of morphine when the patient pressed a request button.[69] Following this, a patient-controlled spring-loaded clamp was described, which controlled the rate of infusion of 500 ml of 5% glucose containing pethidine 300 mg.[70] With advances in electronics, computerized pumps were developed; the first commercially available device was the Cardiff Palliator. Microchip technology has now brought about the development of sophisticated, compact programmable PCAs.

The great advantage of the PCA concept is that it allows patients to titrate their own dose of analgesia, within the limits programmed into the machine, for the amount of pain they feel. This method is the only truly personalized and adaptable regimen for providing pain control. In addition, because PCA eliminates observer bias and nursing bias in analgesic administration, the technique is widely used as a research tool. Methods of analgesia can be compared, and the PCA used to allow the patient to 'top up' analgesia as required. This provides a measure of the effectiveness of the analgesic method under investigation.

Practicalities

The PCA pump allows the delivery of a bolus of opioid, at the push of a button. A further bolus is allowed only after a preset lock-out period. Most pumps can also be programmed to deliver a background infusion of opioid. A maximum dose within a prescribed time period is also set. These variables can all be adjusted individually for each patient.

Using morphine, Owen et al compared bolus doses of 0.5, 1 and 2 mg.[71] They found that the optimal bolus dose of morphine was 1 mg, in that this dose provided the greatest degree of patient satisfaction with least side-effects. A lock-out period of between 5 and 10 min is commonly used, and should allow time for the patient to perceive the analgesic effect of the previous dose before another is allowed. The use of a background infusion provides a constant level of analgesia, which the patient can supplement. However, experimental evidence is lacking to support the suggestion that background infusions improve analgesia,[72] and there is evidence that the risk of oversedation and respiratory depression is increased.

PCA can be used to deliver opioids subcutaneously. Good to excellent analgesia was achieved in up to 93% of subjects using subcutaneous PCA after major orthopaedic and major gynaecological surgery.[73] Patient-controlled epidural analgesia has also been used in the management of postoperative pain; effective pain control was achieved using morphine or pethidine.[74]

Safety aspects and complications

With the increasing use of PCA as a method of postoperative analgesia, a number of complications associated with the technique have become apparent. It has been stated that these problems should not limit the use of PCA,[75] provided that those involved in the care of postoperative patients are aware of the problems, and how to detect and resolve them. The Joint College report on postoperative pain[4] recommends that when PCA is used, the nursing staff should regularly monitor effectiveness of analgesia, ventilation and degree of sedation, and that continuous in-service training is required so that staff may detect rare causes of equipment malfunction.

The complication of paramount concern is that of hypoxaemia related to opioid-induced ventilatory depression. This may occur with the administration of opioids by any route. When PCA was compared to intramuscular and epidural opioid administration, episodes of hypoxaemia (defined as $Sa_{O_2} < 94\%$ for more than 6 min.h^{-1}) occurred with the same frequency in the intramuscular and PCA groups.[76] In this study, epidural opioid administration produced hypoxaemia in more patients, and for longer periods of time.

Problems associated with PCA can result in either failure of analgesia or opioid overdose. The sources of difficulty can be grouped in four categories — the patient, nursing staff, medical staff and the pump and infusion line.

The patient. The patient needs adequate pre- and postoperative instruction on how to use the pump. Children, the disabled and the elderly may be unable to operate the button. Inappropriate administration by concerned nurses or relatives may result in overdose and only the patient should press the button. Deliberate self-administration of excess opioid has been described in more than one habitual drug user.[77]

Nursing staff. Nursing errors may occur during preparation and dilution of opioid PCA infusions. In one case report, a patient received bolus doses of pethidine 100 mg instead of the intended 10 mg.[78] Care must be taken when syringes are replaced, to avoid giving the patient an accidental bolus of opioid. This has been reported with the potent respiratory depressant sufentanil; a patient received an inadvertent bolus dose of 50 μg and severe respiratory depression occurred.[78]

Medical staff. Medical staff must prescribe the correct drug and the correct dilution. They must also programme the PCA pump correctly to deliver the desired bolus with an appropriate lock-out period.

The pump and infusion line. The intravenous cannula may become displaced ('tissued'), resulting in failure of analgesia. If the cannula blocks, the opioid may reflux up 'piggy-backed' intravenous lines; when the cannula is flushed or resited and the intravenous infusion recommenced, a large bolus of opioid may be given unknowingly. This complication can be prevented by using an antireflux valve or by using a dedicated cannula for PCA. An overdose arose in one patient when a cracked glass cartridge containing morphine 150 mg was inserted into a PCA pump;[79] because the machine was situated higher than the patient, the contents of the syringe emptied into the patient under the effect of gravity. Pump malfunction has occurred on more than one occasion. In the cases described, the pump delivered the entire syringe (containing diamorphine 60 mg) in 1 h;[80] these incidents were attributed to electrical interference from power surges or static electricity corrupting the computer programme.

With the expansion of acute pain services (see below), PCA is becoming a useful addition to the analgesic techniques available to anaesthetists. Pain scores may not be lower than with other analgesic methods, but patient satisfaction is high because the patient feels in control, and is able to adjust the administration of drug to achieve an optimum balance between analgesia and side-effects.

Spinal opioids

In this section the term spinal opioids is used to refer to opioids given into either the epidural or subarachnoid space.

Opioid receptors are found in high concentrations in the substantia gelatinosa of the dorsal root of the spinal cord. The use of spinal opioids in humans was first reported in 1979,[81] following demonstrations of a potent analgesic action of extradural opioids in rats. Several advantages of this route of administration were to be predicted:[82]

- segmental analgesia with no sensory or motor block
- no autonomic block, and therefore stable haemodynamics
- avoidance of central opioid-induced respiratory depression
- accidental intravenous injection would not have the serious side-effects associated with intravenous injection of local anaesthetics and
- a specific antagonist, naloxone, exists which could be used in the event of unwanted sequelae.

Subsequent clinical experience has shown that segmental analgesia is possible with relatively low doses of opioid. More importantly, however, clinical experience has shown that the analgesic actions *cannot* be divorced from central respiratory depression; this is due to cephalad spread of opioid in the cerebrospinal fluid (CSF).

Pharmacodynamics of spinal opioids

Spinal opioids produce effective analgesia at much smaller doses than systemically administered opioids. Evidence confirms that the analgesic action of spinal opioids is not related to plasma concentration,[83,84] indicating a direct action at spinal level. The segmental spinal action of morphine has been confirmed in volunteers.[85] It was demonstrated that morphine 3 mg given into the lumbar extradural space produced an increase in pain threshold in the legs but not the forehead. Intramuscular morphine increased the pain thresholds in both areas.

The mechanism of action of spinal opioids is mediated via the opioid receptors at both pre- and postsynaptic sites in the C fibre afferent input into the substantia gelatinosa.[20] Occupation of these receptors by opioids results in inhibition of nociceptive impulses from the C fibre afferents to the relay neurones. Inhibition of relay neurones also damps down wind-up and hypersensitivity occurring in the dorsal column.

Dose–response curves for epidural morphine have been produced.[86] When doses of 0.5, 1, 2, 4 and 8 mg were compared in patients undergoing orthopaedic lower-limb surgery, it was found that doses of 2 mg and greater were equally effective and had comparable durations of action. Generally, as the dose of spinal opioid increases, there is an increase in the incidence of side-effects.

Dose-finding studies have also used epidural PCA to study morphine use in patients after abdominal surgery.[83] When the patient was able to titrate dose according to need, it was found that morphine consumption averaged 12 mg daily. In clinical practice, when intermittent boluses of epidural morphine are used, doses of 2–4 mg 6–8-hourly usually provide satisfactory analgesia.

Intrathecal opioids also provide effective analgesic action, but smaller doses are required. A dose–response study of intrathecal morphine and diamorphine showed an optimal dose of 1.25 mg for both drugs.[87] Increasing the dose above this conferred no additional benefit. Early studies used high doses of morphine (up to 20 mg intrathecally). These doses produced analgesia for up to 48 h.[88] More recently, a study has shown that an intrathecal dose of morphine 0.8 mg given before abdominal aortic surgery produced satisfactory analgesia for up to 24 h.[89]

Virtually all of the available opioids have been used spinally in the management of postoperative pain. They all produce effective analgesia and the differences in rate of onset and duration of action appear to be related to pharmacokinetic properties.

Pharmacokinetics of spinal opioids

To exert their action, opioids given via the epidural or intrathecal route must diffuse into the neural tissue in the dorsal horn, where they interact with the opioid receptors. The area of analgesia established depends on the number of spinal segments affected. This in turn depends on the spread of solution and the region in which the injection is made.

Epidural opioids. When opioids are injected into the epidural space, there are three areas into which the opioid can diffuse:

1. the epidural fatty tissue
2. into the epidural veins and from there into the systemic circulation
3. across the dural membrane into the CSF, whence diffusion into the neural tissue of the spinal cord occurs.

The rate of diffusion into these compartments is dependent on the relative lipid and water solubilities of the opioid used. Epidural morphine is absorbed rapidly into the epidural veins. Peak plasma concentration occurs 15 min after injection of morphine into the epidural space.[90] The amount of morphine crossing the dura into the CSF from the epidural space is relatively small and the bio-availability has been calculated to be only 2%.[91] Due to the hydrophilic nature of morphine, it remains in the CSF, where it slowly migrates cephalad with the flow of CSF. If it reaches the respiratory centre in the midbrain, delayed respiratory depression may occur. This can happen up to 24 h after the original injection. As a result of slow diffusion into the CSF and ultimately neural tissue, onset of analgesia is slow, taking up to 60 min to develop. Initial analgesia may result from systemic absorption from the epidural veins. Once established, the spinal analgesic effect may last for up to 48 h.[84] In addition, because morphine remains in the CSF, it spreads widely. This can be beneficial in thoracic surgery, because lumbar epidural injection provides analgesia in the thoracic dermatomes, although it may take 2 h to establish effective analgesia in that area.[91] The volume in which morphine is injected into the epidural space has not been found to influence CSF concentration.

In comparison with morphine, diamorphine is 200 times more lipid-soluble. As expected, it has a more rapid onset and a shorter duration of action. When injected into the epidural space, rapid uptake into the epidural veins occurs. As with morphine, only a small fraction (<2%) crosses the dura.[92] Due to its lipophilicity, redistribution of diamorphine from the CSF is more rapid and there is less danger of delayed respiratory depression as a result of cephalad spread in the CSF.

Intrathecal opioids. Opioids may be injected directly into the CSF; from this compartment, the opioid may remain in the CSF or diffuse into neural tissue to react with opioid receptors, or back through the dura into the epidural space, where systemic absorption may occur. As the bio-availability of epidural morphine is only 2%, it can be appreciated that very small doses are effective when injected into the subarachnoid space.

Choice of intrathecal or epidural route of administration

The choice of drug and technique depends on the patient and the nature of surgery undertaken. Although morphine is far from the ideal drug, it has been used extensively and a great deal of clinical experience exists with its use.

One advantage of the epidural route is that an indwelling epidural catheter can be inserted, allowing epidural opioid administration to be continued throughout the postoperative period. Intermittent bolus injections are appropriate when long-acting drugs such as morphine are used, but continuous infusion or PCA is more effective with shorter-acting drugs such as fentanyl. Although intrathecal catheters are available in the UK, they have not gained the widespread acceptance of epidural catheters. Intrathecal catheters have been withdrawn from use in the USA because of reports of cauda equina syndrome associated with their use.

It has been suggested that opioids and local anaesthetics have synergistic actions.[93] This principle may be applied to epidural or subarachnoid use of opioids. The use of a combination of opioid and local anaesthetic administered spinally, together with systemic NSAIDs, has been shown to reduce pain scores to zero.[93]

Side-effects and complications

As the use of epidural and subarachnoid opioids has gained popularity, the frequency of side-effects and complications has become clear. (The complications of subarachnoid or epidural injection are discussed elsewhere.) The most serious and potentially life-threatening complication is respiratory depression.

Respiratory depression. Originally, it was hoped that the use of spinal opioids would divorce opioid analgesic action from respiratory depression; this is clearly not so. After intrathecal injection of opioid, respiratory depression can occur at any time between 4 and 24 h.[94] With extradural opioids, a biphasic pattern of respiratory depression is seen.[95] Early respiratory depression occurs within 15–30 min of injection, and results from systemic absorption of opioid via the epidural veins.[96,97] Delayed respiratory depression can occur at any time between 4 and 24 h after injection, depending on the drug used. The greatest delay occurs with the use of morphine;[98] this is a result of cephalad spread of the hydrophilic opioid in the CSF.

From clinical trial results, the incidence of respiratory depression following spinal opioids has been estimated to be between 0.9 and 3.1%.[99,100] A number of factors predispose to respiratory depression:[101]

1. Extremes of age
2. The use of hydrophilic opioids, in particular morphine
3. Concurrent use of parenteral opioids or other central nervous system depressants (including droperidol and the benzodiazepines)
4. Increased intrathoracic pressure (e.g. coughing)
5. Subarachnoid administration in comparison with epidural administration
6. The use of large doses of opioid.

Since delayed respiratory depression occurs as a result of cephalad extension of opioid in the CSF, some investigators have examined the effect of the position of the patient on the incidence of this complication. It was found that, despite nursing the patient in a semirecumbent position, respiratory depression still occurred.[102] The use of hyperbaric morphine has been described,[88] but respiratory depression has been reported following its use.[103]

Minor side-effects. Unlike delayed respiratory depression, these are not life-threatening, but can be very irritating to the patient and can reduce satisfaction with this method of analgesia.

Nausea and vomiting. Reports of the incidence of this range from 12 to >50%.[99] It should be remembered that the incidence of nausea and vomiting is 30% in postoperative patients given conventional intramuscular opioids.

Pruritus. This has been reported to occur in up to 60% of patients given spinal opioids.[86] There is some evidence that the incidence is dose-dependent,[104] although this is not a universal finding. The mechanism of causation of pruritus is not known, but it does not appear to be related to histamine release, as it occurs when fentanyl, a drug which does not release histamine, is administered spinally. In addition, the distribution of itching is not the same as that of analgesia. It frequently occurs around the head, neck and trunk. Itching is particularly troublesome in parturient patients, in whom there is a high incidence of pruritus in association with the use of spinal opioids.[105]

Urinary retention. This troublesome side-effect occurs with varying incidence and has been reported in up to 90% of young males;[105] it may require bladder catheterization. The urodynamic effects of epidural morphine have been studied.[106] Relaxation of the detrusor muscle, with an increase in maximal bladder capacity, was demonstrated. As this does not occur with parenteral morphine administration, it is thought to be secondary to a direct spinal action, possibly at the sacral parasympathetic outflow.

The incidence and severity of all of the minor side-effects can be reduced by administration of intravenous naloxone. This can be given as a low-dose infusion (e.g. 2 mg over 12 h), which does not influence analgesic effects.[107]

Safety aspects

Delayed respiratory depression is a life-threatening complication of spinal opioids. The optimum methods for early detection are unresolved, but have included inductance plethysmography, apnoea alarms, end-tidal carbon dioxide measurements, transcutaneous carbon dioxide electrodes and pulse oximetry. Hourly monitoring of respiratory rate, although widely practised, is an inadequate technique, because slowing of the respiratory rate is an unreliable and late sign of impaired ventilatory function, with no correlation between slow respiratory rate and hypoxaemia.[108] Nursing the patient in an intensive care unit or high-dependency unit provides a high level of nursing input, and is highly desirable. However, the need for routine admission to such units would deprive many patients of this very effective method of analgesia in many hospitals. The setting up of acute pain teams, resulting in increased medical and nurse training, together with the 24-h availability of an acute pain anaesthetist, has permitted the use of spinal opioids on general wards.

Non-steroidal anti-inflammatory drugs

Traditionally, NSAIDs have been used for postoperative analgesia following minor surgery or when opioid analgesia is no longer required after major surgery. With the introduction of newer NSAIDs which can be given parenterally (e.g. ketorolac), these drugs are being used as the sole analgesic in more complicated surgery. In addition, recent clinical trials have shown that the use of NSAIDs in combination with spinal opioid and local anaesthetic produces superior analgesia, to the extent of reducing pain scores to zero.[93]

Classification of NSAIDs

The NSAIDs are a heterogeneous group of compounds, most of which are organic acids. They all possess varying degrees of anti-inflammatory, antipyretic and analgesic actions. They can be classified according to structure (Table 26.3).

Pharmacodynamics

NSAIDs inhibit the formation of prostaglandins from arachidonic acid (Fig. 26.6). Inhibition of prostaglandins may only partly explain the therapeutic effect of NSAIDs.[109] For example, indomethacin and some other NSAIDs inhibit phosphodiesterase.[110] The resultant increase in cyclic adenosine monophosphate levels has been shown to stabilize lysosomal membranes. Stabilization of lysosomal activity results in reduced superoxide generation.

Surgery or other trauma results in release of cellular components such as serotonin, histamine and bradykinin. These directly stimulate peripheral nociceptors, causing afferent neuronal transmission in the nociceptive pathways. In addition, damage to cell membranes

Table 26.3 Classification of non-steroidal anti-inflammatory drugs

Pyrazones
Phenylbutazone

Oxicams
Piroxicam

Carboxyl acids
Salicylates
   Acetylsalicylic acid
Propionic acids
   Ibuprofen
   Naproxen
Anthranillic acids
   Mefenamic acid
Acetic acids
   Indoleacetic acids
     Indomethacin sulindac
   Pyroleacetic acids
     Ketorolac
   Phenylacetic acids
     Diclofenac

activates the synthesis of prostaglandins from arachidonic acid. The prostaglandins PGE_2 and PGI_2 do not cause pain directly but cause hyperalgesia by increasing the sensitivity of the nociceptors.[111] NSAIDs reduce the synthesis of prostaglandins by the inhibition of cyclo-oxygenase (Fig. 26.6). A decrease in nociceptive sensitization occurs and pain reduction is achieved. NSAIDs may also have a central action on pain modulation by mechanisms which remain poorly understood.[112]

Pharmacokinetics

NSAIDs are absorbed rapidly after oral, rectal or parenteral administration. Most are highly protein-bound; they are thus prone to drug interactions by displacing other highly protein-bound drugs such as anticonvulsants, anticoagulants and the oral hypoglycaemics. The majority are metabolized in the liver and excreted renally.

The use of NSAIDs in postoperative pain

Recent editorials have highlighted the potential benefits of the use of NSAIDs in postoperative pain control.[27,112] Particular interest has been expressed in the opioid-sparing effect of NSAIDs, the potential to use NSAIDs as an alternative to opioids and the possible synergistic effects of NSAIDs and opioids used in combination.

The opioid-sparing effect of NSAIDs. Many studies have shown an opioid-sparing effect of NSAIDs.[113–116] Requirements for opioid have been reduced by between 20 and 35%.[117] This effect has been established with diclofenac, indomethacin, ketorolac, ibuprofen, piroxicam and naproxen using a variety of administration schedules including oral, rectal and parenteral routes.

Recent trials have used PCA self-administration of opioid to measure the opioid-sparing effect. For example, Owen et al compared 8-hourly rectal ibuprofen (500 mg) with placebo in 60 patients undergoing abdominal gynaecological surgery.[113] They found reduced morphine consumption in the ibuprofen group compared to the placebo group (39 versus 48.2 mg in 24 h). An earlier study[114] demonstrated that an intravenous infusion of lysine acetyl salicylate 1.8 g over 6 h provided the same level of background analgesia as morphine 10 mg in postoperative thoracotomy patients.

NSAIDs as the sole analgesic. With the advent of day-case admission for minor or intermediate surgery, analgesics without the sedative side-effect of opioids have been sought. With the introduction of parenteral NSAIDs, in particular ketorolac, these drugs have

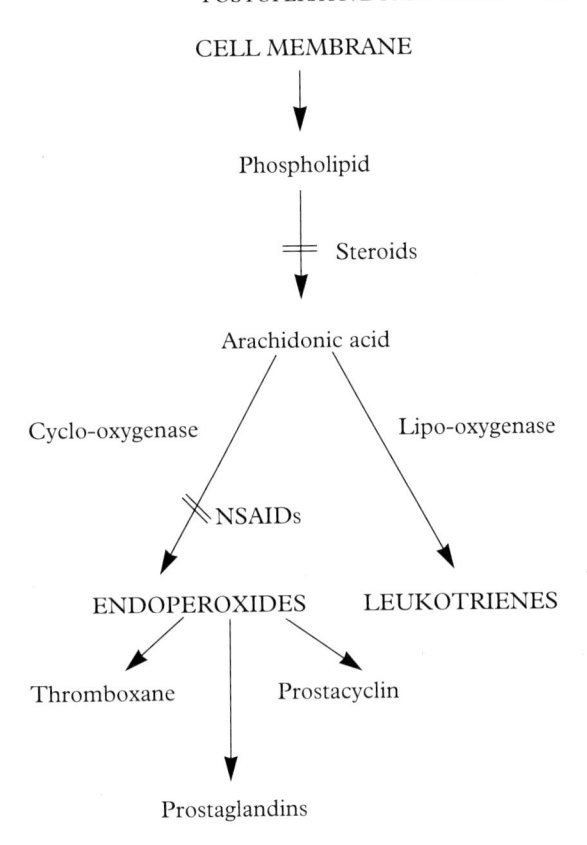

Fig. 26.6 The action of NSAIDs on the cyclo-oxygenase pathway.

been used in place of opioids for peroperative[118] and postoperative analgesia.

In a study of 149 dental patients, Brown et al demonstrated superior analgesia with ketorolac 30 or 10 mg in comparison with pethidine 100 or 50 mg.[119] In addition, the patients in the pethidine group experienced more nausea and vomiting. Previous studies had shown that the analgesic efficacy of ketorolac 30 mg was equivalent to morphine 10 mg.[120]

NSAID–opioid combinations. Because NSAIDs and opioids act via different mechanisms, it has been suggested that the combination of the two drugs results in additive or even synergistic effects.[93] This is a different concept from the opioid-sparing effects discussed above, in that the use of these combinations has been advocated to reduce postoperative pain, rather than reduce the need for opioids. Evidence exists that combinations of an optimal dose of NSAID together with opioid produce an additive analgesic effect greater than that obtained by doubling the dose of each constituent administered alone (synergy).[121,122]

Although the NSAIDs have been promoted on account of opioid-sparing effects and enhanced analgesia when combined with opioids, they are not without side-effects.

Side-effects

These can be categorized into the unpredictable, idiosyncratic reactions such as blood dyscrasias, dermatological, pulmonary and hepatic reactions, and the predictable side-effects related to inhibition of prostaglandins.

Predictable side-effects.

Renal function. In many patients, a proportion of renal blood flow (RBF) is prostaglandin-dependent. This is particularly true in major trauma patients, patients undergoing major surgery, patients with congestive cardiac failure and in the elderly.[123] The use of NSAIDs reduces this portion of RBF. The renal action of NSAIDs is reversible. In a recent editorial,[27] it was emphasized that an estimate of the risk : benefit ratio must be made. The use of NSAIDs in major surgery is not universally accepted[124] because of the risk of acute renal failure. In the elderly, a transient decrease in renal function may be acceptable because a reduction in the opioid requirement by 30% may be achieved.

Gastro-intestinal effects. Upper gastro-intestinal damage is not an infrequent side-effect of chronic use of NSAIDs. The frequency of upper gastro-intestinal damage and bleeding following the acute use of NSAIDs in surgical patients is unknown. The gastropathy occurs because of a reduction in the cytoprotective action of gastric prostaglandins.[125] There is also a decrease in mucosal blood flow and mucus production. The anti-inflammatory action of NSAIDs may also reduce repair of damaged mucosa. As the gastropathy is due to the reduction in prostaglandins, rather than a local irritant effect, it may occur in association with parenteral and rectal administration of NSAIDs.

Platelet adhesion. Due to irreversible inhibition of thromboxane A_2 in platelets, platelet adhesion is reduced by NSAIDs. This is of prime concern in surgical patients and in patients in whom epidural techniques are considered. As a result of the lack of an in vitro test for platelet adhesion, coupled with the fact that it is notoriously difficult to measure operative blood loss accurately, it has been difficult to prove conclusively that pre-operative NSAIDs result in significant blood loss. Most studies have involved only small numbers of patients. Although some studies have demonstrated increased peri-operative blood loss in patients undergoing hysterectomy[126] or abdominal surgery,[127] other studies have shown no increase after hip replacement[128] and transurethral prostatectomy.[129] The reduced platelet adhesion caused by NSAIDs has to be considered if epidural or subarachnoid techniques are contemplated during or after surgery. Once again, the potential risks (especially epidural haematoma) and potential benefits must be considered on an individual basis.[130]

Although the predictable side-effects are well-known because NSAIDs have been used extensively in many types of pain, their clinical significance in relation to the short-term use of the drugs in surgical patients is largely unresolved. The newer drugs and parenteral formulations tend to be employed more commonly than the older agents in the treatment of postoperative pain.

It is pertinent to note that, as a result of 'yellow card' adverse reaction reporting on ketorolac, reduced dosage schedules have been advised[131] following 923 reports (from 16 million prescriptions worldwide) of serious reactions, 97 of which had a fatal outcome. The distribution of reactions is shown in Table 26.4.

Caution has been advocated with the early use of NSAIDs,[124,131] particularly in patients with pre-existing risk factors for developing acute renal failure. These risk factors include pre-existing renal disease, old age, renal or coronary vascular disease, hypertension, congestive cardiac failure (CCF) and diabetes.

Acute pain services

Techniques and drugs are now available to provide satisfactory postoperative pain relief in the majority of

Table 26.4 Adverse reactions reported in association with the use of ketorolac[131]

Reaction	Total no.	Fatal outcome
Gastro-intestinal bleed/ perforation	203	47
Renal impairment	124	20
Haematological	181	4
Hypersensitivity/anaphylaxis	102	7
Neurological	111	
Miscellaneous unexplained	98	19

patients. There is a growing realization within the specialty of anaesthesia that pain relief and/or prevention of pain is a vital part of peri-operative care. Indeed, it is increasingly being suggested that improvements in the quality of postoperative analgesia may lead to a demonstrable improvement in outcome in specific groups of patients, for example those undergoing abdominal aortic surgery.[132] Whereas the choice of anaesthetic agent does not influence outcome,[133–135] the choice of analgesic technique used may do so. If this is demonstrated conclusively, then further review of the provision of postoperative pain, and of the ethical and medico-legal issues involved, will be necessary.

The reasons why conventional analgesic regimens fail to provide adequate postoperative analgesia have been discussed in detail. To a large extent, many of these problems can be overcome by the establishment of an acute pain service along the lines suggested by Bonica, at the annual meeting of the American Society of Regional Anesthesia in 1980.[136] The establishment of an acute pain service formalizes lines of responsibility and accountability for patients treated with PCA and spinal opioids within the hospital. Ready and colleagues at the University of Washington, Seattle, established an acute pain service upon which many others have been based.[137] In the first 36 months, 3500 patients were cared for, with a high measure of success. Patients who had previously undergone surgery and received conventional postoperative analgesia often commented on the superiority of the new service.

The principal aims of an acute pain service[4] are:

- responsibility for the day-to-day management of acute postoperative pain
- responsibility for the organization of services such that the level of care and monitoring is appropriate for each patient and the analgesic technique being employed
- provision of in-service training and education of medical and nursing staff, including recognition and management of complications and hazards associated with specific forms of treatment
- audit of outcome and evaluation of new techniques and equipment
- clinical research into relief of acute pain.

The potential benefits derived from the establishment of an acute pain service are summarized in Table 26.5.

Establishing an acute pain service

There are three essential ingredients for the establishment of an effective pain service: staff, equipment and support services. It is most important that these three components are introduced at the same time. It serves no useful purpose to appoint acute pain specialists without providing adequate resources to purchase equipment or provide adequate staffing.

Acute pain services in the UK have been set up using existing anaesthetic staff.[138] For example, in York District Hospital, the pain service used the existing obstetric anaesthetic service. The only additional member of staff employed was an acute pain sister. A comprehensive acute pain service requires full-time medical and nursing cover, with adequate secretarial and logistical support, and would be considerably more expensive.

Ideally, the service should be established within a department of anaesthesia. This is because of anaesthetists' familiarity with the drugs, equipment and regional techniques employed, together with their expertise in non-invasive respiratory monitoring and the problems of airway management. A senior member of staff should be appointed to head the service and initial discussions should be instigated with the departments of surgery, pharmacy and nursing administration. The importance of a team approach cannot be stressed enough. While many clinicians abhor the modern 'management by committee' approach to

Table 26.5 Potential benefits of an acute pain service

Economic
Reduced hospital stay → increased bed turnover
Reduced complication rate
Cost of treatment reduced

Medical
Reduced complication rate improves outcome

Humanitarian
Relief of pain and suffering
Enhanced patient satisfaction

Professional
Improved standing of anaesthesia as a specialty within the hospital
Improved patient understanding of the role and importance of anaesthesia

medicine, the introduction of new services and new technologies on to the wards cannot be accomplished effectively without a multidisciplinary approach. The issues that have to be addressed are:

- techniques to be employed
- establishment of agreed protocols
- staffing
- funding: initial capital outlay and ongoing costs
- lines of responsibility
- on-call cover
- drug dispensing and storage (ward-based PCA/epidurals)
- respective roles of nursing and medical staff
- proposed methods of audit

Resistance to the introduction of an acute pain service may be encountered from various groups. For example, other departments may object to the funding requirements, and there may be resistance from nursing and surgical departments. Although one study demonstrated an average reduction of 4.3 days spent in hospital when PCA was used for acute postoperative pain,[139] arguing a case for an acute pain service solely on financial grounds is not likely to succeed. There are medical reasons to justify an acute pain service, including a potential reduction in postoperative complications associated with pain and immobility, and the potential to reduce long-term pain syndromes. However, the *major* argument remains a humanitarian one — the relief of suffering. In addition, there is no doubt that, in the future, part of a hospital's reputation will depend on the quality of the postoperative pain relief provided. As patients become more aware of this fact, and begin to indicate a preference, individually or through their general practitioners, provision of pain services will have greater importance. A department of anaesthesia requesting funding for an acute pain service should emphasize these points, especially when hospitals are competing for contracts from purchasers.

With thorough initial consultation, surgical resistance to the new service should be minimal. However, many surgeons regard ongoing management of pain after the initial postoperative period as part of their post-operative management. In addition, in countries such as the USA and Australia, that role is embodied in the fee schedule. It is important that the acute pain service is seen as complementing and assisting in their patients' postoperative pain management, rather than taking patients away from surgical management.

There may also be some resistance from anaesthetic colleagues due to the need for set protocols for dosage regimens and observations. Some practitioners may need to change their practice.

Guidelines for clinical practice and protocols should be established and agreed, prior to the widespread introduction of new analgesic techniques. An initial start date should be set, and the introduction of new methods of pain relief should be targeted to selected wards. These wards should be selected well before the start-up date, and the staff should receive intensive in-service education by the senior nurse on the acute pain service. Problems occurring in the initial pilot pain service should be monitored closely, and addressed before the service is introduced to other wards. By avoiding over-stretching of resources and exhibiting a high profile on a few wards, the value of the acute pain service soon becomes clear to patients, nursing staff and medical staff. The introduction of the service to other wards then becomes easier and desirable, as it is preceded by word-of-mouth comment. In the authors' opinion, the most crucial member of staff in this early stage is the senior nurse on the pain team, who will be liaising with the ward staff on a day-to-day basis and dealing with problems as they arise.

A thorough educational programme for nursing staff, surgical staff, pharmacists, administrators and anaesthetic staff must be implemented before the service is started. This programme is continued after the service has been established, in order to upgrade existing staff and to teach new members of staff. There should be regular quality assurance review and audit. Joint meetings should be held with surgical, anaesthetic and nursing staff.

Pain relief in children

The inadequacies of conventional methods of pain relief in adults apply also to neonates and children. In one study, only 25% of children were pain-free on the first postoperative day.[140] The problem is compounded in neonates and children for many reasons.

1. Pain may be difficult to quantify and assess in children under 5 years of age.
2. It may be difficult to differentiate between pain and anxiety.
3. The response to pain may vary with the child's age and development.
4. It was erroneously hypothesized that neonates did not feel pain due to poorly developed nociceptive pathways. However, more recent studies on crying patterns[141] have not confirmed this.

Neonates pose specific problems in pain management.

Pain relief in neonates

Neonates, especially preterm babies, are more sensitive than adults to the effects of opioids, and particularly the depressant effects. This is due to altered pharmacokinetics, immature metabolizing and excretory capacity and increased permeability of the blood–brain barrier. The management of pain relief in neonates varies according to the surgery performed and whether respiratory support is instituted postoperatively.

In neonates who require mechanical ventilation, the risk of opioid-induced respiratory depression is negated, and an intravenous infusion of opioid may be used. However, the risk of cumulation due to reduced clearance and prolonged half-life must be remembered when it is time to wean the baby from the ventilator. Morphine is used[142] in doses of 10 $\mu g.kg^{-1}.h^{-1}$ In neonates, the elimination half-life of morphine is 6–7 h,[143] compared with 2–3 h in adults. Cumulation may result in high plasma concentrations which may be associated with side-effects such as fitting. In neonates, fentanyl has a much shorter half-life (223 min), and there is less risk of cumulation. Infusions of fentanyl of 2–4 $\mu g.kg^{-1}$ per have been used for sedation and analgesia.[142] This infusion rate is associated with systemic and pulmonary circulatory stability; this is particularly desirable in neonates with pulmonary hypertension.

In neonates breathing spontaneously, morphine and equivalent opioids are not recommended unless the patient is nursed in an intensive care unit.[144] Thus, other methods must be considered. The weaker opioid codeine (1 $mg.kg^{-1}$) is an effective analgesic in neonates. A single dose may be all that is required, and the risk of respiratory depression is small unless further doses are given.[142] Paracetamol is also a valuable mild analgesic at doses of 10 $mg.kg^{-1}$ and can be given orally or rectally.

Regional analgesia and nerve blocks may be used in neonates, and are particularly useful in minor and intermediate surgery. It must be remembered that neonates are at greater risk of local anaesthetic toxicity. This is due to prolonged elimination half-lives (two to three times) resulting from immature microsomal enzyme systems. There are also reduced plasma concentrations of albumin and α_1-acid glycoprotein, resulting in increased free fraction of local anaesthetic. These differences persist until the age of 6 months.[145] The concentration of local anaesthetic required to block nerve conduction is reduced, due to incomplete myelination.[146] The recommended maximum doses for plain bupivacaine (2 $mg.kg^{-1}$) and plain lignocaine (5 $mg.kg^{-1}$) should not be exceeded. Prilocaine should be avoided in neonates, as low levels of methaemoglobin reductase increase the risk of methaemoglobinaemia.

Pain relief in infants and children

Analgesic regimens must be designed to produce efficient analgesia with minimal additional distress and anxiety to the child. Opioids are used commonly in this group. Continuous infusions are popular in paediatric practice and may be given intravenously or subcutaneously. For example, intravenous morphine at a rate of 10–30 $\mu g.kg^{-1}.h^{-1}$ provides satisfactory analgesia with minimal respiratory depression. The same dose may be given subcutaneously. The subcutaneous cannula should be inserted before the child wakes up, and at a central site, to avoid the problems of delayed absorption occurring with peripheral shutdown.

The use of PCA has been described in children as young as 6 years of age.[147] Demand boluses of morphine are set at 10–20 $\mu g.kg^{-1}$ with a lock-out of 5–10 min. A background infusion (5–10 $\mu g.kg^{-1}.h^{-1}$) may be useful in children aged 5–10 years as they may not be able to operate the demand button every time.[148] A longer lock-out time of 10–20 min is required if a background infusion is also employed.

In order to achieve steady-state plasma concentration rapidly, a loading dose of morphine 50–100 $\mu g.kg^{-1}$ is required before intravenous, subcutaneous or PCA morphine infusions.

If intermittent intramuscular injections are used, codeine (1 $mg.kg^{-1}$) or pethidine (1–2 $mg.kg^{-1}$) are appropriate drugs. NSAIDs are particularly useful in minor surgery such as ear, nose and throat and dental extractions. Aspirin should be avoided in children under 12 years, because of the association with Reye's syndrome in this age group.

Local anaesthetic techniques provide very effective analgesia in children, particularly in day-case surgery where the nausea, vomiting and sedation caused by opioids may delay discharge. Epidural analgesia is

Table 26.6 Dose of local anaesthetic given caudally for analgesia

Level of block	Operation	Dose of bupivacaine
L5–S5	Circumcision Hypospadias	0.5 $ml.kg^{-1}$
T9–S5	Herniotomy Orchidopexy	1 $ml.kg^{-1}$

Note: 0.25% bupivacaine is used to a *maximum* volume of 20 ml. Any further volume required after this is achieved by dilution with normal saline.

conveniently applied via the caudal route. This is particularly useful for perineal surgery and hernia repairs. Formulae have been devised to calculate the dose of local anaesthetic required for the desired height of block. The scheme outlined by Armitage is useful[149] (Table 26.6).

The caudal route is not recommended for epidural blocks higher than T9–10, as toxic doses of local anaesthetic are needed. In these situations (such as thoracic surgery), a lumbar epidural may be used. A 19-gauge Tuohy needle with a 23-gauge catheter is commercially available, and has been used in children weighing less than 10 kg.[142]

Peripheral nerve blocks are also useful. The axillary sheath may be cannulated with a 22-gauge cannula to produce peroperative and postoperative brachial plexus block. Finally, simple wound infiltration at the end of surgery provides effective analgesia. This may be the only analgesia that is required after pyloromyotomy. Up to 0.5 ml.kg^{-1} of bupivacaine 0.25% is used.

REFERENCES

1. Leibeskind JC, Melzack R. The international pain foundation: meeting a need for education in pain management. Pain 1987; 30: 1–2
2. Black AMS, Alexander JI. Analgesia for postoperative pain. Rec Adv Anaesth Analg 1991; 17: 119–135
3. Mitchell RWD, Smith G. The control of acute postoperative pain. Br J Anaesth 1989; 63: 147–158
4. The Royal College of Surgeons of England and The College of Anaesthetists. Commission on the provision of surgical services. Report of the working party on pain after surgery. Royal College of Surgeons. London September 1990
5. Burns JW, Hodsman NBA, McLintock TTC, Gillies GWA, Kenny GNC, McArdle CS. The influence of patient characteristics on the requirements for postoperative analgesia. Anaesthesia 1989; 44: 2–6
6. Woolf CJ. Recent advances in the pathophysiology of acute pain. Br J Anaesth 1989; 63: 139–146
7. Merskey H. (ed) Classification of chronic pain: descriptions of chronic pain syndromes and definitions of pain terms. Pain 1986; (suppl 3): S1–S225
8. Raja SN, Meyer RA, Campbell JN. Peripheral mechanisms of somatic pain Anesthesiology 1988; 68: 571–590
9. Marsh SJ, Stansfeld CE, Brown DA, Davey R, McCarthy D. The mechanism of action of capsaicin on sensory c-type neurons and their axons in vitro. Neuroscience 1987; 23: 275–289
10. Davies SN. Dorsal horn of the rat. Brain Res 1987; 27: 402–406
11. Dickenson AH, Sullivan AF. Evidence for the role of the NMDA receptor in the frequency dependent potentiation of deep rat dorsal horn nociceptive neurons following c-fibre stimulation. Neuropharmacology 1987; 26: 1235–1238
12. Woolf CJ, Thompson SWN. The induction and maintenance of central sensitisation is dependant on N-methyl-D-aspartate acid receptor activation; implications for treatment of post-injury pain hypersensitivity states. Pain 1991; 44: 293–299
13. Sher GD, Cartmell SM, Gelgor L, Mitchell D. Role of N-methyl-D-aspartate and opiate receptors in nociception during and after ischaemia in rats. Pain 1992; 49: 241–248
14. Hunt SP, Pini A, Evan G. Induction of C-*fos* like protein in spinal cord neurones following sensory stimulation. Nature 1987; 328: 632–634
15. Pert CB, Snyder SH. Opiate receptor, its demonstration in nervous tissue. Science 1973; 179: 1011–1014
16. Martin WR. History and development of mixed opioid agonists, partial agonists and antagonists. Br J Clin Pharmacol 1979; 7: 2735–2795
17. Pleuvry BJ. Opioid receptors and their ligands: natural and unnatural. Br J Anaesth 1991; 66: 370–380
18. Pleuvry BJ. Opioid receptors and their relevance to anaesthesia. Br J Anaesth 1993; 71: 119–126
19. Stein C, Millan MJ, Shipenberg TS, Peter K, Herz A. Peripheral opioid receptors mediating antinociception in inflammation: evidence for involvement of mu, delta and kappa receptors. J Pharmacol Exp Ther 1989; 248: 1269–1275
20. Dickenson AH. Mechanisms of the analgesic actions of opiates and opioids. Br Med Bull 1991; 47: 690–702
21. Pertovaara A, Kaupplia T, Jyvasjarvi E, Kalso E. Involvement of supraspinal and spinal segmental alpha-2-adrenergic mechanisms in medetomidine induced antinociception. Neuroscience 1991; 44: 705–714
22. Hayashi Y, Maze M. Alpha$_2$ adrenoceptor agonists and anaesthesia. Br J Anaesth 1993; 71: 108–118
23. Bonnet F, Boico O, Rostaing S, Loriferne JF, Saada M. Clonidine induced analgesia in postoperative patients: epidural versus intramuscular administration. Anesthesiology 1990; 72: 423–427
24. Sivilotti L, Nistri A. GABA receptor mechanisms in the central nervous system. Prog Neurobiol 1991; 36: 35–92
25. Krogsgaard-Larsen P, Nielsen L, Madsen U, Nielsen EO. GABA and glutamic acid agonists of pharmacological interest. In: Iversen LL, Goodman E, eds. Fast and slow chemical signalling in the nervous system. Oxford: Oxford Scientific Publications. 1986
26. McQuay HJ, Dickenson AH. Implications of nervous system plasticity for pain management. Anaesthesia 1990; 45: 101–102
27. Murphy DF. NSAIDs and postoperative pain. Br Med J 1993; 306: 1493–1494
28. Schulze S, Roikjaer O, Hasselstrom L, Jensen NH, Kehlet H. Epidural bupivacaine and morphine plus systemic indomethacin eliminates pain, but not systemic response and convalescence after cholecystectomy. Surgery 1988; 103: 321–327
29. Chapman CR, Casey KL, Dubner R, Foley KM, Gracely RH, Reading AE. Pain measurement: an overview. Pain 1985; 22: 1–31
30. Chapman CR. Assessment of pain. In: Nimmo WS,

Smith G, eds Anaesthesia, 2nd edn. London: Blackwell Scientific, 1994; pp 1539–1556
31 McQuay HJ. Pre-emptive analgesia. Br J Anaesth 1992; 69: 1–3
32 Wall PD. The prevention of postoperative pain. Pain 1988; 33: 289–290
33 Dahl JB, Erichsen CJ, Fulgsang-Frederiksen A, Kehlet H. Pain sensation and nociceptive reflex-excitability in surgical patients and human volunteers. Br J Anaesth 1992; 69: 117–121
34 Bach S, Noreng MF, Tjellden NU. Phantom limb pain in amputees during the first 12 months following limb amputation, after preoperative lumbar epidural blockade. Pain 1988; 33; 297–301
35 McQuay HJ, Carroll D, Moore RA. Postoperative orthopaedic pain — the effect of opiate premedication and local anaesthetic blocks. Pain 1988; 33: 291–295
36 Kehlet H, Dahl JB. The value of pre-emptive analgesia in the treatment of postoperative pain. Br J Anaesth 1993; 70: 434–439
37 Tverskoy M, Cozacov C, Ayache M, Bradley EL, Kissin I. Postoperative pain after inguinal herniorrhaphy with different types of anesthesia. Anesth Analg 1990; 70: 29–35
38 Jebeles JA, Reilly JS, Gutierrez JF, Bradley EB, Kissin I. The effect of pre-incisional infiltration of tonsils with bupivacaine on the pain following tonsillectomy under general anaesthesia. Pain 1991; 47: 305–308
39 Ejlerson E, Anderson HB, Eliasen K, Mogensen T. A comparison between preincisional and postincisional lidocaine infiltration and postoperative pain. Anesth Analg 1992; 74: 495–498
40 Dierking GW, Dahl JB, Kanstrup J, Dahl A, Kehlet H. Effect of pre- versus postoperative inguinal field block on postoperative pain after herniorrhaphy. Br J Anaesth 1992; 68: 344–348
41 Richmond CE, Bromley LM, Woolf CJ. Preoperative morphine pre-empts postoperative pain. Lancet 1993; 342: 73–75
42 Pryle BJ, Vanner RJ, Enriquez N, Reynolds F. Can pre-emptive lumbar epidural block reduce postoperative pain following lower abdominal surgery? Anaesthesia 1993; 48: 120–123
43 Dahl JB, Hansel BL, Hjortso NC, Erichsen CJ, Moniche S, Kehlet H. Influence of timing on the effect of continuous extradural analgesia with bupivacaine and morphine after major abdominal surgery. Br J Anaesth 1992; 69: 4–8
44 Katz J, Kavanagh BP, Sandler AN et al. Pre-emptive analgesia: clinical evidence of neuroplasticity contributing to postoperative pain. Anesthesiology 1992; 77: 439–446
45 Murphy DF, Medley C. Preoperative indomethacin for pain relief after thoracotomy: comparison with postoperative indomethacin. Br J Anaesth 1993; 70: 298–300
46 Katz J. Preoperative analgesia for postoperative pain. Lancet 1993; 342: 65–66
47 Egbert LD, Battit GE, Turndorf H, Becker HK. The value of the preoperative visit by an anesthetist: study of doctor–patient rapport. JAMA 1963; 185: 553–555
48 Egbert LD, Battit GE, Welch CE, Bartlett MK. Reduction of postoperative pain by encouragement and instruction of patients. N Engl J Med 1964; 270: 825–827
49 Leigh JM, Walker J, Janaganathan P. Effect of preoperative visit on anxiety. Br Med J 1977; 2: 987–989
50 Burns JW, Hodsman NBA, McLintock TTC, Gillies GWA, Kenny GNC, McArdle CS. The influence of patient characteristics on the requirements for postoperative analgesia: a reassessment using PCA. Anaesthesia 1989; 44: 2–6
51 Dahlstrom B, Tamsen A, Paalzow L, Hartvig P. Patient-controlled analgesic therapy part IV; pharmacokinetics and analgesic plasma concentrations of morphine. Clin Pharmacokinet 1982; 7: 266–279
52 Tamsen A, Hartvig P, Fagerhund C, Dahlstrom B. Patient-controlled analgesic therapy part II; individual analgesic demand and analgesic plasma concentrations of pethidine in postoperative pain. Clin Pharmacokinet 1982; 7: 164–175
53 Cohen FL. Post-surgical pain relief: patient's status and nurses medication choices. Pain 1980; 9: 265–274
54 Cartwright PD. Pain control after surgery: a survey of current practice. Ann R Coll Surg Engl 1985; 67: 13–16
55 Fee JPH, Brady MB, Furness G, Moore J, Dundee JW. Has nalbuphine a place in severe pain? Anesth Analg 1987; 66: S54
56 Slattery PJ, Harmer M, Rosen M, Vickers MD. Comparison of meptazinol and pethidine given IV on demand in the management of postoperative pain. Br J Anaesth 1981; 53: 927–931
57 Bourdle TA. Partial agonist and agonist–antagonist opioids: basic pharmacology and clinical applications. Anesth Pharmacol Rev 1993; 2: 135–151
58 Raffa RB, Friderichs E, Reimann W, Shank RP, Codd EE, Vaught JL. Opioid and non-opioid components independently contribute to the mechanism of action of tramadol, an 'atypical' opioid analgesic. J Pharmacol Exp Ther 1992, 260: 275–285
59 Streisand JB, Stanley TH. Opioids: new techniques in routes of administration. Curr Opin Anaesthesiol 1989; 2: 614–618
60 Duthie DJR, Rowbotham DJ, Wyld R, Henderson PD, Nimmo WS. Plasma fentanyl concentration during transdermal delivery of fentanyl to surgical patients. Br J Anaesth 1988; 60: 614–618
61 Rowbotham DJ, Wyld R, Peacock JE, Duthie DJR, Nimmo WS. Transdermal fentanyl for the relief of pain after upper abdominal surgery. Br J Anaesth 1989; 63: 56–59
62 Ashburn MA, Stephen RL, Ackeman E et al. Iontophoretic delivery of morphine for postoperative analgesia. J Pain Symptom Manage 1992; 7: 27–33
63 Striesand JB, Stanley TH. New delivery systems for analgesia. Anaesth Pharmacol Rev 1993; 1: 199–209
64 Eriksen J, Jensen NH, Kamp-Jensen M. The systemic availability of buprenorphine administered by nasal spray. J Pharm Pharmacol 1989; 41: 803–805
65 Striesand JB, Varvel JR, Stanski DR et al. Absorption and bioavailability of oral transmucosal fentanyl citrate. Anesthesiology 1991; 75: 223–229
66 Ashburn MA, Striesand JB, Tarver SD et al. Oral transmucosal fentanyl citrate for premedication in paediatric outpatients. Can J Anaesth 1990; 37: 857–866
67 Striebel HW, Koenigs D, Kramer J. Postoperative pain management by intranasal demand-adapted fentanyl titration. Anesthesiology 1992; 77: 281–285
68 Helmers JH, Noorduin H, Van-Peer A, Van Leeuwen

68 L, Zuurmond WW. Comparison of intravenous and intranasal sufentanil absorption and sedation. Can J Anaesth 1989; 36: 494–497
69 Sechzer PH. Objective measurement of pain. Anesthesiology 1968; 29: 209–210
70 Scott J. Obstetric analgesia: a consideration of labour pain and a patient-controlled technique for its relief with meperidine. Am J Obstet Gynecol 1970; 106: 959–978
71 Owen H, Plummer JL, Armstrong I, Mather LE, Cousins MJ. Variables of patient-controlled analgesia 1. Bolus size. Anaesthesia 1989; 44: 7–10
72 Owen H, Szekely SM, Plummer JL, Cushnie JM, Mather LE. Variables of patient-controlled analgesia 2. Concurrent infusion. Anaesthesia 1989; 44: 11–13
73 White PF. Subcutaneous PCA: an alternative to IV-PCA for postoperative pain management. Clin J Pain 1990; 6: 297–300
74 Sjostrom S, Hartvig D, Tamsen A. Patient-controlled analgesia with extradural morphine or pethidine. Br J Anaesth 1988; 60: 358–366
75 Rowbotham DJ. The development and safe use of PCA. Br J Anaesth 1992; 68: 331–332
76 Wheatley RG, Somerville ID, Sapsford DJ, Jones JG. Postoperative hypoxaemia: comparison of epidural, intramuscular and patient-controlled opioid analgesia. Br J Anaesth 1990; 64: 267–275
77 Keeri-Szanto M. Drugs or drums: what relieves postoperative pain? Pain 1979; 6: 217–230
78 White PF. Mishaps with patient-controlled analgesia. Anesthesiology 1987; 66: 81–83
79 Thomas DW, Owen H. Patient-controlled analgesia — the need for caution. A case report and review of adverse incidents. Anaesthesia 1988; 43: 770–772
80 Notcutt WG, Knowles P, Kaldas R. Overdose of opioid from patient-controlled analgesic pumps. Br J Anaesth 1992; 69: 95–97
81 Behar M, Magora F, Olshwang D, Davidson D. Epidural morphine in the treatment of pain. Lancet 1979; i: 527–528
82 Morgan M. The rational use of intrathecal and extradural opioids. Br J Anaesth 1989; 63: 165–188
83 Sjostrom S, Hartvig D, Tamsen A. Patient controlled analgesia with extradural morphine or pethidine. Br J Anaesth 1988; 60: 358–366
84 Weddel SJ, Ritter RR. Serum levels following epidural administration of morphine and correlation with relief of post-surgical pain. Anesthesiology 1981; 54: 210–214
85 Torda TA, Pybus DA, Liberman H, Clark M, Crawford M. Experimental comparisons of extradural and IM morphine. Br J Anaesth 1980; 52: 939–942
86 Martin R, Salbaing J, Blaise G, Tetrault J, Tetreault L. Epidural morphine for postoperative pain relief: a dose response curve. Anesthesiology 1982; 56: 423–426
87 Paterson GMC, McQuay HJ, Bullingham RES, Moore RA. Intradural morphine and heroin: dose–response studies. Anaesthesia 1984; 39: 113–117
88 Samii K, Feret J, Harari A, Viars P. Selective spinal analgesia. Lancet 1979; i: 1142
89 Davis I. Intrathecal morphine in aortic aneurysm surgery. Anaesthesia 1987; 42: 491–497
90 Nordberg G, Hedner T, Mellstrand T, Dahlstrom B. Pharmacokinetic aspects of epidural morphine analgesia. Anesthesiology 1983; 58: 545–551
91 Nordberg G, Hedner T, Mellstrand T, Borg L. Pharmacokinetics of epidural morphine in man. Eur J Clin Pharmacol 1984; 26: 233–237
92 Watson J, Moore A, McQuay H et al. Plasma morphine concentrations and analgesic effects of lumbar extradural morphine and heroin. Anesth Analg 1984; 63: 629–634
93 Dahl JB, Rosenberg J, Dirkes WE, Mogensen T, Kehlet H. Prevention of postoperative pain by balanced analgesia. Br J Anaesth 1990; 64: 518–520
94 Gjessing J, Tomlin PJ. Postoperative pain control with intrathecal morphine. Anaesthesia 1981; 36: 268–276
95 Kafer ER, Brown JT, Scott D et al. Biphasic depression of ventilatory responses to CO_2 following epidural morphine. Anesthesiology 1983; 58: 418–427
96 Lomessy A, Magnin C, Viale JP, Motin J, Cohen R. Clinical advantages of fentanyl given epidurally for postoperative analgesia. Anesthesiology 1984; 61: 466–469
97 Scott DB, McClure J. Selective epidural analgesia. Lancet 1979; i: 1410–1411
98 Camporesi EM, Nielson CH, Bromage PR, Durant AC. Ventilatory CO_2 sensitivity after intravenous and epidural morphine in volunteers. Anesth Analg 1983; 62: 633–640
99 Stenseth R, Selvoid O, Breivik H. Extradural morphine for postoperative pain: experience with 1085 patients. Acta Anaesthesiol Scand 1985; 29: 148–156
100 Writer WD, Hurtig JB, Edelist G et al. Epidural morphine prophylaxis of postoperative pain: a report of a double-blind multicentre trial. Can Anaesth Soc J 1985; 32: 330–338
101 Cousins MJ, Mather LE. Intrathecal and epidural administration of opioids. Anesthesiology 1984; 61: 276–310
102 Nolke-Jensen F, Madsen JB, Guldager H, Christensen AA, Eriksen HO. Respiratory depression after epidural morphine in the postoperative period: influence of posture. Acta Anaesthesiol Scand 1984; 28: 600–602
103 Abouleish E. Apnoea associated with intrathecal administration of morphine in obstetrics. Br J Anaesth 1988; 60: 592–594
104 Lanz E, Kehrberger E, Theiss D. Epidural morphine: a clinical double-blind study of dosage. Anesth Analg 1985; 64: 786–791
105 Bromage PR. The price of intraspinal narcotic analgesia: basic constraints. Anesth Analg 1981; 60: 461–463
106 Rawal N, Mollefors K, Axelsson K, Lingardh G, Widman B. An experimental study of urodynamic effects of epidural morphine and of naloxone reversal. Anesth Analg 1983; 62: 641–647
107 Thind GS, Wells JCD, Wilkes RG. The effects of continuous intravenous naloxone on epidural morphine analgesia. Anaesthesia 1986; 41: 582–585
108 Catley DM, Thornton D, Jordan C, Lehane JR, Royston D, Jones JG. Pronounced episodic oxygen desaturation in the postoperative period: its association with ventilatory pattern and analgesic regime. Anesthesiology 1985; 63: 20–28
109 Simon LS, Mills JA. Non-steroidal anti-inflammatory drugs. N Engl J Med 1980; 302: 1179–1184
110 Weiss B, Hait WN. Selective cyclic nucleotide phosphodiesterase inhibitors as potential therapeutic agents. Ann Rev Pharmacol Toxicol 1977; 17: 441–447

111 Rang HP, Bevan S, Dray S. Chemical activation of nociceptive peripheral neurones. Br Med Bull 1991; 47: 534–548
112 Kenny GNC. Ketorolac trometamol — a new non-opioid analgesic. Br J Anaesth 1990; 65: 445–447
113 Owen H, Glavin RJ, Shaw NA. Ibuprofen in the management of postoperative pain. Br J Anaesth 1986; 58: 1371–1375
114 Jones RM, Cashman JM, Foster JMG, Wedley JR, Adams AP. Comparisons of infusions of morphine and lysine acetyl salicylate for the relief of pain following thoracic surgery Br J Anaesth 1985; 57: 259–263
115 Hodsman NBA, Burns J, Blyth A, Kenny GNC, McArdle CS, Rotman H. The morphine sparing effects of diclofenac sodium following abdominal sugery. Anaesthesia 1987; 42: 1005–1008
116 Dueholm S, Forrest M, Hjortso E, Levigh E. Pain relief following herniotomy: a double-blind randomised comparison between naproxen and placebo. Acta Anaesthesiol Scand 1989; 33: 391–394
117 Dahl JB, Kehlet H. Non-steroidal anti-inflammatory drugs: rationale for use in severe postoperative pain. Br J Anaesth 1991; 66: 703–712
118 Murray AW, Brockway MS, Kenny GNC. Comparison of the cardiorespiratory effects of ketorolac and alfentanil during propofol anaesthesia. Br J Anaesth 1989; 63: 601–603
119 Brown CR, Moodie JE, Evans SA, Clarke PJ, Rotherham BA, Bynum L. Efficacy of intramuscular ketorolac and meperidine in pain following major oral surgery. Clin Pharmacol Ther 1987; 43: 161
120 O'Hara DA, Fragen RJ, Kinzer M, Pemberton D. Ketorolac tromethamine as compared to morphine sulphate for treatment of postoperative pain. Clin Pharmacol Ther 1987; 41: 556–561
121 McQuay HJ, Carrol D, Watts PG, Juniper RP, Moore RA. Codeine 20 mg increases pain relief from ibuprofen 400 mg after third molar surgery: a repeat dosing comparison of ibuprofen and an ibuprofen–codeine combination. Pain 1989; 37: 7–13
122 Sushine A, Roure C, Olson N, Laska EM, Zorilla C, Rivera J. Analgesic efficacy of two ibuprofen–codeine combinations for the treatment of post-episiotomy and postoperative pain. Clin Pharmacol Ther 1987; 42: 374–380
123 Clive DM, Stoff JS. Renal syndromes associated with non-steroidal anti-inflammatory drugs. N Engl J Med 1984; 310: 563–572
124 O'Callaghan CA, Andrews PA, Ogg CS. NSAIDs in the postoperative period: many factors threaten renal function. Br Med J 1993; 307: 257
125 Roth SH, Bennet RE. Non-steroidal anti-inflammatory drug gastropathy. Arch Intern Med 1987; 147: 2093–2100
126 Engel C, Lund B, Kristensen SS, Axel C, Nielsen JB. Indomethacin as an analgesic after hysterectomy. Acta Anaesthesiol Scand 1989; 33: 498–501
127 Reasbeck PG, Rice ML, Reasbeck JC. Double-blind controlled trial of indomethacin as an adjunct to narcotic analgesia after major abdominal surgery. Lancet 1982; ii: 115–118
128 Serpell MG, Thomson MF. Comparison of piroxicam with placebo in the management of pain after total hip replacement. Br J Anaesth 1989; 63: 354–356
129 Bricker SR, Savage ME, Hanning CD. Peri-operative blood loss and non-steroidal anti-inflammatory drugs: an investigation using diclofenac in patients undergoing transurethral resection of the prostate. Eur J Anaesthesiol 1989; 4: 429–434
130 Macdonald R. Aspirin and extradural blocks. Br J Anaesth 1991; 66: 1–3
131 Committee on Safety of Medicines. Ketorolac: new restrictions on dose and duration of treatment. Curr Probl Pharmacovigilance 1993; 19: 5–6
132 Hjortso NC, Neumann P, Frosig F et al. A controlled study on the effect of epidural analgesia with local anaesthetics and morphine on morbidity after abdominal surgery. Acta Anaesthesiol Scand 1985; 29: 790–796
133 Slogoff S, Keats A. Randomised trial of primary anesthetic agents on outcome of coronary bypass operations. Anesthesiology 1989; 70: 179–188
134 Tuman KJ. McCarthy RJ, Spiess BD, DaValle M, Dabir R, Ivankovich AD. Does choice of anesthetic agent significantly affect outcome after coronary artery surgery? Anesthesiology 1989; 70: 189–198
135 Leung JM, Goehner P, O'Kelly BF, Hollenberg M, Pineda N, Casson BA. Isoflurane anesthesia and myocardial ischemia: comparative risk versus sufentanil anaesthesia in patients undergoing coronary artery bypass surgery. Anesthesiology 1991; 74: 838–847
136 Bonica JJ. Critical need for better management of acute pain. Presented to Annual Meeting of the American Society of Regional Anesthesia, San Francisco, 1980 (Unpublished.)
137 Ready LB, Oden R, Chadwick HS et al. Development of an anesthesiology-based postoperative pain management service. Anesthesiology 1988; 68: 100–106
138 Wheatley RG, Mandej TH, Jackson IJB, Hunter D. The first year's experience of an acute pain service. Br J Anaesth 1991; 67: 353–359
139 Ready LB. Economic considerations: acute and postoperative pain services. Pain Digest 1991; 1: 17–21
140 Mather L, Mackie J. The incidence of postoperative pain in children. Pain 1983; 15: 271–282
141 Porter FL, Miller RH, Marshall RE. Neonatal pain cries: effect of circumcision on acoustic features and perceived urgency. Child Dev 1986; 57: 790–802
142 Lloyd-Thomas AR. Pain management in paediatric patients. Br J Anaesth 1990; 64: 85–104
143 Lynn AM, Slattery JT. Morphine pharmacokinetics in early infancy. Anesthesiology 1987; 66: 136–139
144 Gauntlet IS. Analgesia in the neonate. Br J Hosp Med 1987; 37: 518–519
145 Mazoit JX, Denson DD, Samii K. Pharmacokinetics of bupivacaine following caudal anesthesia in infants. Anesthesiology 1988; 68: 387–391
146 Wildsmith JAW. Peripheral nerve and local anaesthetic drugs. Br J Anaesth 1986; 56: 692–700
147 Grankroger PB, Tomkins DP, VanDerWalt JH. Patient-controlled analgesia in children. Anaesth Intensive Care 1989; 17: 264–268
148 Lloyd-Thomas AR. Pain relief in children. Continuing medical education day. Association of Anaesthetists of Great Britain and Ireland. London 1992
149 Armitage EN. Caudal block in children. Anaesthesia 1979; 34: 396

27. Cardiopulmonary resuscitation

N. G. Bircher

Cardiopulmonary resuscitation (CPR) ought to comprise an important part of the skills of every health care professional. However, many of the key aspects of CPR are performed poorly by those with limited experience of airway management. Thus, the anaesthetist becomes an essential member of the resuscitation team, for without appropriate airway management, any patient experiencing cardiac arrest will surely die. For each of the interventions discussed below, optimal patient care requires a thorough knowledge of the techniques involved as well as the physiological and pharmacological context for which they are used. Cardiopulmonary resuscitation is divided into three phases, each of which has three steps, as illustrated in Table 27.1. This discussion will include both scientific and clinical principles of resuscitation. This chapter is not designed to present basic skills; these have been reviewed in greater detail elsewhere.[1]

VENTILATION

Emergency airway control

Airway control and assisted ventilation are necessary adjuncts to chest compressions in cardiac arrest since chest compressions do not provide ventilation.[2] Although arterial oxygen tension can remain adequate for up to 30 min during complete cardiac arrest, initiation of chest compression without ventilation results in severe arterial hypoxaemia within minutes.

Manual methods without equipment

In the unconscious patient, backwards tilt of the head and forwards displacement of the mandible will usually prevent hypopharyngeal obstruction by the base of the tongue.[3] Lifting of the chin also prevents hypopharyngeal obstruction and keeps the mouth open.[4-6] Head tilt produced by lifting the chin is not demonstrably different from that produced by lifting the neck.[6,7] However, in some unconscious patients, backwards tilting of the head is not by itself sufficient to open the airway and additional forwards displacement of the jaw may be necessary.[4] The combination of head tilt, forwards displacement of the jaw, and opening of the mouth is termed the *triple airway manoeuvre* or *jaw thrust manoeuvre*. Excessive opening of the mouth can compromise airway patency,[7] as can the epiglottis.[8]

Positive-pressure ventilation attempts

Airway patency is verified by positive-pressure ventilation attempts. At this time, there is no evidence to support the use of 'staircase' ventilation[9] as the initial ventilatory manoeuvre. Furthermore, even a brief period of positive end-expiratory pressure (PEEP) can severely compromise haemodynamics during CPR and high inflation pressures can inflate the stomach.[10] The initial attempts to ventilate an unintubated patient must be of adequate volume but with low inflation pressures.[11] Both inflation of the stomach and passive regurgitation may be reduced by cricoid pressure.[12] Since the chances of successful resuscitation decline rapidly with increasing arrest time,[13-18] the initiation of resuscitation should never be delayed awaiting equipment. Medical personnel who may have to perform resuscitation

Table 27.1 Phases and steps of resuscitation

Phase	Step
Basic life support	A. Airway control B. Breathing support C. Circulation support
Advanced life support	D. Drugs and fluids E. Electrocardiography F. Fibrillation treatment
Prolonged life support	G. Gauging H. Human mentation I. Intensive care

should have a complete array of equipment readily at hand.

Manual methods with equipment

Placement of an oropharyngeal or nasopharyngeal airway may facilitate lifting the tongue off the posterior wall of the pharynx, which is the most common cause of airway obstruction in the comatose or anaesthetized patient. Cuffed pharyngeal tubes[19,20] (e.g. the laryngeal mask) offer a greater likelihood of maintaining a patent airway, although no reduction in the incidence of pulmonary aspiration or improvement in outcome has been demonstrated. Aspiration of stomach contents remains a common complication of conventional ventilatory techniques used prior to tracheal intubation and is associated with a significant incidence of mortality.[21]

Oesophageal obturator airway

This device was designed for use by those not trained to perform tracheal intubation.[22] In a modified form, it allows gastric decompression but does not provide definitive airway control.[23,24] The rate of unrecognized tracheal intubation is up to 3%[25] and a wide range of other complications are associated with the use of this device.[26,27] Although no study has shown a definitive change in outcome compared with tracheal intubation, experts recommend that all hospital personnel and paramedics be trained in the latter, with oesophageal obturator airway or oesophageal gastric tube airway training optional.

Laryngeal mask airway

The laryngeal mask airway (LMA) can be used to secure the airway, at least as a temporary measure. It can be used by those not skilled in tracheal intubation or in patients in whom intubation proves to be difficult or impossible. However, there remains a risk of aspiration, and maintenance of a clear airway is not always possible.

Tracheal intubation

Tracheal intubation remains the definitive means of airway control during resuscitation and should be performed as soon as feasible in all patients for whom CPR is indicated. As indicated above, this should not delay the institution of ventilation by any *immediately* available means. There are no data concerning delay of intubation and its contribution to mortality or morbidity. Aspiration is, however, a common[21] and dangerous, if not fatal, complication. A wide variety of paramedical personnel can be trained to intubate the trachea safely and successfully[28,29] and intubation is a mandatory skill for any physician charged with the care of critically ill patients. Although the data concerning foreign-body obstruction of the airway and difficult tracheal intubation in humans are almost exclusively anecdotal, the unequivocal conclusion is that failure to establish an airway is uniformly fatal and that delay in establishing an airway adversely influences outcome.[16,30] A full spectrum of techniques and equipment should be in the armamentarium of all acute care facilities, especially intensive care units (ICUs).

Emergency ventilation and oxygenation

Ventilation patterns

Intermittent positive-pressure ventilation (IPPV) remains the principal means of artificial respiration during resuscitation. The manual methods of artificial ventilation (Holger-Nielsen, Silvester) are obsolete for the management of cardiac arrest, since they neither control the airway nor provide adequate tidal volume.[31] The use of PEEP is an essential element of the management of most critically ill patients receiving IPPV. However, although hypoxaemia is a frequent antecedent of cardiac arrest[32] and a common occurrence during CPR,[33-35] the use of PEEP during cardiopulmonary resuscitation can either augment[36] or depress cardiac output.[33] The mechanism of the latter effect is not entirely clear, but is probably related to reduction of venous return to the chest. However, pulmonary oedema, which is seen frequently during CPR,[37] may limit resuscitation. As a consequence, 100% oxygen should always be administered during the immediate phase of resuscitation but may subsequently be reduced under controlled circumstances in the ICU.

Ventilation per se may produce some circulation, but it is rarely sufficient to restart the heart once it has arrested. Simultaneous ventilation and compression, whether manually, mechanically or with a vest, have given variable results, which are discussed elsewhere.[38] Independent or asynchronous ventilation (delivered randomly with respect to chest compressions) provides oxygenation and ventilation comparable with interposed or alternating ventilation (delivered in between compressions).[39] The ratio of interposed ventilation to chest compression has little impact on oxygenation or ventilation until the interval between ventilations exceeds 15 s.[40]

Mouth-to-mouth or mouth-to-nose

The superiority of mouth-to-mouth ventilation over the wide variety of alternative manual methods[41,42] has long been recognized.[43-46] The two essential advantages of mouth-to-mouth ventilation are the ability to maintain a patent airway and delivery of positive-pressure ventilation. Exhaled air must be delivered at approximately twice the normal tidal volume in order to maintain satisfactory oxygenation and ventilation. As noted above, ventilation should never be postponed until the arrival of full resuscitation equipment. The essential clinical criterion for adequacy of ventilation is that the chest wall must rise and fall with each and every ventilation attempt. As will be discussed in some detail below, no technique or piece of equipment can be expected to provide ventilation unless used properly. If one technique fails, the problem must be rapidly corrected or another technique rapidly adopted.

Gastric insufflation may be limited by low ventilatory pressure as well as by cricoid pressure.[10–12] Although gastric distension is a real danger in children, it rarely poses a problem in adults.[44] Mouth-to-nose ventilation may be of use in the patient with trismus, arthritic fixation of the jaw, facial or oral scarring, facial fractures or extensive lacerations of the mouth, but is not uniformly successful in the hands of the minimally trained.[3]

Mouth-to-adjunct

Mouth-to-airway ventilation, using any of the airway adjuncts above as well as the S-tube (two Guedel airways connected at their proximal ends), avoids direct contact with the patient, maintains a patent airway, and thereby improves success in ventilation, especially by untrained lay people.[31,47] However, all pharyngeal tubes carry a risk of laryngospasm and the induction of vomiting in the unconscious patient. Mouth-to-mask ventilation also obviates direct patient contact, but does not improve ventilatory efficacy over mouth-to-mouth, and mask leaks may detract from success in ventilation.[48] If equipped with an oxygen nipple, masks will allow delivery of 40–54% oxygen during mouth-to-mask ventilation and 98% during intermittent occlusion of the breathing port of the mask with a 30 l.min^{-1} oxygen inflow.[49]

Bag-valve-mask with oxygen

In inexperienced hands, bag-valve-mask manual ventilation is fraught with hazard, principally due to difficulties in establishing a satisfactory seal with the mask on the face.[50–52] While mouth-to-mask ventilation may be less effective than mouth-to-mouth[53] in the inexperienced, with minimal training and the use of both hands to secure the mask and maintain head tilt, mouth-to-mask becomes clearly more effective than bag-valve-mask. The efficacy of bag-valve-mask ventilation may be improved by enlisting the assistance of a second rescuer[54] by changing masks[55] or by using an oxygen-powered manually triggered positive-pressure ventilation device.[56]

Although the mask seal is the main limitation in the hands of those with limited training, the design of the bag for ventilation is critical in all rescuers. The capability to deliver 100% oxygen during CPR is contingent upon the use of a reservoir of adequate size and flow rates sufficient to keep it filled.[57,58] Paediatric bag-valve units[59] also require higher flows than Mapleson D anaesthetic breathing systems to maintain F_{IO_2} above 90%. The only limitation on the latter is that fresh gas flow must exceed 100 ml.kg^{-1}.min^{-1} to prevent rebreathing. If a pressure-limiting (pop-off) valve is present, F_{IO_2} becomes rate-sensitive[59] and occluding this valve may be necessary to achieve adequate ventilatory pressure and F_{IO_2}. Operator skill does influence delivered tidal volume, even if mask seal is not in question,[60] thus adequate training of providers and adequate supervision of trainees are well-advised. Modern equipment still occasionally malfunctions; back-up equipment should be readily available and, if all else fails, mouth-to-mouth or mouth-to-adjunct ventilation should be initiated.

Mechanical ventilators

Early mechanical ventilators were not adequate for the management of cardiac arrest. However, currently available ventilators can, theoretically, come close to what an operator can do by hand. Unfortunately, this degree of sophistication in equipment, and virtuosity in its use, are rarely available for the treatment of cardiac arrest. However, the vast majority of experimental models of CPR employ mechanical ventilation with satisfactory results. High-pressure ventilation via the tracheal tube results in severe arterial respiratory alkalaemia during CPR in spite of carbon dioxide admixture.[61] At present, the safest approach is manual ventilation guided by frequent arterial blood gas measurement, which allow assessment of both oxygenation and ventilation. Although never studied with respect to outcome, severe hyperventilation carries the risk of exacerbating cerebral ischaemia during CPR.

High-frequency jet ventilation

High-frequency ventilation, delivered by a jet ventilator either transtracheally or via a specially configured tracheal tube to achieve a jet effect, or by a conventional ventilator, all provide adequate ventilation and oxygenation during CPR. This has been investigated for transtracheal ventilation following both ventricular fibrillation[62] and asphyxial cardiac arrest.[63] There was no difference in haemodynamics compared with conventional positive-pressure ventilation and the transtracheal route offers protection against aspiration in the unintubated animal.[64] The necessary techniques and equipment can be mastered by emergency medical technicians[65] and obviate the need to interpose ventilation between compressions. Varying frequencies in jet ventilation do not appear to change ventilation or oxygenation; increased frequency in conventional ventilation results in arterial hypocapnia but does not alter mixed venous blood gases.

EMERGENCY CIRCULATION

No variety of artificial circulation offers adequate perfusion and tissue preservation on an indefinite basis. Resuscitative efforts must therefore be focused on the rapid restoration of spontaneous circulation. This and other resuscitative measures may be facilitated by the use of algorithms or protocols.

Causes of cardiac arrest

The primary and secondary causes of cardiac arrest have been reviewed elsewhere.[66] The cause, if it can be determined, may have very important therapeutic implications[32] but should never delay institution of life-support manoeuvres. The most common electrocardiographic diagnosis associated with cardiac arrest both inside and outside hospitals is ventricular fibrillation. Ventricular fibrillation may be primary, as is common in the pre-hospital setting, or secondary, i.e. associated with non-cardiac disease or injury. Other causes of primary cardiac arrest, in ventricular fibrillation, asystole or electromechanical dissociation, include acute myocardial infarction, heart block, electrical shock to the heart, cardiac toxicity of drugs or cardiogenic shock. Common secondary causes of cardiac arrest include asphyxia and exsanguination as well as severe hypoxaemia or respiratory acidosis from pulmonary disease, metabolic acidosis from septic shock or brainstem failure with intractable systemic arterial hypotension. Sudden arrest of the circulation results in loss of consciousness within 15 s, an isoelectric electroencephalogram in 15–30 s, and agonal gasping for up to 60 s.

Recognition of cardiac arrest

The prompt and accurate diagnosis of cardiac arrest is extremely important. Delay in diagnosis prolongs arrest time, which is among the principal determinants of outcome both experimentally and clinically. Cardiac arrest is defined clinically as the absence of a palpable pulse in a large artery, i.e. the carotid, femoral or brachial artery. If the patient is truly in cardiac arrest, unconsciousness will follow rapidly. However, the patient who is profoundly hypotensive may be able to sustain consciousness.[67] If an arterial line is in place, a pulse pressure of less than 5 mmHg constitutes cardiac arrest, although the prognostic and therapeutic implications of a weakly beating heart have not been thoroughly investigated. The diagnosis of electromechanical dissociation is made imprecise because the absence of a pulse does not necessarily mean cessation of mechanical activity of the heart.[68,69] Fluctuations of intrathoracic pressure such as produced by both positive-pressure ventilation and chest compression[36] may either augment[70] or impede the function of the failing heart.

Closed-chest cardiopulmonary resuscitation

Fundamental physiology

There is now no doubt whatsoever that fluctuations of intrathoracic pressure can cause blood flow during cardiac arrest in a variety of circumstances.[36,71–74] Debate remains about the extent to which direct cardiac compression contributes to flow, and if so, when.[75] Kouwenhoven's hypothesis regarding compression of the heart[76] was challenged almost immediately,[77,78] but it was more than a decade before definitive experimental evidence was amassed.[36] A diffuse rise in intrathoracic pressure cannot, in and of itself, account for blood flow, since it cannot produce a pressure gradient for flow inside the chest. The peripheral vasculature plays a critical role in the generation of pressure gradients giving rise to forward flow during CPR. The valves of the jugular venous system attenuate but do not ablate pressure transmission to the peripheral veins of the head.[36,79–82] The inferior vena cava behaves as a Starling resistor in some[81] but not all[79] animal models. The branches of the aorta are resistant but not impervious to collapse[83,84] and resistance to collapse can be enhanced by adrenaline (epinephrine).[83,85] This allows for a peripheral arteriovenous perfusion gradient and consequent flow.

Relatively few haemodynamic data are available concerning human external CPR. Aortic pressure and cardiac output are less than those attained by direct cardiac massage[86–89] and measurements of arterial and venous pressure tend to support the thoracic pump mechanism of blood flow.[33,78,90] Duration of compression is a major determinant of flow in adult humans.[91] Rate of compression between 40 and 80 compressions per minute does not appear to influence carotid blood flow[91] in adult humans, nor does increasing the compression rate from 60 to 140 alter end-tidal carbon dioxide during CPR.[92] Experimentally, depth of compression shows a threshold of effectiveness,[93] so depth of compression should always be evaluated clinically to ensure that it is sufficient to produce a femoral or carotid pulse.

The brain during CPR

As noted above, high central venous pressures during chest compression are transmitted to peripheral veins and the sagittal sinus is no exception.[71,94] Similarly, the coupling between vena cava pressure and cerebral venous pressure in the steady state was recognized long ago, as was the coupling between intrathoracic pressure and intracranial pressure. During CPR, the large fluctuations in intrathoracic pressure are reflected in the intracranial space,[71,94,95] although intracranial compliance is not altered by cardiac arrest per se. However, in dogs with normal intracranial compliance, intracranial pressure is only modestly elevated by chest compressions,[71,94] through both direct transmission via CSF and non-valved vertebral veins.[95]

Cerebral blood flow during CPR is a critical concern, since the goal in resuscitation is to return the patient home without any neurological sequelae of resuscitation. The maintenance of cerebral perfusion pressure is essential since cerebral autoregulation cannot increase cerebral blood flow if cerebral perfusion pressure is too low and is compromised by hypoxia or by cerebral ischaemia itself. Cerebral perfusion pressure during CPR is the difference between arterial pressure and either intracranial pressure or cerebral venous pressure, whichever is the greater. Arrest time (total circulatory arrest) prior to the institution of CPR is a major determinant of the maximal cerebral blood flow generated by chest compression; maximal cerebral blood flow falls very rapidly with increasing arrest time.[96,97]

Cerebral blood flow during standard CPR can be adequate to maintain cerebral venous oxygen tension[94] above levels thought to cause irreversible damage, but is not reliable in that regard. Although the difference in outcome with complete ischaemia versus very low flow has been debated, the preponderance of evidence suggests that minimal blood flow is better than no flow at all.[98] While cerebral blood flow values as high as 90% of control (spontaneous circulation) have been reported during standard CPR, the majority of reported flows are in the range 0–33% of control. Cerebral perfusion can be improved during standard CPR by adrenaline,[99,100] is improved or unchanged by other α-adrenergic agonists[101,102] and is made worse by isoprenaline (isoproterenol)[99] and by volume loading.[103]

Alternative means of performing CPR variably improve or reduce cerebral blood flow but none has been demonstrated to improve outcome. In particular, despite very promising findings in the laboratory,[73,104,105] simultaneous ventilation–compression CPR failed to improve outcome in a randomized prospective clinical trial.[106] Cerebral blood flow is typically elevated along with intracranial pressure in the immediate post-resuscitation period, but the cerebral hyperaemia is rapidly replaced by cerebral hypoperfusion and normalization of intracranial pressure.[107]

The heart during CPR

Coronary blood flow is usually exceedingly poor during standard CPR.[99–101,108,109] The elevation of right atrial pressure produced by chest compression in humans is nearly equal to the elevation in aortic pressure.[110] Consequently, the perfusion pressure across the heart is nearly zero during chest compression. During the relaxation phase (CPR diastole), perfusion pressures are higher and predict outcome,[111] and coronary perfusion can be markedly improved by adrenaline.

The lung during CPR

Little work has been done to elucidate pulmonary function during CPR. End-tidal carbon dioxide is known to be markedly depressed due to the profound low-flow state,[94,112–114] but no studies have directly measured carbon dioxide production. Dead space is estimated to be quite high[94] and V_D/V_T to be 0.59.[112] In dogs with initially normal lungs, Pa_{O_2} can be maintained around 10.7 kPa (80 mmHg) with room air,[94] but since arterial hypoxaemia is a common finding in clinical resuscitation, 100% oxygen should always be administered when available. Shunt fraction during human CPR has not been studied, although instances in which a satisfactory arterial oxygen tension cannot be achieved with 100% oxygen are rare.

Combinations of ventilation and chest compression

The early investigations in this area established the outer limits of the ratio of compression to ventilation,[40] but did not exhaustively map out optima for this ratio. However, it is clear that chest compressions alone cannot provide ventilation;[2] positive-pressure ventilation is required, and protracted periods between ventilations result in arterial desaturation.

One-rescuer CPR

Current recommendations[9] call for a rate of 80–100 compressions per minute, a ratio of two slow ventilations (i.e. over 1–2 s to minimize peak inspiratory pressure) to every 15 compressions, a minimum tidal volume of 800 ml, and a 50% duty cycle and 4–5 cm (1.5–2.0 in) depth for compressions. This set of recommendations is specifically designed for education of the lay public, who are unlikely to enjoy the luxury of a second trained rescuer. Health care professionals are encouraged to learn both one- and two-rescuer techniques since two or more rescuers are frequently available in both pre-hospital and in-hospital settings.

Recommendations for one-rescuer CPR in infants (the first year of life) and children (age 1–8 years) are similar to those for an adult, except that for infants, the pulse is evaluated in the brachial rather than the carotid artery, the rate of chest compression is greater than 100 min^{-1}, the ratio of compressions to ventilations is 5:1, tidal volume is the minimum required to make the chest rise, and compressions are delivered with the index and middle finger in the middle of the sternum with a depth of 1.5–2.5 cm (0.5–1.0 in). Differences in children are that compressions are performed with the heel of one hand and to a depth of 2.5–3.5 cm (1.0–1.5 in).

Two-rescuer CPR

Current recommendations[9] call for the rate of compression for adult CPR to be 80–100 compressions per min, a brief pause after every fifth compression to deliver slow ventilation as above, and a ratio of five compressions to every ventilation. Since both chest compression and ventilation are physically taxing, rescuers should seek help whenever feasible and know organized means of switching roles in order to avoid interruption of artificial perfusion.[9] The energy cost to the rescuer of performing CPR has never been measured but it is a rapidly fatiguing activity. Once the trachea has been intubated, interposition of ventilation between compressions yields better oxygenation and ventilation[39,40] than ventilation at ordinary pressure simultaneous with chest compression. As discussed above, high-pressure ventilation can overcome this problem but has variable effects on cardiac output and coronary and cerebral perfusion.

Monitoring the effectiveness of CPR

Essential and desirable monitoring equipment

No special devices are required for the evaluation of the effectiveness of artificial ventilation, oxygenation and circulation. However, careful attention must be paid to inspection and palpation. Inspection determines whether or not the chest rises and falls with ventilation, whether the depth of chest compression is adequate, and whether the rescuer's hands are properly positioned. Palpation is essential to establish the clinical diagnosis of cardiac arrest, to locate landmarks and to evaluate the quality of the pulse generated by chest compressions. While simple means of assessing the quality of CPR are useful in avoiding poor performance, they are not reliable, i.e. it is possible to meet the recommended criteria and still have an extremely low cardiac output. For this reason, technological assessment should be employed wherever possible.

Ventilation

The essential clinical criterion is that the chest must rise and fall with every ventilatory effort. Auscultation of breath sounds before and after intubation of the trachea is a useful indicator of air exchange, but neither guarantees adequate ventilation during CPR nor definitively establishes tracheal intubation. Capnography confirms tracheal intubation and provides a useful assessment of cardiac output as well.[113–117] While the absence of arterial blood gas capability does not preclude successful resuscitation, direct measurement of arterial blood gases should be considered an essential item in all in-hospital resuscitation. Abnormalities of oxygenation, ventilation and metabolic acid–base status are common.[23,32,34,35,37,39,43,94,118–124] Repetitive sampling of arterial blood is an indication for arterial cannulation, and since the femoral artery is frequently punctured for this purpose during CPR, placement of an arterial line using the Seldinger technique may be a useful option. Radial artery cut-down is also reliable.[92] The chemically treatable component of acidosis, i.e. the metabolic component, is essentially the same in the arterial and venous sides of the circulation,[118] as is the lactate concentration, even though there may be a substantial difference in pH due to venous hypercapnia. Therefore, use of arterial blood gases should be encouraged, but administration of sodium bicarbonate should be limited to the correction of severe metabolic acidosis (i.e. base deficit greater than 10 $mmol.l^{-1}$). Pulse oximetry relies on delivery of oxygenated blood to tissue in a pulsatile fashion and can be used during CPR to assess adequacy of both oxygenation and circulation, but is not entirely reliable.

Circulation

The clinical assessment of the quality of circulation by palpation of the pulse serves only to ensure that the chest compressions delivered are of sufficient force[93] to generate a palpable arterial pressure wave. Because the intrathoracic perfusion pressures are small and the extrathoracic perfusion pressures difficult to predict, the presence of a pulse may or may not be indicative of flow. Flow is typically too low to allow auscultation of arterial pressure using a sphygmomanometer, although flow may be detectable using a Doppler device. An intra-arterial cannula may be a useful indicator of the adequacy of chest compressions, allows immediate recognition of the return of a pulse pressure, and allows repetitive sampling of arterial blood. Pulse oximetry may give some indication of the quality of circulation but end-tidal carbon dioxide is a much more sensitive indicator. Direct measurement of cardiac output during CPR is feasible but technically difficult due to the profound low-flow state.[86,87]

Neurological function

Neurological assessment during CPR is a very poor predictor of outcome and decisions to continue or stop resuscitative efforts should not be made on this basis. Absence of specific neurological signs during basic life support does not preclude their prompt return on restoration of spontaneous circulation.

Mechanical CPR

Mechanical devices may offer some advantages during clinical CPR. Early versions had a wide variety of problems, but currently available devices offer consistent compressions[125] and higher arterial pressures in humans.[126] However, they have not been shown to influence outcome in patients.

Complications of CPR

The complications of CPR are numerous[127-134] but unavoidable complications are acceptable compared with an otherwise certain death. However, many potentially fatal complications are avoidable. Hepatic trauma, for instance, seems to have been common early in the modern era of CPR and can lead to rapid exsanguination. The recently reported incidence is less. Gastro-oesophageal damage was also a remarkably frequent complication, and carries the risk of fatal mediastinitis or haemorrhage in spite of restoration of circulation and consciousness. Reduced gastric damage may have resulted from attention to landmark location, limiting gastric insufflation by cricoid pressure, earlier tracheal intubation or gastric decompression. Inadvertent oesophageal intubation is not uncommon and is a risk factor for gastric distension and rupture, although pneumoperitoneum does not always indicate visceral rupture. Similarly, trauma to the kidney, pancreas, colon, spleen and mesenteric vessels are rare complications in present-day CPR.

Cardiac trauma presumably falls into the unpreventable category, but this should be tempered by degree. Mild cardiac contusions are routine in the laboratory and clinically, as are small haemopericardia or pericardial effusions, but laceration or rupture of the heart or the great vessels is rare, as is papillary muscle rupture, atheromatous emboli and subclavian thrombosis. Direct mechanical trauma to the lung is ordinarily limited to the hilum but barotrauma tends to be parenchymal. Rupture of the diaphragm is fortunately rare. However, aspiration of gastric contents or blood, pneumonia and adult respiratory distress syndrome[37] are common.

Body trauma is very common and typically involves ribs and sternum, and rarely vertebrae. However, not all patients receiving chest compressions have rib fractures. Haemothoraces secondary to rib fractures can be substantial and may contribute to the relative or absolute hypovolaemia of the patient. Bone marrow emboli are common sequelae of CPR but may arise from other causes.

Infectious complications of CPR related to rescuers contracting disease from those they have attempted to resuscitate have received a great deal of attention in the lay press. While there is no sound epidemiological basis to conclude that the risk is anything other than minimal, common-sense precautions are justified during CPR because of the possibility of cross-infection.

PHARMACOLOGY

Routes for drugs and fluids

Virtually any secure peripheral intravenous route permits successful resuscitation.[135] Central venous access is not a necessity during CPR but offers the advantages of more rapid drug delivery[136,137] and higher peak concentrations, although these are not consistent findings.[138,139] Delay in restarting the heart should not be caused by lack of intravenous access. Alternatives include intratracheal,[140-145] intra-osseous,[146-148] intra-arterial and intracardiac administration. The intramuscular, sublingual and intralingual routes have no role during CPR. The intra-osseous route requires similar doses to those administered intravenously, but intratracheal doses are 2-2.5 times the intravenous dose (usually diluted in 10 ml of saline or distilled water).

Drugs

Adrenaline

With the exception of oxygen, adrenaline is the single most useful drug currently available for the treatment of cardiac arrest. There is now an enormous body of evidence supporting the use of adrenaline during CPR[33,101,131,141,149–167] and withholding this drug if CPR and defibrillation fail to restore spontaneous circulation can only rarely be justified. Optimal use of adrenaline requires that all other components of active resuscitation be conducted efficiently as both metabolic and respiratory acidosis limit the effectiveness of adrenaline, as does hypoxia. Although adrenaline does not alter the rate of successful defibrillation after brief periods of cardiac arrest, it does increase the rate of return of spontaneous circulation.[168] This effect appears to be primarily due to the increased myocardial perfusion provided during CPR (and the increase in aortic diastolic pressure caused by adrenaline), as well as the increase in myocardial contractility which accrues immediately after restarting the heart.[168] Although there is an increase in coronary perfusion pressure and thus myocardial blood flow with adrenaline (an α-adrenergic effect), the β-adrenergic effects may be deleterious. This is because β-effects can limit the degree of improvement in the ratio of subendocardial to epicardial blood flow[169] or myocardial oxygen supply to demand.[170] Alternative α-adrenergic agents that have been compared with adrenaline include noradrenaline,[171,172] phenylephrine,[100,101,163,167,173–175] metaraminol[161,162] and methoxamine.[155,161,163,166,176–179] None of these has been clearly demonstrated to offer any overall advantage in outcome compared with adrenaline. Coronary vasoconstriction remains a risk with any agent with α-adrenergic activity, as is an excessive hypertensive response after restarting the heart. The latter may influence cerebral outcome for better or for worse, or may precipitate re-arrest from coronary ischaemia. However, higher doses of adrenaline may be more efficacious than those presently used clinically.[151,180–185] In pigs, raising the dose from 0.02 to 0.2 mg.kg^{-1} improves myocardial blood flow.[149] Clearly, increasing the dose from 0.01 to 0.1 mg.kg^{-1} causes a much more dramatic increase of adrenaline concentrations compared with those available endogenously.[186] However, when 10 mg vials were made available for human resuscitation, retrospective analysis showed an increase in dose but no change in outcome.[187]

Adrenaline is the drug most commonly administered via the tracheal tube during CPR. While this route appears to be effective in some beating-heart experimental models,[188] it is generally regarded as not reliable[140,156,189] and is not the route of choice. The results during both experimental[151] and clinical CPR[183] have been variable; however, in the absence of intravenous access, adrenaline should be administered in twice the intravenous dose diluted in 10 ml of normal saline or distilled water.

Adrenaline may also change end-tidal carbon dioxide during CPR,[190] so even though capnography can be a useful tool at the bedside during resuscitation, interpretation may be influenced by administration of drugs other than sodium bicarbonate.

Atropine

Atropine is an essential adjunct to the resuscitation of children, in whom profound bradycardia, even in the presence of a pulse, signals a near complete cessation of circulation. The higher degree of vagal tone in children renders them more susceptible than adults to rate-dependent circulatory compromise. Atropine has no known haemodynamic effects during CPR. It is reportedly efficacious in adrenaline-refractory asystole,[191] although its effect is not consistent.[192,193] It is of no value in experimental electromechanical dissociation.[164] It can be administered intravenously, intra-osseously or tracheally.

Sodium bicarbonate

Unfortunately, recent investigations of carbon dioxide transport during CPR[92,113–117] have been widely interpreted to mean that there is no indication for the administration of sodium bicarbonate during CPR. Selective venous hypercapnia[124] is a necessary result of a profound low flow state;[120,194] it follows directly from the Fick principle that if carbon dioxide production remains constant and cardiac output is diminished, the arteriovenous difference in carbon dioxide content must rise. While it is erroneous to use bicarbonate automatically, especially for arrests of brief duration,[195] or in an attempt to correct acidosis of respiratory origin,[118] the correction of severe metabolic acidosis after prolonged periods of complete circulatory arrest does improve outcome in animals.[122,196–198] Severe metabolic acidosis is well-documented to exist in some patient populations[119,199,200] and to depress the myocardium.[201] However, the vast majority of cardiac arrests in in-hospital critical care areas are witnessed and therefore unlikely to be associated with severe metabolic acidosis.

Experimentally, if CPR is initiated after a brief period of arrest, pH falls slowly in dogs.[94,202,203] However, prolonged arrest time can lead to a substantial acidosis.[204] Unwitnessed cardiac arrest associated with severe acidosis is a frequent phenomenon on hospital wards[118,119,200,205] and in the pre-hospital setting.[121] Retrospectively, although patients receiving sodium bicarbonate did develop mild hypernatraemia, their outcome was no worse despite longer CPR times and a wider spectrum of presenting rhythms.[206] Similarly, prolonged resuscitation efforts require bicarbonate to maintain physiological blood gases in spite of early CPR and aggressive hyperventilation.[206] In very rare situations, ventilator therapy fails to correct respiratory acidosis even with a beating heart, and bicarbonate is required to prevent cardiac arrest.[207]

It was shown long ago that severe acidosis of either respiratory or metabolic origin depresses the myocardium[33,208–210] although the beating heart can tolerate extreme hypercapnia remarkably well,[211] and mild metabolic or respiratory acidosis may slightly improve haemodynamics, protect the hypoxic myocardium or prevent hypoxic and post-hypoxic myocardial contracture.[33] In animals with an initially normal pH, bicarbonate infusion produces a decrease followed by an increase in myocardial contractility.[212] Metabolic acidosis renders the heart more susceptible to ventricular fibrillation,[213,214] whereas mild metabolic alkalosis protects against fibrillation and respiratory alteration of pH may have little effect.[213] Mild acidosis and hypoxaemia do not influence the rate of successful defibrillation in animals,[215] but may do so in clinical cardiac arrest.[216]

Although it has long been known that changing the extracellular bicarbonate concentration does change intracellular pH, even if carbon dioxide is held constant, the optimum treatment of metabolic acidosis of ischaemic or hypoxic origin remains controversial.[133,195,217–223] Exogenous infusion of lactic or other acid (extracellular metabolic acidosis) and exogenously administered carbon dioxide (extracellular respiratory acidosis, for which the time-frame for resolution of the extra- to intracellular gradient is very short) are fundamentally different from acidosis which is generated by ischaemia or hypoxia (intracellular metabolic acidosis). In the last instance, the intracellular pH is considerably less than the extracellular pH, and this may produce damage to cellular components by itself. Second, when exogenous metabolic acid is used to bathe normal cells with an intact cell membrane, the cell membrane provides the intracellular components with substantial protection since the acid gets into the cell slowly compared with carbon dioxide. However, although carbon dioxide gets into the cell very quickly, it does relatively little damage to cells by itself.[211]

Risks of bicarbonate therapy include hyperosmolarity, exacerbation of pre-existing hypoventilation, alkalosis, hypernatraemia,[221,223] haemodynamic compromise[218] (especially if hypoxia remains uncorrected[219]) and mixed venous hypercapnia.[223] However, in Mattar and colleagues' series, only 1 of the patients with pH less than 7.3 had a metabolic acidosis; all patients received bicarbonate none the less.[221] Furthermore, only 1 had a normal osmolarity prior to bicarbonate administration. Cerebrospinal fluid acidosis accrues during CPR if bicarbonate is administered every 5 min irrespective of arterial pH,[217] but not if one or two doses are given[123,224] Moreover, after 6 min of ventricular fibrillation during adrenaline-supported CPR, cerebral intracellular pH recovers.[225] Severe alkalosis can cause cardiac arrest by itself,[226] even in previously healthy patients. Clinical administration of sodium bicarbonate must therefore be undertaken judiciously, and titrated to the correction of severe metabolic acidosis documented by arterial blood gases. It cannot be given tracheally, but can be given intravenously or intraosseously.[147]

Alternative buffering agents include 2-amine, 2-hydroxymethyl-1,3-propanediol (also known as tris-(hydroxymethyl) aminomethane (THAM), and tris buffer[208]), dichloro-acetate, sodium lactate,[208] and carbicarb.[227] None has been shown to yield outcome superior to bicarbonate in severe metabolic acidosis due to cardiac arrest and resuscitation. Dichloro-acetate does accelerate clearance of lactate after resuscitation from asphyxial cardiac arrest when compared with saline, but the therapeutic implication of this result remains unclear.[33]

Anti-arrhythmics

Lignocaine (lidocaine) is not known to alter the haemodynamics of CPR. However, it does increase the energy requirement for defibrillation in experimental models,[228] but this effect is modulated by the anaesthetic used.[229] It can facilitate treatment of refractory ventricular fibrillation[230,231] administered by either the intravenous or tracheal route.[232] In the setting of myocardial infarction, it may decrease the incidence of primary or recurrent fibrillation,[233,234] but can also cause asystole.[235,236] Hepatic blood flow is inadequate during CPR to clear lignocaine; thus, infusions should not be initiated until after the heart has been restarted. The anti-arrhythmic efficacy of lignocaine is determined by concentrations of lignocaine in ischaemic myocardium rather than blood levels, so that a higher dose may be required.

The haemodynamic effects of procainamide during CPR have not yet been investigated. After brief periods of cardiac arrest, it does not facilitate successful defibrillation compared with adrenaline alone.[162] Bretylium is known to have a biphasic effect on the sympathetic nervous system during spontaneous circulation.[237] It cannot be relied upon to produce chemical defibrillation. It does not significantly alter defibrillation threshold[229] and does not offer any advantage over lignocaine in the management of cardiac arrest.[238-242]

Adrenergic agonists other than adrenaline

Noradrenaline can provide more cerebral blood flow during CPR than adrenaline,[243,244] but improved outcome after CPR has yet to be demonstrated. It functions best in a non-acidotic milieu, but is currently regarded as a last resort in the pharmacological support of the ischaemic heart. Dopamine and adrenaline are equally effective in the treatment of both asphyxial and fibrillatory cardiac arrest in dogs.[167] However, the principal utility of dopamine is in the support of the beating heart[245,246] and this requires correction of severe metabolic acidosis for optimal effect[247]. Since dobutamine is essentially a pure β-adrenergic agonist, it offers no advantage during CPR, and may worsen outcome compared with α-adrenergic agents.[167] Multiple comparisons of isoprenaline and adrenaline have shown that the latter is vastly superior for the treatment of cardiac arrest.[154,161,167] During CPR, isoprenaline shunts blood away from vital organs.[99] Catecholamine cardiomyopathy is a real risk with isoprenaline; thus its use in the setting of myocardial ischaemia should be such that it is carefully titrated to the desired chronotropic effect in atropine-refractory block and bradycardia. Even asthmatics with a healthy heart can experience fatal myocardial damage during isoprenaline infusion.[248]

Calcium chloride

Ever since Ringer's serendipitous discovery of calcium's inotropic effect,[249] there has been interest in its use for resuscitation. It proved an essential adjunct to direct cardiac massage for fibrillation controlled with potassium salts and the reversal of peri-operative myocardial depression.[250] It has also long been known to be of only moderate efficacy in other resuscitative circumstances.[153,161] In the critical care and peri-operative settings, ionized calcium is an important determinant of myocardial function.[251] Low levels of ionized calcium are observed in patients in the pre-hospital setting[252] more commonly than intensive care arrests. It does not appear to be of any value in asystole[253-256] or experimental electromechanical dissociation.[164,257] The response to calcium is limited to clinical electromechanical dissociation but it appears to be effective in some patients in the pre-hospital setting.[253,258] Administration of calcium has risks both in the patient with a beating heart[259] and during cardiac arrest.[260] The effect of adrenaline is dependent on available calcium, but is impaired only at very low calcium levels.

Calcium antagonists

Calcium antagonists are, in general, negative inotropes and vasodilators.[261,262] Consequently, they have no role during standard CPR and serve to impair the therapeutic advantages offered by adrenaline. Although cardioprotective and antifibrillatory, they are of no value in the treatment of asystole or electromechanical dissociation.[263] They may be of value in refractory ventricular tachycardia or hypercalcaemia, but carry the risk of profound hypotension in recently resuscitated patients and of inducing ventricular fibrillation in patients with Wolff–Parkinson–White syndrome.[264]

REFERENCES

1. Safar P, Bircher NG. Cardiopulmonary cerebral resuscitation: an introduction to resuscitation medicine. London: WB Saunders. 1988
2. Safar P, Brown TC, Holtey WJ, Wilder RJ. Ventilation and circulation with closed-chest cardiac massage in man. JAMA 1961; 176: 574
3. Safar P, Aguto-Escarraga L, Chang F. Upper airway obstruction in the unconscious patient. J Appl Physiol 1959; 14: 760
4. Elam JO, Greene DG, Schneider MA et al. Head-tilt method of oral resuscitation. JAMA 1960; 172: 812
5. Guilder CW. Resuscitation — opening the airway. A comparative study of techniques for opening an airway obstructed by the tongue. JACEP 1976; 5: 588
6. Ruben H, Elam JO, Ruben AM et al. Investigation of the upper airway problems in resuscitation. I. Studies of pharyngeal x-rays and performance by laymen. Anesthesiology 1961; 22: 271
7. Morikawa S, Safar P, DeCarlo J. Influence of the head–jaw position upon upper airway patency. Anesthesiology 1961; 22: 265
8. Boidin MP. Airway patency in the unconscious patient. Br J Anaesth 1985; 57: 306
9. Montgomery WH, Donegon J, McIntyre KM et al. Standards and guidelines for cardiopulmonary resuscitation (CPR) and emergency cardiac care (ECC). JAMA 1986; 255: 2905
10. Ruben H, Knudsen EJ, Carugati G. Gastric inflation in relation to airway pressure. Acta Anaesthesiol Scand 1961; 5: 107

11. Melker RJ. Alternative methods of ventilation during respiratory and cardiac arrest. Circulation 1986; 74 (suppl IV): IV-63
12. Sellick BA. Cricoid pressure to control regurgitation of stomach contents during induction of anaesthesia. Lancet 1961; ii: 404
13. Abramson NS, Safar P, Detre K et al (Brain Resuscitation Clinical Trial I Study Group). Randomized clinical study of thiopental loading in comatose survivors of cardiac arrest. N Engl J Med 1986; 314: 397
14. Bedell SE, Delbanco TL, Cook EF, Epstein FH. Survival after cardiopulmonary resuscitation in the hospital. N Engl J Med 1983; 309: 569
15. Eisenberg M, Bergner L, Hallstrom A. Paramedic programs and out-of-hospital cardiac arrest: I. Factors associated with successful resuscitation. Am J Public Health 1979; 69: 30
16. Redding JS, Pearson JW. Resuscitation from asphyxia. JAMA 1962; 182: 283
17. Sanders AB, Kern KB, Bragg S, Ewy GA. Neurological benefits from the use of early cardiopulmonary resuscitation. Ann Emerg Med 1987; 16: 142
18. Yakaitis RW, Ewy GA, Otto CW et al. Influence of time and therapy on ventricular defibrillation in dogs. Crit Care Med 1980; 8: 157
19. Frass M, Frenzer R, Zdrahal F et al. The esophageal tracheal combitube: preliminary results with a new airway for CPR. Ann Emerg Med 1987; 16: 768
20. Niemann JT, Rosborough JP, Myers R, Scarberry EN. The pharyngeotracheal lumen airway: preliminary investigation of a new adjunct. Ann Emerg Med 1984; 13: 591
21. Lawes EG, Baskett PJF. Pulmonary aspiration during unsuccessful cardiopulmonary resuscitation. Intensive Care Med 1987; 13: 379
22. Don Michael TA. The role of the esophageal obturator airway in cardiopulmonary resuscitation. Circulation 1986; 74 (suppl IV): IV-134
23. Hammargren Y, Clinton JE, Ruiz E. Standard comparison of the esophageal obturator airway and endotracheal tube ventilation in cardiac arrest. Ann Emerg Med 1985; 14: 953
24. Shea SR, MacDonald JR, Gruzinski G. Prehospital endotracheal tube airway or esophageal gastric tube airway: a critical comparison. Ann Emerg Med 1985; 14: 102
25. Gertler JP, Cameron DE, Shea K et al. The esophageal obturator airway: obturator or obtundator? J Trauma 1985; 25: 424
26. Auerbach PS, Geehr EC. Inadequate oxygenation and ventilation using the esophageal gastric tube airway in the prehospital setting. JAMA 1983; 250: 3067
27. McCabe CJ, Browne BJ. Esophageal obturator airway, ET tube, and pharyngeal-tracheal lumen airway. Am J Emerg Med 1986; 4: 64
28. Jacobs LM, Berrizbeitia LD, Bennett B, Madigan C. Endotracheal intubation in the prehospital phase of emergency care. JAMA 1983; 250: 2175
29. Pepe PE, Copass MK, Joyce TH. Prehospital endotracheal intubation: rationale for training emergency medical personnel. Ann Emerg Med 1985; 14: 1085
30. Crile G, Dolley DH. An experimental research into the resuscitation of dogs killed by anesthetic and asphyxia. J Exp Med 1906; 8: 713
31. Safar P, Escarraga LA, Elam JO. A comparison of the mouth-to-mouth and mouth-to-airway methods of artificial respiration with the chest-pressure arm-lift methods. N Engl J Med 1958; 258: 671
32. Camarata SJ, Weil MH, Hanashiro PK, Shubin H. Cardiac arrest in the critically ill. I. A study of predisposing causes in 132 patients. Circulation 1971; 44: 688
33. Bircher NG. Physiology and pharmacology of standard cardiopulmonary resuscitation. In: Kaye W, Bircher NG, eds. Cardiopulmonary resuscitation. New York: Churchill Livingstone, 1989: pp 55–86
34. Fillmore SJ, Shapiro M, Killip T. Serial blood gases during cardiopulmonary resuscitation. Ann Intern Med 1970; 72: 465
35. Gilston A. Clinical and biochemical aspects of cardiac resuscitation. Lancet 1965; ii 1039
36. Rudikoff MT, Maughan WL, Effron et al. Mechanisms of blood flow during cardiopulmonary resuscitation. Circulation 1980; 61: 345
37. Ornato JP, Ryschon TW, Gonzalez ER, Bredthauer JL. Rapid vascular change in pulmonary vascular hemodynamics with pulmonary edema during cardiopulmonary resuscitation. Am J Emerg Med 1985; 3: 137
38. Niemann JT. Alternatives to standard CPR. In: Kaye W, Bircher NG, eds. Cardiopulmonary resuscitation. New York: Churchill Livingstone, 1989; pp. 103–116
39. Wilder RJ, Weir D, Rush BF, Ravitch MM. Methods of coordinating ventilation and closed chest cardiac massage in the dog. Surgery 1963; 53: 186
40. Harris LC, Kirimli B, Safar P. Ventilation–cardiac compression rates and ratios in cardiopulmonary resuscitation. Anesthesiology 1967; 28: 806
41. Gordon AS, Affeldt AE, Sadove M et al. Air-flow patterns and pulmonary ventilation during manual artificial respiration on apneic normal adults. II. J Appl Physiol 1951; 4: 408
42. Gordon AS, Sadove MS, Raymon F, Ivy AC. Critical survey of manual artificial respiration. JAMA 1951; 147: 1444
43. Elam JO, Brown ES, Elder JD et al. Artificial respiration by mouth-to-mask method. A study of the respiratory gas exchange of paralyzed patients ventilated by operator's expired air. N Engl J Med 1954; 250: 749
44. Gordon AS, Frye CW, Gittleson L et al. Mouth-to-mouth versus manual artificial respiration for children and adults. JAMA 1958; 167: 320
45. Safar P. Ventilatory efficacy of mouth-to-mouth artificial respiration. Airway obstruction during manual and mouth-to-mouth artificial respiration. JAMA 1958; 167: 335
46. Safar P. Failure of manual respiration. J Appl Physiol 1959; 14: 84
47. Safar P, McMahon M. Mouth-to-airway emergency artificial respiration. JAMA 1958; 166: 1459
48. Breivik H, Ulvik NM, Blikra G, Lind B. Life-supporting first aid self-training. Crit Care Med 1980; 8: 654
49. Safar P. Pocket mask for emergency artificial ventilation and oxygen inhalation. Crit Care Med 1974; 2: 273
50. Elling R, Politis J. An evaluation of emergency medical

51 Harrison RR, Maull KI, Keenan RL, Boyan CP. Mouth-to-mask ventilation: a superior method of rescue breathing. Ann Emerg Med 1982; 11: 74
52 Hess D, Baran C. Ventilatory volumes using mouth-to-mouth, mouth-to-mask, and bag-valve-mask techniques. Am J Emerg Med 1985; 3: 292
53 Safar P, Redding J. The 'tight-jaw' in resuscitation. Anesthesiology 1959; 20: 701
54 Jesudian MCS, Harrison RR, Keenan RL, Maull KI Bag-valve-mask ventilation; two rescuers are better than one: preliminary report. Crit Care Med 1985; 13: 122
55 Stewart RD, Kaplan R, Pennock B, Thompson F. Influence of mask design on bag-mask ventilation. Ann Emerg Med 1985; 14: 403
56 Pearson JW, Redding JS. Evaluation of the Elder demand valve resuscitator for the use by first-aid personnel. Anesthesiology 1967; 28: 623
57 Barnes TA, Watson ME. Oxygen delivery performance of old and new designs of the Laerdal, Vitalograph, and AMBU adult resuscitators. Respir Care 1983; 28: 1121
58 Campbell TP, Stewart RD, Kaplan RM et al. Oxygen enrichment of bag-valve-mask units during positive-pressure ventilation: a comparison of various techniques. Ann Emerg Med 1988; 17: 232
59 Finer NN, Barrington KJ, Al-Fadley F, Peters KL. Limitations of self-inflating resuscitators. Paediatrics 1986; 77: 417
60 Augustine JA, Seidel DR, McCabe JB. Ventilation performance using a self-inflating anesthesia bag: effect of operator characteristics. Am J Emerg Med 1987; 5: 267
61 Babbs CF, Fitzgerald KR, Voorhees WD, Murphy RJ. High-pressure ventilation during CPR with 95% O_2:5% CO_2. Crit Care Med 1982; 10: 505
62 Brader E, Klain M, Safar P, Bircher N. High frequency jet ventilation versus IPPV for CPR during ventricular fibrillation in dogs. Crit Care Med 1981; 9: 162
63 Brader E, Klain M, Safar P, Bircher N. High frequency jet ventilation versus IPPV in cardiopulmonary resuscitation for asphyxia in dogs. Crit Care Med 1981; 9: 162
64 Klain M, Keszler H, Brader E. High frequency jet ventilation in CPR. Crit Care Med 1981; 9: 421
65 Swartzman S, Wilson MA, Hoff BH et al. Percutaneous transtracheal jet ventilation for cardiopulmonary resuscitation. Evaluation of a new jet ventilator. Crit Care Med 1984; 12: 8
66 Safar P, Bircher NG. Pathophysiology of dying and reanimation. In: Schwartz GR et al, eds. Principles and practice of emergency medicine, 3rd edn. Lea & Febiger. 1992
67 Kovach AGB, Sandor P. Cerebral blood flow and brain function during hypotension and shock. Annu Rev Physiol 1976; 38: 571
68 Bocka JJ, Overton DT, Hauser A. Electromechanical dissociation in humans: an echocardiographic evaluation. Ann Emerg Med 1988; 17: 450
69 Paradis NA, Martin GB, Goetting MG, Rivers EP, Feingold M, Nowak RM. Aortic pressure during human cardiac arrest. Identification of pseudo-electromechanical dissociation. Chest 1992; 101: 123–128
70 Pinsky MR, Summer WR. Cardiac augmentation by phasic intrathoracic pressure support in man. Chest 1983; 84: 370
71 Bircher NG, Safar P, Eshel G, Stezoski W. Cerebral and hemodynamic variables during cough-induced CPR in dogs. Crit Care Med 1982; 10: 104
72 Chandra N, Guerci A, Weisfeldt ML et al. Contrasts between intrathoracic pressures during external chest compression and cardiac massage. Crit Care Med 1981; 9: 789
73 Chandra N, Weisfeldt ML, Tsitlik J et al. Augmentation of carotid flow during cardiopulmonary resuscitation by ventilation at high airway pressure simultaneous with chest compression. Am J Cardiol 1981; 48: 1053
74 Criley JM, Blaufuss AH, Kissel GL. Cough-induced cardiac compression. Self-administered form of cardiopulmonary resuscitation. JAMA 1976; 236: 1246
75 Kuhn C, Juchems R, Frese W. Evidence for the 'cardiac pump theory' in cardiopulmonary resuscitation in man by transesophageal echocardiography. Resuscitation 1991; 22: 275–282
76 Kouwenhoven WB, Jude JR, Knickerbocker GG. Closed-chest cardiac massage. JAMA 1960; 173: 1064
77 Weale FE, Rothwell-Jackson RL. The efficiency of cardiac massage. Lancet 1962; i: 990
78 MacKenzie GJ, Taylor SH, McDonald AH, Donald KW. Hemodynamic effects of external cardiac compression. Lancet 1964; i: 1342
79 Niemann JT, Rosborough JP, Hausknecht M et al. Pressure-synchronized cineangiography during experimental cardiopulmonary resuscitation. Circulation 1981; 64: 985
80 Bircher NG, Safar P. Intracranial pressure and other variables during simultaneous ventilation–compression cardiopulmonary resuscitation. In: Miller JD, Teasdale GM, Rowan JO et al, eds. Intracranial pressure VI. Berlin: Springer Verlag 1986: p 747
81 Lesser R, Bircher N, Safar P, Stezoski W. Venous valving during cardiopulmonary resuscitation (CPR). Anesthesiology 1980; 53 (suppl 3): S153
82 Fisher J, Vaghaiwalla F, Tsitlik J et al. Determinants and clinical significance of jugular venous valve competence. Circulation 1982; 65: 188
83 Brown CG, Taylor RB, Werman HA et al. Carotid artery collapse during CPR — the importance of cardiac versus thoracic pump mechanisms demonstrated with cineangiography. Ann Emerg Med 1987; 16: 513
84 Yin FCP, Cohen JM, Tsitlik J et al. Role of carotid artery resistance to collapse during high-intrathoracic-pressure CPR. Am J Physiol 1982; 243: H259
85 Michael JR, Guerci AD, Koehler RC et al. Mechanisms by which epinephrine augments cerebral and myocardial perfusion during cardiopulmonary resuscitation in dogs. Circulation 1984; 69: 822
86 Del Guercio LRM, Coomaraswamy RP, State S. Cardiac output and other hemodynamic variables during external cardiac massage in man. N Engl J Med 1963; 269: 1398
87 Del Guercio LRM, Feins NR, Cohn JD et al. Comparison of blood flow during external and internal

88. Gurewich V, Sasahara AA, Quinn JS et al. Aortic pressures during closed-chest cardiac massage. Circulation 1961; 23: 593
89. Nixon PGF. The arterial pulse in successful closed-chest cardiac massage. Lancet 1961; ii: 844
90. Paradis NA, Rosenberg JM, Martin GB et al. Simultaneous aortic, jugular bulb, and right atrial pressures during standard external CPR (SE-CPR). Ann Emerg Med 1988; 17: 393
91. Taylor GJ, Tucker WM, Greene HL et al. Importance of prolonged compression during cardiopulmonary resuscitation in man. N Engl J Med 1977; 296: 1515
92. Ornato JP, Gonzalez ER, Garnett AR et al. Effect of cardiopulmonary resuscitation compression rate on end-tidal carbon dioxide concentration and arterial pressure in man. Crit Care Med 1988; 16: 241
93. Babbs CF, Voorhees WD, Fitzgerald KR et al. Relationship of blood pressure and flow during CPR to chest compression amplitude: evidence for an effective compression threshold. Ann Emerg Med 1983; 12: 527
94. Bircher NG, Safar P, Stewart R. A comparison of standard, 'MAST'-augmented, and open-chest CPR in dogs. A preliminary investigation. Crit Care Med 1980; 8: 147
95. Guerci AD, Shi AY, Levin H et al. Transmission of intrathoracic pressure to the intracranial space during cardiopulmonary resuscitation in dogs. Circ Res 1985; 56: 20
96. Lee SK, Vaagenes P, Safar P et al. Effect of cardiac arrest time on the cortical cerebral blood flow generated by subsequent standard external CPR in rabbits. Resuscitation 1989; 17: 105–117
97. Szmolenszky T, Szoke P, Halmagyi G et al. Organ blood flow during external heart massage. Acta Chir Acad Sci Hung 1974; 15: 283
98. Steen PA, Michenfelder JD, Milde JH. Incomplete versus complete cerebral ischemia: improved outcome with a minimal blood flow. Ann Neurol 1979; 6: 389
99. Holmes HR, Babbs CF, Voorhees WD et al. Influence of adrenergic drugs upon vital organ perfusion during CPR. Crit Care Med 1980; 8: 137
100. Schleien CL, Dean JM, Koehler RC et al. Effect of epinephrine on cerebral and myocardial perfusion in an infant animal preparation of cardiopulmonary resuscitation. Circulation 1986; 73: 809
101. Brown CG, Werman HA, Davis EA et al. The effect of high-dose phenylephrine versus epinephrine on regional cerebral blood flow during CPR. Ann Emerg Med 1987; 16: 743
102. Brown CG, Davis EA, Werman HA, Hamlin RL. Methoxamine versus epinephrine on regional cerebral blood flow during cardiopulmonary resuscitation. Crit Care Med 1987; 15: 682
103. Ditchey RV, Lindenfeld J. Potential adverse effects of volume loading on perfusion of vital organs during closed-chest resuscitation. Circulation 1984; 69; 181
104. Koehler RC, Chandra N, Guerci AD et al. Augmentation of cerebral perfusion by simultaneous chest compression and lung inflation with abdominal binding after cardiac arrest in dogs. Circulation 1983; 67: 266
105. Luce JM, Ross BK, O'Quin RJ et al. Regional blood flow during cardiopulmonary resuscitation in dogs using simultaneous and non-simultaneous compression and ventilation. Circulation 1983; 67: 258
106. Krischer JP, Fine EG, Weisfeldt ML, Guerci AD, Nagel E, Chandra N. Comparison of prehospital conventional and simultaneous compression–ventilation cardiopulmonary resuscitation. Crit Care Med 1989; 17: 1263
107. Synder JV, Nemoto EM, Carroll RG, Safar P. Global ischemia in dogs: intracranial pressures, brain blood flow and metabolism. Stroke 1975; 6: 21
108. Bellamy RF, DeGuzman LR, Pederson DC. Coronary blood flow during cardiopulmonary resuscitation in swine. Circulation 1984; 69: 174
109. Ditchey DV, Winkler JV, Rhodes CA. Relative lack of coronary blood flow during closed-chest resuscitation in dogs. Circulation 1982; 66: 297
110. Sanders AB, Ogle M, Ewy GA. Coronary perfusion pressure during cardiopulmonary resuscitation. Am J Emerg Med 1985; 3: 11
111. Sanders AB, Ewy GA, Taft TV. Prognostic and therapeutic importance of the aortic diastolic pressure in resuscitation from cardiac arrest. Crit Care Med 1984; 12: 871
112. Bircher N, Safar P. Cerebral preservation during cardiopulmonary resuscitation. Crit Care Med 1985; 13: 185
113. Sanders AB, Atlas M, Ewy GA et al. Expired $P\text{CO}_2$ as an index of coronary perfusion pressure. Am J Emerg Med 1985; 3: 147
114. Sanders AB, Ewy GA, Bragg S et al. Expired $P\text{CO}_2$ as a prognostic indicator of successful resuscitation from cardiac arrest. Ann Emerg Med 1985; 14: 948
115. Dohi S, Takeshima R, Matsumiya N. Carbon dioxide elimination during circulatory arrest. Crit Care Med 1987; 15: 944
116. Falk JL, Rackow EC, Weil MH. End-tidal carbon dioxide concentration during cardiopulmonary resuscitation. N Engl J Med 1988; 318: 607
117. Garnett AR, Ornato JP, Gonzalez ER, Johnson EB. End-tidal carbon dioxide monitoring during cardiopulmonary resuscitation. JAMA 1987; 257: 512
118. Chazan JA, Stenson R, Kurland GS. The acidosis of cardiac arrest. N Engl J Med 1968; 278: 360
119. Kirby BJ, McNicol MW. Results of cardiac resuscitation in 100 patients: effects on acid–base status. Postgrad Med J 1967; 43: 75
120. Nowak RM, Martin GB, Carden DL, Tomlanovich MC. Selective venous hypercarbia during human CPR: implications regarding blood flow. Ann Emerg Med 1987; 16: 527
121. Ornato JP, Gonzalez ER, Coyne MR et al. Arterial pH in out-of-hospital cardiac arrest: response time as a determinant of acidosis. Am J Emerg Med 1985; 3: 498
122. Sanders AB, Ewy GA, Taft TV. Resuscitation and arterial blood gas abnormalities during prolonged cardiopulmonary resuscitation. Ann Emerg Med 1984; 13: 676
123. Sessler D, Mills P, Gregory G et al. Effects of bicarbonate on arterial and brain intracellular pH in neonatal rabbits recovering from hypoxic lactic acidosis. J Pediatr 1987; 111: 817
124. Weil MH, Rackow EC, Trevino R et al. Difference in acid–base state between venous and arterial blood

during cardiopulmonary resuscitation. N Engl J Med 1986; 315: 153
125 Kaye W, Bircher NG. Access for drug administration during cardiopulmonary resuscitation. Crit Care Med 1988; 16: 179
126 Hedges JR, Barsan WG, Doan LA et al. Central versus peripheral intravenous routes in cardiopulmonary resuscitation. Am J Emerg Med 1984; 2: 385
127 Kuhn GJ, White BC, Swetnam RE et al. Peripheral vs central circulation times during CPR: a pilot study. Ann Emerg Med 1981; 10: 417
128 Barsan WG, Levy RC, Weir H. Lidocaine levels during CPR: differences after peripheral venous, central venous, and intracardiac injections. Ann Emerg Med 1981; 10: 73
129 Dalsey WC, Barsan WG, Joyce et al. Comparison of superior vena caval versus inferior vena caval access using a radioisotope technique during normal perfusion and cardiopulmonary resuscitation. Ann Emerg Med 1984; 13: 881
130 Quinton DN, O'Byrne G, Aitkenhead AR. Comparison of endotracheal and peripheral intravenous adrenaline in cardiac arrest. Is the endotracheal route reliable? Lancet 1987; i: 828
131 Ralston SH, Voorhees WD, Babbs CF. Intrapulmonary epinephrine during prolonged cardiopulmonary resuscitation: improved regional blood flow and resuscitation in dogs. Ann Emerg Med 1984; 13: 79
132 Ralston SH, Tacker WA, Showden L et al. Endotracheal versus intravenous epinephrine during electromechanical dissociation with CPR in dogs. Ann Emerg Med 1985; 14: 1044
133 Roberts JR, Greenberg MI, Knaub M, Baskin SI. Comparison of the pharmacological effects of epinephrine administered by the intravenous and endotracheal routes. JACEP 1978; 7: 260
134 Roberts JR, Greenberg MI, Knaub MA et al. Blood levels following intravenous and endotracheal epinephrine administration. JACEP 1979; 8: 53
135 Roberts JR, Greenberg MI, Baskin SI. Endotracheal epinephrine in cardiorespiratory collapse. JACEP 1979; 8: 515
136 Smith RJ, Keseg DP, Manley LK, Standeford T. Intraosseous infusions by prehospital personnel in critically ill pediatric patients. Ann Emerg Med 1988; 17: 491
137 Spivey WH, Lathers CM, Malone DR et al. Comparison of the intraosseous, central, and peripheral routes of sodium bicarbonate administration during CPR in pigs. Ann Emerg Med 1985; 14: 1135
138 Spivey WH, Unger HD, McNamara RM et al. The effect of intra-osseous sodium bicarbonate on bone in swine. Ann Emerg Med 1987; 16: 773
139 Brown CG, Werman HA, Davis EA et al. The effect of graded doses of epinephrine on regional myocardial blood flow during cardiopulmonary resuscitation in swine. Circulation 1987; 75: 491–497
140 Brown CG, Taylor RB, Werman HA et al. Effect of standard doses of epinephrine on myocardial oxygen utilization during cardiopulmonary resuscitation. Crit Care Med 1988; 16: 536–539
141 Brown CG, Werman HA. Adrenergic agonists during cardiopulmonary resuscitation. Resuscitation 1990; 19: 1–16
142 Koehler RC, Michael JR, Guerci AD et al. Beneficial effect of epinephrine infusion on cerebral and myocardial blood flows during CPR. Ann Emerg Med 1985; 14: 744
143 Niemann JT, Adomian GE, Garner D, Rosborough JP. Endocardial and transcutaneous cardiac pacing, calcium chloride, and epinephrine in postcountershock asystole and bradycardias. Crit Care Med 1985; 13: 699
144 Niemann JT, Haynes KS, Garner D et al. Postcountershock pulseless rhythms: response to CPR, artificial cardiac pacing and adrenergic agonists. Ann Emerg Med 1986; 15: 112
145 Olson DW, Thakur R, Stueven H et al. Randomized study of epinephrine versus methoxamine in prehospital ventricular fibrillation. Ann Emerg Med 1987; 16: 494
146 Orlowski JP, Gallagher JM, Porembka DT. Endotracheal epinephrine is unreliable. Resuscitation 1990; 19: 103–113
147 Otto CW, Yakaitis RW, Redding JS, Blitt CD. Comparison of dopamine, dobutamine, and epinephrine in CPR. Crit Care Med 1981; 9: 366
148 Otto CW, Yakaitis RW, Blitt CD. Mechanism of action of epinephrine in resuscitation from asphyxial arrest. Crit Care Med 1981; 9: 364
149 Paradis NA, Koscove EM. Epinephrine in cardiac arrest. A critical review. Ann Emerg Med 1990; 19: 1288–1301
150 Pearson JW, Redding JS. Epinephrine in cardiac resuscitation. Am Heart J 1963; 66: 210
151 Pearson JW, Redding JS. Influence of peripheral vascular tone on cardiac resuscitation. Anesth Analg 1965; 44: 746
152 Redding JS, Pearson JW. Evaluation of drugs for cardiac resuscitation. Anesthesiology 1963; 24: 203
153 Redding JS, Pearson JW. Resuscitation from ventricular fibrillation. Drug therapy. JAMA 1968; 203: 255
154 Redding JS, Haynes RR, Thomas JD. Drug therapy in resuscitation from electromechanical dissociation. Crit Care Med 1983; 11: 681
155 Spivey WH, Schoffstall JM, Davidheiser S, Kirkpatrick R. Correlation of plasma catecholamines with blood pressure during cardiac arrest. Ann Emerg Med 1988; 17: 413
156 Turner LM, Parsons M, Luetkemeyer RC et al. A comparison of epinephrine and methoxamine for resuscitation from electromechanical dissociation in human beings. Ann Emerg Med 1988; 17: 443
157 Yakaitis RW, Otto CW, Blitt CD. Relative importance of alpha and beta adrenergic receptors during resuscitation. Crit Care Med 1979; 7: 293
158 Otto CW, Yakaitis RW, Ewy GA. Effect of epinephrine on defibrillation in ischemic ventricular fibrillation. Am J Emerg Med 1985; 3: 285–291
159 Livesay JJ, Follete DM, Fey KH et al. Optimizing myocardial supply/demand balance with alpha-adrenergic drugs during cardiopulmonary resuscitation. J Thorac Cardiovasc Surg 1978; 76: 244
160 Ditchey RV, Lindenfeld JA. Failure of epinephrine to improve the balance between myocardial oxygen supply and demand during closed-chest resuscitation in dogs. Circulation 1988; 78: 382
161 Lindner KH, Ahnefeld FW. Comparison of epinephrine and norepinephrine in the treatment of

asphyxial or fibrillatory cardiac arrest in a porcine model. Crit Care Med 1989; 17: 437–441

162 Robinson LA, Brown CG, Jenkins J et al. The effect of norepinephrine versus epinephrine on myocardial hemodynamics during CPR. Ann Emerg Med 1989; 18: 336–340

163 Brillman JA, Sanders AB, Otto CW et al. Outcome of resuscitation from fibrillatory arrest using epinephrine and phenylephrine in dogs. Crit Care Med 1985; 13: 912

164 Brillman JA, Sanders AB, Otto CW et al. Comparison of epinephrine and phenylephrine for resuscitation and neurological outcome of cardiac arrest in dogs. Ann Emerg Med 1987; 16: 11

165 Brown CG, Taylor RB, Werman HA et al. Myocardial oxygen delivery/consumption during cardiopulmonary resuscitation: a comparison of epinephrine and phenylephrine. Ann Emerg Med 1988; 17: 302

166 Bleske BE, Chow MSS, Zhao H et al. Epinephrine versus methoxamine in survival postventricular fibrillation and cardiopulmonary resuscitation in dogs. Crit Care Med 1989; 17: 1310–1313

167 Brown CG, Katz SE, Werman HA et al. The effect of epinephrine versus methoxamine on regional myocardial blood flow and defibrillation rates following a prolonged cardiorespiratory arrest in a swine model. Am J Emerg Med 1987; 5: 362

168 Redding JS, Sullivan FM, Minard RB, Thomas JD. Bretylium or methoxamine for resuscitation from ventricular fibrillation. Anesthesiology 1983; 59 (suppl 3): A123

169 Roberts D, Landolfo K, Dobson K, Light RB. The effects of methoxamine and epinephrine on survival and regional distribution of cardiac output in dogs with prolonged ventricular fibrillation. Chest 1990; 98: 999–1005

170 Brunette DD, Jameson SJ. Comparison of standard versus high-dose epinephrine in the resuscitation of cardiac arrest in dogs. Ann Emerg Med 1990; 19: 8–11

171 Goetting MG, Paradis NA. High dose epinephrine in refractory pediatric cardiac arrest. Crit Care Med 1989; 17: 1258–1262

172 Gonzalez ER, Ornato JP, Garnett AR et al. Enhanced vasopressor response after 3- and 5-mg doses of epinephrine during CPR in humans. Am J Emerg Med 1986; 4: 418

173 Gonzalez ER, Ornato JP, Garnett AR et al. Dose-dependent vasopressor response to epinephrine during CPR in human beings. Ann Emerg Med 1989; 18: 920–926

174 Koscove EM, Paradis NA. Successful resuscitation from cardiac arrest using high-dose epinephrine therapy. Report of two cases. JAMA 1988; 259: 3031

175 Martin D, Werman HA, Brown CG. Four case studies: high-dose epinephrine in cardiac arrest. Ann Emerg Med 1990; 19: 322–326

176 Taylor GJ, Rubin R, Tucker WM et al. External cardiac compression: a randomized comparison of mechanical and manual techniques. JAMA 1978; 240: 644

177 McDonald JL. Systolic and mean arterial pressures during manual and mechanical CPR in humans. Ann Emerg Med 1982; 11: 292

178 Baringer JR, Salzman EW, Jones WA, Friedlich AL. External cardiac massage. N Engl J Med 1961; 265: 62

179 Bedell SE, Fulton EJ. Unexpected findings and complications at autopsy after cardiopulmonary resuscitation (CPR). Arch Intern Med 1986; 146: 1725

180 Bjork RJ, Campion BC, Synder BD, Loewenson RB. Medical complications of cardiopulmonary arrest. Circulation 1980; 62 (suppl III): III-338

181 Clark DT. Complications following closed-chest cardiac massage. JAMA 1962; 181: 127

182 Glasser SP, Harrison EE, Amey BD, Straub EJ. Echocardiographic incidence of pericardial effusion in patients resuscitated by emergency medical technicians. JACEP 1979; 8: 6

183 Morgan RR. Laceration of the liver from closed-chest cardiac massage. N Engl J Med 1961; 265: 82

184 Silverberg B, Rachmaninoff N. Complications following cardiac massage. Surg Gynecol Obstet 1964; 119: 16

185 Thaler MM, Krause VW. Serious trauma in children after external cardiac massage. N Engl J Med 1962; 267: 500

186 Schoffstall JM, Spivey WH, Davidheiser S et al. Endogenous and exogenous plasma catecholamine levels in cardiac arrest in swine. Resuscitation 1990; 19: 241–251

187 Martens PR, Mullie A, Belgian Cerebral Resuscitation Study Group. The availability of 10 mg epinephrine vials for cardiac arrest: a retrospective analysis. Resuscitation 1991; 22: 219–228

188 Chernow B, Holbrook P, D'Angona DS et al. Epinephrine absorption after intratracheal administration. Anesth Analg 1984; 63: 829–832

189 Schneider SM, Yealy DM, Michaelson EA et al. Endotracheal versus intravenous epinephrine in the prehospital treatment of cardiac arrest. Prehosp Disaster Med 1990; 5: 341–348

190 Martin GB, Gentile NT, Paradis NA et al. Effect of epinephrine on end-tidal carbon dioxide monitoring during CPR. Ann Emerg Med 1990; 19: 396–398

191 Brown DC, Lewis AJ, Criley JM. Asystole and its treatment: the possible role of the parasympathetic nervous system in cardiac arrest. JACEP 1979; 8: 448

192 Coon GA, Clinton JE, Ruiz E. Use of atropine for brady-asystolic prehospital cardiac arrest. Ann Emerg Med 1981; 10: 462–467

193 Stueven HA, Tonsfeldt DJ, Thompson BM et al. Atropine in asystole: human studies. Ann Emerg Med 1984; 13: 815

194 Wiklund L, Soderberg D, Henneberg S et al. Kinetics of carbon dioxide during cardiopulmonary resuscitation. Crit Care Med 1986; 14: 1015

195 Guerci AD, Chandra N, Johnson E et al. Failure of sodium bicarbonate to improve resuscitation from ventricular fibrillation in dogs. Circulation 1986; 74 (suppl IV): IV-75

196 Bircher NG. Sodium bicarbonate improves cardiac resuscitability, 24 hour survivorship and neurological outcome after 10 minutes of cardiac arrest in dogs. Anesthesiology 1991; 75 (suppl 3A): A246

197 Vukmir RB, Bircher NG, Safar P. Effect of sodium bicarbonate on survival in a canine 15-minute cardiac arrest model. Ann Emerg Med 1991; 20: 491

198 Ledingham IMcA, Norman JN. Acid–base studies in experimental cardiac arrest. Lancet 1962; ii: 967

199 Henneman PL, Gruber JE, Marx JA. Development of acidosis in human beings during closed-chest and open-chest CPR. Ann Emerg Med 1988; 17: 672
200 Smith HJ, Anthonisen NR. Results of cardiac resuscitation in 254 patients. Lancet 1965; i: 1027
201 Clowes GHA, Sabga GA, Konitaxis A et al. Effects of acidosis on cardiovascular function in surgical patients. Ann Surg 1961; 154: 524
202 Bishop RL, Weisfeldt ML. Sodium bicarbonate administration during cardiac arrest. Effect on arterial pH, $P{CO_2}$, and osmolality. JAMA 1976; 235: 506
203 Sanders AB, Otto CW, Kern KB et al. Acid–base balance in a canine model of cardiac arrest. Ann Emerg Med 1988; 17: 667
204 Carden DL, Martin GB, Nowak RM et al. Lactic acidosis as a predictor of downtime during cardiopulmonary arrest in dogs. Am J Emerg Med 1985; 3: 120
205 Stewart JSS. Management of cardiac arrest, with special reference to metabolic acidosis. Br Med J 1964, 1: 476
206 Aufderheide TP, Martin DR, Olson DW et al. Prehospital bicarbonate use in cardiac arrest: a 3-year experience. Am J Emerg Med 1992; 10: 4–7
207 Menitove SM, Goldring RM. Combined ventilator and bicarbonate strategy in the management of status asthmaticus. Am J Med 1983; 74: 898
208 Clowes GHA, Alichniewicz A, Del Guercio LRM, Gillespie D. The relationship of postoperative acidosis to pulmonary and cardiovascular function. J Thorac Cardiovasc Surg 1960; 39: 1
209 Darby TD, Aldinger EE, Gadsden RH, Thrower WB. Effects of metabolic acidosis on ventricular isometric systolic tension and the response to epinephrine and levarterenol. Circ Res 1960; 8: 1242
210 Wexels JC, Mjos OD. Effects of carbon dioxide and pH on myocardial function in dogs with acute left ventricular failure. Crit Care Med 1987; 15: 1116
211 Steinhart CR, Permutt S, Gurtner GH, Traystman RJ. Beta-adrenergic activity and cardiovascular response to severe respiratory acidosis. Am J Physiol 1983; 244: H46
212 Clancy RL, Cingolani HE, Taylor RR et al. Influence of sodium bicarbonate on myocardial performance. Am J Physiol 1967; 212: 917
213 Gerst PH, Fleming WH, Malm JR. A quantitative evaluation of the effects of acidosis and alkalosis upon the ventricular fibrillation threshold. Surgery 1966; 59: 1050
214 Gerst PH, Fleming WH, Malm JR. Increased susceptibility of the heart to ventricular fibrillation during metabolic acidosis. Circ Res 1966; 19: 63
215 Yakaitis RW, Thomas JD, Mahaffey JE. Influence of pH and hypoxia on the success of defibrillation. Crit Care Med 1975; 3: 139
216 Kerber RE, Sarnat W. Factors influencing the success of ventricular defibrillation in man. Circulation 1979; 60: 226
217 Berenyi KJ, Wolk M, Killip T. Cerebrospinal fluid acidosis complicating therapy of experimental cardiopulmonary arrest. Circulation 1975; 52: 319
218 Cooper DJ, Worthley LIG. Adverse haemodynamic effects of sodium bicarbonate in metabolic acidosis. Intensive Care Med 1987; 13: 425–427
219 Graf H, Leach W, Arieff AI. Evidence for a detrimental effect of bicarbonate therapy in hypoxic lactic acidosis. Science 1985: 227: 754
220 Hindman BJ. Sodium bicarbonate in the treatment of subtypes of acute lactic acidosis: physiologic considerations. Anesthesiology 1990; 72: 1064–1076
221 Mattar JA, Weil MH, Shubin H, Stein L. Cardiac arrest in the critically ill. II. Hyperosmolal states following cardiac arrest. Am J Med 1974; 56: 162
222 Stacpoole PW. Lactic acidosis: the case against bicarbonate therapy. Ann Intern Med 1986; 105: 276
223 Weil MH, Ruiz CE, Michaels S, Rackow EC. Acid–base determinants of survival after cardiopulmonary resuscitation. Crit Care Med 1985; 13: 888
224 Sanders AB, Otto CW, Kern KB et al. The effect of bicarbonate on cerebral spinal fluid acidosis during cardiac arrest. Ann Emerg Med 1987; 16: 1102
225 Eleff SM, Schleien CL, Koehler RC et al. Brain bioenergetics during cardiopulmonary resuscitation in dogs. Anesthesiology 1992; 76: 77–84
226 Mennen M, Slovis CM. Severe metabolic alkalosis in the emergency department. Ann Emerg Med 1988; 17: 354
227 Bersin RM, Arieff AI. Improved hemodynamic function during hypoxia with Carbicarb, a new agent for the management of acidosis. Circulation 1988; 77: 227
228 Babbs CF, Yim GKW, Whistler SJ et al. Elevation of ventricular defibrillation threshold in dogs by antiarrhythmic drugs. Am J Heart 1979; 98: 345
229 Kerber RE, Pandian NG, Jensen SR et al. Effects of lidocaine and bretylium on energy requirements for transthoracic defibrillation: experimental studies. J Am Coll Cardiol 1986; 7: 397
230 Harrison EE. Lidocaine in prehospital refractory ventricular fibrillation. Ann Emerg Med 1981; 10: 420
231 Haynes RE, Chinn TL, Copass MK, Cobb LA. Comparison or bretylium tosylate and lidocaine in management of out of hospital ventricular fibrillation. Am J Cardiol 1981; 48: 353
232 McDonald JL. Serum lidocaine levels during cardiopulmonary resuscitation after intravenous and endotracheal administration. Crit Care Med 1985; 13: 914
233 DeSilva RA, Lown B, Hennekens CH, Casscells W. Lignocaine prophylaxis in acute myocardial infarction: an evaluation of randomised trials. Lancet 1981; ii: 855
234 Horwitz RI, Feinstein AR. Improved observational methods for studying therapeutic efficacy. Suggestive evidence that lidocaine prevents death in acute myocardial infarction. JAMA 1981; 246: 2455
235 Applebaum D, Halperin E. Asystole following a conventional therapeutic dose of lidocaine. Am J Emerg Med 1986; 4: 143
236 Freed CR, Freedman MD. Lidocaine overdose and cardiac bypass support. JAMA 1985; 253: 3094
237 Koch-Weser J. Bretylium. N Engl J Med 1979; 300: 473
238 Hanyok JJ, Chow MSS, Kluger J, Fieldman A. Antifibrillatory effects of high dose bretylium and a lidocaine–bretylium combination during cardiopulmonary resuscitation. Crit Care Med 1988; 16: 691
239 Harrison EE, Amey BD. The use of bretylium in

240 Holder DA, Sniderman AD, Fraser G, Fallen EL. Experience with bretylium tosylate by a hospital cardiac arrest team. Circulation 1977; 55: 541

241 Olson DW, Thompson BM, Darin JC, Milbrath MH. A randomized comparison study of bretylium tosylate and lidocaine in resuscitation of patients from out-of-hospital ventricular fibrillation in a paramedic system. Ann Emerg Med 1984; 13: 807

242 Stang JM, Washington SE, Barnes SA et al. Treatment of prehospital refractory ventricular fibrillation with bretylium tosylate. Ann Emerg Med 1984; 13: 234

243 Brown CG, Robinson L, Jenkins J et al. Cerebral blood flow during CPR — a comparison of norepinephrine versus epinephrine. Ann Emerg Med 1988; 17: 393

244 Brown CG, Robinson LA, Jenkins J et al. The effect of norepinephrine versus epinephrine on regional cerebral blood flow during cardiopulmonary resuscitation. Crit Care Med 1989; 7: 278–282

245 Brandl M, Pasch T, Kamp HD, Grimm J. Comparison of the effects of dopamine and dobutamine during continuous positive-pressure ventilation. Intensive Care Med 1983; 9: 61

246 Francis GS, Sharma B, Hodges M. Comparative hemodynamic effects of dopamine in patients with acute cardiogenic circulatory collapse. Am Heart J 1985; 103: 995

247 Tajimi K, Kosugi I, Hamamoto F, Kobayashi K. Plasma catecholamine levels and hemodynamic responses of severely acidotic dogs to dopamine infusion. Crit Care Med 1983; 11: 817

248 Kurland G, Williams J, Lewiston NJ. Fatal myocardial toxicity during continuous infusion intravenous isoproterenol therapy of asthma. J Allergy Clin Immunol 1979; 63: 407

249 Ringer S. A further contribution regarding the influence of the different constituents of the blood on the contraction of the heart. J Physiol 1883; 4: 29

250 Kay JH, Blalock A. The use of calcium chloride in the treatment of cardiac arrest in patients. Surg Gynecol Obstet 1951; 93: 97

251 Desai TK, Carlson RW, Thill-Baharozian M, Geheb MA. A direct relationship between ionized calcium and arterial pressure among patients in an intensive care unit. Crit Care Med 1988; 16: 578

252 Urban P, Scheidegger D, Buchmann B, Barth D. Cardiac arrest and blood ionized calcium levels. Ann Intern Med 1988; 109: 110

253 Harrison EE, Amey BD. The use of calcium in cardiac resuscitation. Am J Emerg Med 1983; 3: 267

254 Stueven H, Thompson BM, Aprahamian C, Darin JC. Use of calcium in prehospital cardiac arrest. Ann Emerg Med 1983; 12: 136

255 Stueven HA, Thompson BM, Aprahamian C, Tonsfeldt DJ. Calcium chloride: reassessment of use in asystole. Ann Emerg Med 1984; 13: 820

256 Stueven HA, Thompson B, Aprahamian C et al. Lack of effectiveness of calcium chloride in refractory asystole. Ann Emerg Med 1985; 14: 630

257 Blecic S, De Backer D, Huynh CH et al. Calcium chloride in experimental electromechanical dissociation: a placebo-controlled trial in dogs. Crit Care Med 1987; 15: 324

258 Stueven HA, Thompson B, Aprahamian C et al. The effectiveness of calcium chloride in refractory electromechanical dissociation. Ann Emerg Med 1985; 14: 626

259 Carlon GC, Howland WS, Goldiner PL et al. Adverse effects of calcium administration. Arch Surg 1978; 113: 882

260 Dembo DH. Calcium in advanced life support. Crit Care Med 1981; 9: 358

261 Kubo SH, Olivari MT, Cohn JN. Calcium antagonists in heart failure. In: Vanhoutte PM, Paoletti R, Govoni S, eds. Calcium antagonists. Pharmacology and clinical research. Ann NY Acad Sci 1988; 523: 553

262 Martin GB. Use of calcium entry blockers in electromechanical dissociation. Ann Emerg Med 1984; 13: 846

263 Martin GB, Nowak RM, Emerman CL, Tomlanovich MC. Verapamil in the treatment of asystolic and pulseless idioventricular rhythm cardiopulmonary arrests: a preliminary report. Ann Emerg Med 1984; 13: 221

264 Gulamhusein S, Ko P, Klein GJ. Ventricular fibrillation following verapamil in the Wolff–Parkinson–White syndrome. Am Heart J 1983; 106–145

28. Safety in clinical anaesthesia

A.R. Aitkenhead

The anaesthetized patient is at risk of complications resulting from the actions, or inaction, of the anaesthetist, from the actions of the surgeon, and from failure or malfunction of anaesthetic equipment. The state of anaesthesia may be considered to be intrinsically unsafe. Patients are subjected to the administration of drugs which have side-effects, particularly on the cardiovascular and respiratory systems. Unconsciousness carries with it risks of airway obstruction, soiling of the lungs and inability to detect peripheral injury. Pharmacological muscle paralysis necessitates the use of artificial ventilation, making the patient dependent on the anaesthetist and equipment for the fundamental functions of oxygenation and excretion of carbon dioxide. In addition, the anaesthetist may deliberately alter physiological functions, for example by inducing systemic arterial hypotension or ventilating only one lung.

Recognition of the risks associated with anaesthesia is the first step to improving safety. This is not a new concept. In 1949, Professor (later Sir) Robert Macintosh drew attention to the dangers of suppressing information about fatal accidents in anaesthetic practice, with the result that similar accidents occurred elsewhere which could have been avoided if the causes of earlier incidents had been publicized.[1] However, this lesson was learnt only slowly. Major improvements in safety have been driven in many countries by the financial consequences of compensating patients injured during anaesthesia, although fortunately, the measures introduced in these countries have also been adopted in countries where resort to the law is relatively uncommon. Safety and risk management in anaesthesia have become major areas of interest to national and international anaesthesia societies, as well as to individual anaesthetists.

In order to improve safety in anaesthesia it is important to quantify the risks and anaesthetists have been at the forefront among medical specialties in undertaking national studies of mortality, in introducing audit of clinical practice, and in critical incident reporting. There is a need to understand the psychology underlying the human role in accidents, and in this respect, much of the knowledge acquired from the aviation industry can be applied to anaesthesia. In order to reduce the number of accidents, there must be:

1. Careful selection of doctors entering anaesthetic practice.
2. Adequate education and experience for trainees.
3. Continuing education of specialist anaesthetists.
4. Improvements in design of anaesthetic equipment.
5. Regular maintenance of all equipment.
6. Adequate checking of equipment before use.
7. Continued revision and extension of standards of training and clinical practice.
8. Proper conditions of service, including adequate provision for education and rest.[2]

ASSESSMENT OF RISK

Estimates of mortality

Mortality is a vital, although somewhat crude, estimate of risk associated with anaesthesia. During the three decades up to 1980, a number of investigators in various countries had attempted to estimate the frequency with which death was associated with anaesthesia (Table 28.1). There was a general trend towards reduced mortality during this period, but the same principal causes of death continued to be identified: aspiration of gastric contents, airway obstruction, drug overdose, inadequate supervision of trainees, lack of postoperative care, insufficient monitoring and drug mistakes. One of the problems which renders comparison between these studies difficult is that different criteria were used to define anaesthetic death.

The Association of Anaesthetists of Great Britain and Ireland (AAGBI) had addressed the issue of mortality in 1956 and 1960, but these studies lacked denominator data. The AAGBI acquired funding from

686   CLINICAL ANAESTHESIA

Table 28.1 Estimates of the incidence of mortality due to anaesthesia between 1954 and 1980

Authors	Year of publication	Number of anaesthetics	Primary cause	Primary and associated cause
Beecher & Todd[3]	1954	599 548	1 : 2680	1 : 1560
Dornette & Orth[4]	1956	63 105	1 : 2427	1 : 1343
Schapira et al[5]	1960	22 177	1 : 1232	1 : 821
Phillips et al[6]	1960		1 : 7692	1 : 2500
Dripps et al[7]	1961	33 224	1 : 852	1 : 415
Clifton & Hotten[8]	1963	295 640	1 : 6048	1 : 3955
Memery[9]	1965	114 866	1 : 3145	1 : 1082
Gebbie[10]	1966	129 336		1 : 6158
Minuck[11]	1967	121 786	1 : 6766	1 : 3291
Harrison[12]	1968	177 928		1 : 3068
Marx et al[13]	1973	34 145		1 : 1265
Bodlander[14]	1975	211 130	1 : 14 075	1 : 1703
Harrison[15]	1978	240 483		1 : 4537
Hovi-Viander[16]	1980	338 934	1 : 5059	1 : 1412

the Nuffield Provincial Hospitals Trust for a major study of mortality in five regions in the UK. An anonymous and confidential system was established to report deaths which occurred within 6 days of surgery. Voluntary reports were assessed by a committee of expert reviewers, who included anaesthetists, surgeons and epidemiologists. During the study period, an estimated 1 147 362 operations took place in the five regions.[17] The overall peri-operative mortality (calculated from data supplied by the Department of Health and Social Security) was 0.53%, and 61.6% of these deaths were reported to the investigators; 10% of these were examined in detail. It was considered that anaesthesia was totally responsible for death in fewer than 1 : 10 000 operations, but that it may have contributed to death in 1 : 1700 operations, although it was recognized that there was great difficulty in identifying accurately the contribution of anaesthesia in deaths in which surgery had played a pivotal role. Death totally attributable to anaesthesia tended to occur in younger patients than death attributable to other causes. The conclusions of the authors are summarized in Table 28.2.

Because of the importance of the findings of Lunn and Mushin's study, and because of the difficulty in separating anaesthetic and surgical factors when reports came only from anaesthetists, the AAGBI initiated the first Confidential Enquiry into Perioperative Deaths (CEPOD) in conjunction with the Association of Surgeons of Great Britain and Ireland. For the first time, an attempt was made to distinguish between deaths related to surgery and those caused by anaesthesia. Three regions in the UK were studied over a 12-month period. The overall peri-operative mortality was 0.7%.[18] The CEPOD report identified 410 deaths associated with anaesthesia out of a total of 2928 deaths after 555 258 anaesthetics; factors which were believed to have contributed to death are shown in Table 28.3. However, expert assessors considered that only 3 deaths resulted solely from anaesthesia—an incidence of 1 in 185 086 anaesthetics. The reason for the vast improvement in comparison to the 1982 study was not explained, and is difficult to rationalize simply on the basis that surgeons were involved in analysing the causes of death.

The CEPOD studies have continued in the UK, although the emphasis on determining causation has been abandoned. Instead, the national CEPOD studies, which are now funded by the Department of Health, try to uncover issues of quality in the delivery of anaesthesia and surgery. Brief sets of data are collected on all deaths within 30 days of a surgical operation. Each year, a different sample is chosen for detailed study and a report published which highlights areas of concern which appear to have been associated with postoperative death and which indicate spheres of medical practice where improvement could be made. These studies also provide a valuable source of inform-

Table 28.2 Summary of Lunn & Mushin's conclusions in relation to peri-operative death related to anaesthesia[3]

- The overwhelming message is that the process of anaesthesia is remarkably safe
- Although the incidence of death attributable totally to anaesthesia is low, it is equivalent to approximately 280 deaths per year in the UK, the majority of which are probably avoidable
- In approximately 1800 deaths per year, anaesthesia may contribute; this also could largely be avoided
- The events which caused these deaths have not changed much over the past 30 years
- Mistakes occur in the hands of all grades of anaesthetists
- Trainee anaesthetists are often unsupervised and abandoned by their assistants
- The provision of essential monitoring instruments is inadequate, and where they are available, they are not always used
- Clinical anaesthetic records are not always kept
- There appears to be insufficient consultation between surgeon and anaesthetist
- A high proportion of patients suffer from intercurrent disease, and the implications for the anaesthetist are often ignored
- There are still hospitals where proper recovery facilities are not available
- Anaesthesia may contribute to deaths which occur more than 24 h after its administration
- Autopsy reports alone are of limited value in explaining deaths associated with anaesthesia

Table 28.3 Factors involved in deaths attributable in part to anaesthesia, in decreasing order of frequency

Failure to apply knowledge
Lack of care*
Failure of organization
Lack of experience
Lack of knowledge
Drug effect
Failure of equipment
Fatigue

*Including failure of a trainee to consult a more senior anaesthetist, grossly inadequate monitoring, inappropriate drug doses or other clear indication of a poor standard of practice.
Adapted from Buck et al.[18]

ation regarding current patterns of practice; for example, the degree of compliance with national guidelines on monitoring and the frequency with which anaesthetists undertake a pre-operative visit can be determined, at least in patients who have died in the postoperative period. Attempts have been made to gather comparator data from patients who survived surgery, but these proved to be difficult and unrewarding. Nevertheless, the feedback which is derived from the CEPOD and national CEPOD studies remains an invaluable form of quality audit from which improvements in surgical and anaesthetic care should result.

Studies from other countries have suggested higher incidences of death related to anaesthesia than that reported in the CEPOD study. From 1978 to 1982, the French Health Ministry conducted a prospective nationwide survey of major complications during anaesthesia. A representative sample of 198 103 anaesthetics was analysed from 460 institutions selected at random; this represented approximately 8% of the total estimated number of anaesthetics undertaken in France.[19] During anaesthesia, or within 24 h, 268 major anaesthesia-related complications occurred (1 in every 739 anaesthetics). There were 67 deaths within 24 h, and 16 patients suffered coma which persisted after 24 h. The incidence of death and coma attributable totally to anaesthesia was 1 : 7924; death due solely to anaesthesia occurred with an incidence of 1 : 13 207. In half of all the patients who died or suffered coma, postoperative respiratory depression was responsible; almost all of these patients had received narcotics and muscle relaxants during anaesthesia, neither of which had been reversed. Another striking feature was the high proportion of patients who were returned directly to the ward after anaesthesia because of the infrequent use of recovery rooms.

In New South Wales in Australia, a system has been in place since 1960 to undertake a confidential investigation of deaths related to anaesthesia. Deaths are categorized as anaesthetic, surgical, inevitable, fortuitous or unassessable. Deaths attributable to anaesthesia are assessed in detail for errors in management. The incidence of death attributable to anaesthesia decreased by a factor of 5 between 1960 and 1985, from 1 : 5500 to 1 : 26 000,[20] although the exact number of anaesthetics administered during each study period is uncertain. However, with the exception of delivery of a hypoxic mixture of gases, the pattern of errors of management by anaesthetists remained largely unchanged during the 25-year period (Table 28.4). The proportion of deaths attributable to anaesthesia in which no error could be found in management increased from 2.8% in the period 1960–1969 to 10% in the period 1983–1985. However, over the same period, the proportion of specialist anaesthetists involved in deaths attributable to anaesthesia increased from 27 to 62%.

In the Netherlands, a retrospective study of faults,

Table 28.4 Errors of management associated with death attributable to anaesthesia in New South Wales, Australia, between 1960 and 1985, ranked according to frequency

Error	1960–1969 No.	Rank	1970–1980 No.	Rank	1983–1985 No.	Rank
Inadequate preparation	102	3=	93	1	23	1
Wrong choice*	120	2	65	3	13	4
Overdose	127	1	34	7	14	3
Inhalation†	41	9	18	11	1	9=
Inadequate resuscitation	63	7	49	4	6	5=
Hypoxic mixture	14	12	0	–	0	–
Inadequate ventilation	68	5=	21	9	1	9=
Inadequate monitoring	22	11	19	10	6	5=
Technical mishap	25	10	40	6	1	9=
Inadequate crisis management	102	3=	80	2	4	8
Inadequate reversal‡	52	8	22	8	5	7
Inadequate postoperative management	68	5=	43	5	16	2
Total errors	804		484		90	
Errors per death	2.4		2.0		1.8	

* Wrong choice of agent or technique.
† Inhalation of gastric contents.
‡ Inadequate antagonism of neuromuscular block.
From Holland,[20] with permission.

accidents, near accidents and complications associated with anaesthesia in one institution was conducted between 1978 and 1987.[21] During that period, 113 074 anaesthetics were administered (97 496 for non-cardiac procedures). Cardiac arrest during non-cardiac surgery occurred with an incidence of 1 : 3362 anaesthetics, and mortality from cardiac arrest in these patients had an incidence of 1 : 5417 anaesthetics. Anaesthesia was considered to have contributed to cardiac arrest in 1 : 7500 anaesthetics (fatal outcome in 1 : 16 250 anaesthetics). Failure to check, lack of vigilance and carelessness were the most frequently associated human factors.

In Canada, the risk factors associated with death within 7 days of anaesthesia were analysed in a study involving 100 000 surgical procedures.[22] There were 71 deaths per 10 000 patients, and differences in anaesthetic practice were of much less importance in contributing to death than were other factors such as age, physical status and the type of surgery (Table 28.5). This is not surprising in view of the other evidence which has demonstrated that most deaths are not related to anaesthesia. Nevertheless, some anaesthetic factors were found to increase risk.

A study conducted in Denmark[23] examined the mortality and morbidity rates associated with anaesthesia. Mortality attributable to anaesthesia occurred with a frequency of 1 : 2500 (0.04%). The overall peri-operative mortality rate was 1.2%, and 0.05% of patients died during anaesthesia. Mortality in patients who developed postoperative cardiovascular complications was 20%. Two-thirds of the patients who developed an acute myocardial infarction in the peri-operative period died; half of these patients had received spinal or epidural anaesthesia and had suffered cardiovascular complications during the procedure. Hypotension before induction of anaesthesia was associated with a high risk of cardiopulmonary morbidity and mortality.

In the USA, an incidence of 1.7 cardiac arrests per 10 000 anaesthetics was reported in 1985,[24] although not all were fatal. The study involved 163 240 anaesthetics administered over a 15-year period. Of 449 cardiac arrests, 27 were judged to be attributable solely to anaesthesia, and mortality was 0.9 per 10 000 anaesthetics. Three-quarters of these cardiac arrests were considered to be preventable. Two major mechanisms led to cardiac arrest: overdose (55%) and failure of adequate ventilation (45%). Cardiac arrest was six times

Table 28.5 Risk factors associated with operative mortality within 7 days in Canada

Variable	Description	Relative odds of dying
Patient factors		
Age	>80 years versus <60 years	3.29
Sex	Female versus male	0.77
Physical status	ASA III–IV versus ASA I–II	10.65
Surgical factors		
Operation type	Major versus minor	3.82
Duration	>2 h versus < 2 h	1.08
Urgency	Emergency versus elective	4.44
Anaesthetic factors		
Techniques	Inhalation + opioids versus inhalation alone	0.76
	Opioid alone versus inhalation alone	1.41
	Opioid + inhalation versus inhalation alone	0.79
	Spinal versus inhalation alone	0.53
	Number of anaesthetic drugs: 1–2 versus 3+	2.94
Experience of anaesthetist	>600 procedures/year for 8+ years versus <600 procedures/year for <8 years	1.06

From Cohen et al,[22] with permission.
ASA III–IV = American Society of Anesthesiologists grade III–IV.

more likely during emergency anaesthesia than during elective procedures. Cardiac arrest was preceded by bradycardia in 26 of the 27 cases, but the bradycardia was frequently misinterpreted as being of cardiac origin, and was treated inappropriately. In 1991, the same authors published results relating to 241 934 anaesthetics over a 20-year period from 1969 to 1988.[25] They considered the incidences of cardiac arrest attributable to anaesthesia in the two decades 1969–1978 and 1979–1988; during the second decade, pulse oximetry and capnography were introduced. Cardiac arrest related to anaesthetic causes decreased from 2.1 per 10 000 anaesthetics in the first decade to 1.0 per 10 000 in the second decade. Most of this difference was due to a decrease in cardiac arrests from preventable respiratory causes, from 0.8 to 0.1 per 10 000 anaesthetics; the rates for preventable non-respiratory and for non-preventable arrests did not change significantly.

In 1989, Eichhorn[26] reported an incidence of death of 1 in 200 200 following the introduction of modern monitoring standards in nine hospitals. However, there is a crucial difference in methodology between Eichhorn's study and other mortality studies; only deaths reported to the hospitals' insurers were included. Thus, the incidence recorded was that of death associated with the *potential* for litigation. This may be a significant statistic in its own right, but it may overestimate or underestimate the true mortality rate which, on close analysis, can be attributed to anaesthesia.

Estimates of morbidity

Reference has been made above to some studies which have estimated the frequency of serious morbidity as well as mortality. The Multicenter Study in the USA[27–29] was conducted in an attempt to analyse predictors of severe peri-operative adverse outcome related to general anaesthesia. A total of 17 201 patients were studied, and randomized to receive enflurane, fentanyl, halothane or isoflurane for general anaesthesia. They were followed up for 7 days for the occurrence of 14 specified outcomes (Table 28.6). The major risk factors for severe outcome were: cardiovascular surgery, thoracic surgery or abdominal surgery; history of cardiac failure, myocardial infarction, myocardial ischaemia or hypertension; age over 50 years; American Society of Anesthesiologists (ASA) status III or IV; and type of anaesthetic. However, this study dealt very superficially with anaesthesia, and was biased towards an influence of concomitant disease because patients undergoing cardiac and cardiovascular surgery were included. The study was too small to detect important differences (if they exist) between the anaesthetic techniques.

In Canada, data have been collected since 1975 relating to adverse outcomes from anaesthesia. The Canadian Four-Centre Study was based on data from 27 184 patients who underwent anaesthesia and surgery between 1987 and 1989.[30,31] One of the purposes was

Table 28.6 Adverse outcomes defined in the Multicenter Study

Hypotension
Hypertension
Tachycardia
Ventricular arrhythmia
Bradycardia
Atrial arrhythmia
Cardiac failure
Myocardial ischaemia
Myocardial infarction
Bronchospasm
Respiratory failure
Secretions
Any severe myocardial outcome
Any severe respiratory outcome

From Forrest et al,[27-29] with permission.

to identify whether measurement of morbidity was a satisfactory method of comparing quality of anaesthetic care in different institutions. A panel of experts defined 115 major events, and classified them into anaesthesia-related, surgery-related or disease-related categories. There was an anaesthetic involvement in 10.3% of major events. There were no anaesthetic deaths. The authors concluded that measuring quality of care in anaesthesia by comparing major outcomes is unsatisfactory because the contribution of anaesthesia to outcome is often uncertain, and because variations among hospitals may be explained by institutional differences which are beyond the control of the anaesthetist. While the author's reasons for rejecting this method of study may be justifiable in respect of comparisons among hospitals, their general rejection of measurement of major morbidity as an index of quality of care in anaesthesia must be questioned seriously.

Pedersen[9] reported a very high incidence (9%) of intra-operative cardiopulmonary complications associated with anaesthesia *or* surgery, and requiring intervention during the procedure. These were most common in patients aged 70 years or more, in those with pre-operative signs of ischaemic heart disease or a recent myocardial infarction, in patients with chronic cardiac failure or chronic obstructive airways disease, and in those undergoing emergency procedures involving major abdominal surgery. There was a trend suggesting that regional anaesthesia was safer in elderly patients with chronic obstructive airways disease who underwent major orthopaedic surgery. One-third of all complications were considered to be preventable.

The incidences of uncommon major events, such as malignant hyperthermia, anaphylaxis and anaesthetic-associated hepatic necrosis are also important, and have been documented in specific studies. Minor complications are often dismissed by doctors as of little relevance, but are an important source of discomfort, distress and dissatisfaction of patients. Edmonds-Seal & Eve[32] conducted a small study (513 patients) in an attempt to quantify the incidences of minor sequelae. Most patients reported a dry mouth. Vomiting and sore throat were the commonest of the other complications, but patients reported a wide variety of complaints which were mostly temporary, but which affected almost half of all the patients studied (Table 28.7).

Cohen et al[33] reported the incidence of non-fatal complications in a survey of 112 000 anaesthetics administered over a 9-year period, although the majority did not lead to morbidity. One or more anaesthetic complications occurred in 17.8% of patients. Most were minor. Arrhythmias were the most frequent intra-operative complication (365 per 10 000 anaesthetics), but the intra-operative incidence of cardiac arrest was only 7 per 10 000 anaesthetics, so that most arrhythmias appear to have had little impact on outcome. Nausea, vomiting and sore throat were the commonest postoperative complications. An interesting observation was that the incidence of arrhythmias, hypotension and hypertension appeared to increase during the study

Table 28.7 Minor complaints reported by 241 of 531 patients interviewed in the postoperative period

Complaint	Percentage of patients
Dry mouth	>50.0
Vomiting	22.0
Bruises	14.2
Sore throat	
Slight	10.5
Severe	1.9
Loss of voice or hoarseness	1.6
Backache	4.9
Pain at side of jaw	3.1
Headache	2.7
Pain in the heels	2.1
Cough	2.1
Pain around knee	1.7
Pain at elbow	1.7
Dental trauma	1.2
Bruising over upper lip	0.9
Muscle pains	0.7
Pain in the eye	0.6
Pain over bridge of nose	0.4
Laceration of tongue	0.2
Temporary deafness	0.2
Weakness/numbness of hand	0.2
Pain in antecubital fossa	0.2

From Edmonds-Seal & Eve,[32] with permission.

period. In the first 4-year period, 7.6% of patients had one or more intra-operative complications, and post-operative complications occurred in 3.1%; in the second 4-year period, the corresponding figures were 10.6 and 5.9%. This difference was probably related to the increased use of monitoring. In the first period, there was a 9.4% chance of patients suffering a postoperative complication which was related to anaesthesia, and the probability of morbidity was 0.45%; in the second period, the risks were 8.9 and 0.4%. The incidence of complications was (unsurprisingly) higher in patients who were seen in the postoperative period than in those discharged early from hospital; thus, the total incidence of complications was almost certainly underestimated.

Cooper et al[34] studied patients admitted to an intensive care unit (ICU) as a result of serious complications of anaesthesia. Over a 5-year period, 81 780 operative procedures were performed, and a total of 2651 patients were admitted to the ICU. Fifty-three patients (1 in 1543 procedures; 2% of ICU admissions) were admitted as a result of complications of anaesthesia. The majority of complications (62%) occurred in the recovery period, and just over half of all complications involved emergency surgery, although only 12% of procedures were of an emergency nature. As would be expected in this type of study, most complications involved the respiratory or cardiovascular systems. One-quarter of the complications were judged to have been avoidable, and 17% of the patients died.

Critical incident reporting

Critical incident reporting is a technique which was developed by psychologists to evaluate aspects of human behaviour and to study the causes of good and bad performance. An incident is any observable human activity that is sufficiently complete in itself to permit inferences and predictions to be made about the person performing the act. A critical incident is an incident whose purpose or intent is clear to the observer and the consequences of which are sufficiently definite to leave little doubt about its effect. The technique was first described in 1954,[35] but had been used extensively by the US Air Force during the Second World War. Trained observers collected large numbers of factual observations which made an important positive or negative contribution to the activity being studied (for example, the reasons for failure of bombing missions). When these critical incidents were studied, they could be categorized, and steps could be taken to improve success (for example, in guiding recruitment policy so that pilots with good performance could be predicted) and to reduce failure (for example, by improving cockpit design).

In medicine, the critical incident technique has been applied to identifying the causes of errors in administration of drugs by nurses,[36] the quality of care by paediatricians, obstetricians, physicians and surgeons[37] and analysis of professional behaviour in doctors involved in child health.[38] The first report of its use in anaesthesia was in 1978. Cooper et al[39] examined errors and equipment failures in anaesthetic practice. Their definition of a critical incident was:

an occurrence that could have led (if not corrected and discovered in time) or did lead to an undesirable outcome ranging from increased length of hospital stay to death. It must also involve error by a member of the anaesthetic team or a failure of the anesthetists' equipment to function; occur while the patient is under anaesthetic care; be described in clear detail by an observer or member of the anesthetic team; and be clearly preventable.

The large majority of critical incidents do not lead to an adverse outcome. The technique is therefore valuable because much larger quantities of data can be collected than by identification of adverse outcomes and analysis of the causes. In their first study, Cooper et al[39] employed an interview technique; anaesthetists were asked to describe preventable happenings which they had observed involving either equipment failure or human error. The interviews lasted between 60 and 90 min, and a total of 72 interviews were conducted. Staff anaesthetists reported an average of seven incidents, and trainees reported an average of eight; more than half of the incidents had occurred within the previous 6 months, but one-fifth had occurred more than 3 years earlier. The most frequent events involved breathing system disconnections, inadvertent changes in gas flows, errors with syringes, problems with gas supply and disconnection of intravenous lines. Inadequate experience, unfamiliarity with equipment, poor communication, haste, inattention, fatigue and failure to perform equipment checks were cited as associated factors.

In subsequent studies,[40–42] the same group collected data prospectively, using anonymized reporting, produced a more specific analysis of mishaps with substantive negative outcomes and evaluated the effectiveness of some monitoring devices. The early studies can be criticized on the basis that retrospective reporting is prone to error because memory decays rapidly, but their early work was, nevertheless, invaluable, and was instrumental in the routine adoption of the use of low-pressure alarms in ventilator circuits.

Critical incident reporting has been adopted widely over the last decade. Many anaesthetic departments collect data internally,[43] using the data to identify and correct faults with specific items of equipment, to modify protocols, guidelines and training, and to provide feedback at departmental meetings. One of the largest studies is the Australian Incident Monitoring Study,[44] which, in 1993, reported in detail the findings from analysis of the first 2000 incident reports. The commonest incidents cited in reports of such studies are shown in Table 28.8, and the most commonly quoted associated factors in Table 28.9. There is a close similarity with the factors which contributed to death in the CEPOD study[18] (Table 28.3). Cooper et al[41] reported that 70 patients suffered a substantive negative outcome (death, cardiac arrest, cancelled operation, extended stay in the recovery room, ICU or hospital) from 1089 critical incidents. There was an average of 2.5 critical incidents in patients with a negative outcome and 3.4 associated factors. There was also a higher frequency of moderately or severely ill patients among those who had a negative outcome (71%) in comparison to the overall frequency of similar patients in whom critical incidents were reported (41%). In the Australian Incident Monitoring Study, minor physiological changes occurred in association with 30% of incidents, major physiological changes but no injury followed 18%, physical morbidity occurred in 6%, awareness in 1% and death was associated with 1.5%.[45]

Critical incident techniques have an important place in identification of risk and improvement of safety by drawing the attention of anaesthetists to potential errors and by identifying deficiencies in equipment design and function. However, there are potential disadvantages associated with continuous critical incident reporting. An individual anaesthetist who is conscientious in reporting critical incidents in a departmental system, or an individual department in a national scheme, may be regarded as a poor performer if there is any breach of anonymity, and this may encourage under-reporting. Similarly, an apathetic individual or department not only causes under-reporting, but may appear (justifiably or not) to be a good performer. Continuous reporting may result in loss of enthusiasm with time, causing progressively increasing under-reporting; limiting reporting to specific areas of anaesthetic practice in rotation might help to maintain enthusiasm. In addition, it is necessary to define the term 'critical incident' carefully; some authors have used Cooper's original definition, but others have used the term to describe events which may or may not be preventable, which may or may not include anaesthetic error or equipment failure, and which may include only incidents which result in an adverse outcome. The term 'real or potential adverse event' has been proposed[46] as a self-explanatory and unambiguous alternative.

Table 28.8 Examples of the most commonly quoted critical incidents

Problems with breathing system
Disconnections
Misconnections
Leaks

Problems in administration of drugs
Overdosage
Underdosage
Wrong drug

Problems with intubation and control of airway
Failed intubation
Oesophageal intubation
Endobronchial intubation
Accidental or premature extubation
Aspiration

Failure of equipment
Laryngoscopes
Intravenous infusion devices
Breathing system valves
Monitoring devices

Table 28.9 Examples of the commonest factors associated with critical incidents

Inattention/carelessness
Inexperience
Haste
Failure to check equipment
Unfamiliarity with equipment
Poor communication
Restricted visual field or access
Failure of planning
Distraction
Lack of skilled assistance
Lack of supervision
Fatigue and decreased vigilance

Litigation

Because of the high rate of litigation against anaesthetists in some countries, analysis of claims for compensation has been used to examine the pattern of injury which patients may suffer, or believe that they have suffered, as a result of the actions of anaesthetists. There is a risk of bias in analysing claims for compensation, in that the complaints relate predominantly to events which the patient does not expect. For example, totally inept treatment of postoperative pain is very unlikely (at present) to result in a claim for compensa-

Table 28.10 Causes of anaesthetic-related death or cerebral damage in 750 cases reported to the Medical Defence Union between 1970 and 1982

Mainly misadventure		Mainly error	
Coexisting disease	14%	Faulty technique	43%
Unknown	6%	Failure of postoperative care	9%
Drug sensitivity	5%	Drug overdosage	5%
Hypotension/blood loss	4%	Inadequate preoperative assessment	3%
Halothane-associated hepatic failure	3%	Drug error	1%
Hyperpyrexia	2%	Anaesthetist's failure	1%
Embolism	2%		

From Utting,[47] with permission.

tion, because the patient expects to experience postoperative pain. In addition, the pattern of claims is influenced by the personality of the patient, and, in some countries, by the availability of free legal advice. However, anaesthesia is probably less subject to the effects of bias than most other medical specialties because the majority of patients who undergo elective surgery are healthy. While patients are prepared to accept that surgery may not be entirely successful, or may be associated with a small incidence of complications, they anticipate perfection from the anaesthetist and are often unwilling to acknowledge that any consequence which they attribute to anaesthesia, or the anaesthetist, is acceptable. In one extreme example, a patient attempted to sue her anaesthetist for failing to diagnose breast cancer at the pre-operative visit when she underwent cystoscopy; the tumour was diagnosed 6 months later.

Causes of complaint

Table 28.10 lists the causes of death or cerebral damage in cases reported to the Medical Defence Union between 1970 and 1982;[47] the majority were associated with errors. Table 28.11 shows the detailed causes of the incidents which resulted from errors. Recently, death attributable to negligence by anaesthetists has resulted in convictions for manslaughter[48] as well as civil litigation. Less serious incidents may result in distress or physical injury to patients, and may be followed by claims for compensation. The most common events reported to the Medical Defence Union between 1970 and 1982 are shown in Table 28.12. Damage to teeth was by far the single most common complaint, accounting for 52% of reports. The pattern of more serious injuries leading to litigation, or threatened litigation, in a recent review[49] is shown in Table 28.13. The most common single group of complaints in this series related to damage to the brain or spinal cord. Allegations of negligence causing death during anaes-

Table 28.11 Causes of anaesthetic-related death or cerebral damage reported to the Medical Defence Union between 1970 and 1982 in 326 cases thought to be the result of errors in technique

Cause	% of total
Errors associated with tracheal intubation	31
Misuse of apparatus	23
Inhalation of gastric contents	14
Errors associated with induced hypotension	8
Hypoxia	4
Obstructed airway	4
Accidental pneumothorax/haemopericardium	4
Errors associated with extradural analgesia	3
Use of nitrous oxide instead of oxygen	2
Use of carbon dioxide instead of oxygen	2
Errors associated with Bier's block	2
Underventilation	1
Use of halothane with adrenaline	1
Mismatched blood transfusion	<1
Vasovagal attack	<1

From Utting,[47] with permission.

Table 28.12 Untoward anaesthetic-related events (other than death or cerebral damage) in 1501 cases reported to the Medical Defence Union between 1970 and 1982

Event	% of total
Damage to teeth	52
Peripheral nerve damage	9
Extradural foreign bodies (needles, catheter tips)	7
Superficial thrombophlebitis and minor injuries (e.g. abrasions)	7
Awareness	7
Spinal cord damage	4
Pneumothoraces	3
Extravasation of injected drugs	2
Lacerations, falls from table	2
Impaired renal function (mismatched blood transfusion)	1
Burns	1
Others	5

From Utting,[47] with permission.

Table 28.13 Categories of injury alleged in a series of 150 claims of negligence related to anaesthesia reviewed in 1989 and 1990

Alleged injury	% of claims
Brain/spinal cord damage	23.8
Death in postoperative period	17.0
Awareness during general anaesthesia	12.2
Death during anaesthesia	11.6
Pain during regional anaesthesia	7.5
Peripheral nerve damage	4.1
Miscellaneous injuries	23.9

From Aitkenhead,[49] with permission.

thesia were less common than those associated with death in the postoperative period; most of the latter related to death within the first 12 h after anaesthesia. The miscellaneous injuries referred to in Table 28.13 are detailed in Table 28.14. Table 28.15 shows common sources of litigation relating to management by staff of the ICU.

In the USA, the Committee of Professional Liability of the ASA began a structured evaluation of adverse anaesthetic outcomes with the purpose of improving safety by devising strategies to prevent anaesthetic mishaps. Data were extracted from closed claims files of 17 insurance organizations which indemnify doctors. The files normally include the hospital and other relevant medical records, witness statements, expert opinions, reports on the outcome of the case and, if the claim has been successful, the cost of settlement or

Table 28.14 Details of miscellaneous injuries referred to in Table 28.13

Fetal damage
Suxamethonium pains
Fractured ribs
Tissued infusions
Skin necrosis
Ischaemic legs
Laryngeal damage
Retropharyngeal abscess
Halothane hepatitis
Enflurane intoxication
Pneumothorax
Inhaled rubber glove
Post-spinal headache
Unnecessary tracheostomy
Tracheal stenosis
Myocardial infarction
Blood transfusion to Jehovah's Witness
Retained epidural catheter tip
Renal failure

Modified from Aitkenhead.[49]

Table 28.15 Common allegations against anaesthetists relating to management of patients in the intensive care unit (ICU)

Delay in recognizing need for transfer to ICU
Delay in instituting treatment before transfer
Delay in transfer
Complications during transfer (especially between hospitals)
Complications of tracheal intubation
Complications of mechanical ventilation
Unnecessary tracheostomy
Complications of tracheostomy
Complications of vascular catheterization
Inadequate monitoring
Inadequate sedation and/or analgesia
Excessive sedation
Hypoxaemia
Inadequate treatment of hypotension
Inadequate treatment of hypertension
Undertransfusion
Overtransfusion
Skin necrosis
Inadequate measures to protect the brain following cardiac arrest
Undue haste in weaning from mechanical ventilation/extubation/discharge
Deterioration following discharge/delay in re-admission

jury award. Each claim is analysed by an anaesthesiologist who has been specially trained for the closed claim study.

In the first report[50] in 1988, Caplan et al reviewed 14 cases of unexpected cardiac arrest in healthy patients who had received spinal anaesthesia. In a number of these cases, it was postulated that respiratory insufficiency had occurred in relation to administration of sedatives. In others, death was related to cardiovascular insufficiency which had often been treated inappropriately. The second report[51] assessed the potential role of monitoring devices for the prevention of anaesthetic mishaps. It was considered by reviewers that 31.5% of negative outcomes in 1097 claims could have been prevented by the use of additional monitors, particularly pulse oximetry and capnography. In addition, it was noted that the injuries which were, in the reviewers' opinion, preventable by this mechanism were more severe in terms of injury and cost of settlement. These findings applied to adverse outcomes associated with regional as well as general anaesthesia. However, the conclusions of the investigators can be questioned (see the section on monitoring, below).

The third closed claim report[52] concerned specifically adverse respiratory events, which constituted the single largest category of injury (dental damage was excluded from the studies), accounting for 34% of

1541 closed claim files examined. Adverse respiratory events accounted for the worst outcomes; death or brain damage occurred in 85% of cases compared with 30% of non-respiratory events (Table 28.16). The percentage of claims in which the management was considered to have been substandard was much higher for respiratory than non-respiratory events, and particularly in cases of inadequate ventilation and oesophageal intubation (Fig. 28.1). A subsequent report[53] focused on five less frequent respiratory events in 300 claims:

1. *Airway trauma* most frequently involved the larynx, pharynx and oesophagus. Less than half of the cases occurred in association with difficult intubation, but these patients were more likely to suffer perforation of the pharynx or oesophagus, leading to mediastinitis. Other injuries included vocal cord paralysis, arytenoid dislocation, granuloma formation and injury to the temporomandibular joint.

2. *Pneumothorax* was related predominantly to intercostal block, supraclavicular brachial plexus block and airway instrumentation; only 16% of cases involved barotrauma and 7% insertion of a central venous catheter.

3. *Airway obstruction* involved predominantly the upper airway; laryngospasm accounted for more than 25% of cases. In 9% of patients, obstruction involved a tracheal tube. Airway obstruction was commoner in children than in adults.

4. *Aspiration* occurred most commonly during maintenance of anaesthesia with a face mask, but a significant proportion of episodes of aspiration occurred during either induction or emergence. More than half of the cases occurred during elective procedures.

5. *Bronchospasm* occurred principally during induction of general anaesthesia. In half of the patients, there was no history of pulmonary disease or smoking. In a significant proportion of cases, there was difficulty in

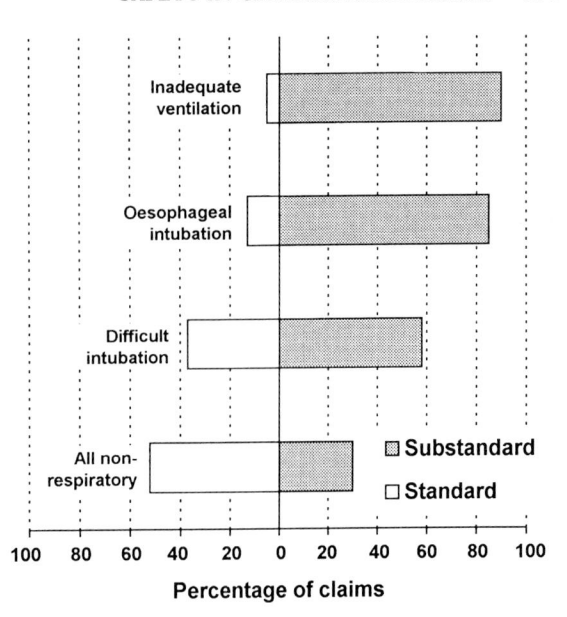

Fig. 28.1 Percentage of claims in which reviewers considered management by the anaesthetist to be substandard or acceptable in relation to events involving respiratory and non-respiratory causes of injury. Data from the American Society of Anesthesiologists closed claim study.[52]

Table 28.16 Outcome, payment and payment frequency for respiratory and non-respiratory events analysed in the American Society of Anesthesiologists closed claim study

	All respiratory events (n = 522)	Inadequate ventilation (n = 196)	Oesophageal intubation (n = 94)	Difficult tracheal intubation (n = 87)	All non-respiratory events (n = 1019)
Outcome (% of cases)					
Death	66	71	81	46	22
Permanent brain damage	19	23	17	10	8
Other permanent injury	5	1	1	18	25
Temporary injury	9	4	1	24	39
No injury	1	1	0	1	6
Payment (in $1000)					
Median	200	240	217	76	35
Range	1–6000	1.5–6000	30–3400	1–4700	<1–5400
Payment frequency (% of claims settled)	72	73	82	67	51

From Caplan et al,[52] with permission.

differentiating bronchospasm from oesophageal intubation or pneumothorax.

Other reports from the ASA closed claim study have examined the pattern of injury in obstetric and paediatric patients. In 1991,[54] 190 claims from a total of 1351 related to obstetric practice. The commonest injuries were maternal death (22% compared with 39% in non-obstetric patients), neonatal brain damage (20%) and headache (12%). There was a larger number of minor injuries (headache, backache, pain during anaesthesia, emotional injury) than in non-obstetric patients (32 versus 4%). Claims involving general anaesthesia were more frequently associated with severe injury than those associated with regional anaesthesia. In 1993,[55] 238 of a total of 2400 claims related to children (under 15 years of age). Respiratory events were commoner (43 versus 30%) and mortality higher (50 versus 35%) than in adults. These increased frequencies were explained predominantly by the higher incidence of inadequate ventilation (23 versus 9%) in children. Reviewers considered that 89% of cases involving inadequate ventilation could have been prevented by the use of pulse oximetry and capnography; however, in only one of the seven claims in which a pulse oximeter was used did it prevent a poor outcome from inadequate ventilation. A subsequent report[56] analysed 54 claims for burns. The commonest causes were related to the use of bags or bottles of fluids warmed in an oven and then placed in contact with the patient to encourage rewarming, or warming mattresses.

A worrying report from Japan[57] found that, in analysing in detail 64 lawsuits relating to anaesthesia, there were a large number of deaths from cardiac arrest or hypotension during spinal anaesthesia administered by non-anaesthetists—a practice which is still common in that country. Human error was the most frequent cause of injury among cases involving anaesthetists, but in the non-anaesthetist cases, there was usually a lack of, or gross omission of, intra-operative monitors.

COMMON INJURIES AND ERRORS

Cerebral damage and death

Damage to the central nervous system during anaesthesia and in the postoperative period may result in death, a variable degree of disability or complete recovery. Causes related to anaesthesia itself, or to administration of drugs in the postoperative period, are associated almost exclusively with arterial hypoxaemia or cerebral ischaemia. In addition, cerebral damage may occur as a result of treatment in the ICU.

Hypoxaemia

This is the commonest reason for cerebral damage and death during anaesthesia and the postoperative period. It may arise from failure to deliver an adequate inspired oxygen concentration, an abnormality of the lungs which impairs oxygenation of pulmonary capillary blood or a failure of ventilation.

Inspired oxygen concentration

Oxygen supply. Occasionally, errors have occurred in the connections of pipelines at source, and nitrous oxide has been delivered through the oxygen pipeline; this is particularly hazardous, as the first instinct of the anaesthetist presented with a hypoxaemic patient is to supply 100% oxygen. Although the pipeline system in the operating theatre is provided with fittings designed to prevent misconnection, there have been instances in which the nitrous oxide pipeline has been connected to the oxygen inlet of the machine and vice versa; these have occurred when hospital staff attempt to use non-standard or damaged equipment, or when old anaesthetic machines without pin-index systems or colour coding were serviced in haste.[58] Faulty air/oxygen mixers may allow contamination of one pipeline gas with the contents of the other. If the pressure in the air pipeline is higher, air leaks into the oxygen pipeline, reducing the oxygen concentration with the potential for delivery of a dangerously low inspired oxygen concentration when the 'oxygen' is mixed with nitrous oxide.[59]

Flowmeters. Rotameter bobbins may give erroneous readings if the rotameter tube becomes contaminated with dirt, or if static electricity collects on the glass walls. The glass tubes are fragile, and occasionally break; if a leak develops above the bobbin either because of a fractured tube or a faulty O-ring seal, the flow rate of oxygen delivered is less than that indicated by the bobbin, especially if the nitrous oxide rotameter is positioned closer to the patient than the oxygen rotameter, and a hypoxic gas mixture may be delivered to the patient. Leaks in other flowmeters (e.g. carbon dioxide, cyclopropane) may also cause leakage of oxygen and a reduced concentration in the inspired gas mixture.[60] In some machines, oxygen may be lost from the anaesthetic gas mixture if a blanking plug, which is positioned adjacent to the top of the oxygen rotameter tube and unscrewed during servicing to measure pressure in the back-bar in order to detect leaks, is not replaced securely.[61] Other gases, for example carbon dioxide, may be delivered in the gas mixture in error, especially if the needle valve is fully open and the bobbin is at the top of the rotameter tube, where it may not be seen by the anaesthetist. The UK is almost now the only country in the world in which the potentially lethal incorporation of a carbon dioxide supply on the anaesthetic machine exists.

Breathing systems. A hypoxic gas mixture may be delivered when a circle system is supplied with low flow rates of oxygen and nitrous oxide because, after the first few minutes of anaesthesia, oxygen is absorbed from the lungs at a greater rate than nitrous oxide. An inappropriately low flow rate of anaesthetic gases to other breathing systems, a leak within the breathing system at its connection with the anaesthetic machine or a leak within the back-bar of the anaesthetic machine may cause rebreathing of gases and inhalation of a progressively hypoxic gas mixture.

Inadequate ventilation. Inadequate ventilation, or total failure of ventilation, results in a decrease in alveolar and arterial oxygen tension and an increase in carbon dioxide tension; the absolute value of oxygen tension depends principally on the alveolar minute ventilation and the inspired oxygen concentration, although the presence of pyrexia may influence the values because of increased oxygen consumption and carbon dioxide production. In addition, hypoxaemia occurs more rapidly if the functional residual capacity (FRC) is low (e.g. pregnant or obese patients). Total failure of ventilation in a normal patient who has been breathing 33% oxygen results in significant arterial hypoxaemia ($PaO_2 < 6.5$ kPa) in about 5 min, but this occurs in less than 2 min in a patient who has been breathing air (e.g. immediately after induction of anaesthesia) and in 1–1.5 min, and sometimes less, in a patient with reduced FRC or pulmonary disease.

Pharmacological depression. Hypoventilation, or apnoea, may be caused by a relative overdose of anaesthetic agent or opioid in the spontaneously breathing patient, and a degree of hypoxaemia may result during anaesthesia. In the immediate postoperative period, the residual effects of these drugs may cause hypoventilation or apnoea because of the absence of surgical stimulation. In the later postoperative period, excessive doses of opioid analgesics given to treat wound pain may cause ventilatory depression and hypoxaemia, especially in elderly patients. This is likely to occur particularly if a continuous infusion of an opioid is employed, as accumulation may take place.[62] Respiratory arrest may be of relatively rapid onset. There has been an increase in popularity of intrathecal or epidural administration of opioids to provide postoperative pain relief after major surgery. Although these techniques are often more effective than conventional systemic administration, there is a documented risk of sudden depression of ventilation many hours after the last administration of analgesic. This is particularly true when lipid-insoluble drugs such as morphine are used, but can occur after administration of any opioid in the vicinity of the spinal cord. In the early postoperative period, residual neuromuscular blockade may cause hypoventilation, or occasionally complete paralysis and apnoea, even if an anticholinesterase drug has been given at the end of the operation. This is most likely when a long-acting relaxant has been given, or if renal function is impaired. Hypoventilation or apnoea may occur in association with the injection of local anaesthetic drugs for subarachnoid or extradural anaesthesia.

Obstruction of equipment. Anaesthetic breathing sytems and connecting tubes may become kinked, or obstructed by a foreign body or manufacturing fault. An amazing variety of objects have obstructed anaesthetic apparatus, including insects, items of equipment used for intravenous access and spinal needles; in some cases, only sabotage could explain the presence of the obstruction. Most anaesthetic tubing is kink-resistant, but standard tracheal tubes may kink in the pharynx, particularly if the neck is flexed or rotated during surgery; reinforced tubes should be used for operations in which such movements are predictable. Breathing system tubing may be compressed by the wheel of the anaesthetic machine or monitoring trolley, or by the feet of unobservant operating department personnel. Overinflation of a tracheal tube cuff, or a weakness in the wall of the cuff, may result in its herniation beyond the end of the tracheal tube, where it may obstruct the tube lumen. The lumen may also become obstructed if the bevel abuts against the wall of the trachea; this may cause a ball-valve effect which will eventually prevent inflation of the lungs.

Upper airway obstruction. In the patient whose trachea is not intubated, airway obstruction may occur in the pharynx because of collapse of the pharyngeal wall during inspiration. The pattern of ventilation is usually monitored closely during anaesthesia by observing the movement of the reservoir bag. However, monitoring is more difficult in the recovery room, where partial obstruction of the airway is a frequent occurrence, and total obstruction not uncommon. Laryngospasm may cause total upper airway obstruction in association with anaesthesia, especially shortly after induction and during recovery. Severe laryngospasm results in the rapid development of hypoxaemia if appropriate measures are not taken; occasionally, hypoxaemia may occur later as a result of fulminant pulmonary oedema (see below). Upper airway obstruction may be one of the presenting complaints of a patient undergoing anaesthesia, e.g. inhaled foreign body, acute epiglottitis. A skilled anaesthetist is required in the management of these patients because not only may tracheal intubation be extremely difficult, but total airway obstruction may occur as soon as consciousness is lost. Use of an inappropriate anaesthetic technique may increase the risk of hypoxaemia. Rarely, upper airway obstruction may result from inhalation of solid material (food or clotted blood) regurgitated from the stomach of the anaesthetized patient before a tracheal tube has been introduced.

Lower airway obstruction. Lower airway obstruction is usually the result of bronchospasm. This is commoner in the asthmatic patient, in whom it may be precipitated by administration of drugs which release histamine, or by the introduction of a tracheal tube. However, it may occur with no apparent precipitating factor, and can be so severe that ventilation of the lungs is impossible. Bronchospasm may occur in non-asthmatic patients as a result of aspiration of gastric contents, in response to irritation of the tracheobronchial tree by an airway or tracheal tube, or as part of an adverse drug reaction.

Misplacement of the tracheal tube. This is the commonest single cause of serious hypoxaemia resulting in death or cerebral damage (see Table 28.11). Oesophageal intubation occurs most frequently in the hands of the inexperienced, and particularly non-anaesthetists who attempt to intubate the trachea at a cardiac arrest or in the emergency department. However, virtually every anaesthetist intubates the oesophagus inadvertently from time to time. In some patients, it is impossible to visualize the larynx at direct laryngoscopy, and blind intubation is necessary. Oesophageal intubation is not always easy to detect.[63] Observation of the chest or auscultation of the lungs may be misleading, especially in the obese patient. The stomach may inflate *and* deflate in some patients when artificial ventilation is applied, although the pattern of refilling of the anaesthetic reservoir bag is seldom normal; however, when a self-inflating bag (e.g. Ambu bag) is employed, as often happens at a cardiac arrest or in the emergency department, the abnormal expiratory pattern is difficult to detect. Similarly, if the tracheal tube is immediately connected to a mechanical ventilator, ventilation may appear to be taking place normally. Small movements of the reservoir bag may occur during attempts at spontaneous ventilation when the oesophagus is intubated. Oesophageal intubation in the paralysed patient causes a progressive reduction in alveolar oxygen tension as the oxygen in the lungs is taken up by blood in the pulmonary capillaries. However, if the lungs have been pre-oxygenated, it may be up to 10 min before alveolar oxygen tension decreases below normal and arterial oxygen saturation starts to fall; saturation then decreases very rapidly. If the effect of pre-oxygenation is not appreciated, the anaesthetist may waste valuable time looking for other causes when hypoxaemia eventually becomes apparent.

Disconnection or ventilator failure. This was one of the common causes of critical incidents identified in Cooper's early studies.[39] Most mechanical ventilators are robust and reliable, but occasionally they malfunction and fail to deliver gas to the patient. More commonly, a disconnection occurs at some point between the ventilator and the tracheal tube; it is common, particularly with the incorporation of monitoring devices, to have 10 or more sites at which disconnection could occur. A loose connection may cause gas to leak from the system, resulting in hypoventilation. However, the positive pressure in the system may cause a loose joint to become completely disconnected, resulting in total failure of ventilation. Disconnections may occur because the tubing has been assembled carelessly, or if one of the operating theatre personnel dislodges a tube inadvertently while moving in the vicinity of the ventilator.

Other causes. Ventilation may be impaired by increased diaphragmatic pressure during spontaneous ventilation, particularly if the abdomen is distended (e.g. during laparoscopy) or if the patient is placed in a steep head-down position. Occasionally, ventilation may be inadequate because of the presence of air or fluid in the pleural cavity.

Pulmonary disease. Patients with pulmonary disease may become hypoxaemic during anaesthesia unless a high inspired oxygen concentration is provided. During one-lung anaesthesia, arterial oxygen saturation is often subnormal even when 100% oxygen is administered; it is possible for the bronchial portion of the double-lumen tube to occlude one or more lobes of the ventilated lung,[64] resulting in severe hypoxaemia.

Pulmonary oedema may develop during or after anaesthesia. The commonest cause is cardiac disease, but excessive fluid administration may result in accumulation of fluid in the alveoli, and occasionally acute upper airway obstruction (e.g. laryngospasm) may result in pulmonary oedema because of the hydrostatic gradient generated across the pulmonary capillary membrane by the highly negative intra-alveolar pressures which occur when the patient attempts to breathe.[65]

Failure of oxygen delivery

Reduced tissue blood flow. This may result from impairment of cardiac output or extreme hypotension for some other reason.

Cardiac contractility. Most anaesthetic agents decrease cardiac contractility in a dose-related manner. This may result in a critical reduction of cardiac output if excessive concentrations, particularly of inhaled anaesthetics, are given or if the patient has received other drugs (e.g. β-blockers) with a negative inotropic effect. Inadvertent intravascular injection of local anaesthetics may reduce contractility, as does high (mid-thoracic or above) spinal or epidural anaesthesia. Patients with pre-existing cardiac disease may be more sensitive to the negative inotropic effects of anaesthetic drugs. Patients with ischaemic heart disease may suffer a reduction of cardiac contractility in the presence of otherwise innocuous degrees of hypoxaemia, tachycardia, hypertension or hypotension.

Cardiac arrhythmias. Probably the commonest arrhythmia during anaesthesia is sinus bradycardia, which usually results from vagal stimulation induced by surgical procedures, and which may be exacerbated by the vagal effects of some anaesthetic agents; halothane is particularly associated with this complication, but it may occur after administration of other anaesthetic or analgesic drugs, and is more likely in the presence of β-blockers. Cardiac output may be reduced by atrial or ventricular arrhythmias. However, these rarely result in serious hypotension unless a severe tachycardia is present. Hypoxaemia also predisposes to abnormal cardiac rhythm or conduction, as do electrolyte abnormalities. Death or cerebral damage may occur if it is not appreciated that, in the presence of an arrhythmia which severely impairs cardiac output (including severe bradycardia), external cardiac massage may be required to support the circulation; frequently, cardiac massage is not started until after asystole or ventricular fibrillation has developed.

Cardiac arrest. Cardiac arrest during anaesthesia is unusual in the absence of a non-anaesthetic cause (e.g. profound hypovolaemia). Asystole may occur as a result of vagal stimulation, usually preceded by sinus bradycardia. It is also the usual terminal event in severe hypoxaemia. Ventricular fibrillation is less common, but may occur as a result of gas embolism, after the administration of adrenaline in a patient receiving halothane, in association with hypoxaemia or because of acute myocardial ischaemia or infarction. Cardiac arrest may also result from intravascular injection of local anaesthetics, particularly bupivacaine, either inadvertently or in association with Bier's block if the tourniquet is applied inadequately or released prematurely, or if the drug is injected rapidly into a large vein. Electrolyte abnormalities, especially related to potassium, may precipitate cardiac arrest; abnormalities of serum potassium concentration may be exaggerated by acid–base changes induced by hypercapnia or hypocapnia. Pulmonary embolism may cause total failure of the circulation without causing cardiac arrest. Electromechanical dissociation may precede asystole in patients with severe hypovolaemia, pneumothorax or prolonged hypoxaemia. It should be treated by external cardiac compression and, if possible, immediate diagnosis and correction of the cause.

Hypotension. Almost all anaesthetic drugs produce some hypotension, by reducing cardiac output, promoting vasodilatation, or both. Hypotension is more marked in the absence of surgical stimulation (e.g. between induction of anaesthesia and the start of surgery) and in the presence of relative hypovolaemia (e.g. after haemorrhage or in the dehydrated patient). However, the presence of low blood pressure is not linked automatically to reduced tissue perfusion or oxygenation, provided that cardiac output is maintained. In the presence of a normal macrocirculation, autoregulation maintains flow despite moderate decreases in arterial pressure. Normally, cerebral autoregulation occurs down to a mean arterial pressure of 60 mmHg; below that value, cerebral blood flow decreases progressively. However, the threshold is increased in chronically hypertensive patients, and flow may be pressure-dependent in patients with atherosclerosis of cerebral arteries; care must be exercised in these groups of patients to prevent profound hypotension. Tissue flow is reduced to a greater degree when hypotension is associated with reduced cardiac output and accompanied by vasoconstriction.[66] Excessive hyperventilation causes profound hypocapnia, which also results in vasoconstriction,[67] and may impair tissue perfusion further in the hypotensive patient. Inadvertent hypotension during anaesthesia may be the result of a relative overdose of general anaesthetic agents, high spinal or epidural anaesthesia or inadequate replacement of blood and plasma losses.

Induced hypotension to reduce surgical blood loss has become less popular, but the technique is still used by a proportion of anaesthetists, particularly for middle ear, pelvic and plastic operations. Anaesthetists vary in their enthusiasm for deliberate hypotension, and there have been cases of cerebral damage, myocardial infarction and death attributable to its use. There is no sudden cut-off value of blood pressure below which serious complications occur predictably. However, there does appear to be an increased risk of complications if deliberate hypotension is used; the incidence of non-fatal complications has been estimated as 2.5%.[68] A large proportion of these complications can be prevented if deliberate hypotension is avoided in patients with pre-existing hypertension, cerebrovascular or ischaemic heart disease, hypovolaemia or anaemia. Hypotensive techniques associated with myocardial depression (by administration of high concentrations of volatile anaesthetic agents or β-blockers) are associated with more complications than those that employ vasodilatation. The complication rate is also increased if mean arterial blood pressure is reduced to less than 70 mmHg, or if the anaesthetist is inexperienced. However, there may be some surgical procedures in which the risk of excessive blood loss warrants the use of lower values of blood pressure in otherwise healthy young patients and there is evidence that an adequate cerebral blood flow can be maintained in such patients at systolic blood pressures of 60 mmHg or slightly less.[54]

Anaemia. Tissue oxygenation may be impaired despite a normal arterial oxygen saturation if the total amount of oxygen carried by blood is decreased by severe anaemia. The most common cause is massive haemorrhage, with replacement of blood volume by artificial solutions. It is a potential problem in any Jehovah's Witness who undergoes major surgery and refuses permission for blood transfusion.

Embolism. Embolism of air or thrombus may result in cerebral ischaemia. Massive venous embolism causes a great reduction in, or cessation, of cardiac output. Arterial emboli may cause focal or generalized cerebral lesions. Massive pulmonary embolism is unusual during anaesthesia, but may occur in patients who have been immobile, or occasionally after release of a pneumatic tourniquet on the leg; postoperative embolism is much more common. Arterial thrombi may originate in the heart or great vessels, and are usually neither predictable nor preventable by the anaesthetist. Air embolism may occur during neurosurgery or operations in the pelvis if the patient is positioned in such a way that the operation site is above the heart. Oxygen emboli have caused cardiac arrest after instillation of hydrogen peroxide into surgical wounds.[69] Fatal carbon dioxide emboli have occurred during laparoscopy.[70] Emboli of air or clot, or reduced cerebral perfusion pressure, may cause focal or global ischaemia after cardiopulmonary bypass;[71] microemboli of platelets, air bubbles or other substances result in a high incidence of minor neurological and psychological sequelae, the majority of which are of little clinical significance and some of which are temporary.

Consequences of cerebral hypoxia or ischaemia

The effects of these two insults are not identical. In the presence of an intact cardiovascular system, the brain is able to adjust for temporary episodes of even severe hypoxaemia by a compensatory increase in cerebral blood flow, thereby minimizing the reduction in oxygen delivery.

If arterial P_{O_2} decreases to less than 6.5 kPa without circulatory arrest, there are increases in intracellular and extracellular brain lactate concentrations. More profound hypoxaemia results in a decrease in intracerebral phosphocreatine concentrations. However, even very severe hypoxaemia is not associated with a significant decrease in adenosine triphosphate concentrations because of a rapid compensatory vasodilatation, a resultant increase in blood flow (in excess of four times normal) and a sixfold increase in glucose metabolism.[72] As long as increased cerebral blood flow is maintained, hypoxaemia must be very severe to threaten neuronal survival, although cerebral function may be impaired during the episode of hypoxaemia. However, prolonged moderate or severe hypoxaemia also affects the cardiovascular system. There is an initial increase in heart rate and stroke volume as a result of sympathetic nervous system stimulation, but bradycardia or other arrhythmias, followed by cardiac arrest, supervene and permanent cerebral changes ensue. In severe hypoxaemia with circulatory inadequacy, the sequelae are similar to those caused by primary cerebral ischaemia.

Global ischaemia, as occurs in severe hypotension or cardiac arrest, results much more rapidly in neuronal damage. Brief episodes of ischaemia are often followed by complete recovery. However, as the duration of ischaemia increases, progressively more permanent damage occurs. Resulting lesions are more likely to affect grey matter than white matter, and are frequently bilateral and symmetrical; they may be confined to the parietal and occipital areas of the cerebral hemispheres, but in most cases involve both the supratentorial and infratentorial compartments.[73] Fits may develop during or shortly after the ischaemic episode. A wide range of residual deficits may result, ranging from mild psychological symptoms or personality changes to a vegetative state or brain death. Cortical blindness is not uncommon. Outcome is influenced by the duration and extent of ischaemia and by age. Paradoxically, incomplete ischaemia (e.g. severe hypotension) may result in a worse outcome than a similar period of complete ischaemia; this is thought to be the result of continued delivery of glucose with an inadequate supply of oxygen in incomplete ischaemia, which causes increased lactate production and a lower intracellular pH. Patients with cerebrovascular disease may develop localized neurological lesions attributable to ischaemic damage in the area of impaired perfusion.

Attempts at reducing the neurological sequelae of hypoxaemia or ischaemia have been disappointing.[74] No specific treatment has been shown to ameliorate the condition in humans. However, it is likely that prompt restoration of the circulation reduces secondary ischaemic damage caused by the reperfusion syndrome[75] and moderate hyperventilation may be of theoretical benefit if there are signs of cerebral oedema. There is no clinical evidence that the use of routine artificial ventilation after cardiac arrest influences neurological outcome. Steroids are of no benefit.

Awareness during anaesthesia

Awareness is almost invariably the result of provision of inadequate concentrations of anaesthetic drugs in the paralysed patient. A common explanation of awareness is that a predictably inadequate anaesthetic technique has been used; some anaesthetists continue to employ techniques in which nitrous oxide is used without supplementation with a volatile or intravenous anaesthetic agent. The commonest time for awareness to occur is at, or shortly after, the time of skin incision. This is often because, either as a result of failure of understanding of the pharmacokinetics of anaesthetic agents or due to fears of producing cardiovascular depression before surgery starts, insufficient concentrations of inhaled agents have been administered to provide adequate anaesthesia for surgery as the effects of the intravenous induction agent decline (Fig. 28.2). Awareness may also occur during difficult intubation if the initial induction dose of anaesthetic is not supplemented, if air is entrained into mechanical ventilators or if vaporizers become empty during anaesthesia. The anticipated concentrations of anaesthetic agents are not delivered to the patient if vaporizers with a Selectatec fitting are not locked on to the Selectatec block, because anaesthetic gases leak to atmosphere. Cases of awareness have occurred because, following modest decreases in arterial oxygen saturation measured by a pulse oximeter to 90–95%, and caused usually by modest cardiovascular depression after induction of anaesthesia, the anaesthetist (usually a trainee) has increased the inspired concentration of oxygen to 50% or more, with a corresponding reduction in the concentration of nitrous oxide, but has not increased the concentration of volatile anaesthetic agent.

Total intravenous anaesthesia has increased in popularity, partly because of commercial pressure, but also because of concerns regarding pollution of the atmosphere of the operating theatre with inhaled anaesthetic agents. The commonest cause of awareness during total intravenous anaesthesia is an interruption of the supply of drug, caused either by disconnection of, or obstruction to, the infusion.[76] However, a number of cases have arisen as a result of confusion on the part of the anaesthetist concerning infusion regimens. The commonest mistake is the failure to appreciate that most published infusion regimens[77,78] were

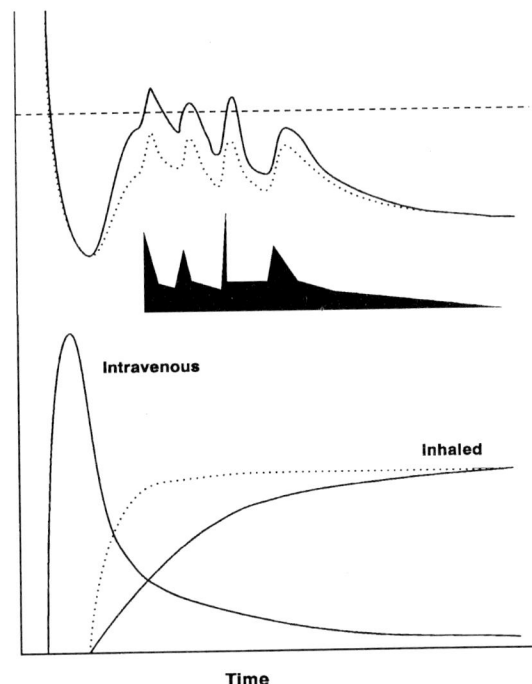

Fig. 28.2 Diagrammatic representation of depth of anaesthesia during and after induction of anaesthesia as the effects of the intravenous anaesthetic agent decrease and those of the inhaled agent(s) increase. Bottom: the brain concentrations of intravenous and inhaled anaesthetic drugs. Top: the resulting depth of anaesthesia; the dotted line represents adequate anaesthesia, and the solid line inadequate anaesthesia, in this case as a result of administration of an inhaled agent at too low an inspired concentration in relation to its solubility. The blocked area represents surgical stimuli, and the horizontal dashed line the depth of anaesthesia at which awareness is likely to occur. Although depth of anaesthesia is adequate before surgery starts, the effect of surgical stimulation is to cause increased arousal and thus awareness.

effective because nitrous oxide and/or large doses or infusions of an opioid were also given; if these regimens are used without nitrous oxide or an appropriate dose of opioid, they are associated with a significant risk of awareness. Another cause of awareness is the failure to appreciate that, in order to achieve a stable blood concentration of intravenous agent, the infusion must be started immediately after the induction dose; delay until after the patient has been transferred into the operating theatre is likely to result in periods in which the brain concentration of anaesthetic agent is less than that which produces effective anaesthesia.

In obstetric anaesthesia, concerns regarding the effects

of anaesthetic agents on the newborn baby and on the risk of haemorrhage from the uterus resulted in the use of anaesthetic techniques which would not be regarded as adequate in other areas of surgery. The perceived risks to the baby and the uterus have almost certainly been overemphasized, and a substantial reduction in the incidence of awareness has been achieved since the introduction of improved techniques.[79] However, the incidence of awareness remains higher in obstetric anaesthesia than in other areas of anaesthetic practice. Most episodes of awareness now occur between skin incision and the delivery of the baby, and result from the short period between induction of anaesthesia and the start of surgery, and reluctance to use overpressure to achieve a rapid increase in the concentration of volatile agent in the blood and brain.[80] A small proportion of patients who complain of intra-operative awareness have experienced events in the immediate postoperative period, but interpreted the events as having occurred during operation.[81]

Patients who have been aware during anaesthesia, and who have experienced pain and distress, may develop the post-traumatic stress disorder. Advice to anaesthetists confronted with a patient who claims to have been aware during anaesthesia has been published.[82]

Regional anaesthesia

Spinal cord/nerve root damage

The commonest reason for complaint in patients who have suffered damage to the spinal cord or nerve roots relates to the use of subarachnoid or epidural anaesthesia. Damage may result from the insertion of a spinal or epidural needle at an inappropriate level of the vertebral column. The early signs of contact between a needle tip and nerve root are masked if the block is performed after induction of general anaesthesia, and thus the likelihood of more severe and permanent damage is probably increased; in the author's opinion, it is prudent to perform spinal or epidural block before inducing general anaesthesia if a combination of regional and general anaesthesia is to be employed. There have been instances in which an inappropriate substance has been injected inadvertently into the epidural or subarachnoid space, causing extensive neurological damage. A number of substances are known to cause neurotoxicity, including potassium chloride and calcium chloride.[83] Most local anaesthetic drugs used in the UK are not associated with neurotoxicity, although there are concerns about their intrathecal use with adrenaline, and their administration through a subarachnoid catheter.[84] There have also been reports of neurotoxicity associated with the use of chloroprocaine, related probably to toxicity of a preservative.[85] However, a substantial proportion of injuries to nerve roots have no obvious cause. There is increasing suspicion that inadvertent subdural injection of local anaesthetic may be responsible for a proportion of unexplained neurological lesions in patients who have undergone epidural anaesthesia;[86] injection of radioopaque dye through a catheter placed inadvertently in the subdural space has demonstrated that fluid may produce compression of nerve roots and the spinal cord.[87] In the ASA closed claim study,[88] 2.5% of claims against anaesthetists related to alleged damage to the lumbosacral nerve roots.

Damage to the spinal cord may also occur as a result of ischaemic lesions, either because of systemic hypotension, or local occlusion of the blood supply (the latter usually in association with coeliac plexus block). Injection of steroids into the epidural space (without a product licence) has been claimed to cause damage to nerve roots in a number of cases;[89] this is a controversial issue.[90]

Pain during surgery

Up to 25% of patients experience pain or discomfort during operations performed under regional anaesthesia, and particularly during Caesarean section. A proportion of these patients suffer severe pain. It is essential that the degree and extent of block are tested adequately before surgery starts, and that the anaesthetist is prepared to take appropriate steps, including induction of general anaesthesia, if the block becomes inadequate during the operation. Consequently, preparation of patients for major regional techniques must be the same as that for patients scheduled to undergo general anaesthesia, and the anaesthetist must remain available to monitor the effects of the block, and intervene if necessary, during the procedure.

There have been a number of recent cases in which patients have claimed to have been assaulted because regional or local techniques were employed without specific consent, and performed under general anaesthesia. In a recent claim,[91] a patient who suffered localized damage to lumbar and sacral nerve roots unilaterally claimed that the caudal anaesthetic to which she attributed the injury should not have been performed during general anaesthesia without her specific consent. In finding against the patient, the judge indicated that, in his opinion, it was inappropriate to expect that patients should be told every detail of the proposed procedure, and that there was no realistic distinction between omitting to tell a patient that she would receive a caudal block for provision of intra-operative analgesia and postoperative pain relief, and omitting to tell her that a tube would be placed in her trachea or that an intramuscular injection of morphine would be given during emergence from the anaesthetic. However, it cannot necessarily be assumed that a similar judgement would be given in respect of a potentially more hazardous block, such as subarachnoid, or lumbar or thoracic epidural.

Backache

Current evidence[92] suggests that there is a substantial increase in the incidence of long-term backache if epidural analgesia is provided during labour (18.2 versus 10.2%) or for instrumental delivery or emergency Caesarean section (19.2 versus 11.2%), in comparison to the incidence in patients who do not receive epidural analgesia, but no increase in the incidence if epidural anaesthesia rather than general anaesthesia is used for elective Caesarean section. The authors concluded that the most likely explanation was that the presence of epidural analgesia during labour might result in abnormal stresses on the ligaments and muscles of the back. Other investigators have also found backache to be a relatively common sequel to the use of regional anaesthesia in obstetrics.[54,93] These findings have important implications in respect of information given to patients when seeking consent for epidural analgesia in obstetric practice.

Peripheral nerve damage

Peripheral nerve damage is usually the result of compression or stretching of the nerve. In a few cases, nerves are damaged by direct trauma from needles or extravasated drugs. Most lesions involve demyelination at a point of localized compression. In most cases, remyelination results in recovery in 6–8 weeks, but in some patients recovery is more prolonged, and in a few, the injury is permanent. In the ASA closed claim study,[88] 15% of claims against anaesthetists related to peripheral nerve injury. Injury to the ulnar nerve represented about one-third of these claims, brachial plexus injury 23% and damage to the lumbosacral roots 16%. Frequently, a cause could not be identified clearly.

The ulnar and common peroneal nerve are particularly susceptible to damage because they lie, at some point, in a very superficial position close to bony promontories. However, there is evidence that many patients have pre-existing subclinical lesions of these nerves related to normal posture, often occupational, such as sitting with the legs crossed or leaning habitually on an elbow. In these patients, a brief period of normally innocuous stretching or compression may result in a clinical lesion. Often, electrophysiological studies in patients who develop a lesion in the postoperative period reveal that the nerve on the contralateral side is also abnormal.[94] Patients with a pre-existing general neuropathy are also at increased risk. The presence of a neuropathy, and any history of regular paraesthesiae on waking from normal sleep, should be elicited at the pre-operative visit, and special care taken during the peri-operative period.

The brachial plexus may suffer injury if the arm is placed in any extreme position during anaesthesia, but particularly if it is abducted and externally rotated. In the supine position, the risk is highest if both arms are abducted; if an arm is abducted beyond 90°; if the arm is abducted and the head is extended and rotated to the opposite side; and if the arm lies below the horizontal plane of the body. In the prone position, there is a risk of damage to the brachial plexus if the arms are abducted excessively; this is most easily prevented by keeping the arms at the side of the body. There is also a risk of damage to the brachial plexus if shoulder braces are used to prevent a patient slipping from a steep head-down position on the operating table. Brachial plexus injury can also complicate cardiac surgery, as a result of stretching during median sternotomy.

Damage to the radial nerve in the upper arm usually occurs as a result of compression, for example under a pneumatic tourniquet.[95] The sciatic nerve is at risk in thin patients placed on a hard operating table for a long operation, but may also be damaged by stretching in the lithotomy position, or by compression by a hard pad placed under the pelvis when patients are placed in the Lloyd-Davies position. Lumbosacral nerve root injuries are associated most commonly with pain or paraesthesiae accompanying a regional anaesthetic technique.[88] Nerves injured less commonly include the tibial, femoral, obturator, saphenous, pudendal, supra-orbital and facial.

Anaphylaxis

An anaphylactic reaction is an exaggerated response of an organism to a foreign protein (or other substance to which it has become sensitized) associated with the liberation of histamine, serotonin and other vasoactive substances. The clinical manifestations are shown in Table 28.17 and 28.18.[96] An anaphylactoid reaction is a term that encompasses all reactions that are clinically indistinguishable from anaphylactic reactions but in which other mechanisms are involved. Examples include histamine-mediated transient hypotension following

Table 28.17 Clinical features reported in 206 patients with severe anaphylactic reactions during anaesthesia. Numbers represent percentage of patients in whom a clinical feature was noted

Clinical features	Induction agents	Muscle relaxants	Other drugs
Number of patients	44	115	47
Cutaneous features			
Rash	14	8	13
Urticaria	9	8	28
Flush	50	41	53
Bronchospasm			
Transient	16	23	17
Severe	7	15	11
Cardiovascular features			
Tachycardia	93	90	83
Bradycardia	5	7	15
Other arrhythmia	9	11	19
Hypotension	93	92	72
Vasodilatation	86	86	79
Vasoconstriction		4	
Oedema			
Pulmonary		16	11
Angioedema	16	33	17
Generalized	9	9	6
Gastrointestinal	20	10	6

From Fisher & Baldo,[96] with permission.

high-dose opioid administration and most cases of pruritus or urticaria after small doses of opioids. The incidence of anaphylactic reactions associated with anaesthesia has been estimated to be approximately 1 : 6000 in France[97] and 1 : 10 000 to 1 : 20 000 in Australia.[96] Reactions are more common in female patients. Anaphylactic reactions may occur to any drug given intravenously during anaesthesia. A history of previous exposure to the drug is not always necessary, particularly in relation to neuromuscular blocking drugs where the absence of a history of previous exposure may be as high as 80%; this may be due to sensitization by some foods and cosmetics, and is also related to the fact that patients may be sensitized to a number of muscle relaxants by previous administration of one drug of this class.

There are three important factors which influence the risk of damage associated with a severe anaphylactic reaction:

1. *History*. It is essential at the pre-operative visit to elicit any history of an adverse event associated with previous anaesthesia which might indicate an anaphylactic reaction. Patients should be asked specifically if they have ever been told that they are allergic to any anaesthetic drug. If a positive history is obtained, the previous records should be scrutinized if they are available. If they are not available, then unless the operation is a dire emergency, it may be advisable to undertake skin testing for the drugs which the anaesthetist proposes to use.[98]

2. *Prompt recognition and appropriate treatment*. The diagnosis of anaphylaxis is made on clinical grounds. A serious anaphylactic reaction starts rapidly after the causative drug is injected, and can be detected almost immediately if appropriate monitoring is employed.

Table 28.18 The first clinical feature of an anaphylactic reaction in 206 patients

Clinical feature	Percentage of patients
No pulse detected	27.6
Flush	26.7
Difficulty in inflation of lungs	23.8
Cough	5.3
Rash	3.9
Urticaria	3.4
Cyanosis	3.4
Subjective feeling	2.9
Oedema	2.4
Hypotension	0.4
No bleeding	0.4

From Fisher & Baldo,[96] with permission.

Various treatment regimens have been recommended.[98] Prompt recognition and appropriate treatment are associated with a successful response and outcome in most patients, even after a severe anaphylactic reaction. Because anaphylactic reactions are uncommon, it has been recommended that anaesthetists and operating room personnel should rehearse a simulated anaphylaxis drill at regular intervals.[98]

3. *Investigation.* It is essential to attempt to identify the cause of an anaphylactic reaction and any patient who has a suspected anaphylactic reaction should be investigated fully. Current recommendations in the UK[98] are that serum tryptase concentration should be measured in a sample of blood taken 1 h after the onset of the reaction; an elevated concentration is a sensitive indicator of the existence of an anaphylactic reaction. If the serum tryptase concentration is elevated, or if the reaction was severe, then skin prick tests should be performed 4-6 weeks later. All drugs administered intravenously during anaesthesia, and *all* neuromuscular blockers, should be tested; it is preferable also to test for other anaesthetic agents, and for allergy to latex. Positive *and negative* reactions should be documented clearly, and the patient should be given a letter, and if possible a warning bracelet, indicating the drugs which showed a positive reaction.

No drug which is proved, or strongly suspected, to have caused an anaphylactic reaction should be administered again.

Damage to teeth

As noted above (Table 28.12), dental damage is the most frequent cause of claims against anaesthetists, although it is often overlooked because the claims are not usually expensive. Lockhart et al[99] surveyed 133 anaesthesia training programmes and estimated the incidence of dental damage to be 1 per 1000 anaesthetics which involved tracheal intubation. Difficult or emergency intubation accounted for about half of the cases of dental damage, but 25% of injuries occurred during extubation or in the recovery room. The upper left incisor tooth was most frequently involved. In 62% of cases in one study, dental damage occurred in teeth which had been restored previously or damaged by peri-odontal disease.[100] A plastic dental shield is used routinely by some anaesthetists, and is claimed to minimize the risk of injury. However, Burton & Baker[100] found that 'the vast majority' of anaesthetists did not use a protective guard routinely, and that 45% of anaesthetists never used one. In another study, 55% of incidents of dental damage were related to the use of an oral airway, and not to tracheal intubation.[101]

Fear of damaging teeth may lead some anaesthetists to take unreasonable risks of other complications.[101] Dental damage was avoided in one vulnerable, obese patient who required Caesarean section; a face mask was used, and she died after massive aspiration of gastric fluid.[102]

Eye injuries

Injuries to the eye during anaesthesia can result in corneal abrasions or blindness.[103-105] The ASA closed claim study found[106] that eye injuries accounted for 3% of total claims. Corneal abrasion occurred in 35% of these cases, and was most probably the result of the eye opening and the cornea drying during anaesthesia, or trauma from the anaesthetic face mask, laryngoscope or surgical drapes. In most cases (84%), injury was temporary. The second commonest source of injury (30%) was related to movement during ophthalmic anaesthesia, usually due to coughing or bucking; in 81% of cases, the reviewers considered that the standard of care was inadequate. Another potential source of blindness is pressure applied to the eye as a result of inappropriate positioning in the prone position, particularly during neurosurgical procedures.

Miscellaneous injuries

Examples of other injuries are shown in Tables 28.7, 28.12 and 28.14. Generalized muscle pain related to administration of suxamethonium is a very common complaint, and patients should be warned of the possibility at the pre-operative visit. Fractured ribs and other injuries have resulted from patients being dropped from the operating table on to the floor. Tissued intravenous infusions may result in damage to skin or nerves and, in rare circumstances, ischaemic damage to an entire limb because of compartment syndrome. Skin necrosis may occur if irritant drugs intended for deep intramuscular injection are delivered instead into the subcutaneous tissues. Skin damage may occur also as a result of burns, pooling of disinfectant and pressure.

Laryngeal damage may be minor (e.g. granulomata) or major (e.g. dislocation of cartilages, or damage to nerves); prolonged and strenuous attempts to intubate the trachea may result rarely in perforation of the pharynx or oesophagus, resulting in retropharyngeal abscess formation or potentially fatal mediastinitis.

The potential risks of hepatitis associated usually with repeated administrations of halothane are well-recognized. Between 1978 and 1985, the Committee on Safety of Medicines (CSM) received 84 reports of hepatotoxicity; adequate histories were available from 62 of the patients, 41 of whom had received halothane more than once. The mortality rate was 29% in those exposed on one occasion, compared with 41% in patients exposed twice and 56% in those exposed on more than two occasions. The CSM has made the following recommendations[107] relating to repeated administrations of the drug, and these should be heeded.

- A careful anaesthetic history should be taken to determine previous exposure and previous reactions to halothane.
- Repeated exposure to halothane within a period of at least 3 months should be avoided unless there are overriding clinical circumstances.
- A history of unexplained jaundice or pyrexia in a patient following exposure to halothane is an absolute *contra-indication* to future use in that patient.

Development of pneumothorax in the peri-operative period is associated most commonly with attempts to insert central venous or pulmonary artery catheters. While this is a recognized risk in a small proportion of patients, the risk is increased if multiple attempts have been made, or if an inexperienced operator has made the attempts with inadequate supervision. Bilateral attempts at cannulation of the internal jugular or subclavian veins should be avoided unless absolutely necessary, because of the potentially catastrophic consequences of bilateral tension pneumothoraces. The anaesthetist must always have a high index of suspicion for the development of pneumothorax in the peri-operative period, particularly if a central venous catheter has been inserted, or if supraclavicular brachial plexus block, intercostal block or intrapleural injection of local anaesthetic has been performed.

Injury related to the use of electrical equipment is also an important issue; the literature on electrical safety is vast, and detailed discussion is beyond the scope of this chapter.

PSYCHOLOGY OF ACCIDENTS

An understanding of the causes of errors is an essential first step to a reduction in the incidences of incidents and accidents. Human error is common to all walks of life. In most cases, errors are mundane and acceptable. However, in medicine, errors may lead to potential or actual injury. In anaesthetic practice, the short time scales involved in the genesis of some types of injury increase the probability of actual injury because of the reduced time available for recognition of the error and for institution of remedial action.

The anaesthetist is part of a complex, interactive system involving the patient, the anaesthetist, other hospital personnel both inside and outside the operating theatre, and a large array of equipment. Consequently, analysing the causes of errors, and preventing their occurrence, is intricate. However, studies of human error have demonstrated that errors often follow predictable patterns, and that there are identifiable mechanisms which can help to explain why they occur.[108]

At least 90% of aviation accidents and industrial fatalities can be attributed to human error or behavioural factors.[109,110] In anaesthesia, human error rates are of a similar order.[39,111] Even when human error is not directly involved in an accident, it is often possible to identify errors in design, manufacture, inspection, installation or maintenance of some part of the system which was the result of an earlier human error.

Errors, incidents and accidents

It is necessary first to consider the ways in which goals and intentions are converted into actions (Fig. 28.3). An anaesthetist may, for example, have the goal of securing the airway after induction of anaesthesia. An intention is then formed; for example, the anaesthetist may decide to secure the airway using a tracheal tube. A specific sequence of actions is then planned. The plan may involve obtaining and unwrapping a tracheal tube of the anticipated size; checking the cuff; cutting the tube to an appropriate length; inserting the connector into the proximal end; lubricating the tube; ensuring that alternative sizes of tube are immediately available; checking that the laryngoscope functions correctly; ensuring that a spare, working laryngoscope is immediately to hand; and checking that equipment for unexpected difficult intubation is available. These actions are then executed and the outcome compared with the intended outcome so that it can be confirmed that the intention has been achieved. Following induction of anaesthesia, the trachea is intubated and the outcome compared with the original goal (to secure the airway). A reasonable plan will usually result in an acceptable outcome.

An error is a flawed plan or action, and results in either an incident or an accident. An incident may be defined as an unintended event or outcome which could have, or did, reduce the safety margin for the patient (i.e. it could have resulted, but did not result, in an adverse outcome). An accident is an adverse or negative outcome. The relationships between acceptable actions,

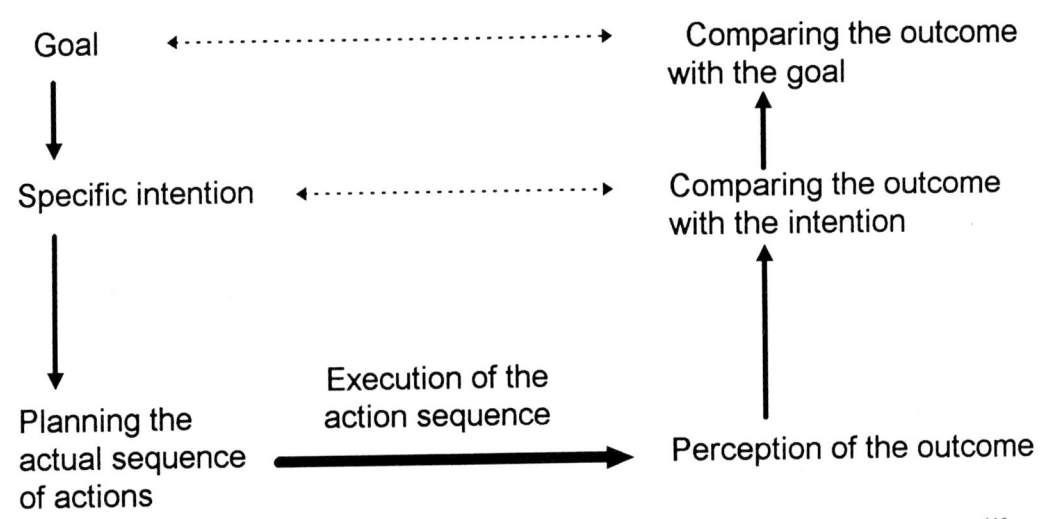

```
Goal  ←·································→  Comparing the outcome
 ↓                                            with the goal
                                                    ↑
Specific intention  ←···················→  Comparing the outcome
 ↓                                            with the intention
                                                    ↑
                  Execution of the
Planning the      action sequence
actual sequence  ──────────────────────→   Perception of the outcome
of actions
```

Fig. 28.3 Schematic representation of how goals and intentions are converted into actions. After Norman.[112]

acceptable outcomes, errors, incidents and accidents are shown in Figure 28.4. The normal result is shown by arrow 1. Errors are common, but most lead to incidents rather than accidents. Using the example of preparing for tracheal intubation, failure to check that the laryngoscope is functioning correctly might lead to an incident (for example, a delay in achieving intubation, with the potential risks which such a delay involves) or an accident (for example, if the patient unexpectedly regurgitates and aspirates during the delay incurred). Acceptable actions sometimes lead to incidents and occasionally to accidents (arrows 4 and 5). For example, delay in intubation may occur despite an appropriate plan and appropriate actions if it transpires that the patient has an unpredictable anatomical abnormality which renders intubation difficult. Even more rarely, chance may intervene; for example, the larygoscope bulb may fail in use despite having worked normally when tested.

Thus, not all accidents are associated with errors. It is also important to recognize that not all errors are culpable, although they may appear to be so with the benefit of hindsight. It has been suggested[113] that errors constitute an inevitable subset within the normal range of human performance and that culpability should be reserved for extreme departures from accepted practice when there are no extenuating circumstances. It is unreasonable to expect every plan and every action of the anaesthetist to be perfect or ideal.

Classification of errors

Errors may be categorized into active errors, which are usually immediate precursors to an incident or accident, and latent errors or shaping factors which often occur long before the event and which may influence the outcome of intentions and plans (see Fig. 28.4).

Active errors. These may be classified as contextual (describing specific actions in specific environments) or modal (categorizing errors into, for example, errors of omission, substitution, etc.). However, in anaesthesia, it is generally considered more useful to classify errors according to the underlying mechanisms, a technique which permits errors of the same type to be analysed together even though the specific events may be very different. This has proved to be more useful than alternative classifications in suggesting ways in which errors in anaesthesia can be prevented.[114]

Knowledge-based errors. These result from forming an inappropriate intention or the development of an inappropriate plan because of inadequate knowledge or experience. An example of an inappropriate intention would be a decision to induce anaesthesia in a hypovolaemic patient who has not received fluid resuscitation. An example of an inappropriate plan would be a decision to use spinal anaesthesia instead of general anaesthesia in the hypovolaemic patient in the erroneous belief that spinal anaesthesia is safer in high-risk patients.

Rule-based errors. These are errors which involve failure to apply a rule designed to avoid error or minimize the risk of an adverse outcome, those which involve application of a bad or inadequate rule, or those which involve misapplication of a rule in some problem-solving situation. An example of the first category is failure to use cricoid pressure in a patient with a high risk of

708 CLINICAL ANAESTHESIA

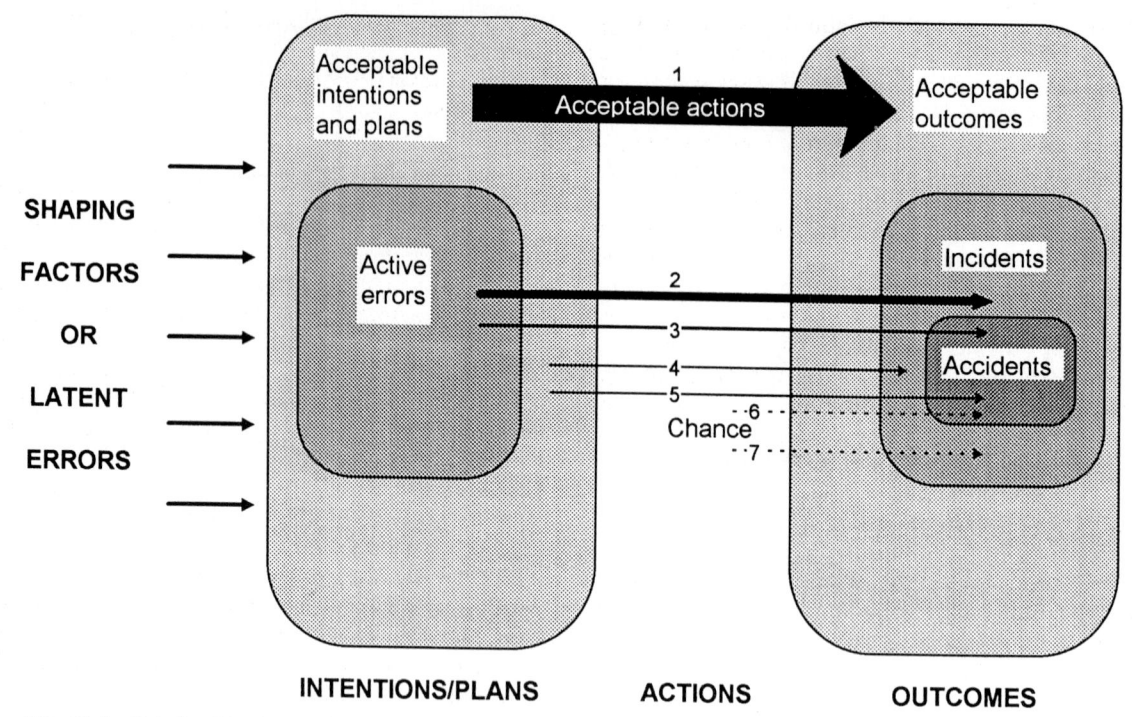

Fig. 28.4 Relationships between errors, incidents and accidents. The thickness of the arrows is related to the relative frequency with which each pathway occurs. Acceptable actions leading to acceptable outcomes (arrow 1) are by far the most frequent. Errors are relatively common, but most commonly lead to an incident (arrow 2), which is unacceptable but causes no injury. A proportion of errors lead to accidents (arrow 3), in which injury occurs. Occasionally, acceptable actions lead to an incident (arrow 4) or an accident (arrow 5), and very occasionally, accidents or incidents may result from chance occurrences (arrows 6 and 7). Redrawn from Runciman et al.[114]

regurgitation. The second type may be exemplified by reliance on auscultation of the chest as the only check for correct insertion of a tracheal tube in an obese patient. An example of the third category is treatment of intra-operative hypertension and tachycardia by a β-blocker drug without considering inadequate anaesthesia as the cause.

Skill-based errors. These are also known as slips or lapses, and are likely to occur during activities at which the individual is skilled and experienced. They may be considered to result from temporary dissociation between automatic and conscious control modes for human action.[112] The automatic control system comprises stored action patterns based on skill and experience, which can be executed rapidly and efficiently with very little attention. The conscious control system is used to check that actions do not deviate from the normal automatic pattern, and is employed also in novel situations. It is slower but more flexible. However, from time to time, the conscious system fails to be an effective monitor of the automatic system (absent-mindedness). An example of a slip would be attempting to induce anaesthesia with an antibiotic instead of thiopentone when both drugs are in 20-ml syringes but are correctly labelled. An example of a lapse would be omitting to administer neostigmine at the end of the procedure despite having drawn the drug into a syringe, because of distraction by other activities required simultaneously.

Technical errors. These arise when an outcome fails to occur or the wrong outcome is produced because the execution of an action was imperfect, despite the intentions and plan being correct, the rules appropriate and the actions undertaken without a skill-based error. An example of the first would be failure to achieve satisfactory anaesthesia of the arm with brachial plexus block, and of the second, production of a pneumothorax while inserting a central venous catheter using an accepted approach. In many cases, these are not really errors, but are the natural consequence of imperfections intrinsic in procedures which involve seeking deep structures blindly with needles introduced percutaneously in patients whose anatomy is not uniform.

Latent errors. These errors are usually hidden in

the system within which the individual works, and may influence the plans, intentions and actions of the individual. The following are examples relevant to anaesthesia.

Task requirements. The perceptual-motor and cognitive skills required for a task influence the type of error and its frequency. Tasks which require long periods of sustained vigilance punctuated by periods of high workload are susceptible to error. Figure 28.5 illustrates two ideas which have been proposed to describe the relationship between arousal level and task performance.[115] The first concept is that there is an optimum arousal level for any task; the second is that easy tasks require higher arousal levels than difficult tasks for satisfactory performance. Variations in arousal level alter performance by changing attentional capacity and processing speed. At low levels of arousal, as may occur after long periods of sustained vigilance of a relatively monotonous nature, responses take longer and lapses of attention and omissions are more likely to occur. With sufficient motivation, apparently normal levels of efficiency can be achieved, but the less important tasks may be neglected. At high levels of arousal, such as may be precipitated by a crisis, information must be processed rapidly but control of attention becomes more difficult. Thus, the efficiency in performing difficult tasks is impaired although easy tasks can be performed well. This is of particular relevance to modern anaesthesia, in which some cues to the presence of a crisis are very non-specific (e.g. rapidly decreasing oxygen saturation) and require considerable cognitive activity to determine the cause or causes in the complex relationships between the anaesthetist's equipment and the various physiological systems of the patient.

Physiological state. Fatigue, illness or emotional stress related either to work or domestic circumstances may influence behaviour and the probability of committing errors.[117]

Design of equipment. Much equipment is poorly designed, resulting in an increased risk of error. Critical incident reporting has identified clusters of incidents related to specific aspects of equipment design, such as the shape of the oxygen flow control,[39] the design of the common gas outlet,[39] design of ventilator disconnection alarms,[114] design of ventilator controls and design of alarms on monitoring apparatus. While enormous effort has been devoted to elimination of potential dangers associated with anaesthetic apparatus by incorporation of safety devices and careful attention to controls and displays,[118] design flaws continue to cause errors.

Workspace layout and design. The anaesthetic room and operating theatre may be designed or laid out in such a way that the anaesthetist cannot see the anaesthetic machine controls or monitor displays clearly from the position adopted for optimal access to the patient. The surgeon may wish lights to be dimmed for some procedures, resulting in the anaesthetist's inability to see the anaesthetic machine controls or the patient clearly. In some procedures, it may be very difficult to see, or gain access to, the patient; this is becoming an increasing problem as the quantity of surgical equipment increases and during imaging in the X-ray department.[119] Noise, inadequate space and disorganization in the working environment also contribute to errors.

Product design. Poor labelling and packaging are a common source of errors in anaesthesia. This is true particularly with generic drugs; some companies produce several drugs in packages and ampoules which are identical except for the name of the drug, which may be printed in very small lettering. Some central venous catheters are of the catheter-through-needle design, and inadvertent withdrawal of the catheter during the process of insertion can sever the catheter. Some makes of breathing tubes are more prone than others to disconnection.

Training. Training of anaesthetists is based on a combination of theoretical and practical training. Many crises in anaesthesia occur rarely, and frequently the individual has never encountered the situation before. Unusual problems tend to be dealt with badly by an individual who is trying to think from first principles in an emergency situation.[120] Training is discussed in more detail below.

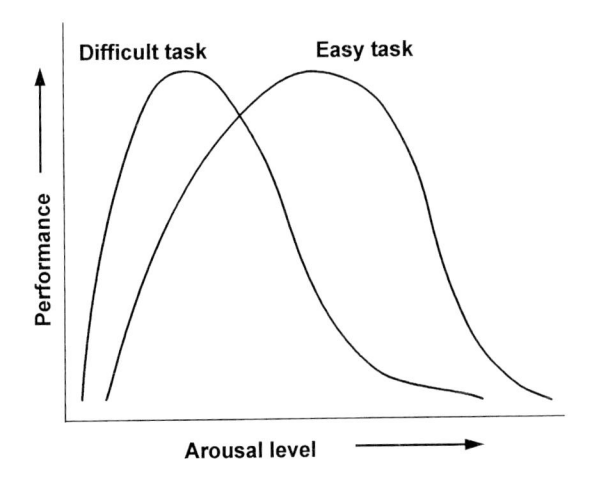

Fig. 28.5 The Yerkes Dodson law[116] relating arousal level to level of performance. See text for details.

Policies and procedures. The anaesthetic department may adopt policies or procedures which increase the risk of errors. For example, in some institutions, patients are assessed pre-operatively by trainee anaesthetists who may not be involved in administration of anaesthesia to the same patients. The practice of changing anaesthetists during an operation is another potential source of error because of inadequate communication.[40] In some departments, 'recipes' of drugs are used for specific categories of patient or for specific surgical procedures; these may be inappropriate for an individual patient. Policies and procedures may become outdated. The anaesthetist also works in an environment in which policies and procedures laid down by other groups (nurses, surgeons, operating theatre manager) are implemented. In some institutions, there is no indication on the operating theatre list when a patient is scheduled for a simple local anaesthetic block performed by the surgeon; frequently, the patient is unaware of the nature of the intended anaesthetic, and the anaesthetist may induce general anaesthesia inadvertently. The anaesthetist has joint responsibility with the surgeon for ensuring that the correct operation is undertaken on the correct patient (because the anaesthetist is responsible for the well-being of the unconscious patient), but in many institutions there is no formal mechanism for this check. The layout of the anaesthetic equipment and drugs in an individual operating room is often delegated to anaesthesia assistants, and may vary from room to room within one institution. The policies and procedures for employing anaesthetists, particularly locum appointments, are often lax.

Assistance and supervision. The qualifications and experience of anaesthesia assistants vary widely, and the anaesthetist may be required to work with a poorly qualified or inexperienced assistant, or, because of shift patterns and internal rotations, with an assistant whose experience and qualifications are unknown. Inexperienced anaesthetists may be rostered to undertake procedures which are inappropriate, either because of the planned surgical procedure or because of factors related to the individual patient, with inadequate supervision; thus, while inexperience may result in knowledge-based human error, there may have been a system failure in permitting the inexperienced anaesthetist to get into a situation in which he or she was unable to cope. Departments may not have the resources to provide

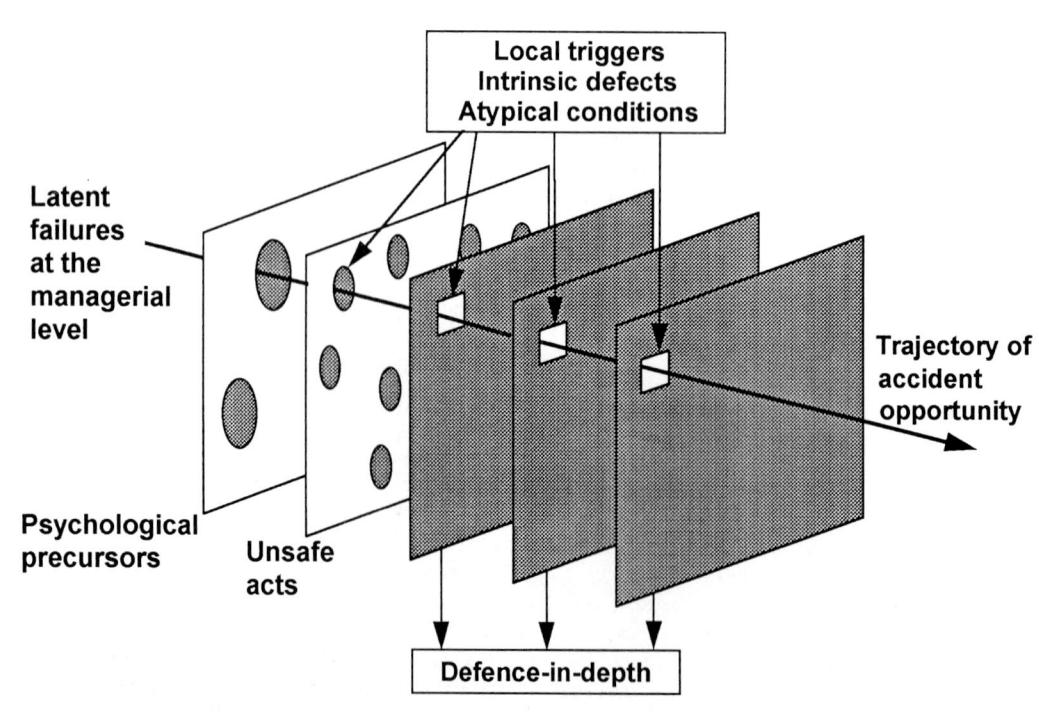

Fig. 28.6 Diagrammatic representation of mechanisms by which latent failures in the organizational system can interact with combinations of human errors, intrinsic defects and atypical conditions to elude defensive strategies, resulting in an accident. Adapted from Reason.[108]

adequate relief for breaks during long procedures, resulting in the anaesthetist leaving the patient unattended.

Social and cultural factors. Some anaesthetists are overconfident and unwilling to seek help either in anticipation of difficulty or when difficulties arise (see below). Errors may arise when anaesthetists of different grade or seniority work together; the senior anaesthetist may be reluctant to demonstrate a gap in knowledge and may proceed inappropriately, while the junior anaesthetist may be unwilling to intervene because to do so would cause embarrassment to the senior colleague.[121]

Reason[108] has argued that these latent or system-based errors may be involved in up to 85% of accidents in complex processes such as that of the operating theatre environment. Although defences are built into the system (Fig. 28.6), they are incomplete. The anaesthetist is at the 'sharp end' and a latent error which escapes the defences of the system may contribute to, or combine with, human error on the part of the anaesthetist to produce an incident or accident.

Frequency of errors. One of the largest detailed studies of the relative frequencies of the various categories of error is the Australian Incident Monitoring Study (AIMS). In a report of the first 2000 incidents, the causes of error, as determined by the anaesthetist reporting the incident, were analysed (Table 19).[122,123] Human factors (types 1–4) were identified as contributory factors in 61% of incidents, and system-based factors in 49% (more than one factor was involved in some incidents). However, system-based factors (principally monitor detection, skilled assistance and supervision) were judged to have minimized the risk of an adverse outcome in 66% of incidents. Corrective strategies which, it was believed, could have reduced the risk if incorporated into the system were suggested in a number of the reports; these are shown in Table 28.20.

Studies of the anaesthetist's tasks and behaviour

There have been several studies of the anaesthetist's intra-operative activities. The earliest studies used time-lapse photography with a frame-by-frame analysis of tasks. One major finding of the first such study[124] was that 'the anesthesiologist's attention was often directed away from the patient–surgical field'. In subsequent studies, it was found that the anaesthetist's gaze was directed away from the patient or surgical field for 40–50% of the time. McDonald and Dzwonczyk[125] classified a direct patient activity as 'one during which the anaesthetist had contact with the patient and a view of the surgical field'; examples were observation of skin colour, palpation of the pulse and auscultation of heart and breath sounds. Observing the arterial pressure monitor or electrocardiogram, and observing or adjusting the anaesthetic machine or

Table 28.19 Contributing factors in 2000 critical incidents reported to the Australian Incident Monitoring Study ranked according to the frequency with which they were reported. More than one factor was reported in some cases

Contributing factor	Type*	Percentage
Error of judgement	1	16
Failure to check equipment	2	13
Fault of technique	4	13
Other system factor	5	13
Equipment problem	5	13
Inattention	3	12
Haste	3	12
Inexperience	1	11
Communication problems	5	9
Inadequate pre-operative assessment	2	7
Monitor problem	5	6
Inadequate pre-operative preparation	2	4
Unfamiliar environment/equipment	1	4
Inadequate assistance	5	3
Fatigue	3	3
Drug label	5	3
Stress	3	2
Lack of facility	5	2
Staff change	5	1
Illness	3	1

* Type 1: knowledge-based error.
  Type 2: rule-based error.
  Type 3: skill-based error.
  Type 4: technical error.
  Type 5: system-based problem.
From Williamson et al,[122] with permission.

Table 28.20 Strategies suggested by reports to the Australian Incident Monitoring Study which might have prevented incidents if incorporated into the system

Equipment design improvement
Additional training
Quality assurance activity
Specific protocol development
Improved communication
Equipment maintenance discipline
Additional equipment
Improved supervision
More staff
Improved environment
Fatigue alleviation routine

From Runciman et al,[123] with permission.

intravenous infusion were classified as indirect patient activities. In their study, 83% of the anaesthetist's time was spent on activities that were not 'direct patient activities'. In a subsequent study by the same group,[126] there was a much higher rate of direct patient monitoring (44.8 versus 16.8% of time); this change was attributed to a change from manual ventilation in 1980, which took up a lot of the anaesthetist's visual attention, to the use of mechanical ventilators in 1985, which freed the anaesthetist to watch the patient. Many anaesthetists would find the late change from manual to automatic ventilation surprising. In addition, many of the activities categorized as indirect were of direct clinical relevance. Differentiation between clinical and non-clinical activities would be considered by many to be more important. The authors found that only about 2% of anaesthetists' time was idle or unclassified.

Boquet et al[127] studied the gaze of anaesthetists using a sophisticated eye-tracking system, and also analysed manual activities recorded on film. The patient or the surgical field took up approximately 60% of the anaesthetists' visual activity time; the breathing system reservoir bag was observed next most frequently (about 10% of time). Less than 1% of visual activity time was considered to be idle. However, the anaesthetists were idle in terms of manual activity for 72% of the time. Drui et al[124] found that 40% of the anaesthetist's time was idle (i.e. no obvious task was seen on that frame on film). However, the authors recognized that the absence of visually apparent activity did not mean that the anaesthetist was truly idle; indeed, they postulated that this time was used by anaesthetists to make the decisions on which the observable tasks were based.

Detailed task analysis studies have been performed in California.[128] These studies have shown that a small number of tasks, repeated frequently, occupy the majority of the anaesthetist's time in the operating theatre. In one study, four tasks (observe monitors, recording, conversation with consultant [for new trainees] and adjusting monitors) accounted for 50.1% of time spent in the operating theatre. Specific activities such as airway management (bag ventilation, laryngoscopy, etc.) occurred in short but intense clusters.

Automation

The early task analysis studies identified as candidates for automation a number of repetitive tasks which did not appear to offer substantial information content or therapeutic benefit; examples were filling out anaesthesia records, measuring the blood pressure and adjusting intravenous infusions. Many of these tasks have now been automated. The impact of automation on task distribution is uncertain. The change to mechanical ventilation did affect the analyses of McDonald and Dzwonczyk, as described above.[125,126] A recent study by Dzwonczyk et al[129] showed no reduction in time spent in recording when automated record-keeping devices were used. However, the Californian investigators have published preliminary data[130] demonstrating a significant reduction in the time spent recording, and a trend towards a higher frequency of direct patient care activities when automated record-keeping is used during cardiac anaesthesia.

Fatigue

It is well known that doctors work long hours and are subject to the effects of fatigue (the tiring effects of continuous work) and sleep deprivation. The subjective symptoms of both factors are commonly referred to as 'fatigue'. Duty periods for anaesthetists for over 24 h are commonplace and it is still not uncommon to have work periods of 36 h or longer. Sleep deprivation and fatigue have been implicated in many industrial and transportation accidents. The best known examples are the explosion of the Space Shuttle Challenger and the nuclear disasters at Three Mile Island and Chernobyl, all of which involved personnel suffering from both acute and chronic fatigue.[131] Doctors are probably less willing than most other groups in society to admit to fatigue because it impairs their 'macho' image and their perception of their own indispensability; this may explain why fatigue is rarely cited as a contributory factor to medical accidents.

Circadian rhythms

Many physiological processes, such as temperature regulation and hormone secretion, are characterized by a 24-h day–night cycle. Normal circadian rhythms are biphasic and reveal a lull in the level of alertness and performance twice in the 24-h period (in the early morning, between about 02.00 and 06.00 h, and in the afternoon, between about 14.00 and 18.00 h).[132] In addition to prolonged work or sleep deprivation, symptoms of fatigue can be related to the disruption of the circadian clock as a result of having a sleep–wake cycle that is out of phase with the individual's natural rhythm.

Effects of fatigue on performance

Small but repeated deficits in sleep accumulate, forming a sleep debt that can only be repaid by recovery sleep. The most obvious results of sleep deprivation are an increased tendency to fall asleep or to remain asleep, and an increased rapidity of sleep onset. The effects of sleep deprivation and fatigue on performance have been studied extensively.[133] There is general agreement that performance deteriorates after 18–24 h without sleep and that a more severe deterioration occurs after about 30–36 h without sleep. The impairment of performance is more severe at the times of the circadian lull.

Fatigue and sleep deprivation are important aspects of the 'out-of-hours' service provided by anaesthetists. Two surveys have shown that fatigue has led to errors in patient care. In the study conducted by Gravenstein et al,[134] trainees in anaesthesia estimated that their average working week was almost 70 h. The longest continuous period of administering anaesthesia without a break averaged 7.7 h, and the longest continuous period with short breaks was 20 h. Respondents considered that a safe limit for continuous work without a break was 5.2 h, and that with breaks, this could be extended to 15 h. In all, 61% of respondents agreed with the statement that they had made an error in anaesthetic administration that they attributed to fatigue. However, the response rate was low (6%) and this may have biased the results. Howard et al[135] conducted a survey of more than 600 anaesthetists, with a response rate close to 50%. They reported that 20% of respondents came under pressure to work when fatigued, that 70% admitted to fatigue at work sometimes or often, and that 21% stated that they were frequently required to work on the day after a night on call. In this study, 54% of respondents agreed or strongly agreed with the statement: 'I have made an error in clinical management which I attribute to fatigue'.

Illness and drug abuse

Every anaesthetist is vulnerable to transient and to chronic medical conditions which could, directly or indirectly, affect performance. For similar reasons to those which may cause doctors to ignore fatigue, or sometimes for financial reasons, they often continue to work with illnesses that would cause others to stay at home or to seek medical advice. The degree to which illness and self-medication affect anaesthetists' performance is unknown.

Drug abuse is a potentially serious problem for anaesthetists.[136] It has been estimated that up to 8% of doctors could be classified as alcoholics. In an anonymous survey of anaesthetists,[137] 75% of respondents reported drinking alcohol on a regular basis. Almost 10% reported that they had undertaken clinical work while hung-over. Although 40% indicated that they had anaesthetized patients within 12 h of consuming alcohol, 84% believed that alcohol use never had an adverse influence on their clinical performance.

The degree to which small doses of alcohol or a hangover affects performance of complex tasks is uncertain. Studies of pilots[138] suggest that hangover effects can degrade performance to a statistically significant degree even when more than 8 h have elapsed since alcohol consumption and there is no detectable blood alcohol level, but the absolute level of impairment was small. The natural history of serious abuse of alcohol, cocaine, sedatives or opioids by anaesthetists is such that cognitive performance is ultimately compromised, although addiction specialists suggest that job performance is one of the last areas of life to become impaired.[136]

In a large survey of training programmes,[139] 73% of respondents submitted at least one report of substance abuse among recent trainees. In all, 180 case reports were submitted to the investigators; this was equivalent to an incidence of drug abuse among trainees of 2%.

REDUCTION OF RISK

Selection of anaesthetists

Anaesthetists are recruited from medical graduates, and their selection is therefore influenced by the methods of selection of medical students. The qualities which have been suggested as ideal in those seeking to embark on a career in anaesthesia are aptitude as a physician, academic ability, enthusiasm and energy, humanity, team membership concept, health, mental stability, sense of humour and conscientiousness.[140] Most of those who sit on selection committees to assess potential undergraduates would be seeking a similar set of qualities, as would those who seek recruits to most other specialties (with the possible exceptions of team membership and sense of humour, in a few specialties!). The first meeting of the International Society on Preventable Mortality and Morbidity in 1984 identified undesirable qualities among anaesthetists; some can be absent-minded, arrogant, careless, deceitful, disorderly, forgetful, headstrong, irresponsible, lazy, obnoxious and quarrelsome. Of course, these are undesirable traits in any group, specialty or profession. Reeve[141] found that, in comparison with the population as a whole, and compared with a group of general practitioners, anaesthetists were more reserved, more intelligent, more serious, more conscientious, more self-sufficient, more tense, less socially able and less self-assured. Anaesthetists have been described as 'loners'.[142]

It is known that specific personality traits are associated with different levels of skill under different circumstances. Extroversion and neuroticism can be assessed by questionnaires. Extroverts require more stimulation than introverts to excite the central nervous system. They are active, sociable and impulsive, whereas introverts are passive, reserved and thoughtful. Introverts tend to work in a methodical, and therefore slow, manner, but tend to make fewer mistakes than extroverts. Stimulants and threatening circumstances raise arousal level, and tend to be detrimental for introverts, whereas they may improve the performance of extroverts. The introvert performs better when sustained vigilance is required. A high neuroticism score has implications for performance in threatening circumstances, as anxiety may divert mental resources into unproductive worry, thereby degrading performance. Psychosomatic illness may result from prolonged exposure to stressful situations.

There is some evidence from aviation and road safety that neuroticism and high extroversion scores are associated with higher rates of accidents.[143] However, not all studies have found such associations, and it is possible that there are only certain types of accident to which individuals with these personality traits are more prone. Although formal assessment of personality is used to guide recruitment in business and aviation, it has not gained acceptance within medicine. It may be worthy of further exploration.

Attitudes are an important component of ability. Psychologists studying judgement in aviators have identified five attitude types as being particularly hazardous, and they have developed specific antidote thoughts for each hazardous attitude.[144] These are shown in Table 28.21. The aviation psychologists instruct pilots physically to verbalize the antidote thought whenever they find themselves thinking in a hazardous way. The invulnerability and macho attitudes are particularly dangerous in anaesthetists, and may be compounded by pressure from surgeons, heads of department or hospital managers to do more cases in less time with fewer cancellations and with less opportunity for pre-operative evaluation. The belief that accidents only happen to other people, and that skill and knowledge will enable the individual to retrieve every situation successfully, can lead to cavalier behaviour and poor planning.

Training and education

Trained people behave more appropriately in all relevant professional circumstances. They have greater cognitive skills; put simply, they know more, and performance becomes more effective. They possess the relevant motor skills, so that practical performance becomes more effective. They have the ability to make reasoned judgements and implement decisions based on their knowledge and skills. Effective training seeks to develop all three of these aspects, although the usual forms of examination test only cognitive skills and, to some extent, the ability to make judgements and decisions. Motor skills can be assessed during training, but formal assessment is often neglected in training programmes. The use of simulators in training (see below) enables all three forms of behaviour to be assessed. The behaviour of anaesthetists is also influenced by

Table 28.21 Examples of hazardous attitudes and their antidotes

Hazardous attitude	Antidote
Anti-authority 'Don't tell me what to do. The policies are for someone else'	'Follow the rules. They are usually right'
Impulsivity 'Do something quickly — anything'	'Not so fast. Think first'
Invulnerability 'It won't happen to me. It's just a routine case'	'It *could* happen to me. Even routine cases develop serious problems'
Macho 'I'll show you I can do it. I can intubate anybody'	'Taking chances is foolish. Plan for the future'
Resignation 'What's the use? It's out of my hands. It's up to the surgeon'	'I'm not helpless. I can make a difference. There is always something else to try that might help'

Adapted from *Aeronautical Decision Making*.[144]

instinctive beliefs and attitudes, but these are difficult to assess.

In some countries, there is a tendency to train anaesthetists in accordance with an examination syllabus. In many ways, this is inappropriate because such a syllabus rapidly becomes outdated, because it discourages the active search for knowledge beyond that specified by the syllabus, and because it diminishes interest in clinical learning. Training programmes should include teaching of basic sciences (particularly pharmacology, physiology and physics), although it is preferable if this teaching is clinically oriented so that the trainee is made aware of their clinical applications. Clinical experience forms an essential part of training because, as well as permitting the development of manual dexterity and reinforcing theoretical knowledge, it contributes to the development of diagnostic and problem-solving skills. However, an important part of any training programme should be the development of appropriate attitudes towards learning and towards patient care. The trainee should want to learn, should want to acquire practical skills, and should want to become a safe anaesthetist.

The aims of a trainee in anaesthesia are shown in Table 28.22.[145] Training may be achieved in several ways: clinical training, academic courses, personal study, and through investigation and research. In recent years it has become necessary for trainees who intend to become specialist anaesthetists to learn also about aspects of management of clinical services, financial resources and assessment of personnel. Standards are important in any discipline, including training. In order to achieve a uniformly high standard of training, it is essential that the importance of education is recognized by those who manage the health delivery system so that adequate provision is made for the necessary time and resources, and that a professional body sets standards and ensures that these standards are achieved (Table 28.23). In the UK, the Royal College of Anaesthetists supervises training programmes in anaesthesia. Training is categorized as basic specialist training (BST) and higher specialist training (HST). BST can be achieved in about 3 years (although its duration is frequently longer), and leads to acquisition of the Diploma of Fellow of the Royal College of Anaesthetists (FRCA) if the trainee is successful in (currently) a three-part examination. Standards of BST are maintained by recognition of hospitals as training establishments; each hospital or hospital group is assessed with regard to the number of trainees who can be educated within the resources provided and in respect of the extent of training which is available. Representatives of

Table 28.22 Aims of trainees in anaesthesia

- Regard the patient's welfare as pre-eminent
- Become a safe, competent, practical anaesthetist
- Acquire such knowledge, practical skills and attitudes applicable to anaesthesia, analgesia and intensive care as will most effectively promote the health of the community
- Become competent in those aspects of medicine, surgery, paediatrics, obstetrics and intensive care and other disciplines which are relevant to the practice of a specialist anaesthetist
- Assign priorities to clinical problems and the resources for the management of these problems in the interests of the patients, their relatives and the community
- Be able to act appropriately as a member or leader of a therapeutic team
- Develop good judgemental skills
- Be willing and able to continue their own education and contribute to the education of nursing, medical and paramedical staff
- Be eager to enquire into clinical and scientific problems, adopting a critical attitude to available information
- Seek to recognize those changes in the specialty, medicine or society which should modify their practice and adapt skills accordingly
- Adopt a critical attitude to their own practice and participate in peer reviews of practice and medical audit

From Adams,[145] with permission.

Table 28.23 Internationally accepted standards for training

Professional organization
Anaesthetists should form appropriate organizations at local, regional and national levels for the setting of standards of practice, supervision of training and continuing education with appropriate certification and accreditation and general promotion of anaesthesia as an independent professional specialty

Teaching, certification and accreditation
Adequate time and facilities must be available for professional training, both initial and continuing, to ensure that an adequate standard of knowledge, expertise and practice is attained and maintained. Formal certification of training and accreditation to practice is recommended

Workload
A sufficient number of trained anaesthetists must be available so that individual doctors may practise to a high standard. Time must be allocated for professional development, administration, research and teaching

From *International standards for a safe practice of anaesthesiology*,[146] with permission.

the College visit each training esablishment at regular intervals, and assess the quality of training by interviewing all trainees and by considering the facilities, standard of staffing, adequacy of teaching programmes and provision of learning material such as books, journals and library facilities.

The quality of HST, which currently is achieved in the final 2 years of training, is supervised by a committee (Joint Committee for the Higher Training of Anaesthetists; JCHTA) with representatives from the Royal College and a number of other professional bodies. Representatives of the JCHTA undertake regular hospital visits, make recommendations to the Committee with regard to the number of higher trainees who can be accommodated and recommend improvements which will support the consultants in each department in achieving a satisfactory standard of training. While the purpose of BST is, as its name suggests, to provide training in the fundamental aspects of anaesthetic practice, HST is intended to equip trainees with the additional skills required of a specialist anaesthetist and to permit development of specialist interests. Currently, a certificate of accreditation is issued by the JCHTA when HST has been achieved.

However, this system imposes an additional tier of training beyond that required in most countries of the European Community, and thus impedes the free movement of specialist anaesthetists from other European countries to the UK, as their certificates of specialist training are not recognized as equivalent to the certificate of accreditation in respect of appointments to consultant posts. In addition, the current system of training in the UK is often very prolonged, unstructured and inefficient.[147] A working group set up by the Chief Medical Officer has proposed changes to the current training structure in the UK in order to overcome this difficulty.[148,149] The working party recommended establishment of a single training grade, a more structured, intensive and shorter training period, and the introduction of a new Certificate of Completion of Specialist Training to be awarded by the General Medical Council on the advice of the relevant Royal College.

In most other European countries, the standard of training is also overseen by a professional body. In most countries, there is a greater emphasis on local assessment of competence than on examinations, although examinations may form part of the appraisal process. The total duration of training is usually shorter than in the UK, but training tends to be more structured, and less unsupervised clinical service work is undertaken by trainees. In an attempt to harmonize standards of training in Europe, the European Academy of Anaesthesiology has established a hospital recognition programme and a Diploma in Anaesthesiology and Intensive Care. The hospital recognition programme is similar in concept to that employed in the UK by the Royal College of Anaesthetists. Visitors representing the Academy, and including a representative from another country, visit training hospitals which apply for recognition, assess the training programme, and report to the Academy; a letter of guidance is then issued, suggesting improvements if appropriate. The examination is in two parts. Part One comprises two multiple-choice papers covering basic sciences, clinical anaesthesia and intensive care. Part Two is an oral examination taken 6–9 months after Part One. Both examinations are held in a number of languages. Part One can be used by recognized training hospitals as an in-training assessment examination, and the results are made available to the department in the context of national and European averages, with a breakdown of performance in each of several categories, enabling the trainers to concentrate on improving training in areas of demonstrated weakness. The Diploma of the European Academy of Anaesthesiology is intended as an exit examination, and is taken when anaesthetists are eligible for specialist status.

The role of examinations

The principal benefits of examinations are that they have a positive influence on motivation and study and that, within certain limitations, they provide an objective and uniform standard for assessment of knowledge. However, they have a number of disadvantages. Written papers are useful tests of factual knowledge but are poor at assessing clinical skills. Oral examinations test factual knowledge, and can assess judgement, problem-solving ability and attitudes. Clinical skills are more difficult to assess formally. In recent years, there has been interest in the objective structured clinical examination[150] (OSCE) in anaesthesia. The objectives of the test are identified and recorded, and the OSCE designed to cover all required areas. The candidates rotate around a series of 'stations'; at each, they are required to perform a clinical task or to answer questions related to material provided. An assessor is present at appropriate stations to assess the candidate's performance, using a standardized checklist. It is possible to incorporate mock patients to assess history-taking or clinical examination, and to test judgement and knowledge using case histories, laboratory results, X-rays, etc. However, it is not practical to test complex motor skills. An OSCE examination now forms part of the assessment in the final FRCA examination, and will be transferred to the new Part One examination in 1996.

Continuing medical education

Completion of a training programme, or possession of a specialist qualification, does not equip individuals with all the skills or knowledge required for the duration of professional life. While this has been recognized for many years by other professions, it is only in recent years that the medical profession has taken steps to address this issue. For many specialist anaesthetists, the scope of practice narrows. Specialists may lack expertise in new fields, and may fail to keep up to date within their own field. This is perhaps more likely in anaesthesia than in many other medical specialties because anaesthetists often work alone, and outdated practices may not be apparent either to the individual or to other members of the department. Anaesthetists working in subconsultant grades are also at risk of becoming out of date; most work unsupervised, and they may not have access to (or may not take advantage of) opportunities for postgraduate education.

Methods of keeping up to date are considered in detail in Chapter 30. In the UK, the Conference of Medical Royal Colleges and their Faculties has debated the question of re-accreditation and re-certification, which may be voluntary, contractual or mandatory, and which may be required every 3–5 years. At present, it is envisaged that, within each specialty, the relevant Royal College will introduce systems for continuing medical education (CME) to ensure that specialists keep up to date with advances in the basic sciences and in clinical practice relevant to their field of work. Areas in which CME points might be accrued are listed in Table 28.24. It is envisaged that, among other possible sanctions, the Royal College of Anaesthetists would not recognize as trainers any consultants who failed to reach the requisite number of CME points within a specified time period. If a voluntary scheme organized by the Royal Colleges proves to be ineffective, then it is possible that listing on the General Medical Council's register of specialists would be dependent on evidence of accumulation of a satisfactory number of CME points, or that evidence of CME would be a condition for employment. The need for increased CME has resource implications, which must be addressed by hospital managers and by governments.

Training devices and anaesthesia simulators

Many life-threatening emergencies occur during anaes-

Table 28.24 Possible sources of continuing medical education (CME) points

Self-learning
Personal reading
Clinical scenarios
Visits to other centres
Preparation of lectures
Editing a book
Publications
   Original research
   Review articles
   Chapters
   Case reports
   Editorials
MD, MSc or PhD thesis
Monograph
Completion of ATLS, ACLS, etc.

Audience participation in CME meeting
Regional society meeting
Meetings of national societies/colleges
International meeting
Locally organized national meeting
National meetings organized by non-anaesthetic bodies

Locally organized meetings
Case conference
Medical grand round
Formal lecture
Guest lecture
Audit and critical incident meeting

From *Continuing Medical Education: Report of a Working Party*,[151] with permission.

thesia with a frequency of 1 in 10 000 or less. An anaesthetist can complete his or her training without being exposed to these situations. Some emergencies are so rare that an anaesthetist may encounter only one during a working lifetime. Attention has been drawn above to the difficulties of assessing clinical skills in trainee anaesthetists, even during routine anaesthesia; an anaesthetist with poor clinical skills may generate life-threatening emergencies, with risk to patients.

The use of simulators was pioneered in aviation; the first effective aircraft simulator was developed in 1929, and they are now an essential part of training, certification and recertification of pilots. Simulators improve the efficiency of pilot training by allowing repetition of routine activities such as take-off and landing, and offer the possibility to practise rare emergencies, or to assess performance during simulated critical incidents, without risk. Simulators can also be used to screen candidates for a particular risk, and to acquaint an individual with new equipment; most pilots are trained in flying new models of aircraft exclusively on a simulator.

In anaesthesia, clinical skills are learned primarily through apprenticeship. Although much of this apprenticeship is undertaken under direct supervision, errors of judgement or practical errors constitute a risk to patient safety. Training devices and simulators can be used to learn practical skills or rehearse clinical actions without risk. *Training devices* focus on specific skills.[152] Examples which involve practical skills include intubation manikins and devices for practising central venous cannulation. Educational computer programs which use only a screen display may also be classified as training devices; examples include programs which simulate uptake and distribution of intravenous or inhalational anaesthetics, fluid and electrolyte balance, or respiratory and cardiovascular physiology, and the Anesthesia Simulator Consultant,[153] a screen-based model of a patient's responses to anaesthetic and other drugs, and to pathological changes. A true *simulator* mimics the environment and phenomena as they appear in the real world, providing a learning experience that has the look and feel of a real operating theatre and real patient. Simulators are valuable for training and expert practice but are not necessarily good for systematic learning of new skills and knowledge. Advantages of simulators are listed in Table 28.25.

Few true simulators have been developed, but these have excited considerable interest. The first realistic simulator was SIM 1, developed by Denson & Abrahamson in the 1960s.[154] It had an anatomically correct airway and palpable pulses. It breathed normally and responded appropriately to administration of a small number of drugs. It was controlled either automatically by a (primitive) computer, or manually from an instructor's console. Trainees who learned tracheal intubation achieved performance criteria in real patients in less time, and with half the number of intubation attempts, than other trainees.[155]

The Gainsville Anesthesia Simulator was developed initially to teach trainees to develop a systematic approach to detecting and correcting equipment failure. Sensors and actuators were added to an anaesthetic machine, breathing system and ventilator to generate 13 equipment malfunctions, including breathing system leaks, valve failure, exhausted carbon dioxide canister and hypoxic gas mixture. It has since evolved to include a patient manikin with pulses, lung and heart sounds, muscle twitch responses and spontaneous breathing, together with an anaesthetic machine, ventilator and standard monitoring equipment supplied with signal and waveform generators by a computer. It has been employed for training anaesthesia residents in basic skills and for continuing education of practising specialists.[156]

The Comprehensive Anesthesia Simulation Environment (CASE) simulator was developed by Gaba & DeAnda in California.[157] This simulator, a modified and updated version of which is now commercially available,* uses a manikin, and standard anaesthesia and monitoring equipment. Computers are used to feed signals to the monitors. The manikin produces carbon dioxide, can be intubated and its breath sounds can be auscultated. The simulator director (an experienced anaesthetist) and operator instruct the system to change monitor and manikin values in real time, based on the anaesthetist's responses and according to written scripts describing the intended crisis scenario. Simulation takes place in a mock operating theatre, with the role of surgeon and theatre nurses adopted by members of the team. The simulator sessions are recorded and video-taped for later review and debriefing.

The Leiden Anaesthesia Simulator is one of two devices developed in Europe.[158] The manikin allows both spontaneous and mechanical ventilation, and compliance, resistance, tidal volume and respiratory rate can be altered by the computer. Carbon dioxide production and oxygen consumption are simulated. Physiological signals are generated by the computer, and supplied to standard monitors. Non-invasive blood pressure measurement and pulse oximetry can be simulated. The computer contains algorithms for calculating the effects of drug administration and various physiological insults on the cardiovascular and respiratory systems. In a preliminary study, the simulator was used to test the responses of a group of 28 trainees.[159] Thirteen of the trainees were allocated to undergo training on the simulator in the management of anaphylactic shock, and 15 in the management of malignant hyperthermia. Four months later, all of the trainees underwent blinded evaluation of their performance in managing malignant hyperthermia. Those

Table 28.25 Advantages of simulators in anaesthesia

No risk to patient
Scenarios involving uncommon but serious problems can be presented
Same scenario can be presented to many trainees
Scenarios can be repeated
Errors can be allowed without any risk to patient
Simulation can be stopped for teaching, and restarted
Recording, replay and critique of performance are facilitated

*Virtual Anesthesiology Training Simulation System; CAE-Link Corporation, Binghamton, New York, USA.

who had been trained in the management of this condition during the first session responded more rapidly, and treated the condition more appropriately and with fewer deviations from the protocol, than the trainees who had undergone training only in management of anaphylactic shock.

The role of simulators in training and assessment of competence. Regular programmes of training using simulators have been instituted in Belgium, the Netherlands and the USA. In principle, the anaesthesia simulator should be a useful tool for evaluating the performance of trainees and others. However, scoring or certifying competence using the simulator is more difficult. Even simulators which contain physiological and pharmacological models cannot represent the patient perfectly, and there is no way to validate their operation objectively. Thus, the precise actions taken by an anaesthetist using a simulator may not reproduce exactly the outcome which would result in real life. In this respect, the actions themselves may not be as important as the processes of observation, decision, action and re-evaluation.

Using the simulator as a tool for examinations would require independent evaluation of the simulated scenarios and of the predictive power of the subjective judgements made by experts scoring the candidate. Despite these difficulties, it is likely that, if the use of anaesthesia simulators does become more widespread, anaesthetists will become more interested in using them to assist in evaluating performance. The existing system of performance evaluation uses a relatively haphazard system of subjective judgements of clinical competence by a large number of trainers with widely different expectations, together with written and oral examinations, and this conventional system has never been validated. Simulation could offer candidates the ability to demonstrate their clinical abilities in a controlled and standardized clinical situation.

The field of anaesthesia simulation is new and it is inevitable that there will be many changes over the next few years. The simulators themselves will probably become more sophisticated, although there is a trade-off between fidelity and cost. The physiological and pharmacological models used in the simulators may become more sophisticated, supported by ever-improving computer hardware. However, medical simulators will always remain less reliable than those used in aviation because, unlike an aircraft, patients respond in different ways to the same set of actions. A development which is being pursued in a number of centres is the use of virtual-reality simulators which allow the subject to be completely immersed in a simulated situation without physically replicating the operating theatre environment; these devices will be less realistic, but much cheaper both to purchase and to maintain.

Fatigue

It is widely accepted that 24–36 h of continuous duty is an absolute limit for anaesthetists. It is already common in many anaesthetic departments to limit duty to a maximum of 24 h, followed by a full day off for recuperation. However, this practice is not followed uniformly. Furthermore, significant acute and chronic fatigue may still develop even with the day off duty, because sleep will probably be disturbed during the recuperation period and many individuals will not take full advantage of the time to sleep because of other demands of their life. It is important that individuals are taught to recognize serious fatigue in themselves. Periods of microsleep (brief periods of sleep, lasting only for seconds) are familiar to most people; they occur when an individual is seriously fatigued and are immediate harbingers of a complete lapse into sleep. Any anaesthetist who experiences periods of microsleep during clinical work must increase the level of stimulation (work or conversation), and attempt to secure assistance or relief. There are strict rules to control the total number of hours of continuous work, and the hours worked each week, for lorry drivers and airline pilots because of the perceived dangers of fatigue. While many countries have introduced restrictions to an average of 48–56 h per week for trainee doctors, few countries have produced legislation to limit the working hours of qualified specialists.

Illness and drug abuse

The specialty of anaesthesia has recognized the risks associated with impairment of function as a result of illness or drug abuse, and has implemented mechanisms of dealing with those who are detected. Methods of managing doctors who are found to be abusing drugs have been recommended but the question of whether to return these individuals to clinical practice in anaesthesia is controversial. Menk et al[139] conducted a survey of teaching hospitals, and found that 113 trainees in whom drug abuse had been detected were re-admitted to the training programmes. The success rate associated with re-admission was 34% for opioid abusers and 70% for those who had abused other groups of drugs. Fourteen of the trainees committed suicide or died as a result of a self-administered drug overdose. In 13 of 79 opioid abusers re-admitted to training programmes, death was the first sign of relapse. The authors concluded that drug rehabilitation followed by redirection into an alternative specialty was the most prudent course of action for trainee anaesthetists in whom opioid abuse was recognized. Although the main risk appears to be to the individual's own safety, concerns about patient safety can never be eliminated.

Audit

Medical audit is a relatively new term, which entails monitoring practice, reviewing the data collected, identifying areas where improvement is required, devising strategies for improvement, implementing these strategies and repeating the cycle. The term encompasses activities such as national collection of information regarding death related to anaesthesia, large studies of morbidity and critical incident reporting. However, local audit is an important activity within each department as a means of identifying problems related to techniques used by individuals or groups, and working practices within the institution. The subject is dealt with in detail in Chapter 29.

Checklists, guidelines and protocols

Anaesthetists are required to rely heavily on memory for essential facts when carrying out routine and emergency procedures. In aviation, pilots use checklists to ensure that the aircraft is safe before every flight, and to deal with emergency conditions. Several studies[17,43] have indicated that, in up to 33% of cases in which death or misadventure occurred in association with anaesthesia, no pre-operative check of the anaesthetic machine had been undertaken.

Checklists for anaesthetic and monitoring equipment have been published by a number of individuals and professional bodies,[160-164] but some are very time-consuming. The checklist procedure published by the AAGBI[165] has the following features:

- Check that the oxygen analyser detects incorrectly filled cylinders, contamination of the oxygen pipeline and inadvertent pipeline crossover.
- Check vaporizer mounting, gas or liquid leakage and back-bar pressure relief valve.
- Check integrity and configuration of breathing system, adjustable pressure-limited valve function and leakage from breathing system.
- Check the operation of the ventilator and its controls, function of the pressure relief valves, disconnect valve and availability of an emergency ventilator or resuscitator.
- Check suction equipment.

In one study,[166] this checklist was completed in a mean time of 8.9 min (range 5–19 min). Faults were detected in 60% of the machines checked (significantly more were detected in machines in the anaesthetic room than in the operating theatre), and of these, 18% were deemed to be serious. Thus, the checklist appears to justify the expenditure of time. In order to ensure compliance, it is recommended that a logbook is kept for each anaesthetic machine, and that it is signed each day when the machine is checked. The anaesthetist is solely responsible for ensuring that the anaesthetic equipment functions correctly at the start of every operating session, and for rechecking the equipment if any alteration is made to its configuration during an operating session.

Protocols and guidelines regarding clinical practice are eschewed by many anaesthetists as contrary to 'clinical freedom'. There are also concerns that any deviation from a published guideline may be interpreted by lawyers as representing an inadequate standard of care. In some countries, relatively strict guidelines are established by the head of department. In most countries, protocols and guidelines are developed within a department to inform trainees about standard methods of dealing with specific clinical problems (e.g. routine practices in the obstetric department) and to establish the limits of unsupervised practice (e.g. the minimum age of children who can be treated without reference to a consultant). These documents are usually drawn up locally, and thus their scope and content vary widely from centre to centre. Protocols for management of rare emergency situations (e.g. severe anaphylaxis or malignant hyperthermia) are valuable, as anaesthetists of all grades are likely to benefit from a checklist because most will value the cues, and because, for reasons discussed above, performance is often impaired in a crisis if the individual needs to work from first principles. Although such protocols are available, their distribution is often patchy, even within an institution. There is scope for standardization of protocols and guidelines for trainees, and in respect of emergency situations.

Monitoring

This subject is discussed in detail in Chapter 5. Minimal monitoring standards in anaesthesia have been recommended by most national professional bodies, and in some states in the USA the use of these standards has become mandatory by law and enforced by state inspectors.[167] The adoption of improved monitoring has led to reduced premiums for malpractice insurance in the USA and Canada. It has been assumed that this has been the result of improved safety, although better monitoring in conjunction with good record-keeping makes claims for compensation defensible in situations in which there was no fault and in which injury was not related to anaesthesia, but where absence of adequate monitoring and records might have made it impossible to demonstrate that anaesthesia or the anaesthetist was not responsible. For example, anaesthesia was responsible for between 3 and 5% of malpractice claims handled by one American insurer,[168] and for 11% of the total sum of money paid in compensation in 1974; by 1989, the number of claims remained at 3.5%, but the total cost had dropped to 3.6% of the total. It is therefore important to examine closely the evidence which relates improvements in monitoring to improvements in *safety* rather than reductions in insurance premiums.

Eichhorn et al[169] compared two groups of patients anaesthetized at the Harvard group of hospitals. From 1976 until 1985, 757 000 patients were studied; there were 10 serious accidents and 5 deaths. From 1985, when minimal monitoring standards were introduced, there was 1 accident and no deaths among 244 000 patients. However, this difference is not statistically significant, there was no control group, and over the period studied there had been many changes in technique and training other than the introduction of (predominantly) pulse oximetry and capnography. Keenan & Boyan[24] also compared two periods of anaesthetic practice before and after the introduction of monitoring standards. Between 1969 and 1983, there were 27 cardiac arrests during anaesthesia, from which 14 patients died, in 163 240 cases. After adoption of monitoring standards, there were no cardiac arrests in a study of 25 000 cases. However,[25] the incidence of cardiac arrests was decreasing before the standard of monitoring was improved. In addition, the authors indicated that bradycardia was detected commonly in the earlier period using existing monitoring devices, but that the cause was misinterpreted; it can be argued that increased complexity of monitoring increases the risk of misinterpretation of data.

Cullen et al[170] reported a decrease in the number of patients admitted unexpectedly to the ICU following the introduction of pulse oximetry during anaesthesia. However, this finding was not replicated by Moller et al[171,172] who conducted a randomized, controlled investigation of the impact of pulse oximetry in the peri-operative period in over 20 000 patients from five Danish hospitals. In both the operating theatre and the recovery ward, significantly more patients in the oximetry group had at least one 'respiratory event', a result of a 19-fold increase in the incidence of diagnosed hypoxaemia. Pulse oximetry failed in 2.5% of patients overall, and in 7.2% of those graded as ASA IV. Myocardial ischaemia occurred in 12 patients in the oximetry group, and 26 in the non-oximetry group (patients undergoing cardiac surgery were excluded from the study). The use of oximetry in the recovery ward was associated with the use of higher flow rates of oxygen, an increase in the frequency of patients being discharged to the ward with continued administration of oxygen and an increase in the use of naloxone. However, there were no differences between the groups in respect of death, duration of hospital stay or postoperative complications; 10% of patients in the oximetry group developed one or more postoperative complication compared with 9.4% in the non-oximetry group. The only benefit was to the anaesthetists, 80% of whom felt 'more secure' when oximetry was available.

The ASA closed claims study[53] concluded that the use of better monitoring (almost invariably pulse oximetry or capnography) would have prevented more than 90% of claims related to inadequate ventilation or oesophageal intubation, and that the standard of care was inadequate in approximately 85% of such claims compared with 30% in claims related to non-respiratory events. The large majority of these respiratory complications resulted in death or permanent brain damage, compared with a minority of non-respiratory events. However, the authors drew attention in a separate publication[173] to the fact that reviewers were more likely to find an inappropriate standard of care in cases involving brain damage than in those in which the patient recovered. In addition, in 305 of 346 cases which were considered to be preventable, at least one clinical sign of abnormality was indicated by existing monitors, but was ignored or misinterpreted. Further, the closed claims study found later that cases were being considered which previously would have been classed as inadequate ventilation, but in which, because pulse oximeters were being used, it was known that the oxygen saturation was normal, and another cause had to be postulated;[174] how accurate were the reviewers' analyses in the initial report?

Keats[174] has questioned the benefits of improved monitoring, and suggested that it is possible that mortality from anaesthesia has not decreased because we create new mechanisms of mortality at the same rate as we solve old ones. For example, there is little evidence of benefit from the use of pulmonary artery catheters, and a suggestion that mortality may be increased in some circumstances.[175] There are risks that anaesthetists rely entirely on numbers generated by monitoring devices, even if they are incompatible with the clinical condition of the patient. There are also risks that anaesthetists treat 'abnormal' numbers generated by monitoring devices, even when the degree of abnormality is so small that no injury can result, but when the treatment itself may result in injury. For example, as indicated above, there have been cases of awareness resulting from a reduction in inspired nitrous oxide concentration by trainee anaesthetists who were responding to arterial oxygen saturations of 92–93% shortly after induction of anaesthesia. Many trainee anaesthetists reduce the minute volume of ventilation to 3 l.min^{-1} using a non-rebreathing mechanical ventilator in order to generate a 'normal' end-tidal carbon dioxide concentration, failing to appreciate the alteration in arterial to end-tidal carbon dioxide difference which accompanies anaesthesia and positive-pressure ventilation. As noted above, the ASA closed claims study comparing paediatric with adult patients[41] found that, although reviewers considered that 89% of claims relating to inadequate ventilation could have been prevented by better monitoring, an adverse outcome was avoided in only 1 of the 7 cases in which a pulse oximeter was used. It has been suggested that increased dependence on monitoring may induce a sense of complacency and decrease vigilance. In one study,[176] the oesophageal stethoscope was occluded with a clamp following a staged distraction (conversation, or a loud noise). Residents who had been trained in a department equipped with automated blood pressure measurement devices detected the occlusion considerably later than those who were trained to measure blood pressure manually, suggesting that the former group were less vigilant.

In view of the range of injuries which patients suffer at the hands of anaesthetists, it is foolish to assume that improved monitoring can abolish risk, because some errors (e.g. administration of an inappropriate drug) are likely to cause damage irrespective of the standard of monitoring, and because, although monitors are connected, they are not always heeded. The author has encountered a number of cases in which patients have been seriously injured because the anaesthetist either was totally unable to interpret the mass of data presented by the monitors, or had switched off all the alarms (or both).

There can be few anaesthetists trained before the advent of modern monitors who would wish to return to the 'finger on the pulse' and the occasional measurement of blood pressure using a mercury sphygmomanometer. The AIMS study found that 52% of critical incidents were detected first by a monitor; the pulse oximeter and capnograph detected the first changes in more than half of these cases, and electrocardiogram, blood pressure monitor or low-pressure breathing system alarm in a further 39%.[177] A theoretical analysis predicted that a pulse oximeter, on its own, would have detected 82% of applicable incidents (nearly 60% before any potential for organ damage), and that a combination of pulse oximetry, capnography and blood pressure monitoring would have detected 93% of applicable incidents. However, the study also identified a number of instances in which monitors failed or provided misleading information.

If monitors are to achieve their full potential in improving safety, they must be used wisely, alarms must be set at appropriate levels, and the information provided by the monitors must be scanned regularly and interpreted in conjunction with the results of clinical observation. Monitors must not be used as an alternative to vigilance by the anaesthetist, but as an adjunct.

CONCLUSION

Modern anaesthesia is very safe, but is still not without risk. Although many claims have been made that the risk associated with anaesthesia has decreased substantially in recent years, there is little hard supportive evidence. Many assumptions have been based on retrospective analysis of events which 'could have been prevented', but numerous studies have demonstrated that the same pattern of errors, incidents and accidents continues to occur. The safety of patients does not depend solely on application of standards of practice, the purchase of new equipment and the institution of new monitoring techniques. Safety can be increased only by combining the use of modern technology with improvements in education, training, supervision, attitudes, standards of clinical practice, audit and vigilance.

REFERENCES

1. Macintosh RR. Deaths under anaesthetics. *Br J Anaesth* 1949; 21: 107–136
2. Adams AP. Safety in anaesthetic practice. In: Atkinson RS, Adams AP (eds) *Recent advances in anaesthesia and analgesia 17*. Edinburgh: Churchill Livingstone, 1992: pp 1–24
3. Beecher HK Todd DP. *A study of the deaths associated with anesthesia and surgery*. Springfield, Illinois: Charles C Thomas, 1954
4. Dornette WHL, Orth OS. Death in the operating room. *Anesth Analg* 1956; 35: 545–551
5. Schapira M, Kepes ER, Hurwitt ES. An analysis of deaths in the operating room and within 24 hours of surgery. *Anesth Analg* 1960; 39: 149–152
6. Phillips OC, Frazier TM, Graff TD, DeKornfeld TJ. The Baltimore anesthesia study committee. A review of 1024 postoperative deaths. *JAMA* 1960; 174: 2015–2020
7. Dripps RD, Lamont A, Eckenhoff JE. The role of anesthesia in surgical mortality. *JAMA* 1961; 178: 261–266
8. Clifton BS, Hotten WIT. Deaths associated with anaesthesia. *Br J Anaesth* 1963; 35: 250–259
9. Memery HN. Anesthesia mortality in private practice. *JAMA* 1965; 194: 1185–1188
10. Gebbie D. Anaesthesia and death. *Can Anaesth Soc J* 1966; 13: 390–396
11. Minuck M. Death in the operating room. *Can Anaesth Soc J* 1967; 14: 197–204
12. Harrison GG. Anaesthetic contributory death—its incidence and causes. *S Afr Med J* 1968; 42: 514–518, 544–549
13. Marx GF, Matteo CV, Otkin LR. Computer analysis of post anesthetic deaths. *Anesthesiology* 1973; 39: 54–58
14. Bodlander FMS. Deaths associated with anaesthesia. *Br J Anaesth* 1975; 47: 36–40
15. Harrison GG. Death attributable to anaesthesia: a 10 year survey (1967–1976). *Br J Anaesth* 1978; 50: 1041–1046
16. Hovi-Viander M. Death associated with anaesthesia in Finland. *Br J Anesth* 1980; 52: 483–489
17. Lunn JN, Mushin WW. *Mortality associated with anaesthesia*. London: Nuffield Provincial Hospitals Trust, 1982
18. Buck N, Devlin HB, Lunn JN. *Report on the confidential enquiry into perioperative deaths*. London: Nuffield Provincial Hospitals Trust/The Kings Fund Publishing House, 1987
19. Tiret L, Desmonts JM, Hatton F, Vourc'h G. Complications associated with anaesthesia—a prospective survey in France. *Can Anaesth Soc J* 1986; 33: 336–344
20. Holland R. Anaesthetic mortality in New South Wales. *Br J Anaesth* 1987; 59: 834–841
21. Chopra V, Bovill JG, Spiderdijk J. Accidents, near accidents and complications during anaesthesia: a retrospective analysis of a 10-year period in a teaching hospital. *Anaesthesia* 1990; 45: 3–6
22. Cohen MM, Duncan PG, Tate RB. Does anesthesia contribute to operative mortality? *JAMA* 1988; 260: 2859–2863
23. Pedersen T. Complications and death following anaesthesia. A prospective study with special reference to the influence of patient-, anaesthesia-, and surgery-related risk factors. *Dan Med Bull* 1994; 41: 319–331
24. Keenan RL, Boyan CP. Cardiac arrest due to anesthesia: a study of incidence and causes. *JAMA* 1985; 253: 2373–2377
25. Keenan RL, Boyan CP. Decreasing frequency of anesthetic cardiac arrests. *J Clin Anesth* 1991; 3: 354–357
26. Eichhorn JH. Prevention of intraoperative anesthesia accidents and related severe injury through safety monitoring. *Anesthesiology* 1989; 70: 572–577
27. Forest JB, Rehder K, Goldsmith CH et al. Multicenter study of general anesthesia.I. Design and patient demography. *Anesthesiology* 1990: 72: 252–261
28. Forrest JB, Cahalan MK, Rehder K et al. Multicenter study of general anesthesia. II. Results. *Anesthesiology* 1990; 72: 262–268
29. Forrest JB, Rehder K, Cahalan MK, Goldsmith CH. Multicenter study of general anesthesia. III. Predictors of severe perioperative adverse outcomes. *Anesthesiology* 1992; 76: 3–15
30. Cohen MM, Duncan PG, Tweed AW et al. The Canadian four-centre study of anaesthetic outcomes. I. Description of methods and populations. *Can J Anaesth* 1992; 39: 420–429
31. Cohen MM, Duncan PG, Pope WDB et al. The Canadian four-centre study of anaesthetic outcomes. II. Can outcomes be used to assess the quality of anaesthesia care? *Can J Anaesth* 1992; 39: 430–439
32. Edmonds-Seal J, Eve NH. Minor sequelae of anaesthesia: a pilot study. *Br J Anaesth* 1962; 34: 44–47
33. Cohen MM, Duncan PG, Pope WDP, Wolkenstein C. A survey of 112 000 anaesthetics at one teaching hospital (1975–83). *Can Anaesth Soc J* 1986; 33: 22–31
34. Cooper AL, Leigh JM, Tring IC. Admissions to the intensive care unit after complications of anaesthetic techniques over 10 years. *Anaesthesia* 1989; 44: 953–958
35. Flanagan JC. The critical incident technique. *Psychol Bull* 1954; 51: 327–358
36. Safren MA, Chapanis A. A critical incident study of hospital medication errors. *Hospitals* 1960; 34: 32–66
37. Sanazaro PJ, Williamson JW. Physician performance and its effect on patients: a classification based on reports by internists, surgeons, pediatricians and obstetricians. *Med Care* 1970; 8: 299–308
38. Waterson T. A critical incident study in child health. *Med Educ* 1988; 22: 27–31
39. Cooper JB, Newbower RS, Long CD, McPeek B. Preventable anesthesia mishaps: a study of human factors. *Anesthesiology* 1978; 49: 399–406
40. Cooper JB, Long CD, Newbower RS. Philip JH. Critical incidents associated with intraoperative exchanges of anesthesia personnel. *Anesthesiology* 1982; 56: 456–461
41. Cooper JB, Newbower RS, Kitz RJ. An analysis of major errors and equipment failures in anesthesia management: considerations for prevention and detection. *Anesthesiology* 1984; 60: 34–42
42. Newbower RS, Cooper JB, Long CD. Failure analysis—the human element. In: Gravenstein JS, Newbower RS, Ream AK, Smith NT (eds) *Essential*

non-invasive monitoring in the operating room. New York: Grune & Stratton, 1980: pp 269–281
43 Craig J, Wilson ME. A survey of anaesthetic misadventures. *Anaesthesia* 1981; 36: 933–936
44 Holland R. Symposium—the Australian incident monitoring study. *Anaesth Intensive Care* 1993; 21: 501
45 Webb RK, Currie M, Morgan CA et al. The Australian incident monitoring study: an analysis of 2000 incident reports. *Anaesth Intensive Care* 1993; 21: 520–528
46 Derrington MC. Critical incidents in anaesthesia. In: Walker JS (ed) *Quality and safety in anaesthesia.* London: British Medical Journal, 1994: pp 105–128
47 Utting JE. Pitfalls in anaesthetic practice. *Br J Anaesth* 1987; 59: 877–890
48 Brahams D. Medicine and the law. Two anaesthetists convicted of manslaughter. *Lancet* 1990; 336: 430–431
49 Aitkenhead AR. Anaesthesia. In: Jackson JP (ed) *A practical guide to medicine and the law.* Springer-Verlag, London, 1991: pp 45–75
50 Caplan RA, Ward RJ, Posner K, Cheney FW. Unexpected cardiac arrest during spinal anesthesia. A closed claims analysis of predisposing factors. *Anesthesiology* 1988; 68: 5–11
51 Tinker JH, Dull DL, Caplan RA, Ward RJ, Cheney FW. Role of monitoring devices in prevention of anesthetic mishaps: a closed claims analysis. *Anesthesiology* 1989; 71: 541–546
52 Caplan RA, Posner KL, Ward RJ et al. Adverse respiratory events in anesthesia: a closed claims analysis. *Anesthesiology* 1990; 72: 828–833
53 Cheney FW, Posner KL, Caplan RA. Adverse respiratory events infrequently leading to malpractice suits: a closed claims analysis. *Anesthesiology* 1991; 75: 932–939
54 Chadwick HS, Posner K, Caplan RA, Ward RJ, Cheney FW. A comparison of obstetric and nonobstetric anesthesia malpractice claims. *Anesthesiology* 1991; 74: 242–249
55 Morray JP, Geiduschek JM, Caplan RA, Posner K, Gild WM, Cheney FW. A comparison of pediatric and adult anesthesia closed malpractice claims. *Anesthesiology* 1993; 78: 461–467
56 Cheney FW, Posner KL, Caplan RA, Gild WM. Burns from warming devices in anesthesia: a closed claims analysis. *Anesthesiology* 1994; 80: 806–810
57 Shimada Y, Kato Y. Anesthesia mortality and morbidity in Japan: a study of lawsuit cases. *J Anesth* 1994; 8: 1–5
58 Bonsu AK, Stead AL. Accidental cross-connexion of oxygen and nitrous oxide in an anaesthetic machine. *Anaesthesia* 1983; 38: 767–769
59 Thorp, JM, Railton R. Hypoxia due to air in the oxygen pipeline: a case for oxygen monitoring in theatre. *Anaesthesia* 1982; 37: 683–687
60 Cole AGH, Thompson JB, Fodor IM, Baker AB, Sear JW. Anaesthetic machine hazard from the Selectatec block. *Anaesthesia* 1983; 38: 175–177
61 Hanning CD, Kruchek D, Chunara A. Preferential oxygen leak—an unusual case. *Anaesthesia* 1987; 42: 1329–1330
62 Notcutt WG, Morgan RJM. Introducing patient-controlled analgesia for postoperative pain control into a district general hospital. *Anaesthesia* 1990; 45: 406–408

63 Pollard BJ, Junius F. Accidental intubation of the oesophagus. *Anaesth Intensive Care* 1980; 8: 183–186
64 Smith GB, Hirsch NP, Ehrenwerth J. Placement of double-lumen endobronchial tubes: correlation between clinical impressions and bronchoscopic findings. *Br J Anaesth* 1986; 58: 1317–1320
65 Jackson FN, Rowland V, Corssen G. Laryngospasm-induced pulmonary edema. *Chest* 1980; 78: 819–821
66 Adams AP. Techniques of vascular control for deliberate hypotension during anaesthesia. *Br J Anaesth* 1975; 47: 777–792
67 Alexander SC, Smith TC, Strobel G, Stephen GW, Wollman H. Cerebral carbohydrate metabolism of man during respiratory and metabolic alkalosis. *J Appl Physiol* 1968; 24: 66–71
68 Lindop MJ. Complications and morbidity of controlled hypotension. *Br J Anaesth* 1975; 47: 799–803
69 Timperley AJ, Bracey DJ. Cardiac arrest following the use of hydrogen peroxide during arthroplasty. *J Arthroplasty* 1989; 4: 369–370
70 Beck DH, McQuillan PJ. Fatal carbon dioxide embolism and severe haemorrhage during laparoscopic salpingectomy. *Br J Anaesth* 1994; 72: 243–245
71 Smith PLC, Treasure T, Newman SP et al. Cerebral consequences of cardiopulmonary bypass. *Lancet* 1986; 1: 823–825
72 Siesjö BK, Ljunggren B. Cerebral energy reserves after prolonged hypoxia and ischemia. *Arch Neurol* 1973; 29: 400–407
73 Garcia JH, Conger KA. Ischemic brain injuries: structural and biochemical effects. In: Grenvik A, Safar P (eds) *Brain failure and resuscitation. Clinics in critical care medicine,* vol 2. New York: Churchill Livingstone, 1981: pp 35–54
74 Aitkenhead AR. Cerebral protection after cardiac arrest. *Resuscitation* 1991; 22: 197–202
75 Safar P. Resuscitation after brain ischemia. In: Grenvik A, Safar P (eds) *Brain failure and resuscitation. Clinics in critical care medicine,* vol 2. New York: Churchill Livingstone, 1981: pp 155–184
76 Sandin R, Nordström O. Awareness during total i.v. anaesthesia. *Br J Anaesth* 1993; 71: 782–787
77 Roberts FL, Dixon J, Lewis GTR, Tackley RM, Prys Roberts C. Induction and maintenance of propofol anaesthesia: a manual infusion scheme. *Anaesthesia* 1988; 43: S14–S17
78 Schüttler J, Kloos S, Schwildern H, Stoeckel H. Total intravenous anaesthesia with propofol s and alfentanil by computer-assisted infusion *Anaesthesia* 1988; 43: S2–S7
79 Lyons G, Macdonald R. Awareness during Caesarian section. *Anaesthesia* 1991; 46: 62–64
80 McCrirrick A, Evans GH, Thomas TA. Overpressure isoflurane at Caesarean section: a study of arterial isoflurane concentrations. *Br J Anaesth* 1994; 72: 122–124
81 Taylor v Worcester and District Health Authority. *Med Law Rep* 1991; 2: 215–231
82 Aitkenhead AR. Awareness during anaesthesia: what should the patient be told? *Anaesthesia* 1990; 45: 351–352
83 Shanker KB, Palkar NV, Nishkala R. Paraplegia following epidural potassium chloride. *Anaesthesia* 1985; 40: 45–47
84 Rigler ML, Drasner K, Krejcie TC et al. Cauda equina

syndrome after continuous spinal anesthesia. *Anesth Analg* 1991; 72: 275–281
85 Ravindran RS, Bond VK, Tasch MD et al. Prolonged neural blockade following regional anesthesia with 2-chloroprocaine. *Anesth Analg* 1980; 59: 447–451
86 Reynolds F, Speedy HM. The subdural space: the third place to go astray. *Anaesthesia* 1990; 45: 120–123
87 McMenemin IM, Sissons GRJ, Brownridge P. Accidental subdural catheterization: radiological evidence of a possible mechanism for spinal cord damage. *Br J Anaesth* 1992; 69: 417–419
88 Kroll DA, Caplan RA, Posner K, Ward RJ, Cheney FW. Nerve injury associated with anesthesia. *Anesthesiology* 1990; 73: 202–207
89 Nelson DA. Intraspinal therapy using methylprednisolone acetate. Twenty-three years of clinical controversy. *Spine* 1993; 18: 278–286
90 Walsh EM. Steroid epidurals for low back pain and sciatica: still safe and effective after all these years? *J Pain Soc* 1992; 10: 21–24
91 Davis v Barking, Havering and Brentwood Health Authority. *Med Law Rep* 1993; 4: 85–91
92 MacArthur C, Lewis M, Knox EG, Crawford JS. Epidural anaesthesia and long term backache after childbirth. *Br Med J* 1990; 301: 9–12
93 Ong B, Cohen MM, Cumming M, Palahniuk RJ. Obstetrical anaesthesia at Winnipeg Women's Hospital 1975–83: anaesthetic techniques and complications. *Can J Anaesth* 1987; 34: 294–299
94 Alvine FG, Schurrer ME. Postoperative ulnar-nerve palsy. *J Bone Joint Surg* 1987; 69-A: 255–259
95 Fletcher TR, Healy TEJ. The arterial tourniquet. *J R Coll Surg Engl* 1983; 65: 409–417
96 Fisher MM, Baldo BA. Anaphylactoid reactions during anaesthesia. *Clin Anaesthesiol* 1984; 2: 677–692
97 Laxenaire MC, Mouton C, Moneret-Vautrin DA et al. Drugs and other agents involved in anaphylactic shock occurring during anaesthesia. A French multicenter epidemiological inquiry. *Ann Fr Anesth Réanim* 1993; 12: 91–96
98 Suspected anaphylactic reactions associated with anaesthesia. Report of the second working party. London: Association of Anaesthetists of Great Britain and Ireland, 1995
99 Lockhart PB, Feldbau EV, Gabel RS et al. Dental complications during and after tracheal intubation. *J Am Dent Assoc* 1986; 112: 480–483
100 Burton JF, Baker AB. Dental damage during anaesthesia and surgery. *Anaesth Intensive Care* 1987; 15: 262–268
101 Clokie C, Metcalf I, Holland A. Dental trauma in anaesthesia. *Can J Anaesth* 1989; 36: 675–680
102 Endler GC, Marion FG, Sokol RJ, Stevenson LB. Anesthesia-related maternal mortality in Michigan, 1972–1984. *Am J Obstet Gynecol* 1988; 159: 187–193
103 Terry HR, Kearns TP, Love JG, Orwoll G. Untoward ophthalmic and neurologic events of anesthesia. *Surg Clin North Am* 1965; 45: 927–929
104 Snow JC, Kripke BJ, Norton ML et al. Corneal injuries during general anesthesia. *Anesth Analg* 1975; 54: 465–468
105 Batra YK, Bali IM. Corneal abrasions during general anesthesia. *Anesth Analg* 1977; 56: 863–866
106 Gild WM, Posner KL, Caplan RA, Cheney FW. Eye injuries associated with anesthesia. *Anesthesiology* 1992; 76: 204–208
107 *British national formulary* 28. London: The Pharmaceutical Press, 1995
108 Reason JT. *Human error*. Cambridge: Cambridge University Press, 1990
109 Nagel DC. Human error in aviation operations. In: Weiner EL, Nagel DC (eds) *Human factors in aviation*. New York: Academic Press, 1988
110 Williamson AM, Feyer A. Behavioural epidemiology as a tool for accident research. *J Occup Accidents* 1990; 12: 207–212
111 Webb RK, Currie M, Morgan CA et al. The Australian incident monitoring study: an analysis of 2000 incident reports. *Anaesth Intensive Care* 1993; 21: 520–528
112 Norman DA. The psychology of everyday things. New York: Basic Books, 1988
113 Allnutt MF. Human factors in accidents. *Br J Anaesth* 1987; 59: 856–864
114 Runciman WB, Sellen A, Webb RK et al. Errors, incidents and accidents in anaesthetic practice. *Anaesth Intensive Care* 1993; 21: 506–519
115 Eysenck HJ, Eysenck SBG. Manual of the Eysenck personality inventory. Sevenoaks: Hodder & Stoughton, 1964
116 Yerkes RM, Dodson JD. The relation of strength of stimulus to rapidity of habit formation. *J Comp Neurol Psychol* 1908; 18: 459–482
117 Gaba DM. Human error in anesthetic mishaps. *Int Anesthesiol Clin* 1989; 27: 137–147
118 Greenbaum R. Design of equipment for safety. In: Walker JS (ed) Quality and safety in anaesthesia. London: British Medical Journal, 1994: pp 154–172
119 Westhorpe RN. Ergonomics and monitoring. *Anaesth Intensive Care* 1988; 16: 71–75
120 Runciman WB. Crisis management. *Anaesth Intensive Care* 1988; 16: 87–88
121 Schaefer HG. Safety in the operating theatre environment. *Clin Anaesth Intensive Care* 1995 (in press)
122 Williamson JA, Webb RK, Sellen A, Runciman WB, Van der Walt JH. Human failure: an analysis of 2000 incident reports. *Anaesth Intensive Care* 1993; 21: 678–683
123 Runciman WB, Webb RK, Lee R, Holland R. System failure: an analysis of 2000 incident reports. *Anaesth Intensive Care* 1993; 21: 684–695
124 Drui AB, Behm RJ, Martin WE. Predesign investigation of the anesthesia operational environment. *Anesth Analg* 1973; 52: 584–589
125 McDonald JS, Dzwonczyk RR. A time and motion study of the anaesthetist's intraoperative time. *Br J Anaesth* 1988; 61: 738–742
126 McDonald JS, Dzwonczyk R, Gupta B, Dahl M. A second time-motion study of the anaesthetist's intraoperative period. *Br J Anaesth* 1990; 64: 582–585
127 Boquet G, Bushman JA, Davenport HT. The anaesthetic machine, a study of function and design. *Br J Anaesth* 1980; 52: 61–67
128 Weinger MB, Hendon OW, Zornow MH, Paulus MP, Gaba DM, Dallen LT. An objective methodology for task analysis and workload assessment in anesthesia providers. *Anesthesiology* 1994; 80: 77–92
129 Dzwonczyk R, Allard J, McDonald JS et al. The effect

of automatic record keeping on vigilance and record keeping time. *Anesth Analg* 1992; 74: S79

130 Herndon OW, Weinger MB, Zornow MH, Gaba DM. The use of automated record keeping saves time in complicated anesthetic procedures. *Anesth Analg* 1993; 76: S140

131 Mitler MM, Carskadon MA, Czeisler CA, Dement WC, Dinges DF, Graeber RC. Catastrophes, sleep, and public policy: consensus report. *Sleep* 1988; 11: 100–109

132 Hoddes E, Zarcone V, Smythe H et al. Quantification of sleepiness: a new approach. *Psychophysiology* 1973; 10: 431–435

133 Krueger GP. Sustained work, fatigue, sleep loss and performance: a review of the issues. *Work Stress* 1989; 3: 129–141

134 Gravenstein JS, Cooper JB, Orkin FW. Work and rest cycles in anesthesia practice. *Anesthesiology* 1990; 72: 737–742

135 Howard SK, Gaba DM, Jump B. A survey of anesthesiologists' attitudes towards production pressure. *Anesthesiology* 1993; 79: A1110

136 Spiegelman WG, Saunders L, Mazze RI. Addiction and anesthesiology. *Anesthesiology* 1984; 60: 335–341

137 Herndon OW, Weinger MB, Englund C. Indices of substance abuse and psychological disturbances in a population of anesthesia providers. *Anesthesiology* 1992; 77: A1047

138 Yesavage JA, Leirer VO. Hangover effects on aircraft pilots 14 hours after alcohol ingestion: a preliminary report. *Am J Psychiatry* 1986; 143: 1546–1550

139 Menk EJ, Baumgarten RK, Kingsley CP, Culling RD, Middaugh R. Success of re-entry into anesthesiology training programs by residents with a history of substance abuse. *JAMA* 1990; 263: 3060–3062

140 Adams AP. Safety in anaesthetic practice. In: Atkinson RS, Adams AP (eds) *Recent advances in anaesthesia and analgesia 17*. Edinburgh: Churchill Livingstone, 1992: pp 1–24

141 Reeve PE. Personality characteristics of anaesthetists. *Anaesthesia* 1983; 38: 395–396

142 Editorial. The gasman goeth. *Lancet* 1980; ii: 409

143 Chappelow J. Psychology and safety in aviation. In: Walker JS (ed) *Quality and safety in anaesthesia*. London: British Medical Journal, 1994: pp 87–104

144 *Aeronautical Decision Making*. Advisory circular number 60-22. Washington, DC: Federal Aviation Administration, 1991

145 Adams AP. Standards and postgraduate training. In: Walker JS (ed) *Quality and safety in anaesthesia*. London: British Medical Journal, 1994: pp 27–47

146 International standards for a safe practice of anesthesiology. *Eur J Anaesthesiol* 1993; 10 (suppl 7): 12–15

147 Healy TEJ. *Plan for assessment and structured training of anaesthetists. Training methods working party*. London: Royal College of Anaesthetists, 1992

148 *Report of a working group on specialist medical education. Hospital doctors: training for the future*. London: HMSO 1993

149 *Report to the chief medical officer's working group to advise on specialist training in the United Kingdom. Training for specialist practice*. London: HMSO, 1993

150 Harden RMcG, Stevenson M, Downie WW, Wilson GM. Assessment of clinical competence using objective structured clinical examination. *Br Med J* 1975; 1: 447–451

151 *Continuing medical education: report of a working party*. London: Royal College of Anaesthetists, 1993

152 Andrews DH. Relationships among simulators, training devices, and learning: a behavioral view. *Educ Technol* 1988; 28: 48–54

153 Schwid HA, O'Donnell D. Anesthesiologists' management of simulated critical incidents. *Anesthesiology* 1992; 76: 495–501

154 Denson JS, Abrahamson S. A computer-controlled patient simulator. *JAMA* 1969; 208: 504–508

155 Abrahamson S, Denson JS, Wolf RM. Effectiveness of a simulator in training anesthesiology residents. *J Med Educ* 1969; 44: 515–519

156 Good ML, Gravenstein JS. Training for safety in an anesthesia simulator. *Semin Anesth* 1993; 12: 235–250

157 Gaba DM, DeAnda A. A comprehensive anesthesia simulation environment: re-creating the operating room for research and training. *Anesthesiology* 1988; 69: 387–394

158 Chopra V, Engbers FHM, Geerts MJ, Filet WR, Bovill JG, Spierdijk J. The Leiden anaesthesia simulator. *Br J Anaesth* 1994; 73: 287–292

159 Chopra V, Gesink BJ, de Jong J, Bovill JG, Spierdijk J, Brand R. Does training on an anaesthesia simulator lead to improvement in performance? *Br J Anaesth* 1994; 73: 293–297

160 *Protocol for checking an anaesthetic machine before use*. Faculty of Anaesthetists of the Royal Australasian College of Surgeons, 1980

161 Kestin IG, Chapman JM, Crosse MM, Edwards JC. Guidelines for trainees during the first 8 weeks of anaesthetic training. *Today's Anaesthetist* 1989; 4: 26–36

162 Cundy JF, Baldock G. Safety check procedures in anaesthetic machines. *Anaesthesia* 1982; 37: 161–169

163 FDA checkout procedure. Anesthesia apparatus checkout recommendations. *Anesth Patient Safety Found Newslett* 1986; 1: 15

164 *Guidelines to the practice of anaesthesia as recommended by the Canadian Anaesthetists' Society*. Toronto: The Canadian Anaesthetists' Society, 1987

165 *Checklist for anaesthetic machines: a recommended procedure based on the use of an oxygen analyser*. London: Association of Anaesthetists of Great Britain and Ireland, 1990

166 Barthram C, McClymont W. The use of a checklist for anaesthetic machines. *Anaesthesia* 1992; 47: 1066–1069

167 Moss E. New Jersey enacts anesthesia standards. *Anesth Patient Safety Found Newslett* 1989; 4: 13–18

168 Pierce EC. Anesthesia: standards of care and liability. *JAMA* 1989; 262: 773

169 Eichhorn JH, Cooper JB, Cullen DJ, Maier WR, Philip JH, Seeman RG. Standards of patient monitoring during anesthesia at Harvard Medical School. *JAMA* 1986; 256: 1017–1020

170 Cullen DJ, Nemaskal JR, Cooper JB, Zaslavsky A, Dwyer MJ. Effect of pulse oximetry, age, and ASA physical status on the frequency of patients admitted unexpectedly to a post-operative intensive care unit. *Anesth Analg* 1992; 74: 181–188

171 Moller JT, Pedersen T, Rasmussen LS et al. Randomized evaluation of pulse oximetry in 20 802 patients. I. Design, demography, pulse oximetry failure rate, and overall complication rate. *Anesthesiology* 1993; 78: 436–444

172 Moller JT, Johannessen NW, Espersen K et al. Randomized evaluation of pulse oximetry in 20 802 patients. II. Perioperative events and postoperative complications. *Anesthesiology* 1993; 78: 444–453

173 Caplan RA, Posner K, Ward RJ, Cheney FW. Peer review of anesthetic mishaps; effect of severity of injury. *Anesthesiology* 1988; 69: A722

174 Keats AS. Anesthesia mortality in perspective. *Anesth Analg* 1990; 71: 113–119

175 Gore JH, Goldberg RJ, Spodick DH, Alpert JS, Dalen JE. A community-wide assessment of the use of pulmonary artery catheters in patients with acute myocardial infarction. *Chest* 1987; 92: 721–727

176 Kay J, Neal M. Effect of automatic blood pressure devices on vigilance of anesthesia residents. *J Clin Monit* 1986; 2: 148–150

177 Webb RK, Van der Walt JH, Runciman WB et al. Which monitor? An analysis of 2000 incident reports. *Anaesth Intensive Care* 1993; 21: 529–542

29. Audit and quality assurance

W. B. Runciman

Health care consumes a substantial proportion of the resources of most countries (approximately 6, 8 and 11% of Gross Domestic Product in the UK, Australia and the USA respectively), and an increasingly more sophisticated, better informed and less complacent public is demanding that identifiable mechanisms be put into place to ensure that these substantial funds are well spent. These mechanisms, and the philosophies underlying them, are evolving rapidly. Recently, much has been written in this area and much new jargon has been introduced. Concepts and terms are being used in the medical 'quality assurance' literature which have been borrowed from this rapidly developing area in industry; some terms with which we are familiar (e.g. 'audit') are used in different contexts in industry, and others which are well established in industry are just entering the medical lexicon (e.g. 'Total Quality Management' or TQM). Thus, before considering some of the specific activities which may be undertaken, it is necessary to define some of these terms and to discuss the evolving perspective of medical audit and quality assurance.

AUDIT

The word 'audit' is derived from the Latin verb '*audire*', to hear, and means 'hearing'; a more specific meaning relevant to its use in the context of this chapter is 'to make an official, systemic examination.'[1] It is used commonly in industry in a commercial context, where its use implies a financial audit, the aim of which is to present a true and fair account of the financial state of a company or organization, usually with details of income and expenditure over the previous year. 'Medical audit' has been defined in a National Health Service (NHS) Review White Paper '*Working for patients*' (1989) as 'the systematic critical analysis of the quality of medical care, including the procedures used for diagnosis and treatment, the use of resources, and the resulting outcome and quality of life for the patient'.[2] In the UK, participation in medical audit is one of the conditions that must be met before a hospital can obtain recognition from the Royal College of Anaesthetists for suitability for specialist training. This is also required by the Australian and New Zealand College of Anaesthetists. It is evident that this NHS definition of 'medical audit' is so broad that, in practical terms, it has become a generic term embracing most systematic quality assurance activities.

QUALITY ASSURANCE

'Quality Assurance' is a somewhat unfortunate term which seems now to be in widespread use and refers to measures by which it is intended and hoped (rather than assured) to improve the quality of the activity in question (in this case anaesthesia and related activities). A single, simple definition for the word 'quality' is difficult to supply as its meaning is somewhat context-dependent, but notions of 'excellence' or at least of 'a high standard', of 'appropriateness', 'efficiency', 'cost-effectiveness' and of 'consumer satisfaction' may all be implied, depending on the circumstances. Quality assurance activities may be directed towards individuals or groups of people (e.g. trainees, anaesthetic technicians), to structure (e.g. gas supplies, monitoring equipment), to medical or administrative processes (e.g. pre-operative assessment, management of operating theatres), or to outcomes from the perspective of the various groups involved (e.g. cost and efficiency for administrators, effectiveness and ease of implementation for clinicians, or convenience and satisfaction for patients and their relatives). In the jargon of quality assurance these groups are known as 'internal' and 'external' customers. It is clear that the meaning of quality will depend on the context in which it is used, and that 'quality assurance' may cover a wide range of activities (Table 29.1). Each of these activities will be considered later in this chapter; some of these are best carried out at departmental level, whereas others are

Table 29.1 Scope of audit/quality assurance activities

Morbidity and mortality meetings
Reviews of peri-operative deaths
Confidential Enquiry into Perioperative Deaths (CEPOD)
National CEPOD
Reviews of incident reports
Reviews of staff members
Audits of efficiency and resource utilization
Audits of anaesthetic records
Audits of clinical indicators
Audits of selected clinical techniques
Reviews of teaching activities
Audits of research activities
Audits of selected patient groups
Audits of patients' opinions and attitudes
Audits of 'internal customer' opinions and attitudes
Audits of factors influencing the clinical practice of anaesthesia (see Fig. 29.3)
    Personnel
    Drug supplies
    Patients
    Equipment
    Infrastructure
    The process of clinical anaesthesias
Audits of policies and guidelines (see Tables 29.2–29.4)

best co-ordinated at a national level. What is envisaged by the term 'quality assurance' in the medical context has been influenced by the main thrust of activities to date, and tends to vary from country to country.[3] In the UK, for example, 'quality assurance programmes' have tended to be derived from management concerns for consumer satisfaction and their direction by nurses has largely determined their content (e.g. waiting times, patient privacy), whereas medical audit has tended to refer to activities designed to improve diagnosis, management and outcome. Nevertheless, the two terms may be considered virtually synonymous, and a general model may be proposed for the process of quality assurance or audit (Fig. 29.1).[4-6] This process may apply to a full range of activities ranging from the review of a single incident or individual to systematic studies involving the whole department.

The evolving perspective

Traditionally, it has been assumed that if a person was properly educated and trained, underwent a period of scrutiny during an 'apprenticeship' (hospital training and specialization), was successful in the various selection processes and attended some continuing education and morbidity and mortality meetings, then good intentions and due care would ensure a high quality of clinical practice.[7] The occasional deviant was expected to be identified by peers and counselled by the head of department or by senior colleagues (the 'three wise men' concept), or failing that, be subject to a complaints procedure or have to answer to an ombudsman. It was assumed that only a recalcitrant few would end up facing disciplinary action by a Medical Registration body or be involved in a malpractice law suit.

The main emphasis was on getting the right person into the system, and then assuming that that person would maintain motivation and keep up with advances in the discipline. Indeed, great care has always been taken in the selection process, as experience has shown that it is exceedingly difficult to remove people once they have been granted 'tenure'. Out of this system grew a notion that the vast majority of practitioners would be beyond reproach, but that there would be a few 'bad apples' who would behave carelessly, take short-cuts and generally defy sound practice.

People-based problems — the 'bad apple' theory[8]

When the 'quality assurance' banner was originally raised, it was perceived that the challenge lay in finding these 'bad apples' and bringing them to account. With this approach, standards have to be defined, and it is also necessary to have sensitive, specific methods for measuring performance to identify whether or not they are being met. These methods must then be systematically used to document the behaviour of individuals with respect to these standards.

This is clearly an awesome task in the area of clinical medicine. It is extremely difficult to set standards for many aspects of clinical care, given the heterogeneous nature of both disease processes and the patient population, and the imposition of additional documentation can rapidly alienate even the most conscientious practitioner. Implicit in this 'bad apple' theory is that people are the cause of any problem, which implies carelessness, venality or incompetence.[8] It is now being recognized that this approach to quality assurance leads to a disaffected work force, is very difficult to implement and is often ineffective.[8,9]

Nevertheless, it is obvious, with the rapid rate of the evolution of our specialty, that it is not sufficient simply to leave people to their own devices for the 30 years or more of their career as a consultant. It has been proposed that an alternative, more constructive

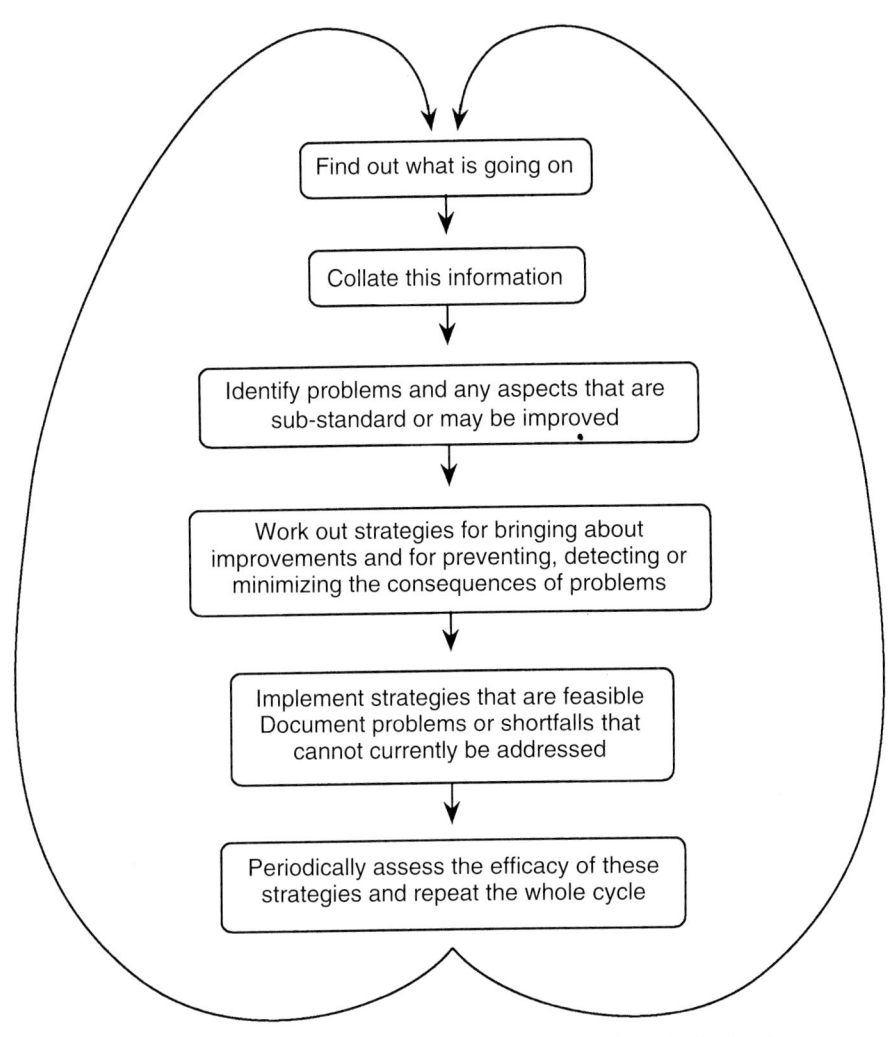

Fig. 29.1 A general model for the process of quality assurance. This may be applied to individual incidents, departmental projects or national surveys.

approach be adopted, based on the premise that most problems are inherent in the whole 'system', and are not necessarily directly attributable to individuals.

SYSTEM-BASED PROBLEMS

The notion that problems may arise from the system rather than from individuals had its origins in the 1920s when an American statistician, Walter Shewhart, began to study the 'philosophical basis of quality'.[10] His emphasis was on studying the total system from inputs to outputs and trying to elucidate cause and effect mechanisms within the process. This led to the development of 'statistical process control' for improving quality control, eliminating waste and enhancing cost-effectiveness. This was applied to sections of the manufacturing industry in the USA in the 1930s and was used in World War II to enhance quality and reliability for the 'war machine'. However, upon emergence from World War II, the USA entered a period of rapid growth and the emphasis shifted from quality, durability and reliability to maximizing output to meet an ever-increasing demand. Frequent changes to production processes were made for commercial reasons, and the concept of planned obsolescence became acceptable as a tool for ensuring ongoing profitability. Quality and reliability were no longer primary goals, and the emphasis on orienting the whole management of the system towards these aims was lost.

In contrast, Japan entered the post-war period in a completely different state. Without raw materials and with a severely damaged infrastructure, Japan had to start again from the basics. It was in this environment that Americans such as Deming and Juran were able to introduce their concept, based on the original ideas of Shewhart, that poor quality or quantity of output is seldom due to lack of motivation or skill on the part of the worker, but is much more likely to be due to defects in the layout, processes and systems of the work place (typically, problems are 85% 'system-based' and only 15% 'people-based'.[11,12] In implementing this concept, the theory of 'continuous quality improvement' evolved.

CONTINUOUS QUALITY IMPROVEMENTS[8]

The idea of continuous quality improvement is that the system can be improved every day by identifying the causes of any problems no matter how small, and putting into place mechanisms for preventing them in the future. The epigram 'every defect is a treasure' sums up this approach and provides a basic mechanism for 'Kaizen'. 'Kaizen' basically translates as a 'continuous striving to achieve improvements in all the processes and in the performance of all the people in any system'.

The theory of continuous improvement concentrates on small improvements in the performance of every aspect of the system on an ongoing basis. It concentrates on improving the entire quality–quantity curve by a small amount each year, rather than on trying to chop off the trailing edge (Fig. 29.2). It does not assume, when there is an adverse outcome, that some individual necessarily made a mistake, or was careless; indeed, the concept that not all accidents or adverse outcomes are caused by errors is an important one.[13]

Kaizen, coupled with the Japanese predilection for a team approach in the work place (the *han* system) paved the way for the post-war development of Japanese industry to its pre-eminent economic position today. The explicit recognition and promotion of the team concept in this context led to the 'Total Quality Management' movement.

TOTAL QUALITY MANAGEMENT (TQM)

This term is used when an organization takes specific measures to embrace the concepts outlined by Shewhart, Deming and Juran, and has been described as 'a structured, systematic process for creating organization-wide participation in planning and implementing continuous improvements in quality'.[14] It is proposed that everyone in the organization should be involved and that it is vital that the concepts be fully and enthusiastically accepted by 'management'. The aim is to change the 'corporate culture' so that the whole process starts to operate in a decentralized way. The person at 'the end of the line' interacting with the various internal and external 'customers' (e.g. referring surgeons and patients, respectively) is most likely to be able to identify problems and may also be the person who will have to implement corrective measures. It is generally accepted, however, even with the enthusiastic implementation of a system-wide programme, that the time required for TQM to be implemented is usually at least 3–5 years.

THE SCOPE OF AUDIT ACTIVITIES

A list of possible audit activities is presented in Table 29.1; each of these will be considered briefly. This list is not comprehensive but comprises most of the important areas that should be reviewed regularly. A schematic representation of how personnel, drugs, equipment, infrastructure and the process of clinical anaesthesia all impinge on the patient undergoing anaesthesia is shown in Figure 29.3. Each of the components of this diagram may be subjected to audit, and will also be reviewed briefly. Some components may need to be reviewed relatively infrequently (e.g. adequacy of gas supplies and alarms), whereas others (e.g. the fraction of patients who receive pre-operative assessment) may need annual review. Another approach is to review 'guideline' and 'policy documents' regularly

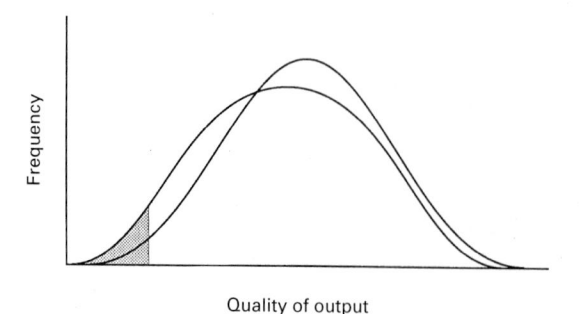

Fig. 29.2 The left-hand curve shows the normal distribution of quality of output; the shaded portion is that notionally represented by the performance of a few 'bad apples'. The right-hand curve represents the situation after introducing 'continuous quality improvement'. The curve has become narrower (indicating less variation in performance), has shifted to the right (better overall performance) and only a small amount of activities remain 'substandard' (smaller shaded area).

AUDIT AND QUALITY ASSURANCE 733

PERSONNEL	DRUGS	PATIENT	EQUIPMENT	INFRASTRUCTURE
⇓	⇓	⇓	⇓	⇓
- ODA/Anaesthetic Nurse - Recovery Ward Nurse - Trainees - Consultants	- Routine - Emergency - Backup/standby	- Selection - OPD appointment - Admission - Clerking	- Selection - Funding - Purchase	- Design of OT, recovery ward - Gas supplies/ suction - Electricity - Climate control - Communications
⇓	⇓	⇓	⇓	⇓
- Training - Certification - Accreditation	- Selection - Purchase - Stock control (central)	- Pre-anaesthetic assessment - Investigations - Information/consent	- Acceptance testing - Commissioning - Deployment	- Construction - Testing - Commissioning
⇓	⇓	⇓	⇓	⇓
- Selection - Appointment	- Delivery to OT - Storage in OT - Imprest/layout - Stock control in OT	- Pre-anaesthetic preparation - Documentation & results	- Preventative maintenance - Education in use - Documentation of problems	- Maintenance - Routine checks - Testing backups
⇓	⇓	⇓	⇓	⇓
- Orientation - Continuing education - Rostering	- Choice of drugs - Draw-up, preparation - Labelling/coding	- Acceptance to OT (checks) - Holding in OT - Checks pre-induction	- Pre-use testing - Calibration - Check lists	- Pre-use checks - Pre-use tests

Induction of anaesthesia

Maintenance of anaesthesia

Emergence from anaesthesia

Recovery Ward

| Home | Ward | High Dependency Unit | Intensive Care Unit |

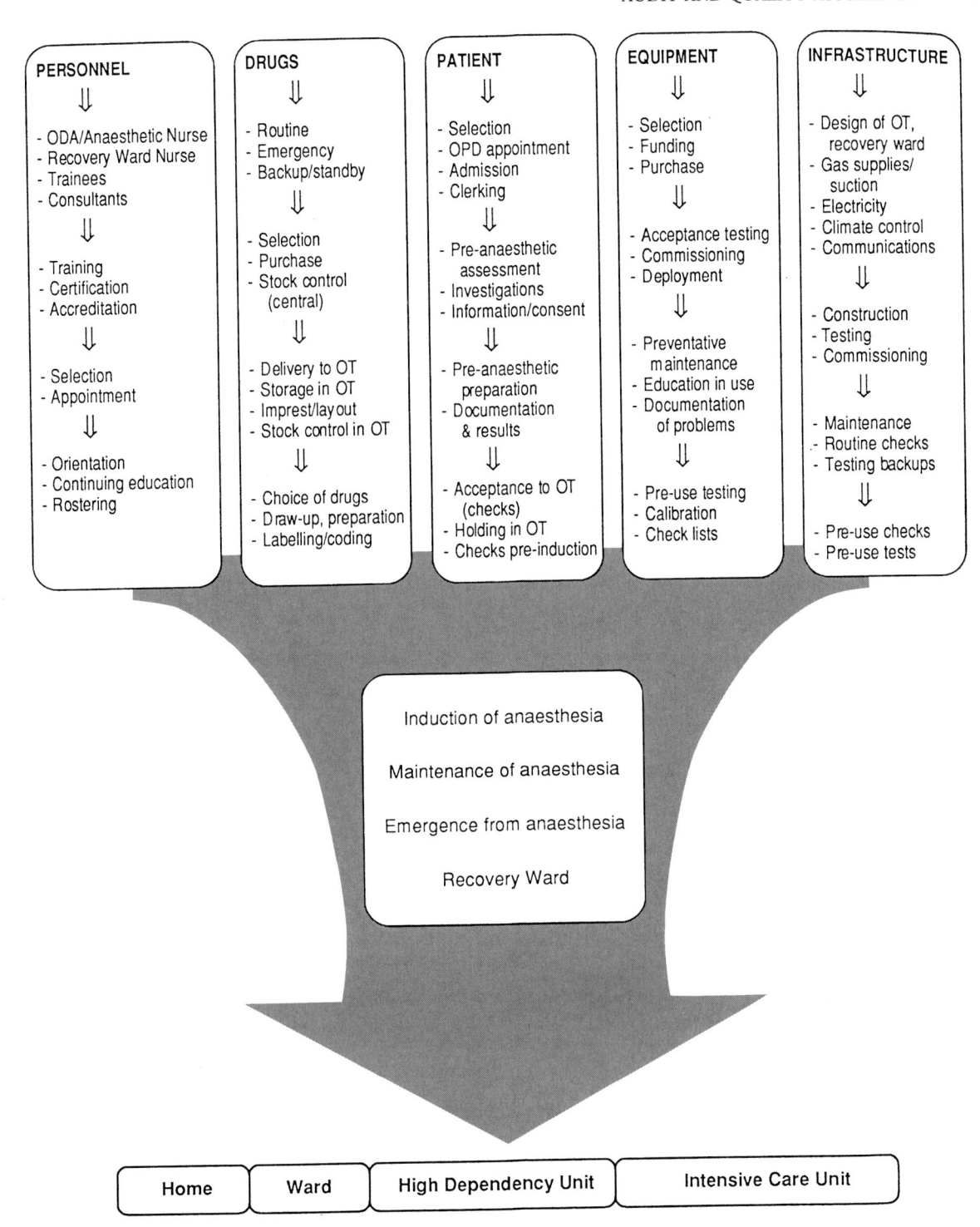

Fig. 29.3 A schematic representation of some factors which may influence the clinical practice of anaesthesia. The anaesthetist conducting an anaesthetic relies on many 'upstream' processes. Each of these should be reviewed from time to time to ensure that they are being properly carried out. Nearly all adverse outcomes require several failures in this system; the unfortunate anaesthetist may simply constitute the final common pathway through which a composite misadventure may pass, all too often travelling at speed and with considerable momentum. The shaded portion represents the sea of variables through which the anaesthetist is required to navigate. ODA = operating department assistant; OT = operating theatre; OPD = outpatient department.

Table 29.2 Booklets published by the Association of Anaesthetists of Great Britain and Ireland

Publication	Date published
Anaesthetic Services for Obstetrics — a Plan for the Future	October 1987
AIDS and Hepatitis B — Guidelines for Anaesthetists	April 1988
Guidelines on Duties of Chairmen of Division of Anaesthesia	July 1988
Assistance for the Anaesthetist	November 1988
Consultant : Trainee Relationships — A Guide for Consultants	May 1989
Recommendations for Standards of Monitoring During Anaesthesia and Recovery	October 1989
Checklist for Anaesthetic Machines	July 1990
Work Load for Consultant Anaesthetists	July 1990
Anaphylactic Reactions Associated with Anaesthesia	September 1990
The High Dependency Unit — Acute Care in the Future	February 1991
The Role of the Anaesthetist in the Emergency Service	July 1991

Table 29.3 Booklets published by the Australian and New Zealand College of Anaesthetists: educational matters

Publication	Date published
Clinical Review	1987
Duties of a Regional Education Officer	1987
Supervisors of Training in Anaesthesia and Intensive Care	1988
Formal Project	1989
Secretarial Services to Departments of Anaesthesia and Intensive Care	1989
The Supervision of Trainees in Anaesthesia	1989
Guidelines for hospitals seeking Faculty Approval of Training Posts in Intensive Care	1990
The Duties of the Anaesthetist	1990
The Supervision of Vocational Trainees in Intensive Care	1990
Guidelines for Hospitals seeking Faculty Approval of Training Posts in Anaesthesia	1991
Guidelines for the Provisional Fellowship Year	1991
The Duties of an Intensive Care Specialist in a Hospital with Approved Training Posts	1991

Table 29.4 Booklets published by the Australian and New Zealand College of Anaesthetists: technical matters

Publication	Date published
Recommended Minimum Facilities for Safe Anaesthetic Practice in Operating suites	1989
Recommended Minimum Facilities for Safe Anaesthetic Practice in Organ Imaging Units	1989
Recommended Minimum Facilities for Safe Anaesthetic Practice in Electro-Convulsive Therapy (ECT)	1989
Recommended Minimum Facilities for Safe Anaesthetic Practice in Dental Surgeries	1989
Recommended Minimum Facilities for Safe Anaesthetic Practice in Delivery Suites	1989
Protocol for Checking an Anaesthetic Machine before Use	1990

Table 29.5 Booklets published by the Australian and New Zealand College of Anaesthetists: professional matters

Publication	Date published
Protocol for the Use of Autologous Blood	1986
Endoscopy of the Airways	1987
Guidelines for the Care of Patients Recovering from Anaesthesia Related to Day Surgery	1987
Guidelines for the Conduct of Epidural Analgesia in Obstetrics	1987
Major Regional Anaesthesia	1987
Continuous Intravenous Analgesic Infusions	1988
Guidelines for the Care of Patients Recovering from Anaesthesia	1989
Minimum Assistance Required for the Safe Conduct of Anaesthesia	1989
The Pre-Anaesthetic Consultation	1989
Minimum Requirements for the Anaesthetic Record	1990
Monitored Care by an Anaesthetist	1990
Monitoring During Anaesthesia	1990
Responsibilities of Anaesthetists in the Post-Operative Period	1990
Sedation for Dental Procedures	1990
Statement on Patients' Rights and Responsibilities	1990
Essential Training for General Practitioners Proposing to Administer Anaesthetics	1991
Management of Cardio-Pulmonary Bypass	1991
Minimum Standards for Intensive Care Units	1991
Privileges in Anaesthesia Faculty Policy	1991
Statement on Principles for the Care of Patients who are given Drugs Specifically to produce Coma	1991
Statement on Smoking	1991
The Use of Sedation for Diagnostic and Minor Surgical Procedures	1991

and determine to what extent individuals or departments comply with these (Tables 29.2–29.5).

Morbidity and mortality meetings

In many departments, morbidity and mortality meetings have constituted the main audit activity; cases in which there was any adverse outcome are collected and presented at a departmental meeting. An advantage is that because these cases are real and pertain to that specific department, problems of particular relevance to that system may be identified. Analysis of each case is enhanced if a structured approach is used and the evolution of the event is traced carefully. Predisposing factors may be identified, alternative approaches which might have been used can be discussed and possible ways of preventing such an outcome in future may be proposed. However, there are also some major disadvantages. Because there was, by definition, an adverse outcome, care must be taken that opinions passed at the meeting cannot be exploited medicolegally. Although proceedings relating to quality assurance are nonadmissible in courts in most states of the USA, this is not the case in the UK and Australia. It is prudent, therefore, to avoid identifying features such as patient name, age and sex and even the surgical procedure, if it is not relevant to the particular problem. Recommendations arising from the meeting should be documented (and disseminated, if necessary), but these should be general in nature and should be aimed at putting into place measures to avoid repetition of such a problem.

Another disadvantage, when the individual involved in the problem presents the case, is that there may be public criticism of his or her actions. In many instances this may be made by individuals using the wisdom of hindsight, and may cause resentment if the criticisms are perceived to be harsh or unjust. This tendency to be more judgemental the worse the outcome is manifested even in systematic 'impartial' reviews. It has been shown that reviewers from 'closed-case' insurance claims are more likely to judge care inappropriate when there was a serious and/or permanent adverse outcome.[15] A solution is for another person always to present the case, and for the person who was involved to remain anonymous. However, it is often difficult to conceal the identity of individuals, especially in small departments or when the case involves an unusual sequence of events. Morbidity and mortality meetings are valuable, but it is most important that cases be carefully selected, that suggestions be constructive and reasonable, and that identifying features be avoided when possible.

REVIEW OF PERI-OPERATIVE DEATHS

The first systematic study of relevance to anaesthetists in this respect was the Confidential Enquiry into Maternal Deaths, which was set up in the 1930s by the Royal College of Obstetricians and Gynaecologists; this is the longest-standing study of its kind, and continues to have considerable influence on the practice of anaesthesia in this area. The first large-scale systematic reviews of deaths attributable specifically to anaesthesia were undertaken in the 1950s. In the USA, Beecher & Todd studied over half a million 'anaesthesias',[16] Greene et al surveyed over 120 000 cases in Connecticut,[17] and Dripps & Vandam followed up 10 000 spinal anaesthetics.[18] In the UK, Edwards et al reported on over 1000 deaths;[19] this was followed up by a report of a further 600 deaths in 1964 by Dinnick.[20] Systematic studies were set up in several other countries from the 1960s onwards, including an ongoing confidential reporting system in Australia.[21–25] The next major mortality study in the UK in 1982 made the point that further progress could be made only if a surgical element was included in a study, as many of the deaths involved problems arising from both surgery and anaesthesia.[26] This led to the setting up of the Confidential Enquiry into Perioperative Deaths (CEPOD).

CEPOD

CEPOD represents a most important quality assurance initiative. It was started in 1982 as a joint venture between the Associations of Surgeons and Anaesthetists of Great Britain and Ireland, as a result of the recommendation by Lunn & Mushin.[26] It reviewed surgical and anaesthetic practice over 1 year in three NHS regions during 1985 and 1986; 1300–1400 deaths were reviewed in each region. Over 95% of surgeons, gynaecologists and anaesthetists participated, resulting in a comprehensive report which was published in 1987.[27]

One of the striking outcomes was the evidence provided of very substantial variability between regions. Although, inevitably, there were some criticisms of the methodology, this ambitious project resulted in some important recommendations. Significantly, it led to the Secretary of State for Health immediately granting further funding for the work to be continued.

This was followed by Wales, Northern Ireland, the Department of Defence and major hospital groups from the private sector also deciding to participate and provide some funding. Further discussions led to the formation of the independent National Confidential Enquiry into Perioperative Deaths (NCEPOD) with the support of the associations and colleges of the relevant medical specialties.[28]

NCEPOD

NCEPOD was established to enquire into clinical practice and to identify remediable factors in the practice of anaesthesia and surgery. All the important features of CEPOD were retained and certain criticisms in methodology were addressed. It was decided to compare deaths with a random sample of matched patients. Only 0.2% of all consultant surgeons, gynaecologists and anaesthetists declined to participate in NCEPOD.[1] The long-term aim is to review 6000 peri-operative deaths each year, which represents about 1 in 5 of the estimated 30 000 deaths occurring within 30 days of surgical procedures in Great Britain and Ireland. It was decided in the first year to choose a manageable task, namely to investigate fully all deaths of children aged 10 years and under. The first report of NCEPOD into this group of patients was published in 1989.[28] The task of analysing approximately 6000 deaths each year, along with 6000 matched survivor cases and up to 5000 index cases (a larger sample of all surgical practice), is now proceeding. A large quantity of information has been gathered, and the major task of providing feedback to hospitals and attempting to institute corrective measures is in progress.

Reviews of incident reports

Although morbidity and mortality meetings have been valuable in identifying where attention should be directed to prevent similar problems from occurring again, the progressive reduction in the incidence of adverse outcomes as well as the difficulties outlined above have limited the benefits of this activity at a local level. Pooled confidential mortality data also provide very valuable information, but as individual incidents in each institution are rare and conclusions tend to be general, much of the riveting detail of a 'blow-by-blow' account is inevitably lost.

An anonymous incident-reporting system overcomes many of these drawbacks. With such a system all incidents which did or could have reduced the safety margin for the patient are reported. Reporting is voluntary and anonymous, and as most reports are 'near-misses', and there was no adverse outcome, the information is usually of high quality. By reporting incidents in which there was no adverse outcome, about 20 times more incidents are reported than with morbidity and mortality meetings;[29] in addition, most clinicians identify closely with detailed accounts of individual incidents.

The technique was described originally in 1954 by Flanagan in relation to pilot training in World War II,[30] and has since undergone further refinement and validation. The first application to increasing patient safety in anaesthesia was by Jeffrey Cooper and colleagues at Harvard University,[31] and the technique has now been applied in various formats in several other countries.[32-34] These studies all report critical incidents; an essential component of the definition of this term is the implication of error and preventability. An important feature of an Australia-wide system which started in 1988 the Australian Incident Monitoring Study; (AIMS) is that any incident may be reported without consideration of whether there may or may not have been error.[29] Thus, staff are requested to report incidents of anaphylaxis, for example, as well as of giving the wrong drug.

This emphasizes that there is no interest in culpability. Implicit in the design of the structured component of the reporting form is the recognition that several 'system-based' as well as 'operator-based' factors usually contribute to such incidents.

When a hospital or private practice group joins AIMS, a 'Starter Kit' is sent. This requires, first of all, that an individual be identified at the relevant institution to act as co-ordinator or 'person on the spot' (POS). The POS is responsible for explaining the philosophy and practicalities of the AIMS study to the department, for ensuring that reporting forms are available in every anaesthetizing location (usually on each anaesthetic machine), and for ensuring that the locations of the locked post boxes for the incident reports are known (usually in convenient places such as the operating theatre tea rooms). The POS is also available to help to fill in the AIMS report, which has both a free narrative and structured component. In practice, most reporters are perfectly happy to discuss their incident with other people, particularly if there was no adverse outcome. At some institutions, there are weekly meetings at which all the incidents from the previous week are presented. At others, reviews may be held monthly, or even less frequently. In any event, all the incident forms are forwarded to a central location, where the information is entered into a database. At this stage it is ensured that any identifying features which may inadvertently have been included are removed.

At regular intervals, trends from this database are summarized, and are sent to each participating institution. The computer software for creating similar summaries is supplied to each institution upon request. Thus, if a department so chooses, it can compare its own incident profile with the national profile, and can thus address local problems which may be causing an unusually high incidence of specific events.

At a national level, the incidents are analysed and results are published. Feedback has been provided to manufacturers and distributors of equipment, to the College of Anaesthetists, and to the Therapeutic Goods Branch of the Commonwealth Department of Health. Many trends and clusters of problems have become evident when the total database is examined, and changes have been made at local and national levels as a result of the analysis of this database. Major advantages of incident reporting are universal applicability, low cost and the wealth of relevant information provided.[35]

Reviews of staff members

The greatest asset of any department is its staff. A quick calculation of the annual salary budget and the capital sum that would need to be invested to provide this amount each year reveals the massive investment in personnel. It is eminently logical that all reasonable steps should be taken to gain the maximum benefit from this investment by having staff who are happy and active. If aspirations and attributes can be matched and each individual has a reasonable prospect of working largely in areas of his or her choice, performance is likely to be maintained at a high level. In an ideal department each person would have his or her desired work pattern and the make-up of the department would be such that all the work would be covered by people who wished to do it. In reality, some less desirable tasks are left over, and these should be shared out in as equitable a manner as possible.

Meetings should be held with each staff member as regularly as necessary but at least once every 1-2 years. These should be informal but structured two-way discussions with the aim of creating the best possible conditions for enhancing motivation and promoting development. The professional aspirations, interests and difficulties of each staff member should be discussed and related to the requirements of the department. The meeting provides an opportunity to encourage self-review of the extent to which the goals of the previous period were met and to clarify responsibilities and work assignments. Feedback on the perceptions of medical students and trainees on the teaching of each staff member may be provided.

At this meeting, plans should be made for the forthcoming period, including those for study and conference leave, and for any planned research and teaching. Further meetings may be needed to plan specific aspects of the individual's proposed activities, such as the preparation of research grant applications. Such a meeting is also an opportunity for the head of the department to express appreciation for the work that has been carried out in the previous period. It is surprising how often one is able to discover areas of interest not previously recognized in an individual, and how often promoting activity by the individual in that area can lead to enhancement of both the individual's working life and the activities of the department. Most individuals are keen to make their own special contribution to a department, but often lack specific ideas on how to go about this.

Audits of efficiency and resource utilization

A critical examination of aspects of efficiency and resource utilization may allow substantial improvements and savings to be made without compromising patient care; indeed, not infrequently, improvements in patient care result. These are sometimes best carried out by a new appointee or by someone who has worked recently in a different system. It is more difficult for a long-term incumbent to come up with radical changes. A change from morning and afternoon to all-day lists, using one instead of two nursing shifts, may, for example, result in substantial reductions in expenditure on nursing salaries. The use of a 'booking theatre' during the day to prevent low-priority cases from being operated on in the middle of the night may provide substantial savings as well as increasing patient safety. Savings may include those which result from structural changes (e.g. changing from banks of cylinders to a bulk oxygen supply), procedural changes (e.g. chest X-rays being ordered by anaesthetists only for highly specific indications), changing the pattern of use of certain disposable items and changes in work practices.

It is clear that motivation and rewards are required if major changes are to be implemented which may alter well-established work practices. Activities in these areas are obviously best carried out as part of a department-wide, or preferably a hospital-wide, TQM programme. With such programmes, a substantial proportion of the savings can usually be spent at the discretion of the department in which the savings were made, thus providing ongoing incentives for new ideas and further improvements. Although arrangements to do this are easier to implement in the USA, there is evidence that systems providing incentives have been implemented effectively in the UK.[36] A note of caution must be sounded in pursuing savings overenthusiastically. Arguments that a change is 'cost-effective' must be examined carefully, especially when it has been proposed by those with a vested interest in the change (e.g. administrators, equipment suppliers, single-theme lobbyists). Low cost and high effectiveness may be mutually exclusive in some cases.[37]

Audits of anaesthetic records

Regular audits of anaesthetic records can be useful to identify deficiencies in the system as well as in the practices of specific individuals. In 1982, Holland suggested 10 criteria that could be used; in 1986, three more were added in a study designed to determine whether the use of a new anaesthetic form had improved practice as judged against these 13 criteria (Table 29.6).[38] A number of 'system-based' problems were identified; for example, 'fluids lost and given' were noted to be recorded poorly in both the original study and in the follow-up study because of a requirement to use inappropriate forms, and measures were planned to remedy this. Practice had improved in respect of most other criteria. For example, evidence of the preoperative visit had increased from 32 to 90%; nevertheless, it was concluded that there was still room for improvement in that area. Examining relatively small

Table 29.6 Anaesthetic record criteria

Patient identification
Evidence of pre-operative assessment
Premedication given and effect
Operation performed
Drugs administered
Doses of drugs administered
Duration of anaesthesia
Record of airway invasion
Record of monitoring used
Fluids lost and given
Postoperative note
Anaesthetist's name
American Society of Anesthesiologists classification

From Gayland & Williams,[38] with permission.

samples of records can yield useful qualitative information about individual practices; up to 40% of all records may contain serious errors.[39] As would be expected, some individuals keep very comprehensive, clear records. In the case of others, several reminders may be needed that a full anaesthetic record not only contains useful clinical information, but that it may constitute their best defence in any medicolegal case.[40]

Audits of 'clinical indicators'

A clinical indicator has been defined as 'a measure of the clinical management and outcome of care', and may thus be directed towards process (e.g. the percentage of patients who had a satisfactory pre-operative visit) or to outcome (e.g. the frequency of unplanned admission to hospital after outpatient surgery).[41] Requirements of clinical indicator are that the data be available, that the indicator be relevant and appropriate, and that the measure be achievable and acceptable to the relevant health care workers. Of course, there may be valid reasons for a particular institution scoring different values (e.g. patient referral base, type of surgery). Absolute figures by which institutions may be compared with each other should not generally be made available publicly. Nevertheless, in spite of the difficulties and potential political risks of publishing differences in outcome between institutions, there is evidence that doctors are voluntarily prepared to do this in the interest of improving quality of care.[42] The Joint Commission of Accreditation of Hospitals in the USA has moved away from its traditional reliance on structural measures, and has formally taken up quality assessment based on severity-adjusted outcomes as the basis of its future strategy for monitoring hospitals.[43] The Australian Council for Health Care Standards, which since 1974 has accredited hospitals on the basis of their structural and organizational elements, has also recently been commissioned to conduct trials of a clinical indicator programme on behalf of various specialist colleges. Five clinical indicators were chosen by the Australian and New Zealand College of Anaesthetists and a trial was started in selected private and public hospitals in late 1990 (Table 29.7).[41] It is evident that some of these indicators may be more valuable than others. For example, although it is likely that the programme will have a positive effect on the rate of pre-operative visiting, it is also conceivable that patients who are still somewhat compromised may be discharged from the recovery area early, to beat an arbitrary deadline.

Much effort has been expended in the USA on collecting clinical data that will allow comparisons of risk-adjusted outcome among hospitals; this has even become a statutory requirement in some states. However, evidence is mixed as to the sensitivity and specificity of this approach, with some studies showing no correlation between poor performance judged by outcome and other measures of quality. In general, the defensiveness engendered by comparing outcomes between institutions negates any benefits.[9] Nevertheless, there is objective evidence that a reduction in morbidity and improvement in performance can result from carefully designed outcome studies.[44] It is likely that there will be specific parameters which will lend themselves well to the clinical indicators approach. It remains to be determined whether, for a given clinical indicator, the best cost–benefit lies in a continuous process, or in taking appropriate samples at regular intervals.

Table 29.7 Clinical anaesthesia indicators

Percentage of patients admitted for elective surgery who have a pre-operative visit by an anaesthetist

Mortality within 24 h of administration of an anaesthetic

Unplanned admission to an ICU/HDU within 24 h of administration of an anaesthetic

Failure to be discharged from the recovery area within 5 h

Unplanned admission to hospital after anaesthesia for an outpatient procedure

ICU = Intensive care unit; HDU = high-dependency unit. From Collopy,[41] with permission.

Audits of selected clinical techniques

Valuable information may be obtained by carrying out audits of selected clinical techniques. These are best carried out on a prospective basis using a carefully designed protocol. For example, a simple form can be completed by everyone who inserts a central venous catheter. Information about the indication, technical difficulties and complications can then be collated and related to factors such as supervision and experience of the operator. When setting up new services in a department, it may be possible to design the record system in such a way that specific aspects of the service can be audited from time to time simply by accessing a suitably designed database. In this way, for example the incidence of respiratory depression and side-effects of postoperative epidural analgesia may be examined regularly.[45] Useful information may be obtained when almost any aspect of clinical practice is subjected to systematic study.

Reviews of teaching activities

An annual audit of teaching activities provides useful feedback for teachers. One system is for all medical students and trainees to be provided with a form on which they can score their degree of exposure to each staff member, the effort each staff member appears to put into their teaching, and their perception of the value of each staff member as a teacher. Space is also left on the form for comments about aspects of the department which are thought to be valuable, and aspects of the department which are thought to be deficient; suggestions for improvements are invited. The distribution of these scores may be presented at a departmental meeting, together with the identity of one or two of the most highly rated teachers. It is obviously most important that only one or two members of the department have access to all of the scores, and that feedback should be provided privately to all except the highest scorers. Highly consistent trends may be obtained from year to year. In this way, good teachers receive encouragement to continue to put the necessary effort into their teaching, and people about whom students are highly critical may be encouraged to improve their performance. It is most important that the forms are collected in a way that preserves the anonymity of the students or trainees. To survey all trainees annually and to survey medical students after a group has had a 'block' of exposure to anaesthesia constitutes an adequate safeguard in most institutions.

Audits of research activities

It is valuable to set aside adequate time for departmental research activities to be reviewed and for plans for the coming period to be presented. Such a review may be best carried out annually, at a time when the various granting bodies have come to their decisions about any research grant applications which may have been submitted. Having in place some prospective system of documentation is most useful. A brief one-page summary of each research project may be all that is required for such a review. This can contain the names of the researchers, the title of the project, the aims and the significance, with details of ethics consent and any resources required, a brief timetable for the research programme, and a list of the proposed authors and titles of any anticipated publications. Such sheets can then be presented by each individual or research team, and reviewed by the group; new sheets for the coming year can be lodged at the same meeting.

Clinicians are notorious for failing to follow up research projects with publications, and this process can provide a valuable stimulus. A calculation of the cost of each research publication may reveal that even a simple study has cost in excess of £10 000 if all the time of all participants is taken into consideration.

The question of how to carry out a quantitative evaluation of the research activities of an academic department has become topical with funding moving away from a formula basis towards a competitive system. This is a contentious issue, but most academics accept the need for some sort of evaluation. Volume of research output, bibliometric citation analysis and esteem indicators are all considered to have a role, but the general consensus is that these performance indicators are most acceptable as a means of strengthening peer review judgements rather than as substitutes for them.[46] Success in obtaining externally reviewed grant applications may also be used as a measure, but caution is needed in correlating success with the sums allocated. Some excellent research can be conducted with very modest resources, whereas other projects, by their very nature, require substantial personnel, maintenance and equipment funding. A major dilemma is to distinguish between quantity and quality. There is no doubt that this debate will continue, but it is also likely that specific comparative measures will be necessary to provide a basis for allocation of whatever funds may be available. Certainly, regular review of the research activities of both individuals and departments is a fundamental requirement and is greatly facilitated by having a regularly updated database of projects, funding and publications.

Audits of selected patient groups

Audits of selected patient groups may best be carried out in conjunction with other disciplines (e.g. an endocrinologist for an audit of all diabetics presenting for surgery, or specialist surgeons for specific types of surgical patient).[27] Such audits usually require considerable planning and resources to be worthwhile. An audit may be undertaken because it is perceived that a specific group of patients may be subject to significant morbidity or mortality, or because it seems possible that an alternative approach or new technique may be feasible. Anaesthetists may be concerned about issues related to patient selection and informed consent, whereas surgeons may be concerned about the impact of new anaesthetic techniques on operating time and aspects of immediate postoperative care. Such audits generally lead to a far better appreciation by each group of the problems of the other and may lead to a more consistent approach to the management of complex problems. Indeed, auditing groups of patients such as those undergoing carotid endarterectomy or gastro-oesophageal resection frequently leads to plans for a prospective randomized study on the impact of some aspect of management on these patients. The protocol-based approach necessary for such a study often leads to better patient management.

Audits of patients' opinions and attitudes

The most important 'customers' of all are the patients. Regular surveys of their opinions and attitudes can reveal problems which should be addressed; in many cases considerable improvements can be made with relatively little effort. There is a growing appreciation that instruments based on subjective data from patients can provide important information in respect of outcome that is just as relevant as, or more relevant than, many of the biochemical or physiological indices upon which doctors have traditionally relied.[43] In setting up new services (e.g. day-stay surgery, acute pain service), it may be possible to build some patient survey components into a computer database which records all aspects of the service. Then, regular audits of specific aspects become very easy. Prior to setting up an acute pain service, funding was obtained to conduct a comprehensive survey of the attitudes, not only of patients, but of medical and nursing staff, as well as to determine the incidence and severity of postoperative pain.[47-50] Results of this survey formed the basis for a variety of initiatives developed specifically to address the problems identified; education programmes were put into place for student nurses, registered nurses, medical students, interns and registrars and specific steps were taken to make sure that a number of myths prevalent in patient opinions could be dealt with during pre-operative patient education about the use of the patient-controlled analgesia devices. It is intended to carry out follow-up surveys every 3 years.

There is a good argument for following up every patient who has had an anaesthetic. Indeed, this is widespread practice amongst some anaesthetists and in a number of departments of anaesthesia. However, there are also institutions in which virtually no patient is followed up unless there is a major problem. Even if it is not possible to follow up every patient, regular structured surveys of patients' opinions and attitudes should be carried out at regular intervals so that it can be determined whether progress is being made in addressing some of the problems identified.

Audits of 'internal customer' opinions and attitudes

There are several groups who can be regarded as the 'internal customers' of a department of anaesthesia. The attitudes of medical students and trainees have already been considered. Surveys can be carried out of any other group that interfaces with a department of anaesthesia (e.g. surgical clinics, radiologists, disciplines requiring a pain service). It is surprising how often certain points which have caused dissatisfaction over a long time can be addressed relatively easily by a change in administrative arrangements.

Audits of factors influencing the clinical practice of anaesthesia

Some of the factors which influence the clinical practice of anaesthesia have been depicted in a flow chart in Figure 29.3. Any of the components of this chart may be subject to audit. An advantage of visualizing the factors which influence the clinical practice of anaesthesia in this way is that the importance of the overall system is emphasized rather than that of the individual.[13] In effect, the anaesthetist, when inducing anaesthesia, is relying on the assumption that many factors have been properly managed 'upstream', as well as on his or her immediate pre-operative check.

Personnel

Regular audits may be held on any aspect of the topics listed under this heading in Figure 29.3. There are great regional variations in the quantity and quality of anaesthetic and recovery room assistants and/or nurses. In some regions, the majority of those who assist the anaesthetist may have a qualification obtained after a 3-year course. In others, a brief orientation of a few days is all that is allowed, and from then on it is a matter of 'learning on the job'. A systematic review of the circumstances pertaining in a particular department, followed by a formal recommendation arising from an audit, will at least start the process of upgrading the system. Even if there is likely to be a long 'lead-time' before the basic qualifications of such people are improved, much can be done in the department itself. The orientation of new staff members can be upgraded, and a weekly continuing education programme initiated.

Regular reviews of rostering practices are also recommended. No staff member who has been working for most of the previous night should be expected to take clinical responsibility for patients. Flexible arrangements may be made whereby a competent trainee rostered for teaching can be redeployed if a consultant has had to come into the hospital after midnight.

It is important that overall policies are not degraded by forces operating within the system which may have other objectives. This is another area in which anonymous feedback by trainees can provide useful information about how well the system works. In particular, it must be ensured that trainee staff are not expected to proceed with major cases under suboptimal circumstances due to pressure by nursing staff, surgeons or any other group. Ample support for this approach has been provided by both the CEPOD and AIMS studies.[27–29] The only way in which this can be properly safeguarded is by feedback to a properly constituted audit.

Drug supplies

The quality of drugs available in the UK, Australia and the USA is strictly regulated. However, the chain of supply between the wholesaler and the anaesthetist should be subjected to regular audit. In Australia, an 'epidemic' of errors involving the administration of the wrong drug was precipitated by a manufacturer who changed the packaging and labelling of a commonly used drug:[51] A national workshop on this subject revealed that it was possible for the suppliers of drugs to be changed so that drugs with totally different packaging, sometimes similar to that of other commonly used drugs, appeared suddenly in the work place without any notification of anaesthetists by the hospital pharmacy. Ampoules are frequently unpacked into 'galley pots' in some institutions to facilitate rapid access, and the layout of drug storage drawers or trays in operating theatres frequently varies even within the same hospital. Personal practices with respect to 'coding' and labelling of syringes vary widely, even though anaesthetists may relieve each other for periods of time. A national audit in Australia has revealed the need for a systematic approach. Over 100 'wrong drug' errors have been reported over the last 3 years and one anaesthetist in New Zealand has been convicted of manslaughter as a result of administration of a wrong drug during a clinical emergency.[52] Regular audit of the chain of drug-handling from purchase to injection and the introduction of standard layout, labelling and checking protocols are likely to reduce the incidence of such errors.

Patients

Regular audits should be held on aspects pertaining to patient management which are listed in Figure 29.3. Although fundamental to the practice of anaesthesia, the pre-anaesthetic assessment varies greatly in the reliability with which it is performed, and in its quality. It requires a persistent, dedicated anaesthetist to perform pre-anaesthetic assessments on every patient despite the obstacles that may need to be overcome. Recent surveys of pre-operative investigations in the author's hospital revealed that up to one-fifth of all chest X-rays ordered pre-operatively were not available at the time that the patient went to the operating theatre, and that nearly four-fifths of chest X-rays were ordered specifically because the patient was undergoing anaesthesia, but were regarded by the department of anaesthesia as being unnecessary. It is clear that there is much room for restructuring in this area.

It is surprising how poorly many of the processes which affect the patient in the immediate pre-operative period are actually performed. In one survey, it was shown that only 40% of pre-operative orders were carried out.[53] Audits of activities in this area are of particular importance.

Equipment

The purchase, acceptance testing, preventive maintenance, calibration and pre-operative checking of monitors and equipment such as warming blankets, humidifiers and blood warmers should all be subjected to review from time to time.[54–56] An audit of the ability of trainees to operate new 'menu-driven' electronic monitors in the author's department revealed that some individuals had very poor knowledge and abilities in this area; this led to a programme of orientation and testing for new trainees. This programme is to be extended to consultants. Another audit of the frequency with which a proper check of the anaesthetic machine and ancillary equipment was carried out has revealed that a number of individuals routinely default in this area. This led to debate about whether a standard checking process should always be carried out by two individuals in a manner analogous to the pre-flight check that is carried out by pilot and co-pilot. The fact that nearly one-fifth of all incidents (see section on reviews of incident reports, above) would have been prevented by proper checking provides substantial weight to arguments in favour of this proposal.

Infrastructure

Audit of any of the areas shown under this heading in Figure 29.3 constitutes a suitable project for a trainee; some of these audits may need formal funding and the attention of several people. New facilities should be constructed and equipped to comply with relevant standards.[57] However, it is also necessary, from time to time, to review the arrangements that are in place for safeguarding basic services such as gas supplies, suction and electricity. This should be done in conjunction with appropriate biomedical engineers after any relevant standards, recommendations or guidelines have been obtained and the literature reviewed. Regular audits of each of the topics listed under 'infrastructure' have revealed several deficiencies in the author's hospital. Many suction outlets have been shown to provide substandard suction (due to kinking, gradual blocking or contamination of hoses) and in one suite of three operating theatres the piped oxygen supply failure alarms, although fitted some 30 years ago, had never been connected. The anaesthetic machines in this area had not been fitted with low-pressure oxygen alarms, and the oxygen analysers which had been supplied had been stored in the cupboard. Pulse oximeters were not available at this stage. When rectifying these defects, it was discovered that gas regulators on the anaesthetic machines were set at inappropriate pressures. It was calculated that some 60 000 patients may have been at risk of undetected exposure to hypoxic mixtures in these three operating theatres over the previous 20 years. Plans for regular checks were made, and procedures for maintenance work and for corrective measures in the event of failure were updated.

The process of clinical anaesthesia

There are many aspects of the process of clinical anaesthesia which may be reviewed. The processes of checking the patient, the equipment and drugs may all be subjected to systematic review, as well as aspects of induction, maintenance, emergence and recovery from anaesthesia. For example, data from the AIMS study suggested that respiratory complications in the recovery ward constitute a major preventable cause of potential morbidity and mortality: 1000 consecutive recovery patients were therefore subjected to systematic audit. This confirmed that virtually all problems occurred after general anaesthesia with a relaxant, and that the incidence of problems increased markedly with increasing age of the patient. Although such a survey frequently does not reveal any new qualitative information, it may provide a valuable stimulus to improving clinical practice when it has been confirmed that there is a major problem in that department. Recommendations such as increasing the use of short-acting muscle relaxants, and always waiting for signs of recovery from neuromuscular blockade before attempts at reversal, have far greater impact if the data have been obtained in the same department, and if there are plans for the study to be repeated in the future.

Audits of policies and guidelines

Examples of policies and guidelines which are in use in the UK, Australia and New Zealand are shown in Tables 29.2–29.5. Determining whether a department complies with any of these guidelines constitutes a simple audit project suitable for medical students or trainees. In spite of the apparent simplicity of this process, valuable information is often obtained which results in defects being corrected.

THE DESIGN OF AUDIT ACTIVITIES

This depends on the subject of the audit, but some general principles apply (Fig. 29.4). The first stage is

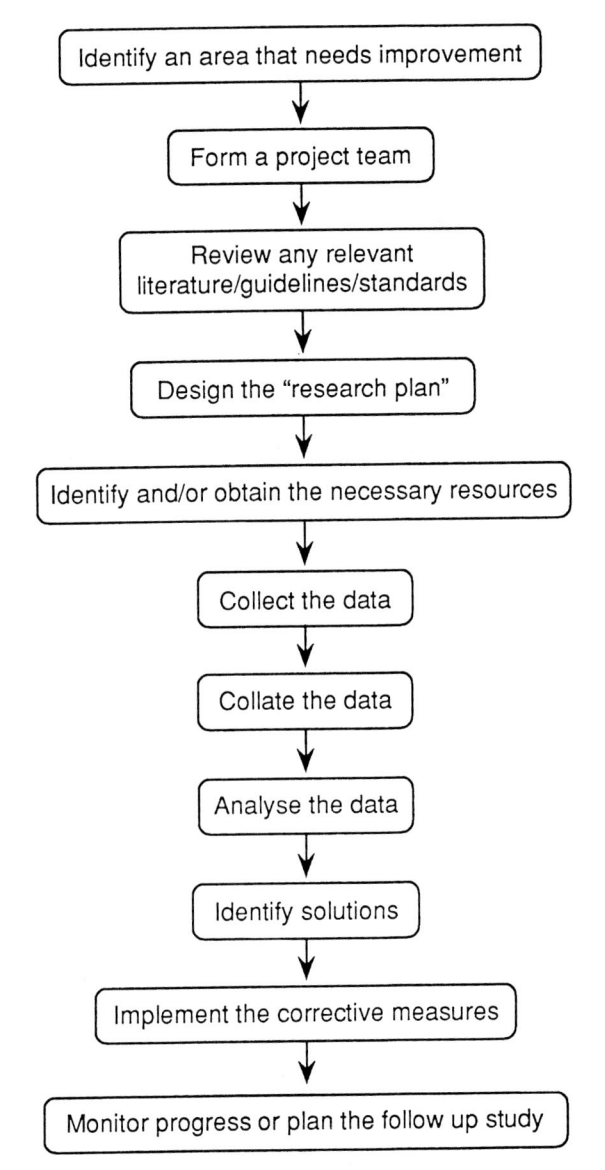

Fig. 29.4 Stages in designing and carrying out an audit or quality assurance project.

to identify the subject for audit. This may be selected from any of those considered above, or may simply occur to an individual who has been involved in a specific incident or who has a special interest. The person or people involved should then be identified and their roles delineated. Even for a simple audit on, for example, determining whether the equipment necessary for compliance with the recommended guidelines for patient monitoring is available, it is desirable to have a senior person advising the person carrying out the project. The supervisor/s may help by providing advice about where to look for the relevant literature and policy documents. The next stage involves making a detailed plan of how the data collection is to be carried out. It is important that a defined plan is laid out clearly at the beginning, and that it is confirmed by an experienced supervisor that the project can be completed in the intended time with the resources available. It may be necessary to make plans at this stage to acquire any additional resources that may be required. The design of forms and the compilation of checklists usually increase efficiency and ensure complete data sets. Another advantage is that these forms and checklists may be suitable for use in a follow-up study.

After the information has been collected, it should be assembled in a form which renders it amenable to display and statistical analysis, if necessary. Ideally, the layout of the forms on which the original data were collected should be such that analysis is facilitated. The use of a desk-top computer with appropriate statistics and graphics software may allow the whole process to be completed with minimal handling of the data. Once the data have been collected they can be displayed and subjected to analysis with statistics if necessary.

Analysis is made much easier if display formats such as histograms and scattergrams are readily available. Having analysed the problem, a list of contributing factors should be made, with possible solutions for each. A set of recommendations should be constructed, and after approval by those responsible for the area, the executive arm of the department should implement them. At this stage, it may be decided that some aspects of the problem and its implementation should be monitored. If this is impractical, a plan should be made for a follow-up study to determine if the exercise was successful. The follow-up study should be designed in the light of data obtained in the initial study, as it is frequently possible to eliminate measures which did not prove to be useful, and to predict the sizes of the data sets necessary to detect a change with acceptable statistical power. Ideally, a network of interested people in different departments should collaborate to develop a bank of standardized projects, thus facilitating not only longitudinal studies within departments, but comparisons between departments.

There is a tendency for some people to institute projects which gather statistics on an ongoing basis (see the section on audits of clinical indicators, above). There are a number of problems inherent in this approach. It is frequently necessary to delegate data collection to front-line workers with no specific interest in the project. If a small number of people are involved, it may be possible to continue to motivate them (e.g. an acute pain service). However, when large numbers are involved (e.g. a project involving all patients going through a large recovery ward), this tends to result in incomplete, and sometimes inaccurate, information. The danger is that a considerable amount of time can be consumed collecting a large mass of low-grade information which contains insufficient detail to allow analysis of mechanisms, contributing factors, and so on. There is a trade-off between the amount of information which it is practicable to record and how long the necessary collective effort can be sustained.

It is generally better to plan a specific project to 'biopsy' the system from time to time by taking a statistically adequate sample than to try to monitor many parameters on an ongoing basis.

LEVELS OF QUALITY ASSURANCE ACTIVITY

Activities at a local and regional level

Many of the activities listed in Table 29.1 and dealt with above can and should be undertaken at a local or departmental level. Some may be carried out at a regional level. For example, each state in Australia has Mortality Committee legislation to ensure that all information supplied to this Committee cannot be subpoenaed. Thus, classification and feedback to individuals take place at a regional or state level in Australia. Recently, arrangements have been made for a representative of each of these Committees to attend national meetings under the auspices of the National Health and Medical Research Council. The aim of these is to try to standardize classifications so that, ultimately, a national database can be developed.

ACTIVITIES AT A NATIONAL LEVEL

United Kingdom

The Association of Anaesthetists of Great Britain and Ireland commissioned the reviews of anaesthetic deaths published by Edwards et al[19], Dinnick[20] and Lunn &

Mushin.[26] The last of these led to the formation of CEPOD, as described above, and then the independent NCEPOD, which is still supported by the Association, but which also receives funds from other associated organizations. This constitutes a very ambitious national quality assurance activity which has had, and will continue to have, a major impact on the quality of care. It has also put into place a mechanism which will gradually evolve and which will exert a powerful influence on practice (e.g. the type, quality and content of medical records).

The Association of Anaesthetists of Great Britain and Ireland has also published a series of booklets which essentially set standards by providing a well-thought-out, thoroughly referenced set of recommendations (Table 29.2); these provide the basis for audit activities designed to determine whether or not an institution meets specific standards.

The Royal College of Anaesthetists formed a Quality of Practice Committee after its Audit Committee published its first report in 1989. The activities of the Audit Committee were subsumed into those of the new committee at that time. Membership consists of nine council members, representatives of interested organizations (e.g. the Association of Anaesthetists, NCEPOD, the Pain Society, the Intensive Care Society and the Department for Health) and a full-time administrative assistant funded jointly by the College and the Department for Health.

This provides a national focus for activities relating to quality of practice. The Committee has instituted a national enquiry into brain damage and/or cardiac arrest occurring during and/or within 6 h of completing an anaesthetic, and has supported a pilot study into methods of reporting and reviewing critical incidents with the aim of developing a national critical incident register. A joint study into the incidence of neurological complications of obstetric epidural anaesthesia has been started with the Royal Colleges of Obstetricians and Gynaecologists and of General Practitioners. Advice has been provided to several Fellows on audit methodology, and the Committee is currently organizing or supporting a range of audit activities. The College is investigating methods for computerized perioperative record keeping, and has also decided that trainees should keep a log book of their activities.

Other European countries

The origins and progress of quality assurance activities are, not surprisingly, quite different in each European country. Nevertheless, the sudden recent progression towards a requirement for quality assurance activities and the tendency for the diverse pre-existing activities to be co-ordinated under 'umbrella' organizations is quite striking. For example, both Belgium and Germany enacted legislation in 1988 mandating co-ordinated quality assurance programmes. A review of this complex area is beyond the scope of this chapter; the interested reader is referred to an international comparative study published in 1990.[3]

Australia and New Zealand

The Australian and New Zealand College of Anaesthetists (ANZCA) formed a Clinical Review Committee about 10 years ago, which generated a document outlining how the clinical review process was to take place at the departments of anaesthesia accredited for training by the College. The Committee started to direct its attention towards broader issues of quality assurance, and in 1991 changed its name to the 'Quality Assurance Committee'. Its membership includes representatives of the College Council from the Education Committees representing both Anaesthesia and Intensive Care, and it has a representative from the Australian Society of Anaesthetists. It has recently published a quality assurance document which provides advice on how to implement quality assurance in departments of anaesthesia. This is a comprehensive document. Each department is required to appoint a co-ordinator of Quality Assurance to monitor and evaluate quality and appropriateness of patient care and clinical performance of staff, to identify and implement changes where improvements are desirable, and then to monitor these changes. Audits are designed prospectively and suggested topics include most of those listed in Table 29.1; the final requirement is that the quality-assurance programme itself should be subjected to audit from time to time.

ANZCA also publishes a number of 'Guidelines' which constitute *de facto* standards; these are updated regularly (see Tables 29.3–29.5), and provide a valuable resource for Heads of Departments.

United States of America

The situation in the USA is complex and is evolving rapidly; only selected aspects are considered here. In the USA, most hospitals are accredited by the Joint Commission for Accreditation of Hospitals (JCAH), which replaced a similar body in 1952, in order to be eligible for government funding. Prior to the 1970s, a requirement for morbidity and mortality review and random audits of records comprised the quality assurance requirements. This was replaced by a formal requirement for audits using written objective criteria, but in 1979 this was judged ineffective and the requirement was rescinded; each hospital was required only to establish an organized quality assurance programme. Since then, 'generic screening' (a systematic determination of the incidence of adverse occurrences or outcomes) has been a major activity. This approach has significant limitations; nevertheless, it has provided much useful information. A critique of generic screening has been provided recently.[58] The JCAH has now indicated that hospital accreditation will be based on 70 adjusted outcomes;[43] it is likely that there will be much activity in developing the necessary methodology in the next few years.

The American Society of Anesthesiologists (ASA) has a major commitment to quality assurance, and has recently levied its members so that all are members of the Anesthesia Patient Safety Foundation, which has been responsible for several initiatives and a number of recent projects in this area. The ASA also provides films, videos and written material designed to enhance quality of care.

CONCLUSIONS

One of the functions of the Royal College of Physicians of London which was incorporated in its original charter of 1578 is to uphold the standards of medicine 'both for their own honour and public benefit'.[5] For over 450 years, it seems that education, training, participation in meetings at intervals and informal peer review were regarded as adequate mechanisms for safeguarding this function. Although there have been some notable forerunners in the field of quality assurance in anaesthesia,[16-26] widespread interest is a relatively recent phenomenon.[39] It is likely that 'total quality improvement' and TQM notions will invade the domain of the anaesthetist from their current strongholds in industry.

Most industries produce a limited range of products, and do so under fairly controlled conditions. To set quality control standards is, in many instances, a relatively simple task. Thus, at least the mechanistic aspects of the TQM process are amenable to accurate assessment by well-accepted methods. However, even for industry, the challenge has proved to be a substantial one, although there are now few major successful companies which have not addressed the question of introducing TQM, either overtly or under some guise.

The challenge for medicine is far greater. We have a diverse set of working environments, an enormous number of disease processes, a wide range of patients and a variety of end-points. Furthermore, we have poor control over many of the variables in the systems in which we presently operate. Nevertheless, the time has come when the public is demanding that the health care system must provide good value for money, and it seems rational to proceed along a path now well-defined by industry. The proven outcomes from industry of improved productivity, reduced costs, fewer defects and greater consumer satisfaction are all attractive to the practitioner, the patient, the administrator and the public. The challenge lies in application of the lessons learnt in industry to the very complex area of clinical medicine. Advice on methods by which these lessons may be applied in the medical context is starting to appear in the literature,[59,60] but much needs to be done before appropriate methods become well-established in clinical medicine.

CEPOD and NCEPOD have highlighted the fact that there are substantial differences in practice between regions. An objective demonstration that variation in processes and outcomes had been reduced would constitute progress as defined by statistical process control criteria. To achieve this, it would be necessary for each department to engage in as many of the audit activities listed in Table 29.1 as could be achieved with available resources and time; whether there should be some co-ordinated timetable or sequence is open to debate. Any such plan may represent an undesirable and unachievable degree of overregulation; however, some may argue that a systematic approach is overdue.

Many of the activities listed in Table 29.1 are complementary. Morbidity and mortality meetings, NCEPOD reports and incident monitoring reviews all provide qualitative information about what is going wrong and identify where excessive variability exists in the system. Specific audits can then be designed to biopsy (take statistically useful samples) aspects of the system to determine the incidence of identified problems in an institution. Follow-up studies can then determine if any progress has been made in addressing problem areas; examples have been given above of this approach with an acute pain service and for postoperative respiratory difficulties in a recovery ward.[45,58] It is conceivable that a number of standardized studies could be developed, and that these could then be undertaken at departmental level from time to time.

An attempt has been made to give an overview of the system in which the anaesthetist operates, and to identify specific activities that can be undertaken to start individuals and departments along the way to continuous quality improvement. It is likely, in the next decade, that all anaesthetists will become conscious of the need to introduce quality assurance into their everyday practice and thinking, and that departments and institutions will embark on TQM programmes. If anaesthetists continue their tradition of supporting activities to enhance the quality of their practice, and become involved and support such programmes, it is likely that increases in job satisfaction and sense of achievement will be at least commensurate with the improvements that will result in quality and outcome of patient care.

REFERENCES

1. Friedrichsen GWS. (ed) The shorter Oxford dictionary. London: Oxford University Press. 1973
2. Working for patients. Working paper 6. Command 555. London: HMSO. 1989
3. Jost TS. Assessing the quality of medical practice — an international comparative study. London: King Edwards Hospital Fund for London. 1990
4. Shaw CD. Introducing quality assurance. London: King Edward Hospital Fund for London, Kings Fund Centre. 1986
5. Shaw C. Medical audit — a hospital handbook. London: King's Fund Centre. 1990
6. Brown EM. Quality assurance in anesthesiology — the problem-oriented audit. Anesth Analg 1984; 63: 611–615
7. Fowkes FGR. Quality assurance in clinical practice in the United Kingdom: medical audit In: Lunn JN ed. Quality of care in anaesthetic practice. London: Royal Society of Medicine/Macmillan Press, 1984: pp 1–28
8. Berwick DM. Sounding board. Continuous improvement as an ideal in health care. N Engl J Med 1989; 320: 53–57
9. Jencks SF. Quality assurance. JAMA 1990; 263: 2679–2681
10. Shewhart WA. The application of statistics as an aid in maintaining quality of a manufactured product. J Am Stat Assoc 1925; 20: 546–548
11. Juran JU, Gryna FU Jr, Bingham RS Jr. Quality control handbook. New York: McGraw-Hill. 1979
12. Deming WE. Out of the crisis. Cambridge, MA: Massachusetts Institute of Technology Centre for Advanced Engineering Study. 1986
13. Runciman WB, Sellen A, Webb RK, Williamson JA, Currie M, Morgan C, Russell WJ. Errors, Incidents and Accidents in Anaesthetic Practice. Anaesth Intensive Care 1993; 21: 506–519
14. Hume SK. Total quality management. Health Prog 1990; 16: 16–19
15. Caplan RA, Posuer KL, Cheney FW. Effects of outcome on physician judgements of appropriateness of care. JAMA 1991; 265: 1957–1960
16. Beecher HK, Todd DP. A study of the deaths associated with anesthesia and surgery based on a study of 599 428 anesthesias in 10 institutions 1948–52 inclusive. Ann Surg 1954; 140: 2–35
17. Greene NM et al. Survey of deaths associated with anesthesia in Connecticut; a review of 120 935 anesthetics. Conn Med 1959; 23: 512–518
18. Dripps RD, Vandam LD. Long-term follow-up of patients who received 10 098 spinal anesthetics: failure to discover major neurological sequelae. JAMA 1954; 156: 1486–1491
19. Edwards G, Morton HJV, Pask EA, Wylie WD. Deaths associated with anaesthesia. Anaesthesia 1956; 11: 194–220
20. Dinnick OP. Anaesthetic deaths. Anaesthesia 1964; 19: 125
21. Gebbie D. Anaesthesia and death. Can Anaesth Soc J 1966; 13: 390–396
22. Harrison GG. Anaesthetic contributory deaths — its incidence and causes. S Afr Med J 1968; 42: 514–518, 544–549
23. Hovi-Viander M. Death associated with anaesthesia in Finland. Br J Anaesth 1980; 52: 483–489
24. Holland R. Special committee investigating deaths under anaesthesia: report on 745 classified cases, 1960–68. Med J Aust 1970; 1: 573–594
25. Holland R. Anaesthesia-related mortality in Australia. Int Anaesthesiol Clin 1984; 22: 61–71
26. Lunn JN, Mushin WW. Mortality associated with anaesthesia. London: Nuffield Provincial Hospitals Trust. 1982
27. Buck M, Devlin HB, Lunn JM. The report of a confidential enquiry into perioperative deaths. London: Nuffield Provisional Hospitals Trust. 1987
28. Campling EA, Devlin HB, Lunn JM. The report of the national confidential enquiry into perioperative deaths 1989
29. Webb RK, Currie M, Morgan CA, Williamson JA, Mackay P, Russell WJ, Runciman WB. The Australian Incident Monitoring Study: An Analysis of 2000 Incident Reports. Anaesth Intensive Care 1993; 21: 520–528
30. Flanagan JC. The critical incident technique. Psychol Bull 1954; 51: 327–358
31. Cooper JB, Newbower RS, Long CD, McPeek B. Preventable anesthesia mishaps: a study of human factors. Anesthesiology 1978; 49: 399–406
32. Currie M, Pybus DA, Torda TA. A prospective survey of anaesthetic critical events: a report on a pilot study of 88 cases. Anaesth Intensive Care 1988; 16: 103–107
33. Tiret L, Desmonts JM, Hatton F, Vourc'h G. Complications associated with anaesthesia — a prospective survey in France. Can Anaesth Soc J 1986; 33: 336–344
34. Harrison GG. Critical incidents. S Afr Med J 1990; 77: 412–415
35. Williamson JA, MacKay P. Incident reporting. Med J Aust 1991; 155: 340–344
36. Wickings I. Putting it together; the patient, the purse, and the practice. Lancet 1977; 239–240
37. Doubilet P, Weinstein MC, McNeil BJ. Use and misuse of the term 'cost effective' in medicine. N Engl J Med 1986; 314: 253–255
38. Gayland D, Williams K. Criteria audit of anaesthetic records. Aust Clin Rev 1986; (23) 220–221
39. Orkin FK, Hirsh RA. Reports of scientific meetings. Anesthesiology 1981; 54: 93–94
40. Mackay P. The anaesthetic record — an essential monitor. Anaesth Intensive Care 1988; 16: 25–27
41. Collopy RT. Developing clinical indicators. Bull Fac Anaesth R Aust Coll Surg Melbourne 1991; 2: 41–42

42 Berwick DM. The double edge of knowledge. JAMA 1991; 266: 841–842
43 Epstein AM. The outcomes movement — will it get us where we want to go? N Engl J Med 1990; 323: 266–269
44 Gruer R, Gordon D, Gunn AA, Ruckley CB. Audit of surgical audit. Lancet 1986; 23–26
45 Macintyre P, Runciman WB, Webb RK. An acute pain service in an Australian teaching hospital: the first year. Med J Aust 1990; 153: 417–421
46 Collins PMD. Quantitative assessment of departmental research — A survey of academics' views. SEPSU policy study No 5. London: Science and Engineering Policy Studies Unit of the Royal Society and The Fellowship of Engineering, The Royal Society. 1991
47 Hart L, Lavies N, Katsikitis M, Winefield H, Rounsefell B, Runciman WB. Identification of patient, medical and nursing staff attitudes to postoperative opioid analgesia: stage 1 of a longitudinal study of postoperative analgesia. Pain 1990; (suppl 5): S237
48 Katsikitis M, Winefield H, Hart L, Rounsefell B, Runciman WB. Post surgical assessment of pain following cholecystectomy: stage 1 of a longitudinal study of post-operative analgesia. Pain 1990; (suppl 5): S293
49 Winefield HR, Katsikitis M, Hart L, Rounsefell B, Runciman WB, Lavies N. Patient perceptions of post cholecystectomy pain: stage 1 of a longitudinal study of postoperative analgesia. Pain 1990; (suppl 5): S237
50 Southall EG, Macintyre PE, Webb RK, Semple TJ, Runciman WB. A structured response to objectively identified barriers to pain relief: stage 1 of a longitudinal study of postoperative analgesia. Pain 1990; (suppl 5): S236
51 Currie M, Mackay P, Morgan C, Runciman WB, Russell WJ, Sellen A, Webb RK, Williamson JA. The "Wrong Drug" Problem in Anaesthesia: An Analysis of 2000 Incident Reports. Anaesth Intensive Care 1993; 21: 596–601
52 Collins D. Medical manslaughter in New Zealand. Aust J Med Defence Union 1991; 5: 58–59
53 Wild R, Nimmo WS. Do fasting patients receive their prescribed medications? Br J Anaesth 1987; 59: 1329
54 Phillips GD, Germann PAS. Selecting and purchasing clinical equipment. Anaesth Intensive Care 1988; 16: 18–20
55 Ilsley A, Runciman WB. Assessment and evaluation of devices: an analysis of organisations providing information of comparative evaluation studies. Anaesth Intensive Care 1988; 16: 16–18
56 Robson JB, Ilsley AH. Hospital acceptance checking, maintenance, calibration and documentation of electromedical devices. Anaesth Intensive Care 1988; 16: 20–22
57 Russell WJ. Monitoring supplies of compressed gas and electricity for anaesthesia and intensive care. Anaesth Intensive Care 1988; 16: 28–31
58 Sanazaro PJ, Mills DH. A critique of the use of generic screening in quality assessment. JAMA 1991; 265: 1977–1981
59 Laffel G, Blumenthal D. The case for using industrial quality management science in health care organizations. JAMA 1989; 262: 2869–2873
60 Kritchevsky SB, Simmons BP. Continuous quality improvement — concepts and applications for physician care. JAMA 1991; 266: 1817–1823

30. The quest for quality — how to keep up to date

J. N. Lunn

The essence of a profession (apart from self-governance) is that professionals always do their best. This best is beyond the basic requirements of the service offered for clients. The application of this ideal to medicine involves, amongst other things, regular attempts by doctors to keep their knowledge, and thus their practice, up to date. There is, however, an important consideration to recognize before critically evaluating methods of keeping up to date. Deterioration associated with age is a phenomenon which is well-understood in theory but sometimes allowance for it is not made in practice. It is at least possible to argue that a doctor who has just reached a point in training where a permanent post is the next to be sought is probably at the peak of the learning curve. It is common experience that slow and progressive decline then occurs; this chapter examines some of the strategies which may be available to minimize what may, even so, be inevitable.

READINESS TO CHANGE

There is the inherent presupposition in this argument that professionals are ready to change their behaviour in response to an appropriate stimulus; that is a considerable assumption and not one which is amenable to a rigorous test. There does not seem to be much evidence that medical students are selected with this, or indeed any other, single criterion in mind; nevertheless, such an elementary human characteristic seems desirable for professionals, and if not in all doctors, then at least in anaesthetists!

The development of this characteristic may need to start at a much earlier stage than mature adulthood; one significant feature of Japanese culture is the philosophy of kaizen, and this is taught at, or even before, school age. Kaizen is the quest for quality; quality is defined as that which may be improved. Lifetime training for this naturally starts early but, in the manufacturing industry for example, continues by means of regular participation in quality assurance programmes at all levels of staff, not just for those in training but also for those at the highest levels on the board of management. There is a clear need for western educational bodies to improve their efficacy since failure is so catastrophic. It is at least arguable that an emphasis in this, and in many other spheres upon encouragement rather than punishment might be more efficacious.

Medical education in most countries is based on scientific method and is taught in the university environment. This desirable process may not last for ever and it is worth re-iterating that, were responsibility ever to pass from the university to another authority, this important early training would be lost irretrievably. We may not instil the idea of continuous improvement (kaizen) very effectively but at least the skill to question, to seek for evidence and to evaluate critically is not neglected.

The practice of anaesthesia may not seem, to the onlooker, to be an intellectual one. Nevertheless it is. The number of diagnoses which an anaesthetist may be called upon to make are relatively few compared, for example, with a physician or a surgeon. However, the time interval available for an anaesthetist, if disaster is to be avoided, is measured in seconds or minutes, rather than hours, days or weeks. Thus an anaesthetist must not only remain alert, but also keep up to date.

The recurrent needs of most anaesthetists for intellectual stimulation will be met by talking, reading and listening in a variety of different ways and proportions.

READING

It is assumed that the readers of this chapter will be those who, like its author, strive to keep up with the burgeoning literature. There is no external pressure on this reader; examinations are passed and finished and reading is now to be more pleasurable, not compulsory but selective. The problem now is choice. Even the relatively disciplined world of anaesthesia has spawned six new journals in the last few years and the number of new titles of books is ever-increasing. Cynics opine that the only beneficiaries are the publishers, and with that view it is easy to agree.

Selection of reading matter is not therefore likely to be simple. It is a personal matter and advice about it should not be authoritarian. How, therefore, should one choose? It is certainly no bad approach to read *book reviews*; the writers of these accounts should, if the editor of the journal has done his or her job, know something about the subject or be amongst the target audience for the book. It is easy enough to discern whether the review has any internal validity and if you are told anything more than can be discovered from a quick scan of the contents page, then perhaps the reviewer's comments are worth something. However, reading is a notoriously subjective matter and what appeals to the reviewer may not do so to you. Previous experience of the individual reviewer may help you to make a choice which does not disappoint you; otherwise *caveat emptor* (let the buyer beware) obtains. Another approach is to consult the book in the library.

READING MATERIAL

The most obvious sources of information are *books* and *journals*. There must be very few anaesthetists who can claim to sit down to read entire books for their continuing education, whatever an author may hope! Indeed this author has often suffered acute annoyance because his words in books have received such slight attention; this is not really to be wondered at since fewer than 50% of all published papers are ever quoted. Journals thus fare little better than books. However, some familiarity with modern editions of standard texts seems a reasonable aim. It is sometimes quite revealing to note how few of the errors are corrected in successive editions and this is itself an educative experience.

The choice of monograph naturally depends upon current interests but subscription to a regular series may stimulate reading beyond this. The choice of journals is, to some extent at least, forced because most professional societies provide one with the other benefits of membership; thus all members of the Association of Anaesthetists of Great Britain and Ireland and of the American Society of Anesthesiologists receive copies of the relevant journal, *Anaesthesia* or *Anesthesiology*; fellows of the Royal College of Anaesthetists also receive the *British Journal of Anaesthesia*. It is by no means certain that this automatic availability has increased the amount of professional reading, and many anaesthetists maintain their loyalty to those journals which they perceive to satisfy their recurrent needs. The result of this widespread practice is that when these doctors are themselves driven to write, they can only quote their 'own' journal, with the result that international ignorance is perpetuated. It is possible that modern literature retrieval systems will lessen this undesirable behaviour. It is not confined to one country, but size does have an effect.

One of the medical profession's least attractive modern features is the 'throwaway' magazine. These often start as free items of advertising material which masquerade as science. Some editors even advertise them as suitable for 'that article of yours which was rejected'. Readers should understand very clearly that these papers are not subject to any form of rigorous peer review and may be worthless.

There is also the need to be conversant with developments outside one's own limited field and this is the role of the general journals such as the *New England* and *British Medical* journals and the *Lancet*. It is somewhat disturbing to learn how few anaesthetists read even one of these. The fact that anaesthesia is such a far-reaching discipline is readily acknowledged and, as a direct result of this, many early findings may be interesting to disciplines other than our own. Authors submit their articles to general journals in order to reach a wider audience than anaesthesia; thus the well-read anaesthetist needs to be aware of the contents of general journals.

The government and consumer organizations provide several both useful and regular publications which often contain material which is relevant to anaesthetists. *Prescriber's Journal*, the *Drugs and Therapeutics Bulletin* and the *Emergency Care Research Institute* reports come into this category.

There are several hazards for the unwary when a scientific report is to be read. Authors, advisers and editors ought to prevent the worst excesses of unjustified extrapolations; the most widespread of these is the misuse of statistics, including the common confusion between the demonstration of a statistically significant difference and the claim by authority that this means the same as clinical significance. Interested readers are referred to a succinct account of this subject by Yancey.[1]

DISCUSSIONS AND MEETINGS

One of the recognized disadvantages of small departments of anaesthetics is that the members may not see much value in local meetings. There is some embarrassment about their structure and formality. However, there is little doubt that the opportunity to talk about recent clinical events can be helpful to all concerned and the discipline of a meeting can encourage exchange of views. Anaesthetists do not see a great deal of their colleagues in the operating room and often are in complete ignorance about what another's work entails (but they nevertheless insist at interviews that the new member of a department should be compatible with everyone!). If there are meetings, then the task of preparation of a talk, however informal, does act as a stimulus to the presenter both to read and to evaluate information. This sequence of events is particularly fruitful when individuals occasionally are forced to work outside their customary field and then have to explain what and why to others who regularly undertake this clinical work; everyone benefits.

Representatives of the drug industry

The days when these individuals came to anaesthetists to learn for themselves have long passed; they are, nowadays, often science graduates and quite capable of giving the latest information to us in an expert manner. Some anaesthetists readily acknowledge that their appreciation of recent advances in drug development comes from these sources but surely it is not appropriate for this to be the sole mechanism of education.

A certain degree of scientific scepticism is desirable. A few anaesthetists sometimes deceive themselves that they are up to date by their ready acceptance of information from drug companies in an uncritical manner. This is particularly the case with individuals who wish to acquire a reputation for clinical investigation; they then rush to use the new drug and, subject to the availability of suitable blandishments from the drug company, seek to act as advocates for the drug. Their advocacy is eventually counterproductive for the individual firm but the harm is done. Anaesthesia, that is the specialty as a whole, is thereby besmirched. It might be preferable for us to be less keen to embrace the novel drug and to concentrate on proven drugs. The contrast between this readiness to use new drugs with the reluctance to employ therapies, particularly those which are designed to increase patient safety, is a remarkable behavioural characteristic of anaesthetists. The natural and laudable desire to be modern may thus sometimes need to be held in check.

USE OF LIBRARIES

Most hospitals today have libraries for use by their staff. The section devoted to anaesthesia is sadly not always very extensive, despite the best efforts of the Royal College of Anaesthetists or other regulatory bodies to insist that there should be an appropriate library for trainees to use. Those who inspect hospital training programmes can hardly fail to be unimpressed when a library contains only a few books; does this reflect on the local status of the senior anaesthetists? It is perhaps a little surprising that there is no prescriptive advice issued to departments about which books and journals are expected by the hospital visitors; implicit criteria are applied and therefore there is neither uniformity nor standardization in the provision. Three journals in the English language (at least) and one comprehensive modern textbook for reference at night is all that is sought. Such provision cannot be regarded as sufficient to give anyone a real opportunity to keep up to date.

All libraries are linked to regional or university libraries and facilities usually exist for staff to make use of them at a distance. They may have recommended book lists for trainees but not for others.

Computer technology can provide information very quickly. The ease with which this can be achieved is improving rapidly; laser technology exists so that the world medical literature can be scanned readily and the information transferred through the telephone system easily. The library information officer should be able to help. (Each system is different, so it is better to consult.) You need, however, to have a clear idea of the question to which you seek an answer before you ask for advice. *Key words* are often required. These are terms applied consistently to describe items or subjects within the article; they are often supplied by the author and are intended to assist the reader to gain access to the subjects in which he or she is interested quickly and accurately. The key words should be those used by *Index Medicus* and Medlars/Medline to enable the officer and the computer to understand what you want quickly. There are now several data banks in addition to Medline; *Excerpta Medica* and *Current Contents* are two. They are all expensive.

These retrieval systems are very useful; individuals can arrange for items about their particular interest to be listed automatically and then to be transferred to their own personal computer. Key words or words in the title may need to be specified precisely but after that the process is automatic.

TEACHING

There is no doubt that the opportunity to teach is a great stimulus, if not to the student then to the teacher! A well-researched lecture does not happen by chance and much is revealed to the audience by a speaker who has not bothered to prepare the material fully. Audiences do not often leave the room but some members may indicate their lack of approval by going to sleep! This is not the place to explore the topic of preparation except to restate the fact that teaching needs to be prepared and that most teachers find this process a source of stimulation. Routine lectures need to be kept up to date by regular revision. New items of information do not suddenly come to mind when the moment for the lecture arrives but they need to be noted when they are first read and then incorporated at the next revision of the lecture.

The invitation to give a lecture on a relatively unfamiliar subject is one which many people naturally are inclined to reject although, if one can overcome one's disinclination to undertake the new work required, the preparation can be very worthwhile. It is most probable that considerable advances in knowledge have occurred since the last occasion on which the subject was studied and the process of reading around it again is very instructive. Nevertheless, many anaesthetists, particularly those in large departments (the author included), tend almost never to undertake a new subject and are content merely to do what they have always done; they do not take advantage of this opportunity for stimulation. Other anaesthetists are often forced by the circumstances of a small department to teach to a very wide syllabus and when they are able to do this conscientiously they rapidly become very well-informed about many subjects.

A lecture is a somewhat stereotyped event and the more demanding teaching event is the *seminar*, particularly when this is for an audience which still has a spirit of question, doubt and enquiry. *Tutorial* teaching by question and answer is hard for the teacher and the student but is certainly believed to be the most effective; it would be impossible to be effective in either of these without proper preparation.

Individual, one-to-one teaching, in the operating room, intensive care unit or pain clinic, is a Hippocratic obligation. The extent to which this is a source of stimulation often depends more upon the trainee than the teacher. The effect of an astute question can be dramatic: why has the expired carbon dioxide decreased, doctor? The patient may benefit if the disconnection has not been recognized, the trainer is stimulated and the trainee seldom forgets because his or her brain was active in the learning process.

ABSTRACT JOURNALS AND REVIEW ARTICLES

Many anaesthetists rush towards these when they are faced with the prospect of a presentation. Abstract journals may be quite useful but the original article should always be consulted should quotation be indicated. The summaries are usually those of the original article and often do not contain all caveats of the whole article. *Reviews* are sometimes extremely useful but it needs to be remembered that they are often written with a particular bias which should be recognized before the contents are accepted with blind faith by any reader. Indeed, it is this author's view that review articles should not be accepted for publication unless the writer already has an established place as, at least, a worker in the field; this will usually be because of experience gained by personal research and would not include merely the experience derived from one patient. Informed criticism is an essential part of a review and this is somewhat insubstantial on some occasions. The literature is already full enough without unnecessary and unhelpful additions.

CHANGE IN CLINICAL PRACTICE

The problems posed by the need to change are well-known but it is sometimes surprising how reluctant individual anaesthetists are to change their practice. The best manner in which this point can be made is by way of a true story. A senior trainee was responsible for a regular operating list. The ward sister approached the author with the complaint that all the patients on the list were vomiting after their operations and that this was not the usual sequence of events. Fentanyl was used in the anaesthetic but no anti-emetic was prescribed. The fact that opioids cause vomiting was of course known to the anaesthetist but he had not thought to add a change to his customary practice when he started to use a new drug with opioid properties.

The suggestion that all patients might benefit from oxygen inhalation after general anaesthesia is not new but it has taken a long time for this simple suggestion to be accepted as reasonable and for it to become routine practice. It is possible that the current emphasis on audit may cause improvements to be brought into common use more quickly than previously.

Total quality assurance systems are well-known in industrial circles. Equipment is randomly inspected to ensure that all standards (dimensions, strength, purity, etc.) are met. This type of activity is spreading into medicine, and several countries, particularly the USA, the Netherlands and Australia, have developed intricate systems. Anaesthetists have, by the nature of their practice, always had an interest in the subject but only recently has this reached a point when, in the UK, some specific effort is being expended to promote quality assurance. The entire *raison d'être* of such programmes is that the participants should be helped to keep themselves up to date.

AUDIT

This is not the place for a complete review of audit but the opportunity must be taken to explain how it will help anaesthetists keep up to date. The traditional division of audit into structure, process and outcome will be used. Many hospitals still allow surgery in locations which are out of date, unsatisfactory and poorly staffed or equipped. Some hospital authorities appear to be reluctant to do anything to put the matter right. However, when the reports of the National Confidential Enquiry into Perioperative Deaths are published, comparison with the adjoining region is possible and any hospital's shortcomings are immediately obvious. If the structure is not up to standard, the possibility exists for the hospital to change.

If an individual consultant anaesthetist sees in the above report that most other consultant anaesthetists directly supervise trainees for emergency procedures, see their own patients before anaesthesia, complete proper anaesthetic records and do all the other things that modern anaesthetists do in the *process* of anaesthesia, then there is at least hope that he or she will be stimulated to keep up to date with them. Unfortunately, it is probable that this anaesthetist will neither see nor read the report but it is possible that the hospital manager may express some interest in his or her reluctance. The philosophy of kaizen (see above) is particularly applicable to matters of structure and process because these involve improvement in the environment of the workers. Changes in work patterns are more readily achieved when everyone is perceived to benefit.

Outcome data (complications, morbidity or even mortality) carry the greatest potential for assisting anaesthetists in their desire to keep abreast of modern practice. The provision of proper pain relief services after surgery will undoubtedly be noted by patients. Hospitals which do not provide appropriate services may not receive contracts; anaesthetists who do not take part in national audit schemes may find that their managers want to review their work programmes. Details about the practice of anaesthesia in other hospitals are very illuminating to the percipient reader.

Thus it is likely that participation in these audit processes will affect everyone's behaviour and help us all keep up to date.

RESEARCH

The processes of research involve several stages. The first is usually that a question be posed. The answer is sought from books, journals, colleagues and eventually an experiment is designed in the attempt to answer the question. The origin or nature of the question is almost irrelevant since the ensuing process usually follows the same course; however, for those who find ideas difficult to generate, it is those notions which spring from everyday work which seem to be most fruitful. The search for the published evidence for efficacy of a specific management can be very illuminating; often this so-called evidence is scanty or at least questionable, and this revelation prompts the enquirer to ask more questions.

Many inexperienced anaesthetists neglect the literature at this stage; it is at least partly because this fundamental lesson needs to be learnt that some experience in investigation is often sought at interview for promotion. Established workers do not make this error and therefore gain the benefit from the impetus which the involvement in research brings.

The stage of a research project at which another stimulus occurs is when the item has to be prepared for publication. The absolute requirement, that all references be checked before they are quoted, is not obviously fulfilled by all writers; it is not only that the journal references should be quoted precisely but also that the authors should not be misquoted, that is, stated erroneously to have demonstrated an effect or event when close perusal of their article reveals that they did no such thing. The effort in this process is quite considerable and certainly provokes anyone who does it to be kept up to date.

Motivation in research takes many forms; the need for continual provocation is at least one and many anaesthetists recognize this for what it is.

EDITORS AND PUBLICATION

The different types of journal have already been noted; they have different functions and editors attempt to fulfil these by the selection of material for publication which meets these aims. General interest journals are for everyone and must not have a predominant specialist flavour. Specialist journals, to some extent at least, may reflect the particular bias of the editor; some try to be universal in their appeal but they usually fail in some respect. Most editors seek to provide their readers with reliable material on which they may be able to base their practice. Novelty by itself is not necessarily the criterion by which a manuscript is judged, although most editors find an article with a new idea an attractive proposition.

It is not merely the editor who makes these decisions. The editor is supported by a number of others who advise in an expert or general manner. No one has to follow the advice that is offered and, indeed, that of an expert may sometimes be so flagrantly biased that a wise editor ignores it. Some journal editors make a fetish of selection and always obtain two or three other opinions. The decision between these views, which often vary widely, is neither made any more easy nor more valid by their number. Peer review is debated by editors regularly and the absence of a clear conclusion in the matter suggests that we just do not know the ideal method of selection. Meanwhile, all editors make mistakes and the correspondence columns exist for readers to challenge their selection.

The request for the provision of an opinion about a manuscript is another incentive to keep up to date. This privilege must not be abused; the knowledge gained from a manuscript is at least confidential and at best secret. The temptation to advise the editor to reject an article from publication and then to use the information gained for a piece of personal research must be strenuously resisted. It seems probable to this writer that unconscious breaches in this code of behaviour must occur; when one sees a large number of manuscripts each day it becomes increasingly difficult to recall where a particular item was seen and leaks are almost inevitable. Advisers (note that the term is not referees) are asked to express their opinion about the ethics of the project, its novelty, the methods, the data handling, the statistics, the discussion and the conclusions. Note also that they are not usually asked to give a view about whether or not the paper should be published. Editors make that decision themselves. Some system always exists to tell authors about the views of the advisers. Receipt of these comments by the authors is another method by which anaesthetists can keep abreast of modern attitudes.

Many anaesthetists start their writing career by means of a *case report*. These have a very important role in medicine and they should not be disparaged. Editors will seek evidence of new techniques or drugs in the manuscript. The occurrence of a rare syndrome with potential, but unrealized, interactions with anaesthesia is unlikely to enthuse the usually sceptical editor. An episode with an unexpected complication, particularly if this is also uncommon or even new, may well cause interest to be expressed since this will also appeal to readers.

Small catastrophes may sometimes be worth publication in the *letters* column; unfortunately, they may not always be noticed in that location but this is a risk that the author must take. Key words are not usually allocated to correspondence and so letters may be omitted from indices and databases; there is no easy way to avoid this disadvantage. Editors do, however, tend to be more benign towards letters than to other submitted material. The provision of a forum for debate about articles which are already published is a very important function of the correspondence column and editors are thus inclined to be generous. There is, however, one limitation; the interval between publication of the article and the letter of repudiation must be as brief as possible, otherwise everyone has forgotten about the subject. This interval is about 6 weeks for weekly journals and is unlikely to exceed 3 or 4 months for monthly journals; overseas writers to journals foreign to them have thus to be particularly prompt.

Authors have sometimes to be disappointed. *Rejection* is unpleasant but most well-balanced individuals recognize it for what it is: robust criticism delivered in order that the next submission, perhaps of the same manuscript elsewhere, will be accepted. This happens very often, although sometimes the opportunity for revision is ignored, and the article appears unaltered. The *British Medical Journal* states that this occurs with or without modification to about 90% of their rejected articles but the incidence with other journals is not known. One perhaps should not worry overmuch since, as has already been stated above, about 50% of published articles are never referred to again. Furthermore, it is said of all publications that a 1% rule applies: that is, 1% of the people who read a title read the summary and 1% of the latter go on to read the entire article (10 000 : 100 : 1).

EFFICACY OF CONTINUING MEDICAL EDUCATION

Considerable expense is involved in continuing medical education but there has never been any satisfactory assessment of its efficacy. The problem is that its aims have not always been clearly defined and understood by doctors. It should be possible to assess any scheme if the aim and objectives of that scheme are clearly stated. It is customary to state that programmes are designed to provide participants with the latest review of the topic in question. Do these many assemblies of anaesthetists, for instance, achieve this aim? We cannot know. When the question is posed in committee the answer is often given in terms of monetary profit and loss. Postgraduate course organizers sometimes invite attendees to grade the lecturers but the objectivity of this approach is not very stringent. Incentives to attend courses are frequently provided (food, fees); some find the assumption that such inducements are required slightly offensive and others that they simply do not work. The possibility exists that a form of recertification of specialist qualification may be issued after a certain number of 'credits' have been earned by the doctor. This system is used in the USA for anaesthesiologists and in the UK for general practitioners but the advantages do not seem to exceed the disadvantages; attendance is no guarantee that anything is learnt. It is estimated that one-third of the relevant population comes regularly to meetings, one-third comes occasionally and one-third never attends any postgraduate function. There is neither information about the quality of the latter group's practice nor that the former's is superior.

The American Society of Anesthesiologists provides a *self-assessment* programme, based on its Refresher Course Lectures, and uses a large series of multiple choice questions; answers are provided with references to the supporting literature. Completion of this is a daunting task but the plan certainly has the potential for self-improvement.

Another American idea in this field is the potential for interactive models or *simulators* to be used in the initial training of recruits to the specialty. These could also be employed when a practitioner needs to refresh his or her knowledge after a break as a result of illness or a period of enforced leave. These systems seem particularly attractive to anaesthetists because of our need to respond promptly, precisely and accurately in the face of a rapidly changing situation.

PENALTIES

The public is demanding, in this writer's view correctly, a greater degree of accountability on the part of the medical profession. Evidence of attendance at postgraduate functions could be required in the event of *legal* action against an anaesthetist, but such a use of the legal process would be a cumbersome method to ensure attention to personal educational needs. It could legitimately be argued in rebuttal that not everyone learns in the same way and that other methods were favoured by the defendant. The important matter for doctors is that we should ourselves want to keep up to date without any coercion, particularly that from fear of legal action. It is interesting, but not perhaps surprising, that there is no statistical evidence of a causal relationship between fear of litigation and change in clinical practice,[2] although there were changes in practice (fields of practice, drugs, monitoring) during the relevant period.

It is possible, but unlikely, that employing authorities may suggest that an anaesthetist requires additional educational opportunities before privileges are continued. Crown indemnity in National Health Service hospitals may cause some managers to pursue this approach and one could hardly criticize them for such action. Insurance companies in the USA are similarly disposed to encourage doctors to change their practice in conformity with modern developments, and hospital boards there require evidence of continuing medical education.

REWARDS

The ambition to be the best at one's job is, in many ways, the most attractive form of inducement. Recognition by one's peers is *the* motivating force for many, but not all, individuals. Healthy competition is one way for individuals to force themselves to achieve more and it is hoped that this chapter will help at least one reader to do so.

REFERENCES

1 Yancey JM. Ten rules for reading clinical research reports. Am J Surg 1990; 159: 533–539

2 Cohen MM, Wade J, Wood C. Medicolegal concerns among Canadian anaesthetists. Can J Anaesth 1990; 37: 102–111

Index

Numbers in *italics* refer to illustrations or tables

A-mechano-heat receptors (AMHs) 639
Abdominal
 obesity 66
 surgery 189–200
  see also Aortic: clamping
  aneurysmectomy 206
  gynaecological procedures 276
  lower 189–195
  SSEP monitoring 138
  upper 195–198
Abrupto placentae 353
Acceleration of thumb, evoked response 144
Accidents, psychology of 706–713
Acetylsalicylic acid *see* Aspirin
Achalasia *243*, 261
Acquired immunodeficiency syndrome (AIDS) 70–71, 279
 drugs 102–103
 treatment of infections *104*
Acromegaly 13–14, 66, 521–522
Activated
 clotting time (ACT) 147
  cardiopulmonary bypass 394–395, 403
 partial thromboplastin time (APTT) 100, 147
Active errors 707–708
Acute
 confusional states, elderly patients 72
 intermittent porphyria 166
 pain
  physiological effects *638*
  service 637, 658–660
  and surgical diagnosis 637
 rejection, heart transplant 504, 505
 renal failure 13, 51
Acute Physical and Chronic Health Evaluation (APACHE) 20–21
Adamkiewicz artery 228
Addison's disease 13
Adrenaline 564
 arrhythmias 317
 cardiac arrest 670, 674

Caesarean section 348
 epidural anaesthesia 571
 infusion 340, 346
 epidural/spinal test dose 347
 low-output syndrome 401
Adrenocortical malfunction 13
Adult respiratory distress syndrome (ARDS) 630, 633
Afterload 126, 384–385
Age, postoperative pain relief 648
Air embolism 608–609
 Caesarean section 355
 infratentorial surgery 522–523
Airway 8
 Caesarean section 349
 emergency control 667
  manual methods with equipment 668
  manual methods without equipment 667–668
 ENT and ophthalmology 315–316
 liver transplantation 498
 maxillofacial procedures 290, 291
 obstruction 241, 543–544, 695, 697–698
 mediastinal tumours 257–258
 predicting difficult 21, 22–23
 pressure 134
  increase in 47
 spinal surgery 283
 trauma 695
ALA-synthetase 165, 166
Alanto-occipital subluxation 525
Alarm systems 115–116
 ventilator 135
Alberti regimen 68
Alcohol abuse 7
 cardiomyopathy 492
 intoxication
  head injury 527
  multiple trauma 632
 liver transplantation 491
Aldrete score 620
Alfentanil 289
 cardiac surgery 381, 395
 day-case surgery 421, 425
 labour 336, 340
 neurosurgery 515

Allen's test 120
Allergy
 see also Anaphylaxis
 anaesthetic agents 163–165, 612–613
 history of 4, 6–7
Allografts 485
α-agonists 85, 109, 372, 423, 643
α-antagonists 85
α-stat regulation 394
Alveolar ventilation 157
 uneven emptying 132
Amantadine 95
American Society of Anesthesiologists (ASA) 750
 classification, physical status 20
 Committee of Professional Liability closed claims study 694–696, 703, 721, 722
 Postanesthesia Care Units (PACUs) 619
  admission statement 620
  quality assurance 746
  self-assessment programme 755
Amethocaine 322, 564
Amiloride 83
γ-aminobutyric acid (GABA) 94, 109, 156, 643
ε-aminocaproic acid (EACA) 497
Aminoglycosides 101
 burn injuries 479
Aminophylline 47, 90, 628–629
Amiodarone 88
Amitriptyline 91
Amniotic fluid embolism 355
Ampligen 102
Amrinone 401
Amyloidosis 64
Anaemia 14, 15, 16, 700
 chronic
  haemolytic 69
  renal failure 55–56, 268
 end-stage renal disease 494
 paediatric surgery 543
Anaesthetic history 3, 14
Anaphylaxis 703–705, 718
 anaesthetic agents, anaphylactoid reactions 6, 612–613, 703
 history of atopy 6

757

Anaphylaxis (contd)
  investigation 705
Anastomoses
  intestinal 54, 190, 192, 193
  oesophageal 261
Aneurysm
  aortic
    Adamkiewicz artery 228
    exercise ECG 208
    postoperative complications 211
    ruptured 223
  cerebral artery 518–520
    postoperative management 520
Aneurysmectomy, abdominal 206
Angina 8–9, 31, 32, 33
  aortic stenosis 36, 388
  CABG mortality 369
  lumen diameter 386
  medication 602
  risk assessment, vascular surgery 207
Angiography, cerebral 518
Angioplasty 445
Angioscintigraphy 209–210
Angiotensin-converting enzyme inhibitors 43, 84, 206, 221, 372, 493
Ankle nerve blocks 587
Anorexia nervosa 67
Antacid therapy 350–351
Antepartum haemorrhage 53
Anterior
  spinal artery syndrome 346
  suspension operations 276
Anti-arrhythmic drugs 82, 85–88, 229, 231, 254, 675–676
Anti-emetics 427–428, 624
Antibiotics 95, 101–102
  allergy 6
  burn injuries 478–479
  drugs with potential anaesthetic interaction 5
Antibodies
  anti-CD4 102
  digoxin-specific 89
  IgE to thiopentone 164
  OKT-3 449, 504
Anticholinergic drugs 90, 107, 111, 239, 351, 370, 371, 428
  premedication 109–110
    contra-indications 108
Anticholinesterases 5, 258
  peri-operative 259
Anticoagulants 5, 58, 99–101, 146, 147, 342, 357
  see also Antiplatelet therapy
  cardiopulmonary bypass 394–395, 403–404
  epidural/spinal anaesthesia 575–576, 576–577
  prophylactic low-dose 25, 628
Anticonvulsants 5, 14, 58, 87, 94–95, 177
Antidepressants 91, 448, 602
Antihypertensive agents 602
  see also Calcium antagonists

Antimitotic agents 5
Antiparkinsonian drugs 95–96
Antiplatelet therapy 576
Antipsychotic drugs 93
Antiretroviral therapy 102–103
Antithrombin III (AT-III) 403, 464
  deficiency 394–395
Antithyroid drugs 98, 300–301
Antituberculous therapy 102
Antitumour therapy, AIDS 103
Anxiety
  day-case surgery 414–415
  and postoperative outcome 192
Aortic
  aneurysm see Aneurysm, aortic
  clamping 219, 227–228, 396, 598–599
  coarctation 43
  declamping 228
  regurgitation *10*, 37, 388–389
  stenosis *10*, 36–37, 387–388
  surgery 227–228
    induction 221–223
    risk assessment 210–211
    thoracic epidural analgesia 226
  valve disease, mixed *10*
  valves
    artificial 37
    bicuspid 43
Aortocaval compression, pregnancy 332–333, 358
APACHE scores 20–21
Apert's syndrome 291
Aplastic anaemia 16
Apnoea 697
  following anaesthetic induction 162
  infants 538
    premature 533
  test, brain death 487
Aqueous humour 320–321
Argon lasers 316–317
Armoured tracheal tube 261, 294
Arrhythmias 9, 40–42, 600–601, 690, 699
  see also Bradycardia; Tachycardia
  cardiac surgery 373, 391–392
  ENT surgery 317
  epidural/spinal anaesthesia 348
  extracorporeal shock-wave lithotripsy 269
  incidence 600
    predisposing factors 600, *601*
  malignant 388
  management 601
    anti-arrhythmic drugs 82, 85–88, 229, 231, 254, 675–676
    monitoring 117–118
    respiratory sinus 140
    thoracotomy, postoperative 254
Arterial
  blood gas 19
    continuous monitoring 129
  cannulation 120
  and end-tidal PCO_2 132–133
  hypotension, plastic surgery 454–455
  monitoring, direct 35, 50

  oxygen saturation, obese patients 66
  tonometry 120
Arteriography 443–444
Arteriovenous malformations (AVMs) 520
Artherosclerosis 205–206, 219
Arthroscopic knee surgery 283, 427
Aspiration 24, 61, 62, 350, 416–417, 668, 695
  associated features 602–603
  central venous pressure catheter 523
  emergency colonic surgery 193–194
  gastro-oesophageal reflux 12
  incidence 602
  obesity 66
  pulmonary artery catheter 523
  silent, ketamine anaesthesia 162
  teeth 24
Aspirin 6, 19, 63, 79, 99, 292, 342–343, 426
  bleeding time 99, 343, 576
  cardiac surgical patients 371
  epidural anaesthesia 576
  low dose therapy 19, 99
    pre-eclampsia 354
    regional anaesthesia, Caesarean section 342–343
Association of Anaesthetists of Great Britain and Ireland (AAGBI) 750
  Confidential Enquiry into Perioperative Deaths (CEPOD) 686–687, 745
  equipment checklists 720
  mortality study 685–686
  published booklets *734*, 745
Asthma 11, 46–47, 90, 544, 605
  cardiac surgery 373
Atelectasis 397, 627
  prevention 67–628
Atlanto-axial
  impaction 16
  subluxation 16, 62
    Down's syndrome 281
Atracurium 34, 57, 142, 289, 295, 384, 596
  burns injuries 477
  kidney transplantation 503
  liver transplantation 498
  myasthenia gravis 259
  neurosurgery 515
Atrial
  fibrillation 40–41
  flutter 40
  septal defect 391
Atrioventricular block 595–596
Atropine 109, 111, 239, 351
  cardiac arrest 674
  vagal action, abolition 107–108
Audit and quality assurance 720, 729–747, 752, 753
  anaesthetic records 738–739
  clinical indicators 739
  continuous quality improvements 732

design of audit activities 743–744
efficiency and resource utilization 738
factors influencing clinical practice 741–743
incident reports 736–737
internal customer opinions and attitudes 741
local and regional level 744
national level 744–746
patient's opinions and attitudes 741
people-based problems 730–731
research activities 740
reviews, staff members 737–738
scope of activities *730*, 732–735
selected clinical techniques 739
selected patient groups 740–741
system-base problems 731–732
teaching activities 740
total quality management 732, 746
Auditory
  dysfunction, subarachnoid anaesthesia 568–569
  evoked potentials (AEPs) 138, 182–183, 517
    mid-latency 137, 140
Australia
  Incident Monitoring Study (AIMS) 692, 711, 722, 737, 743
  New South Wales, deaths related to anaesthesia 687, *688*
Australian and New Zealand College of Anaesthetists (ANZCA), booklets published *734–735*
  Clinical Review Committee 745
Automation 712
Autonomic nervous system, functional status 33
Awake intubation 292, 293, 294, 303
Awareness 609–610, 701–702, 722
  Caesarean section 341, 352
  cardiac surgery 380
  rigid bronchoscopy 240
Axillary
  artery 582
  block 553, 581–583
Azathioprine 103

B-cell lymphoma, AIDS patients 103
Back
  pain, spinal cord compression 343
  surgery 281
Backache
  epidural anaesthesia 348, 703
  subarachnoid anaesthesia 568
Bacteraemia 632
Bag-valve-mask ventilation 669
Balloon
  atrial septostomy 445
  catheter, intra-aortic 402–403
  dilatation, bladder tumours 272
Barbiturates 109, 162, 625
  see also Methohexitone; Thiopentone
  induction of anaesthesia
    allergic reactions 163–164

central haemodynamic effects 161
  intracranial pressure 162
  neurosurgery 514
  therapeutic index 155
Baricity, local anaesthetic solutions 564, 565
Baroreflexes 458, 596
  depression 216, 228, 229
  infants 539
Barotrauma
  lungs 240, 608
  middle ear 318
Basal metabolic rate 71
Basic specialist training (BST) 715
Beer's law 127, 128, 132
Benzhexol 95
Benzodiazepines 51, 94, 108–109, 111, 112, 239, 445, 456, 625
  cardiac surgery 380, 383
  CT scanning 441
  dental procedures 288
  induction of anaesthesia 160
    allergic reactions 165
    central haemodynamic effects 161–162
  labour 336
  neurosurgery 515
  paediatric surgery 545
  premedication
    day-case surgery 415
    vascular surgical patients 221
Benztropine 95
Bernouille phenomenon 537
β-agonists 89–90, 335, 387, 400, 628
β-antagonists 80–81, 86, 206, 222, 231, 232, 301, 316, 371, 400, 423, 455
  properties of *81*
Bicuspid aortic valves 43, 387
Bier's block 281, 424
Bifascicular heart block 40
Bifurcating prostheses 242
Biliary reconstruction and drainage 199
Bipolar leads 117
Bladder
  surgery 269–270
    dilatation 271–272
    temperature 146
Bleomycin 258
Blepharocardiac reflex 318
Blinking 322
Blood
  arterial gases 19
    continuous monitoring 120
  chemistry 18–19
  diseases of 68–69
  flow
    cerebral *see* Cerebral: blood flow (CBF)
    local control 459
    renal, subarachnoid anaesthesia 566
  spinal cord 283
  uterine 333
  full count 18

loss, intra-operative 185
  colonic surgery 192–193
  hepatic surgery 197
  liver transplantation 497
  microvascular surgery 462
  orthopaedic surgery 280, 284
  paediatric surgery 542, *543*
  transurethral prostatectomy 272
patch, epidural 344, 568
pressure
  see also Hypertension; Hypotension
  acute changes 597–598
  arterial, cardiac surgery 373–374
  ENT surgery and ophthalmology 316
  humoral control 458–459
  induction of anaesthesia 156
  microvascular surgery 463
  monitoring 119–120, 219, 373–374
  neural control 458
  rHuEpo therapy 56
  systolic 215, *217*, 218
pump units 403
transfusion
  end-stage renal disease 494
  exchange, sickle-cell disease 69
  hepatic surgery 197
  multiple trauma 629–630
  pre-operative 15
vessel distensibility 459, 461
viscosity 193, 461
volume and composition, pregnancy and labour 331
Bone
  cement 280, 609
  marrow failure 16
Boyle's machine, dental use 288
Brachial plexus 581
  block 281, 424
    interscalene 580
  injury during anaesthesia 703
Bradycardia 40, 595–596, 600, 699
  aortic
    regurgitation 37
    stenosis 37
  ophthalmic surgery 318
  vagally induced 107
Brain
  cardiopulmonary resuscitation 671
  death 487–488, 490, 528–529, 535
    signs 528
  diffuse injury 527–529
  partial pressure, anaesthetic agents 173, 174
  protection during CPB 395–396
Brainstem auditory evoked potentials (BAEPs) 138
  etomidate 163
  propofol 162–163
Breast reconstruction 457
Breathing
  mechanics 537
  regulation 536–537

Breathing (contd)
  spontaneous, paediatric anaesthesia 546–547
  systems, errors 697
Breech delivery 338, 355–356
Bretylium 88, 676
British Medical Journal 754
Bromocriptine 93, 95
Bronchiectasis 48
Bronchocath double-lumen tube 246, 247, 248
Bronchoconstriction 47
Bronchodilators 12, 47, 89–90, 628–629
Bronchopleural fistula 254
  repair 255–256
Bronchoscopy *see* Rigid bronchoscopy
Bronchospasm 89, 162, 164, 315, 605–606, 628–629, 695–696, 698
  predisposing causes *606*
  prevention and management 606–607
Brown adipose tissue (BAT) 534–535
Bryce-Smith tube 239
Bubble oxygenators 392, 393
Buccal morphine 651–652
Bumetanide 83
Bupivacaine 270, 335, 346, 423–424, 564, 565
  day-case surgery, postoperative 426
  epidural analgesia 338, 339, 340, 346, 572, 646
    paediatric 552
  interscalene block 580, 581
  spinal analgesia 344
  toxicity in pregnancy 331
Buprenorphine 426, 650, 652
Burns
  ASA closed claims study 696
  ECG monitoring 119
  metabolic effects 465–467
  paediatric 541–542
  pathophysiology, major thermal injury 465
  pulse oximeters and MRI 443
  surgery 466, 470–479
    anaesthetic problems 479
    early assessment and treatment 470–475
    effect of injury on drug use 476–479
    laser 317
  transcutaneous O_2 and CO_2 monitoring 130
Butorphanol 336, 339

C-polymodal receptors (C-PMNs) 639
Caesarean section 329, 333, 334, 338, 341–353
  general anaesthesia 349–353
    effects on fetus and newborn 341, 353
    effects on mother 341
    pre-eclampsia 355
  pre-operative preparation 341
  regional anaesthesia 342–349
    aortic regurgitation 37

  complications 347–349
  epidural procedure *345*
  twins or multiple delivery 356
  urgent 353
Caffeine 90, 568
Calcitonin 64, 298
Calcium
  antagonists 81–82, 229, 232, 254, 387
    as anti-arrhythmic drugs 86
    cardiopulmonary resuscitation 676
    myocardial ischaemia 231
    subarachnoid haemorrhage 518, 519
  chloride
    cardiopulmonary resuscitation 676
    liver transplantation 496–497, 499
Canada
  Four-Centre Study 689, 690
  risk factors, operative mortality 688, *689*
Candidiasis 70
Cannulation
  arterial 120
  central venous 121
Capnography 131–132, 672
  cardiac surgery 372
  clinical uses *133*
Capnometry 131–132
Captopril 84
Carbamazepine 58, 94, 95
Carbidopa 59, 95
Carbimazole 98, 300
Carbon dioxide
  see also Hypercapnia
  arterial partial pressure (Pa_{CO_2}) 513, 604
  lasers 241, 316, 317
  pneumoperitoneum 275, 276
  tension
    intra-ocular pressure 322
    transcutaneous 129–130
Carbon monoxide 7, 130
  poisoning 469, 475
Carboxyhaemoglobin 7
Carcinoid syndrome 54–55
  surgery 199–200
Carcinoma
  gastric 195–196
  head of pancreas 196
  kidney 268
  lung 244–245
    see also Lung: resection
  oesophagus 55, 261
  thyroid gland 305
Cardiac
  see also Heart; Myocardial
  anatomy 126
  arrest 670, 688–689, 699, 721
    ASA closed claims study 694
    epidural/spinal anaesthesia 348, 562–563
  arrhythmias *see* Arrhythmias
  catheterization 444
  compression, tumour 258
  conduction, disorders of 9, 39–40

  congenital malformations 539
  failure
    after CPB 390–391, 400–401, 405
    congestive 84, 492–493
  filling pressures 120–123
  function
    assessment of global 126
    contractility 126, 698–699
    tests 20, *368*
  glycosides 89, 372
  measurements, recovery room *623*
  output 71
    after CPB 399–402
    burns 468
    cardiac surgery 374–376
    inhaled anaesthetics 157–158
    microvascular surgery 458
    monitoring 123–125
    obese patients 66
    thoracotomy 251
  risk
    indices, multifactorial 23, *24*
    vascular surgery 207
  surgery 367–405
    anaesthesia induction and maintenance 378–384
    complications 367–370
    mechanical assistance after 402–403
    monitoring 372–378
    myocardial protection before CPB 384–387
    outcome predictors, pre-operative 367
    postoperative course 405
    re-operations 390
    recovery period 626
    specific valvular diseases 387–390
    ventilatory weaning 404–405
Cardiac Arrhythmia Suppression Trial, 1989: 88
Cardiogenic pulmonary oedema 218
Cardiological electrophysiological testing 445
Cardiology 444–445
Cardiomyopathy 44–46
  dilated 492–493
  hypertrophic 45, 215, 221, 225
Cardioplegia 396–397
Cardiopulmonary bypass (CPB) 147, 367, 392–402
  acid-base management 394
  anaesthesia 395
  anticoagulation during 394–395
  brain protection 395–396
  discontinuation 397–399
    checklist *398*
  extracorporeal systems 392–393
  femoral vein to femoral artery 258
  haemodynamic management 393–394
  heart transplantation 502
  hypothermia 376
  myocardial
    preservation during 396–397

INDEX 761

protection before 384–387
partial 242, 393, 398
Cardiopulmonary resuscitation 667–676
  chest compression/ventilation combinations 672–673
  complications 673
  monitoring effectiveness 672–673
  pharmacology 673–676
    routes for drugs/fluids 673
  physiology 670–671
Cardiorespiratory assessment, PACU 620, 621, 622
Cardiovascular
  complications 595–602
    collapse, epidural/spinal anaesthesia 348
    colonic surgery 191
    lung resection 254
  drugs 80–89
    interactions during anaesthesia 602
    with potential anaesthetic interaction *4–5*
  effects
    inhaled anaesthetics 597–598
    liver disease 50
    subarachnoid anaesthesia 566
  function, laboratory tests, cardiac surgical patient *368*
  monitoring 35, 116–126, 212
    vascular surgical patients 219–221
  system
    disease of heart muscle 44–46
    essential hypertension 43
    examination 8–11
    heart disease 31–43
    paediatric 538–539
    pregnancy and labour 330–331
    recovery period 622
    transplanted heart and lungs 43–44
Cardioversion 444–445
Carigan post-anaesthesia score 620, *621*
Carlen's tube 239, 246
Carotid
  artery surgery 228–229
    clamping, carotid artery 229
    endarterectomy *see* Endarterectomy, carotid
    induction 221–223
    intra-operative functional testing 135–136
    risk assessment 210
  emboli, transcranial Doppler (TCD) 139
Carpal tunnel syndrome 281
Case reports, writing 754
Cataract surgery 322
  intracapsular extraction 324–325
  local anaesthesia 322–323
Cauda equina syndrome 578, 655
Caudal epidural analgesia 274, 424, 570
  children *661–662*
  labour 340–341
  paediatric 552
    high-risk neonates 552

Central
  anticholinergic syndrome 108, 109–110, 371
  temperature monitoring 145–146
  venous pressure (CVP) 44, 121
    cardiac surgery 374–376
    catheter, aspiration 523
    correlation with PAOP 220
Central nervous system
  see also Neurological
  drugs 5, 90–96
  function, paediatric anaesthesia 535–536
  intra-operative complications 609–611
  monitoring 135–140
    vascular surgical patients 220–221
  pregnancy 332
Cephalosporins 101
Cerebral
  artery aneurysm 518–520
  blood flow (CBF) 139–140, 487, 513
    brain death 487
    cardiopulmonary bypass 393–394
    cardiopulmonary resuscitation 671
    paediatric anaesthesia 535–536
    threshold values 611
  damage and death 696–701
  embolism 58
  function
    analysing monitor (CFAM) 136, 516
    monitor (CFM) 136, 516
  haemodynamics and pressures, i.v. induction agent effects 162–163
  hypertension, thoracic aortic clamping 228
  hypoxia 700–701
  ischaemia 137, 163, 517, 611, 700–701
  magnetic resonance imaging spectroscopy 140
  metabolic rate for oxygen ($CMRO_2$) 513
  metabolism 140
  palsy 544
  perfusion pressure (CPP) 488, 535
  thrombosis 58
Cerebrospinal fluid (CSF)
  and epidural venous congestion 333
  pressure, induction agents 162
Cerebrovascular disease 58
Certificate of Completion of Specialist Training 716
Cervix, dilatation and curettage 274
Checklists, equipment 720
Chemonucleolysis 285
Chemotherapy, mediastinal tumours 257, 258
Chest
  drainage
    after CPB 404
    management 252–253
  physiotherapy 194, 254

  trauma 262
  wall compliance, infants 537
  X-ray *see* Radiology: chest
Children
  see also Infants; Paediatric surgery
  cardiopulmonary resuscitation 672, 674
  postoperative pain relief 660–662
  radiotherapy 445–447
  rectal etomidate 159
  URTIs 12
Chloramphenicol 95, 101
Chloroprocaine 345–346, 348
Chlorpromazine 93, 109
Chlorpropamide 97
Cholangiocarcinoma 504–505
Cholecystectomy 198–199
Cholinesterase deficiencies 14
Chronic
  haemolytic anaemia 69
  obstructive airways disease 12, 47–48, 605, 627
  rejection, heart transplant 506
  renal failure 55–57
    causes 55
    management of anaesthesia 57
    pre-operative assessment 55–57
  renal impairment 12–13
Chvostek's sign 304
Cilazapril 84
Cimetidine 79, 95, 110
Circadian rhythms 712
Circulatory control
  deliberate hypotension 454–455
  microvascular surgery 458–461
Circumcision 426, 553
Circumferential burns 470
Cirrhosis, hepatic 50, 196
  Child and Turcotte's risk grading *51, 52*
Clamping
  aorta 219, 227–228, 396, 598–599
  carotid artery 229
Clark electrode sensor 129, 130
Cleft lip and palate 455
Clomipramine 91
Clonazepam 94
Clonidine 85, 109, 372, 423
Closed circuit anaesthesia 176
Closed-chest cardiopulmonary resuscitation 670–671
Closed-loop systems 182–183
Cloward's procedure 525
Co-existing disease
  influence on management 31–72
  orthopaedic surgery 279–280
Coagulation
  burns 467–468
  factors
    liver transplantation *495*, 500
    pregnancy 331
  microvascular surgery, changes 464
  studies 19
  tests of 50, 53, 100, 146–147, 147, 394–395, 403

762 INDEX

Coagulopathy
  disseminated intravascular (DIC) 197
  infants 545
  liver disease 51
    end-stage 497
  multiple trauma 629–630
  renal disease 56
Coarctation of aorta 43
Cocaine, topical 318, 322
Cold potassium cardioplegia 397
Collateral circulation and aortic surgery 227
Colloid, burn injuries 471
Colonic surgery 189–194
  pre-operative preparation 189
  premedication 189
  posture 189–190
  techniques 190
    comments 191
  postoperative
    care 190
    ileus 193
    pulmonary function 194
Colposcopy 274
Coma 488, 528, 687
  see also Consciousness, delayed return
  diffuse brain injury 527
  Glasgow scale *526*
  hepatic failure 491
  myxoedema 301–302
  undetermined cause 487
Committee on Safety of Medicines (CSM), halothane recommendations 3, 706
Complement activation, burns 468
Complications
  cardiac surgery 367–370, 404
  cardiopulmonary 690
    resuscitation 673
  day-case surgery *414*
  diagnosis, acute pain 637
  epidural anaesthesia 347–349, 573–574, 655–656
  estimates of morbidity 689–691
  interscalene block 581
  intra-operative 595–613
  intravenous induction of anaesthesia 163–167
  minor complaints *690*
  paediatric surgery 544
  patient-controlled analgesia (PCA) 653
  postanaesthetic 624–629
  prophylactic measures 26
  subarachnoid anaesthesia 347–349, 562–563, 566–569, 655–656
Comprehensive Anesthesia Simulation Environment (CASE) simulator 718
Compressed spectral array (CSA) 136, 517
Compression
  aortocaval, pregnancy 332–333, 358

cardiac, tumour 258
  intrathoracic vascular structures 258
Computer-driven infusion techniques 180–181
Computerized tomography (CT) 440–441
  mediastinal disease 242, *257*
  stereotactic neurosurgery 524, 525
  thyroid disease 300
Conference of Medical Royal Colleges, re-accreditation 717
Confidential Enquiry into Maternal Deaths 736
Confidential Enquiry into Perioperative Deaths (CEPOD) 80, 193, 686–687, 736, 746
Conjunctival oxygen tension 130
Conn's syndrome 13
Consciousness, delayed return 624–627
  causes *625*
Consent, obtaining 25
Continuous
  ejection fraction monitoring 35
  infusion epidural analgesia 339
  positive airways pressure (CPAP) 48, 251
  spinal block 349
Contrast media, radiology 441
Convulsions *see* Seizures
Coracobrachialis muscle 582
Cormack and Lehane classification, pharyngeal structures 23
Cornea 316
Coronary
  perfusion pressure 385
  sinus catheterization 386
Coronary artery bypass grafting (CABG) 367, 393
  myocardial ischaemia, detection 386
  peri-operative myocardial infarction 369
Coronary artery disease 19, 31–36, 206, 207
  IDDM 67, 68
  management of anaesthesia 33–35
    isoflurane 223–224
    lumbar epidural and spinal analgesia 225–226
    nitrous oxide 224
  monitoring 35
  pathophysiology 32
  peri-operative myocardial infarction 32–33
  postoperative care 35–36
  stenoses 385–386
Cortical auditory evoked potentials 138
Corticosteroids 5, 13, 90, 96, 103, 521
  glucocorticoids 356, 629
Coughing 316, 321
  epidural anaesthesia 570
Cranial nerve palsies, subarachnoid anaesthesia 568–569
Craniofacial malformations 291, 543–544
Cricothyrotomy 350

Critical
  closing pressure 459, 461
  incident reporting 691–692
Crohn's disease 53–54, 189
  causes of malabsorption *53*
Crouzon's syndrome 291
CRST syndrome 60
Cryoanalgesia 253, 427
Crypane Quantiflex mixer valves 288
Crystalloid
  cardioplegia 396
  solution, intra-operative fluid shifts 185, 342
CT scan *see* Computerized tomography (CT)
Cuff size 119
Cushing's disease 13, 65, 521
Cyanide poisoning 469, 475
Cyanotic heart disease, labour 357
Cyclic adenosine monophosphate-specific phosphodiesterase inhibitors 401
Cyclizine 320
Cyclopropane 420
  paediatric radiotherapy 446
Cyclosporin 103, 485, 491, 501
Cystectomy 269, 270
Cystic
  fibrosis 44, 48, 544
  lung disease 256–257
Cysto-urethroscopy 271
Cystoscopy 270
Cytochrome P-450 enzymes 52, 79
Cytomegalovirus 70–71, 504, 505
Cytotoxic drugs 103

Dacrocystorhinostomy 323–324
Dantrolene 93
Day-case surgery 413–430
  dental procedures 287–290
  discharge criteria 428–430
    unexpected hospital admission 430
  general anaesthesia 417–423
    adjuvants to 423
  local anaesthesia 424
  postoperative pain relief 425–427
  pre-operative assessment 413–414
    questionnaires 2, 414
  premedication 111–112
  preparation 414–417
  regional anesthesia 423–424
  sedation-analgesic technqiues 424–425
  techniques 417
  transurethral procedures 271
Defibrillator
  direct current, aortic stenosis 36
  paddles, glyceral trinitrate patches 85
Denmark, mortality and morbidity rates 688
Density spectral array (DSA) 136, 137, 517
Dental
  see also Teeth, damage to
  intervention 24

carious teeth, scleroderma 60
procedures 287–290
 pre-operative considerations 287
 sedative techniques 287–288
 general anaesthetic techniques 288–290
 postoperative recovery 290
 Poswillo report 287, 311–314
Deoxyhaemoglobin 127, 128
Depth of anaesthesia *701*
 alterations, classical signs 155
 monitoring 140, 182–183, 610
 EEG 137, 140, 610
Dermatomes 560
Descending inhibitory neurons 643–644
Desflurane 156, 157, 158, 175, 229, 259, 303, 381
 day-case surgery 420
 visual analogue scales, side effects *421*
 maxillofacial procedures 295
'Designer drugs' 4
Desipramine 91
Desmethyldiazepam 94
Desoxycortisone acetate (DOCA) pellets 545
Detsky's multifactorial cardiac risk index 24
Dexamethasone 521
Dexmedetomidine 109, 423
Dextran
 liver transplantation 499
 microvascular surgery 464
 prophylaxis 342
Dextromethorphan 92
Diabetes mellitus 13, 67–68, 81
 cardiac surgery 372
 insulin 97–98
 labour 358
 paediatric surgery 544
 pregnancy 332
 protamine reactions 403–404
 vascular surgical patients 206–207
Diagnostic mode, ECG monitoring 116–117
Dialysis, renal 13, 55, 56, 57, 493–494, 502
Diamorphine 108, 654, 655
Diaphragm
 congenital hernia 549–550
 neuromuscular blockers 143
Diastolic
 blood pressure, hypertension 9
 dysfunction 216
 heart failure after CPB 400
 pressure-volume relationship, ventricles *374*, 389
Diathermy
 Doppler instruments 523
 near obturator nerve pathway 271
 resection, intraluminal tumours 241
Diazemuls 165
Diazepam 94, 108, 162, 380, 445, 456, 625

allergic reactions 165, 613
 cardiac surgery 370, 383
 day-case surgery 415
 labour 336
Dideoxycytidine (DDC) 102
Diffuse toxic goitre 63
Digital nerve blocks 583
Digitalization, pre-operative, thoracotomy 254
Digitoxin 89
Digoxin 89, 372
Dilated cardiomyopathy 45
Diltiazem 82, 86, 231
Dinamap 119
Diploma in Anaesthesiology and Intensive Care 716
Dipyridamole-thallium scintigraphy 208–209
Direct arterial monitoring
 coronary artery disease 35
 pulmonary hypertension 50
Discharge criteria, PACU 623–624
Disopyramide 87
Dissection of aorta 223
Disseminated intravascular coagulopathy (DIC) 197
Dissociative techniques, facial surgery 456–457
Diuretics 82–84
 implications for anaesthesia 83–84
Dobutamine 401
Donor, organ 488–489
 living, liver 501
Dopamine 59, 92, 401, 499
 cardiac arrest 676
Doppler techniques 124–125
 see also Echocardiography: transoesophageal (TEE)
 colour flow 125
 continuous wave 377
 transcranial (TCD) 139
Dorsalis pedis arterial cannula 463
Dothiepin 91
Double-burst stimulation 142
Double-lumen endobronchial tubes 239, 246, 247–249, 251
 auscultation 248
 left-sided *248*
 right-sided *249*
Down's syndrome 323
 atlanto-axial instability 281
Doxacurium 384
Doxazosin 85
Doxepin 91
Driving after day surgery 429
Droperidol 93, 109, 428
Drug
 abuse 4
  anaesthetic staff 713, 719–720
  premedication 111
  signs and symptoms 6
  withdrawal, multiple trauma patients 632
 history 4, 79
 representatives 751

 supplies 742
Drugs, non-anaesthetic/analgesic
 cardiopulmonary resuscitation 673–676
 chronic, cardiac surgical patients *371*
 colonic surgery 191
 half-life in elderly 71
 inotropic, cardiac surgery 400, *401*, 402
 intercurrent medication 79–104
 labelling and packaging 709
 metabolism in liver disease 51–52
 with potential anaesthetic interaction 4–5, 613, *626*
Duchenne muscular dystrophy 14
Ductus arteriosus 534, 539, 540
Dura mater 559
 post-dural puncture headache 344, 423, 567–568
Duration of blockade, epidural and subarachnoid 558
Dwyer device 284
Dyes, pulse oximetry readings 128

Echocardiography 125–126, 210
 coronary artery disease 31
  intra-operative 35
 mitral stenosis 38
 transoesophageal (TEE) 125–126, 214–215, 216, *217*, 220, *222*, 496, 523, 600, 609
  cardiac surgery 376–377, *378*
  liver transplantation 496
Eclampsia 354–355
Ecothiopate iodide 79
Ecstasy 4
Ectopic pregnancy 275–276
Edrophonium 82, 259
Eduction *see* Recovery
Ehlers-Danlos syndrome 61
Eisenmenger's syndrome 357
Elbow, inadequate blocks 583
Elderly patients 71–72, 315
 day-case surgery 413
 hypothermia 145
 postoperative confusion 282
 premedication 111
 regional anaesthesia 281
 vascular distensibility 219
Electrical burns 465
Electrocardiography (ECG) 19, 116–119, 182
 basic requirements for monitoring 116–117
 CABG patients 369
 cardiac surgery 372–373
  heart transplant rejection 506
 computerized 214
 continuous Holter monitoring 116, *212*
 coronary artery disease 31, 35
 during MRI 443
 hypertrophic cardiomyopathy 45
 lead systems 117, 118, 213, 214
 mitral stenosis 38

Electrocardiography (ECG) (contd)
  prolonged QT syndrome 41–42
  recovery period 622
  ST segment analysis 118–119, 216, 219, 373, 600
  subarachnoid haemorrhage 519
  vascular surgical patients 213–214
    ambulatory 208, 221
    exercise 208
    resting 207–208
Electroconvulsive therapy (ECT) 447–450
  anaesthetic management 448–450
  the patient 448
  physiological impact 447–448
  postanaesthesia care 450
Electroencephalogram (EEG) 136–137
  brain death 487
  cardiac surgery 377–378
  depth of anaesthesia 610
  neurosurgery 516–517
  vascular surgical patients 220
Electrolyte needs, paediatric surgery 541
Electromyography 143–144
  frontalis muscle 140, 610
Eltanolone 161, 419
Embolism 700
  see also Thrombo-embolism
  Caesarean section 355
  cardiopulmonary bypass 396
  cerebral 58
  fat 609
  pulmonary 280, 628, 700
  tumour 268
  venous air 522–523, 608–609
Emergencies
  aortic surgery 223
  Caesarean section 341, 349, 353
  cardiac surgery 378
  cardiopulmonary resuscitation 667–676
    circulation 670–673
    ventilation 667–670, 672
  chest trauma 262
  colonic surgery 193–194
  incidental surgery in pregnancy 358
  neonatal surgery 548–550
  obstetric 329
    ruptured ectopic pregnancy 275
  premedication 110
  revascularization procedures 463
Emla cream 545–546
Emotional response, pain 644
Emphysematous bullae 256–257
Enalapril 84
Encainide 88
End-tidal and arterial PCO_2 132–133
Endarterectomy, carotid 137
  regional cerebral blood flow (r-CBF)
    xenon washout 139, 220
  SSEP monitoring 139, 220–221
  stump pressure 139–140, 220

Endobronchial intubation 246–249
Endocrine
  disease 63–68
    paediatric 544–545
  drugs 96–99
  response to surgery 194–195, 612
Endothelial permeability, large burns 465, 470
  thermal injury, gut 475–476
Endothelium, peripheral vascular control 459
Endothelium-derived contracting factors (EDCF) 459
Energy expenditure, infants 540–541
Enflurane 14, 57, 156, 163, 175, 259, 379, 629
  cardiac surgery 381, 382
  day-case surgery 420
  dental procedures 289
  EEG changes 137
  labour 337
  maxillofacial procedures 295
  neurosurgery 514
ENT surgery 315–320
  autonomic reflexes 317–318
  postoperative recovery 319
  pre-operative assessment 315
Enteral nutrition, burns patients 475–476
Ephedrine 92, 229, *230*
Epidermolysis bullosa 59–60
Epidural
  blood patch 568
  catheter 346
  saline, post-dural puncture headache 568
  space 559, 570
Epidural anaesthesia 558–559, 562–563, 569–577
  abdominal gynaecological procedures 276
  assessment of block 572–573
  colonic surgery 191, 192
  combined with spinal 348–349
  complications 347–349, 573–574, 575–577, 655–656
    failure of technique 573–574
  coronary artery disease 33
  day-case surgery 423
  drugs used 572
  kidney transplantation 503
  loading dose 347
  lumbar 226, 253, 570
    Caesarean section 344–347
    vaginal delivery 338–340
  microvascular surgery 463
  NSAIDS 99
  opioids 653–656
  orthopaedic surgery 281
  paediatric 550, 552
    dosages *551*
  renal surgery 268
  site of needles 559, *560*, *563*
  spinal cord/nerve root damage 702
  test dose 346–347, 574–575

  thoracic 226–227, 253
  thoracotomy 253–254
  transurethral procedures 271
  urinary surgery 270
  vascular surgical patients 225, 226, 229
Epilepsy 14, 58
Epinephrine see Adrenaline
Episiotomy 337
Equilibrium
  inhalation agents 176
  intravenous agents 178
Equipment
  apparatus dead space 132–133
  audit 742
  checklists 720
  design 709
  monitoring see Monitoring
  obstruction of 697
Ergometrine 275, 335, 353
Errors 706–707
  classification 707–709
  latent 708–711
Escharotomy 470
Esmolol 222, 229, 387, 400
  day-case surgery 423
Ethacrynic acid 83
Ethambutol 102
Ethinyloestradiol 25, 98
Etomidate
  allergic reactions 613
  cardiac surgery 382–383
  day-case surgery 418
  electroconvulsive therapy 449
  induction of anaesthesia 159, 288
    allergic reactions 164
    central haemodynamic effects 161
    cerebral haemodynamic and pressure effects 162, 163
    emulsion formation 161
  neurosurgery 514
European Academy of Anaesthesiology 716
Evaporative losses, burn injuries 473–474
Evoked potentials 137–139, 517
  recording of 143–144
Excitatory phenomena 641–642
  intravenous induction agents 163
Expired gas concentrations, measures of 131–133
Extra-ocular procedures 323–324
  examination under anaesthesia 323
Extracellular fluid
  extravascular, pregnancy 331
  infants 539–540
  intra-operative shifts 185
Extracorporeal shock-wave lithotripsy 268–269
  patient position 269
Eyelash reflex 155, 159
Eyes
  diabetes mellitus 68
  injury during anaesthesia 705

lid surgery 322
  penetrating injury 324

Face lift *see* Rhytidectomy
Facial surgery 455–457
  general versus local anaesthesia 455–456
Failed intubation protocol 350, *351*
Fallot's tetralogy 42
Family history 4
Fast transmitter release 641
Fasting, pre-operative 24, 416
  infants 540
Fat
  embolism 609
  group (FG) tissues 173, 173–174
    rate of equilibrium *174*
Fatigue, anaesthetic staff 712–713, 719
Fellow of the Royal College of Anaesthetists (FRCA) diploma 715
Felty's syndrome 282
Femoral nerve 584, 585
Femur, fractured neck 71–72
Fentanyl 92, 93, 161, 223, 625
  aortic surgery 222
  cardiac surgery 379, 380, 395
  day-case surgery 415–416, 422, 425
    postoperative 425
  induced bradycardia 596
  intranasal 652
  labour 336, 340, 344
    epidural 346
  neurosurgery 515
  oral transmucosal 652
  transdermal 651
Fetal
  death 338
  effects
    anaesthetic drugs 335, 356
    caesarean section 341
  heart rate (FHR) 334
  monitoring 334
  surgery, in utero 358
Fibre-optic
  bronchoscopes
    bronchopleural fistula 256
    checking double-lumen tube position 248–249
  catheter, neurosurgery 516
  intubation 292, 293–294, 525
    Caearean section 349
  oesophagoscopy 243
Fibrinolysis, pregnancy 331
Fick cardiac output measurement 123–124
Finapres monitor 35, 119
First stage labour 333
  pain pathways 329
First-degree heart block 39
Fixed-rate infusion, intravenous anaesthetics 180
Flail chest wall 262
Flecainide 87–88

Flexion withdrawal reflex, nociceptive input 642
Flowmeters 696–697
Fluid
  balance
    and energy expenditure, paediatric 539–542
    recovery period 623
  losses, burns 465–466, 471
  requirements
    maintenance of anaesthesia 184–185, 296–297
    microvascular surgery 462
  resuscitation, burn injuries 470–471, 473–474
    assessment of adequacy 474
    calculating requirement 471, 473–474
Fluids, pre-operative oral 416
Flumazenil 160, 424–425, 457
Fluoxetine 91
Fluvoxamine 91
Food-derived monoamines 91–92
Foot, nerve blocks 587
Forced
  expiratory volume (FEV_1)
    pre-lung resection 245
    to vital capacity ratio 47
  vital capacity (FVC), pre-lung resection 245
Forceps delivery 337, 357
Foscarnet 102
Fosinapril 84
Fractures
  depressed skull 526
  femoral 71–72
  hip 282
  maxillofacial 290–291, 297
  ribs 262
France, major anaesthetic complications 687
Frank-Starling curves *374*
  after CPB 399
Frontalis muscle electromyogram 140
Frusemide 83

G-proteins 85
Gainsville Anesthesia Simulator 718
Galvanic fuel cell analyser 134
Gamete intrafallopian transfer (GIFT) 276
Gaseous induction, anaesthesia *see* Inhalation anaesthesia: induction
Gastrectomy 195–196
Gastric
  emptying 24, 416
    emergencies 193–194
    pregnancy 331–332
  intraluminal tonometry and pH 131
  ulcer 195
Gastro-intestinal
  disease 53–55
    scleroderma 60
  effects, NSAIDs 658

  system, pregnancy 331–332
Gastro-oesophageal reflux 12
Gastroschisis 549
Gender, postoperative pain relief 648
Gene expression, dorsal horn neuron 642
General Anaesthesia, Sedation and Resuscitation in Dentistry, Poswillo 287
  Department of Health recommendations 313–314
  principal recommendations 311–312
General health, assessment of 1–2
Genitalia, surgery to male external 273–274
  circumcision 426, 553
Glasgow coma scale *526*
Glaucoma 322
  severe angle-closure 321
Glucocorticoids 629
  preterm labour 356
Glucose solutions 541
Glucose-6–phosphate dehydrogenase deficiency 14
Glucuronidation, liver disease 52
Glyceral trinitrate 84, 85
Glycine irrigation solution 272–273
Glycopyrronium 108, 109
Glycosides, cardiac 89, 372
Goldman's multifactorial cardiac risk index *23*
Graft rejection 44, 464
  heart 504, 505
  kidney 506
Graves disease 63, 299, 300
Guanethidine, intra-arterial 463–464
Guedal's first stage, anaesthesia 288
Gynaecological surgery 274–276

H_2-antagonists 79, 95, 110, 417, 499
Haem synthesis pathways *167*
Haematocrit 461
  and haemodilution 461
  optimal 185
Haematological disorders 15
Haematoma 342, 343, 577
  epidural anaesthesia 575
  intracranial 527
Haemodialysis *see* Dialysis, renal
Haemodilution 193, 461
  hypervolaemic 464
Haemodynamic
  effects
    epidural and spinal blocks, children 553
    extracorporeal shock-wave lithotripsy 269
  indicators, ischaemia 215–216, 599
  monitoring, invasive
    burn injuries 474
    hyperthyroidism 63
    hypothyroidism 64
    mitral regurgitation 39
    mitral stenosis 38
    phaeochromocytoma 65–66

INDEX

Haemoglobin
  anaemia *see* Anaemia
  haemoglobin S 69
  mixed venous saturation
    measurement 129
  pulse oximetry 127, 128
Haemoglobinopathies 14
  see also Anaemia
  screening for 19
Haemophilia 279
Haemorrhage
  antepartum 353
  bleeding time, aspirin 99, 343, 576
  cardiac surgery 370
    after CPB 404
  colonic surgery 192
  epidural anaesthesia 575–577
  gastric ulcer 195
  liver disease 53
  placental separation 331
  post-tonsillectomy 319
  postpartum 353
  subarachnoid 518, 519
  thyroidectomy 304
Haemostasis
  after CPB 403–404
  lumbar puncture or epidural
    analgesia 342
  pregnancy 331
Haloperidol 93
Halothane 37, 65, 82, 156, 157, 175,
    176, 259, 601
  β-adrenoceptor antagonists 81
  burn surgery 478
  cardiac surgery 381
  children 419–420
    paradoxical breathing 537
    radiotherapy 446
  Committee on Safety of Medicines
    recommendations 3, 706
  coronary artery disease 34
  day-case surgery 418
  dental procedures 289
  ENT surgery 316
  hepatitis 420, 446, 705–706
  liver disease 53
  metabolism 176
  neurosurgery 514
  repeat exposure 3
  vascular surgical patients 223
Hanging drop technique 570
Harrington rod 284
Head injuries 526–529
  BAEPs 138
  brain death 487–488
  EEG monitoring 137
  intravenous induction agents 162
Headache
  continuous subarachnoid anaesthesia
    577
  post-dural puncture 344, 423,
    567–568
Heart
  see also Cardiac; Myocardial
  disease 31–43

  congenital 42–43, 391
  maternal, labour 357
  muscle 44–46
  during cardiopulmonary
    resuscitation 671
  rate, changes 155–156, 595–596, 598
  transplantation *see* Transplantation,
    organ: heart
Heat loss 145
HELLP syndrome 343, 354
Henderson-Hasselbach equation 131
Heparin 100–101, 146, 147, 628
  Caesarean section 342
  cardiopulmonary bypass 394–395
    reversal of activity 403–404
  epidural/spinal anaesthesia 576, 577
    low-molecular weight (LMWH)
    575–576
  postoperative, stroke 58
  prophylactic low-dose subcutaneous
    25, 628
  prosthetic heart valves, labour 357
Hepatectomy, partial 501
Hepatic *see* Liver
Hepatitis 12
  halothane 3, 420, 446, 705–706
  liver transplantation 491
Hepatobiliary cancer 491
Hepatoblastoma 491
Hepatorenal syndrome 51, 492, 504
Hereditary coproporphyria 167
Hernia
  congenital diaphragmatic 549–550
  hiatus 243, 244, 261
  inguinal 552
High-frequency jet ventilation (HFJV)
    319
  bronchopleural fistula 256
  bullectomy 256
  cardiopulmonary resuscitation
    669–670
  thoracotomy 252
High-threshold mechanoreceptors 639
Higher specialist training (HST) 715,
    716
Hip
  arthroplasty 282
    pulmonary thrombosis 280, 609
  congenital dislocation 281–282
  fracture 282
Histaminoid wheal 164
Histocompatibility, renal
  transplantation 490
History, patient 2–7, 207
  acute pain 648
  anaphylactic reaction 704
  presenting condition and concurrent
    medical history 2–3
  symptoms and signs, cardiac surgery
    368
Homografts 485
Hormonal responses, intra-operative
    194–195, 612
Hormone replacement therapy (HRT)
    25, 98–99

Horner's syndrome 581
Human error 115
Human immunodeficiency virus (HIV)
    70–71, 102–103
Humidification, microvascular surgery
    462
Hydralazine 355
Hydrocephalus, obstructive 520–521
Hydrocortisone 96
γ-hydroxybutyric acid (GABA) *see*
  γ-aminobutyric acid (GABA)
21-Hydroxylase deficiency 545
Hyoscine 108, 109, 111, 370, 371, 428
Hyperadrenocorticism *see* Cushing's
    disease
Hyperaldosteronism 13
Hyperalgesia 639, *640*, 641, 642, 645
Hyperbilirubinaemia 51
Hypercalcaemia 64
Hypercapnia 513, 604–605
Hypercoagulability, myocardial
    infarction 33
Hyperdynamic
  cardiovascular profile, end-stage liver
    disease 492
  phase, burn injuries 465–466, 470,
    476
Hyperglycaemia 65, 372, 541
Hyperkalaemia 83, 630
  liver transplantation 496, 500
  suxamethonium in burns injuries 477
Hyperoxia, CBF 513
Hyperparathyroidism 64–65, 304–305
  bone disease 56
  end-stage renal disease 494
Hyperpolarization, opioid-induced 642,
    643
Hyperreflexia, autonomic
  spinal cord injury 285
  transurethral procedures 272
Hypersensitivities *see* Allergy;
  Anaphylaxis
Hypertension 9, 13, 23, 43, 80, 387,
    598–599
  ACE inhibitors 84
  chronic renal failure 56
  coronary artery disease 34
  diabetic autonomic neuropathy 68
  end-stage renal disease 494
  obesity 66
  pulmonary arterial 49–50, 60
  rHuEpo therapy 56
  vascular surgical patients 206, 219
    thoracic cross-clamping 228
Hyperthermia 145, 622–623
Hyperthyroidism 13, 63–64, 98,
    299–301, 302
  investigations 300
  treatment 300–301
Hypertrophic cardiomyopathy 45, 215,
    221, 225
  management of anaesthesia 46
Hyperventilation
  carbon dioxide washout 322
  maternal 357

neurosurgery 516, 521
paediatric anaesthesia 535–536
Hyperventilation-hypoventilation sequence, labour 330
Hypocalcaemic tetany 304
Hypocapnia 513
Hypodynamic phase, burn injuries 476
Hypoglycaemia
    see also Oral hypoglycaemic agents
    diabetes mellitus 13, 81, 372
    infants 541
Hypokalaemia 13, 83, 89, 500
Hyponatraemia, dilutional 273
Hypoparathyroidism 304, 305
Hypoplasia, odontoid process 280–281
Hypotension 596, 597, 699–700
    ACE inhibitors 84
    after CPB 399–402
    controlled 57, 699–700
        aneurysmal clipping 519
        ENT surgery 316
        plastic surgery 454–455
    epidural anaesthesia 574
    lung resection, postoperative 254
    myocardial ischaemia 387
    orthostatic 59
    phaeochromocytoma 65
    postural
        haemodynamic response in elderly patients 72
        neurosurgery 522, 524
    subarachnoid analgesia 225, 566–567
    supine hypotensive syndrome 332–333
    vascular surgical patients 229
Hypothermia 145, 146, 513, 611–612, 622
    coronary pulmonary bypass 376, 394, 395, 397
    liver transplantation 496
    microvascular surgery 464
    multiple trauma 630
Hypothyroidism 13, 64, 98, 301–302
Hypoventilation 604–605, 697
Hypovolaemia 216, 218, 232
    burns 465
    systolic blood pressure (SBP) 217
Hypoxaemia 603–604, 696–698
    pharmalogical depression 697
Hypoxia 134, 603–604, 622
    burns injuries 474
    cerebral, consequences of 700–701
    pulse oximetry 127
Hypoxic
    pulmonary vasoconstriction, one-lung anaesthesia 250–251
    ventilatory drive 12
Hysterectomy 276
    pre-emptive analgesia 646–647

Ilio-inguinal block 426, 553
Illness, anaesthetic staff 713, 719–720
Imipramine 91
Immobilization, thrombo-embolism 280
Immunological effects, burns 467–468
Immunosuppression, AIDS patients 70, 71
Immunosuppressive agents 103
Impedance plethysmography 125
In vitro fertilization 276
Indicator dilution cardiac output measurement 124
Indomethacin 84
Induction of anaesthesia 155–167, 174
    agents used 158–162
    aims 155
    Caesarian section 349–352
    cardiac surgery 378–384
    carotid and aortic surgery 221–223
    cerebral artery aneurysm 519
    dental procedures 288
    extra-ocular procedures 323
    liver transplantation 498
    lung resection 245–246
    maxillofacial procedures 292–295
    thyroidectomy 303
Infants
    cardiopulmonary resuscitation 672
    circulation 538–539
    cleft lip and palate 455
    day-case surgery 413
    hypothermia 145
    liver transplantation 501
    neonates
        see also Premature babies
        caudal epidural block 552
        general anaesthetic effects 341, 353
        pain relief 661
        surgical emergencies 548–550
    non-shivering thermogenesis 534–535
    pain relief 661–662
    tracheal intubation 315, 546
    transitional circulation 72
Infection
    organ transplantation 504, 505, 506
    rescuers, from CPR 673
    subarachnoid anaesthesia 568
Inferior vena cava, compression 275, 332
Inflammatory bowel disease 53–54
    extra-intestinal manifestations 54
Information retrieval systems 751
Infrarenal aortic surgery 211
    clamping 228
Infratentorial surgery 522–524
    anaesthesia 523–524
Inguinal
    field blocks, pre-emptive analgesia 646
    hernia, neonates 552
Inhalation anaesthesia
    see also Desflurane; Enflurane; Halothane; Isoflurane; Nitrous oxide; Sevoflurane
    effects on
        circulation 597–598
        heart rate 596
    induction 156–158, 174

factors influencing speed of 157
intra-ocular pressure 322
labour 337
    placental transfer 334
    uterine activity 335
maintenance 173–178
    duration of anaesthesia 177–178
Inherited conditions 14–15
Inhibitory events, spinal cord transmission 642
Inotropic drugs, cardiac surgery 400, 401, 402
Inspiratory-to-expiratory ratio 155
Inspired
    anaesthetic agent concentration 156–157
    oxygen concentration, measurement 134
Insulin 97–98
    pre-operative administration 68
Insulin-dependent diabetes mellitus (IDDM) 67–68
Intensive care unit (ICU)
    admissions following anaesthetic complications 691
    allegations against anaesthetists 694
Intercostal nerve block 253, 268–269
Intercurrent medication 79–104
    see also Drugs, non-anaesthetic/analgesic
α-interferon 103
Intermittent injection, intravenous agents 180
Intermittent positive-pressure ventilation (IPPV)
    cardiopulmonary resuscitation 668
    thoracotomy 250
International normalized ratio (INR) 100
Interscalene block 580–581
Interstitial lung disease 49
Intervertebral disc prolapse 285
Intra-aorta counter-diastolic pressure 402–403
Intra-arterial pressure monitoring 373–374
Intra-ocular
    pressure 320–322
        intravenous agents 321
    procedures 324–325
Intra-uterine dysmaturity 338
Intracardiac air 126
Intracellular fluid, intra-operative shifts 185
Intracranial
    blood flow, brain death 487
    bolts 488
    complications, recovery period 627
    haematoma 527
    haemorrhage 58
    pressure 513
        head injuries 526
        monitoring 496, 516
        paediatric anaesthesia 535, 536
        raised 162, 440

Intragastric pH, raising 416–417
Intramuscular
　anaesthesia, induction 158
　opioids 649
　premedication 110, 111
Intramyocardial electrocardiogram 117
Intranasal opioids 652
Intrapleural regional analgesia 254
Intravascular
　oximetry 130
　volume, assessment 216–218
Intravenous anaesthesia
　see also Benzodiazepines; Ketamine; Methohexitone; Propofol; Thiopentone
　allergic reactions 163–164, 612, 613
　contrast media, radiology 441
　induction
　　central haemodynamic effects 161–162
　　complications 163–167
　　disposition paramenters *157*
　　effects on cerebral haemodynamics and pressures 162–163
　　effects on ventilation 162
　　kinetics and dynamics 156
　　patient recovery 163
　intra-ocular pressure 321
　maintenance 178–183
　　administration techniques 180–181
　　dose calculation 179–180
　　indications 183–184
　placental transfer 334
　premedication 110
Intraventricular catheters 488
　fluid-filled 516
Intrinsic sympathomimetic activity 80
Introducer sheaths 495
Intubation
　awake 292, 293, 294, 303
　awareness 701
　Caesarean section 349–350
　　management of failed 350, *351*
　candidiasis 70
　for CT scan 441
　difficult airway
　　maxillofacial procedures 290, 291
　　prediction 21, 22–23
　endobronchial 246–249
　ENT and ophthalmology 315–316
　fibre-optic 292, 293–294, 349, 525
　nasal 295, 456
　oesophageal 673, 698
　thyroidectomy 303
　tracheal
　　cardiopulmonary resuscitation 668
　　day-case surgery 418
　　intra-ocular pressure 322
　　maxillofacial procedures 292–293, 294–295
　　orthopaedic surgery 280–281, 282
　　plastic surgery 453
　　prolonged attempts 705
　　young children 315
　transplanted organs, response to 44

Invasive
　blood pressure measurement 120
　　indications for *120*
　cardiac output measurement 123–124
Investigations 17–20
　guidelines for pre-operative 17, *18*
Iodide 98, 300, 301, 302
Iodine isotope
　scan 300
　treatment 301
Iontophoresis 426, 651
Ipratropium 90
Ischaemia
　cerebral 611, 700–701
　　EEG monitoring 137, 517
　　induction agents 163
　ECG monitoring 117, 118–119
　liver, transplantation 500
　myocardial *see* Myocardial ischaemia
　postoperative 626–627
　spinal cord 228
Ischaemia-induced metabolic coronary vasodilation 223
Ischaemic heart disease 7, 8–9, 9, 80
Isoflurane 82, 156
　brain concentration, over-pressure 175
　cardiac surgery 381–382
　coronary artery disease 34
　day-case surgery 420
　　visual analogue scales, side effects *421*
　dental procedures 289
　EEG changes 137
　infratentorial surgery 524
　labour 337
　liver disease 52–53
　maxillofacial procedures 295
　myasthenia gravis 259
　neurosurgery 514
　obesity 67
　partial pressure cascade *174*
　radiotherapy, children 324
　thyroidectomy 303
　uptake *173*
　　total body *176*
　vascular surgical patients 223–224, 229
　　aortic surgery 227
Isoflurane-induced coronary vasodilation 224
Isolated forearm technique 352
Isoniazid 102
Isoprenaline 676
Isosorbide
　dinitrate 84
　mononitrate 84

Jaundice, pre-operative 12
Jaw
　thrust manoeuvre 667
　wiring 295, 297
Joint Committee for the Higher Training of Anaesthetists (JCHTA) 716

Journals 750
　abstract 752
　British Medical Journal 754
　letters column 754
Jugular venous oxygen saturation (Sj_{vO_2}) 517–518, 527–528
Junctional
　bradycardia 595
　rhythm 41
Juvenile rheumatoid arthritis 282

Kaizen philosophy 732, 749, 753
Kallikreins 54
Kaposi's sarcoma 70, 71, 103
Kartagener's syndrome 48–49
Keeping up-to-date 749–755
　change in clinical practice 752
　discussions and meetings 750–751
　editors and publication 753–754
　libraries 751
　penalties 755
　readiness to change 749
　reading 749–750
　research 753
　rewards 755
　teaching 751–752
Keratoconjunctivitis sicca 62
Ketamine 90, 156, 449, 456, 607
　burn injuries 478
　cardiac surgery 383
　children
　　intracranial pathology 536
　　radiotherapy 324, 447
　CT scanning 440
　day-case surgery 418, 424
　induction of anaesthesia 160–161
　　allergic reactions 164
　　central haemodynamic effects 162
　　effects on ventilation 162
　　liver function 167
　labour 337
　neurosurgery 515
　restrictive cardiomyopathy 45
　right-to-left intracardiac shunts 42
Ketanserin 55
Ketorolac 658, *659*
Key words 751, 754
Kidney *see* Renal
'Kidney bridge' 267
Klippel-Feil syndrome 285
Knee
　nerve blocks 586
　surgery 283, 427
Knowledge-based errors 707
Kyphoscoliosis, labour 358

Labetalol 232, 316, 455
Labour
　CSF and epidural venous congestion 333
　gastric emptying 332
　hyperventilation-hypoventilation sequence 330
　non-anaesthetic drugs, uterine contractility 335–336

pain pathways 329
placental separation 331
preterm and delivery 356–357
regional anaesthesia 337–341
  progress of, epidural analgesia effects 340
uterine
  activity, progress of labour 333
  blood flow 333
vaginal delivery 336–337
Lactate dehydrogenase$_V$ (LDH$_V$) 167
Laevothyroxine 301
Lambert's law 127, 128, 132
Laparoscopy 275, 276
Laproscopic cholecystectomy 198–199
Laryngeal
  mask
    Caearean section 349–350
    for CT scan 441
    day-case surgery 418
    dental procedures 289
    intra-ocular pressure 322
  muscles 143
Laryngectomy 320
Laryngoscope, fibre-optic *293*, *294*
Laryngoscopy, Caesarean section 349, 352–353
Laryngospasm 316
Laser surgery
  bronchoscopy 241
  ENT surgery 316–317
Latent errors 708–711
Lateral
  decubitus, central blockade 563
  femoral cutaneous nerve 584, 585
  position, renal surgery 267
Law of Laplace 459
Le Fort maxillary fractures 291, 297
Lead systems, ECG monitoring 117, 214
  arrhythmia detection 118
  cardiac surgery 372–373
  pre-operative, awake patient 213
Lean body mass (LBM) 180
Left
  atrial
    catheters 374–375
    pressure measurement 123
  bundle branch block 40
  heart failure after CPB 402
  stellate ganglion block 42
  ventricular
    dysfunction 206, 216
    end-diastolic pressure *see* Preload
    hypertrophy 9
Left-to-right intracardiac shunts 42, 376
Leiden Anaesthesia Simulator 718–719
Leukaemia 16
Levodopa 59, 92, 95
Lid surgery 322
Lidocaine *see* Lignocaine
Ligamentum flavum 570
'Lighted stylet', Caesarean section 349
Lignocaine 87, 456, 564

carbonated 571
cardiopulmonary resuscitation 675
day-case surgery, postoperative 426
epidural anaesthesia 571–572
epidural/spinal test dose 347
interscalene block 580–581
Lincosamines 101
Liquid crystals 145
Lisinopril 84
Lisuride 95
Lithium 93–94
  carbonate 301
  diuretics 84
  heparin 296
Lithotomy position 270–271, 274
Lithotripsy *see* Extracorporeal shock-wave lithotripsy
Litigation 692–696
  causes of complaint 693–696
Liver
  blood flow, subarachnoid anaesthesia 566
  disease 12, 50–53
    assessment of function 52
    children 545
    management of anaesthesia 52–53
  drug metabolism, burn injuries 476
  failure 491
  function
    intravenous induction agents 167
    postoperative abnormalities 629
    pregnancy 332
  surgery 196–197
    anaesthetic considerations 196–197
    surgical considerations 196
  transplantation *see* Transplantation, organ, liver
  trauma, CPR 673
Lloyd-Davies position 189–190, 270
Loading dose, epidural anaesthesia 347
Lobectomy 252
Local anaesthesia 344, 345–346, 348, 557–589, 571, 646
  see also Regional anaesthesia
  advantages, regional versus general 557
  cardiac catheterization 444
  central blockade 558–578
    see also Epidural anaesthesia; Subarachnoid anaesthesia
    clinical aspects 562–563
    fundamental considerations 558–559
    history 558
    positioning 563, 565
  day-case surgery 426
  drug toxicity 573
  pregnancy 331
  epidural in labour
    intermittent bolus injections 338, 339
    with opioids 339–340
  facial surgery 456
  ionization and protein binding 334–335

neurosurgery 516
peripheral nerve blocks 578–587
  rescuing inadequate 583
premedication 112
Lofepramine 91
Long-acting thyroid stimulator (LATS) 299
Loop diuretics 83
Lorazepam 108, 111, 370
  day-case surgery 415
Loss of resistance technique 570
Losses, anaesthetic agents 176
Low-output syndrome, cardiac 400
Lower
  abdominal surgery 189–194
  airway obstruction 698
  oesophageal sphincter (LOS) 243, 332
  tracheal surgery 260
Lower-extremity nerve blocks 583–587
  anatomy 584
  distal 586–587
Lown-Ganong-Levine syndrome 41
Lugol's solution 98, 300
Lumbar
  paravertebral block 585
  plexus 584
Lumbar epidural anaesthesia 570
  labour 338
    Caesarean section 344–347
    dose regimens 338–340
    indications and contraindications, vaginal delivery 338
  paediatric 552
  thoracotomy 253–254
  vascular surgical patients 225, 226
Lumbosacral approach, central blockade 563
Lund and Browder charts, burn injuries 471, *472*
Lung
  see also Respiratory
  barotrauma 240
  cancer 244
    mediastinoscopy 242
  compliance, burn injury 469
  during cardiopulmonary resuscitation 671
  growth and maturation 536
  resection 244–254
    pre-operative assessment 244–245
    positioning patient 249
    one-lung anaesthesia 246, 249–252
    termination of anaesthesia 252
    postoperative management 252–254

McGill Pain Questionnaire (MPQ) 645
Madopar 95
Magill nasotracheal tubes, uncuffed 289
Magnesium sulphate
  liver transplantation 499
  pre-eclampsia 354–355

Magnetic resonance imaging (MRI)
  anaesthesia 441–443
    equipment 442
    practical application 443
  magnetic fields 442
  mediastinal disease 242
  stereotactic neurosurgery 524, 525
  thyroid disease 300
  trachea 260
Magnetoencephalography 137
Main stream analysis, capnography 132
Maintenance of anaesthesia 173–185
  Caesarean section 352
  cardiac surgery 378–384
  cerebral artery aneurysm 519
  liver transplantation 498
  lung resection 246
  maxillofacial procedures 295–297
  thyroidectomy 303
  vascular surgical patients 223–224
Malignant hyperthermia 14, 167, 323, 718–719
Mallampti's classification, pharyngeal structures 22–23, 349
Manual infusion techniques, anaesthetic agents 180
Maprotiline 91
Marfan's syndrome 39
Mass spectrometry 132, 133–134
Maxillary fractures, Le Fort 291, 297
Maxillofacial procedures 290–297
  anaesthetic aims 290
  pre-operative assessment 290–292
  premedication 292
  recovery and postoperative care 297
Maximum breathing capacity (MBC) 245
MDMA 4
Mean arterial pressure (MAP) 597, 611
Mechanical
  cardiopulmonary resuscitation 673
  ventilators 669
Mechanomyography 143
Median nerve 143, 579, 583
Mediastinal tumours 257–258
Mediastinoscopy and medisatinotomy 242–243
Medical Defence Union, cases reported 693–694
MEGX levels, donor 504
Membrane oxygenators 393, 396
Meningioma 521
Mental handicap, premedication 111
Meperidine *see* Pethidine
Meptazinol 650
Metabolic
  acidosis 674, 675
    liver transplantation 496
  effects of burns 465–467
  responses to anaesthesia 459
Metabolism, anaesthetic agents 176–177, 185
Metacarpal nerve blocks 583
Metal implants, MRI 442

Metaraminol 92
Metastases, liver resection 196
Metformin 96, 97
Methadone 92
Methohexitone 14, 58, 612
  cardioversion 444
  electroconvulsive therapy 449
  induction of anaesthesia 158–159
    allergic reactions 163, 164
    day-case surgery 418
    emulsion formation 161
    liver function 167
  maintenance of anaesthesia, day-case surgery 422
  neurosurgery 514
  paediatric surgery 545
  therapeutic index 155
Methoxamine 92
Methoxyflurane 337
Methylamphetamine 92
Methyldopa 85
Mexiletine 87
Mianserin 91
Micro-albuminuria 67
Microlaryngoscopy 319–320
Microspinal catheters 578
Microvascular surgery 457–465
  practical considerations 461–465
    adjuvant techniques 463–464
    postoperative care 464
    selection of technique 463
  theoretical considerations 458–461
Mid-latency auditory evoked potentials 137, 140
Mid-tracheal surgery 261
Midazolam 445, 625
  cardiac surgery 380, 383
  CT scanning 441
  day-case surgery 415
  dental procedures 288
  induction of anaesthesia 160
    central haemodynamic effects 161, 162
    cerebral haemodynamic and pressure effects 162
    effects on ventilation 162
  neurosurgery 515
  paediatric surgery 545
  therapeutic index 155
Middle ear surgery 316, 320
  nitrous oxide 318
Migration, catheter 339, 346–347
  pulmonary 376
Mill-wheel murmur 523, 609
Minimal alveolar concentration (MAC)
  agent tolerance 177, *178*
  body temperature 184
  inhalational agents 184, *379*
  temperature 395
  opioids 183–184
Minimum
  effective analgesic concentration (MEAC) 648–649
  infusion rate (MIR) 156, 178–179
Mithramycin 64

Mitral
  regurgitation *10*, 38, 389–390
  stenosis *10*, 38, 389
  valve
    disease, mixed *10*
    prolapse 39, 357
Mivacurium 259, 289
  day case-surgery 417–418
Mobitz type I and II heart blocks 39–40
Modified bipolar limb leads 117, 118
Monitoring 7, 115–147
  anaesthetic
    agent 133–134
    machine 134
  ASA closed claims study 694
  cardiac surgery 372–378
  cardiopulmonary resuscitation, effectiveness 672–673
  cardiovascular system 116–126
    coronary artery disease 35
    vascular surgical patient, peri-operative 212, 219–221
  central nervous system 135–140
    clinical assessment 135–136
    spinal column surgery 284
    vascular surgical patients 220–221
  coagulation 53, 146–147
  colonic surgery 190
  dental procedures 289–290
  depth of anaesthesia 140, 182–183, 610
  EEG 137, 140, 610
  discontinuing 116
  during MRI 442–443
  extracorporeal shock-wave lithotripsy 269
  fetal 334
  head injuries 527–528
  kidney transplantation 502–503
  liver
    disease 53
    transplantation 495–496
  maxillofacial procedures 295–296
  neuromuscular function 141–145
  neurosurgery 516–518
  plastic surgery 453
  Postanaesthetic Care Unit (PACU) 620–623
  radiotherapy 447
  respiratory system 126–135
    thoracic surgery 246
  standards 115, 720–722
  temperature 144–145
    methods 145–146
  thyroidectomy 303
Monitoring mode, ECG 116–117
Monoamine oxidase inhibitors (MOAI) 79, 91–93, 448, 602
  implications for anaesthesia 92–93
Monochromatic non-dispersive infrared spectrometry 134
Montgomery T-tube 242
Morbidity
  estimates of 689–691
  and mortality meetings 735–736

Morphine 92, 93, 107, 108, 183, 193, 370
  anastomotic breakdown 190, 192
  buccal and sublingual 651–652
  burn injuries 478
  cardiac surgery 380
  day-case surgery, postoperative 426
  epidural 646, 654–655
  intra-ocular pressure 321
  labour 336
    Caesarean section 344, 346
  paediatric, epidural 551–552
  patient-controlled analgesia (PCA) 653
  respiratory depression 655–656
Mortality
  see also Predictive scoring, peri-operative morbidity or mortality
  anaphylactoid reactions 6
    thiopentone 164
  aortic surgery 210, 211
  artificial aortic valves 37
  aspiration 602
  carcinoma of oesophagus 261
  cardiac surgery 367, 369
    re-operations 390
  carotid artery surgery 210
  CEPOD 80, 193, 686–687, 736
  dyrrhythmia surgery 391
  estimates of 685–689
  hip
    fractures 282
    replacement 282
  intra-operative, elderly patients 71
  laser bronchoscopy 241
  liver transplantation 490–491, 504, 505
  lung resection 244
  and morbidity meetings 735–736
  myocardial re-infarction 32
  NCEPOD 20, 736
  obesity 12
  postoperative venous thrombosis 24
  prematurity 533
  review, peri-operative deaths 736
  UNOS one-year survival rates, organ transplantation *507*
Motor
  block 573
  evoked potentials (MEPs) 139, 517
Mouth gags 453
Mouth-to-adjunct resuscitation 669
Mouth-to-mouth resuscitation 668–669
Mouth-to-nose resuscitation 669
MRI *see* Magnetic resonance imaging (MRI)
Mucous membrane, agent losses 176
Multiple
  deliveries 356
  pregnancies 338
  sclerosis 59
Multistep infusion regimen 180, *181*
Muscle
  effect of selected agents *460*
  nociceptors 639

  pain, generalized 705
Muscle group (MG) tissues 173
  rate of eqilibrium *174*
Muscle relaxants 34–35, 80, 142, 240, 246, 289, 295, 596
  see also Suxamethonium
  burns injuries 477
  cardiac surgery 383–384
  day-case surgery 417
  intra-ocular pressure 321–322
  kidney transplantation 503
  liver transplantation 498–499
  myasthenia gravis 259
  neurosurgery 515–516
  vascular surgical patients 223
Musculocutaneous nerve 579, 582, 583
Myalgias 624
Myasthenia gravis 62, 63
  thymectomy 258–260
    postoperative ventilation 259–260
Myasthenic syndrome (Eaton-Lambert) 62
Myocardial
  infarction 80, 206, 219, 626
    incidence of peri-operative 32–33, 369
    previous 8, 32, 626
    risk factors *31*
    thoracotomy, postoperative 254
  ischaemia 35, 206, 599–600
    acceptable time 489
    bronchoscopy 240
    CABG patients 371, 386
    detection 126, 212–216, 386, 599–600
    graft rejection 44
    PAOP 122
    pre-induction 33–34
    prediction 386
    prevention of peri-operative 33
    treatment 230, 231, 386–387
  perfusion scanning, coronary artery disease 31, 33
  preservation during CPB 396–397
  protection before CPB 384–387
  reperfusion injury 397, 398, 399
Myopathies 14, 56
Myotomes 560, *561*, 562
Myotonic dystrophy 61–62
Myxoedema coma 301–302

Nalbuphine 336, 650
Nasal intubation 295
  blind, Caesarean section 349
  facial surgery 456
Nasopharyngeal temperature 145
National Confidential Enquiry into Perioperative Deaths (NCEPOD) 20, 736, 746
Nausea and vomiting 24, 321, 624
  colonic surgery 191
  day-case surgery 427–428
  epidural anaesthesia 656
  subarachnoid anaesthesia 567, 656
Near infrared spectroscopy 140

Needlestick injury, HIV 70
Neohepatic phase, liver transplantation 500
  prostaglandins 504
Neonates *see* Infants: neonates
Neostigmine 82, 144
  intestinal anastomoses 192
Nephrectomy 494
  see also Transplantation, organ: kidney
Nerve
  injury 280, 303–304
  root damage 702
  stimulator 142–143, 582, 585, 587–588
  site of stimulation 143
Netherlands, study of complications 687–688
Neuroleptanalgesia 109
Neuroleptic malignant syndrome (NMS) 93
Neurological
  complications
    cardiac surgery 369–370
    subarachnoid anaesthesia 568
  disease 58–59
  examination 14
  function, CPR 673
Neuromodulator release 641–642
Neuromuscular
  blockers *see* Muscle relaxants
  disorders 14
  function monitoring 141–145
    clinical correlates, non-depolarizing block 144
Neuropathies 14
  peripheral, AIDS patients 71
Neurosurgery 513–529
  effects anaesthetic drugs 513–516
  monitoring 516–518
New York Heart Association (NYHA) classification, angina 8, *9*
Nicardipine 82, 232
Nicotine 7
Nifedipine 82, 232, 387
Nimodipine 82, 518, 519
Nitrates 84–85
Nitroglycerine 222–223, 231, 387
Nitrous oxide 156–157, 183, 193, 498, 626
  cardiac surgery 382
  chronic obstructive airways disease 47
  coronary artery disease 34
  day-case surgery 418, 422
  dental procedures 288
  diffusion to gaseous spaces
    emphysematous bullae 256
    ENT surgery and ophthalmology 318–319
  hepatic surgery 197
  labour 337
  losses through skin 176
  neurosurgery 513–514
  pipeline misconnections 696

Nitrous oxide (contd)
  tolerance to 177
  vascular surgical patients 224
NMDA antagonists, head injury 528
No-flow phenomenom 489
Nociceptive impulses 638, 639
Nociceptors
  peripheral 639
  supraspinal 644
Non-depolarizing neuromuscular block
  clinical correlates 144
  post-tetanic count 142
  tetanic stimulation 142
  train-of-four stimulation 141
Non-insulin-dependent diabetes mellitus 68
Non-invasive measurement
  blood pressure 119–120
  cardiac output 124–125
Non-Q-wave infarcts 8
Non-REM sleep 536
Non-steroidal anti-inflammatory drugs (NSAIDs) 5, 6, 19, 57, 84, 99, 109, 297, 647
  classification 656, *657*
  pharmacodynamics 656–657
  pharmacokinetics 657
  postoperative analgesia 644, 656–658
    day-case surgery 426
  side-effects 658
Non-surgical interventions, anaesthesia 439–450
  equipment 439
  patient factors 439
  personnel 439
  physical environment 439–440
Non-toxic goitre 299
Non-ventilated lung, delivering oxygen 251–252
Noradrenaline 400, 676
Nutritional support
  burn patients 475–476, *477*
  septic shock 633

Obesity 12, 66–67
  labour 357
  operating positions 270–271
Objective structured clinical examination (OSCE) 716–717
Observer assessment, pain 644
Obstetric analgesia and anaesthesia 329–358
  anatomy, physiology and pharmacology 329–336
  ASA closed claims study 696
  awareness 701–702
  Caesarean section 341–353
  complicated obstetrics 353–357
  concomitant medical disorders 357–358
  incidental surgery in pregnancy 358
  premedication 110
  regional anaesthesia 337–341
  vaginal delivery 336–337
Obturator nerve 584, 585

Oculocardiac reflex 317, 318
Odontoid process
  displacement 62–63
  hypoplasia 280–281
  surgery 525
Oedema
  pharyngeal 292
  pulmonary 698
    cardiogenic 218
    spinal cord injury 284, 285
  tissue, burns injuries 471, 473
Oesophageal
  atresia 548, 549
  electrocardiogram 35, 117
  intubation 673, 698
  lower, contractility 140
  obturator airway device 350, 668
  reflux 371
  surgery 261
  temperature 145–146
Oesophagoscopy 243–244
Oesophagus, carcinoma of 55, 261
OKT-3 antibody 499, 504
Oliguria, trauma patients 630
  management 631
Olympus LF-1 fibre-optic bronchoscope 248
Omeprazole 417
Ondansetron 427, 428
One-lung anaesthesia 246, 249–252, 698
  management of ventilation 251–252
  physiological aspects 250–251
One-rescuer CPR 672
Oocyte fertilization, effects of anaesthesia 276
Open circuit anaesthesia 174
Ophthalmological surgery 111, 315–320
  pre-operative assessment 315
  autonomic reflexes 317–318
  intra-ocular pressure 320–322
  local anaesthesia 322–323
  general anaesthesia 323–325
  postoperative recovery 319
Opioid
  agonist/antagonists 650–651
  receptors 642–643
Opioids 92, 93, 107, 161, 223, 310
  allergic reactions 613
  bradycardia, fentanyl-induced 596
  burn injuries 478
  cardiac surgery 222, 379–381, 405
    cardiopulmonary bypass 395
  cholecystectomy 198
  combined with local anaesthetics 564
  day-case surgery 415–416, 422
    postoperative pain 425, 426
  dental procedures 289
  epidural 646, 654–655
  intra-ocular pressure 321
  labour 334, 336, 339, 340
    Caesarean section 344, 346
  liver transplantation 499
  lung resection 246, 253–254
  maintenance of anaesthesia 183–184

male external genitalia, surgery 273–274
neurosurgery 515
novel delivery routes 651–652
paediatric epidural 551–552
patient-controlled analgesia (PCA) 653
pelvic surgery 270
postoperative pain relief 637
  conventional use 649–650
  epiural/subarachnoid catheters 225–226
premedication 108
respiratory depression 653, 655–656, 697
spinal (epidural and subarachnoid) 653–656
  pharmacodynamics 654
  pharmacokinetics 654–655
  safety aspects 656
  side-effects and complications 655–656
Opportunistic infections, AIDS patients 70–71
Optical fluorescence measurements 394
Optical shunting 128
Oral
  contraceptive pill 5, 24–25, 79, 98
  hypoglycaemic agents 96–97
  opioids 649
  premedication 110
  transmucosal fentanyl 652
Organ
  donor 488–489, 501
  failure, multiple trauma 630, 631, 632
  perfusion pressure, monitoring 218–219
  transplantation see Transplantation, organ
Orotracheal tube 289
Orphenidrine 95
Orthopaedic surgery 279–286
  anticipated problems 279–281
  positioning 280
  choice of anaesthesia 281
  postoperative pain management 285–286
Orthotopic liver transplantation see Transplantation, organ: liver
Oscillometric method, blood pressure monitoring 119
Outlet forceps delivery 337, 357
Ovarian surgery 276
Over-pressure 175
  see also Multistep infusion regimen
Oximetry
  see also Pulse oximetry
  catheters, miniature 129, 130
  cerebral 131
Oxygen
  see also Hypoxaemia; Hypoxia
  bag-valve-mask ventilation 669
  consumption and skin temperature, children *535*
  inspired concentration

common errors 696–697
  measurement 134
 myocardial balance 384–386
  aortic stenosis 388
 one-lung ventilation 251–252
 pre-operative, cardiac surgery 371
 resuscitation 668
 saturation, measures of 126–129, 517–518
 tension
  measures of 129–130
  transcutaneous 129–130
 to spinal cord 283
 total body reserve, assessment 219
 transport, burn injury 469–470
Oxygen-derived free radicals (OFR), reperfusion injury 489
Oxygenation, measures of regional 130–131
Oxygenators, cardiopulmonary extracorporeal systems 392–393, 396, 398
Oxyhaemoglobin 127, 128
Oxytocin 335

Pacemakers
 extracorporeal shock-wave lithotripsy 269
 and MRI 441–442
 pre-operative insertion 9, 40, 61
  indications for 11
Pacing electrodes, CPB discontinuation 398
Paediatric circle system 547–548
Paediatric surgery 533–553
  see also Children; Infants; Premature babies
 age-related aspects 546
 blood replacement 542, 543
 burns, Lund and Browder charts 471, 472
 cardiac catheterization 444
 circumcision 426
 congenital heart disease 391
 controlled ventilation 547–548
 day-case surgery 413, 415–416
 dental procedures 287, 288, 289, 290
 emergence and recovery 553
 ENT surgery 315, 319
 fluid balance and energy expenditure 539–542
 head injury, CBF 527
 hepatoblastoma 491
 inhalational anaesthesia 419
 neonatal emergencies 548–550
 ophthalmological surgery 323
 organ
  function and anaesthesia 535–539
  transplantation 487, 500–501
 phaeochromocytoma 545
 physiology 533–535
 plastic surgery 453–454
 postoperative pain relief 660–662
 pre-operative assessment
  complicated children 543–545

normal children 543
 premedication 110–111
  day patients 112, 415–416
  and pre-operative psychological preparation 545–546
 regional anaesthesia 550–553
 rigid bronchoscopy 240
  ventilation 240
  spontaneous breathing 546–547
Paget's disease 279
Pain
 during surgery, regional anaesthesia 702–703
 measurement 644–647
  objective 644
 pathological 638–639
 pathways, labour 329
 physiological 638
Pain relief, postoperative 624, 637–662
 children 660–662
 methods 648–662
  conventional management 648–649
  misconceptions 649
  pharmacodynamics 648–649
  pharmacokinetics 648
  physiological basis, pain management 638–644
Pancreatic surgery 196
Pancreaticoduodenectomy 196
Pancuronium 34, 142, 246, 295, 596
 cardiac surgery 384
 neurosurgery 515
 vascular surgical patients 223
Papaveretum 92, 108
Paracervical block 337, 424
Paracetamol 79
Paradoxical
 air embolism 523
 breathing 537
Paramagnetic oxygen analyser 134
Paraplegia, epidural anaesthesia 575
Parathormone (PTH) 304, 305
Parathyroid glands 304–305, 494
Paravertebral nerve block 253
Parenteral antibiotics, burn injuries 479
Parkinson's disease 59, 95–96
 tremor 524
Paroxetine 91
Paroxysmal
 atrial tachycardia (PAT) 40, 601
 supraventricular tachycardia (SVT) 601
Partial pressure, anaesthetic agents 173, 174, 175–176
Pathological pain 638–639
Patient
 information, providing 25
 management, medical audit 742
 selection, day-case surgery 413, 414
Patient-controlled analgesia (PCA) 637, 652–653, 654
 burn injuries 478
 children 661
 day-case surgery 425–426
 labour 336, 340

practicalities 652–653
 safety and complications 653
Pelvic surgery 267–276
Penetrating eye injury 324
Penicillins 101
Penis, surgery 273, 274, 553
Pentazocine 650
Perfusion pressure, monitoring 218–219
Perineal
 infiltration 337
 surgery 274
Peripheral
 nerve blocks 281, 578–587
  children 662
  rescuing inadequate 583
 nerve damage 703
 nociceptors 639
 temperature monitoring 146
 vascular surgery
  lumbar epidural and spinal analgesia 225–226
  risk assessment 211–212
Peroneal nerve 584, 703
Personality traits, anaesthetic staff 713–714
 hazardous attitudes 714
Personnel
 anaesthesia, non-surgical interventions 439
  CT scan, radiation exposure 441
  MRI 442
 drug abuse and illness 713, 719–720
 fatigue 712–713, 719
 medical audit 741–742
 microvascular surgery 462
Perspiration, infants 540
Pethidine 93, 108, 183, 231
 allergic reactions 613
 labour 334, 336, 337, 356
 effects on fetus 335
Phaeochromocytoma 65–66
 children 545
 surgery 199
Phantom limb pain 558
 pre-emptive analgesia 645–646
Pharmacodynamic interactions 79–80
Pharmacokinetic interactions 79
Pharyngeal
 odema 292
 structures, Mallampti's classification 22–23, 349
Phase I and II block 144
Phenelzine 92
Phenformin 97
Phenobarbitone 58, 94, 95
Phenothiazines 109
Phenoxybenzamine 545
Phentolamine 92
Phenylephrine 92, 229, 230, 564
Phenylpropranolamine 92
Phenytoin 58, 87, 94, 95, 177
Photoluminescence PO_2 sensor 129
Physical examination 7–16
Physiological pain 638

Physiotherapy, chest
  abdominal surgery 194
  thoracotomy 254
Pierre-Robin syndrome 291, 455, 543
Pipecuronium 384
Pirbutarol 89–90
Pituitary surgery 521–522
Placenta
  accreta 353
  manual removal 354
  praevia 353
  separation 331
  transfer, anaesthetic drugs 334
  preterm fetus 356
Plasma
  protein fraction (PPF), burn injuries 473
  renin activity 599
Plaster casts 280
Plastic surgery 453–457
  anaesthetic techniques 454–457
  historical review 453–454
Plasticity, nociceptive impulses 638, 639
  implications, postoperative pain relief 644
Platelet
  see also Thrombocytopenia
  adhesion, NSAID effects 658
  function 19
    after CPB 404
    liver disease 51
  numbers, epidural and subarachnoid blocks 343
Pleura 243, 268
Pleural effusion 628
Pneumococcal
  meningitis 69
  vaccination, renal transplant patient 507
Pneumocystis pneumonia 70
Pneumonectomy 245, 252, 253, 254
Pneumonitis, aspiration 602
Pneumoperitoneum, carbon dioxide 275, 276
Pneumotachograph 135
Pneumothorax 607–608, 695, 706
  tension 268, 608
Poiseuille-Hagen equation 458
Polarographic fuel cell analyser 134
Policies and procedures 710
  audit 743
Polychromatic non-dispersive infrared spectrometry 134
Polycystic kidney disease 58
Polycythaemia 15, 42
Polymethylmethacrylic bone cement 280, 609
Polymyxins 101
Porphyria 14–15
  intravenous induction agents 165–167
Positive end-expiratory pressure (PEEP) 523
  one-lung anaesthesia 251, 252

Positive-pressure ventilation
  cardiopulmonary resuscitation 667–668
  systolic pressure variations 218
Post-dural puncture headache 344, 423, 567–568
Post-systolic shortening 214
Post-tetanic
  count 142
  facilitation 142
Postanaesthesia care 619–634
  the anaesthetist 633–634
  complications 624–629
    delayed 627–629
    intra-operative 626–627
  discharge criteria 623–624
  multiple trauma 629–632
  postoperative orders *621*
Posterior tibial nerve 584, 587
Postoperative pain relief *see* Pain relief, postoperative
Postpartum haemorrhage 353
Poswillo report 287
  Department of Health recommendations 313–314
  principal recommendations 311–312
Power spectral analysis, heart rate variability 33
Prazosin 85
Pre-admission clerking appointments 2
Pre-eclampsia 338, 342, 354–355
Pre-emptive analgesia 645–648
  trial design *647*
Pre-excitation syndromes 41, 86, 391, 392, 601
Pre-induction
  management, vascular surgical patients 221
  myocardial ischaemia 33–34
Pre-operative assessment 1–26
  before hospital admission 2
  decision to operate, factors influencing *1*
  fitness score (PAFS) 21
  overall procedure 2–20
Pre-optic hypothalamic nuclei (POH) 462
Pre-oxygenation, general anaesthesia Caesarean section 351
Precordial Doppler probe 523
Predictive scoring, peri-operative morbidity or mortality 20–24
  non-specific adverse outcome 20–21, 22
  specific adverse events 21–24
Prednisolone 103
Pregnancy 330–336
  aortocaval compression 332–333, 358
  ectopic 275–276
  incidental surgery 358
  physiological changes 330–332
  termination 274–275, 335–336
  thrombocytopenia 343
  toxaemia 354–355
5β-Pregnanolone 161, 419

Preload 120, 122, 126, 384–385, 598
  dilated cardiomyopathy 492–493
Premature babies 533–534
  caudal epidural block 552
  hyperglycaemia 541
  regulation of breathing 536–537
Premedication 26, 107–112
  see also Sedatives
  advantages 107–108
  asthma 46
  bronchopulmonary fistula 255
  cardiac surgery 370–372
  colonic surgery 189
  coronary artery disease 33–34
  day-case surgery 415
  development 107
  drugs used 85, 108–110
    contra-indications 108
  electroconvulsive therapy 448
  epidural/subarachnoid anaesthesia 562
  extra-ocular procedures 323
  liver disease 53
  lung resection 245
  maxillofacial procedures 292
  mitral stenosis 38
  oesophagoscopy 243–244
  paediatric surgery 545–546
    intracranial pathology 536
  radiotherapy 446
  rigid bronchoscopy 239
  route of administration 110
  special situations 110–112
  thyroidectomy 302
  tracheal resection 260
  vascular surgical patients 221
Preparation of patients, pre-operative 24–26
Pressure
  areas, microvascular surgery 462
  transducer system 121
Prilocaine 424
Primidone 94
Problem cases, pre-operative recognition 2
Procainamide 87, 675–676
Procyclidine 95
Product design, errors 709
Promethazine 109
Propanidid, emulsion formation 161
Propofol 109, 156, 183, 295, 422, 428, 562
  burn injuries 478
  cardiac surgery 382
  cardioversion 444
  CT scanning 441
  dental procedures 288, 289
  electroconvulsive therapy 449
  induction of anaesthesia 159–160
    allergic reactions 164–165
    apnoea 162
    central haemodynamic effects 161
    day-case surgery 418, 421
    intracranial pressure 162
    vascular surgical patients 221

INDEX

local and regional anaesthesia 424, 425
multistep infusion regimen 180, *181*
neurosurgery 515
rigid bronchoscopy 240
therapeutic index 155
Propranolol 80, 81
Propylthiouracil 98, 300
Prostacyclin 343, 354
Prostaglandins 335–336, 657
   congenital cardiac malformations 539
   therapy, liver transplantation 504
Prostatectomy
   retropubic 269, 270
   transurethral 272
Prosthetic valves *11*
   labour 357
Protamine 403, 404
Prothrombin time 50
Protocols and guidelines, clinical practice 720
Pruritis, spinal opioids 656
Pseudocholinesterase 144
   deficiency 449
Psoas compartment block 585–586
Psychiatric conditions 14
Psychometric testing 156
Psychomotor tests 429
Pudendal nerve block 337
Pulmonary
   artery
     see also Pulmonary artery catheters
     compression, tumour 258
     hypertension 49–50, 60
     occlusion pressure (PAOP) 215–216, 218, 374, 388, 399
     pressure measurement 121–123
     temperature 146
   capillary wedge pressure (PCWP) 599
   changes from cutaneous burns 468–469
   complications
     cardiac surgery 370
     paediatric surgery 544
     recovery period 627–629
   damage, direct thermal injury 469
   embolism 280, 628, 700
   fibrosis 88
   function
     obese patients 66
     postoperative abdominal surgery 194, 211
   oedema 698
     cardiogenic 218
     spinal cord injury 284, 285
   regurgitation *11*
   shunting 50
   stenosis *11*
   vasoconstriction, hypoxic, one-lung anaesthesia 250–251
Pulmonary artery catheters 35, 65, 218, 219, 220, 599, 721
   cardiac surgery 375–376, 378, 392
     heart transplantation 390–391, 502

complications 122, 123
flotation (PAFC) 122, 125
   indications for 122, *123*
thermal dilution 474
Pulse oximetry 115, 116, 126–129, 721, 722
   carboxyhaemoglobin 7
   cardiac surgery 372
   during MRI 443
   principles of 127–129
   recovery period 621
Pyrazinamide 102
Pyridostigmine 258, 259
Pyridoxine 102

Q-wave infarcts 8
QT syndrome, prolonged 41–42
Quality assurance committees 633, 634
   see also Audit and quality assurance
Questionnaires
   McGill Pain Questionnaire (MPQ) 645
   medical and nursing pain relief misconceptions 649
   pre-operative 2, *3*
Quinapril 84
Quinidine 87

Radial
   arterial pressure, cardiac surgery 373–374
   nerve 579, 583, 703
Radiology
   see also Computerized tomography (CT); Magnetic resonance imaging (MRI)
   anaesthesia 440–444
   cerebral angiography 518
   cervical 16, 62–63, 68
   chest 19
     achalasia, oesophageal *243*
     emphysematous bullae *256*
     mitral stenosis 38
   contrast media 441
   coronary arteriography 31
Radiotherapy
   children 324, 445–447
     pre-operative preparation 446
   mediastinal tumours 257, 258
RAE tracheal tubes 289, 294
Raman analysis 132
Ranitidine 110, 417, 499
Rapid
   eye movement (REM) sleep 536
   Infusion Device (RID), Sorenson 495
   inhaled induction (RII) 157, 158
Rate-pressure product (RRP) 32, 215, 222, 386, 599
Rebreathing system, partial 547, 548
α-receptors 643
Recombinant human erythropoietin (rHuEpo) 56
Recovery 156
   agent elimination 176–177

coronary artery disease 35–36
day-case surgery 420–423, 428–430
intravenous induction agents 163
paediatric surgery 553
postanaesthesia care 619–634
   discharge criteria 623–624
thyroid disease 13
Rectal
   opioids 650
   premedication 110, 111, 545
   route, induction of anaesthesia 158, 159
   temperature 146
Rectum, villous adenomas 189
Reflex bradycardia 596
Regional anaesthesia
   see also Local anaesthesia
   aortic regurgitation 37
   Bier's block 281, 424
   bleeding time test 19
   chronic renal failure 57
   coronary artery disease 34
   day-case surgery 423–424
   epidermolysis bullosa 60
   hypertension 43
   injuries and errors 702–703
   intrapleural 254
   kidney transplantation 503
   labour 337–341
     Caesarean section 342–349
   liver disease 52
   orthopaedic surgery 281
   paediatric 550–553
   premedication 112
   preterm labour 356–357
   scleroderma 61
   sickle-cell disease 69
   vascular surgical patients 224–225
Regional wall motion abnormalties (RWMAs) 377
Rehydration, paediatric anaesthesia 541
Relative analgesia 288
Renal
   blood flow, subarachnoid anaesthesia 566
   disease 12–13, 55–58
     AIDS patients 71
     end-stage 493, 494
     osteodystrophy 56
   failure
     advanced liver disease 492, 504
     trauma patients 631
   function
     aortic aneurysm, surgery 211
     aortic clamping 228
     neonates 540
     NSAID effects 658
     postoperative abnormalities 629
     pregnancy 332
   hepatorenal syndrome 51, 492, 504
   surgery 267–268
     patient position 267, 268
   transplantation 485, 487, 489, 490, 493–494, 502–503

Reperfusion
  injury
    cerebral 611
    myocardial 397, 398, 400
    organ transplantation 489–490
    liver, transplantation 499–500
Reservoir, cardiopulmonary bypass 393
Respiratory
  see also Lung
  acidosis 675
  complications 23–24
    ASA closed claim study 694–696
    thoracotomy 254
  depression, opioid-induced 653, 655–656, 697
  disease 46–50
    vascular surgical patients 207
  drugs 89–90
  effects
    burns 468–470, 474–475
    subarachnoid anaesthesia 566
  function
    liver disease 50–51
    recovery room 622
    tests 19–20
  movements, extracorporeal shock-wave lithotripsy 269
  pattern, paediatric anaesthesia 537–538
  sinus arrhythmia 140
  system
    examination 11–12
    intra-operative complications 602–609
    monitoring 126–135
    pregnancy and labour 330
Restrictive cardiomyopathy 45
Resuscitation, cardiopulmonary 667–676
Retinal detachment 318–319
Retinoblastoma 324
Retinopathy of prematurity 534
Retrograde intubation, Caesarean section 349
Retrosternal pain, post delivery 329
Review articles 752
Rewarming 145, 622
  vascular surgical patients 232
Rhabdomyosarcoma 324
Rheology, altered, microvascular surgery 464
Rheumatic
  fever 38
  heart disease 357, 389
Rheumatoid arthritis 62–63, 279, 282
  knee joint replacement 283
  paediatric 544
  systemic complications 15, 16
Rhytidectomy 456
Ribavirin 102
Ribs, fractures 262
Rifampicin 102
Right
  bundle branch block 40
  heart failure, after CPB 401–402
  ventricular ejection fraction catheter 502
Right-to-left intracardiac shunts 42
Rigid bronchoscopy 239–242
  diagnostic 239–241
  therapeutic 241–242
Rigidity, opioid anaesthesia 380
Rimiterol 89–90
Ringer's solution, lactated, burn injuries 473
Risk
  assessment 685–696
    vascular surgery 207–221
  index, multifactorial, non-cardiac surgery 244
  management committees 633, 634
  predictive scoring, peri-operative morbidity or mortality 20–24
  reduction of 713–722
Robertshaw tubes 239, 246, 249
Rotameter bobbins 696
Royal College of Anaesthetists 750
  Quality of Practice Committee 745
  training programmes 715–716
Ruby lasers 317
Rule of nines, burn injuries 471
Rule-based errors 707–708
Rusch Robertshaw tubes 246, 247, 249

Sacral plexus 584
Saddle block 274
Safety, clinical anaesthesia 685–722
  assessment of risk 685–696
  common injuries and errors 696–702, 696–706
  psychology of accidents 706–713
  reduction of risk 713–722
  selection of anaesthetists 713–714
St Thomas's Hospital cardioplegic solution 396
Salbutamol 47, 89–90
Salivation 107, 162
  rigid bronchoscopy 239
Sanders injector 317
Saphenous nerve 584
Scalene muscles 580
Sciatic nerve 584, 586
  injury during anaesthesia 703
Scleroderma 60–61
Scoliosis surgery 283–284
  lower limb SSEP monitoring 138
  'wake-up' test 136
Scopolamine see Hyoscine
Scrotum, surgery 273
Second
  messengers, dorsal horn neurons 642
  stage labour 333
    pain pathways 329
Second-degree heart block 39–40
Secretions, drying of 107
Sedative techniques
  CT scan 440
  day-case surgery 424–425
  dental procedures 287–288
  facial surgery 456

Sedatives
  burn injuries 478
  labour 336
Segmental anaesthesia, epidural 559
Seizures 58, 59
  see also Electroconvulsive therapy (ECT)
  epidural/spinal anaesthesia 347–348
  propofol 159–160
  rHuEpo therapy 56
Selective serotonin re-uptake inhibitors 91, 92
Selegiline 92
Selegine 95
Self-assessment, pain 645
Sellick manoeuvre 351
Sensory block, epidural anaesthesia 572–573
Sepsis 632–633
Serotonin 199, 200
Serum
  lactate 600
  tryptase 705
Severinghaus carbon dioxide electrode 129
Sevoflurane 157, 158, 175, 229
  day-case surgery 420, 420–421
  maxillofacial procedures 295
Shivering 145, 612, 622, 630
Shock 626, 630
  septic 632, 633
    anastomotic leak 192
  spinal 284–285
Shoulder pain, post delivery 329
Sick sinus syndrome 40
Sickling disorders 14, 68–69, 543
  screening for 19
  tourniquets 280
Side-stream analyser 132
Silent nociceptors 639
SIM 1 simulator 718
Simulators 717–719, 755
  role in training and assessment of competence 719
Sinemet 95
Single twitch 141
Single-lumen endobronchial tubes 239
Sinus
  bradycardia 40, 595, 699
  tachycardia 40, 596–597
Sitting position
  central blockade 563
  neurosurgery 522, 524, 536, 608
Skill-based errors 708
Skin
  loss of agents 176
  and musculoskeletal disorders 59–63
Skull fracture, depressed 526
Sleep, regulation of breathing 536–537
Smoke inhalation, burns injury 468
  assessment and treatment 474–475
Smoking 7
  artherosclerosis 205
  cardiac surgery 370

chronic obstructive airways disease 47
postoperative pulmonary morbidity 627
respiratory dysfunction, vascular disease 207
Social
  and cultural factors, errors 711
  issues, organ transplantation 490
Sodium
  bicarbonate, CPR 674–675
  citrate 350, 351
  nitroprusside 316, 355, 387, 402
  valproate 94, 95
Somatosensory evoked potentials (SSEPs) 138–139
  carotid endarterectomy 220–221
  spinal column surgery 284
  thiopentone 162
Somatostatin 200
  analogue 55
Sore throat 624
Sotalol 86
Spectral edge frequency (SEF) 136, 137, 377, 517
Spinal
  anaesthesia see Subarachnoid anaesthesia
  anatomy 559, 560
  cord
    compression 343
    damage 702
    development 550, 551
    injury 284–285
    ischaemia 228
    pain transmission 639, 640, 641–644
  surgery 283–285, 525–526
Spirometry 19, 134–135
  incentive 48, 194
Spironolactone 83
Splanchnic
  circulation 192–193
  tissue acidosis 131
Splenectomy 197–198
Splenomegaly, liver transplantation 500
Split liver transplantation 500–501
Spontaneous breathing 155
Sputum retention 254
ST segment analysis 118–119, 600
  cardiac surgery 373
  vascular surgical patients 216, 219
Starling's law 468
Static magnetic field, MRI scanner 441–442
Steal-prone anatomy 224, 381, 382
Stereotactic neurosurgery 524–525
Steroids see Corticosteroids
Stesolid 165
Stevens-Johnson syndrome 60
Stiff joint syndrome 68
Still's disease 282
Strabismus surgery 323–324
  oculocardiac reflex 318
Streptomycin 102

Stroke
  CABG patients 370
  volume, aortic regurgitation 389
Subarachnoid
  catheters 577–578, 655
  haemorrhage 518, 519
    grading 518
Subarachnoid anaesthesia 558–559, 562–569
  Caesarean section 343–344
  clonidine 85
  cognitive impairment, elderly patients 72
  colonic surgery 191–192
  combined with epidural 348–349
  complications 347–349, 566–569, 655–656
  continuous 577–578
  contra-indications 569
  day-case surgery 423
  drugs used 564–566
  effects 566
  indications 569
  kidney transplantation 503
  multiple sclerosis 59
  needles 564
    post-dural puncture headache 567
  site of 559, 560, 563
  opioids 653–656
  paediatric 551, 552
  renal surgery 268
  spinal cord/nerve root damage 702
  tourniquet pain 588–589
  transurethral procedures 271
  urinary surgery 270
  vascular surgical patients 225
Subcutaneous
  opioids 650
  oximetry 130
  premedication 110
Subdural haematoma 527
Sublingual
  buprenorphine 652
  morphine 651–652
Subluxation
  atlanto-axial 16, 62
  atlanto-occipital 525
  of atlas 281
Succinylcholine see Suxamethonium
Suction outlets 743
Sufentanil 339, 422
  cardiac surgery 379, 380–381
  intranasal 652
  liver transplantation 499
Sulphonamides 83
Sulphonylureas 96–97
Sulphur hexafluoride, intravitreal 318–319, 325
Super conducting quantum interference devices (SQIDs) 137
Super-oxide dismutase 488, 489
Superior vena cava, tumour compression 258
Supervision 710–711

Supine hypotensive syndrome 332–333
Supraclavicular
  approach, upper-extremity 579–580
  nerve blocks 494
Supramaximal stimulus, muscle fibres 141
Suprarenal aortic clamping 228
Supraspinal nociceptive transmission 644
Suprasternal notch, Doppler measurement 124
Supratentorial surgery 518–522
  tumours 520–521
Sural nerve 584
Surgical
  consultation 1
  diagnosis, acute pain 637
  stress response 194–195, 612
    suppression, subarachnoid anaesthesia 566
Suxamethonium 14, 34, 62, 107, 144, 246, 289, 705
  burn injuries 477
  Caesarean section 351–352
  cardiac surgery 384
  day-case surgery 417
  electroconvulsive therapy 449
  intra-ocular pressure 321–322
  liver transplantation 498
  myasthenia gravis 259
  neurosurgery 515–516
  pregnancy 332
  renal surgery 267–268
  rigid bronchoscopy 240
  treatment of seizures 348
Sweating, inhibition 109
Sympathetic
  block, epidural anaesthesia 573
  nervous system 562
Systemic lupus erythematosus 61
Systolic
  blood pressure (SBP)
    arterial (SAP) 215, 218
    hypovolaemia 217
  dysfunction 216
  function (Frank-Starling) curves, ventricles 374
    after CPB 399
  heart failure after CPB 400
  shortening 214

Tachycardia 40, 41, 596–597, 600, 601
  aortic stenosis 37
  coronary artery disease 32, 34
    recovery period 36
  with ischaemia 387
  mitral regurgitation 39
  supraventricular 86
Tachyphylaxis see Tolerance, anaesthetic agents
Tactile recording, evoked potentials 143
Target-controlled infusion systems 181–182

778 INDEX

Tasks
  requirements and errors 709
  studies of anaesthetist's 711–712
Taylor approach, central blockade 563
Technical errors 708
Teeth, damage to 705
Temazepam 108, 111, 112, 239
  day-case surgery 415
Temperature 513, 611–612
  cardiac surgery 376
  cardiopulmonary bypass 376, 394, 395, 397
  colonic surgery 191
  hyperthyroidism 63
  hypothyroidism 64
  liver
    disease 53
    transplantation 496
  maintenance of anaesthesia 184
  maxillofacial procedures 296
  microvascular surgery 462, 464
  monitoring 144–145
    methods 145–146
  multiple
    sclerosis 59
    trauma 630
  non-shivering thermogenesis 534–535
  recovery period 622–623
Terazosin 85
Terbutaline 89–90
Termination of pregnancy 274–275, 335–336
Test dose, epidural anaesthesia 346–347, 574–575
Tetanic stimulation 142
Tetany, hypocalcaemic 304
Tetracaine see Amethocaine
Tetracyclines 101
Thalassaemia 19
Thallium scan, myocardial ischaemia 31, 33
Theophylline 90, 628
Thermistor 145
Thermocouple 145
Thermodilution technique, cardiac output 124, 376
Thermogenesis, non-shivering 534–535
Thermoregulatory threshold 184
Thiamylal 514
Thiazide diuretics 82–83
Thiopentone 92, 111, 156, 545, 607, 625
  allergic reactions 163–164, 612
  burn injuries 478
  cardiac surgery 382, 396
  cardioversion 444
  EEG changes 137
  electroconvulsive therapy 449
  induction of anaesthesia 158
    Caesarean section 351, 352
    central haemodynamic effects 161, 162
    cerebral haemodynamic and pressure effects 162, 163
  day-case surgery 418
  effects on ventilation 162
  vascular surgical patients 222
  neurosurgery 514
  placental transfer 334
  rigid bronchoscopy 240
  therapeutic index 155
Thoracic
  aortic cross-clamping 227–228
  epidural anaesthesia (TEA)
    thoracotomy 253
    vascular surgical patients 226–227
  surgery 239–262
    lung resection 244–254
    mediastinoscopy and mediastinotomy 242–243
    oesophagoscopy 243–244
    rigid bronchoscopy 239–242
    risk index 244
Thoracotomy 303
  analgesia 253–254
    pre-emptive 646
  emergency 262
  ventilation and perfusion distribution 249–250
Three-in-one block 424
Thrombo-embolism 24–25, 355
  Caesarean section, low-dose heparin 342
  immobilization 280
  pregnancy 331
Thrombocytopenia
  multiple trauma 629–630
  pre-eclampsia 354
Thromboelastography 53, 147, 197, 576
  liver transplantation 497, 498
Thromboxane 343, 354
Thymectomy 258–260
Thyroid
  disease 13, 63–64, 299–302
    'thyroid storm' 13, 63, 299–300, 302
  dysfunction, elderly patients 72
  physiology and normal function 297–298
  regulation of function 298–299
Thyroid-stimulating hormone (TSH) 298, 299, 302
Thyroidectomy 301, 302
  anaesthetic management 302–304
  postoperative problems 303–304
Thyrotoxic crisis 304
Thyrotropin-releasing hormone (TRH) 298, 299
Thyroxine (T_4) 98, 297, 298, 302
Time to first analgesic (TFA) request 646, 647
Tissue
  flaps, oxygen delivery 461
  irritation, intravenous induction agents 163
  oedema, burns injuries 471, 473
  P_{O_2} electrode 130–131

Tocainide 87
Tolerance, anaesthetic agents 177–178
Tonsillectomy 319
Total
  body
    uptake, anaesthetic agents 176
    weight (TBW) 179–180
  intravenous anaesthesia (TIVA) 183, 289, 701
  parenteral nutrition (TPN), burns patients 475
  quality management (TQM) 732, 746
  spinal anaesthesia 348, 574
Tourniquets 280
  pain from 588–589
Toxaemia of pregnancy 354–355
Toxic
  goitre 299
  megacolon 54
Tracheal
  collapse 304
  intubation see Intubation: tracheal
  resection 260–261
  tubes 261, 289, 294–295
    and laser surgery 317
Tracheobronchial stents, insertion 241–242
Tracheomalacia 304
Tracheostomy 260, 292, 295, 303
  laryngectomy 320
  microvascular surgery 463
Train-of-four-stimulation 141–142, 144, 625–626
Training and education 709, 714–719
  continuing medical education 717
  efficacy 754–755
  role of examinations 716–717
  training devices and simulators 717–719
Tramadol 650
Transcranial Doppler (TCD) 139, 517
Transcutaneous oxygen and carbon dioxide tensions 129–130
Transdermal fentanyl 651
Transducer drift, intra-arterial pressure monitoring 373
Transitional circulation, infants 534
Transluminal angioplasty 445
Transmucosal drug administration 651–652
Transoesophageal
  Doppler measurement 124–125
  echocardiography see Echocardiography: transoesophageal
Transplantation, organ 103, 485–507
  future trends 507
  general considerations 486–490
  heart 487, 492–493, 501–502
    pre-operative management 493
    pulmonary artery catheters 390–391, 502
    postoperative management 505–506
  heart and lungs 43–44

kidney 485, 487, 489, 490, 493–494, 502–503
  end-stage renal disease 493
  living related 503
  postoperative management 506–507
liver 147, 485, *486*, 487
  selection and preparation 490–492
  intravenous access 495
  monitoring 495–496
  venovenous bypass 496–498, 500
  anaesthetic tehniques 498–499
  medications 499
  postoperative management 503–505
Transtracheal
  Doppler measurement 125
    liver transplantation 496
  oxygenation 350
Transurethral procedures 270–273
Trauma 279–280
  avoidance during surgery 296
  chest 262
  eye
    injury during anaesthesia 705
    penetrating injury 324
  facial 290, 291
  head injuries 526–529
  multiple 629–632
    CT scanning 441
    drug withdrawal 632
  teeth, during anaesthesia 705
  vertebral column 284, 285
Trazodone 91
Treacher-Collins syndrome 291, 543
Trendelenburg position 270, 567
Tri-iodothyronine (T$_3$) 297, 298, 302
Triamterine 83
Triazolam, day-case surgery 415
Trichloroethylene 177
Tricuspid
  regurgitation *10*, 38, 39, 376
  stenosis *10*
Tricyclic antidepressants 91, 92, 448, 602
Trieger scores *422*
Trifascicular/atrioventricular heart block 40
Trimeprazine 111
Trimetaphan 423
Trimipramine 91
Triple
  airway manoeuvre 667
  fluorescence catheter 129
  index (TI) 215
Trousseau's sign 304
Truncus arteriosus 43
Tuberculosis 70
  antituberculous therapy 102
Tubocurarine 34, 90, 295
TUR syndrome 271, 272–273
Twins, delivery 356
Two-dimensional echocardiography 125
Two-rescuer CPR 672

Tympanic membrane, hypothalamic temperature 145

Ulcerative colitis 53–54
Ulnar nerve 143, 579, 583
  damage to 703
Ultrasound scan
  see also Doppler techniques; Echocardiography
  thyroid 300
Umbilical cord compression 334
Unifasicular heart block 40
Uniform Anatomical Act 486–487
Unipolar leads 117
United Kingdom, quality of practice 744–745
United Network for Organ Sharing (UNOS) 486, 490
  allocation, organ 487
University of Wisconsin (UW) solution 485, 488, *489*
Upper
  abdominal surgery, postoperative pulmonary function 194, 627
  airway obstruction 241, 697–698
  respiratory tract infections (URTIs) 11, 12, 323
  tracheal surgery 260, 261
Upper-extremity
  anatomy 578–579
  nerve blocks 578, 579–583
Uraemia 13, 267
Ureteric surgery 267–268
Urinalysis 17–18
Urinary retention
  epidural opioids 656
  extracorporeal shock-wave lithotripsy 270
  subarachnoid anaesthesia 568
  thoracotomy 254
Urine output
  cardiac surgery 376
  fluid resuscitation, burn injuries 474
Urological surgery 267–274
USA
  see also American Society of Anesthesiologists (ASA)
  cardiac arrest study 688–689
  Joint Commission for Accreditation of Hospitals, (JCAH) 745, 746
  Multicenter Study 689, *690*
Uterine
  activity
    and anaesthetic drugs 335
    progress of labour 333
    suppression, preterm labour 356
  blood flow 333

Vagal block 107
Vaginal
  delivery 336–337
    caudal epidural analgesia 340–341
    epidural analgesia regimen *339*
    general anaesthesia 341
    lumbar epidural analgesia 338–340

  surgery 274–275
Valium 165
Valvular heart disease 36, 387–390
  assessment of patients 9, *10–11*
Valvuloplasty 445
Vaporizer 178
  output 133
Vapour, anaesthetic 176
Variegate porphyria 166–167
Vascular resistance, systemic in burn injury 468
Vascular surgery 205–232
  see also Microvascular surgery
  intra-operative management 221–232
    control of haemodynamics 229–230
  early postoperative care 231–232
  patient characterisitcs 205–207
  risk assessment 207–221
    peri-operative monitoring 212–219
    practical approach to cardiac 212
    type of surgery 210–212
Vasectomy 274
Vasodilators
  microvascular surgery
    local 463–464
    systemic 464
  therapy, end-stage heart disease 390
Vasodilatory coronary vascular reserve 386
Vasopressin 499
Vasospasm, cerebral artery 518, 519
Vaughan-Williams classification, anti-arrhythmic drugs *86*
Vectorcardiography 214
Vecuronium 34, 35, 142, 240, 289, 295, 596
  burn injuries 477
  cardiac surgery 384
  day-case surgery 417
  liver transplantation 498–499
  myasthenia gravis 259
  neurosurgery 515
Vena cava, compression 258, 267, 275
  pregnancy 332–333
Venous
  admixture, one-lung anaesthesia 250
  thrombosis
    postoperative 24–25, 355
    prevention 296
Venovenous bypass 196
  liver transplantation 496–498
  removal of cannulae 500
Ventilation
  bronchoscopy 240
  cardiopulmonary resuscitation 667–670, 672
    ventilation patterns 668
  controlled
    during MRI 443
    paediatric surgery 547–548

Ventilation (contd)
  effects of intravenous induction agents 162
  high-frequency jet (HFJV)
    bronchopleural fistula 256
    bullectomy 256
    thoracotomy 252
    tracheal resection 260, 261
  inadequate 697
  intermittent positive-pressure (IPPV)
    cardiopulmonary resuscitation 668
    thoracotomy 250
  organ donor 488
  positive-pressure, systolic blood pressure variations 218
  tracheal tube 260–261
  Venturi 240, 241, 242, 256
  volumes, paediatric anaesthesia 537–538
  weaning after cardiac surgery 404–405
Ventilation/perfusion (V/Q) mismatch 132
Ventilators
  alarms 135
  disconnection or failure 698
Ventricular
  arrthymias 600
    tachycardia 41
  contractions
    after CPB 400
    premature (PVCs) 41, 601
  fibrillation 670

filling pressures, cardiac surgery 374–376
Venturi ventilation 240, 241, 242, 256
Verapamil 82, 86, 229, 231, 254
Vertebral
  artery 581
  landmarks, spinal levels 559, 560
  venous plexus 283
Vessel-poor group (VPG) tissues 173
  rate of equilibrium *174*
Vessel-rich group (VRG) tissues 173, 176
  rate of equilibrium *174*
Vigabatrin 94
Villous adenomas, rectum 189
Virtual-reality simulators 719
Visual
  analogue scales, pain measurement 645
  dysfunction, subarachnoid anaesthesia 568
  evoked potentials (VEPs) 138, 517
  recording, evoked potentials 143
Vitamin D, parathyroid glands 304
Vitamin K 100
  deficiency 545
Vitrectomy 325
Volume-depletion 84
  liver disease 51
  paediatric anaesthesia 541
Vomiting *see* Nausea and vomiting
Von Willebrand factor 404

Vulvectomy 274

'Wake-up' test 136
Warfarin 100, 342, 576
Water manometer 121
Weight, postoperative pain relief 648
Wertheim's hysterectomy 276
Wheezing, postoperative 628
Whipple's procedure 196
Wilson score 23
Wind-up (action potential discharge) 642, 645, 647
  implications, postoperative pain relief 644
Withdrawal syndrome, alcohol 7
Wolff-Parkinson-White syndrome (WPW) 41, 391, 392, 601
  verapamil 86
Working hours 712, 713, 719, 741
Workspace layout and design 709
Wound infiltration, local anaesthetic 427
Wright's respirometer 135
Wrist nerve blocks 583

Xanthine oxidase 489
Xenografts 485, 507
Xenon washout 139

Yttrium-aluminium-garnet (Nd-YAG) lasers 241, 316

Zidovudine (AZT) 70, 102
Zopiclone 94

Companion to Clinical Anaesthesia Exams

C F Corke and I J B Jackson

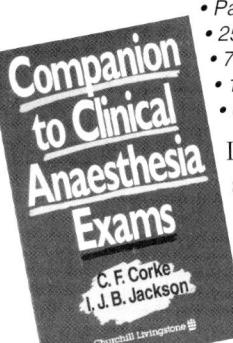

- Paperback
- 256 pages
- 75 line illustrations
- 1994
- 0 443 04962 9

Improve your chances of success in clinical anaesthetic examinations *and* save valuable revision time. This concise revision aid is particularly useful for the new Part III FRCA examination and will help you prepare for the Part I FRCA examination.

✔ **Answer Plans** – highlight key issues on a specific topic to enable you to reproduce all the important points in a logical order. The text features simple line illustrations – easy to reproduce in the exam.

✔ **Practical Clinical Section** – guidance to interpreting ECG traces, chest x-rays, pulmonary function tests, blood gas analysis - avoid pitfalls *and* learn how not to antagonise the examiner.

✔ **Viva Questions** – practice oral examination technique and improve your presentation skills with these questions.

✔ **Core References** – help you pinpoint any weak areas requiring further revision *and* the references are star rated to easily identify essential reading.

Clinical Scenarios in Anaesthesia

W A Chambers and R Patey

- Paperback
- 190 pages
- 20 halftone illustrations
- 1995
- 0 443 05070 8

A practically structured and illustrated study aid aimed at trainees preparing for the **'clinical scenarios' viva** – a vital part of the FRCA final examination.

Forty-seven key clinical scenarios cover a wide range of topics in
- general
- obstetric
- paediatric

anaesthesia, including some rare conditions.

An **essential self-study guide** to help candidates develop and defend a plan of action for each case in preparation for the examination.

Keep up-to-date with Churchill Livingstone's **Anaesthesia programme**

PHONE
Customer Services
Freephone – *UK only*
0500 556 242
Tel: +44(0)131 535 1021

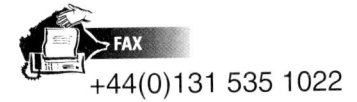

FAX
+44(0)131 535 1022

CHURCHILL LIVINGSTONE